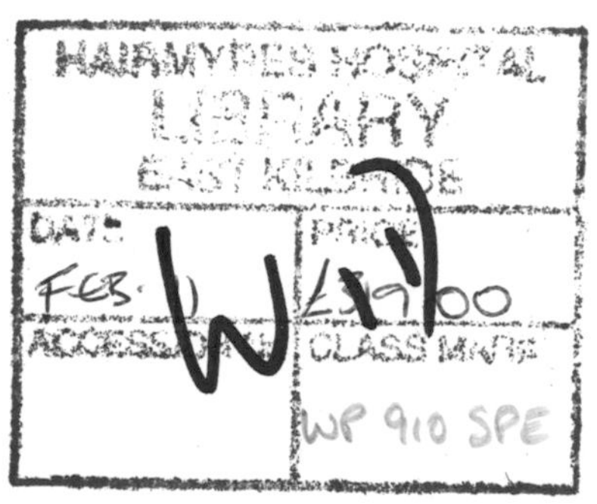

Surgery of the Breast
Principles and Art

Third Edition

Volume Two

Surgery of the Breast
Principles and Art

Third Edition

Editor

SCOTT L. SPEAR, MD, FACS

Professor and Chairman
Department of Plastic Surgery
Georgetown University Hospital
Washington, DC

Associate Editors

SHAWNA C. WILLEY, MD

Director, Betty Lou Ourisman Breast Health Center
Associate Professor of Clinical Surgery
Department of Surgery
Georgetown University Medical Center
Washington, DC

GEOFFREY L. ROBB, MD

Professor and Chair
Department of Plastic Surgery
The University of Texas
M.D. Anderson Cancer Center
Houston, Texas

DENNIS C. HAMMOND, MD

Clinical Assistant Professor
Department of Surgery
Michigan State University College of Human Medicine
East Lansing, Michigan
Associate Program Director
Plastic and Reconstructive Surgery
Grand Rapids Medical Education Partners
Grand Rapids, Michigan

MAURICE Y. NAHABEDIAN, MD

Associate Professor
Department of Plastic Surgery
Georgetown University Hospital
Washington, DC

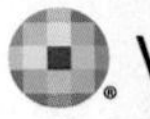
Wolters Kluwer | Lippincott Williams & Wilkins
Health

Philadelphia • Baltimore • New York • London
Buenos Aires • Hong Kong • Sydney • Tokyo

Acquisitions Editor: Brian Brown
Managing Editor: Julia Seto
Marketing Manager: Lisa Lawrence
Production Editor: Alicia Jackson
Senior Manufacturing Manager: Ben Rivera
Designer: Doug Smock
Compositor: Aptara, Inc.

Two Commerce Square
2001 Market Street
Philadelphia, PA 19103

Printed in China

Library of Congress Cataloging-in-Publication Data

Surgery of the breast : principles and art / editor, Scott L. Spear ;
associate editors, Shawna C. Willey . . . [et al.]. – 3rd ed.
p. ; cm.
Includes bibliographical references and index.
ISBN 978-1-60547-577-6 (hardback : alk. paper)
1. Breast—Cancer—Surgery. 2. Breast—Surgery. 3. Mammaplasty.
4. Mastectomy. I. Spear, Scott L.
[DNLM: 1. Breast—surgery. 2. Breast Neoplasms—surgery.
3. Mammaplasty—methods. 4. Mastectomy—methods. WP 910]
RD667.5.S87 2011
616.99′449059—dc22 2010034582

To purchase additional copies of this book, call our customer service department at (800) 638-3030 or fax orders to (301) 223-2320. International customers should call (301) 223-2300.

Visit Lippincott Williams & Wilkins on the Internet: http://www.LWW.com. Lippincott Williams & Wilkins customer service representatives are available from 8:30 am to 6:00 pm, EST.

06 07 08 09 10
1 2 3 4 5 6 7 8 9 10

To my teachers and professors who served as role models and left their indelible marks on how I think and operate: Bob Replogle from the University of Chicago who directed me into a surgical career and helped me grow up as a medical student; Bill Silen and Don Glotzer, both general surgeons from the Beth Israel at Harvard who set the standard of integrity and discipline that I humbly try to emulate to this day; Ralph Millard from the University of Miami who singularly embodies artistic skill, creativity, hard work, and the never satisfied pursuit of beautiful outcomes; and also my colleagues around the country who toil at the same work as I do and inspire me to think smarter and work harder to raise the bar on what we can achieve.

To the women who have allowed me to take care of them, repair them, or enhance them such that their lives have been made more pleasant, comfortable, or even pleasurable. Helping them has enriched my life at least as much as I have enriched theirs.

To Cindy, my wife, who never ceases to amaze with her seemingly unlimited energy, sensitivity, thoughtfulness, compassion, generosity, wisdom, loyalty, and love that flows so easily from her and enriches the lives of everyone that she touches, including me, thankfully.

Contributing Authors

William P. Adams, Jr., MD
Associate Clinical Professor
Department of Plastic Surgery
UT Southwestern Medical Center
Dallas, Texas

Jamal Ahmad, MD
Staff Plastic Surgeon
The Plastic Surgery Clinic
Mississauga, Ontario, Canada

Ali Al-Attar, MD
Department of Plastic Surgery
Georgetown University Hospital
Washington, DC

Wafa Alkhayal, MD
Georgetown University Hospital
Division of Breast Surgery
Washington, DC

Robert J. Allen, MD, FACS
Louisiana State University Health Sciences Center
New Orleans, Louisiana

Rebecca Cogwell Anderson, PhD
Professor
Department of Surgery
Medical College of Wisconsin
Frodfert Memorial Lutheran Hospital
Milwaukee, Wisconsin

Matthew B. Baker, MD, PhD
Baker Center for Plastic Surgery
Staff Surgeon
Division of Plastic Surgery
Littleton Adventist Hospital
Littleton, Colorado

Elisabeth K. Beahm, MD, FACS
The University of Texas M.D. Anderson Cancer Center
Department of Plastic Surgery
Houston, Texas

Michael Beckenstein, MD
Birmingham, Alabama

Hilton Becker, MD, FACS, FRCS
Division of Plastic Surgery
University of Miami Miller School of Medicine
Boca Raton, Florida

Louis C. Benelli, MD
Department of Surgery
Bichat Hospital
University of Paris
Paris, France

Bradley P. Bengtson, MD, FACS
Bengtson Center for Aesthetics and Plastic Surgery
Department of Plastic Surgery
Spectrum Health
Grand Rapids, Michigan

Thomas Biggs, MD
Clinical Professor of Plastic Surgery
College of Medicine
Baylor University
Houston, Texas

Jay Boehmler, MD
Assistant Professor
Division of Plastic Surgery
The Ohio State University
Columbus, Ohio

Mitchell H. Brown, MD
Associate Professor
Department of Surgery
Program Director
Division of Plastic Surgery
University of Toronto
Toronto, Ontario, Canada

Klaus E. Brunnert, MD
Chief
Department of Senology
Klinik Fur Senologie
Osnabruck, Germany

Edward P. Buchanan, MD
Fellow in Plastic Surgery

Celia Byrne, MD
Cancer Genetics and Epidemiology
Lombardi Cancer Center
Georgetown University Hospital
Washington, DC

Paul R. Callegari, MD, FRCS
Private Practice
South Crest Hospital
Tulsa, Oklahoma

Giuseppe Catanuto, MD
Instituto Nazionale per lo Studio e la Cura dei Tumori
Scuola di Oncologia Chirurgica Ricostructtiva
Milan, Italy

Therese Soballe Cermak, MD
Department of Pathology
Georgetown University Hospital
Washington, DC

David W. Chang, MD, FACS
Professor of Plastic Surgery
Department of Surgery
University of Texas M.D. Anderson Cancer Center
Houston, Texas

Constance M. Chen, MD
New York, New York

Pierre M. Chevray, MD, PhD
Adjunct Associate Professor
Department of Surgery
Baylor College of Medicine
The Methodist Hospital
Plastic Surgeon
Houston, Texas

Armando Chiari, Jr., MD
Brazil

Minas T. Chrysopoulo, MD
Plastic, Reconstructive, and Microsurgical Associates of South Texas
San Antonio, Texas

Mark W. Clemens, MD
Department of Plastic Surgery
Georgetown University Hospital
Washington, DC

Costanza Cocilovo, MD
Assistant Professor of Surgery
Department of Plastic Surgery
Georgetown University Hospital
Washington, DC

Mark A. Codner, MD
Clinical Associate Professor
Department of Plastic Surgery
Emory University
Atlanta, Gerogia

Hiram S. Cody, III, MD
Attending Surgeon, Breast Service
Department of Surgery
Memorial Sloan-Kettering Cancer Center
Professor of Clinical Surgery
The Weill Medical College of Cornell University
New York, New York

Michael Cohen, MD
Department of Plastic Surgery
Georgetown University Medical Center
Washington, DC

Sydney R. Coleman, MD
Assistant Clinical Professor
New York University Medical Center
Director, Tribeca Plastic Surgery
New York, New York

Lawrence B. Colen, MD
Professor Department of Surgery
Eastern Virginia Medical School
Norfolk, Virginia

Melissa A. Crosby, MD
Assistant Professor
Department of Plastic Surgery
The University of Texas M.D. Anderson Cancer Center
Houston, Texas

Laurie W. Cuttino, MD
Associate Professor
Department of Radiation Oncology
Virginia Commonwealth University Health System
Richmond, Virginia

Steven P. Davison, MD
DAVinci Plastic Surgery
Washington, DC

Emmanuel Delay, MD, PhD
Department of Plastic and Reconstructive Surgery
Léon Bérard Center
Lyon, France

Daniel Del Vecchio, MD, MBA
Back Bay Plastic Surgery
Boston, Massachusetts

Albert De Mey, MD
Professor
Department of Plastic Surgery
Free University, Brussels
Brussels, Belgium

Richard V. Dowden, MD
Department of Plastic Surgery
Cleveland Clinic Hillcrest Hospital
Mayfield Heights, Ohio

Ivica Ducic, MD, PhD
Professor
Chief, Peripheral Nerve Surgery
Department of Plastic Surgery
Georgetown University Hospital
Washington, DC

Jennifer Eng-Wong, MD, MPH
Assistant Professor
Department of Internal Medicine
Lombardi Comprehensive Cancer Center
Medical Oncologist
Georgetown University Hospital
Washington, DC

Karen Kim Evans, MD
Division of Plastic Surgery
Georgetown University Medical Center
Washington, DC

Elizabeth D. Feldman, MD
Division of Breast Surgery
Georgetown University Hospital
Washington, DC

Neil A. Fine, MD
Clinical Associate Professor
Department of Plastic Surgery
Northwestern University Feinberg School of Medicine
Northwestern Memorial Hospital
Chicago, Illinois

Diane Franck, MD
Resident
Department of Plastic Surgery
Brugmann University Hospital
Brussels, Belgium

Marianne A. Fuller, RN
Clinical Manager
Cleveland Clinic
Cleveland, Ohio

Allen Gabriel, MD
Director of Research
Department of Plastic Surgery
Loma Linda University Medical Center
Loma Linda, California

Onelio Garcia, Jr., MD, FACS
Voluntary Assistant Professor
Division of Plastic Surgery
University of Miami, Miller School of Medicine
Miami, Florida
Chief, Division of Plastic Surgery
Palmetto General Hospital
Hialeah, Florida

Caroline A. Glicksman, MD
Associate Clinical Professor
Department of Plastic Surgery
Jersey Shore University Medical Center
Neptune City, New Jersey

João Carlos Sampaio Góes, MD, PhD
Instituto Brasileiro de Controle do Cancer
São Paulo, Brazil

Jesse A. Goldstein, MD, MPH
Resident
Department of Plastic Surgery
Georgetown University Hospital
Washington, DC

Ruth Maria Graf, MD
Assistant Professor
Department of Plastic Surgery
Federal University of Paraná
Curitiba, Brazil

James C. Grotting, MD
Clinical Professor of Plastic Surgery
University of Alabama at Birmingham
Grotting Plastic Surgery
Birmingham, Alabama

Geoffrey C. Gurtner, MD, FACS
Professor
Department of Surgery
Stanford University
Stanford, California

Elizabeth J. Hall-Findlay, MD, FRCSC
Private Practice
Banff, Alberta, Canada

Moustapha Hamdi, MD, PhD
Professor
Department of Plastic and Reconstructive Surgery
Gent University Hospital
Gent, Belgium
Edith Cavell Medical Institute
Brussels, Belgium

Dennis C. Hammond, MD
Clinical Assistant Professor
Department of Surgery
Michigan State University College of Human Medicine
East Lansing, Michigan
Associate Program Director
Plastic and Reconstructive Surgery
Grand Rapids Medical Education Partners
Grand Rapids, Michigan

Neal Handel, MD, FACS
Associate Clinical Professor
Division of Plastic Surgery
David Geffen School of Medicine
University of California at Los Angeles
Los Angeles, California
Santa Barbara Cottage Hospital
Santa Barbara, California

Catherine M. Hannan, MD
Resident
Department of Plastic Surgery
Georgetown University Hospital
Washington, DC

Barbara B. Hayden, MD
Santa Monica, California

Per Hedén, MD
Associate Professor
Karolinska Instiutet
Chief
Department of Plastic Surgery
Akademikliniken
Stockholm, Sweden

Christopher L. Hess, MD
Division of Plastic Surgery
Georgetown University Medical Center
Washington, DC

Saul Hoffman, MD
Fifth Avenue Center for Aesthetic Surgery
New York, New York

Karen M. Horton, MD
Division of Microsurgery and Department of Plastic Surgery
California Pacific Medical Center
San Francisco, California

Michael A. Howard, MD
Clinical Assistant Professor
Section of Plastic Surgery
University of Chicago Pritzker School of Medicine
Chicago, Illinois
North Shore University Health System
Northbrook, Illinois

Dennis J. Hurwitz, MD
Clinical Professor of Plastic Surgery
University of Pittsburgh Medical School Center
Attending Plastic Surgeon
Magee-Women's Hospital
Pittsburgh, Pennsylvania

Matthew L. Iorio, MD
Department of Plastic Surgery
Georgetown University Hospital
Washington, DC

Claudine J. D. Isaacs, MD
Associate Professor of Medicine
Lombardi Comprehensive Cancer Center
Georgetown University
Washington, DC

F. Frank Isik, MD, FACS
Seattle, Washington

Jeffery M. Jacobson, MD
Department of Plastic Surgery
Georgetown University Hospital
Washington, DC

M. Renee Jespersen, MD
Georgetown University Medical Center
Washington, DC

Mark Jewell, MD
Eugene, Oregon

Marwan R. Khalifeh, MD
Assistant Professor
Department of Surgery
Johns Hopkins University School of Medicine
Baltimore, Maryland
Senior Partner
Ivy Plastic Surgery Associates
Chevy Chase, Maryland

Roger K. Khouri, MD, FACS
Chief Director
Miami Breast Center
Key Biscayne, Florida

R. Michael Koch, MD
Assistant Professor
Department of Surgery
New York Medical College
Attending Surgeon
Division of Plastic Surgery
West Chester Medical Center
Valhalla, New York

Steven J. Kronowitz, MD, FACS
Professor
Department of Plastic Surgery
The University of Texas M.D. Anderson Cancer Center
Houston, Texas

Ethan E. Larson, MD
Department of Plastic Surgery
Georgetown University Hospital
Washington, DC

Claude Lassus, MD
Attending Plastic Surgeon
University Hospital NICE
Saint Paul France

Peter Ledoux, MD
Plastic Reconstructive and Microsurgical Associates of South Texas
San Antonio, Texas

Valerie Lemaine, MD
Memorial Sloan-Kettering Cancer Center
New York, New York

Jason C. Levine, MS
University of Wisconsin, Milwaukee
Milwaukee, WI

Joshua L. Levine, MD
Center for Microsurgical Breast Reconstruction
New York, New York

Joan E. Lipa, MD, MSc, FRCS
Associate Professor
David Geffen School of Medicine at UCLA
Division of Plastic & Reconstructive Surgery
University of California, Los Angeles
Los Angeles, California

Frank Lista, MD
Medical Director
The Plastic Surgery Clinic
Mississauga, Ontario, Canada

J. William Little, MD
Clinical Professor of Surgery
Department of Surgery
Georgetown University Medical Center
Washington, DC

Minetta C. Liu, MD
Associate Professor
Director, Translational Breast Cancer Research
Lombardi Comprehensive Cancer Center
Georgetown University
Washington, DC

Albert Losken, MD, FACS
Associate Professor
Division of Plastic and Reconstructive Surgery
Emory University
Atlanta, Georgia

Maria M. LoTempio, MD
New York, New York

Daniel P. Luppens, MD
Atlantic Plastic Surgery
Salisbury, Maryland

Antonio Luiz V. Macedo
Hospital Israelita Albert Einstein
São Paulo, Brazil

Erini Makariou, MD
Associate Professor and Chief, Breast Imaging
Department of Radiology
Georgetown University Hospital
Washington, DC

Donna-Marie E. Manasseh, MD
Breast Surgery
Betty Lou Ourisman Breast Health Center
Georgetown University Medical Center
Washington, DC

Daniel A. Marchac, MD
Ancien Chef de Clinique a la Faculte
Chirurgien attendant Consultant de l'Hopital Necker
Professeur Associe au College de Medecine des Hopitaux de Paris
Paris, France

Alessandra Marchi, MD
Regional Center for Breast Reconstruction
Verona, Italy

Derek L. Masden, MD
Resident
Department of Plastic Surgery
Georgetown University Hospital
Washington, DC

G. Patrick Maxwell, MD
Baptist Medical
Nashville, TN

James W. May, Jr., MD
Department of Plastic Surgery
Massachusetts General Hospital
Department of Surgery
Harvard Medical School
Boston, Massachusetts

Colleen M. McCarthy, MD
Assistant Professor of Surgery
Plastic and Reconstructive Surgery
Weill Cornell Medical Center
Memorial Sloan-Kettering Cancer Center
New York, New York

John McCraw, MD
Professor of Surgery
Department of Surgery
University of Mississippi Medical Center
Jackson, Mississippi

Juan Diego Mejia, MD
Private Practice
Medellin, Colombia

Nathan G. Menon, MD
Department of Plastic Surgery
Georgetown University Hospital
Washington, DC

Ali N. Mesbahi, MD
Division of Plastic Surgery
Georgetown University Medical Center
Washington, DC

Joseph Michaels V, MD
Monarch Aesthetic and Reconstructive Plastic Surgery
North Bethesda, Maryland

Michael J. Miller, MD
Professor
Division of Plastic Surgery
The Ohio State University
Chief, Division of Plastic Surgery
The Ohio State University Medical Center
Columbus, Ohio

Martin Jeffrey Moskovitz, MD
Image Plastic Surgery
Paramus, New Jersey

Antonio Aldo Mottura, MD
Associate Professor of Surgery
Universidad de Cordoba
Cordoba, Argentina

Jefferson E. C. Moulds, MD
Associate Professor of Clinical Radiation Medicine
Georgetown University
Washington, DC
Radiation Oncologist
Reston Hospital Center
Reston, Virginia

Alexandre Mendonça Munhoz, MD
Assistant Professor
Department of Plastic Surgery
University of Sao Paulo
Sirio-Libanes
Sao Paulo, Brazil

Maurice Y. Nahabedian, MD, FACS
Associate Professor
Department of Plastic Surgery
Georgetown University
Washington, DC

Farzad R. Nahai, MD
Assistant Clinical Professor
Division of Plastic Surgery
Emory University School of Medicine
Department of Surgery
Piedmont Hospital
Atlanta, Georgia

Foad Nahai, MD, FACS
Clinical Professor of Plastic Surgery
Department of Plastic Surgery
Emory University
Atlanta, Georgia

James D. Namnoum, MD
Atlanta Plastic Surgery
Atlanta, Georgia

Chet Nastala, MD, FACS
Plastic Reconstructive and Microsurgical Associates of South Texas
San Antonio, Texas

Maurizio Nava, MD
Instituto Nazionale per lo Studio e la Cura dei Tumori
Milan, Italy

Maria Cecília Closs Ono, MD
Plastic Surgeon
Member of the Brazilian Society of Plastic Surgery
Curitiba, Brazil

Kristina O'Shaughnessy, MD
Plastic Surgery Chief Resident
Department of Surgery
Northwestern University Feinberg School of Medicine
Chicago, Illinois

David Otterburn, MD
Division of Plastic and Reconstructive Surgery
Emory University Hospital
Atlanta, Georgia

Joseph Ottolenghi, MD
Instituto Nazionale per lo Studio e la Cura dei Tumori
Milan, Italy

Pranay M. Parikh, MD
Department of Plastic Surgery
Georgetown University Hospital
Washington, DC

Julie E. Park, MD
Assistant Professor of Surgery
Section of Plastic and Reconstructive Surgery
The University of Chicago
The University of Chicago Medical Center
Chicago, Illinois

Ketan M. Patel, MD
Resident Physician
Department of Plastic Surgery
Georgetown University Hospital
Washington, DC

Christopher Vincent Pelletiere, MD
Private Practice
Barrington Plastic Surgery, LTD.
Inverness, Illinois
Chief, Division of Plastic Surgery
Northwest Community Hospital
Arlington Heights, Illinois

Angela Pennati, MD
Instituto Nazionale per lo Studio e la Cura dei Tumori
Milan, Italy

Beth N. Peshkin, MS, CGC
Associate Professor
Department of Oncology
Georgetown University
Washington, DC

Steven M. Pisano, MD
Plastic Reconstructive and Microsurgical Associates of South Texas
San Antonio, Texas

Jason K. Potter, MD
Southwestern Medical Center
Dallas, Texas

Christian A. Prada, MD
Division of Plastic Surgery
Georgetown University Medical Center
Washington, DC

Julian J. Pribaz, MD, FRCS
Professor Department of Surgery
Harvard Medical School
Department of Surgery
Brigham and Women's Hospital
Boston, Massachusetts

Andrea Pusic, MD
Memorial Sloan-Kettering Cancer Center
New York, New York

Samir S. Rao, MD
Georgetown University Medical Center
Washington, DC

Elan Reisin, MD
Reisin West Institute
Chevy Chase, Maryland

Neal R. Reisman, MD
Clinical Professor of Plastic Surgery
Baylor College of Medicine
Chief, Plastic Surgery
St. Luke's Episcopal Hospital
Houston, Texas

Egidio Riggio, MD
Instituto Nazionale per lo Studio e la Cura dei Tumori
Milan, Italy

Gino Rigotti, MD
Director
Plastic Surgery, Burn Unit, Regional Center for Breast Reconstruction
Azienda Ospedaliera Universitaria di Verona
Verona, Italy

Geoffrey L. Robb, MD
Professor and Chair
Department of Plastic Surgery
The University of Texas M.D. Anderson Cancer Center
Houston, Texas

Julia H. Rowland, MD
Director, Office of Cancer Survivorship
National Institutes of Health
Bethesda, Maryland

J. Peter Rubin, MD
Director, Body Contouring Program
Associate Professor of Surgery
Division of Plastic Surgery
University of Pittsburgh
Pittsburgh, Pennsylvania

James J. Ryan, MD
Cockeysville, Maryland

Amer Saba, MD
Division of Plastic Surgery
Georgetown University Medical Center
Washington, DC

Alesia P. Saboeiro, MD
Attending Physician
Department of Surgery
New York Downtown Hospital
New York, New York

Michael Saint-Cyr, MD
Assistant Professor
Southwestern Medical Center
Dallas, Texas

C. Andrew Salzberg, MD
Associate Professor
Department of Surgery
New York Medical College
Chief, Division of Plastic Surgery
Westchester Medical Center
Valhalla, New York

Anousheh Sayah, MD
Department of Radiology
Georgetown University Medical Center
Washington, DC

Adam D. Schaffner, MD
Clinical Assistant Professor of Otorhinolaryngology
Weill Cornell Medical College
New York, New York

Michael Scheflan, MD
Atidim Medical Center
Tel Aviv, Israel

Jamie Schwartz, MD
Department of Plastic Surgery
Georgetown University Hospital
Washington, DC

Mitchel Seruya, MD
Resident
Department of Plastic Surgery
Georgetown University Hospital
Washington, DC

Minal Shah, MD
Hematologist/Medical Oncologist
St. Mary's Hospital
Leonardtown, Maryland

Kenneth C. Shestak, MD
Associate Professor of Plastic Surgery
Department of Surgery
University of Pittsburgh School of Medicine
Magee-Women's Hospital
Pittsburgh, Pennsylvania

Melvin J. Silverstein, MD
Professor of Surgery
Department of Surgical Oncology
Keck School of Medicine
University of Southern California
Los Angeles, California
Director, Hoag Breast Program
Hoag Memorial Hospital Presbyterian
Newport Beach, California

Baljit Singh, MD, MBBS
Associate Professor
Director of Breast Pathology
Department of Pathology
New York University Langone Medical Center
New York, New York

Navin K. Singh, MD, MBA, PACS
Clinical Assistant Professor
Department of Plastic Surgery
Johns Hopkins University
Sibley Memorial Hospital
Chevy Chase, Maryland

Sumner A. Slavin, MD
Department of Surgery
Beth Israel Deaconess Medical Center
Brookline, Massachusetts

David H. Song, MD, MBA
Professor of Surgery
Section of Plastic Surgery
University of Chicago
Chief, Department of Surgery
University of Chicago Medical Center
Chicago, Illinois

Andrea Spano, MD
Instituto Nazionale per lo Studio e la Cura dei Tumori
Milan, Italy

Scott L. Spear, MD, FACS
Professor and Chairman
Department of Plastic Surgery
Georgetown University Hospital
Washington, DC

Louis L. Strock, MD, FACS
Fort Worth, Texas

Simon G. Talbot, MD
Department of Plastic Surgery
Brigham and Women's Hospital
Boston, Massachusetts

André Ricardo Dall'Oglio Tolazzi, MD
Plastic Surgeon of the Plastic Surgery Unit of Federal University of Paraná
Curitiba, Brazil

Koenraad Van Landuyt, MD, PhD
Associate Professor
Department of Plastic Surgery
Gent University Hospital
Gent, Belgium

Julie V. Vasile, MD
Associate Adjunct Surgeon
Department of Plastic Surgery
New York Eye and Ear Infirmary
New York, New York
Attending Surgeon
Department of Surgery
Stamford Hospital
Stamford, Connecticut

Mark L. Venturi, MD
McLean, Virginia

Frank A. Vicini, MD, FACR
Clinical Professor
Oakland University William Beaumont Hospital School of Medicine
Chief of Oncology
William Beaumont Hospital
Royal Oak, Michigan

Robert L. Walton, MD
Plastic Surgery Chicago
Chicago, Illinois

Justin E. West, MD
Department of Plastic Surgery
Breast Care and Imaging Center
Orange, California

Pat Whitworth, MD
Private Practice
Nashville, Tennessee

Shawna C. Willey, MD
Director, Betty Lou Ourisman Breast Health Center
Associate Professor of Clinical Surgery
Department of Surgery
Georgetown University Medical Center
Washington, DC

Victor W. Wong, MD
Postdoctoral Research Fellow
Stanford University
Stanford, California

Michael R. Zenn, MD
Vice Chief
Department of Plastic and Reconstructive Surgery
Duke University Medical Center
Durham, North Carolina

Christophe Zirak, MD
Resident
Department of Plastic Surgery
Brugmann University Hospital
Brussels, Belgium

Foreword

Dr. Scott Spear has written a phenomenal, one of a kind book on the comprehensive management of all aspects of breast disease from oncologic diseases to all aspects of reconstruction, cosmetic breast surgery and breast reduction – all in one text. This unique text has evolved into the gold standard as it enters its third edition. By using a multidisciplinary approach in the management of complex problems of the breast, this book surpasses what can be done by any one surgical specialty text. Dr. Spear had the foresight to begin this journey over a decade ago when he published his first edition in 1998 as well as his second edition along with superb associate editors Drs. Shawna Willey, Director of Breast Health Center at Georgetown University Medical Center, Department of Surgery; Geoffrey L. Robb, Professor and Chair, Department of Plastic Surgery at the University of Texas M.D. Anderson Cancer Center; Dennis C. Hammond, Center for Breast and Body Contouring, Grand Rapids, Michigan; and Maurice Y. Nahabedian, Associate Professor in the Department of Plastic Surgery at Georgetown University Medical Center.

This textbook has become the bible for specialties dealing with diseases of the breast from breast cancer screening and management and prevention to an oncologic approach to breast surgery as well as the reconstructive aspects and refinements and advancements in breast surgery. This book reveals the paradigm shift in how breast patients are managed and that it is no longer done by one specialty in isolation. A multidisciplinary approach to the management of breast patients definitely improves care and outcomes in breast cancer. Dr. Spear is a uniquely talented surgeon in that he has tremendous organizational and people skills to assemble some of the most well known authors in the world in each area from breast cancer to cosmetic surgery of the breast for this book.

I have known Dr. Spear as a friend and colleague for almost twenty years and have followed his career as he became Chairman of Plastic Surgery at Georgetown University Hospital and developed a superb department with his unique administrative people skills and surgical talents. He has been a tremendous role model for all of us in the field of plastic surgery of how plastic surgery can strive for excellence and thrive in an environment where innovation, ingenuity and discovery are important. Dr. Spear excels in all of these areas.

This book, which contains the new adjunct and promising therapies in the management of breast cancer as well as refinements from perforator flaps for breast reconstruction to minimally invasive procedures for breast reshaping to the evolving new modalities for breast augmentation and refinements in breast implants as well as the potential for lipoaugmentation with fat transfer, has now become a classic text to which all others must be compared in the future.

I, along with the entire specialties of surgery and plastic surgery, applaud Dr. Spear and his associate editors for this truly remarkable, third edition text on surgery of the breast.

Rod J. Rohrich, MD, FACS
Professor and Chairman
Crystal Charity Ball Distinguished Chair in Plastic Surgery
Warren and Betty Woodward Chair in
Plastic and Reconstructive Surgery
Department of Plastic Surgery
University of Texas Southwestern Medical Center
Dallas, Texas

Foreword to 2nd Edition

A decade ago when Dr. Spear asked me to contribute to a new book on breast surgery as associate editor, I demurred. In the first place, did the world really need another textbook on plastic surgery of the breast? It would be a lot of work, especially for him; was he prepared for all the tardy contributors who would have to be coaxed and wheedled and threatened to keep on any sort of publication schedule? And secondly, what could I contribute? I was at a point in my career where my clinical interests had turned away from breast surgery toward the rethinking that was beginning to sweep through the field of facial rejuvenation. Fortunately Dr. Spear persisted, of course, and the final product was indeed a wonderful contribution to the specialty. Here for the first time were all the attendant disciplines concerned with breast disease and deformity included in depth for the convenient review of the practicing plastic surgeon. Here also was a rich compendium of key surgical techniques within each of the various components that make up plastic surgery of the breast, presented by the most respected authorities worldwide. And all this in a single, tidy volume.

Dr. Spear and I both trained with Dr. D. Ralph Millard, Jr., who penned the foreword for the first edition. After leaving Miami, Dr. Spear spent fellowship training in Paris studying craniofacial surgery with Dr. Daniel Marchac. When I invited him to join me at Georgetown, it was with the thought that he would help develop this clinical area. But such is the nature of the diverse field we call plastic surgery that we can never predict where the needs of the specialty will take us, however we try to define our particular interests early in our careers. Such also was the case with Dr. Stephen Kroll, too early taken from us; despite thorough training in otorhinolaryngology before his plastic surgery residency with Dr. Spear and myself at Georgetown, his greatest contributions also fell to the field of breast surgery. Dr. Spear took quickly to the breast surgery program at the Medical Center and became a key contributor and later lead author on the various breast papers that issued from our unit. After I taught myself dermal tattooing for nipple-areolar coloration, for example, it was Dr. Spear who went to the manufacturers to help develop a line of custom, premixed pigments for the convenient use of practicing plastic surgeons. When the silicone breast implant crisis took over the specialty in the early nineties, my reaction to the intrusion of politics into patient care was one of distaste and disillusionment, as I watched my clinical results deteriorate overnight. I was not alone, of course; it was no coincidence, for example, that Dr. Rod Hester and I found ourselves independently developing new interests (and new midface lifts) in the wake of the controversy. But Dr. Spear saw opportunity in adversity, as he continued to labor within the system to make the best of a bad situation. Again he worked with the manufacturers to help develop saline implants of better design, but also to foster the necessary studies to support the return of the silicone implant, a looming if long-delayed reemergence that will ultimately owe a good deal to his individual efforts.

The fact that we so soon have a second and much expanded edition of this valuable work is reflective of Dr. Spear's managerial efficiency. In the little more than a decade since Dr. Spear succeeded me at Georgetown, for example, that same efficiency brought impressive growth to the plastic surgery division, culminating in its recent graduation to departmental status, joining Georgetown to an appallingly small club of plastic surgery departments within the nation's many university medical centers. The associate editors for this second edition, all surgeons directly involved in surgery of the breast, have appropriately grown to four for this much larger offering. The three plastic surgeons, Drs. Robb, Hammond, and Nababedian, are all well-known to the specialty, each bringing a special expertise to the overall project. The general surgeon, Dr. Willey, brings a woman surgeon's insight to overall matters of breast health. The new edition has grown by half, with the total number of chapters more than a hundred, over one-third of which are entirely new . . . reflecting the latest concepts and emergent techniques of the past decade. Most of the remaining chapters have been extensively rewritten as well, to reflect the forward progress of the same period. Two volumes, of course, are now required to contain the added information. I am certain this expanded and timely second edition will immediately prove not only valuable, but indeed indispensable to any practicing plastic surgeon who operates on the breast. And when I contemplate this handsome, well-edited set and finger through the many chapters with their intriguing titles and beautiful clinical photographs and results, I must admit—as a plastic surgeon with a clinical practice now limited to surgical rejuvenation of the face . . . I must admit a certain wistfulness. . . .

J. William Little, MD

Foreword to 1st Edition

This book is one of a kind.

Two of the authors, Editor Scott L. Spear and Associate Editor John William Little, were sought as residents for our Plastic Surgery Division at the University of Miami School of Medicine because of their record of superiority in collegiate leadership, scholarship, and athletics, graduation from outstanding medical schools, and completion of sound training in general surgery at superior medical centers. Bill Little also had completed a plastic surgery residency under the great Cliff Kiehn before coming to our program. During their residency, they both excelled in applying principles to the planning and execution of plastic surgery. It was obvious that both were destined for important roles in their specialty. Bill Little became program chairman of plastic surgery at Georgetown Medical Center and served with distinction for 10 years, at which time Scott Spear took over for him.

During the past 20 years, as evidenced by publications, symposia, and teaching sessions, Drs. Little and Spear have had enormous experience in plastic surgery of the breast at Georgetown University. Despite this, I challenged Dr. Spear to tell me why, specifically, he was writing this book. These are his comments, which give insight into the real purpose and true value of this book.

"As one of your trainees and a descendent of the Gillies-Millard School of plastic surgery, I have wanted to, hoped to, and tried to play my part in passing on to the present and future plastic surgeons the importance of key principles. I have been impressed in a wide range of plastic surgery endeavors, that only a handful of plastic surgeons are able to combine principles and art, particularly in reconstructive surgery. Surgery of the breast as it is performed currently is in need of much of the same focus that cleft lip and palate surgery received with your books, *Cleft Craft*. Also, I borrowed the title of your first book, *The Principles and Art of Plastic Surgery* and will bring principles of plastic surgery into play in a broadly aimed textbook on surgery of the breast, in an attempt to help surgeons do their job and ultimately help patients to get better results.

"In addition, I have been struck that the field of breast surgery needed a textbook which could cover the whole gamut of breast surgery from the surgical point of view. What is available currently in bookstores is focused either on purely cosmetic surgery, reconstructive surgery, or ablative surgery. No one has tied these three together; so we have oncologic surgeons who do not understand aesthetic principles, we have aesthetic surgeons who do not understand oncologic or reconstructive principles, and we have reconstructive surgeons who do not understand aesthetic or oncologic principles. Thus, this book is divided into four sections, including oncologic surgery, reconstructive surgery, and cosmetic surgery. The reason that the book is multiauthored is that no one that I know of can write all three sections authoritatively. I expect that, in the future, breast surgery will become more and more of a specialty by itself with one surgeon working in all three areas rather than having two or three surgeons involved. In that sense, the same surgeon might diagnose breast cancer, perform the biopsy, do the ablation, and finally perform the reconstruction. This trend is beginning to happen already in the United States with Grant Carlson at Emory University. It is also occurring in Europe, in both Italy and Germany. I see this textbook, therefore, as the fundamental text for this next generation of breast surgeons.

"Bill Wood, Chief of Plastic Surgery at Emory University, an expert in breast oncology, was instrumental in helping to organize the content and authors of the oncology section.

"John W. Little's important chapters, by his specific analysis, rely less on scientific discussion and documentation than on surgical art, the personal and empiric accumulation of insight into the operations. His contributions are memorable.

"Marc Lippman, one of the world's leading authorities on breast cancer, is a medical oncologist and was head of that portion at the National Institutes of Health for many years before coming to Georgetown to run the Lombardi Cancer Center. His chapter is concerned with the future trends in management of breast cancer in the next millennium."

Thus, you will find this book complete in its coverage, detailed in its description, and enjoyable in its presentation.

D. Ralph Millard, Jr., M.D., F.A.C.S., Hon. F.R.C.S. Ed, Hon. F.R.C.S. Eng., O.D. Ja.
Light-Millard Professor and Chairman Emeritus
University of Miami School of Medicine
Miami, Florida

Preface

The primary mission of a physician is to help his or her patients. The higher mission of a medical textbook is to help other physicians help even more patients. Although I have been asked before to write other books on other medical subjects, I preferred to wait until I thought I had something truly substantial to add on a subject that would help other surgeons in some special way that other text had not yet accomplished. As mentioned, with the many changes in breast surgery during the last two decades and the increasing need for interspecialty collaboration and cooperation, the seeds of this book were thus sown. I saw an opportunity to write and edit a unifying text/atlas that embraced the plastic surgery principles as espoused by Gilles and Millard and yet span the entire breadth of this discipline from breast oncology to breast augmentation. At the same time, in the Millard tradition, my goal is to show others that beautiful or normal-looking results are not only obtainable but critical for this important area. This book is thus written for plastic surgeons, general surgeons, gynecologists, oncologists, or anyone else who is looking for a unified source of information for practical and principled surgical management of the breast. Although the section dealing with oncology is primary text in nature, most of the remaining chapters are in atlas format, thus allowing the reader to pursue the surgical approach espoused within the text. In total, there are over 130 chapters with over 150 contributing authors. In order to have the most expertise in as many areas as possible, we chose a multiauthored approach to the subject rather than a single-authored text. With a single-author book, the scope necessarily would have been more limited or the tone less authoritative. The atlas format is meant to provide a "how-to" outline for many procedures. The text chapters, on the other hand, are meant as resources regarding important oncologic, reconstructive, or other principles. The first edition of this text was developed with the help of Bill Wood, Chief of Surgery at Emory University in Atlanta, and Bill Little, my predecessor as Chief of Plastic Surgery at Georgetown University. The second edition included some additional new talent, who have returned for the third edition. I am grateful to Shawna Willey, head of the Breast Oncology Section at Georgetown University Hospital; Dennis Hammond, a practicing plastic surgeon in Grand Rapids, Michigan; Maurice Nahabedian, my plastic surgery colleague here at Georgetown; and Geoff Robb, Chief of Plastic Surgery at the M.D. Anderson Hospital, all of whom have helped me tremendously as associate editors of this third edition.

In the preface to the first edition, I mentioned key principles as proposed by Ralph Millard, which I have hoped to carry forward in my practice and in this text. Just to review, some of the most critical and relevant principles that are highlighted in this text include:

- Know the ideal beautiful normal.
- Diagnose before treating.
- Tissue losses should be replaced in kind whenever possible.
- Reconstruct in units.
- Make a plan, a pattern, and a second plan (a lifeboat).
- Consider the secondary donor area.
- Follow up with a critical eye.
- Teaching our specialty is its best legacy.

Although there are other good books written about the breast, none that I know of has tackled this diverse subject so broadly and yet tried to focus on the critical issues in so many different areas. If this text helps other physicians and, in particular, other surgeons treat their patients, then I will feel that it has succeeded.

Acknowledgments

As the work in preparing this third edition of this textbook comes to a close, the task of acknowledging those who have helped along the way certainly becomes more challenging. Where to start? So, let's start with my associate editors who have each given up countless hours and expertise to contribute their own chapters, and shape, edit and discuss the chapters of others in their respective sections. Doctors Hammond, Nahabedian, Robb, and Willey are each well-respected authorities in their respective fields and could, and in fact, have written their own texts. So to each of you: Thank you, really.

Similarly, to the over 150 authors who also contributed to these pages: Thank you. Only those who have ever endeavored to publish or write a medical text can appreciate how much uncompensated work goes into these efforts.

Then there are the residents and fellows who work with me and all the other associate editors. I make no bones about the fact that surgery is not a "one man act." My patients know that I rely heavily on a team of residents and fellows to help with the surgery, help take care of the patients, and even help with scholarly things such as this textbook. Thanks to all of you. I do appreciate it even if I don't always show it.

How about my professional staff of nurses, physician assistants, administrative assistants, and even administrators? So thanks to all of you, especially Sonia Alexander, Lisa Grollman, Mary Beth Brubeck, Cathalene Blake, Joni Douglas, Karen Johnson, Benson Won, and Mark Pollard. You all know that I could not do this work without your tireless efforts, day in and day out.

Finally, let me mention my industry partners and associates. Often maligned or taken for granted, my partners in industry—whether book publishers, implant manufacturers, pharmaceutical companies, or others—create and provide the products that allow us to do our job, and support us with education, grants, and other tools that make our work possible. So a special thanks to Hani Zeini, Lisa Colleran, and Rene Snowden who have helped me so much along the way.

Contents

SECTION I: Oncology and Oncoplastic Surgery

SECTION II: Breast Reconstruction

Volume 2

SECTION III: Reduction Mammaplasty and Mastopexy

SECTION IV: Augmentation Mammaplasty

SECTION

III

Reduction Mammaplasty and Mastopexy

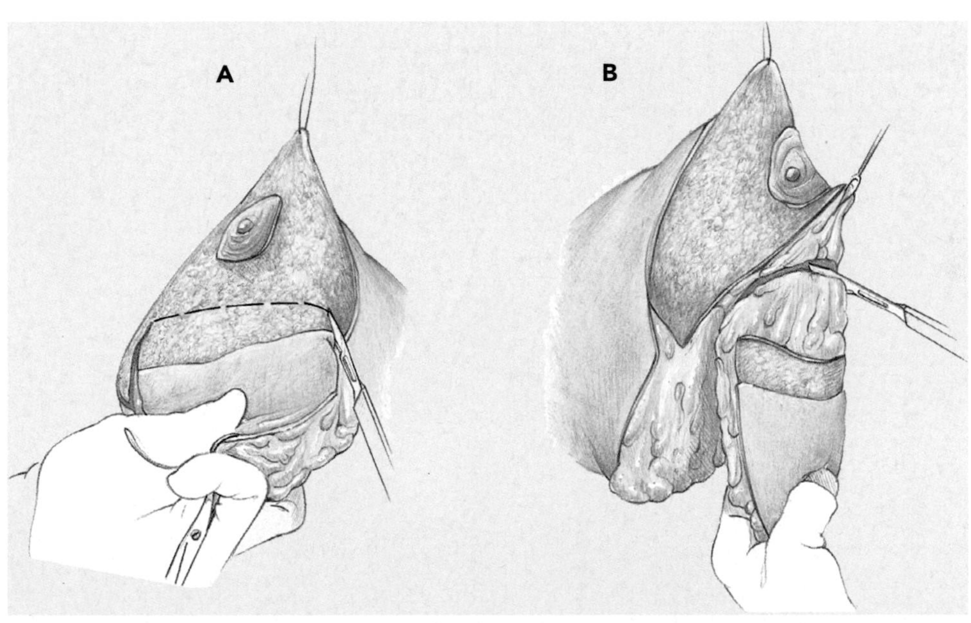

CHAPTER

82

Dennis C. Hammond

Reduction Mammaplasty and Mastopexy: General Considerations

INTRODUCTION

Reduction mammaplasty and mastopexy are two distinct yet interrelated procedures that share many points in common. Both operations result in lifting of the nipple and areola, reduction of the breast skin envelope, and generally an overall improvement in the shape of the breast. As a result, these goals are accomplished for both procedures using similar operative strategies. While recognizing these similarities, it is important to note that the major focus of breast reduction is to reduce the volume of the breast, whereas mastopexy is generally intended to lift and reshape the breast with little or no breast volume change. Typically, the aesthetic concerns in mastopexy are generally more demanding than those in breast reduction. Understanding the basic elements of each procedure is key to developing a successful operative plan that provides the best results possible and yet minimizes potential complications.

OPERATIVE GOALS: REDUCTION

Many different and varied techniques for breast reduction have been described. Several of these procedures have come to be known simply on the basis of the name of the physician who described the operation. In addition, many of these procedures have variably overlapping technical details, all of which can create confusion when attempting to evaluate published results. To assist in organizing and evaluating the multiple techniques of breast reduction, it is helpful to realize that any procedure designed to accomplish breast reduction must consist of the following four interrelated elements: preserving the nipple-areola complex (NAC) blood supply, removing the redundant parenchyma, removing excess skin, and shaping the breast. Understanding how the technical details of each individual procedure satisfy these four cardinal elements allows us to group the various procedures to be grouped. For instance, the superior pedicle procedures can be contrasted with the inferior pedicle procedures. With this as an organizational framework, direct comparison of the different techniques is facilitated and results in a better understanding of these various operations.

NIPPLE-AREOLA COMPLEX VASCULARITY

Inherent in any breast reduction procedure is a strategy to preserve the blood supply to the NAC. Because the vascularity to the NAC has many different and overlapping sources, almost any pedicle can be fashioned to maintain the viability of the NAC after breast reduction. Common variations include the superior pedicle (1–3), inferior pedicle (4,5), lateral pedicle (6), superomedial pedicle (7), central pedicle (8), vertical bipedicle (McKissock) (9,10), and horizontal bipedicle (Strombeck) (11). Each operative strategy facilitates resection of excessive breast parenchyma while maintaining a healthy blood supply to the NAC.

EXCISION OF EXCESS PARENCHYMA

Once the pedicle has been designed, the redundant breast parenchyma is removed from around the pedicle. Typically, this removal takes on the shape of a horseshoe centered on the pedicle. Although many surgeons remove this tissue en bloc, others remove it in sections such that side-to-side comparison can ensure that symmetric removal is accomplished. In addition, removal in segments allows regional identification of any problem areas that may show up later on pathologic examination. If further tissue resection is required, knowledge of which segment of breast tissue was involved can help guide subsequent operative planning.

SKIN ENVELOPE REDUCTION

To accommodate the new and reduced volume of the breast, the skin envelope surface area must also be reduced. Although many different patterns have been described, it is the location and length of the cutaneous scar that come to define the ultimate result. The classic method to manage the skin envelope results in an inverted-T scar pattern (8). More recently, other "short-scar" strategies have been described that limit the scar to the periareolar area and then variably down to the inframammary fold (13–20). Understanding the advantages and disadvantages of each skin envelope management strategy is important in appropriate patient selection.

BREAST SHAPING

Shaping the reduced breast can involve everything from simple skin redraping to more elaborate internal breast flaps (21,22), internal suturing, and even the placement of a supportive mesh framework (23). It is these multiple and varied breast shaping maneuvers that have contributed significantly to the complexity of the various breast reduction procedures. At the same time, the tremendous imagination and artistry that has been brought to breast reduction since the mid-1990s has manifested itself largely in the development of these shaping maneuvers.

OPERATIVE GOALS: MASTOPEXY

Because the procedures for breast reduction and mastopexy are basically similar in design, the described procedures for mastopexy can be evaluated using the same four considerations described previously. However, it should be noted that issues related to scar length and breast shape take on added importance when this analysis is applied to mastopexy. In addition, because little or no parenchyma is removed, the need for developing a true pedicle for the NAC via tissue resection is eliminated. Because the breast is largely being reshaped in mastopexy, internal shaping maneuvers become decidedly more relevant, and it is these shaping maneuvers that distinguish among the various described procedures for mastopexy.

CLINICAL APPLICATION

To more fully understand this organizational strategy, it is helpful to describe several of the more popular techniques of breast reduction and mastopexy based on the four cardinal elements.

Wise Pattern Inverted T

This procedure is the most commonly performed breast reduction operation in the United States. It is based on an inferior pedicle, removes tissue from around the pedicle medially, superiorly, and laterally; removes skin below the medial and lateral breast flaps, including the deepithelialized inferior pedicle; and, most often, simply redrapes the skin around the inferior pedicle to shape the breast (Fig. 82.1).

Vertical Mammaplasty

This procedure has gained in popularity as a method to reduce the length of the cutaneous scars. It is based on a superior or superomedial pedicle, removes tissue from the lower pole of the breast, uses a circumvertical skin resection pattern, and typically does not involve any attempt at internal shaping other than suturing together the medial and lateral pillars of parenchyma created during dissection. Although several variations of this procedure have been described, breaking them down onto the four cardinal elements helps in understanding how they are related (Figs. 82.2 and 82.3).

Short-Scar Periareolar Inferior Pedicle Reduction Mammaplasty

This procedure is a different variation on the strategy used by the classic inverted-T procedure and the vertical mammaplasty.

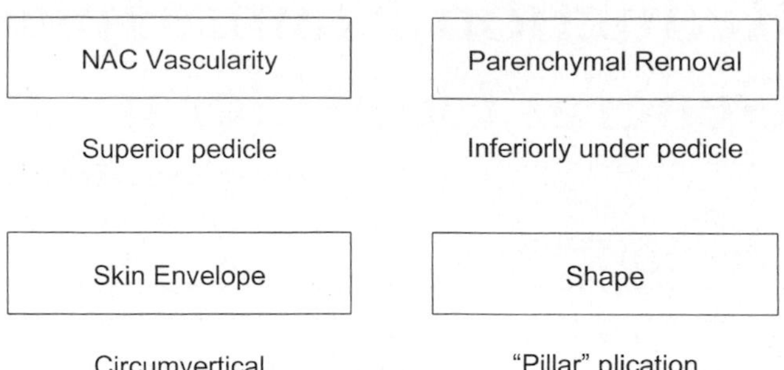

Figure 82.2. Basic elements of the vertical mammaplasty. NAC, nipple-areola complex.

Short-scar periareolar inferior pedicle reduction mammaplasty is based on an inferior pedicle but uses a circumvertical skin resection pattern. In addition, aggressive internal shaping with sutures is used to reposition the breast parenchyma to create a more aesthetic shape than that obtained with simple skin redraping. These technical modifications are readily understood when the operation is described using the four cardinal elements (Fig. 82.4).

In fact, any described procedure designed to accomplish either breast reduction or mastopexy can be broken down into the four basic elements. By analyzing the operative strategies inherent in these procedures in this fashion, vague and confusing terms to describe the procedures are avoided and a more direct and meaningful comparison between procedures can be performed.

INFRAMAMMARY FOLD

Regardless of what technique is used to accomplish breast reduction or mastopexy, accurate preservation or repositioning of the inframammary fold is critical in determining the quality of the final result. It is a common circumstance that the position of the inframammary fold is changed as a result of the dissection

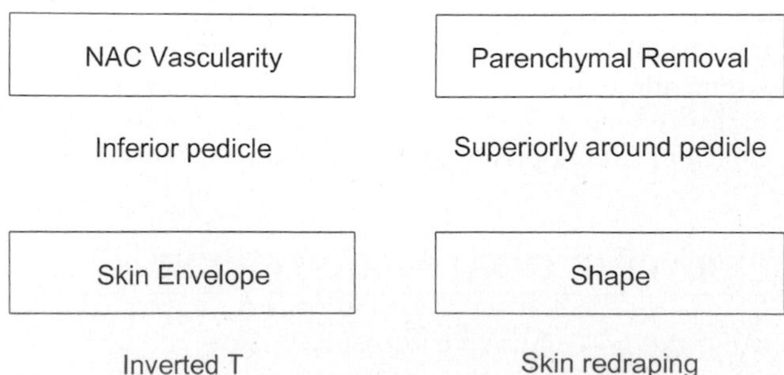

Figure 82.1. Basic elements of the Wise pattern inverted-T inferior pedicle breast reduction. NAC, nipple-areola complex.

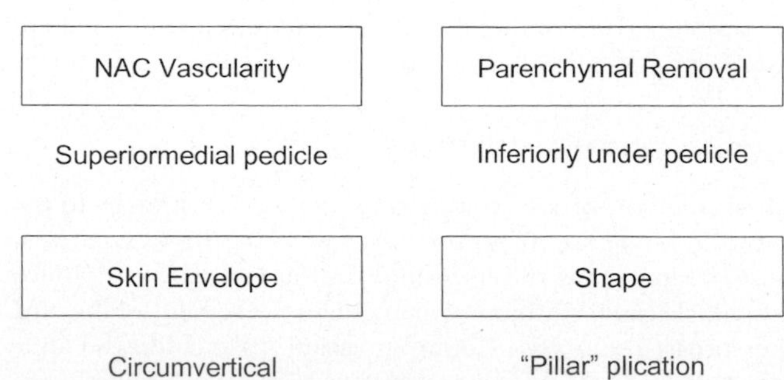

Figure 82.3. Basic elements of the superomedial pedicle vertical mammaplasty. NAC, nipple-areola complex.

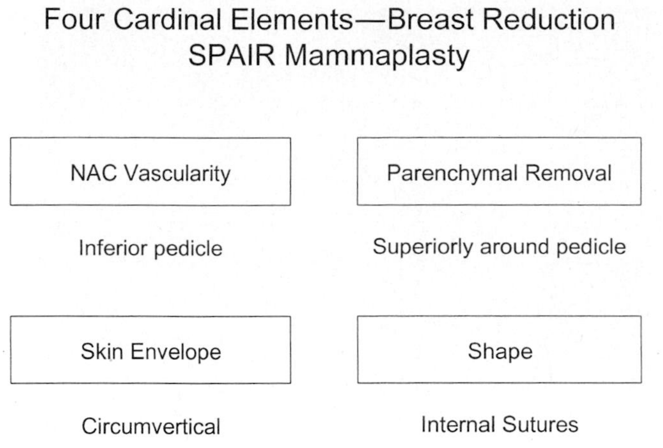

Four Cardinal Elements—Breast Reduction SPAIR Mammaplasty

NAC Vascularity

Inferior pedicle

Parenchymal Removal

Superiorly around pedicle

Skin Envelope

Circumvertical

Shape

Internal Sutures

Figure 82.4. Basic elements of short-scar periareolar inferior pedicle reduction (SPAIR) mammaplasty. NAC, nipple-areola complex.

performed during the procedure. In most instances, the fold position is lowered, which, along with expansion of the lower skin envelope, contributes to the phenomenon of "bottoming out." Here, bottoming out refers to the gradual descent of breast parenchyma below the original inframammary fold location. This results in an NAC position that appears displaced superiorly, an excessive distance between the nipple and the inframammary fold, and, in the case of an inverted-T type of procedure, a riding up of the inframammary fold scar such that it is 2 to 3 cm above the location of the new but lowered fold (Fig. 82.5).

Preventing this postoperative loss of shape can be accomplished in many ways. Perhaps the most straightforward technique is to not violate the attachments of the inframammary fold during the dissection of the breast. If the attachments of Scarpa's fascia to the inferior pole of the breast are kept intact, it is unlikely that the force of the overlying parenchyma will disrupt these attachments postoperatively (20). If these attachments are disrupted during dissection of the breast, they can be sutured back into position to stabilize the position of the fold or if desired, to actually elevate the fold. Alternatively, the breast parenchyma that actually creates the "bottomed out" effect can be removed, with the remainder of the breast subsequently folding together to form the final breast shape. This is the basic strategy of many vertical mammaplasty techniques. However the fold is managed, the importance of predictably positioning a stable fold in the desired location cannot be overstated because it is truly the foundation of the breast. If and when the position of the fold changes, it is usually to the detriment to the overall quality of the final result.

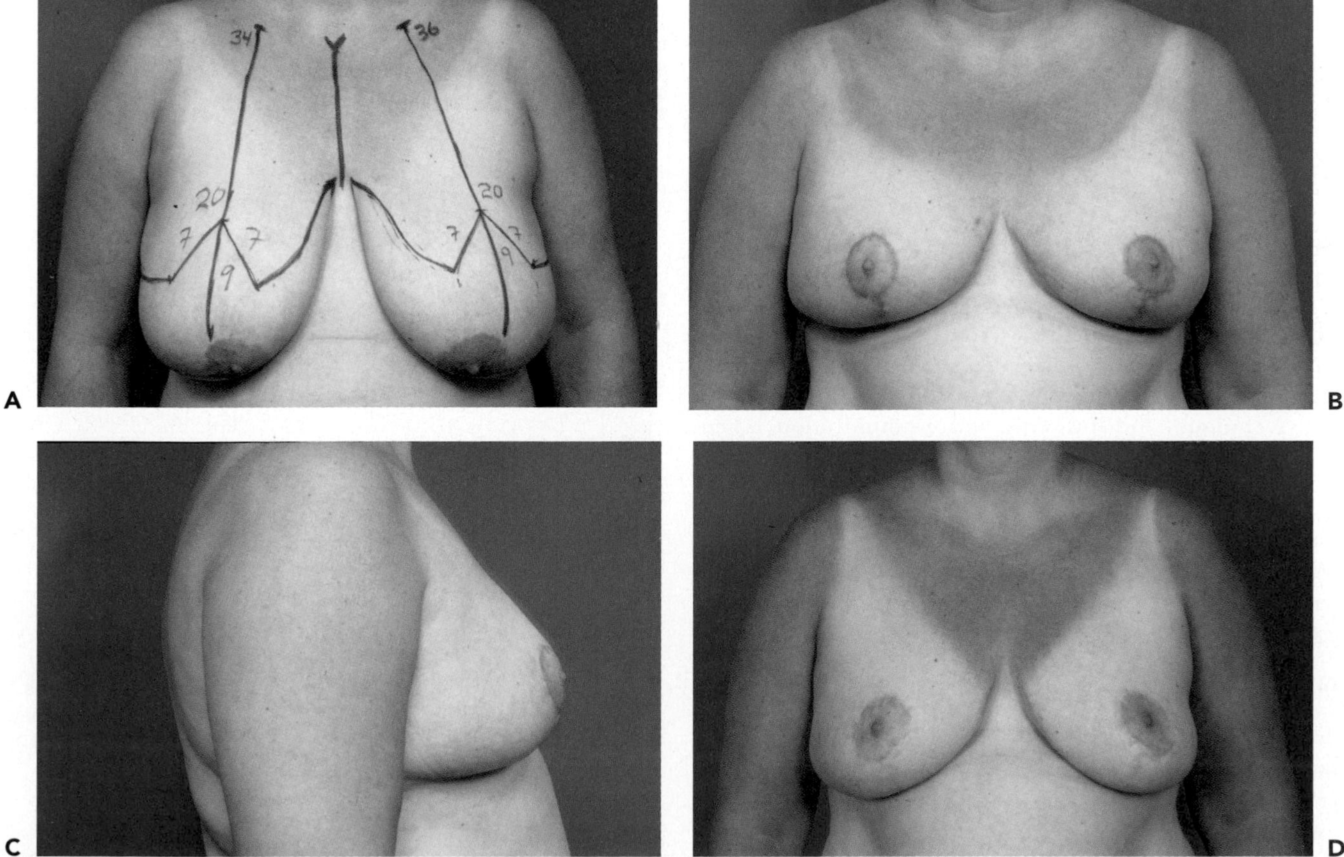

Figure 82.5. **A:** Preoperative marks in preparation for an inverted-T inferior pedicle breast reduction. **B, C:** Anteroposterior and lateral views of the results at 6 weeks. The breast volume appears to be proportionate to the remainder of the body habitus, and it is centered under the nipple-areola complex (NAC), which is positioned directly at the point of maximal projection. **D, E:** Anteroposterior and lateral views of the results at 1 year. There has been a shifting of the breast volume into the lower pole of the breast such that the breast appears hollowed out superiorly and the NAC now rides higher up so it is no longer located at the apex of the breast projection. (*continued*)

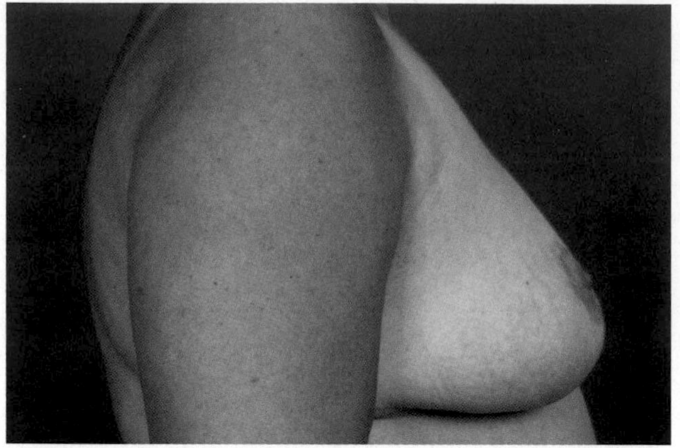
E

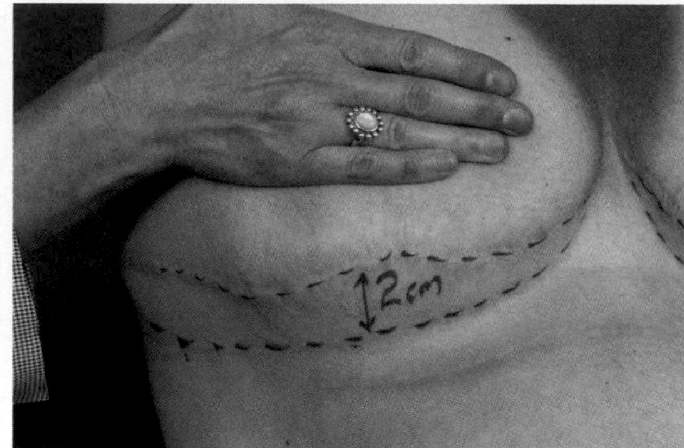

F

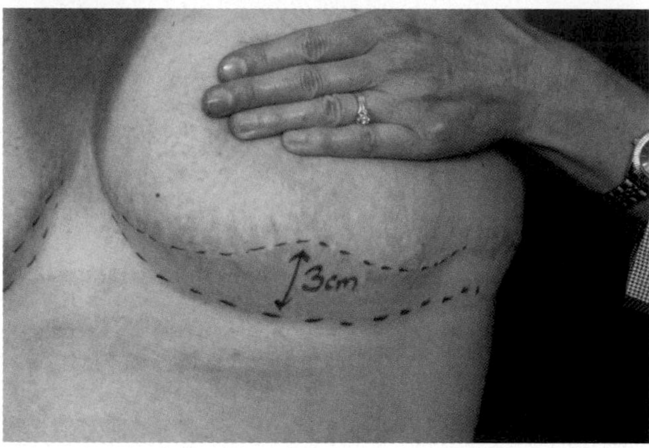

G

Figure 82.5. (*Continued*) **F, G:** As the breasts are lifted, the final location of the inframammary fold can be seen to have settled 2 to 3 cm below the inframammary fold scar. This scar defined the initial location of the fold after surgery. It is the descent of breast tissue below this landmark that contributes to the creation of the classic "bottoming out" phenomenon after breast reduction.

CONCLUSION

There are many described techniques for breast reduction and mastopexy. Despite the widely divergent technical details inherent in many of these procedures, there is a commonality among them that can be summarized in the four common elements. Understanding these elements and how they apply to these procedures allows accurate evaluation of the merits of each technique and prevents miscommunication when attempting to compare results. Such an understanding leads to a better insight into the operative strategy for accomplishing breast reduction and mastopexy.

EDITORIAL COMMENTS

In this chapter, Dr. Hammond reviews the basic principles and concepts of reduction mammaplasty and mastopexy, with an emphasis on similarities and differences. The four cardinal elements for these techniques that are emphasized include preservation of the blood supply to the NAC, removal of excess parenchyma, removal of excess skin, and shaping of the breast. The techniques that are used are ultimately based on characteristics of the breast and on the comfort level of the surgeon with a given procedure. All techniques described can deliver an excellent outcome when women are properly selected and when the operation is properly designed and executed.

Additional information that should be of value to surgeons is provided. Although the list of pedicles described was comprehensive, one pedicle that was not included on the list is the medial pedicle. Although this is similar to the superomedial pedicle and the two names are often used interchangeably, there are differences with respect to their orientation. In their initial description, Orlando and Guthrie oriented the vertical limb of the superomedial pedicle from the 12 o'clock position on the breast and then extended it 75 to 90 degrees clockwise for the right breast and counterclockwise for the left breast. This pedicle was principally used for small-volume breast reduction. With the medial pedicle, the vertical limb is oriented from the 1 o'clock position on the right breast and from the 11 o'clock position on the left breast and then extended roughly 45 degrees in the clockwise and counterclockwise directions, respectively. This allows for an improved arc of rotation and prevents any folds or kinks of the pedicle during the insetting of the NAC. This is especially important in women who require large-volume resection. Other advantages of the medial and superomedial pedicles are that the blood supply originates from the internal mammary and pectoral perforators, the innervation to the NAC is preserved in the majority of women, and the length of the pedicle is usually less for a given breast. Although preservation of blood supply to the NAC on a vascularized pedicle is possible in the majority of women, a free nipple graft may occasionally be necessary in cases of severe mammary hypertrophy (>2,500 g per breast).

M.Y.N.

REFERENCES

1. Weiner DL, Aiache AE, Silver L, et al. A single dermal pedicle for nipple transposition in subcutaneous mastectomy, reduction mammaplasty, or mastopexy. *Plast Reconstr Surg* 1973;51(2):115–120.
2. Weiner D. Breast reduction: the superior pedicle technique (dermal and composite). In: Goldwyn RM, ed., *Reduction Mammaplasty*. Philadelphia: Lippincott Williams & Wilkins; 1990:233–238.
3. Arufe HN, Erenfryd A, Saubidet M. Mammaplasty with a single, vertical, superiorly-based pedicle to support the nipple-areola. *Plast Reconstr Surg* 1977;60(2):221–227.
4. Courtiss EH, Goldwyn RM. Reduction mammaplasty by the inferior pedicle technique. An alternative to free nipple and areola grafting for severe macromastia or extreme ptosis. *Plast Reconstr Surg* 1977;59(4):500–507.
5. Robbins TH. A reduction mammaplasty with the areola-nipple based on an inferior dermal pedicle. *Plast Reconstr Surg* 1977;59(1):64–67.
6. Skoog TD. A technique of breast reduction: transposition of the nipple on a cutaneous vascular pedicle. *Acta Chir Scand* 1963;126:453–465.
7. Orlando JC, Guthrie RH Jr. The superomedial dermal pedicle for nipple transposition. *Br J Plast Surg* 1975;28(1):42–45.
8. Hester TR Jr, Bostwick J III, Miller L, et al. Breast reduction utilizing the maximally vascularized central breast pedicle. *Plast Reconstr Surg* 1985;76(6):890–900.
9. McKissock PK. Reduction mammaplasty with a vertical dermal flap. *Plast Reconstr Surg* 1972;49(3):245–252.
10. McKissock PK. Reduction mammaplasty by the vertical bipedicle flap technique. Rationale and results. *Clin Plast Surg* 1976;3(2):309–320.
11. Strombeck JO. Mammaplasty: report of a new technique based on the two pedicle procedure. *Br J Plast Surg* 1960;13:79.
12. Wise RJ. A preliminary report on a method of planning the mammaplasty. *Plast Reconstr Surg* 1956;17(5):367–375.
13. Lassus C. A technique for breast reduction. *Int Surg* 1970;53(1):69–72.
14. Lassus C. Breast reduction: evolution of a technique—a single vertical scar. *Aesthetic Plast Surg* 1987;11(2):107–112.
15. Lassus C. A 30-year experience with vertical mammaplasty. *Plast Reconstr Surg* 1996;97(2):373–380.
16. Lejour M, Abboud M, Declety A, et al. Reduction of mammaplasty scars: from a short inframammary scar to a vertical scar. *Ann Chir Plast Esthet* 1990;35(5):369–379.
17. Lejour M. Vertical mammaplasty and liposuction of the breast. *Plast Reconstr Surg* 1994;94(1):100–114.
18. Lejour M, Abboud M. Vertical mammaplasty without inframammary scar and with breast liposucution. *Perspect Plast Surg* 1996;4:67–90.
19. Hall-Findlay EJ. A simplified vertical reduction mammaplasty: shortening the learning curve. *Plast Reconstr Surg* 1999;104(3):748–759.
20. Hammond DC. Short scar periareolar inferior pedicle reduction (SPAIR) mammaplasty. *Plast Reconstr Surg* 1999;103(3):890–901.
21. Benelli L. A new periareolar mammaplasty: the "round block" technique. *Aesthetic Plast Surg* 1990;14(2):93–100.
22. Graf R, Biggs TM. In search of better shape in mastopexy and reduction mammoplasty. *Plast Reconstr Surg* 2002;110(1):321–322.
23. Góes JC. Periareolar mammaplasty: double skin technique with application of polyglactin or mixed mesh. *Plast Reconstr Surg* 1996;97(5):959–968.

CHAPTER

83

Louis C. Benelli

Periareolar Benelli Mastopexy and Reduction: The "Round Block"

Whatever type of mammaplasty is performed, the main concerns are to limit scars and create a nice breast shape. Ideally, scarring is confined to the periareolar circle.

The indications for various periareolar plasty techniques have been limited (1–6). Only moderate cases of small breast ptosis should be treated using periareolar mastopexy, owing to the risk of enlargement and distortion caused by tension on the areola. The "round block" technique helps eliminate this complication, making feasible the treatment of many cases of breast ptosis and hypertrophy by periareolar mastopexy (7,8).

One of the principal elements of our technique is to treat ptosis and hypertrophy by using a blocked circular dermal suture passed in a purse-string fashion. The round block constitutes a cerclage, fixing a solid circular dermodermal scar block around the areola (Figs. 83.1 and 83.2).

To obtain a nice breast shape, it is necessary to separate the work on the gland (creating the conic shape) from the work on the skin (removing the excess skin around the areola). The skin must cover the cone shape obtained by the work on the gland without any tension. Excess tension on the skin will flatten the shape.

To achieve the greatest anterior projection of the breast, we perform a criss-cross T-inverted technique on the gland, which provides good coning and support without cutting the skin. The skin is simply detached to cover the glandular cone without irregularity.

This control of the periareolar scar gives us a number of new possibilities in breast surgery because the periareolar approach provides easy access to the whole gland, minimizing the required incision. The periareolar approach thus allows us to perform diverse operations, such as mastopexy, mastopexy with reduction or augmentation, tumorectomy, subcutaneous mastectomy, and total mastectomy with reconstruction.

The image of the breast as a symbol of femininity plays an essential role in the way a woman looks at herself. It also contributes to her personal and social development. This image is shaped by the ethnocultural context or sometimes just by the fashion of the moment—the same patient may find herself simultaneously offered a breast augmentation by a North American surgeon and a breast reduction by a Brazilian surgeon. The surgeon must set aside his or her personal taste and listen carefully to the patient's demands, keeping in mind that these demands must be considered with regard to anatomic harmony because certain patients want to pass from one extreme to the other regarding the size of their breasts.

The progress made in endoscopic surgery and other areas has permitted the reduction of scars in many operations. By the use of an axillary or periareolar approach, breast augmentation patients can obtain a satisfying result, with very discreet or invisible scars. Because fashion uncovers rather than covers a woman's body, the long scars resulting from mammaplasty are less accepted now than they were in the past—more so because the scar quality is unforeseeable. Even if the scars are generally discreet when the patient is sitting upright, they may be more visible when the patient is lying supine.

The scars may be less important for a mature woman but might have negative consequences for a young woman in whom scars are sometimes hypertrophic. The scar can be minimized simply by making the incision only around the circumference of the areola.

Mammaplasty via periareolar incisions has the aesthetic advantage of a short scar, but the surgeon should be alert to other potential obstacles inherent to this procedure. It is important to prevent reduction of the scar, which can detrimentally affect the shape of the breast and the quality of the periareolar scar itself.

In this chapter, I analyze the technical elements that make it possible to avoid these potential obstacles to a successful result and to judiciously select the periareolar technique that is suitable for the particular patient. Each technique can yield outstanding results when it is executed in the appropriate case.

EVOLUTION OF PERSONAL TECHNIQUE

In 1983, we started performing periareolar mastopexy with dermal cerclage of the areola via a purse-string suture to prevent postoperative enlargement of the areola and the scar. In view of this procedure's effectiveness, we extended its application, calling it the *round block*. This name was used because of the solidity of the dermodermal circular scar block reinforced by the cerclage, with a nonresorbable suture passed in a purse-string manner through the edge of the periareolar dermis. This procedure has enabled us to treat more serious cases of ptosis and thereby extend the indications of periareolar mastopexy that in the past had been reserved only for moderate ptosis or hypertrophy, essentially because of the postoperative risk of enlargement of the areola and periareolar scar.

Our use of the round block technique has progressed with prudence. In the beginning, we obtained the best results in the correction of hypotrophic ptosis by using periareolar mastopexy with round block and simultaneous placing of a breast implant, ensuring the shape and the anterior projection of the breast.

To obtain breast conization in the treatment of simple ptosis and hypertrophy, simple plication and invagination of the base of the breast has yielded satisfactory results for small breasts but unsatisfactory results for larger breasts, with some leading to long-term shape flattening and recurrence of ptosis.

Therefore, we applied the techniques classically used for reduction mammaplasty in an inverted T. Yet, we practiced them only on the mammary gland without cutting the skin, which

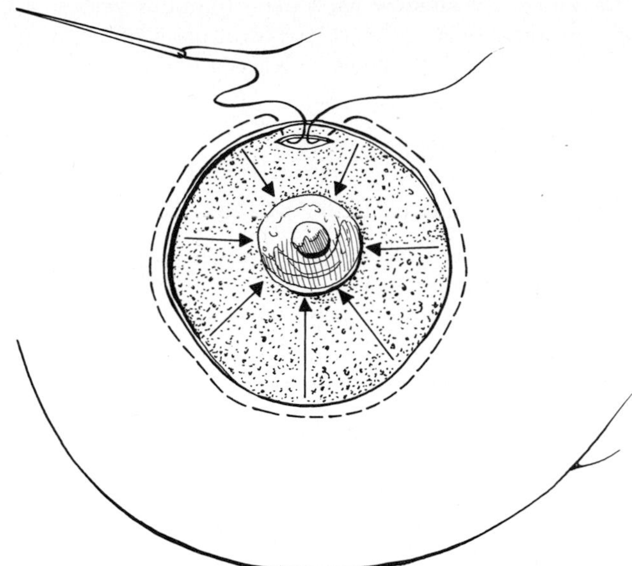

Figure 83.1. Round block cerclage stitch of 2/0 Mersilene made with a long, straight needle passed in a purse-string method. This stitch is passed in a regular plane in the deep dermis 5 mm beyond the edge of deepidermization. This round block cerclage facilitates good control of the areola and scar and can be used in many aesthetic tumoral and reconstructive periareolar operations.

was redraped around the areola without tension using a round block on the skin aperture. We then reduced and reshaped the breast in the manner of an internal inverted T to the breast alone.

The inverted-T techniques that give maximum coning and the best long-term hold are those that are characterized by a crossing and overlapping of two flaps (lateral and medial), which ensures a maximum of anterior projection to the areola (9).

To ensure the breast keeps its shape, we found it equally useful to perform a fixation, at least temporarily, of the glandular cone to the pectoralis major muscle (10).

Concerning work on the breast itself, our goal has been to limit its detachment as much as possible to maximize the vitality of the glandular flaps and to ensure the conical shape. Concerning the skin, the trend has been to limit the amount of resection of the ellipse of the periareolar deepithelialization. This helps prevent complications such as bad scarring and flattening of the breast owing to excess tension in the periareolar area.

PATIENTS AND METHODS

Since 1983, we have performed this surgical procedure on more than 386 patients in aesthetic, tumoral, and reconstructive surgeries (Table 83.1). We have been progressive in our advancement of this procedure for cases of serious ptosis or

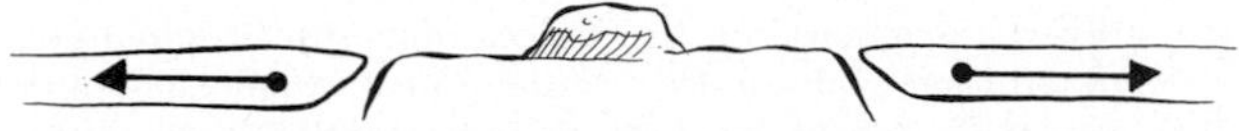

Figure 83.2. Cross-section view showing that the round block cerclage stitch does not produce tension on the areola and scar.

TABLE 83.1 Clinical Series (January 1983 to January 1997)

Breast reductions	51%	198
Mastopexies	19%	73
Mastopexies and augmentations	18%	69
Tumoral and reconstructive surgeries	12%	46
Total number of cases	100%	386

hypertrophy. Breast reductions have entailed an average resection of 220 g (maximum 1,200 g) on each breast.

The principle of the operation is to perform an internal inverted-T mastopexy, with a large, superiorly based dermoglandular pedicle supporting the areola, and to redrape the skin without tension around the areola on the glandular cone by "round block," just like a glove covers a hand. The skin will naturally retract itself on the new breast cone once the postoperative edema has disappeared, a few weeks after the operation. The breast skin has a remarkable capacity to retract, programmed by nature to adapt itself to the considerable changes of volume occurring during pregnancy and lactation, during which the areola easily adapts itself to various changes in diameter.

On the breast, we distinguish between (a) the thin and elastic periareolar skin, whose function is to adapt itself to the breast volume changes and which generally produces fine scars and is easily stretched by the weight of the gland, and (b) the skin of the base of the breast and of the submammary fold. This thick skin's function is to support the breast, and the scars it produces are potentially much larger.

For support of the breast, the periareolar technique is used to remove the thin and elastic stretched skin around the areola, which does not have any supportive value, and to conserve the thick skin at the base of the breast and submammary fold. However, other techniques producing an inverted-T scar involve skin removal at the base of the breast, whereby the vertical skin suture, underneath the areola, is the former thin and elastic periareolar skin that was transposed to reshape the breast. This fact explains the good scars generally seen with this vertical scar, as well as its tendency to stretch and elongate in the postoperative period. This segment is usually fixed at 5 cm during the operation because it is known to stretch out afterward.

Vascularization and innervation of the areola and mammary gland are addressed in the same manner as for an inverted-T technique, with a vertical dermoglandular flap supporting the areola with a superior pedicle. This pedicle will be larger because it occupies the whole length of the ellipse, whereas in the design of an inverted-T mammaplasty the pedicle will be narrower, passing through the edge of the areola, where a straight liberation of the adjacent tissue is required to allow the lift. For this reason, the vitality, breast-feeding ability, and innervation of the areola seems to be better preserved by the round block technique.

Subdermal vascularization is preserved with skin excision done with scissors close to the gland. At the time of the dermal incision within the wide deepithelialized ellipse, we conserve a 1-cm strip of dermis to protect the vascularity of the ellipse's skin edge, especially in its lower part.

The entire operation thus preserves the blood supply and innervation of the breast. This advantage is essential to the improved control of the scar and vitality of the tissues constituting the remodeled breast.

PATIENT SELECTION AND PREPARATION

Consultation before surgery is essential to understand the patient's expectations; these expectations often extend beyond the possibilities of surgery. The patient should be informed that the result of the operation depends on the anatomic quality of tissue. Thus, patient selection and surgery preparation must be performed with care.

In planning the operation, we must consider three factors: the psychological context, the anatomy, and our experience with the technique.

Psychological Context

This is the most important element. Patients must be willing to accept a less-than-perfect shape in favor of a reduced scar. Therefore, one should paint a realistic picture of such possible postoperative difficulties to test the patient's motivation to limit the scar.

Patients should be made aware of the potential postoperative inconveniences of mastopexy, in general, and periareolar mastopexy, in particular, such as the wrinkling and scalloping of the periareolar skin, which may last for weeks or even months, the need to wear a bra night and day for 2 months, the possible need to revise the scar in case of poor scarring, persistence of cutaneous irregularities, and, in case of complete failure, the possible need to undergo an inverted-T mastopexy after all.

The patient's reaction to this warning allows identification of those who probably could not emotionally tolerate the postoperative difficulties. "Impatient patients" are generally excluded, as are those with unrealistic expectations or exaggerated narcissistic suffering. Patients who demand a short-scar technique usually want to obtain a natural appearance and are generally satisfied with the result of the operation, appreciating the shape as well as the discreet nature of the scar.

Anatomy

The best indications are moderate ptosis or hypertrophy in a young patient. In these patients, the skin has a good retracting potential and the breast tissue is firmer, which is important because the scar of a young woman's skin is more likely to become hypertrophic, so we want to limit the extent of the scar.

However, contraindications include breasts that are essentially fat or have a lot of additional skin. Surgeons should exercise caution when considering patients who are overweight, elderly, or smokers.

The morphology of the thorax and the breast shape are also important: Tubular breasts are a good indication, but very large breasts are more difficult to treat.

Experience With the Technique

It is preferable for surgeons unfamiliar with this technique to start by operating on patients with moderate ptosis, where the vertical axis of the planned periareolar ellipse does not exceed 10 cm. After gaining some experience, the surgeon may choose to extend the indications to more severe cases of ptosis or hypertrophy. The degree of difficulty mostly depends on the degree of ptosis. The resection is performed on the distal part of the glandular flaps, cut out like a reduction mammaplasty in inverted-T fashion but without cutting the skin.

We would thus be more likely to perform this procedure in a young patient, even in severe cases of hypertrophy, if the psychological and anatomic conditions are favorable.

SURGICAL TECHNIQUE

STEP 1: PLANNING AND MARKING

We have no standard pattern. Each surgery is specific to the individual patient. The marking begins with the patient standing, then lying supine, and finally back in the standing position.

Marking in the Standing Position

The midline is marked to maintain symmetry (Fig. 83.3). The breast meridian is marked at the beginning on the clavicle, 6 cm from the midline. The meridian is not the meridian of the ptotic breast, but the meridian of the manually reshaped breast. This new meridian will not necessarily cross the ptotic nipple because the mammary ptosis is generally a lateralization of the breast due to chest wall convexity.

The new meridian is often more medial than that of the ptotic breast. The lower part of the breast meridian is not marked while the patient is standing but while she is lying supine.

The New Areola Vertical Position. The superior border of the areola (point A) is marked on the breast meridian, 2 cm higher than the anterior projection of the submammary crease. Reshaping the breast manually, the surgeon verifies that point A is marked in the correct position. Contralateral point A is marked by measuring the distance to the sternal notch.

Symmetry. For a more precise evaluation, the surgeon observes the patient standing in the anatomic position. The

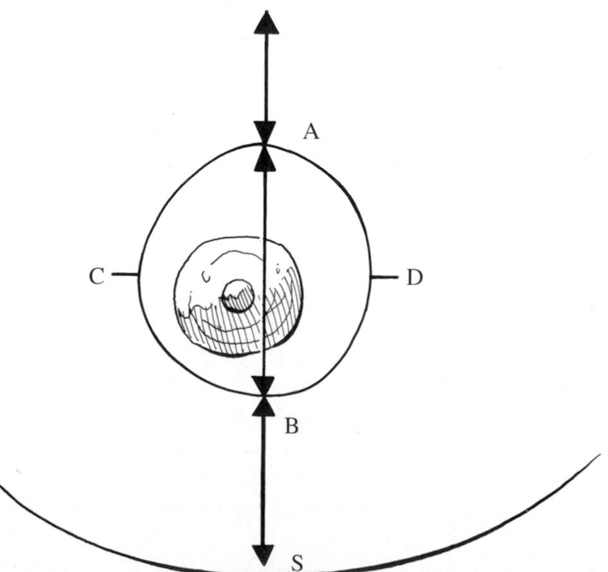

Figure 83.3. Skin marking. The four cardinal stitches should be selected to reduce the ellipse size to its minimum. A large amount of skin is needed to cover the glandular cone, and the skin will retract after surgery. Any skin over the resection can create serious complications. For descriptions of points A, B, C, D, and S, see text.

best position for the observer is facing the patient at a minimum of 3 to 6 feet. During this inspection, the surgeon also checks for any other breast asymmetry.

In cases of volume asymmetry, this preoperative evaluation in the standing position is useful for estimating the possible variation in reduction specimen weight from one side to the other.

Marking the Patient Who Is Lying Supine

The lower part of the marking is done while the patient is lying supine, with the arms lying symmetrically at the patient's sides.

Marking of the Submammary Crease and of the Gland Limits. Point S is the point where the breast meridian crosses the submammary crease. It usually crosses the crease roughly 10 cm from the midline.

Point B is the inferior border of the new areola. It is marked on the breast meridian, and its position is determined by the estimated final breast volume to be covered and by the potential for the breast skin to retract. The distance between point B and point S (BS) may vary from 5 to 12 cm.

Leaving an Ample Distance BS Has Two Advantages. Covering the glandular cone without skin tension prevents flattening of the breast shape, allowing the skin to retract in a more natural adaptation to the height of the new glandular cone obtained by internal shaping of the gland. Reducing the size of the excised skin facilitates better skin adaptation to the final size of the areola during periareolar skin suturing.

Points C and D are the lateral and medial limits of the ellipse, respectively. These points are marked symmetrically, using the breast meridian as a guide and aiming to mark the minimal size of the ellipse because ample skin is needed to cover, without tension, the new glandular cone, lifted and projected earlier. For this reason, point C, the lateral limit of the ellipse, is usually near the lateral border of the areola.

The medial limit of the ellipse (point D) is symmetric to point C, using the breast meridian as a guide, and is located 8 to 12 cm from the midline following the width of the chest wall, the breast implantation, and the breast volume to cover. The medial border of the contralateral ellipse is marked symmetrically, referring to the midline.

Checking the markings is done by pinching together A and B, then C and D, to verify that the remaining skin will be adequate to cover the glandular cone without tension. Finally, the ellipse is marked with a dotted line that joins points A, B, C, and D. At this point, the ellipse shape should be almost round when the patient is lying supine.

A final check of the ellipse design is done with the patient standing, in which case gravity gives a vertical shape to the ellipse. The surgeon should check the symmetry and note and photograph the measurement of the marking.

STEP 2: PREPARATION

With the patient sitting partly upright, the arms are affixed to the body using adhesive bands around the thighs. The region is infiltrated with a dilution of physiologic saline (1,000 mL), epinephrine (0.25 mg), and Xylocaine 2% (20 mL). The area that will be detached is subcutaneously infiltrated, except for the ellipse and surrounding 3 cm, so as to preserve the vascularity of the skin edges. The prepectoral space is also infiltrated in the area of glandular resection and in the area in which the gland will be fixed on the pectoralis major muscle.

STEP 3: INCISION AND DISSECTION

Deepithelialization of the periareolar ellipse is performed by pulling on a concentric epidermal flap (Fig. 83.4). The areola is marked with a tube on the tensed skin at 1-cm-diameter more than the desired final diameter to compensate for stretching and retracting afterward.

An incision on the deepithelialized dermis is made from 2 to 10 o'clock, 1 cm inside the skin edge to improve the subdermal vascular support of the epidermal edge.

Subcutaneous dissection is performed with consideration for the blood supply to the skin. Dissection extends from the ellipse to the submammary fold limits (Fig. 83.5). In the upper-outer quadrant, the dissection has to be more superficial to preserve the vessels extending from the lateral thoracic artery, which is superficial in this glandular area. For good exposure, good retraction is necessary.

At this stage, the surgeon incises the gland to constitute the dermoglandular flap that will be supporting the areola. This incision does not follow the edge of the dermis because it is often too near the areola, especially on the lateral side.

The glandular incision is semicircular at 3 cm from the inferior areola's edge to preserve innervation and blood supply to the areola. This incision facilitates opening the prepectoral space, which we dissect only in the avascular central space, preserving the peripheral blood supply, where the breast is more adherent to the fascia and where the perforators are located.

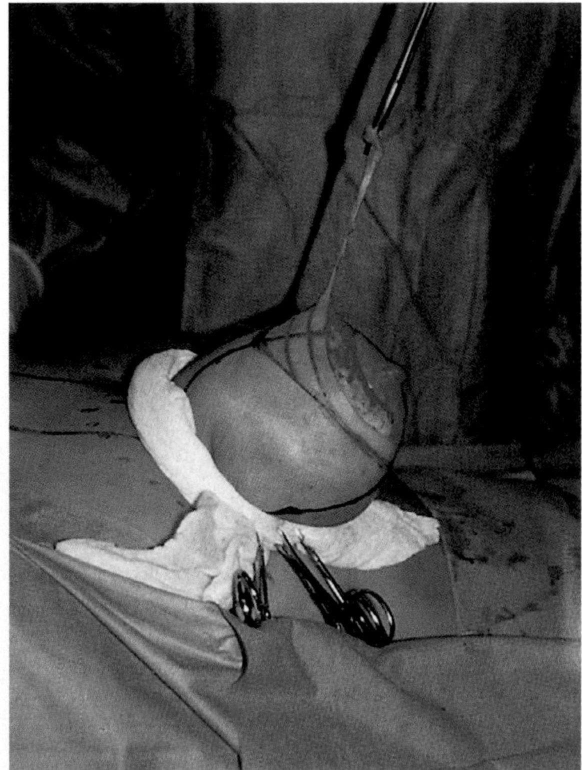

Figure 83.4. Deepithelialization. The periareolar epidermis can be removed quickly by simple traction of a concentric epidermal flap.

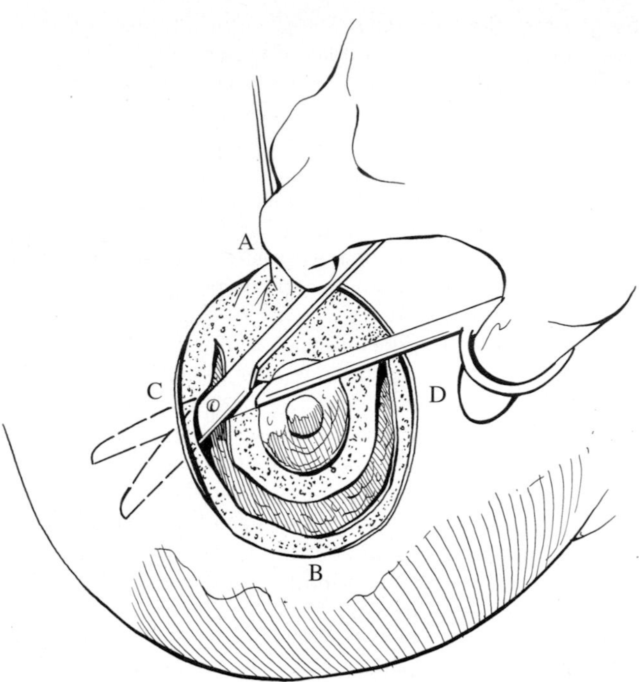

Figure 83.5. The cutaneoglandular detachment is extended at the minimum to facilitate even skin distribution over the new glandular cone.

The inferior glandular flap is then elevated between two clamps and cut vertically beyond the breast meridian up to the fascia.

As a result of this dissection, four flaps will have been created (Fig. 83.6):

- A superior dermoglandular flap supporting the areola
- A glandular medial flap
- A glandular lateral flap
- The detached skin flap

Work on the glandular flaps will facilitate a reduction in volume, if necessary, and will reshape the breast by fixation of the flaps in a new position, forming a glandular cone on which the skin will be redraped with the round block closing.

STEP 4: RESECTION OF GLAND

Depending on the case, resection can be executed on the different glandular flaps. To reduce the upper pole, a Pitanguy keel-like resection can be performed (Fig. 83.6). To reduce the lateral lower pole, the resection on the lateral flap is performed as for a T-inverted reduction (Fig. 83.6). If the lateral flap remains too thick, the reduction can be extended to the posterior side of the flap in the prepectoral space to obtain the desired thickness.

To reduce the medial lower pole, the resection can be performed on the distal part of the medial flap. If the volume to resect is large, the resection can be performed as in a T-inverted technique. In other cases, the medial flap reduction is not extended medially, so as to leave the necessary volume to refill the inner pole of the breast.

STEP 5: GLANDULAR MODELING

Depending on the anatomy of each patient, the glandular flaps are situated to achieve a nice shape with a minimal detachment to prevent fat necrosis. If a good-quality gland and ample volume are not present, we do not create glandular flaps. Instead,

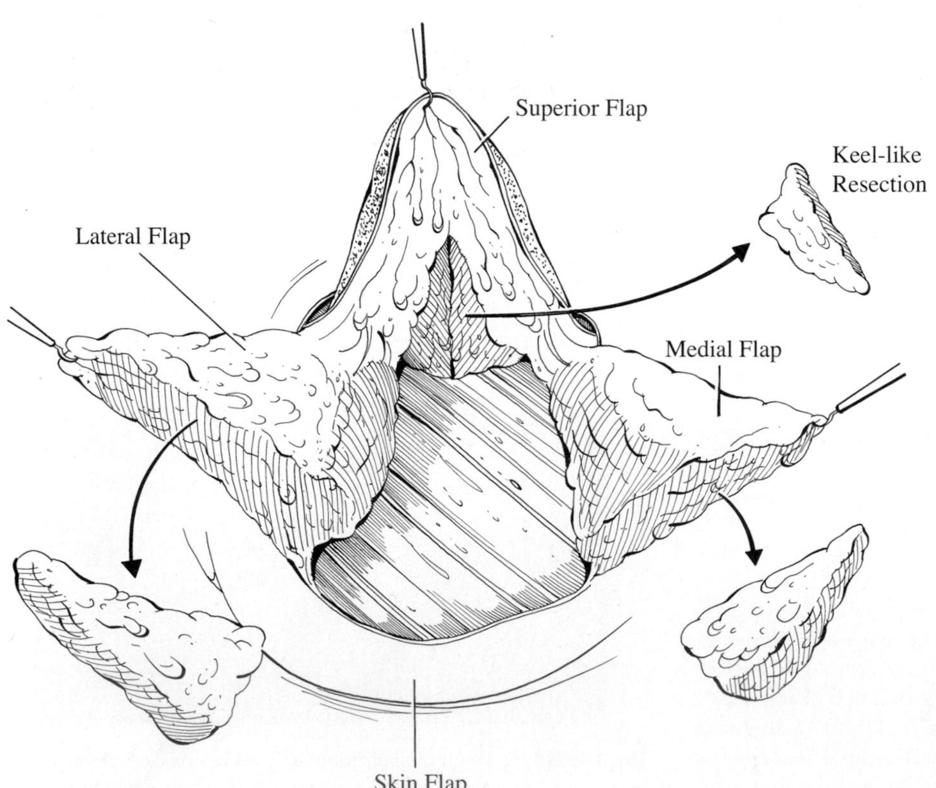

Figure 83.6. The cut of the glandular flaps and, if necessary, their reduction are similar to those used in a T-inverted technique: a vertical dermoglandular, superiorly based flap supporting the nipple-areola complex, a lateral and medial glandular pillar, and a skin flap.

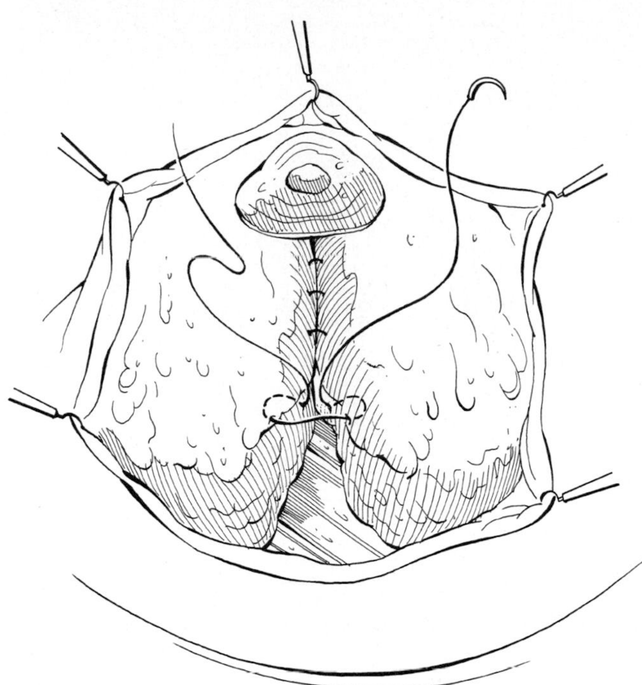

Figure 83.7. Plication invagination of the gland inferior pole allows conization and elevation of the breast shape with minimal glandular devascularization because the retromammary space is not detached. This method is useful for small breasts and in cases of poor-quality glandular tissue.

we perform a simple plication invagination of the gland on the meridian axis without any posterior detachment of the gland (Fig. 83.7). This type of plication invagination nicely cones small breasts, whereas for larger breasts long-term support of the conical shape is better with a criss-cross mastopexy.

The glandular flaps are assembled to reduce the base of the breast, providing a conical shape and the best long-term support. The criss-cross mastopexy often works well to accomplish these goals.

We begin reducing the upper base of the breast using a plication, closing the keel-like reduction with a stitch. This stitch of plication is not cut but is directly fixed to the pectoralis muscle at the top of the retroglandular undermining, allowing at the same time coning and elevation of the breast upper pole. This elevation is temporarily exaggerated, creating a hyperconvexity of the upper pole.

If the upper pole is not hypertrophic, the keel-like reduction is not performed, and a simple posterior fixation to the pectoralis major muscle is performed to elevate the upper pole (Figs. 83.8 and 83.9). During healing, with gravity, the hyperconvexity created by the elevation of the upper pole disappears within a few weeks.

The lower base of the breast is reduced by crossing the two lower glandular flaps (lateral and medial). The flap that is crossed over the other has the biggest amplitude of translation. Because ptosis involves a sagging of the breast but also generally a lateralization of it, we generally prefer crossing the lateral flap over the medial one to medialize the breast shape. In the rare cases in which we want to lateralize the breast, we cross the medial flap over the lateral one.

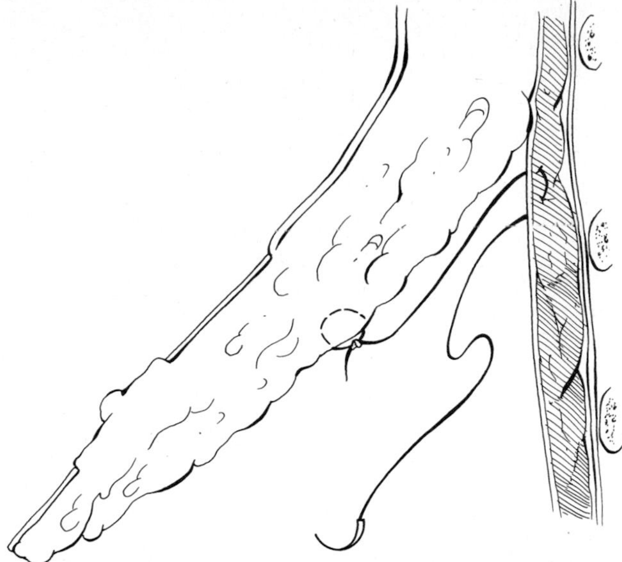

Figure 83.8. Elevation of the upper pole and fixation to the pectoralis. To avoid strangulation of the glandular tissue using this stitch, we first tie a knot on the glandular grip without tension and then tie a knot of fixation to the pectoral grip.

In most cases, we begin the criss-cross mastopexy by rotating and folding the medial flap behind the areola, fixing its distal part to the pectoralis muscle using a U point (Fig. 83.10). The lateral flap is crossed over and fixed to the medial flap by additional U points (Fig. 83.11). Moving these flaps reduces the base of the breast and creates a glandular cone on which we place the areola.

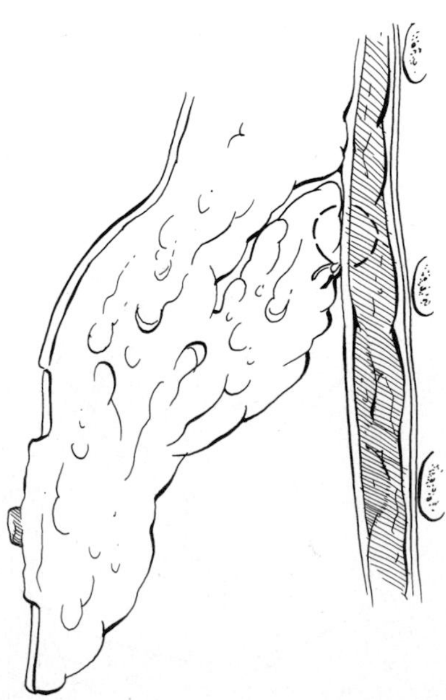

Figure 83.9. Lifting of the pectoral point elevates the areola and breast upper pole. This prevents recurrence of ptosis after healing. The immediate hyperconvexity of the upper pole is common, regardless of the type of scar or mammoplasty performed.

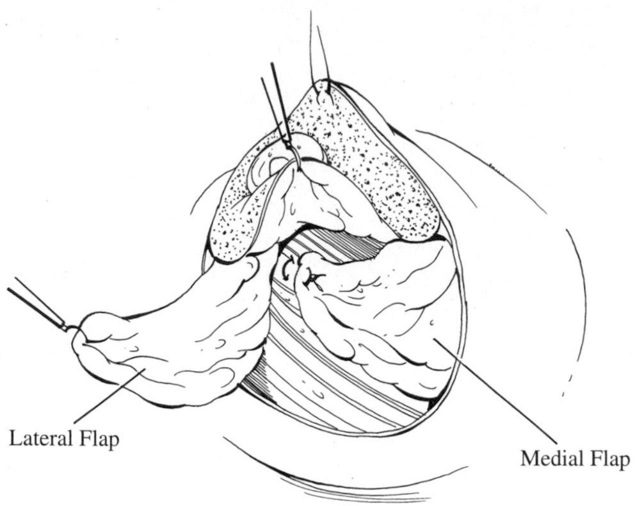

Figure 83.10. Medial flap rotation, folding, and fixation using a U point on the pectoral. The position of the fixation on the pectoral must be evaluated according to the anatomy of each patient. Most of the time, the medial flap is sutured behind the areola to ensure a better support of the areola anterior projection.

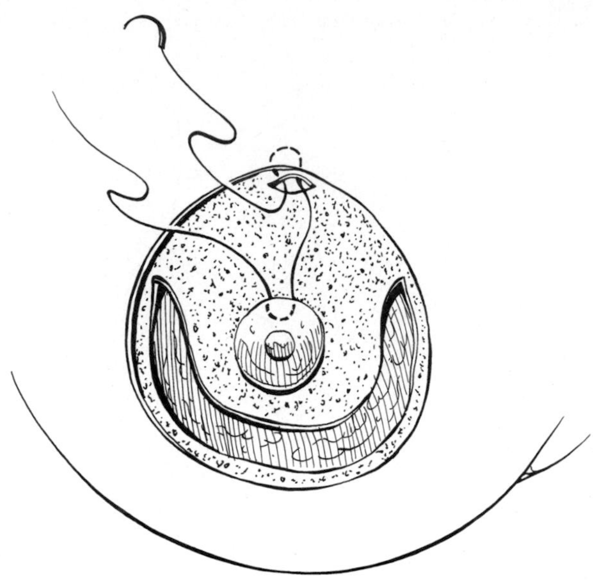

Figure 83.12. The dermal window prevents enlargement of the scar by strong fixation of the areola's superior border through the window and allows the surgeon to bury the round block cerclage knot.

STEP 6: THE DERMAL WINDOW FOR AREOLA FIXATION

The fixation of the areola to the superior border of the ellipse is facilitated by a dermal window that we open with a 1-cm incision of the dermis (Fig. 83.12), 5 mm from the edge. Through this window, we create a small subdermal pocket in which we will lift and suture the supra-areolar dermis to the deep dermis of the pocket. This fixation supports the areola without tension on the skin edge.

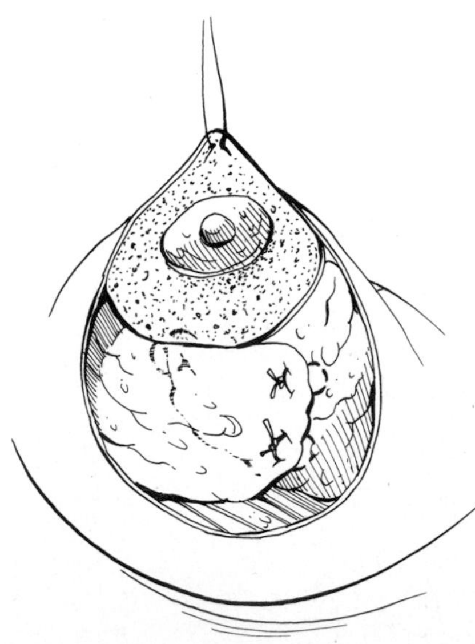

Figure 83.11. The lateral flap is crossed over the medial flap, and the crossing line is sutured using some superficial U points, grasping the Cooper's ligaments to prevent any constriction of the flap vascularization. Strong support of the new conic shape will be achieved after full breast lacing (step 7).

STEP 7: THE FULL BREAST LACING

Optimally, the glandular cone will be well shaped, with the areola at the top of the cone. The quality of the tissue determines whether this result can be maintained long term. To provide the best support of the shape, we prefer to use full breast lacing of braided polyester 2/0 applied with a long, straight needle (Fig. 83.13). This type of lacing is useful in case of poor-quality glandular tissue, especially in patients with adipose involution.

This lacing is created by some large inverted stitches, with moderate tension traversing the entire thickness of the breast diameter to maintain the crossing of the glandular flaps. This lacing, at its superior part, also passes through the areola dermoglandular flap. This passage allows control of the anterior projection of the nipple-areola complex and prevents any protrusion of it. It is important that these full breast lacing stitches be applied without tension to avoid strangulating the gland and creating fat necrosis. The role of the full breast lacing is to provide passive support of the conical shape obtained by the superficial stitches of the glandular modeling (see step 5).

STEP 8: ROUND BLOCK CERCLAGE STITCH

The detached skin is redraped on the glandular cone, and complementary detachment may be necessary to free some skin to obtain an easy elevation and even distribution of the skin all around the areola.

The round block cerclage stitch is passed like a purse-string in the deep dermis, 5 mm beyond the edge of the ellipse (Fig. 83.14). The suture begins through the dermal window over the suture fixing the areola, follows a regular plane in the deep dermis, and finishes at its starting point (Fig. 83.1). We use Mersilene 2/0 applied with a 7-cm-long straight needle, allowing a regular plane in the dermis.

Pulling on the suture elevates the detached skin around the areola, whereas a sliding of the skin on the stitch allows

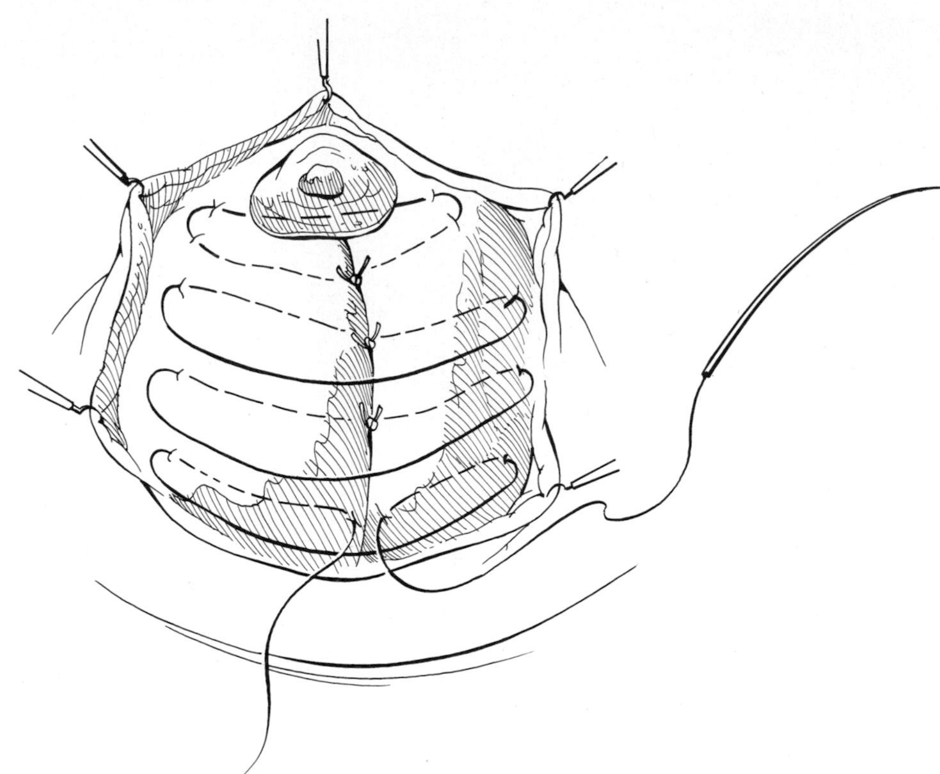

Figure 83.13. Using a long, slightly curved needle, full breast lacing strongly supports the conic shape by using large inverted stitches of Mersilene 2/0. The first stitch is transareolar and allows control of the nipple-areola complex anterior projection. The other stitches traverse the entire thickness of the breast diameter. All these stitches are tied without any tension.

an even distribution of the pleats. A tube of the desired diameter is inserted, and the suture is tied onto it (Fig. 83.15). The knot is buried behind the skin through the dermal window and receives a drop of Betadine. Before use, the suture receives an impregnation of Betadine. We prefer a braided polyester suture because the scar penetrates the fiber of the stitch, avoiding a sliding of the skin on the suture when moving the breast.

Before applying the suture, we improve the distribution of the pleats around the areola. We avoid deep pleats. Instead, we try to have more numerous superficial pleats. This is more a compression than a plication of the skin excess. The round block allows the elevation and the even distribution of the skin flap over the new glandular cone (Fig. 83.16).

STEP 9: REGULATION OF AREOLA PROJECTION

The conization of the gland gives a strong anterior projection to the nipple-areola complex, sometimes generating its protrusion. Therefore, we propose some specific sutures to control the anterior projection of the nipple-areola complex:

- The full breast lacing transareolar first stitch (Fig. 83.13) is the first control of the nipple-areola complex anterior projection, performed after glandular modeling (step 7).
- Inverted dermoareolar stitches take a large vertical grip in the areola's thickness and a large horizontal grip in the edge of the dermal ellipse. The location of these stitches is also useful for an even distribution of the skin excess (like Cardinal stitches) (Fig. 83.17).

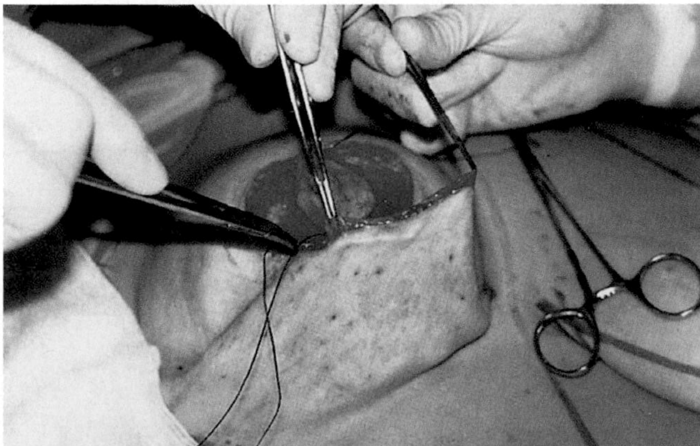

Figure 83.14. View of the long, straight needle passing in a regular plane in the deep dermis 5 mm beyond the ellipse edge. The round block cerclage stitch is buried behind the entire thickness of the skin and is not superficially exposed below the scar.

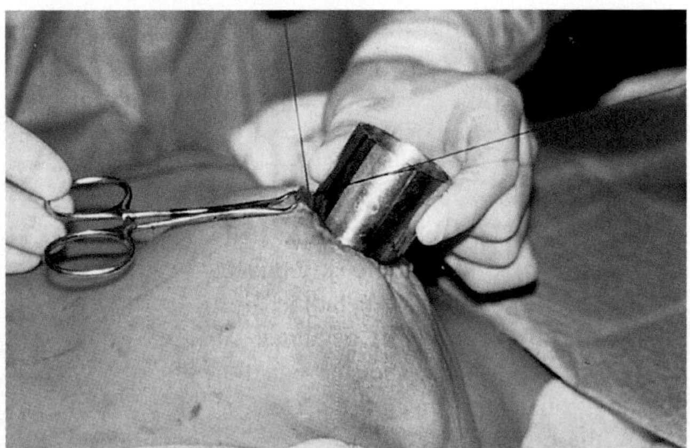

Figure 83.15. The round block cerclage stitch is pulled and tied onto a tube, facilitating exact measurement and symmetry of the diameter of the two areolas.

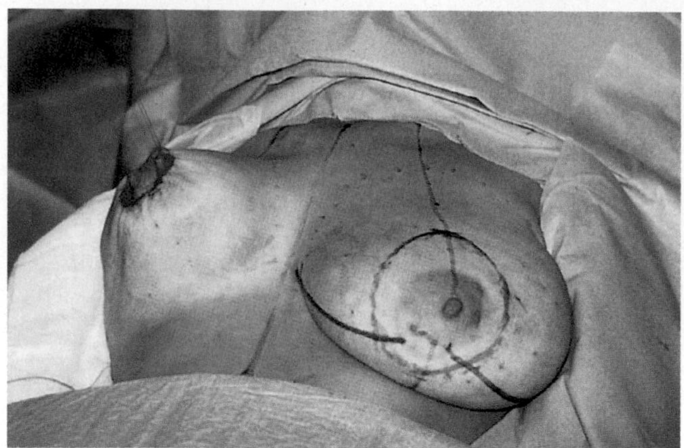

Figure 83.16. The round block allows the surgeon to lift and drape the detached skin regularly over the reshaped glandular cone, with an even distribution of the skin excess.

- Diametric transareolar U points are passed with 2/0 braided polyester using a straight needle. To cover the knot, the suture begins and finishes buried behind the areola (Fig. 83.18). This U point is also useful to give a circular shape to the areola; in some cases, the areola tends to take on an oval form. This diametric U point is put in place in the great diameter of the oval areola. A little tension on the stitch gives a circular shape to the areola.

All these stitches allow control of the size, shape, and projection of the nipple-areola complex.

STEP 10: THE SKIN COMPENSATION SUTURE

Accommodation of the big ellipse to the small areola requires a compensation suture. We use Vicryl 4/0 intradermal sutures starting at the top of the areola, taking a large horizontal bite on the edge of the ellipse and a vertical bite on the edge of the areola. This suture is performed to avoid creating deep pleats but to have an even distribution of superficial pleats. The suture is left in place and will resorb; only the knot will be cut after 3 weeks.

STEP 11: THE DRESSING AND POSTOPERATIVE CARE

The first dressing is a wet compress on the areola and dry compresses on the detached skin. They are maintained with an adhesive bandage of moderate compression to prevent hematoma formation. Vacuum drainage exits below the axilla.

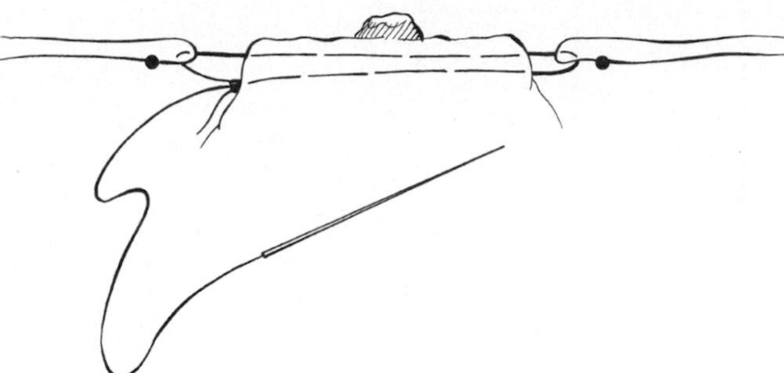

Figure 83.18. Diametric transareolar U points constitute a barrier, preventing the areola's protrusion and giving a circular shape to the areola when it has a tendency to be ovoid.

The second day after surgery, the patient leaves the clinic. The vacuum drainage and all the dressings are usually removed. We check the vitality of the flaps and clean the skin with antiseptic solution, and later with ether, to facilitate the adhesion of an adhesive pad. This is a sterile, ultrathin, highly conformable, semiocclusive polyurethane foam adhesive pad. This dressing covers the areola and scar and maintains all the detached skin. The patient leaves the clinic wearing a simple brassiere that maintains the breast and the adhesive pad.

This adhesive polyurethane foam pad has many advantages. For example, it:

- Prevents tension on the scar
- Absorbs exudate
- Protects against trauma and bacteria
- Controls nipple-areola anterior projection during the swelling period
- Is simple for the patient, who does not have to remove the dressing and who will only have to visit the office for a weekly control and change of the adhesive pad

Use preoperative and postoperative antibiotherapy for 6 days with parenteral or oral analgesia when necessary.

The patient must wear a brassiere night and day for 2 months.

CASE

Results are shown in Figure 83.19.

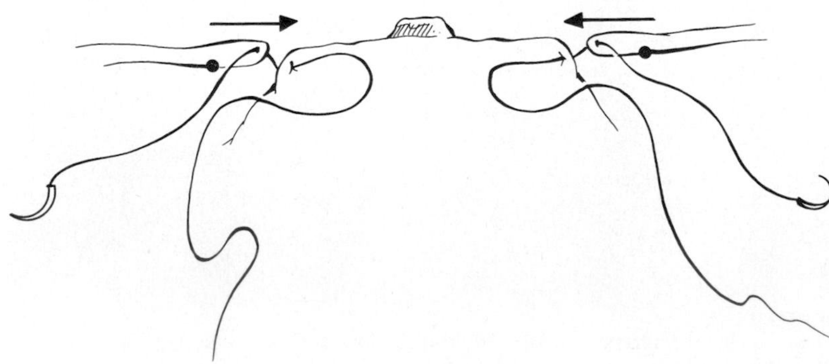

Figure 83.17. Inverted dermoareolar stitches facilitate control of the areola's protrusion through the round block cerclage and prepare the even distribution of the pleats around the areola like cardinal stitches.

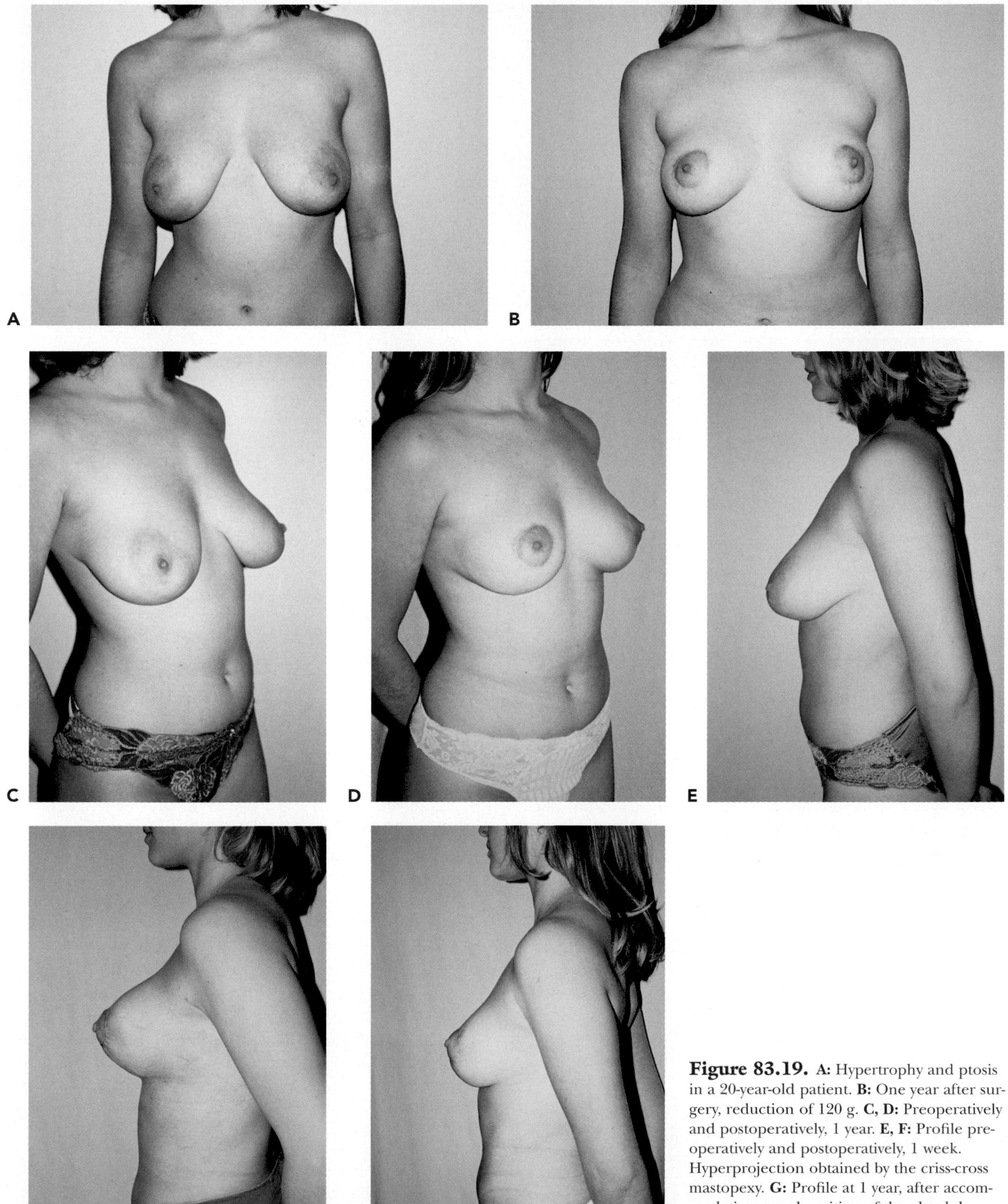

Figure 83.19. **A:** Hypertrophy and ptosis in a 20-year-old patient. **B:** One year after surgery, reduction of 120 g. **C, D:** Preoperatively and postoperatively, 1 year. **E, F:** Profile preoperatively and postoperatively, 1 week. Hyperprojection obtained by the criss-cross mastopexy. **G:** Profile at 1 year, after accommodation; good position of the glandular cone maintained by the breast lacing, and anchored to the pectoralis by permanent suture Mersilene. (*continued*)

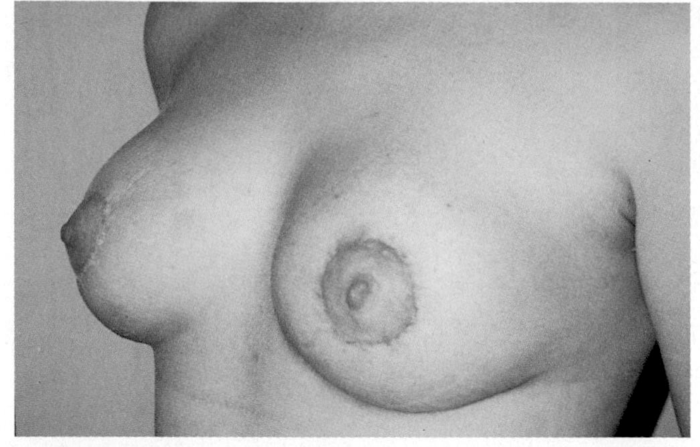
H

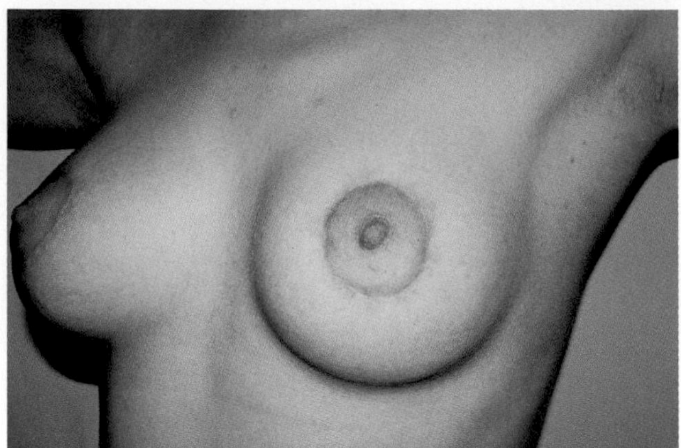
I

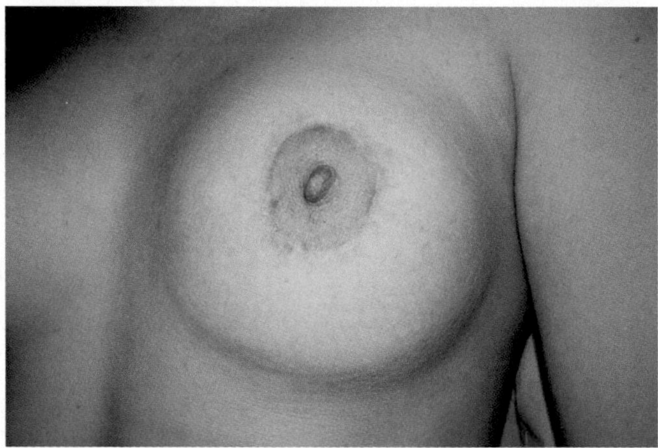
J

Figure 83.19. (*Continued*) **H:** Areola at 1 month; even distribution of excess skin by the round block stitch, avoiding deep pleats. **I:** Areola at 1 year; the round block stitch avoids enlargement of the areola and scarring. **J:** Areola in the supine position at 1 year, disappearance of the pleats, and the natural aspect of the original submammary crease preserved by the dissection.

COMPLICATIONS

The same complications as those occasioned by the traditional mammaplasty (Table 83.2) are apparent. Cutaneoglandular detachment eases the problems of cutaneous necrosis and glandular cytosteatonecrosis. To avoid those complications, some precautionary measures must be observed. For good cutaneous vascularization:

- Avoid tension by resecting as little skin as possible.
- Do not infiltrate the edge of the deepithelialized ellipse.
- During subcutaneous dissection, preserve subdermal vascularization.
- Restrict the subcutaneous detachment to its sufficient minimum. This makes it possible to redrape skin over the glandular cone, such as in a subcutaneous facelift done in conjunction with working on the superficial musculoaponeurotic system.
- Delicately manipulate the flap by only pinching the deepithelialized dermis margin.

For a good glandular vascularization:

- Do not infiltrate the glandular flap basis.
- Restrict the subcutaneous and prepectoral detachment to its sufficient minimum to allow the necessary glandular mobilization and to reduce and reshape the mammary cone. Execute volume reduction over the distal parts of the flaps to limit their length.

The first assembling stitches of the criss-cross mastopexy should be superficial to avoid strangulation of the flaps. The full breast lacing stitches extend through the thickness of the reshaped glandular cone and are set without any tension. Their only role is one of passive contention of the mammary cone. For that lacing, we prefer to use a braided polyester thread because the penetration of the scar within the braided fibers of the thread allows the best contention of tissues.

One case of infection involved a 16-year-old girl with thoracic acne. She had taken hot baths with her dressings and had kept them wet, not changing them for the whole week after surgery. The result was a sudden worsening of the acne underneath the wet dressings, in addition to staphylococcal cellulitis of each breast. The infected tissues then needed to be surgically cleaned. After spontaneous healing, she again underwent surgery, but this time with the T-inverted technique, which yielded a satisfactory result.

TABLE 83.2 Complications in 340 Cases of Mastopexies, Reduction, or Augmentation

Hematoma	6	1.7%
Seroma	1	0.2%
Infections	3	0.8%
Cytosteatonecrosis cysts	6	1.7%
Total or marginal areola necrosis	0	0.0%
Areola sensitivity loss	0	0.0%
Skin flap partial necrosis	3	0.8%
Hypertrophic scar	1	0.2%

Two other cases of infection involved a severe polycystic mastosis and cytosteatonecrosis of the glandular flaps owing to tight, strangulating glandular stitches on a fatty breast in adipose involution, respectively. In these two cases, the healing was delayed but was finally satisfactory. Scar revision was undertaken using local anesthesia, but the scar remained periareolar.

LONG-TERM PROBLEMS

Scar and areola enlargement are prevented via minimal periareolar skin resection, the correct use of the round block cerclage stitch (see step 8), and the anchoring of the areola through the dermal window (see step 6).

Flattening of the shape and ptosis recurrence are prevented by good criss-cross mastopexy or glandular plication invagination maintained by the full breast lacing (see steps 5 and 7).

The persistence of pleats is avoided by passing the round block cerclage stitch in a regular plane inside the deep dermis, by even distribution of the skin excess all around the areola, by making the skin slide over the round block cerclage stitch (see step 8), and by applying a final intradermal compensation suture (see step 10).

Protrusion of the areola is prevented via use of the transareolar full breast lacing first stitch (see step 7), inverted dermoareolar stitches, or transareolar diametric U points (see step 9).

CONCLUSION

The starting point of the round block technique is the use of a deep dermal periareolar cerclage stitch passed like a purse string to treat mastopexies and hypertrophies, resulting in only a simple periareolar scar with no widening of the areola or the scar itself.

The critical analysis of the results obtained allowed us to elaborate, step by step, a whole range of solutions for each obstacle encountered. With these improvements and the judicious selection of patients, the round block technique allows us to regularly achieve consistent and satisfying results, including a discrete scar and a satisfactory breast shape, all with a minimum rate of complications.

The surgeon should apply this technique at first to cases in good anatomic condition with small ptoses or hypertrophies. To achieve good results, each detail of the operation—from the preoperative markings to the cutaneous sutures—requires meticulous care.

It is hoped that the diverse and potential application of the round block technique in aesthetic or reconstructive tumoral surgery, aided by the improvements brought by other interested clinicians, will lead to improvement of patients' wellbeing as a result of reduced scar sequelae.

EDITORIAL COMMENTS

Many thanks to Louis Benelli for contributing this chapter on the round block approach to the periareolar mastopexy. Certainly, Dr. Benelli gets credit for popularizing and reenergizing the concept of periareolar surgery without the addition of vertical or transverse scars on the breast. His chapter expresses the same message as that of Dr. Góes in this book: In properly selected patients, a periareolar mastopexy or periareolar surgery can achieve excellent cosmetic results without resorting to additional scars on the breast. However, careful attention to patient selection and operative detail are critical in performing this procedure.

S.L.S.

REFERENCES

1. Dartigues L. Etat actuel de la chirurgie esthétique mammaire. *Monde Med* 1928;38:75.
2. Erol O, Spira M. Mastopexy technique for mild to moderate ptosis. *Plast Reconstr Surg* 1980; 65:603.
3. Faivre J, Carissimo A, Faivre JM. La voie péri-aréolaire dans le traitement des petites ptoses mammaires. In: *Chirurgie Esthétique.* Paris: Maloine; 1984.
4. Gruber RP, Jones HW Jr. The "donut" mastopexy: indications and complications. *Plast Reconstr Surg* 1980;65:34.
5. Hinderer U. Plastia mammaria modelante de dermopexia superficial y retromammaria. *Rev Esp Cirurg Plast* 1972;5:521.
6. Kausch W. Die operationen der mammahypertrophie. *Zentralbl Chir* 1916;43:713.
7. Benelli L. Technique de plastie mammaire le "round block." *Rev Fr Chir Esthet* 1988; 13:7–11.
8. Benelli L. A new periareolar mammaplasty: round block technique. *Aesth Plast Surg* 1990;14:99.
9. Vinas J. The double breasted breast. *Rev Soc Argentina Cirurg Estet* 1974;1:25.
10. Vogt T. Mammaplasty: the Vogt technique. In: Georgiade NG, ed. *Aesthetic Surgery of the Breast.* Philadelphia: WB Saunders; 1990:271–290.

CHAPTER

84

Ruth Graf
Thomas Biggs
André Ricardo Dall'Oglio Tolazzi
Maria Cecília Closs Ono

Mastopexy With Chest Wall–based Flap and Pectoralis Muscle Loop

INTRODUCTION

The evolution of all surgery, including breast surgery, is persistent and ongoing (1–14). The great advances by Wise (15), Pitanguy (16), Lassus (17–19), Lejour (20–23), Benelli (24), and others have not only simplified the operative plan, but have also contributed to a shorter scar and a more aesthetic breast. This chapter describes a maneuver designed to give a better shape. This maneuver involves the use of a chest wall–based flap of breast tissue that is moved into the upper pole of the breast and held in place by a loop of pectoral muscle under which it is passed. The technique can be used with different kind of incisions: standard inverted T, short T, L-shaped incisions, or periareolar-vertical incisions. Our choice, and the maneuver described in this chapter, is a vertical incision with whatever redundant skin remains after excising the vertical ellipse removed from around the nipple and closed with a round block suture. This is best described as a circumvertical excision. If reduction is necessary, it can easily be carried out in this maneuver by removing the desired amount from under the breast and in the most appropriate location for resection. There is no limit to the amount of breast tissue that can be removed.

TECHNIQUE

Marking is done with the patient in the upright position. Lines are drawn first straight down the midline from the suprasternal notch to the xiphoid process and second from a point 5 cm from the suprasternal notch at the clavicle to the nipple-areola complex (NAC) and then straight down to the areola. A point at 17 to 20 cm on the suprasternal–NAC line is marked (point A), which will be the top of the areola. A point is made (point D) on the line through the middle of the breast and 2 to 4 cm above the inframammary fold. This distance varies between 2 and 4 cm depending on the size of the breast (Fig. 84.1). The breast is then gently displaced laterally (as in the technique described by Lejour), and a line is drawn parallel to the midline and connected to point D. A similar line is drawn with the breast displaced medially. A distance of 5 to 8 cm is measured from point D on the medial and lateral lines (points B and C). It should be pointed out that the tension resulting from this displacement should be firm enough to allow adequate skin resection but not so tense as to create difficulty with closure. This distance varies also in accordance with the size and laxity of the breast. Gently curved lines are drawn from point A to point B and C. Line A–B should never be closer than 9 cm to the midline and line A–C never less than 10 cm from the anterior axillary line.

The variation in distances of point D to the inframammary fold and of lines B–D and C–D allows the surgeon the latitude of adjustments, depending on the size of the breast. The larger the breast is to be, the greater are these distances; however, the distances should never exceed 4 and 8 cm, respectively.

One additional item in the markings is to move points B and C slightly closer together so that when they are closed there will be no significant tension.

OPERATIVE PROCEDURE

The patient is placed supine on the operating table, and, after induction with general or epidural anesthesia (local is possible) and preparation and draping, the incision markings are infiltrated subdermally (except superior to the areola), with a dilute epinephrine-in-saline solution (1:100,000). The area of the skin demarcated by lines A–B, A–C, B–D, and C–D is deepithelialized (Fig. 84.2), leaving the NAC (4.5 to 5 cm in diameter) in place. An incision is made in the dermis transversely along lines B–D and C–D, passing 1 cm below NAC. This is the beginning of the creation of the chest wall–based flap (Fig. 84.3). Along the vertical lines this incision is beveled inward for 1 to 2 cm to preserve tissue on the medial and lateral pillars for closure later. After preserving this tissue, the incisions continue inward and away from the flap so the base is broad. This dissection is carried to the chest wall, with a minimal amount of subcutaneous tissue being left on the skin as dissection is carried to the inframammary fold.

After this dissection has been performed laterally and medially a large hook is placed in the NAC and the breast is lifted straight up. Then, an incision is made in the breast tissue from point B to point C, proceeding to the pectoral fascia. Great care must be taken at this point not to undercut the flap (chest wall pedicle). The flap is now freely mobile and is based on vessels from the fifth and sixth intercostal spaces, as a perforator flap (Figs. 84.4 and 84.5). The flap is free from all of the four sides: superior, lateral, inferior, and medial. It is very important that the flap not be restrained; if it is, continuous dissection should be extended to the pectoral fascia. This freely mobile, totally chest wall–based flap is made up of the tissue that in other procedures "bottoms out," but in this procedure it is being transposed into the upper pole, where it will remain permanently.

The breast tissue is retracted upward and cephalad and dissected off the pectoral fascia up to the second intercostal space, creating a space in the upper pole of the breast into which the flap will be fixed. Before this, however, a strip of pectoral muscle approximately 8 to 10 cm long and 1.5 to 2 cm wide is marked with methylene blue. Its caudal or inferior line is at the cephalad end of the flap base (Fig. 84.6).

This muscle strip is elevated incorporating no more than one half of the muscle (the posterior fascia of the muscle is not

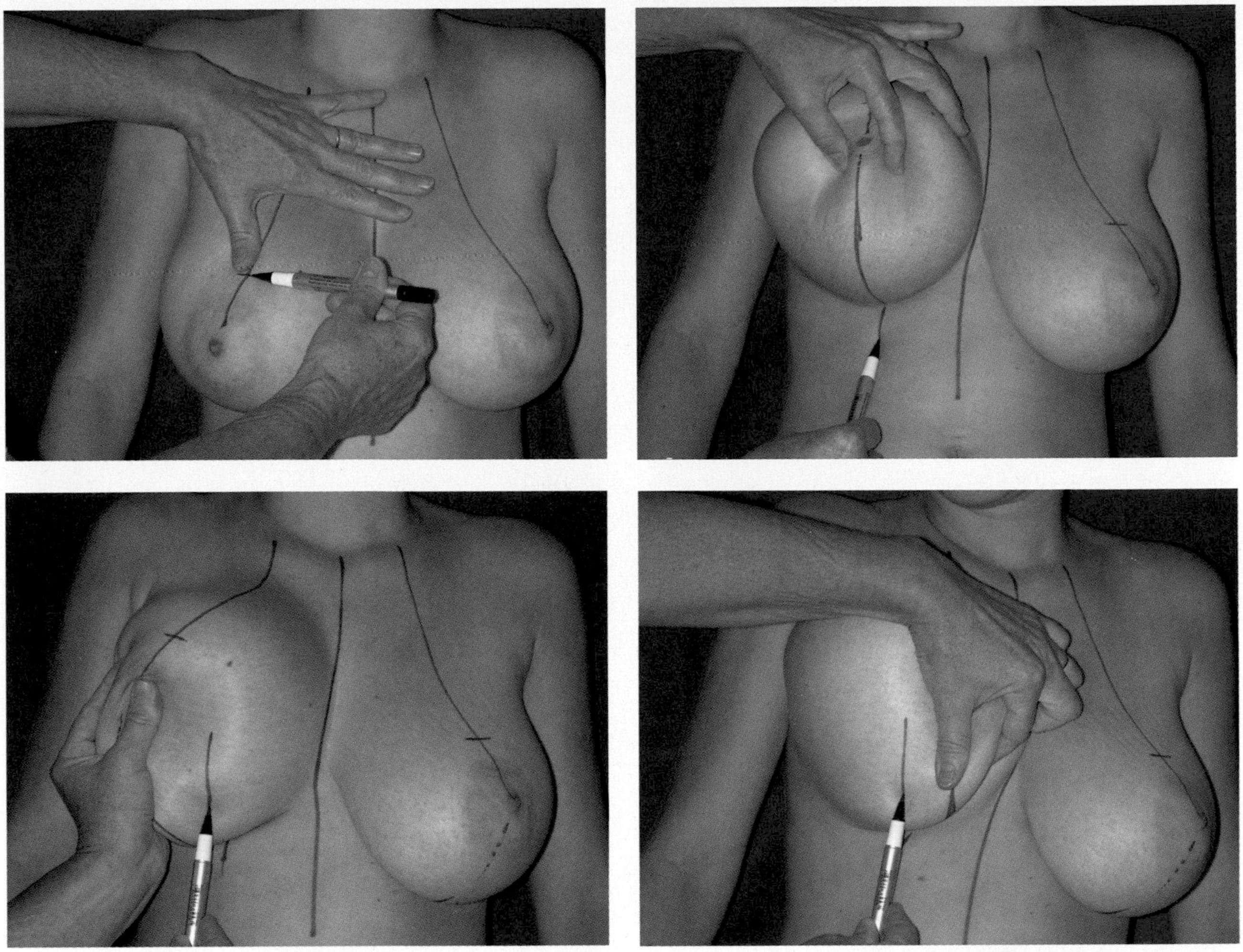

Figure 84.1. Basic markings of the vertical technique. Lines are drawn straight down the midline from the suprasternal notch to the nipple-areola complex (NAC). Point A, 20 cm from the clavicle, will be the top of the areola **(A)**, from a point 5 cm from the suprasternal notch at the clavicle to the NAC and then straight down parallel to the midline line, crossing the inframammary crease, not less than 11 cm **(B)**. The breast is gently, with the Lejour maneuver, displaced laterally **(C)** and medially **(D)** to obtain the vertical lines. The suprasternal notch is noted to be at the cephalad edge of the bone, not down into the notch.

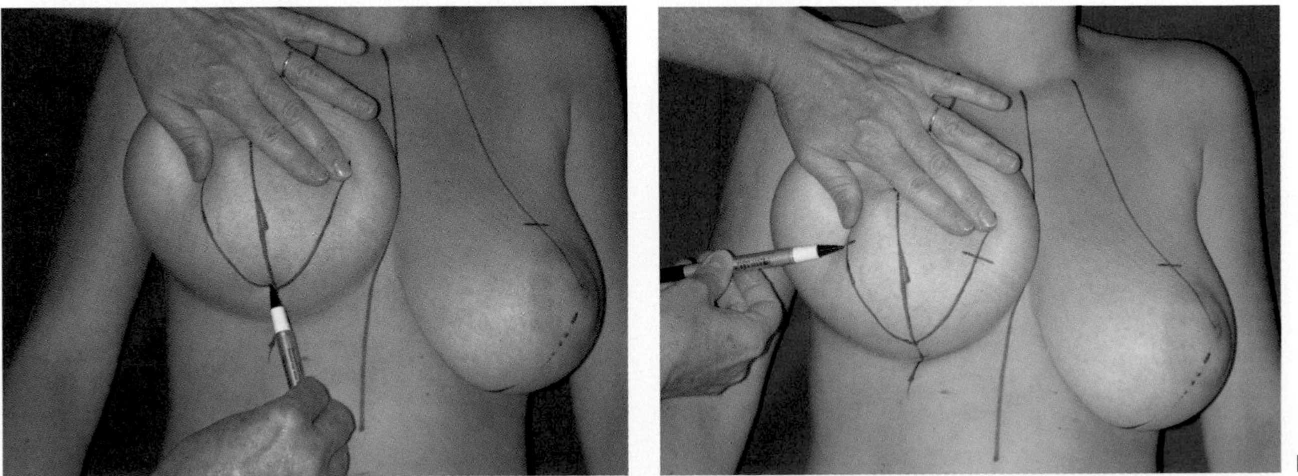

Figure 84.2. **A:** The vertical lines cross at the midbreast line, 2 to 4 cm above the inframammary fold, and point D is made. **B:** A distance of 5 to 8 cm is measured on the medial and lateral lines, and points B and C are placed, respectively. A gently curved line is drawn from point A to point B **(C)**, and again from point A to point C **(D)**. *(continued)*

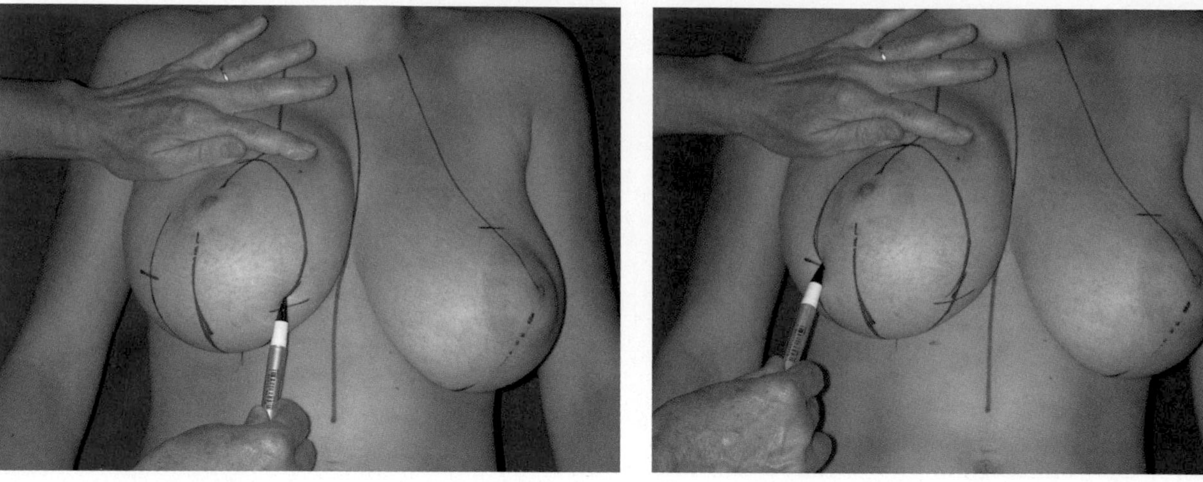

Figure 84.2. (*Continued*) Line A–B should never be closer than 9 cm to the midline, and line A–C should never be less than 10 cm from the anterior axillary fold.

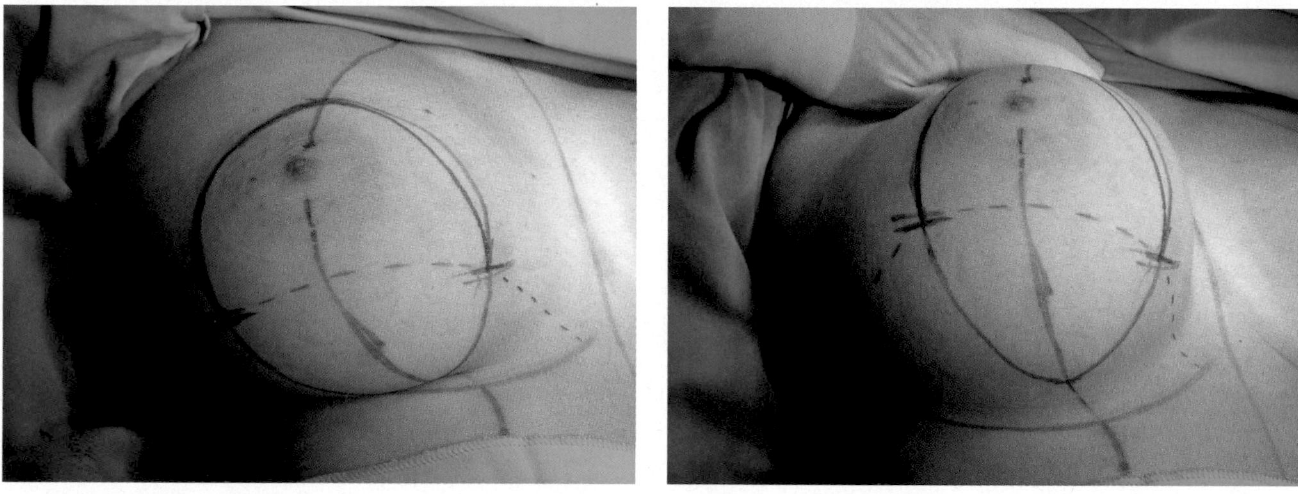

Figure 84.3. **A, B:** Patient on the operating table. Skin demarcated with vertical lines and the chest wall–based flap.

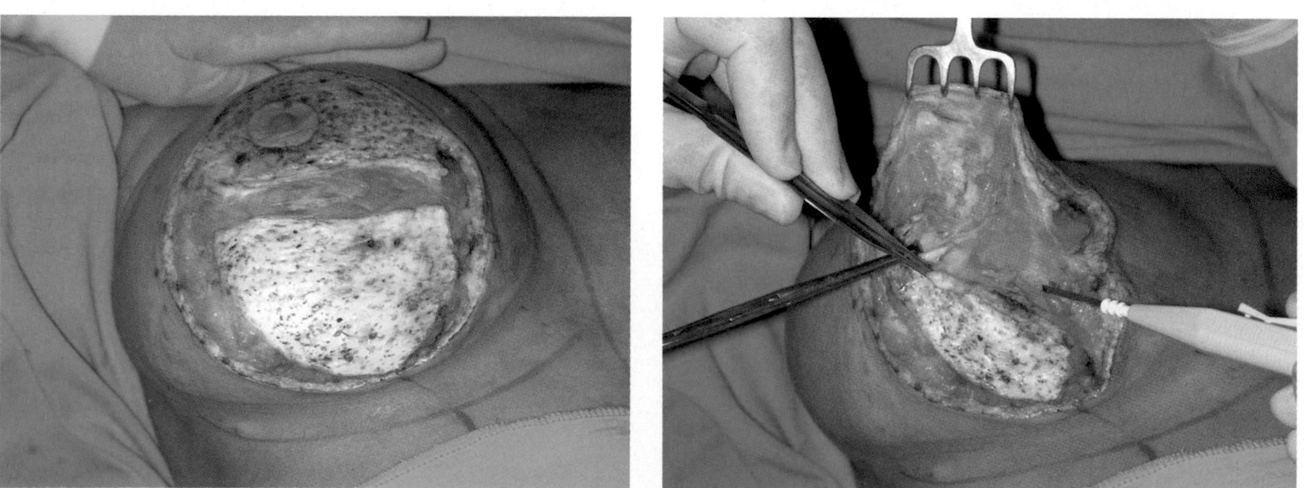

Figure 84.4. **A:** Deepithelization and dermis incision following demarcation, to 2 cm above points B and C. Along the vertical lines, this incision is beveled inward for 1 to 2 cm to preserve tissue on the medial **(B)** and lateral **(C)** pillars, preserving this tissue for closure later. **D:** A large hook is placed in the nipple-areola complex, the breast is lifted straight up, and dissection of the breast tissue from point B to point C is carried out 1 cm below the areola, proceeding to the pectoral fascia. (*continued*)

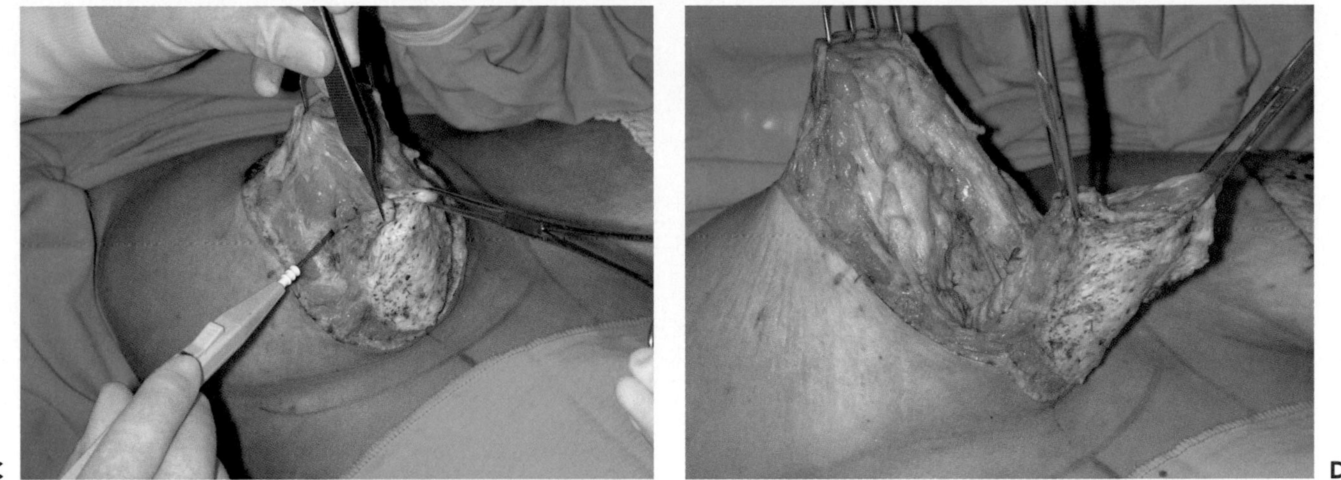

C D

Figure 84.4. *(Continued)*

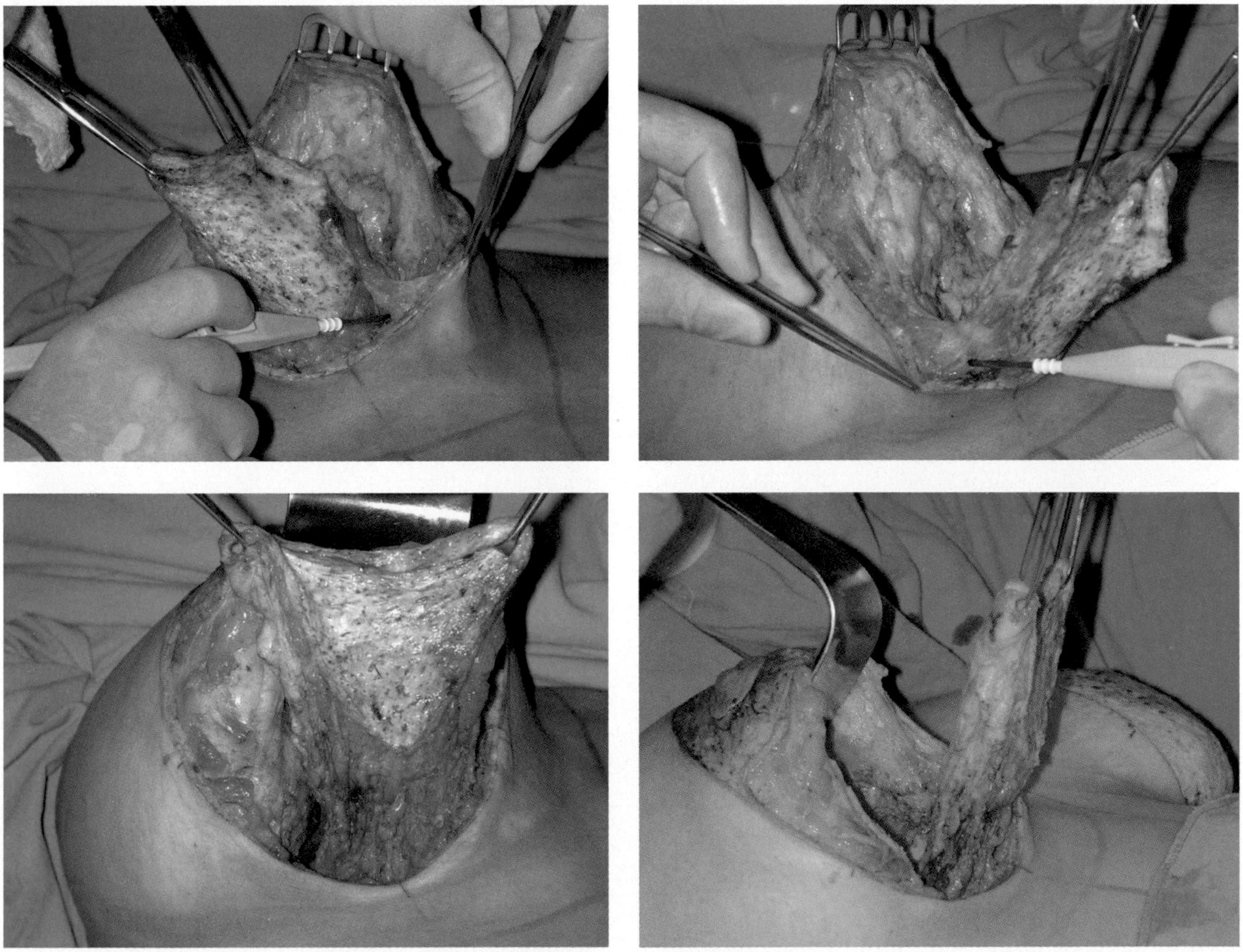

A B

C D

Figure 84.5. **A, B:** The incisions continue inward and away from the flap so the base is broad. This dissection is carried to the chest wall with a minimal amount of subcutaneous tissue being left on the skin as dissection is carried to the inframammary fold. **C, D:** Undermining of chest wall–based flap maintaining the large base.

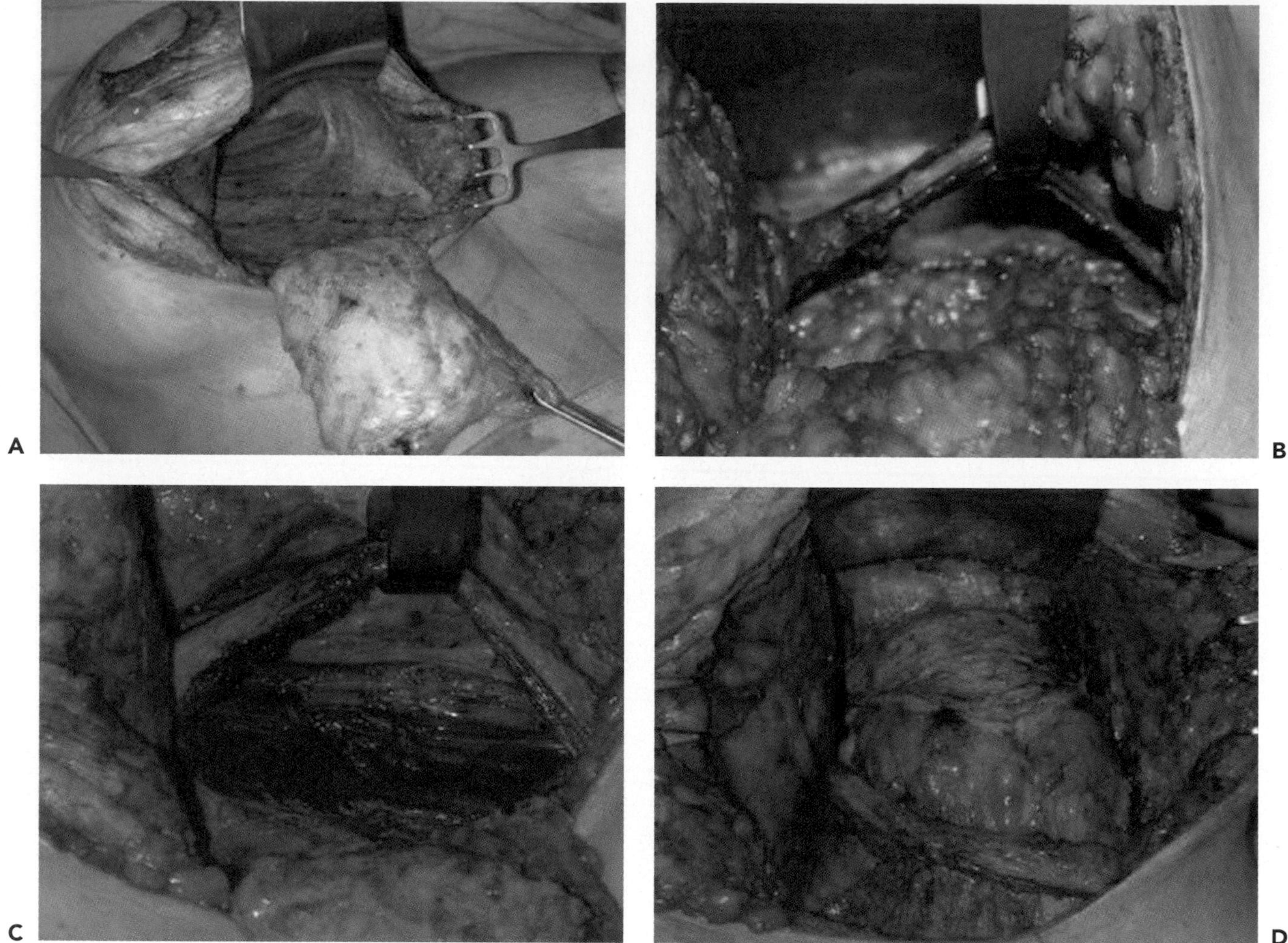

Figure 84.6. A strip of pectoral muscle approximately 8 to 10 cm long and 1.5 to 2 cm wide is marked with methylene blue just superior to the base of the chest wall–based flap **(A)** and elevated leaving the deep half of the muscle intact **(B)**. Passage of chest wall–based flap under the bipedicled muscular flap, closure of the donor site **(C)**, and suture of the flap to the second intercostal space **(D)**.

violated), and the donor site is close with 2-0 nylon. This loop will be used to help hold the flap in position in the upper pole. The flap is then passed under the pectoral loop into the space of the upper pole of the breast. It is very important that all dermal elements on the flap be completely passed under this loop. The dermis of the flap is then sutured to the pectoral fascia with a running 2-0 nylon suture, starting laterally and finishing medially. If, after passing the flap under the loop, there seems to be excessive tension on the loop causing pressure on the flap, the loop can be released by a small amount of dissection laterally (medial dissection could disrupt the origin of the pectoralis) (Fig. 84.6).

With the flap in the correct position and the breast suspended by the hook in the NAC, breast tissue excess is removed. At this step of the surgery the reduction is made in accordance with the breast's size and the desire of the patient. The main block of tissue is removed as an inverted central kill, from the base of the breast laterally and a lesser amount centrally to reduce the base and the excessive projection of the breast. The highest reduction with this technique (vertical incision and circumvertical closure) is 800 to 1,000 g, including the suction in the lateral aspect of the breast, although the chest wall–based flap can be used in any breast size.

After reducing the excessive breast tissue (Fig. 84.7), one interrupted suture of 2-0 nylon is placed in the superior breast tissue and the pectoral fascia just cephalad to the flap (at the second intercostal space) in order to lift the undermined breast tissue and improve upper pole projection.

Closure starts with suturing the pillars with 2-0 nylon in several layers. It is preferable to place the needle laterally deeper than medially to preserve more fullness medially. Deep dermis of the superior vertical wound is sutured placing together the subareolar points B and C.

A round block suture is done around the NAC to homogeneously distribute the periareolar skin and to reduce tension on the NAC (Fig. 84.8). Eight cardinal points are marked in the periareolar skin and in the areola. The running suture is done using a 3-0 colorless nylon. Passing through the deep dermis of the outer skin and the areolar deep tissue, the suture takes small amount of tissue between the markings in the areola and large bites right on the markings of the periareolar skin. Tensioning the suture reduces the periareolar circumference up to the desired diameter for NAC (about 4.5 cm).

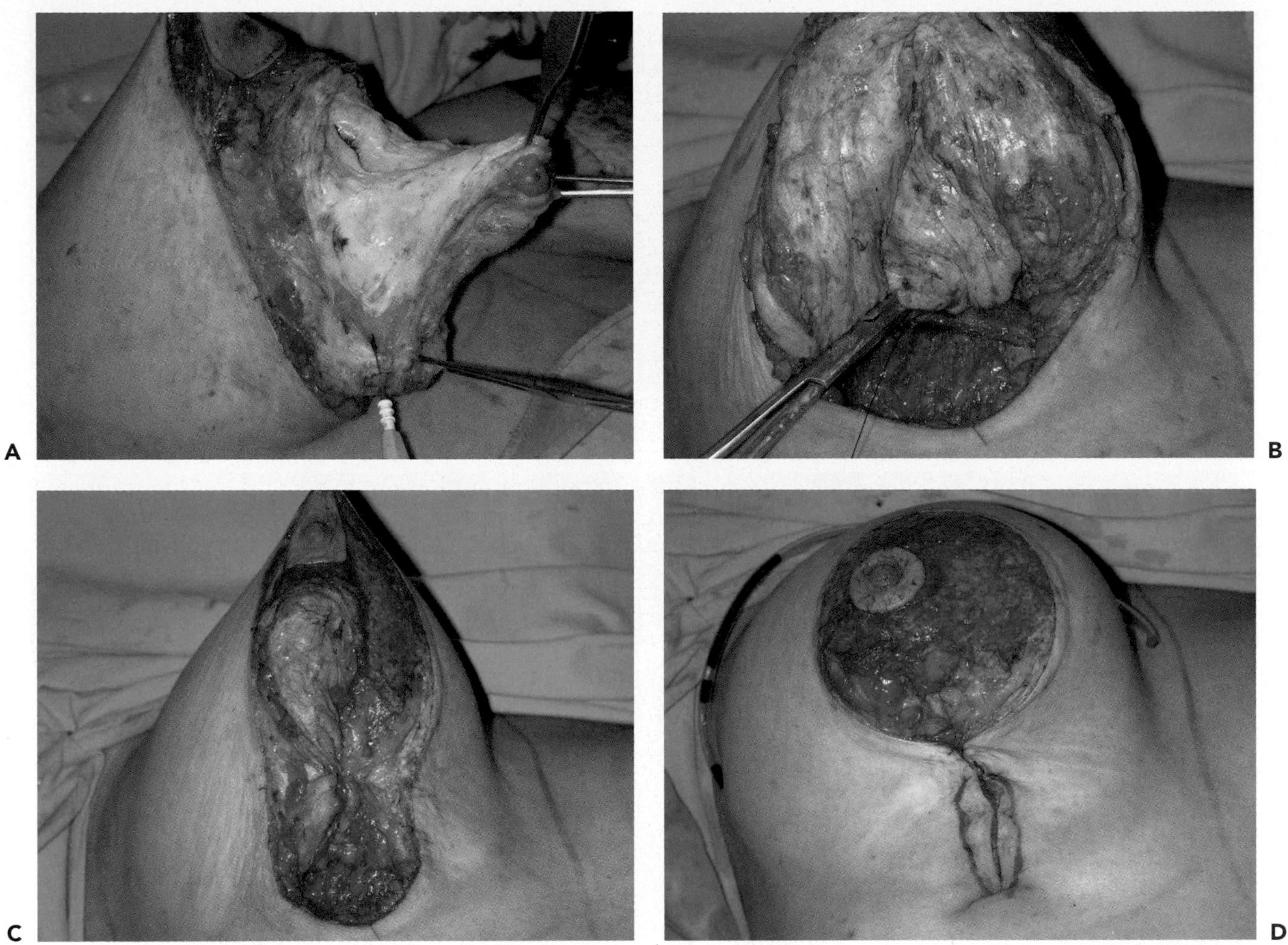

Figure 84.7. **A:** Resection of the excessive breast tissue. **B:** Suture the upper breast tissue to the pectoral muscle superior to the flap. **C:** Suture of the medial and lateral breast columns. **D:** Dermal and skin closure removing the skin excess.

Starting from point D, vertical skin is closed with interrupted sutures of 3-0 Monocryl. Anchoring the deep dermis to the underneath pillars, these sutures elevate the whole vertical component, placing the point D at the level of the new inframammary fold. So, the final vertical scar will end up at the level of or slightly above the new inframammary crease. Final skin closure is done with a running intradermic suture of 4-0 Monocryl (Fig. 84.9). No drains are routinely used.

DISCUSSION

Although the classic inverted-T incision mammaplasties are easily learned techniques for less experienced plastic surgeons and give more reproducible results on the operating table, they have several drawbacks that should be reassessed (25,26). The short-vertical-limb dogma (near 5 cm) associated with the inferior horizontal pattern resection of the skin and parenchyma leads to a breast with a broad and flat cone shape, with poor projection, and which tends to worsen with time (25,27,28). All of these issues and the concern about scar length promoted the development of new techniques for breast surgery.

Although the history of vertical mastopexy dates back to Lotsch (29) and Dartigues (30) and was later extended to breast reduction by Arié (4), it was otherwise lost to surgical history until Lassus (17–19) resumed interest in the 1960s. Using adjustable markings, an upper pedicle for the areola, and central breast reduction, Lassus employed vertical reduction mammaplasty in a wide range of breast hypertrophies. It was then modified and popularized by Lejour (20–23) and several other authors (27,31–38). In 1990, Levet (39) described a pure posterior pedicle flap for breast reduction. During this time, many authors observed that breast descent and loss of upper pole fullness ("bottoming out") was often seen in their work and the work of others. Ribeiro's technique (40,41), which uses an inferior pedicle flap transposed into the upper pole, provided improvement of this problem. Daniel (42) associated a bipedicled flap of major pectoralis muscle to keep Ribeiro's flap in a higher position, further minimizing the bottoming-out phenomenon. We have proposed some modifications to the mammary flap, describing it as totally based on the chest wall and held in place by the pectoral loop (33–36). There are also other flaps described in the literature (43).

Since 1994, these flaps have been performed in inverted-T, oblique, L-scar, and, more recently, vertical scar mammaplasties. The approach was switched from inferior pedicle flaps to flaps based only in the thoracic wall vasculature, completely

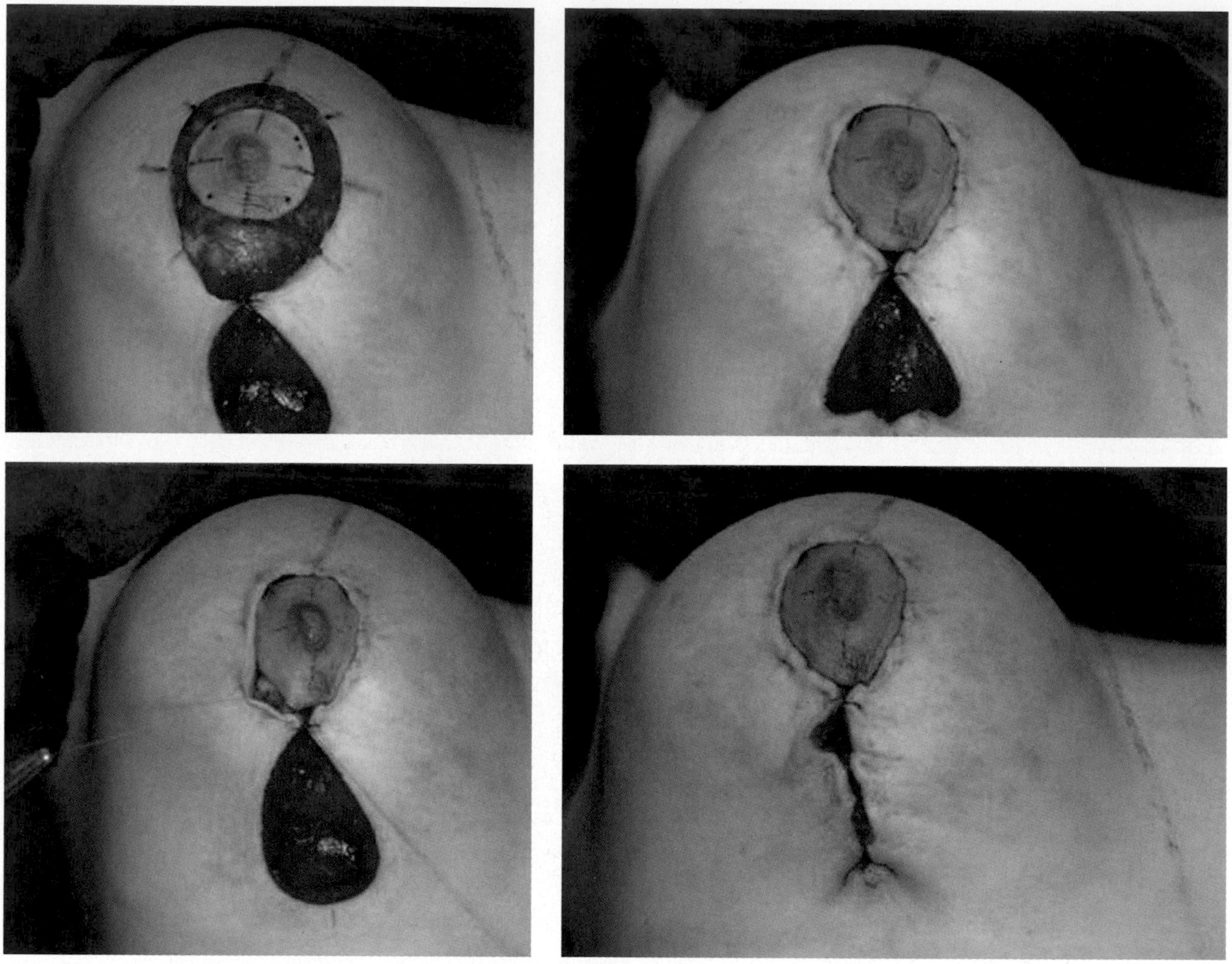

Figure 84.8. **A, B:** The round block is done around the nipple-areola complex (NAC). Eight cardinal points are marked at the skin and at the areola to spread regularly the areola. To close the skin and reduce wound tension around the areola, a round block suture is made all the way around the periareolar skin with 3-0 colorless nylon. This is a running suture passing through the deep dermis of the outer skin and the areolar deep tissue. In the external skin the suture is passed on the markings, taking a large amount of tissue, and at the areola the suture is passed between the markings, taking a small amount of tissue. Tensioning the suture reduces the circumference up to the desired diameter accommodating a 4.5-cm NAC. **C, D:** Starting from point D, skin is closed with 3-0 Monocryl in the deep dermal tissues with interrupted sutures, anchoring the vertical wound to the deep pillar tissue, continuing suturing until reaching the subareolar skin, so the vertical scar is kept at the same level as the new inframammary crease.

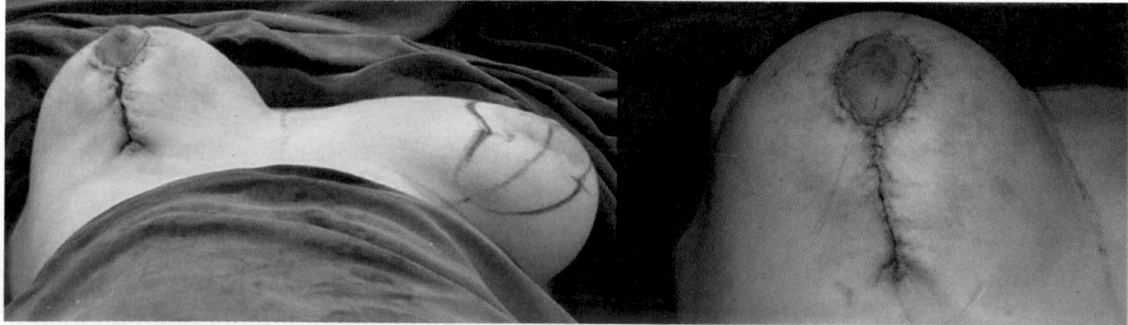

Figure 84.9. Final skin closure with shortening of the vertical incision and round block suture around the areola.

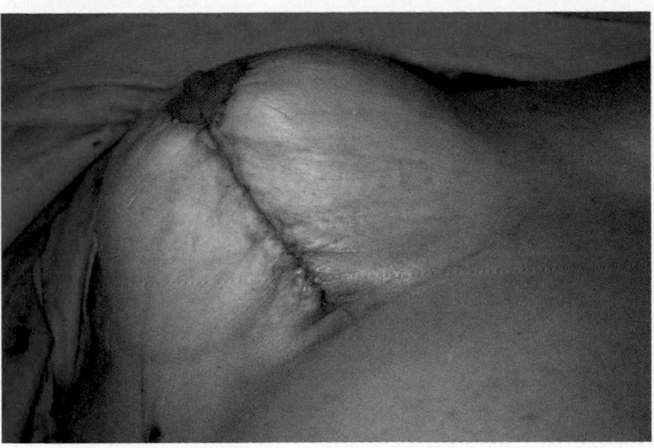

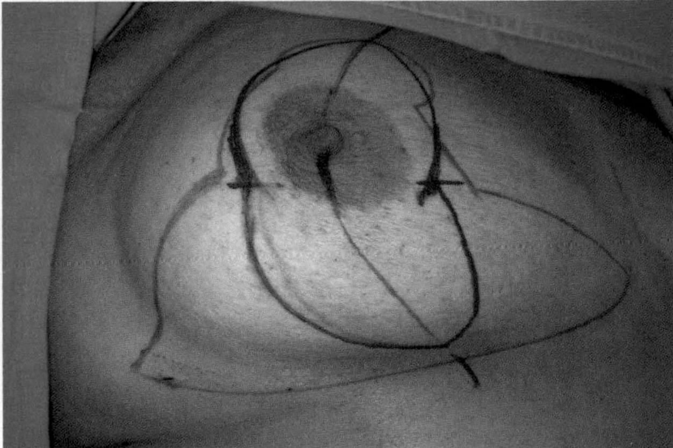

Figure 84.10. Skin markings of the vertical technique. Comparison of skin resection between the vertical scar technique (red ink) and an inverted-T or Wise pattern (blue ink).

detached from surrounding structures, maintaining the overlying dermis in order to give better support and shape to the flap after fixation to the underlying pectoralis. Figure 84.10 demonstrates minimization of the scar in the vertical technique when compared with a technique using a Wise pattern (15).

The upper pole of the breast maintains good volume, and the vertical scar is placed above or at the level of the new inframammary crease with a minimal breast descent.

The length of the chest wall–based flap changes according to the distance between the areola and the inframammary crease. Its upper limit is located 1 cm below the inferior edge of the areola, and the lateral borders extend to the medial and lateral breast contours. Its base extends to the inframammary crease with width 6 to 8 cm and thickness 4 cm, with its vascular pedicle based on the intercostal vessels of the fifth and sixth intercostal spaces. The bipedicled muscle flap (pectoralis loop) is situated immediately above the base of the breast tissue flap, with width 1.5 to 2 cm and length 8 to 10 cm. It should be dissected in the same direction as the muscle fibers, with the caution to elevate no more than one half of the muscle thickness superficially. The posterior fascia of the muscle is not violated, leaving intact the ganglion chain between the minor and the major pectoralis muscles, which is responsible for part of the lymphatic drainage of the breast.

It is possible to use this combination of techniques for mastopexy only, when there is no breast tissue in excess to be removed, or for breast reduction, when the resection of excessive breast tissue is done in the columns or base of the breast, after the thoracic wall flap is fixed. With this technique we observed that we remove less breast tissue than techniques that do not use the chest wall–based flap and that the breasts have a narrower base. In our experience, the average amount of breast tissue resected was 250 g, less than in other techniques we have used without the thoracic flap. In great hypertrophies or severe ptosis, the point D should be marked higher above inframammary fold, up to 4 cm. This maneuver is done to leave skin and subcutaneous tissue of the lower breast pole as part of the thoracic wall, with a higher new inframammary crease. Redundant skin is removed in the vertical excision and the circumareolar round block excision.

The exceeding skin in the vertical branch observed during surgery can be closed with a subcuticular suture that shortens this scar. During the first 2 months of the postoperative period, there is an accommodation with no need to remove skin horizontally in the inferior portion of this scar, as suggested by Marchac and Olarte (44). A round block suture is done around the areola to reduce even more the length of the vertical scar by compensating skin excess around the areola.

Some advantages of this technique are as follow (Figs. 84.11–84.14):

1. Long-lasting breast projection and upper pole fullness with the patient in both supine position and decubitus. The areola remains in a good location, and very little breast descent occurs (no bottoming out).
2. A vertical scar that does not cross the new inframammary crease, and with better quality due to less skin tension, which was achieved through internal sutures of breast tissue.
3. A narrower breast base, due to the vertical principle of parenchyma resection and approximation of breast pillars.

CONCLUSIONS

The achievement of a good aesthetic result in mammaplasty requires an adequate shape, minimal scar, NAC complex on the top of the breast projection, and a relatively narrow base. With the traditional techniques, breast shape has been accomplished with dermal sutures that would relax over the years, resulting in a descent of all breast tissue ("skin stretches with time").

By performing the vertical scar technique associated with a chest wall–based flap and holding it in position in the upper pole with a bipedicled major pectoralis muscle flap, it is observed in long-term follow-up that a minimal scar results, the shape is better, and there is maintenance of upper pole fullness and no bottoming out (thus keeping the NAC in the optimal position of breast projection) (Fig. 84.15).

This technique accomplishes this with a vertical scar that does not extend below the inframammary fold. In older techniques, breast shape was determined by skin tightening, and as the skin stretched, the shape was lost. By this technique, breast tissue is divided and moved into its desired position and fixed by the pectoral loop, thus ensuring maintenance of the shape, in that it does not depend on skin closure for contour, and the specific tissue that "bottoms out" is that which is transposed into the new position in the upper pole. This is another step in the evolution of breast surgery.

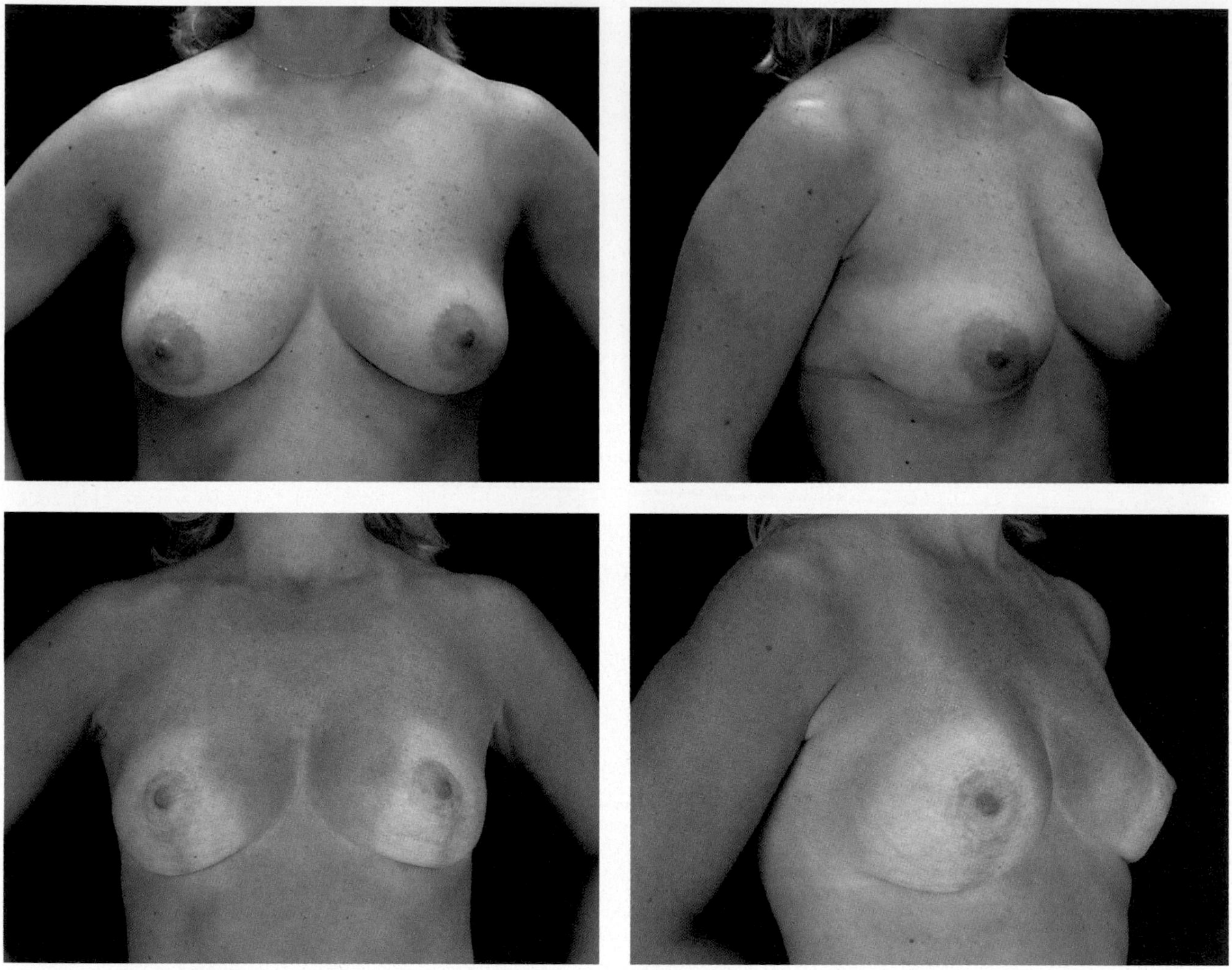

Figure 84.11. **A, B:** Preoperative view of a 30-year-old patient with breast ptosis. **C, D:** Six months postoperative mastopexy with vertical scar and use of the chest wall–based flap.

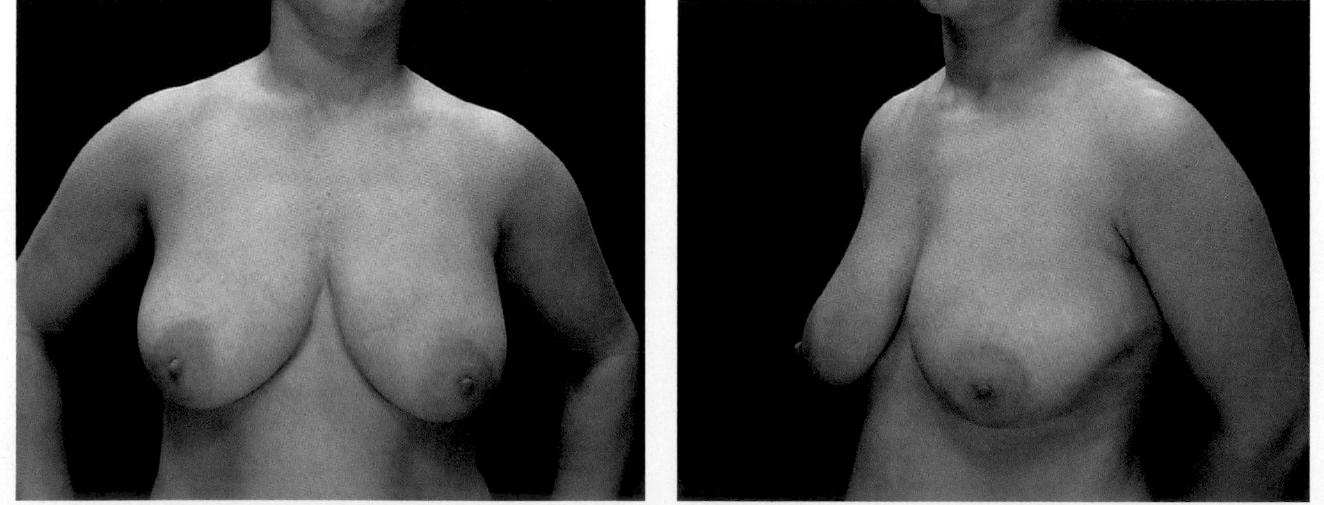

Figure 84.12. **A, B:** Preoperative view of a 38-year-old patient with breast hypertrophy and ptosis. (*continued*)

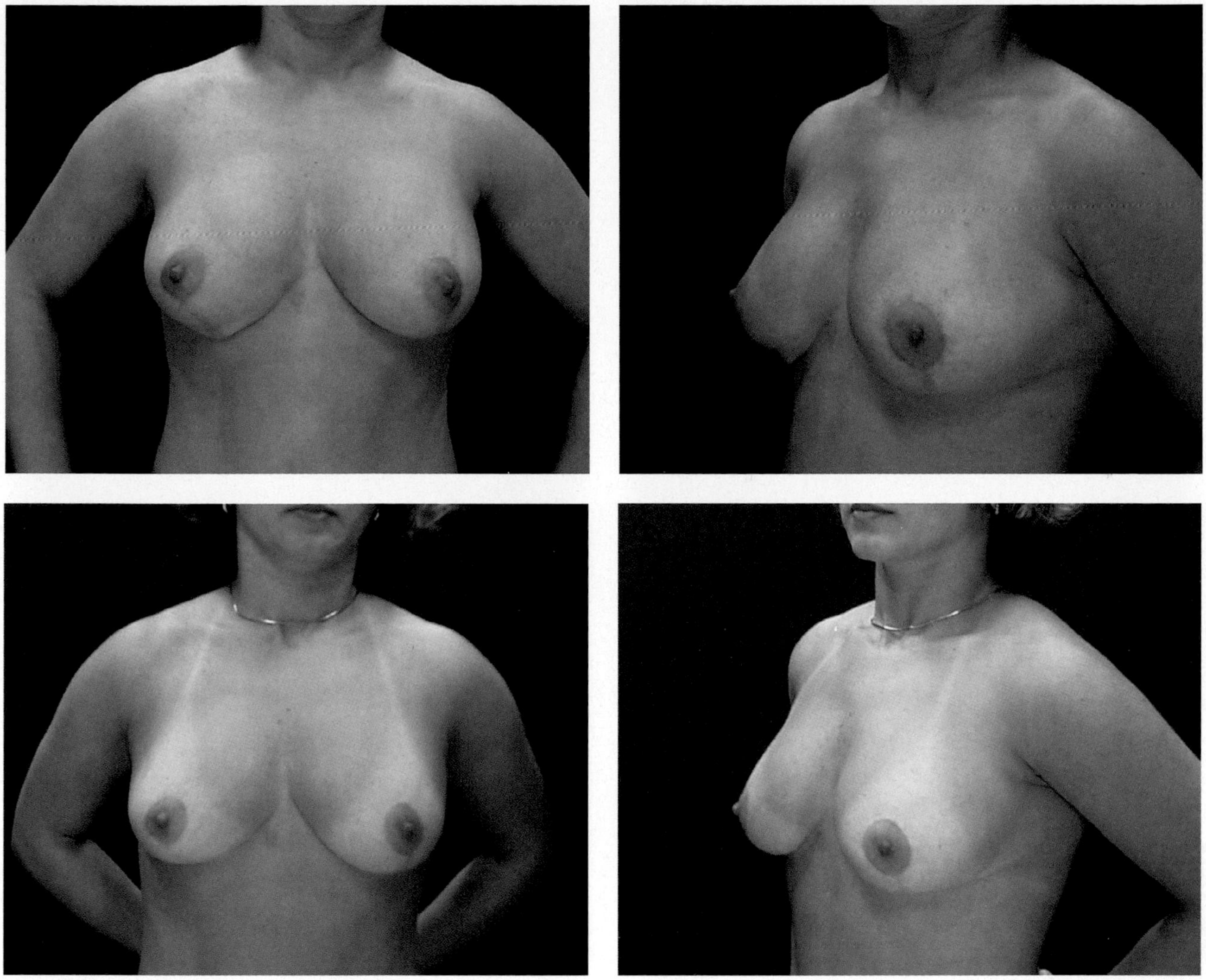

C D

E F

Figure 84.12. (*Continued*) **C, D:** One year after vertical mastopexy and breast reduction of 300 g for each breast. **E, F:** Two years after scar revision with a short horizontal scar.

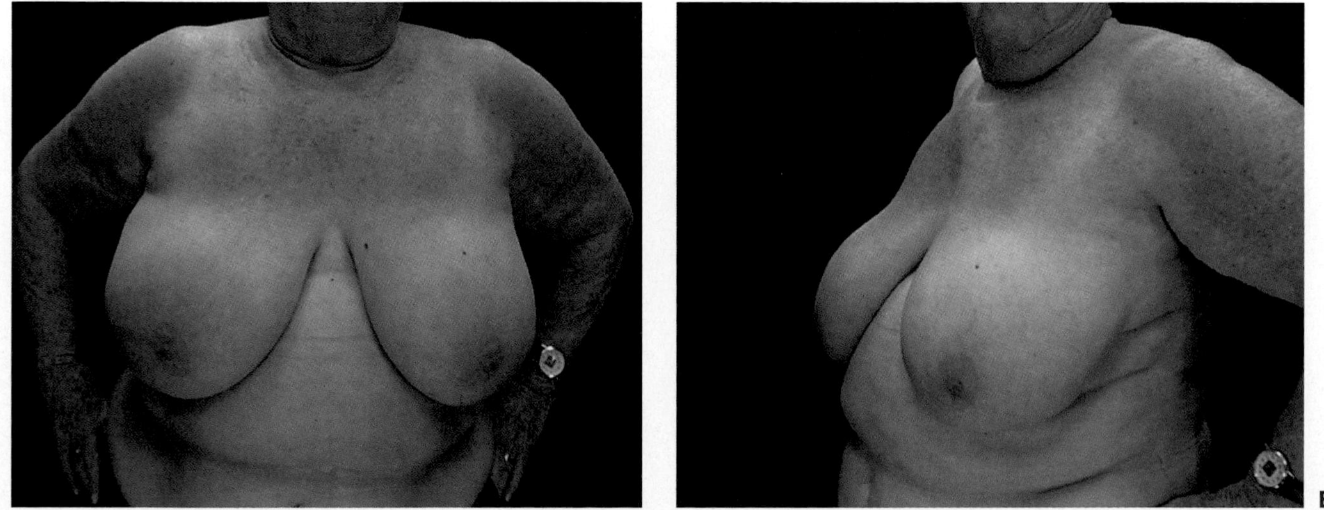

Figure 84.13. **A–C:** Preoperative view of a 71-year-old patient with breast hypertrophy and ptosis (left, middle, and top right). (*continued*)

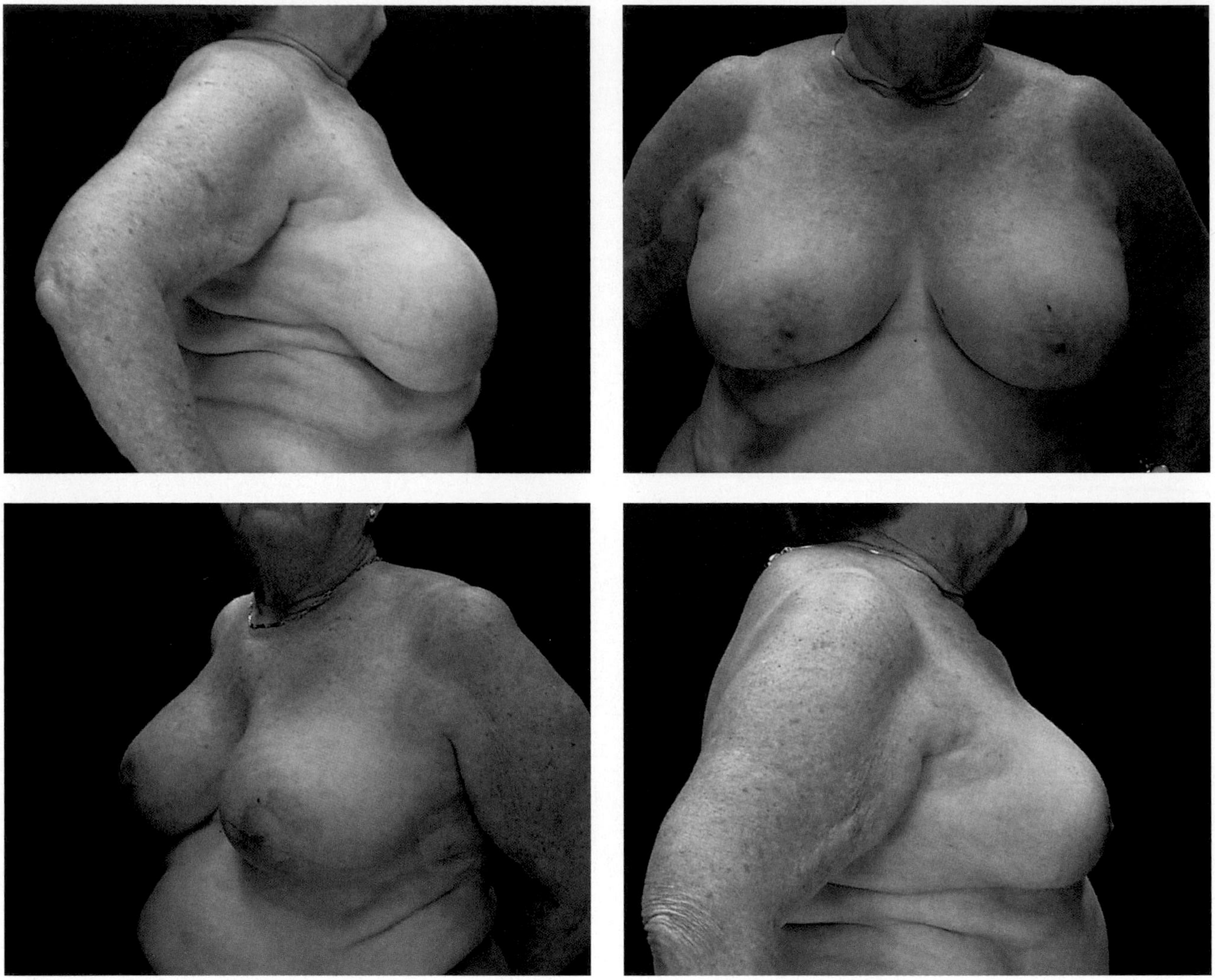

C D

E F

Figure 84.13. (*Continued*) **D–F:** One year after vertical mastopexy and 900 g for each breast reduction and the use of the chest wall–based flap (medial, middle, and bottom right).

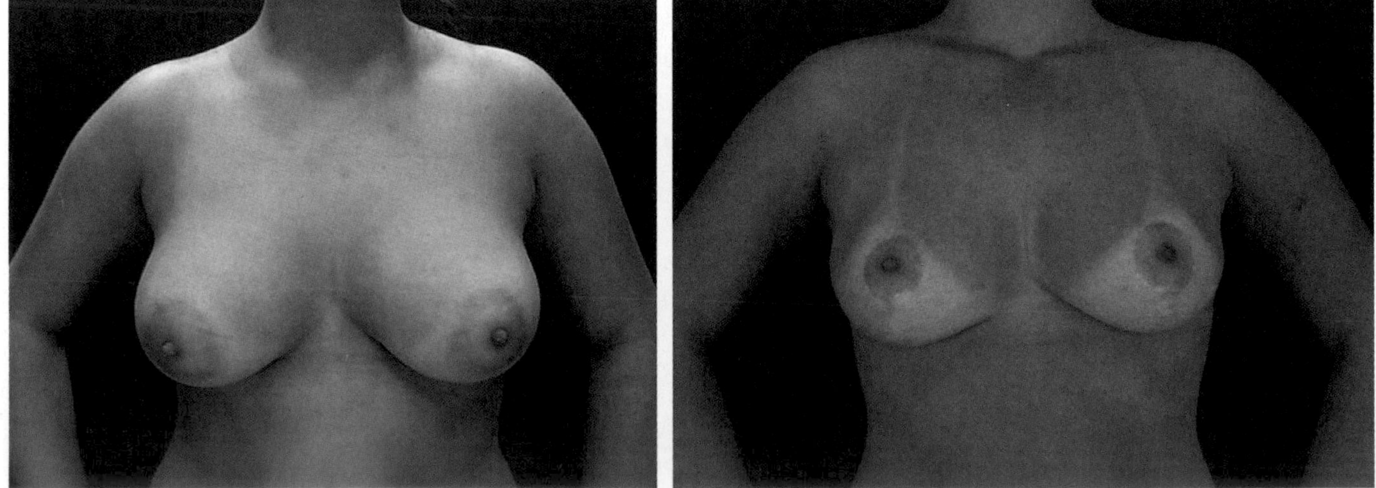

Figure 84.14. Preoperative and 10-year postoperative views. (*continued*)

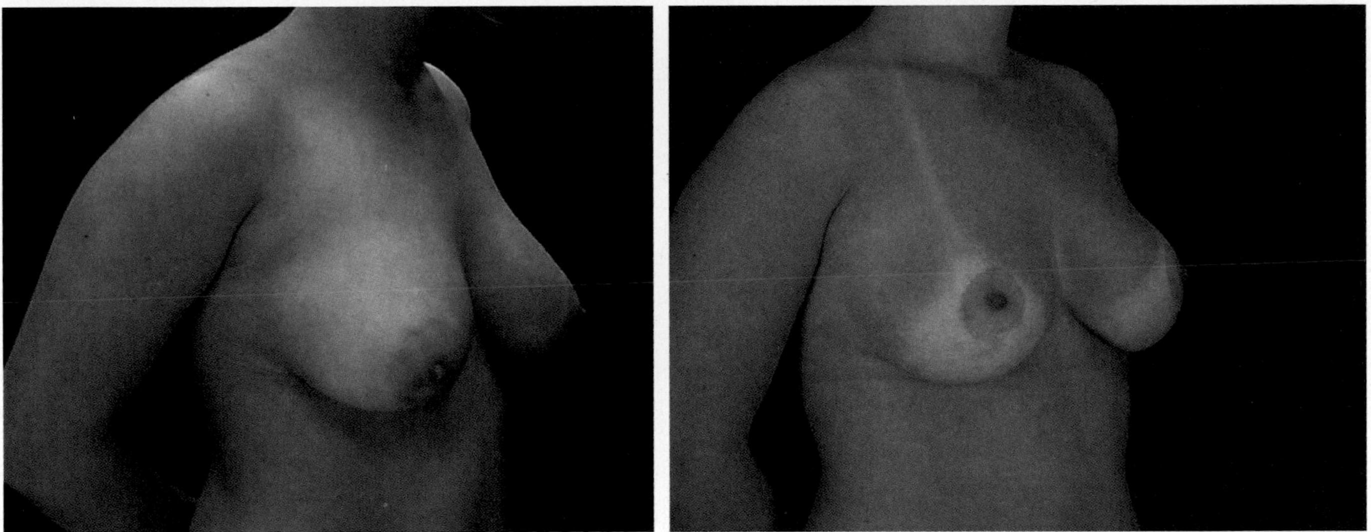

Figure 84.14. (*Continued*)

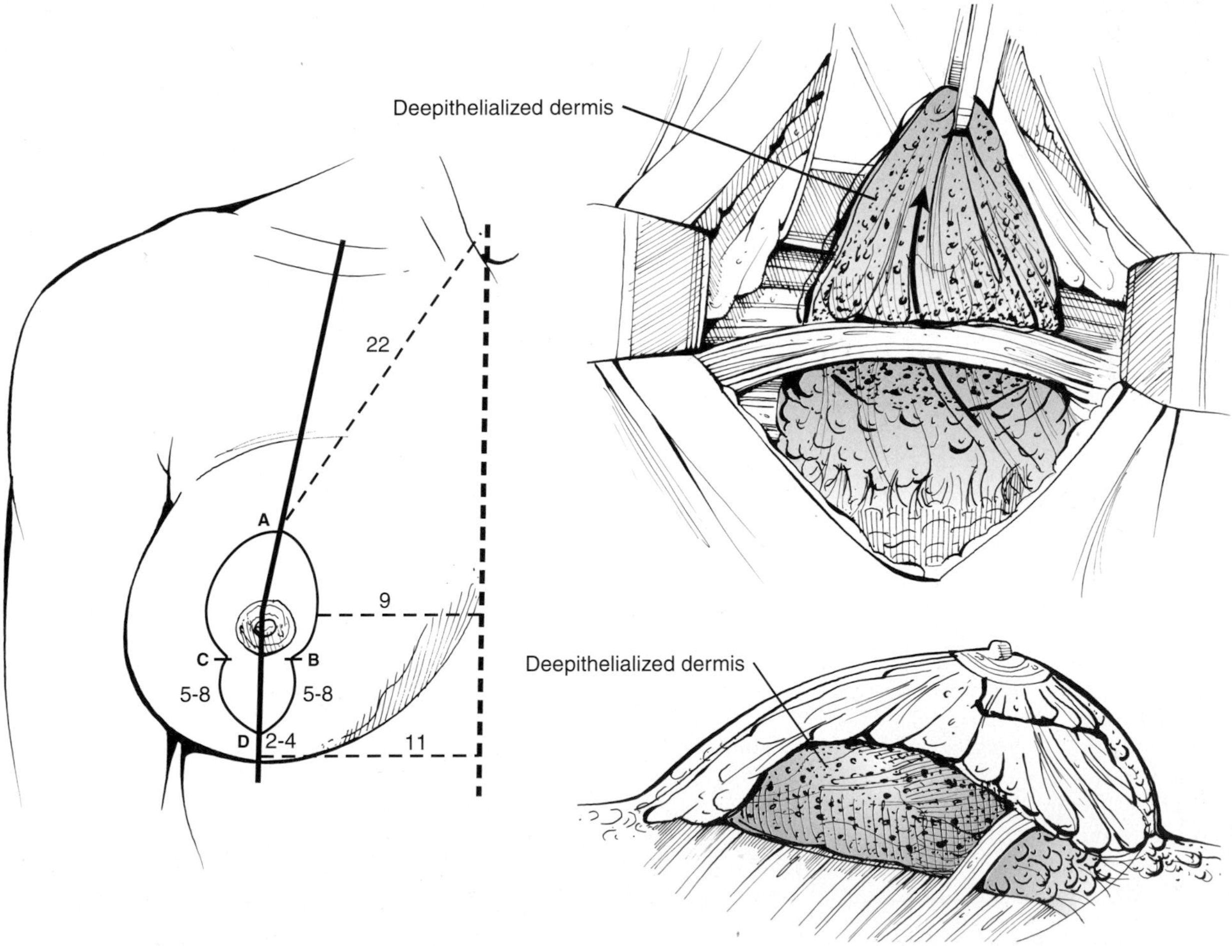

Figure 84.15. Skin markings of the vertical technique. Passing the chest wall–based flap under the pectoral loop. Schematic lateral view of the flaps.

EDITORIAL COMMENTS

As techniques for breast reduction and mastopexy have evolved, imaginative efforts to improve the shape of the breast have been developed. The procedure described in this chapter certainly falls into this category. Several aspects of this technique merit specific comment. As stated, this strategy of creating an inferiorly based dermoparenchymal flap can be used with any skin pattern, whether it is vertical, circumvertical, or an inverted T. The only limitation is that some other pedicle is used for maintaining neurovascular support to the NAC. In the vast majority of cases, this will be with a superior or superomedial pedicle. That being stated, the vascular patterns of the breast as described by Wuringer et al. (1) and Wuringer (2) have particular relevance to this technique. It is true that intercostal, and more important, internal mammary (3) perforators will supply the inferior pedicle, even when the dermis is divided, as long as the inferior portion of the transversely oriented deep septum of the breast is not violated. It is along this septum that these perforators are located. Recognizing and preserving this septum will prevent inadvertent interruption of the vascular supply to this tissue. In the past, concerns related to the viability of this flap buried deep within the breast have been raised. If significant fat necrosis develops in the buried inferior pedicle, it would likely be difficult to detect, depending on the size of the breast. However, findings on mammogram could raise suspicions that would be difficult to differentiate from malignancy.

As a shaping maneuver, including this flap in the overall design of any breast lifting and reshaping procedure is an extremely powerful technique. The ability to provide upper pole fullness and centralize the breast volume allows beautiful shapes to be created. This ability has everything to do with the design and location of the flap and, in my opinion, little to do with the inclusion of the pectoralis loop. I believe the same benefits described by the author could be obtained by simply suturing the flap to the pectoralis fascia. Regardless of whether the muscle loop is used, bottoming out will be restricted using this technique. The secured inferior pedicle, along with its attachments to the inframammary fold, functions as a tether holding the position of the fold in place, even if it has been violated during other portions of the dissection. Although other variables may be involved, this support helps at least limit the "bottoming out" phenomenon.

As breast surgery continues to evolve, it is incumbent on any serious breast surgeon to be able to incorporate techniques such as this into his or her armamentarium. Used wisely, these techniques can provide outstanding results in properly selected patients.

COMMENTARY REFERENCES

1. Wuringer E, Mader N, Posch E, et al. Nerve and vessel supplying ligamentous suspension of the mammary gland. *Plast Reconstr Surg* 1998;101:1486.
2. Wuringer E. Refinement of the central pedicle breast reduction by application of the ligamentous suspension. *Plast Reconstr Surg* 1999;103:1400.
3. van Deventer PV. The blood supply to the nipple-areola complex of the human mammary gland. *Aesthet Plast Surg* 2004;28:393.

REFERENCES

1. Lexer E. Ptosis operation. *Clin Monatsbl Augenh* 1923;70:464.
2. Holländer E. Die operation der mamahypertrophie und der hangebrust. *Deutsche Med Wochenschr* 1924;50:1400.
3. Lotsch GM, Gohrbandt E. Operationen an der weibliche brustdrüse. *Chir Oper Leipzig* 1955.
4. Arié G. Una nueva técnica de mastoplastia. *Rev Lat Am Cir Plast* 1957;3:23–28.
5. Dufourmentel C, Mouly R. Plastic mammaire par la méthode oblique. *Ann Chir Plast* 1961;6:45.
6. Elbaz JS, Verheecke G. La cicatrice en L dans les plasties mammaires. *Ann Chir Plast* 1972;17:283–288.
7. Regnault P. Reduction mammaplasty by the "B" technique. *Plast Reconstr Surg* 1974;53(1):19–24.
8. Meyer R, Kesselring UK. Reduction mammaplasty with an L-shaped suture line. *Plast Reconstr Surg* 1975;55:139–148.
9. Horibe K, Spina V, Lodovici O. Mamaplastia redutora: nuovo abordaje del método lateral oblícuo. *Cir Plast Ib Latinoam* 1976;11(1):7–15.
10. Ely JF. Guidelines for reduction mammaplasty. *Ann Plast Surg* 1981;6(6):424–429.
11. Bozola AR, Mamoplastia em "L"-contribuição pessoal. *Rev AMRIGS* 1982;26(3):207–214.
12. Chiari AJ. The L short-scar mammaplasty: a new approach. *Plast Reconstr Surg* 1992;90(2):233–246.
13. Góes JCS. Periareolar mammaplasty with mixed mesh support: the double skin technique. *Plast Reconstr Surg* 1992;2:575–576.
14. Góes JCS. Periareolar mammaplasty: double skin technique with application of polyglactine or mixed mesh. *Plast Reconstr Surg* 1996;97(5):959–966.
15. Wise RJ. A preliminary report on a method of planning the mammaplasty. *Plast Reconstr Surg* 1956;17:367–375.
16. Pitanguy I. Surgical treatment of breast hypertrophy. *Br J Plast Surg* 1967;20:78.
17. Lassus C. Breast reduction: evolution of a technique. A single scar. *Aesthet Plast Surg* 1989;11:107.
18. Lassus C. A technique for breast reduction. *Int Surg* 1970;53:69–72.
19. Lassus C. Update on vertical surgery. *Plast Reconstr Surg* 1999;104:2289–2298.
20. Lejour M, Abboud M, De Clety A, et al. Reduction des cicatrices de plastie mammaire: de l'ancre courte a la verticale. *Ann Chir Plast Esthet* 1990;35:369–379.
21. Lejour M. *Vertical Mammaplasty and Liposuction of the Breast.* St. Louis, MO: Quality Medical Publishing; 1993.
22. Lejour M. Vertical mammaplasty and liposuction of the breast. *Plast Reconstr Surg* 1994;94(1):100–114.
23. Lejour M. Vertical mammaplasty: early complications after 250 personal consecutive cases. *Plast Reconstr Surg* 1999;104(3):746–770.
24. Benelli L. A new periareolar mammaplasty: round block technique. *Aesthet Plast Surg* 1990;14(2):99–100.
25. Ramirez OM. Reduction mammaplasty with the "owl" incision and no undermining. *Plast Reconstr Surg* 2002;109:512.
26. Atiyeh BS, Rubeiz MT, Hayek SN. Refinements of vertical scar mammaplasty: circumvertical skin excision design with limited inferior pole subdermal undermining and liposculpture of the inframammary crease. *Aesthet Plast Surg* 2005;29:519–531.
27. Pallua N, Ermisch C. "I" Becomes "L": modification of vertical mammaplasty. *Plast Reconstr Surg* 2003;111:1860.
28. Daane SP, Rockwell WB. Breast reduction techniques and outcomes: a meta-analysis. *Aesthet Surg J* 1999;19:293.
29. Lotsch F. Uber Hangebrustplastik. *Zentralbl Chir* 1923;50:1241.
30. Dartigues L. Traitement chirurgical du prolapsus mammaire. *Arch Franco Belg Chir* 1925;28:313.
31. Hall-Findlay E. A simplified vertical reduction mammaplasty shortening the learning curve. *Plast Reconstr Surg* 1999;104:748–759.
32. Hall-Findlay E. Vertical breast reduction with a medially-based pedicle. *Aesthet Plast Surg* 2002;22:185–194.
33. Graf R, Biggs TM, Steely RL. Breast shape: a technique for better upper pole fullness. *Aesthet Plast Surg* 2000;24:348–352.
34. Graf R, Auersvald A, Bernardes A, et al. Reduction mammaplasty and mastopexy with shorter scar and better shape. *Aesthet Surg J* 2000;20:99–106.
35. Graf R, Biggs TM. In search of better shape in mastopexy and reduction mammoplasty. *Plast Reconstr Surg* 2002;110(1):309–317.
36. Graf R, Reis de Araujo LR, Rippel R, et al. Reduction mammaplasty using the vertical scar and thoracic wall flap technique. *Aesthet Plast Surg* 2003;27(1):6–12.
37. Mottura AA. Circumvertical reduction mastoplasty: new considerations. *Aesthet Plast Surg* 2003;27(2):85–93.
38. Peixoto G. Reduction mammaplasty: a personal technique. *Plast Reconstr Surg* 1980;65(2):217–225.
39. Levet Y. The pure posterior pedicle procedure for breast reduction. *Plast Reconstr Surg* 1990;86(41):67–75.
40. Ribeiro L, Backer E. Mastoplastia com pediculo de seguridad. *Rev Esp Cir Plast* 1973;6:223–234.
41. Ribeiro L. A new technique for reduction mammaplasty. *Plast Reconstr Surg* 1975;55:330–334.
42. Daniel M. Mammaplasty with pectoral muscle flap. In: *Transactions of the 64th Annual Scientific Meeting of the American Society of Plastic and Reconstructive Surgeons, Montreal, Canada*; 1995:293–295.
43. Cerqueira AA. Mammoplasty: breast fixation with dermoglandular mono upper pedicle under the pectoralis muscle. *Aesthet Plast Surg* 1998;22:276–283.
44. Marchac D, Olarte G. Reduction mammaplasty and correction of ptosis with a short scar. *Plast Reconstr Surg* 1982;69:45.

CHAPTER

85

Barbara B. Hayden

A Mastopexy Technique Without Implants: Superolaterally Based Rotation Flap

This chapter reviews some of the procedures currently used for mastopexy without implants. I discuss my preference for mastopexy without implants in patients requiring soft tissue augmentation of the chest/breast upper inner quadrant, narrowing of breast base width, and repositioning of the inframammary fold. The described procedure is one of many emerging procedures that use tissue in unwanted areas to autoaugment areas of the volume-depleted ptotic breast.

INTRODUCTION

One of the oldest adages in surgery is that the more solutions there are to a problem, the less likely it is that any one of them is consistently successful in all situations. Each mastopexy procedure aspires to lift, shape, and support the ptotic breast and to maintain that result for a meaningful postoperative period. The ideal procedure should minimize scarring and maximize breast cancer surveillance.

To date, there is no singular approach that can achieve these goals to the exclusion of others. Instead it is generally accepted that the type of mastopexy and its associated risks should be paired with degree and type of the patient's problem and the surgeon's facility with the technique. A patient with minimal ptosis and thick breast tissue does not necessarily merit a complex procedure that involves rotation flaps, tissue advancement, fascial or muscle slings, and accessories such as meshes (synthetic and absorbable), dermal grafts, or allogeneic and xenogeneic dermal matrices. However, there is no doubt that there are patients with problems that may require one or more of these options. An understanding of and a comfort with these more aggressive approaches allow each surgeon to customize his or her solution for each patient.

HISTORY OF MASTOPEXY WITHOUT IMPLANTS

Mastopexy has evolved from skin and tissue resection to parenchymal modification, implants (1,2), local advancement flaps, rotation flaps (3), stacked flaps (4) supported flaps using dermal suspension (5), fascial suspensions (6–8), pectoralis muscle suspensions (9), meshes (10–12), allografts, and xenografts (13,14). With increased parenchymal rearrangement and internal support, mastopexy techniques have moved away from inverted-T incisions to the smaller scars of a vertical mastopexy (15,16), periareolar mastopexy skin incisions (15,17–22), and limited inframammary fold incisions (23). An excellent overview of the history of mastopexy is provided elsewhere in this textbook and has been summarized by many authors (3,4,6,7).

Breast augmentation has been a facile ancillary tool for treating the depleted ptotic breast. As mastopexy procedures have evolved to more complex parenchymal rearrangements, the advisability of pairing the procedure with breast augmentation has been questioned. Arterial and venous insufficiency, nipple necrosis, sensory loss, malposition of the implant, and unpredictable results have been sited as serious risks when combining breast implantation with mastopexy, particularly when implants are placed in a subglandular position (1,2). Without the crutch of implants, mastopexy procedures are often unable to provide upper-pole soft tissue augmentation.

Some of the more aggressive mastopexy procedures have been proposed as solutions to the loss of volume as well as to the significant problems exhibited in postbariatric surgery patient (24–28). The massive weight loss with which patients present is an extreme version of problems that are also apparent in the postpartum and the aging breast. Redundant tissue lateral to the anterior axillary line has invited many proposals for mobilizing this tissue to augment the central mound. It is from this desire (to use redundant tissue that might otherwise be discarded) that my preferred technique had evolved.

PREFERRED TECHNIQUE

The superolaterally based rotation flap (SLBRF) has evolved as a technique that can address several concerns in the ptotic breast:

- Depletion of the upper breast
- Poor projection
- Loose and fluid breast parenchyma
- Widening of breast base width
- Loosening and lowering of inframammary fold (IMF)
- Breast tissue below the IMF
- Excessive lateral chest wall tissue
- Redundant skin

This procedure strives to autoaugment the upper medial chest and cleavage, rebuild the IMF, and improve the thickness of the breast tissue by rotating and advancing tissue that was below the IMF and lateral to the anterior axillary line. The SLBRF pedicle takes advantage of the well-described blood supply to the nipple provided by the upper outer quadrant of the breast. The rotation of the flap not only augments the upper inner quadrant, but it also decreases the base width of the breast and gives improved projection while shortening the medial and lateral extent of the IMF scars. Scars can be expected to heal nicely since they are closed without any tension.

INDICATIONS AND FAVORABLE SITUATIONS

The patient best suited for this procedure is typically postpartum and or post massive weight loss. There is a significant depletion of tissue in the upper inner quadrant. The procedure works best when there is excessive length to the breast, the nipples point outward, and the breast and fatty tissue extend lateral to the anterior axillary fold.

This procedure is particularly valuable when there is a need to elevate or rebuild a ptotic or detached inframammary fold. Rejuvenation of the inframammary fold is often neglected in many mastopexy procedures. This is unfortunate since it is a major concern for most women who might look acceptable in nude postoperative photographs but still look frumpy in off-the-rack clothing with high-riding darts and a "short waist."

CONTRAINDICATIONS

This procedure is not for patients with minimal true ptosis unless the fold is very low and requires a several-centimeter elevation and the breast is wide enough to give length to the flap. If the length of the breast is inadequate, there will not be enough tissue to rotate the flap up into the upper inner quadrant of the breast for autoaugmentation of the upper inner quadrant. If the nipple-areolar complexes (NAC) are medially displaced preoperatively and the pedicle is short, it can be difficult to rotate the NAC into an aesthetically pleasing position without risking kinking of the venous outflow from the NAC.

This procedure should not be used in secondary breast surgery unless the surgeon is confident that the superolateral pedicle is intact and there is adequate venous egress.

PREOPERATIVE PLANNING AND MARKING

The patient is marked in a standing position. Landmarks are boldly indicated, as they provide orientation for intraoperative tailoring. These landmarks include a midline extending from the sternal notch to the umbilicus. The anterior axillary fold and existing IMFs are also marked. The axis of each breast is determined and typically runs from the midclavicular line to the NAC. Markings are altered as needed to correct for asymmetry.

In addition, markings include the planned transverse incision, which is placed several centimeters higher than the existing IMF to achieve a youthful new fold. To accommodate women's clothing, the IMF is best positioned halfway between the sternal notch and umbilicus or halfway between the acromion and the elbow. Having the patient demonstrate issues with clothing may help to clarify the best location for the rejuvenated fold and projecting breast.

The estimated ideal location for the NAC is marked, but the surgeon is advised against extending the vertical incision too high. The vertical incision can be extended superiorly intraoperatively as needed once the flap has filled the upper and lower inner quadrants.

OPERATIVE TECHNIQUE

The patient is placed in a supine position on the operative table. The patient's arms and legs are draped in a lounge chair position and the patient's positioning is reevaluated in a sitting position to be sure that there are no areas of hyperextension, abduction, or excessive pressure. The endotracheal tube is carefully supported and checked in supine and sitting positions to guarantee adequate redundancy in the tubing. The Foley catheter is similarly evaluated prior to draping. These simple steps before draping minimize the risk for adverse outcomes that result from positioning errors hidden during these long cases.

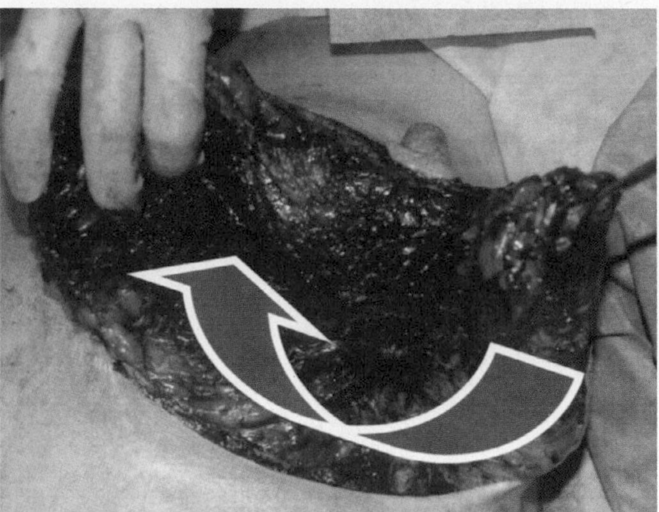

Figure 85.1. The central pedicle is deepithelialized.

The patient is prepped and draped, exposing the superior edge of the umbilicus and giving adequate access to the lateral chest wall back to the posterior axillary line. Inadequate visualization of these important landmarks will impede the surgeon's ability to tailor the breast on the table.

The central pedicle is deepithelialized as shown in Figure 85.1.

MEDIAL FLAP DISSECTION

The medial breast skin flap is incised along the planned vertical and limited horizontal incisions. The dissection is beveled toward the pectoralis fascia, and a pocket is opened to receive the SLBRF. Care is taken to avoid any dissection down to the pectoralis lateral to the midclavicular line (Fig. 85.2).

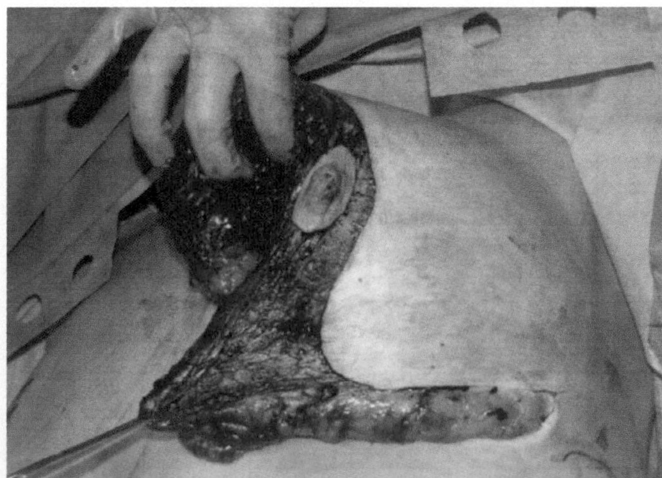

Figure 85.2. The left breast medial pocket is opened to receive a superolaterally based rotation flap. All attachments are preserved lateral to the midclavicular line.

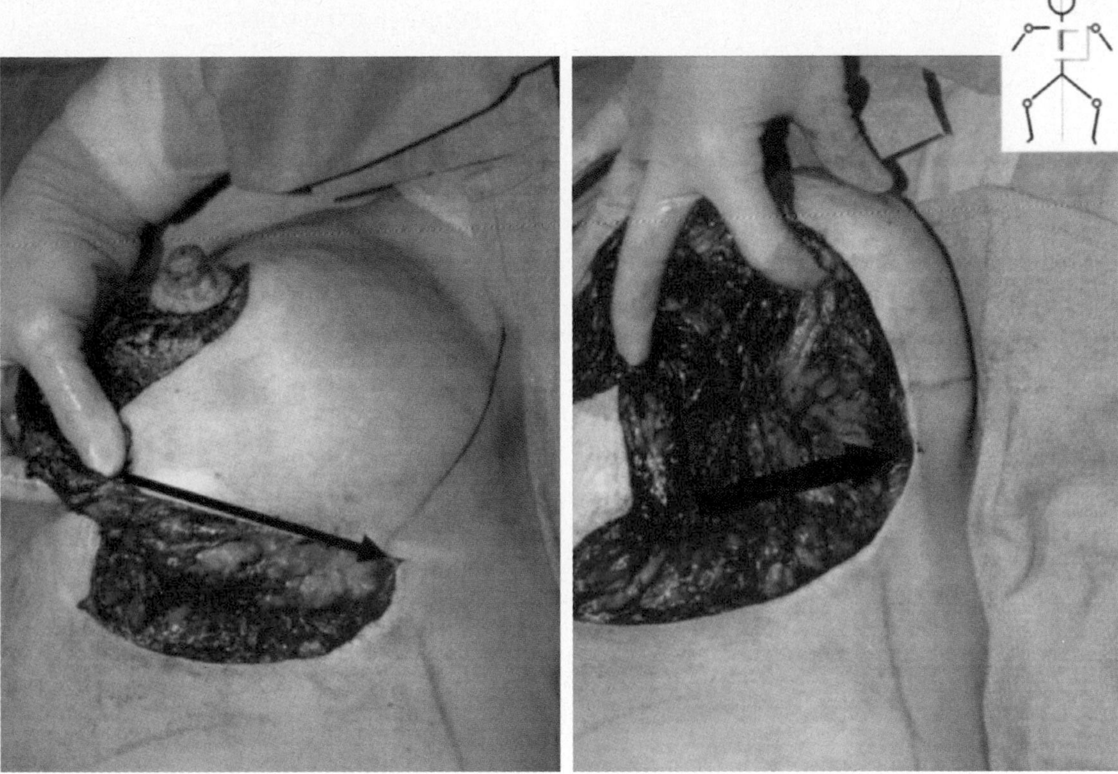

Figure 85.3. Medial tension on the flap reveals parenchymal tissue that must be released laterally.

SUPEROLATERALLY BASED ROTATION FLAP DISSECTION

The SLBRF is designed to use as much of the lower, inner deepithelialized flap as possible. An Allis clamp is used to distract the medial edge of the flap toward the midline, revealing tissue that is restricting mobilization of the flap (Fig. 85.3). The parenchyma is divided along the fold, beveling superiorly up to the inferior border of the pectoralis major. Care is taken to preserve any possible support tissue or ligaments that run from the inferior border of the pectoralis to the ptotic IMF. The skin incision can be limited, but the parenchymal dissection typically extends posterior to the anterior axillary line (Fig. 85.3). This extended dissection is needed to release the flap and allow it to rotate anteriorly and superiorly into the previously dissected medial breast pocket.

No dissection or liposuction is performed in the upper outer quadrants. However, redundant tissue that does not rotate anterior to the fold can be carefully removed as long as the excised tissue is inferior to the axilla and posterior to the anterior axillary fold.

RECONSTRUCTION OF THE INFRAMAMMARY FOLD

Prior to positioning the SLBRF, the patient is placed in a sitting position and the IMF is reconstructed. The subcutaneous tissue below the transverse incision is advanced superiorly to the chest wall using preserved IMF ligaments and/or by restoring the ligaments using dermal grafts, allografts, or xenografts as needed (Fig. 85.4). Restoring the integrity of the fold is crucial to achieving a long-lasting result. Permanent sutures are recommended.

SUPEROLATERALLY BASED ROTATION FLAP ROTATION AND FIXATION

Rotating the flap into the pocket can require some ingenuity, particularly if the base of the flap is stiff or if the length of the flap is short (Fig. 85.5). When the flap can rotate greater than 100 deg the breast achieves a nicely projecting cone shape and the NAC rocks out laterally to give a pleasing appearance. Finesse moves such as finger debridement of fatty tissue above

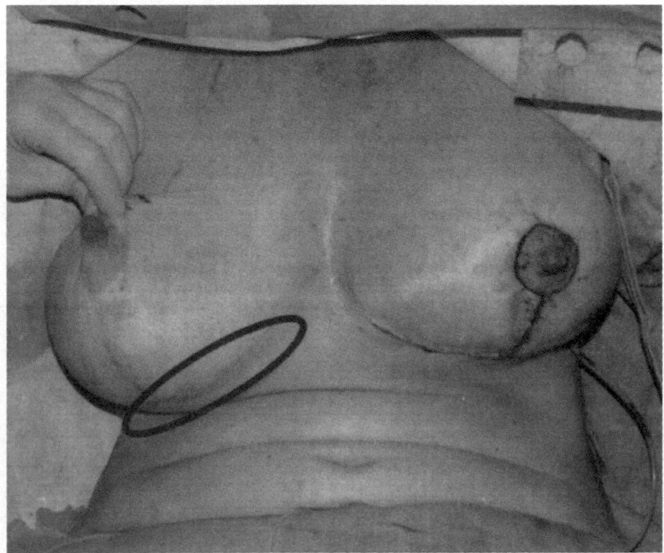

Figure 85.4. Restoring the integrity of the inframammary fold is crucial to achieving a long-lasting result.

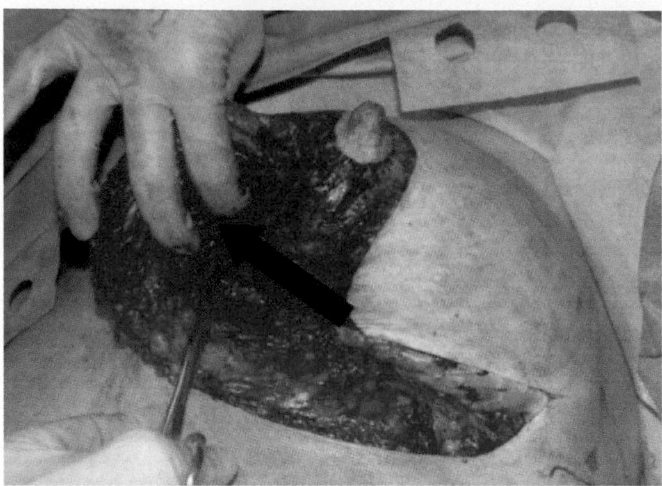

Figure 85.5. A shorter, laterally based rotation flap pedicle resists rotation into pocket and may require further release along the inframammary fold and lateral chest wall.

the NAC can allow the flap to rotate without disrupting venous outflow.

Once the flap is positioned in an appealing way without tension, the flap is secured along the medial border of the sternum with fixation sutures. The inferior edge of the rotated flap is then secured to the reconstructed fold and chest wall (Fig. 85.6).

EDITORIAL COMMENTS

Barbara Hayden introduces us to an alternative method of reshaping and lifting the breast when performing a mastopexy. She gets it right when she writes that whenever there are multiple accepted techniques for something, it usually means that none is either ideal or suited to every situation. One thing is clear. The more powerful techniques include glandular reshaping and go beyond just skin reduction. The SLBRF that she describes follows in the footsteps of other glandular remodeling procedures such as those described by Lassus, Graf, and others. Dr. Hayden brings some interesting and special perspectives to this topic, in that she has a special empathy and understanding for the needs of her Southern California patient population. Thus she emphasizes not just how things look in medical photographs, but also how clothes fit. In addition, raising the inframammary fold, narrowing the breast, maintaining sensation, and filling out the upper-inner quadrant without an implant are all stressed.

I perform a similar procedure to Dr. Hayden, except that I usually leave the nipple attached to a flap based superiorly and rotate the glandular tissues without the nipple on a separate, laterally based flap. Both of these techniques and others have their place, and thus proper patient selection as described by Hayden becomes critical. Clearly there are patients for whom these procedures are not appropriate because their breast tissues are not located in

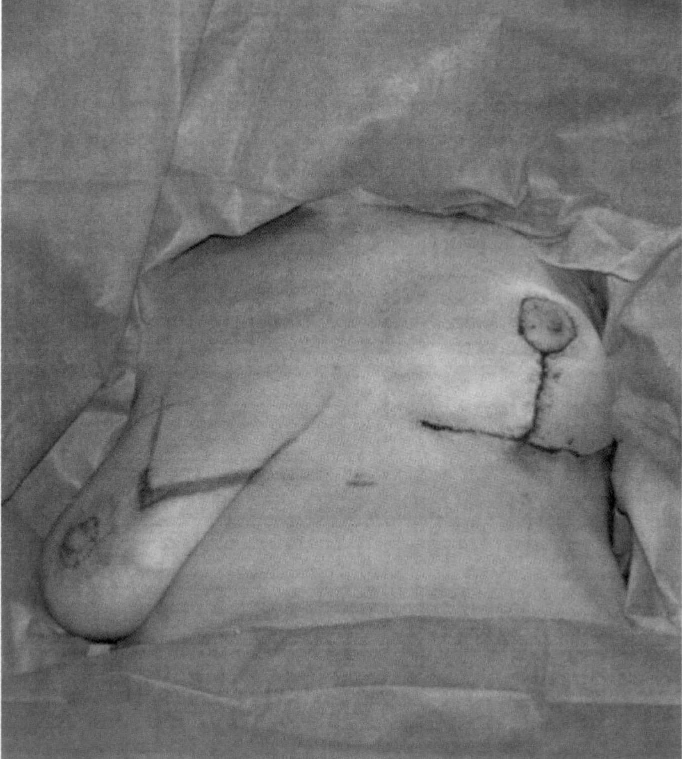

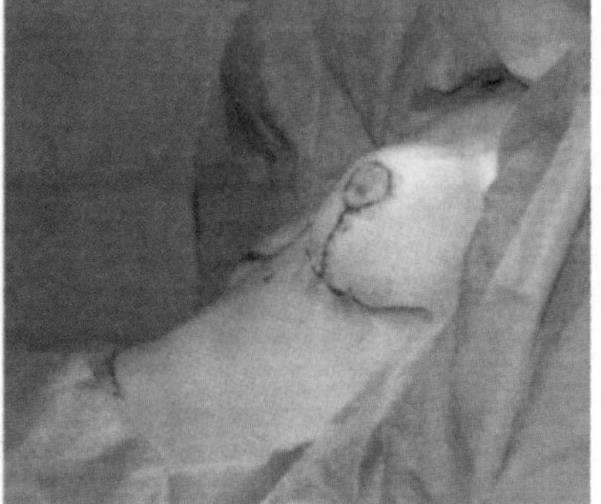

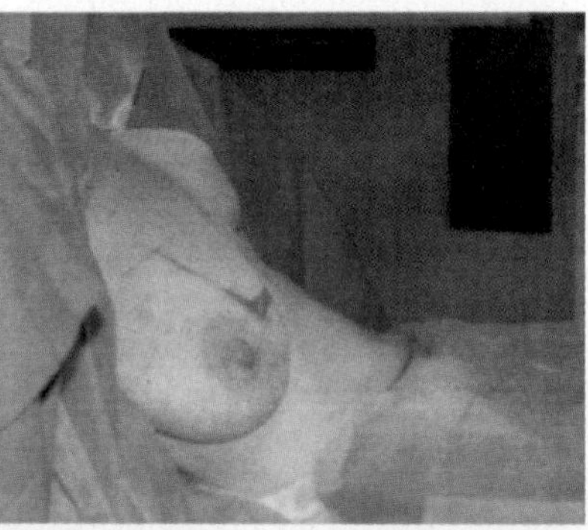

Figure 85.6. Appearance after parenchymal closure. Note lack of tension on skin prior to skin closure. Also note the degree of autoaugmentation of the upper inner quadrant, narrowed base width, projection, and elevated intramammary fold.

a suitable location to allow rotation of the nipple and parenchymal flaps as needed.

While skin-only mastopexies may still have a place in breast surgery, parenchymal reshaping procedures are the more powerful alternative and are destined to become more popular as time goes by.

S.L.S.

REFERENCES

1. Spear S. Augmentation/mastopexy: "surgeon, beware." *Plast Reconstr Surg* 2003;112(3): 905–906.
2. Handel N. Secondary mastopexy in the augmented patient: a recipe for disaster. *Plast Reconstr Surg* 2006;118(7S):152S–161S.
3. Losken A, Holtz DJ. Versatility of the superomedial pedicle in managing the massive weight loss breast: the rotation-advancement technique. *Plast Reconstr Surg* 2007;120(4):1060–1068.
4. Foustanos A, Zavrides H. A double-flap technique: an alternative mastopexy approach. *Plast Reconstr Surg* 2007;120(1):55–60.
5. Rohrich RJ, Gosman AA, Brown SA, et al. Mastopexy preferences: a survey of board-certified plastic surgeons. *Plast Reconstr Surg* 2006;118(7):1631–1638.
6. Lockwood T. Reduction mammaplasty and mastopexy with superficial fascial system suspension. *Am Soc Plast Surg* 1999;103(5):1411–1420.
7. Ritz M, Silfen R, Southwick G. Facial suspension mastopexy. *Plast Reconstr Surg* 2006;117(1):86–94.
8. Wuringer E. Refinement of the central pedicle breast reduction by application of the ligamentous suspension. *Plast Reconstr Surg* 1999;103(5):1400–1410.
9. Graf R, Biggs T. In search of better shape in mastopexy and reduction mammoplasty. *Plast Reconstr Surg* 2002;110(1):309–317.
10. Goes JC, Landecker A, Lyra EC, et al. The application of mesh support in periareolar breast surgery: clinical and mammographic evaluation. *Aesthetic Plast Surg* 2004;28(5):268–274.
11. de Bruijn HP, Johannes S. Mastopexy with 3D preshaped mesh for long-term results: development of the internal bra system. *Aesthetic Plast Surg* 2008;32(5):757–765.
12. Goes JC. Periareolar mammaplasty: double skin technique with application of polyglactine or mixed mesh. *Plast Reconstr Surg* 1996;97(5):959–968.
13. Panettiere P, Marchetti L, Accorsi D. The underwire bra mastopexy: a new option. *J Plast Reconstr Aesthet Surg* 2009;62(7):e231–e235.
14. Colwell AS, Breuing KH. Improving shape and symmetry in mastopexy with autologous or cadaveric dermal slings. *Ann Plast Surg* 2008;61(2):138–142.
15. Hidalgo DA. Y-scar vertical mammaplasty. *Plast Reconstr Surg* 2007;120(7):1749–1754.
16. Pechter EA, Roberts S. The versatile helium balloon mastopexy. *Aesthet Surg J* 2008;28(3): 272–278.
17. Spear S, Giese SY, Ducic I. Concentric mastopexy revisited. *Plast Reconstr Surg* 2001;107(5): 1294–1299.
18. Lassus C. A 30-year experience with vertical mammaplasty. *Plast Reconstr Surg* 1996;97(2):373–380.
19. Hammond DC. Short scar periareolar inferior pedicle reduction (SPAIR) mammaplasty. *Plast Reconstr Surg* 1999;103(3):890–901.
20. Lejour M. Vertical mammaplasty: early complications after 250 personal consecutive cases. *Plast Reconstr Surg* 1999;104(3):764–770.
21. Rohrich RJ, Thornton JF, Jakubietz RG, et al. The limited scar mastopexy: current concepts and approaches to correct breast ptosis. *Plast Reconstr Surg,* 2004;114(6):1622–1630.
22. Hammond DC, Alfonso D, Khuthaila DK. Mastopexy using the short scar periareolar inferior pedicle reduction technique. *Plast Reconstr Surg* 2008;121(5):1533–1539.
23. Corduff N, Taylor GI. Subglandular breast reduction: the evolution of a minimal scar approach to breast reduction. *Plast Reconstr Surg* 2004;113(1):175–184.
24. Rubin JP, Gusenoff JA, Coon D. Dermal suspension and parenchymal reshaping mastopexy after massive weight loss: statistical analysis with concomitant procedures from a prospective registry. *Plast Reconstr Surg* 2009;123(3):782–789.
25. Graf RM, Mansur AE, Tenius FP, et al. Mastopexy after massive weight loss: extended chest wall-based flap associated with a loop of pectoralis muscle. *Aesthetic Plast Surg* 2008;32(2): 371–374.
26. Hamdi FA. A mastopexy with lateral intercostal artery perforator (LICAP) flaps for patients after massive weight loss. *Ann Plast Surg* 2007;58(5):588.
27. Kwei S, Borud LJ, Lee BT. Mastopexy with autologous augmentation after massive weight loss: the intercostal artery perforator (ICAP) flap. *Ann Plast Surg* 2006;57(4): 361–365.
28. Rubin JP, Gusenoff JA, Coon D. Dermal suspension and parenchymal reshaping mastopexy after massive weight loss: statistical analysis with concomitant procedures from a prospective registry. *Plast Reconstr Surg* 2008;123(3):782–789.
29. Strauch B, Elkowitz M, Baum T, et al. Superolateral pedicle for breast surgery: an operation for all reasons. *Plast Reconstr Surg* 2005;115(5):1269–1277.
30. Goes JC, Landecker A, Lyra EC, et al. The application of mesh support in periareolar breast surgery: clinical and mammographic evaluation. *Aesthetic Plast Surg* 2004;28(5): 268–274.

CHAPTER

86

Claude Lassus

Vertical Scar Breast Reduction and Mastopexy Without Undermining

In 1964, I performed a breast reduction on a patient with unilateral breast hypertrophy (Fig. 86.1) using a procedure that combined four principles (Fig. 86.2):

1. A central vertical wedge resection to reduce the size of the breast
2. Transposition of the areola on a superiorly based flap
3. No undermining
4. A vertical scar to finish off

I first published this technique in 1969 and then again in 1970. More than 40 years after this first operation, I am still using vertical mammaplasty, even though some modifications have been made to avoid the vertical scar appearing below the inframammary fold.

WHY THE VERTICAL MAMMAPLASTY?

For many years, most of the candidates for breast reduction were only concerned with the diminution of the size of their breasts. This was also the main concern for plastic surgeons, who did not give much thought to scarring. However, more recently, candidates for this operation have been demanding better results.

Most important, they want beautiful breasts. What is a beautiful breast? What is considered beautiful is certainly different in Europe than in North and South America, Asia, and Africa. In France, a breast is considered beautiful if it has a good size with fullness in the upper part, good projection, and good position of the nipple (Fig. 86.3). Patients want their results to last over the years. They also want a safe procedure with minimal scarring.

In France, the results of a recent poll showed that 78% of patients are anxious about the complications of any aesthetic operation. It is obvious that we must always use safe procedures, particularly in mammaplasty because the breast is so important to women.

IS VERTICAL MAMMAPLASTY A SAFE PROCEDURE?

Neither the surgeon nor the patient likes to see bleeding, infection, skin necrosis, glandular necrosis, nipple loss, or loss of nipple sensation after reduction mammaplasty. One of the principles of the operation is to reduce the size of the breast through a central wedge "en bloc" resection at the lower part of the breast (skin, fat, and gland) and only fat and gland beneath the areolar flap (Fig. 86.2A). When this resection has been achieved, the breast cone is reconstructed by drawing centrally each lateral part of the amputated breast (Fig. 86.2B). Because no undermining has been performed (the skin is not elevated from the gland, and the gland is not separated from the muscle), at the end of the operation no dead space is present in the breast. So, if accurate hemostasis has been achieved, no hematoma will be seen in the postoperative course. Drains are unnecessary (Fig. 86.4).

The central vertical wedge resection does not impair the blood supply to the gland or to the skin (Fig. 86.5). Moreover, because the gland has not been separated from the muscle, the flow of blood through the perforators remains undisturbed. With a vertical mammaplasty, there should be no skin necrosis or glandular necrosis.

An important principle of mammaplasty is the safe transposition of the nipple-areola complex. Since 1964, I have generally used a superiorly based pedicle. Why? If we look at the three main possible patterns of blood distribution to this anatomic complex as described by Marcus in 1934 (Fig. 86.6), it is clear that the superior pedicle flap does not impair any of these different patterns. That explains why this flap is safe. However, when the nipple-areola complex has to be moved too high (greater than 10 cm), the pedicle is folded back on itself so much so that the venous blood return can be disturbed and an areolar necrosis may occur. In such instances, I use a lateral flap as advocated by Skoog in 1963 or a medial dermoglandular flap such as the one I have described (Fig. 86.7).

The nipple is innervated from many sources, not just from the anterior branch of the fourth lateral intercostal nerve. The superiorly based flap preserves most of the sources, and because the skin has not been separated from the gland, the anterior branch of the fourth lateral intercostal nerve is also preserved (Fig. 86.8). Nipple sensation is rarely disturbed after a vertical mammaplasty.

My vertical mammaplasty produces excellent long-lasting results. Large breasts can be reduced through a horizontal amputation, a vertical amputation, or a combination of these types of resection. It is well known that a horizontal amputation produces a flat breast (Fig. 86.9). In contrast, a vertical amputation gives projection to the breast. When the central wedge resection has been performed as previously described, the breast cone is reconstructed by joining the lateral parts of the amputated breast. This maneuver moves the remaining breast tissues upward and forward, as does the pinching of the inferior pole with the fingers. Vertical mammaplasty employing a vertical amputation yields the same result (i.e., a nice projection and fullness at the upper pole) (Figs. 86.10 to 86.12).

When the central wedge resection is performed, most of the pendulous portion of the breast is removed (Fig. 86.13). To reconstruct the breast cone, the lateral portions of the amputated breast are drawn centrally toward each other; however, because these lateral parts are not ptotic, there is no need to anchor them in a higher position by suturing them to the muscle. This

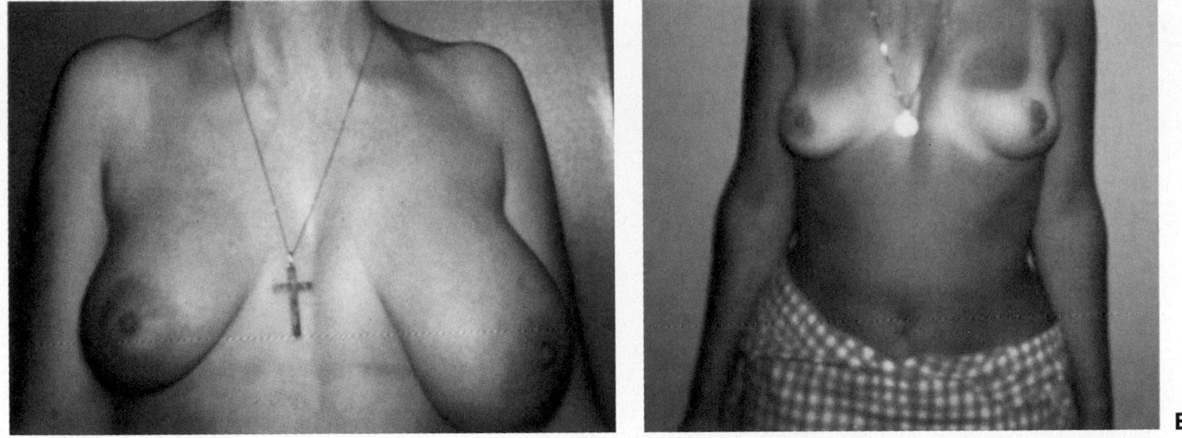

Figure 86.1. First case of vertical mammaplasty: before (**A**) and after 2 years (**B**).

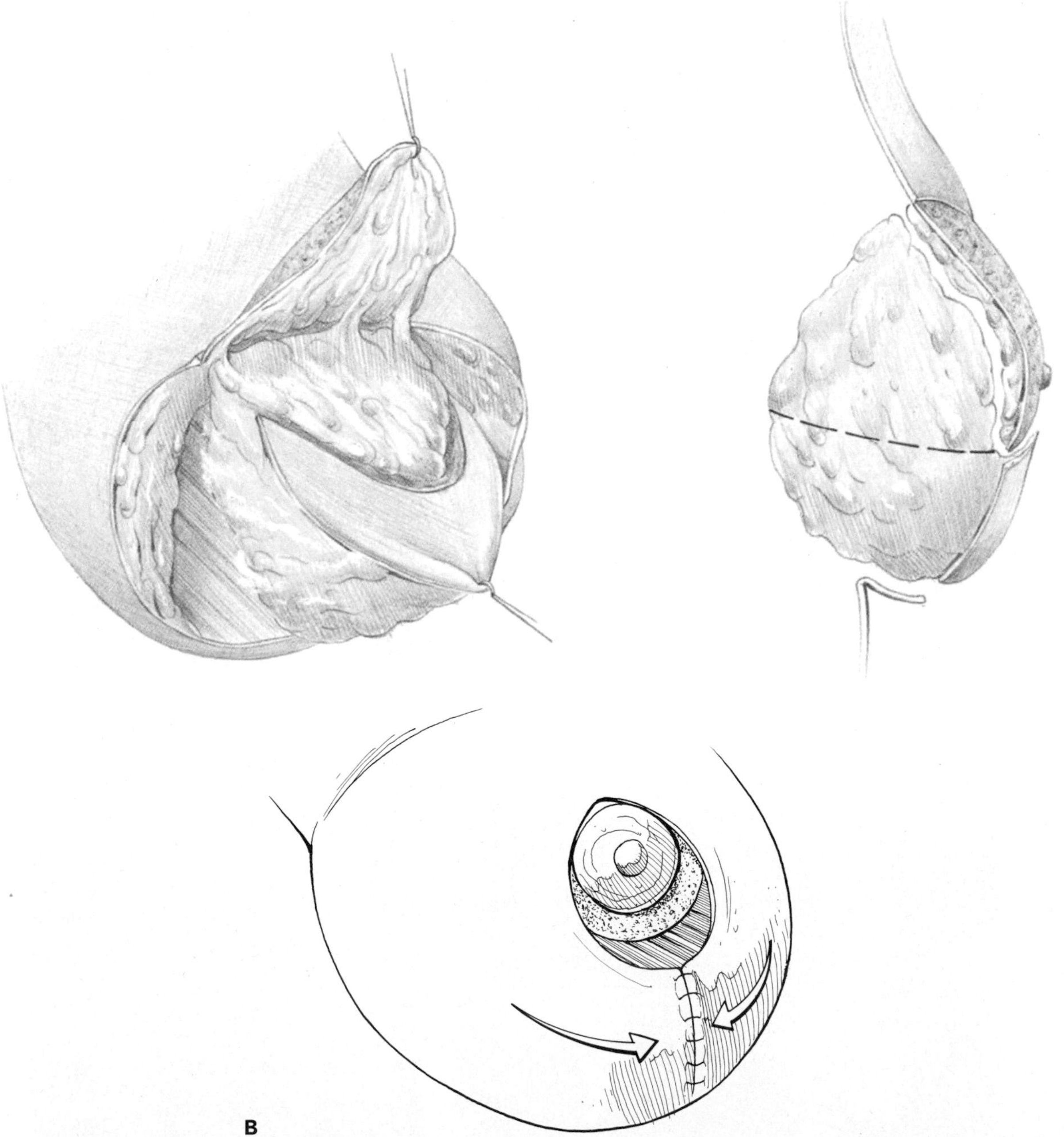

A

B

Figure 86.2. Principle of vertical scar breast reduction and mastopexy without undermining. **A:** The breast size is reduced using a central wedge resection en bloc at the lower part of the breast (skin, fat, and gland) and only fat and gland beneath the areolar flap. **B:** After resection, the breast cone is reconstructed by repairing centrally each lateral part of the amputated breast.

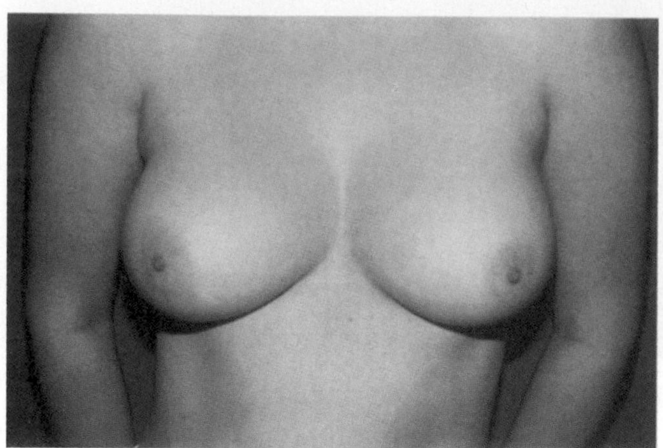

Figure 86.3. A beautiful breast in a young woman.

makes the results longer lasting. Avoiding undermining also helps.

THE VERTICAL SCAR IS NOT THE MINIMAL SCAR THAT CAN BE LEFT AFTER A MAMMAPLASTY

Although a periareolar scar is the shortest possible scar, my experience is that in average or large hypertrophies the vertical scar is the shortest scar that is practical. This type of scar has several advantages. It is barely visible in the standing position, it usually vanishes over the years, and it rarely becomes hypertrophic, even in women with darker skin.

Many surgeons have long said that the vertical scar should not exceed 5.5 cm in length at the end of surgery. Why? If we measure the distance between the inferior border of the areola and the inframammary fold in a variety of different breasts that are considered beautiful, we see that this distance is variable according to the size of the breast. It ranges from 4.5 to 10 cm or even more. Therefore, the appropriate length of the vertical scar is not fixed. The only important point is that at the end of the operation the inferior extremity of the vertical scar must be situated above the existing submammary fold. If the scar is positioned above or at the limit of this fold, its inferior part will not show afterward.

The vertical mammaplasty, as I perform it, allows a significant reduction of breast volume, but this does not mean converting extremely large breasts into very small ones. Vertical mammaplasty can only reduce about 50% of the existing volume.

Careful patient selection with this procedure is crucial. A good choice is a young woman with good elastic skin and a firm, glandular breast, not too big and not too ptotic (Fig. 86.14). After having performed several operations of this type, the surgeon can progressively extend its indications (Fig. 86.15).

I do not believe it is possible to draw exact preoperative markings for a reduction mammaplasty, just as it is impossible to draw out the plan in a rhinoplasty or a face lift. Why should it then be possible in breast reduction? To me, surgery of the breast is just like rhinoplasty, that is, sculpture. The surgeon is working in three dimensions and must have an artistic feeling to achieve beautiful breasts. A sculptor needs landmarks to achieve his or her work; the surgeon also needs landmarks to accomplish a vertical mammaplasty.

Point A is no longer the new nipple position. It marks the new position of the upper border of the areola. I do it as shown in Figure 86.16: I measure the acromion–olecranon distance. I take the midpoint of this distance and another point located 2 cm below. From this last point, I draw a horizontal line that

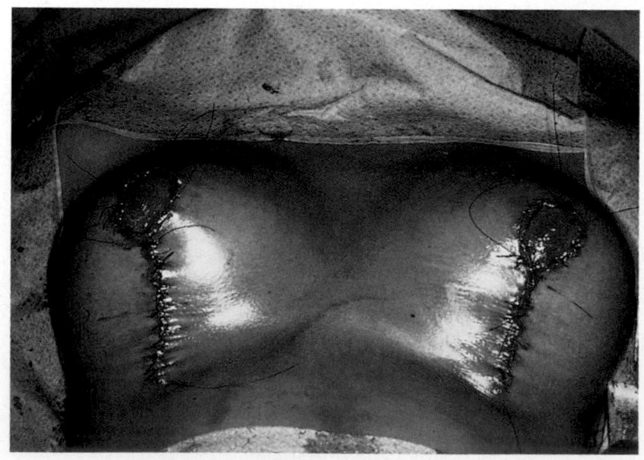

A

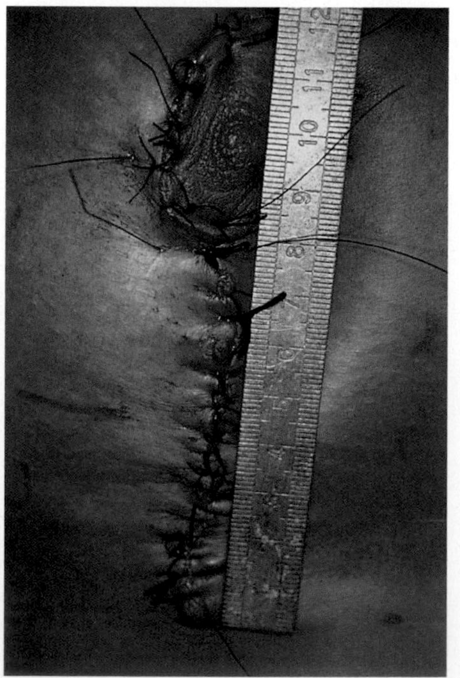

B

Figure 86.4. A: The suturing is completed. **B:** The length of the scar is 8 cm.

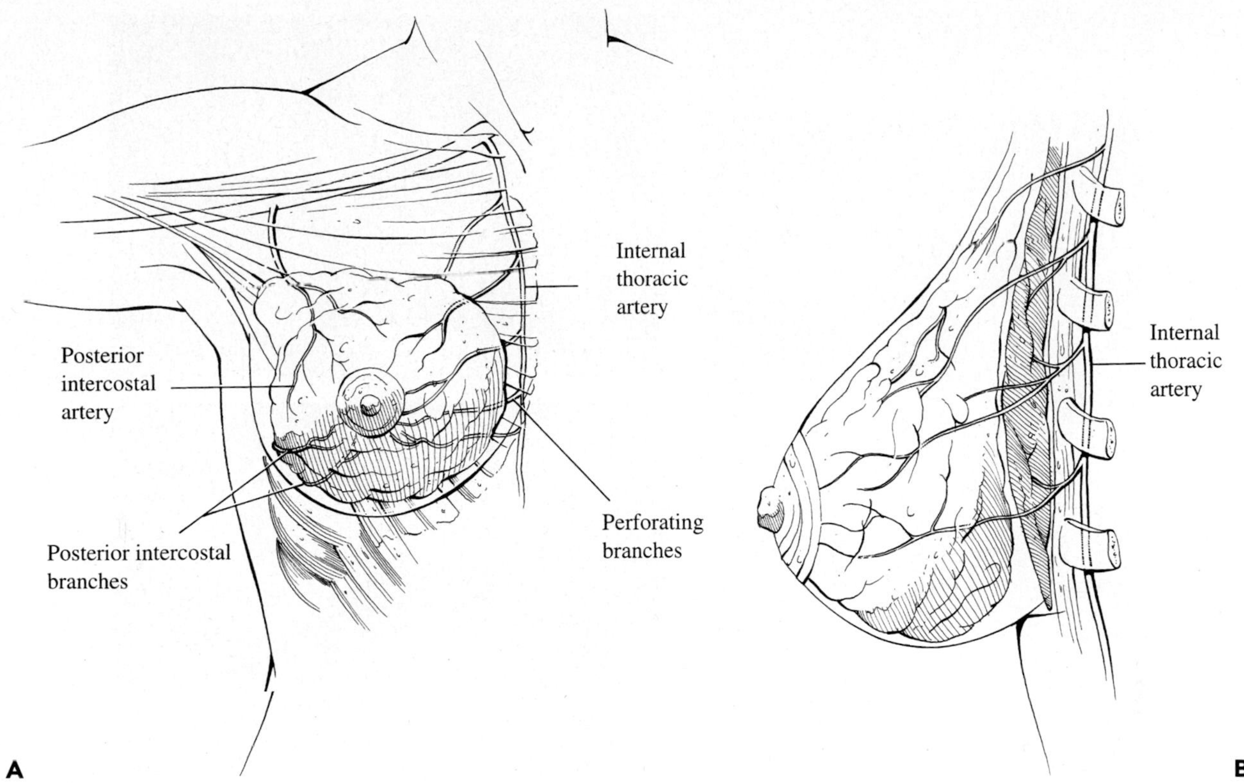

Figure 86.5. The block of resection does not impair the blood supply to the remaining gland and skin. Because the gland remains attached to the muscle, the blood coming through the perforators remains intact.

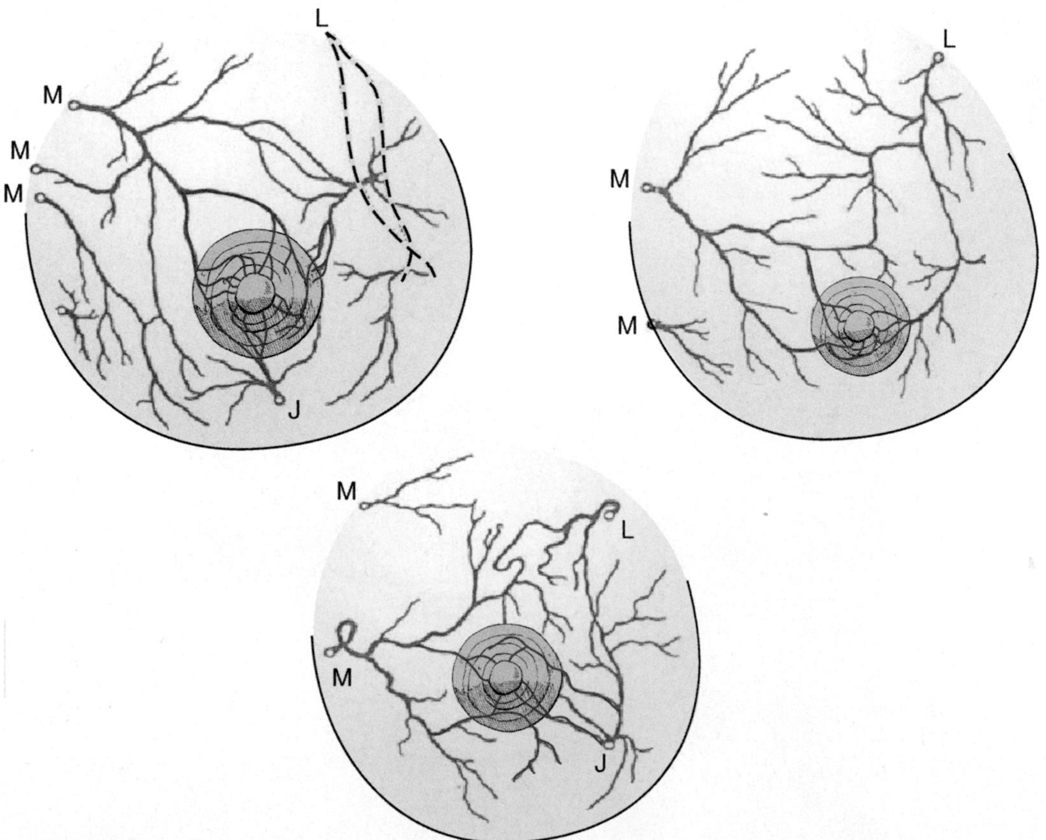

Figure 86.6. The block of resection does not impair the blood supply to the remaining gland and skin.

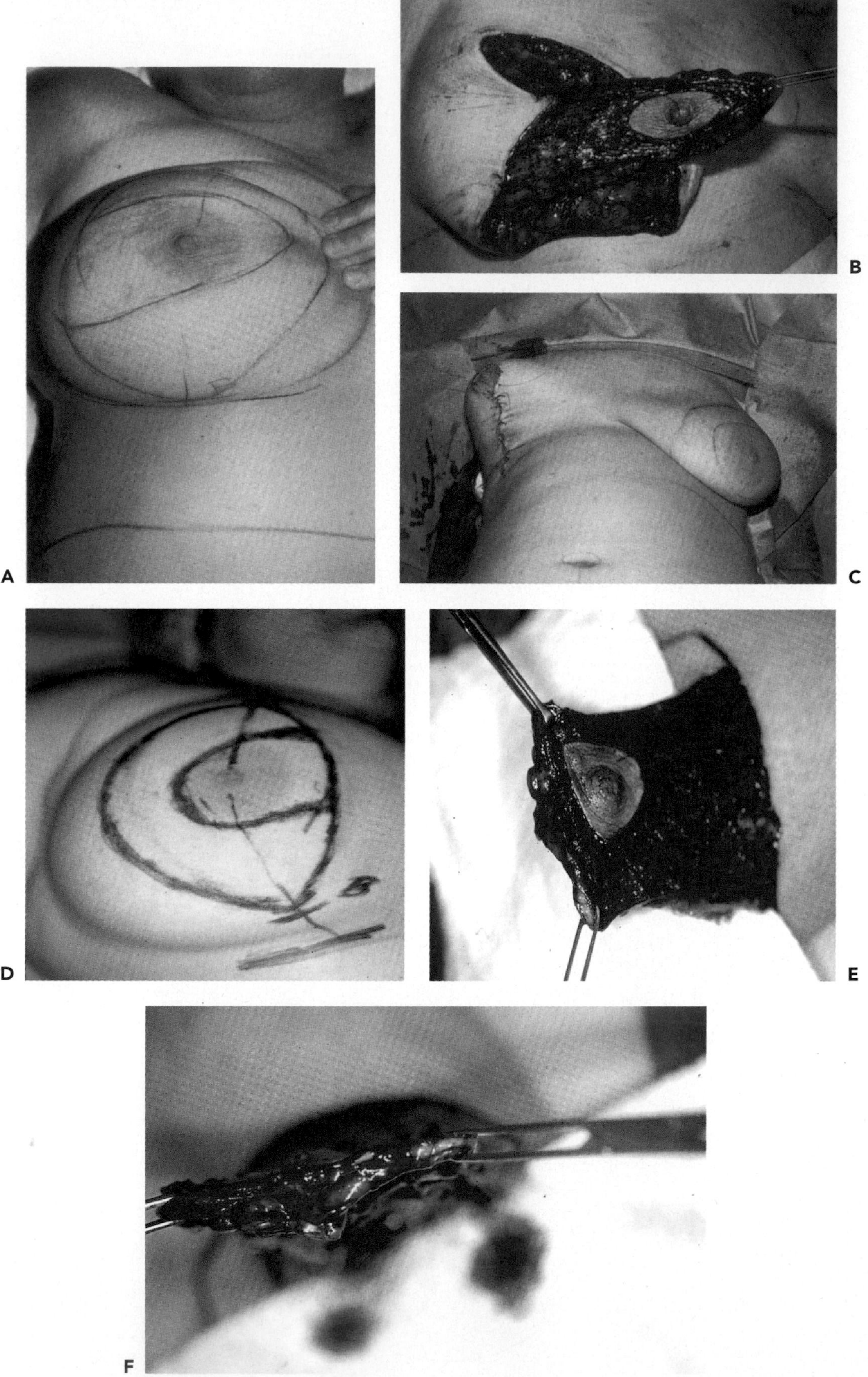

Figure 86.7. **A:** Drawing of the lateral flap. **B:** The flap has been raised. **C:** One side completed. **D:** Drawing of the medial flap. **E:** The flap has been raised. **F:** Thickness of the flap.

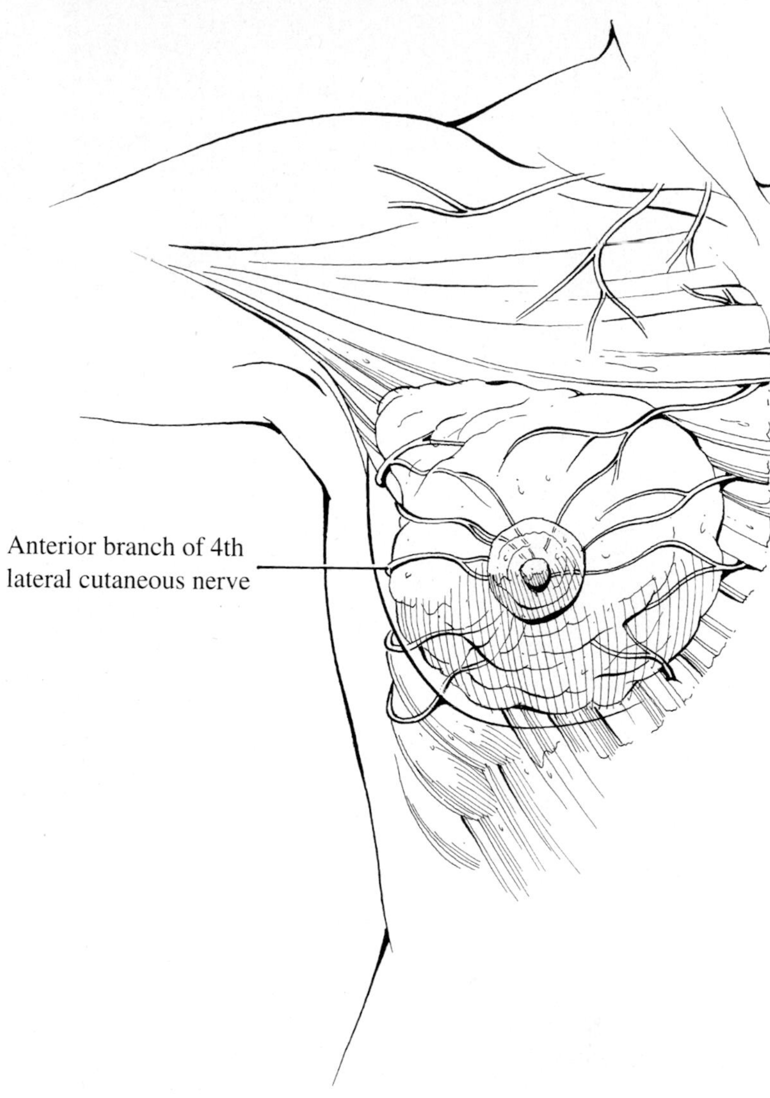

Figure 86.8. The superiorly based flap preserves most of the sources of sensibility to the nipple-areola complex. The anterior branch of the fourth lateral intercostal nerve remains intact because no subcutaneous undermining has been done.

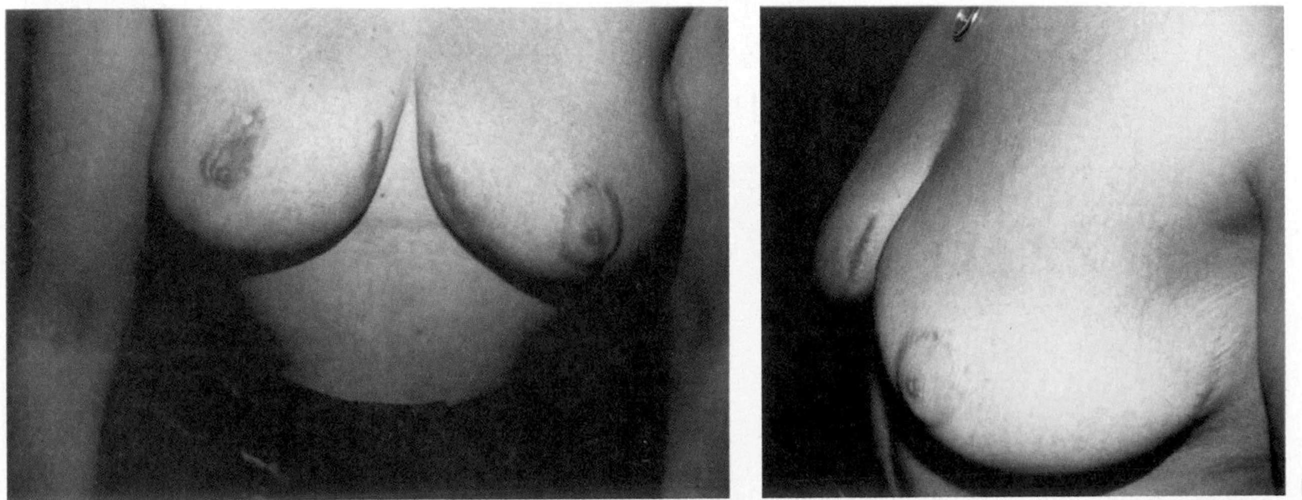

Figure 86.9. Flat breast after a horizontal amputation. **A:** Front view. **B:** Oblique view.

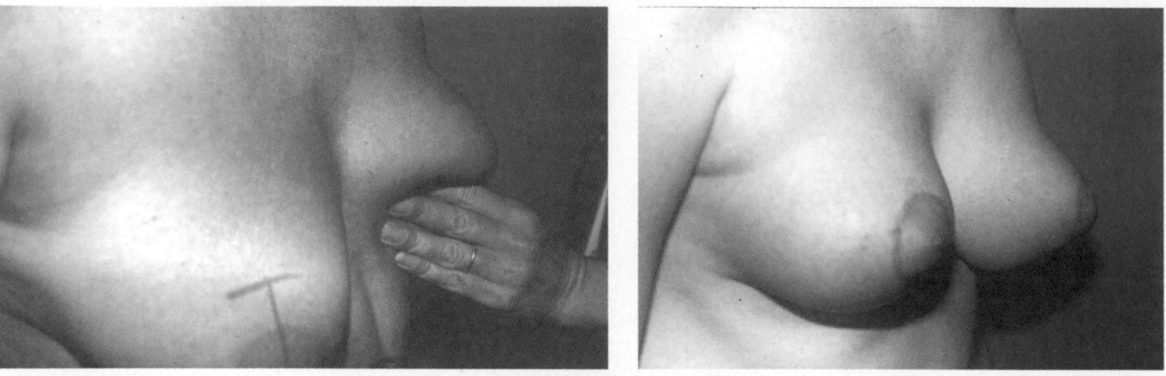

Figure 86.10. The vertical mammaplasty achieves fullness at the upper pole and projection to the breast, as does the pinching of the inferior pole with the fingers.

A

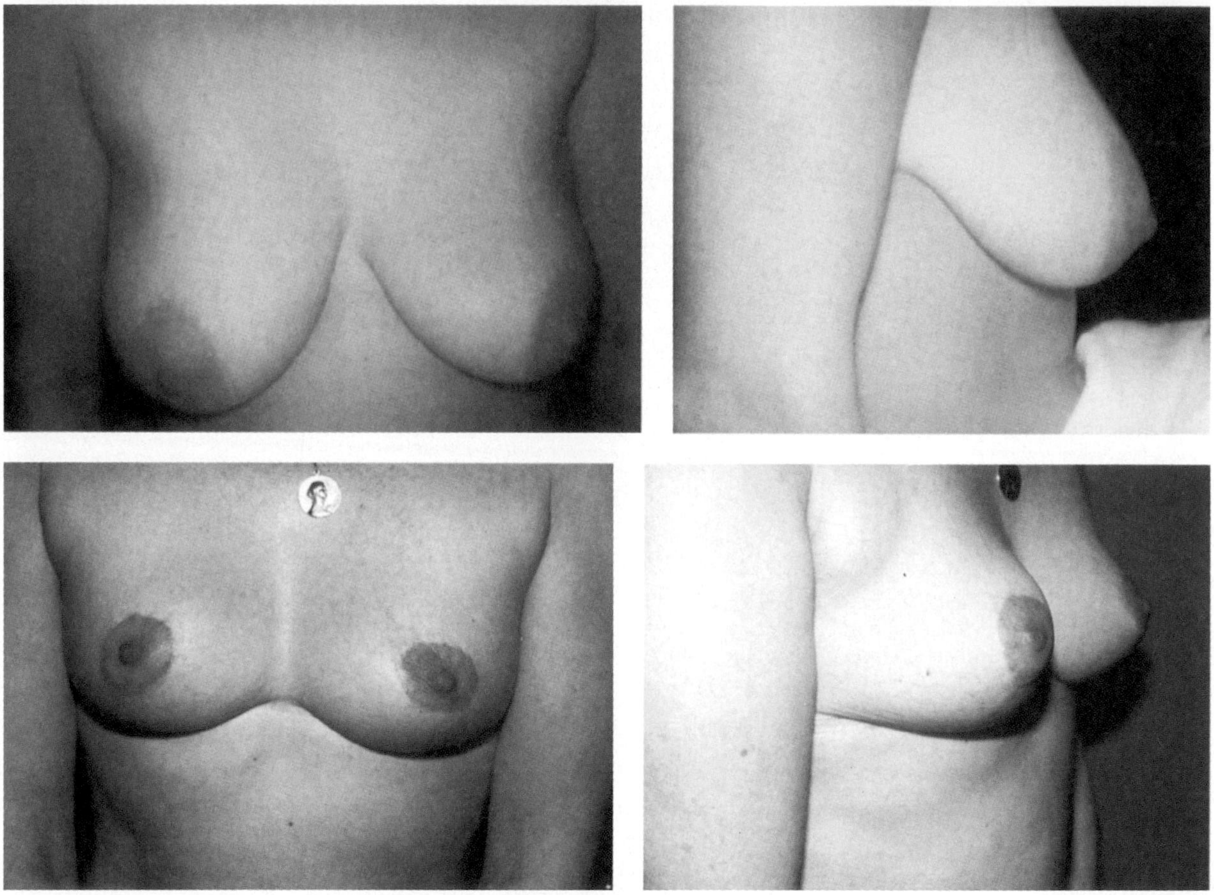

B

Figure 86.11. Before **(A)** and after 20 years **(B)**.

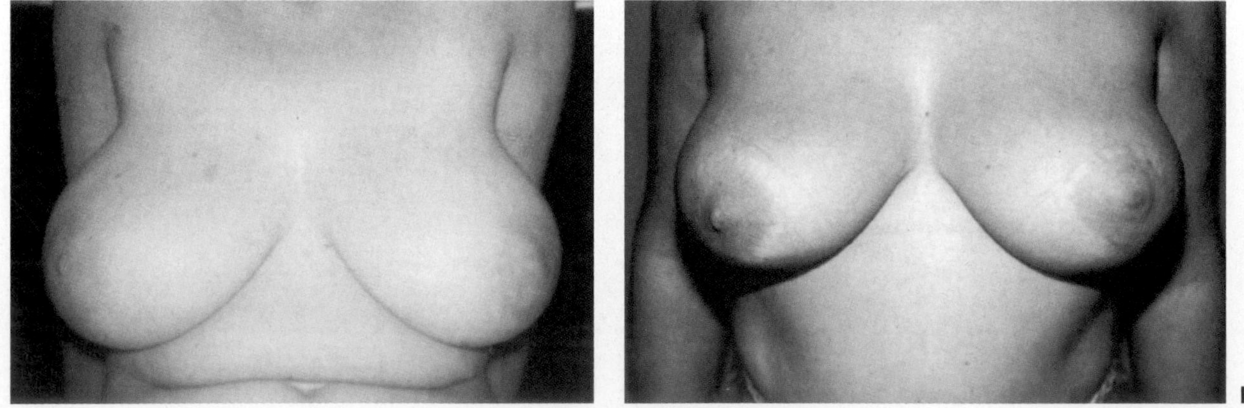

A B

Figure 86.12. Before **(A)** and after 18 years **(B)**.

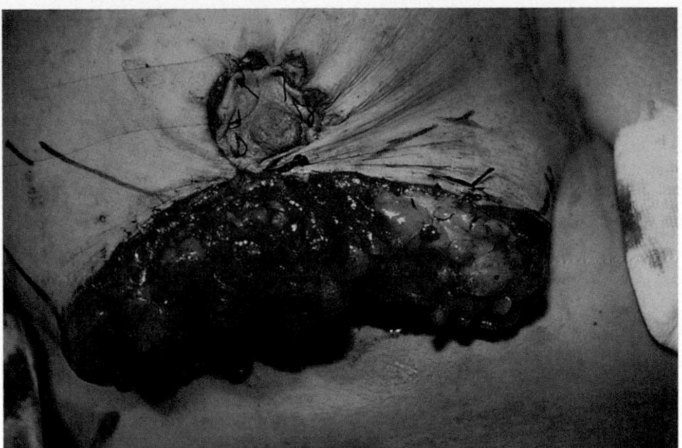

Figure 86.13. Most of the pendulous part of the breast has been removed. The lateral parts of the remaining breast, which are a composite block of skin, fat, and gland, are not ptotic; they do not need to be anchored to the muscle in an upward position.

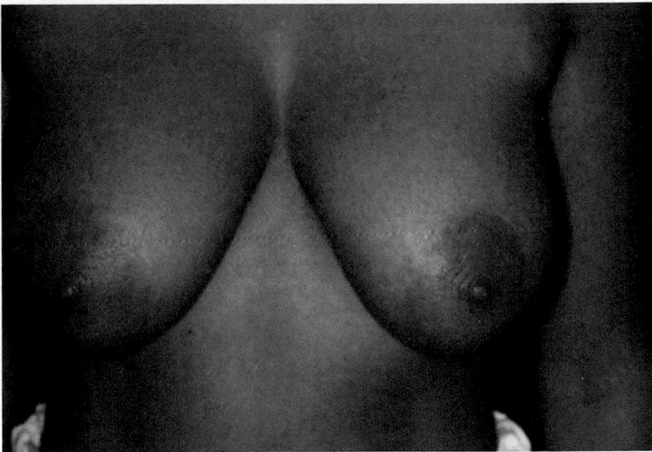

Figure 86.14. A good candidate to begin with the vertical mammaplasty: good elastic skin, firm, glandular breast, and moderate hypertrophic ptotic skin.

crosses a vertical line coming from the nipple; at the intersection of these two lines is point A.

The second key point is point B, located above the crossing of the inframammary fold with the vertical line coming from the nipple (Fig. 86.17): It is at 3 cm in small hypertrophies and ptosis; at 4.5 cm in average cases; and at 6 to 9 and even 10 cm in very large hypertrophic ptotic breasts. The estimated amount of resection is then determined. By pushing the breast medially and then laterally, one joins A and B (Fig. 86.18). This area may also be determined by pinching the breast with the fingers. Two points are then marked where the fingers touch each other, and then A and B are joined through these two points. Figure 86.19 shows the approximate area of resection and how the superior flap is drawn.

These markings indicate the area to be deepithelialized in the superior flap and the en bloc resection to be performed on the lower part of the breast. The patient is situated on the operating table in a semisitting position. This is very important for the success of the procedure. Vertical mammaplasty is a customized operation tailored to the patient. The patient must be in the semisitting position to facilitate every component of the procedure: the shape of the breast, the length of the vertical scar, the symmetry in the resection, the position of the nipples, and the form of the two breasts. If some difference is noticed,

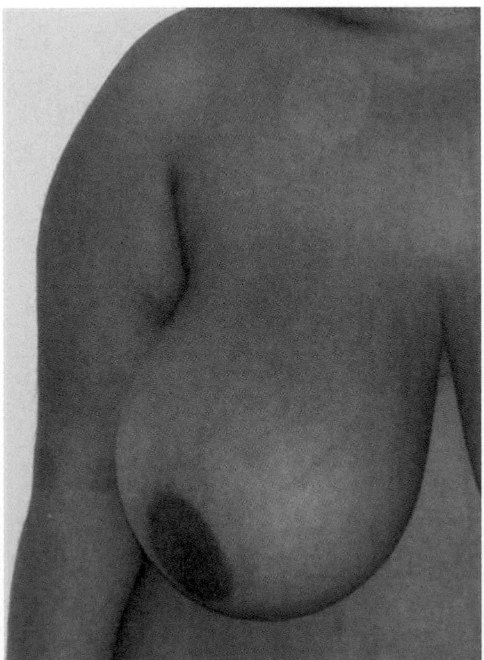

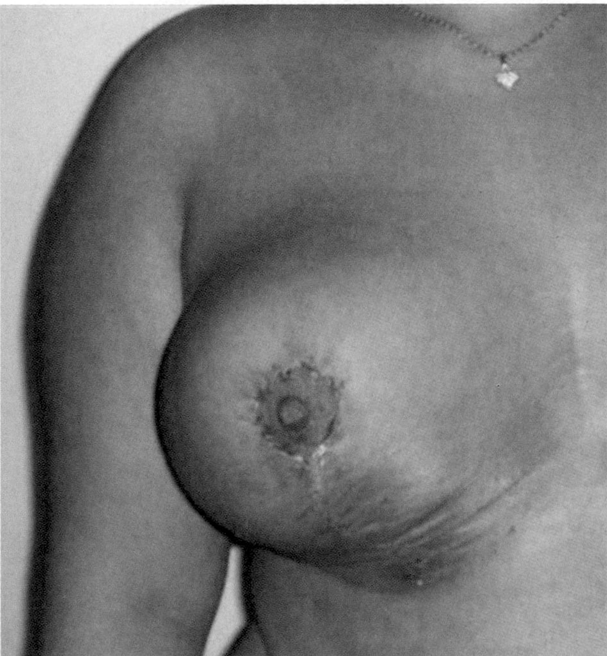

Figure 86.15. After the surgeon has performed several operations, he or she can consider more indications.

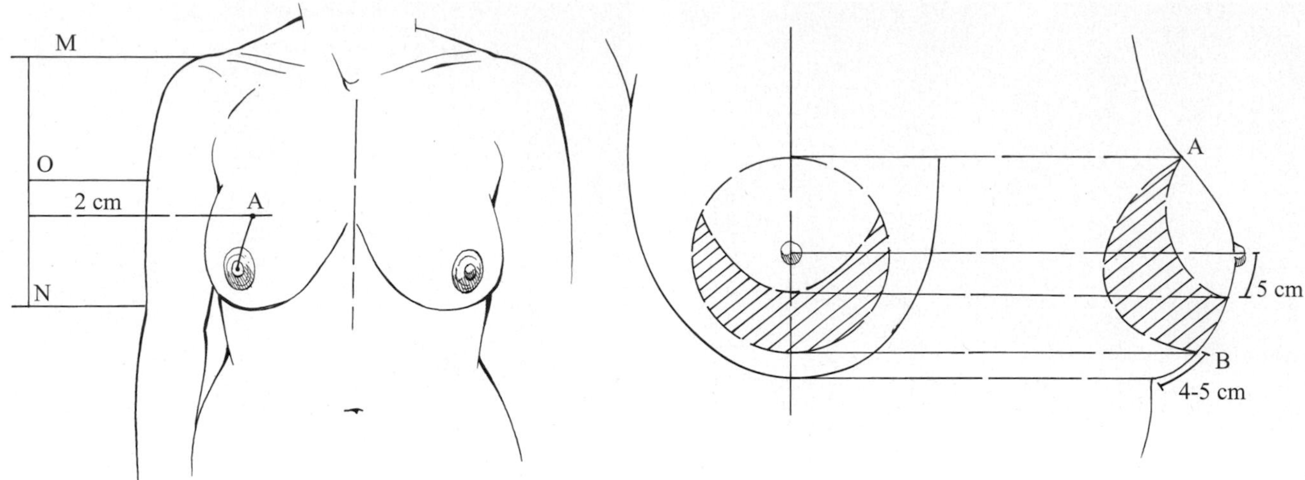

Figure 86.16. Method of determining nipple position.

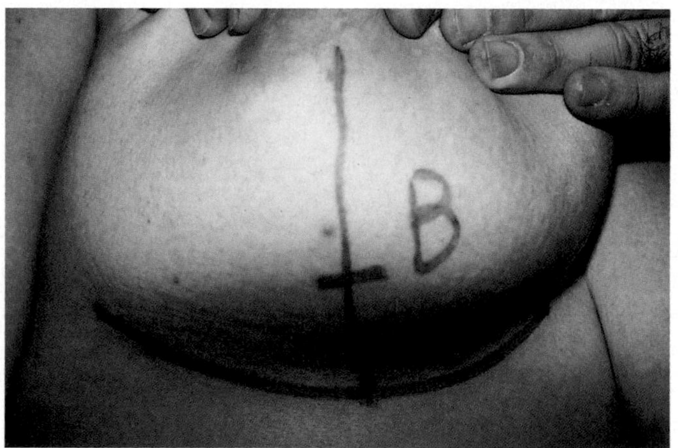

Figure 86.17. Point B.

we have to readjust immediately on the operating table to finish in a satisfactory manner. For me, this is the only way to achieve beautiful, symmetric breasts.

The procedure begins with the deepithelialization of the superior flap. The lateral margin markings below the nipple flap are then incised to the pectoralis fascia. This lower central part of the breast is elevated from the chest wall at the level of the submammary fold (Fig. 86.20). After the inferior border of the areolar flap is cut to a depth of 7 to 8 mm, dissection proceeds upward to point A, leaving a glandular lining underneath the flap (Fig. 86.21). Resection is completed by cutting the lateral margins of the glandular tissue located underneath the areolar flap. The central wedge resection is then achieved. It is divided into two portions: the inferior portion, composed of the en bloc resection (skin, fat, and gland), and

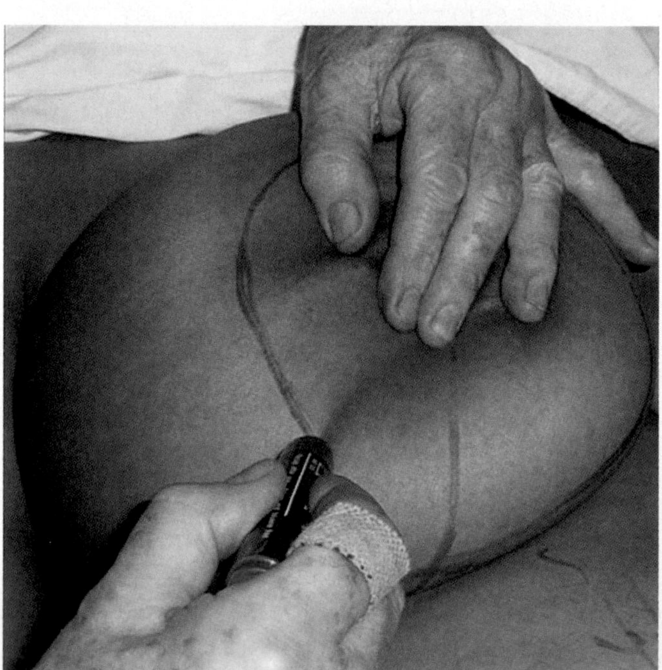

Figure 86.18. Determination of the amount of resection.

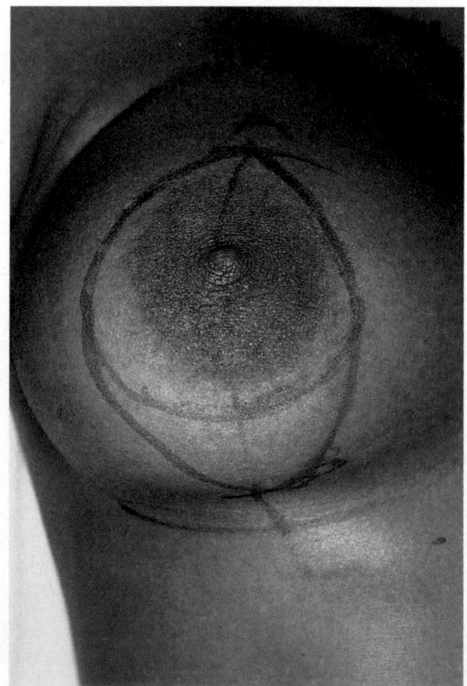

Figure 86.19. Area of resection and superior flap.

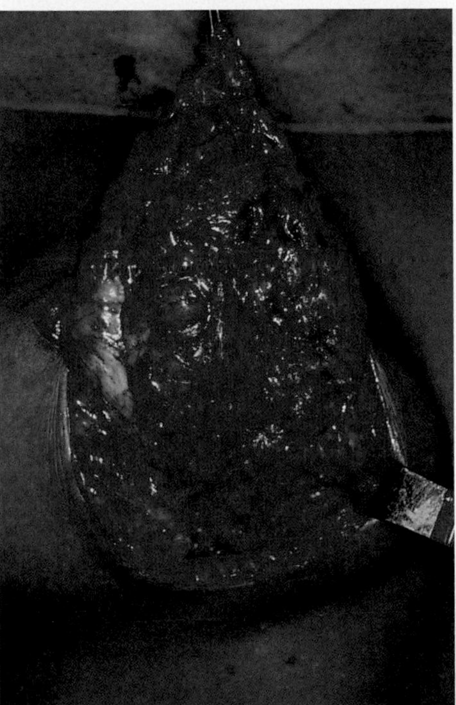

Figure 86.20. Elevation of the gland from the chest wall between the lateral margin markings. The only undermining of the operation.

the superior portion, composed of fat and gland only. No more undermining will be performed. This is a key feature of the technique. The skin remains attached to the gland, and the remaining gland remains attached to the pectoralis. These principles make the vertical mammaplasty a safe procedure. The breast is then reshaped by drawing together the lateral portions of the amputated gland with skin framing stitches from downward to upward to chase the excess tissue of the inferior pole to the superior pole. Sometimes more resection is needed. The stitches are cut, and a complementary resection is performed where it is needed. At this point, the form of the breast is suboptimal (Fig. 86.22). Therefore, the breast is reshaped with skin stitches until a satisfactory form is created (Fig. 86.23).

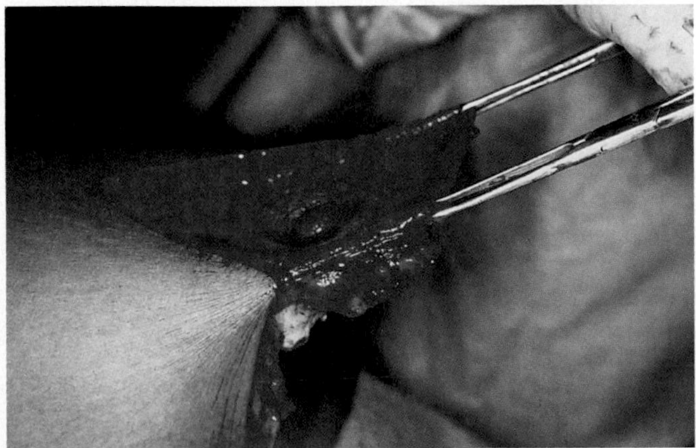

Figure 86.21. The superior flap.

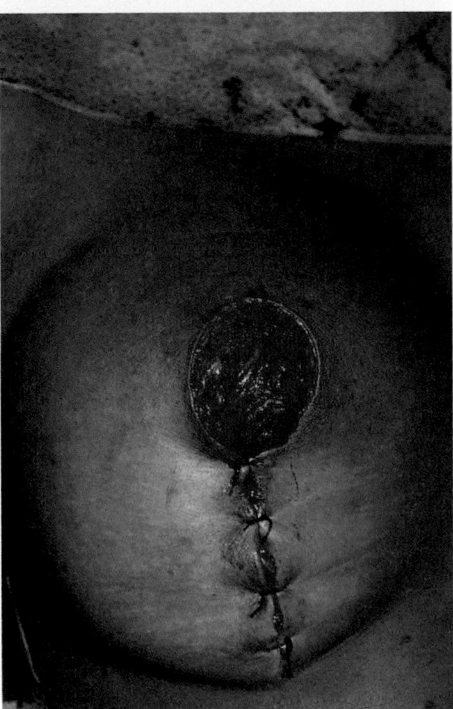

Figure 86.22. Unsatisfactory shape of the breast, demonstrating that my vertical technique produces two "dog ears": an inferior one and a superior one. The superior one is fine. It allows me to inset the nipple-areola complex without any preoperative marking. In contrast, the inferior dog ear has to be removed. It could be done by a horizontal resection, leaving a short horizontal scar. I prefer to remove it with a vertical excision, reshaping the breast with skin stitches.

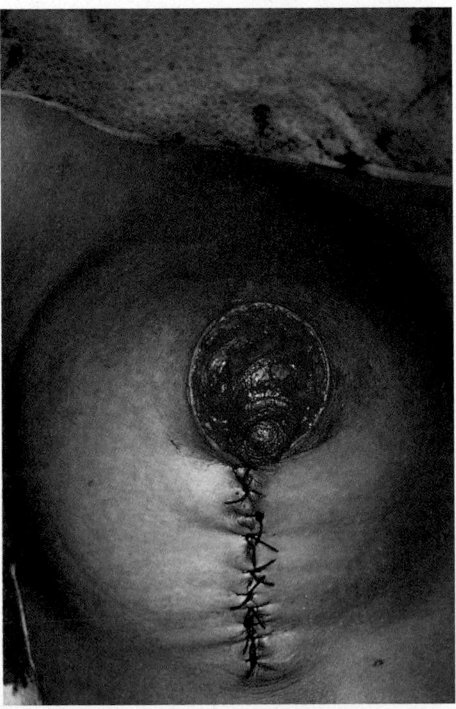

Figure 86.23. Reshaping of the breast cone with skin sutures.

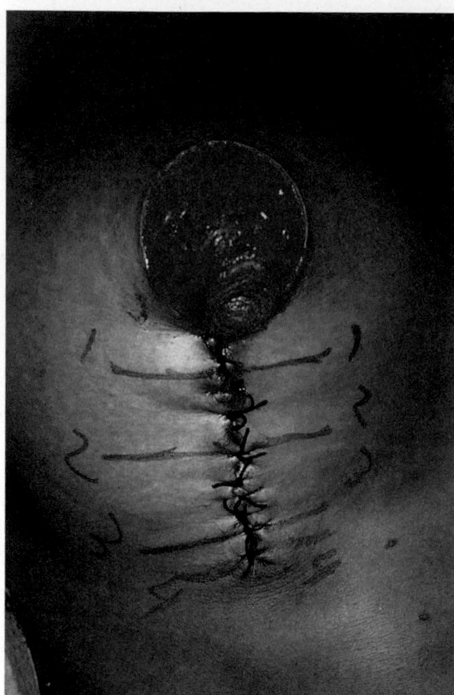

Figure 86.24. Application of methylene blue along the new suture line and drawing of horizontal lines with a number on each of them.

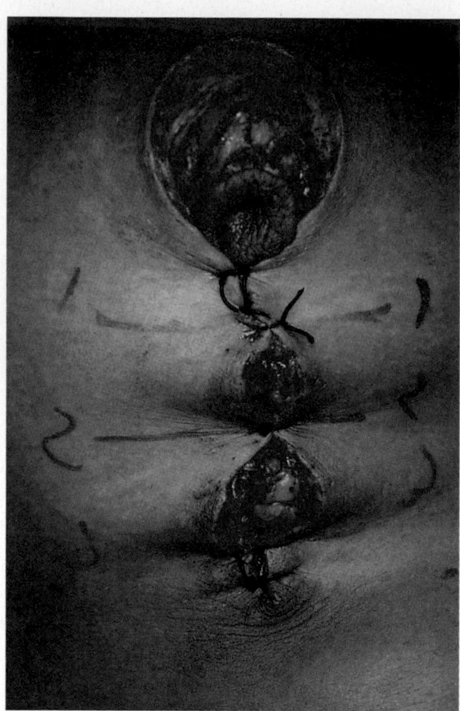

Figure 86.26. The skin edges are reapproximated, uniting 1 to 1, 2 to 2, and 3 to 3.

After a satisfactory form has been achieved, this new suture line is marked with methylene blue, and three or four lines are drawn on both sides. Each has a number, the same on the left as on the right (Fig. 86.24). The stitches are cut, and these new markings indicate the exact amount of the complementary resection to be performed (Fig. 86.25). When cutting the stitches, it is imperative to verify that the methylene blue marking shows up adequately; otherwise, it must be reapplied more precisely. The new resection is then performed following these new markings. Afterward, the skin edges are reapproximated, uniting 1 to 1, 2 to 2, 3 to 3, and so on (Fig. 86.26). Using this method saves time and prevents mistakes in the reshaping of the breast. Suturing is completed on two planes: a row into the deep dermis of a nonabsorbable monofilament suture, and superficial subcutaneous tissues and a second row of subcuticular running sutures (Fig. 86.4). I do not suture the deep tissues in the lateral part of the breast because more often there is almost only fat. Giving a bite into fat will not hold for long, and the constrictive action of the stitches can produce fat necrosis. Therefore my vertical mammaplasty does not rely on the skin for support. The skin does not act as a brassiere, so this procedure does not result in scar dehiscence. This fibrous solid band provides ample support for good projection to the breast and long-lasting results. Because no undermining has been performed during the procedure, drainage is usually not necessary.

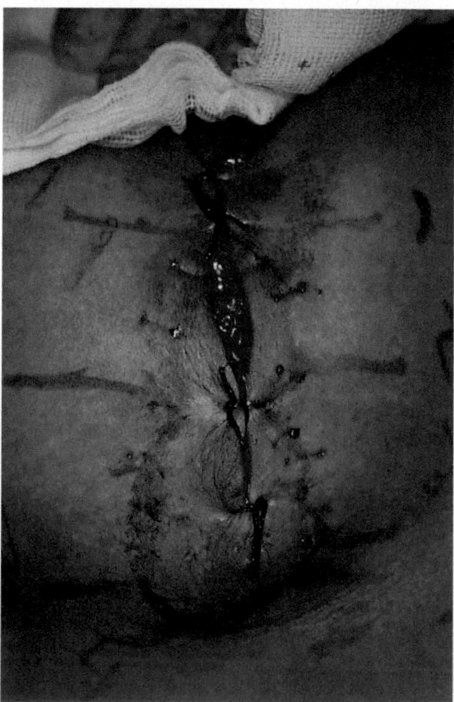

Figure 86.25. The skin sutures have been removed, and the new resection appears.

The patient can be discharged in the evening of the day of surgery or the next morning. The intradermal running sutures are removed 2 weeks later. No brassiere is worn for 3 months until the breasts have taken their final shape. Figure 86.27 shows this patient's results 2 months postsurgery.

Since the late 1960s, I have operated on 1,350 breasts (439 mastopexies, 911 reductions), the results of which have demonstrated that the vertical technique is a safe procedure that provides excellent, long-lasting results if the guidelines as already discussed are heeded. However, some complications are possible.

The vertical scar can become hypertrophic, which is a serious problem. In my series, 4 severe cases led to a terrible result, whereas 16 severe cases improved over the years. In large

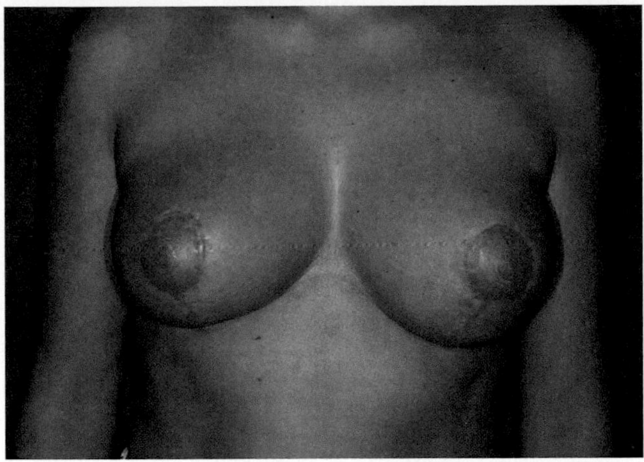
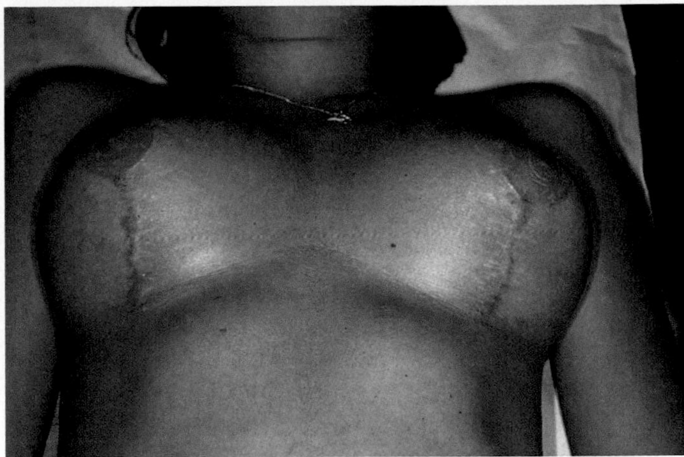

Figure 86.27. Result on this patient 2 months postsurgery.

hypertrophic ptotic breasts, the inferior part of the vertical scar may appear below the inframammary fold. This can also occur in less severe cases because of a mistake made during the procedure. In my opinion, it is better to wait 3 or 4 months after the operation, when the postoperative descent of the breast will have occurred. A small triangular skin resection effectively addresses this problem, resulting in only a short horizontal scar.

Unsatisfactory breast shape may result after vertical mammaplasty. Here, too, it is better to ask the patient to wait 3 months postsurgery. By this time, the shape of the breast will usually have improved. If after this interval the shape of the breast is still unsatisfactory, the situation must be reevaluated. In most cases, the unsatisfactory shape is attributable to a lack of tightening at the inferior pole of the breast. Under local anesthesia, the breast is reshaped with skin sutures in the same way as during the original operation, that is, from downward to upward. Methylene blue is then applied along this new suture line in such a way that it is possible under local anesthesia to resect the amount of skin, fat, and gland shown by these new drawings. I have revised 56 cases in this way.

In my series, no necrosis of the areola has been observed because I stopped transposing the nipple-areola complex on a superiorly based flap when it has to be moved superiorly more than 9 cm. Before that, I had 2 cases of total areolar necrosis and 17 partial losses.

MASTOPEXY

The vertical mammaplasty technique for mastopexy is similar. The estimated skin resection is drawn in the same way as for the breast reduction, but here of course there is no removal of breast tissue (Fig. 86.28). Only the skin is excised within the lateral markings (Fig. 86.29). Then, as for a reduction mammaplasty, the lateral markings are cut perpendicular to the pectoralis muscle. The gland within this incision is detached centrally from the muscle to the upper pole (Fig. 86.30). The inferior part of the glandular flap is then folded back on itself and the inferior extremity is anchored to the pectoralis muscle at the level of the upper part of the breast (Fig. 86.31). Afterward, the skin edges are approximated (Fig. 86.32).

I check the shape of the breast as I do in the reduction mammaplasty procedure. Generally, I have to reshape the breast cone with skin sutures and perform maneuvers as in a reduction.

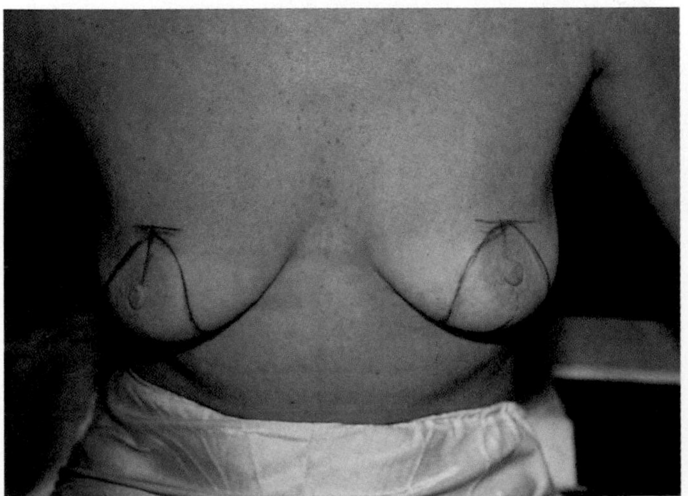
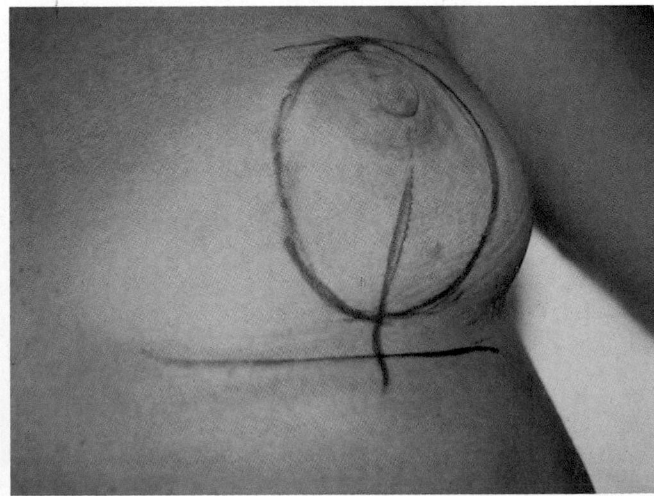

Figure 86.28. Preoperative drawings.

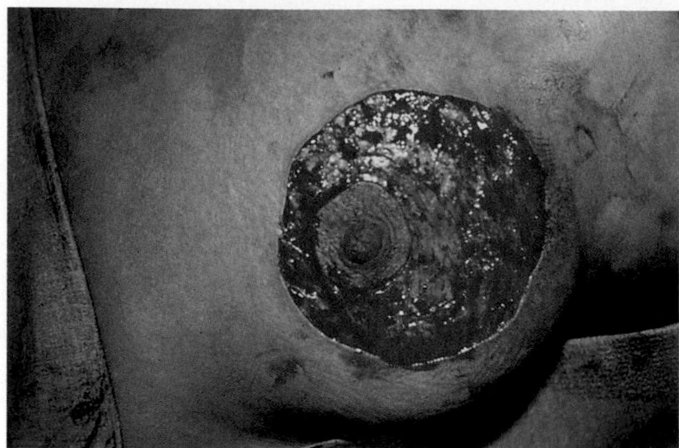

Figure 86.29. Deepithelialization within the lateral markings.

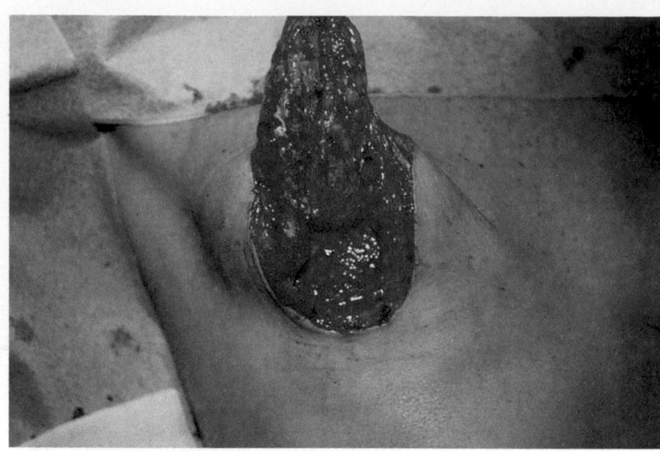

Figure 86.30. The lateral markings are cut to the pectoralis muscle, creating a glandular flap.

In mastopexy, the folding of the central lower portion of the breast creates good projection (as in breast reduction) because it brings tissue from the lower pole to the upper pole, and (as after a central wedge resection) the lateral borders are brought centrally toward each other, giving the rest of the breast tissue fullness at the upper pole, projection, and long-lasting results.

At the end of the operation and for the first few days postsurgery, the breast may have a surprising shape, resembling the nose of a Concorde (Fig. 86.33). It generally takes 2 to 2.5 months for the breast to acquire a satisfactory appearance. In the immediate postoperative period, the vertical scar may appear below the new submammary fold, but within 2 or 3 months, with the descent of the breast, the scar is usually no longer apparent (Figs. 86.34 and 86.35).

This procedure is also useful for reshaping a breast when a prosthesis that has been present for many years has been removed (Fig. 86.36). It also can be used in combination with a breast implant to solve the problem of excess skin in patients with deficient breast tissue (Fig. 86.37).

LONG-LASTING RESULTS

Many procedures achieve excellent results in the short term, but long-lasting results remain a challenge. To achieve long-lasting results, we must first understand the reasons for "bottoming out." Gravity is evident, and there is nothing we can do about it, but gravity produces bottoming out because of concomitant reasons. What are they? To understand these reasons, one must remember some anatomic features. The mammary gland is more intimately connected with the skin than with the muscle. The adherent skin plays a dominant role, mainly in the young, preventing gravity from bringing down the breast. The skin of the breast adheres closely to the underlying structures. It supports the organ both by its elasticity and by virtue of the fibrous connections between it and the gland. Cooper's ligaments are numerous strong fibrous elements that link the skin to the gland, the gland to the nipple, and the various portions of the gland to one another (Fig. 86.38). Once the skin and the Cooper's ligaments have been stretched and weakened, they never regain their supportive role.

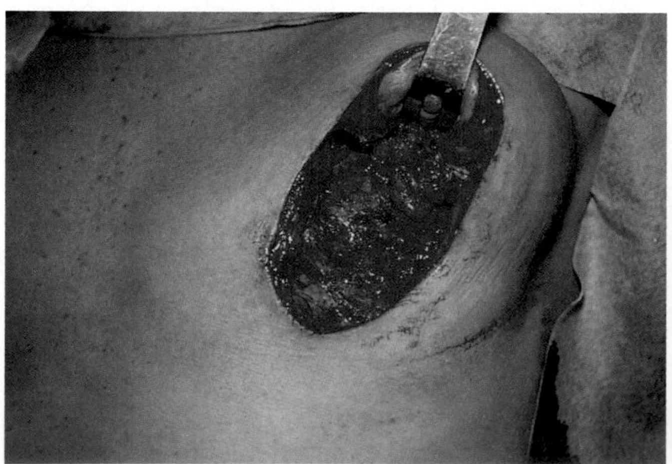

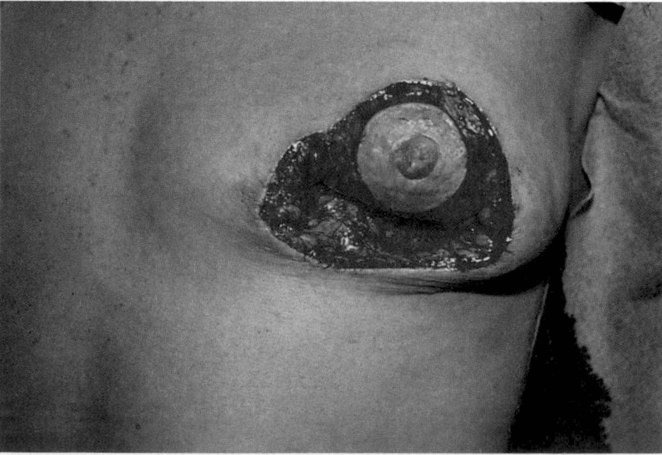

Figure 86.31. Anchoring of the inferior part of the glandular flap to the pectoralis muscle at the upper part of the breast.

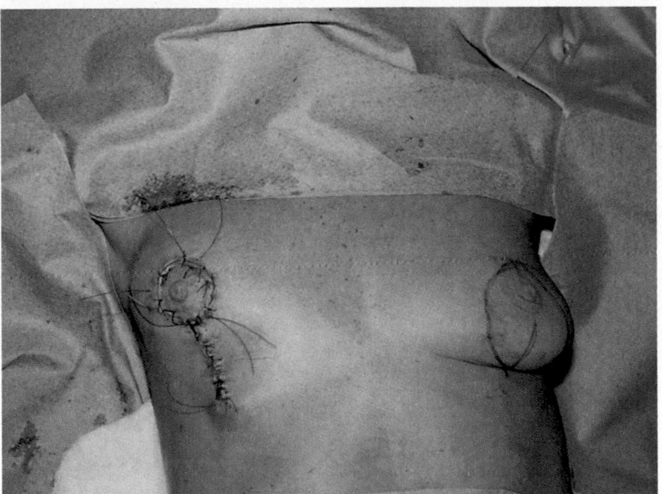

Figure 86.32. Skin edges are approximated, and the operation is completed on one side.

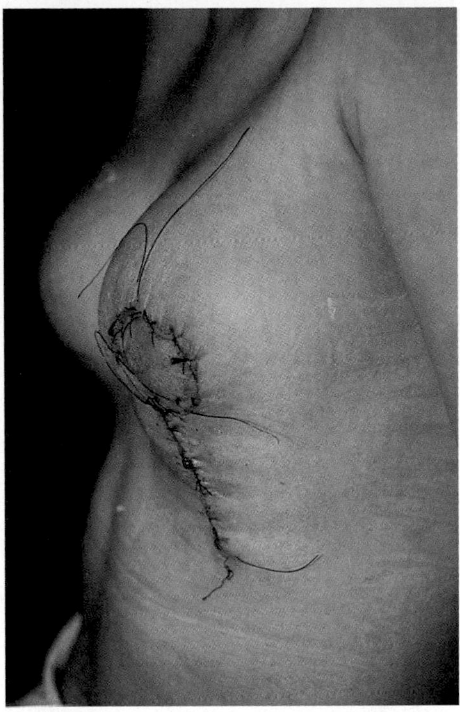

Figure 86.33. Five days postsurgery, the breast has the look of the nose of the Concorde.

Bottoming out can be caused by poor skin and/or damaged Cooper's ligaments. Nothing can help to restore the skin or damaged Cooper's ligaments, but one must protect the remaining ligaments. Even if their supportive role is reduced, they still help support the breast. In 1970, I wrote "skin undermining is nonsense because it cuts the fibrous crests which are the main suspension of the mamilla." My operation does not rely on the skin.

A CENTRAL VERTICAL WEDGE RESECTION

As stated earlier in the chapter, large breasts can be reduced through a horizontal amputation, a vertical amputation, or a combination of these types of resection. A horizontal amputation produces a flat breast (Fig. 86.9). In contrast, a vertical amputation gives projection to the breast. Pinching the inferior midbreast with the fingers gives projection to the breast and fullness at the upper pole (Fig. 86.10). My technique uses a vertical wedge amputation (Fig. 86.2); it yields the same result—a full upper pole and good projection (Fig. 86.11). Most of the techniques reduce the size of the breast with a Wise resection, which combines the horizontal and vertical amputations, giving less-projected breasts.

For me, the aim of mammaplasty is projection. So a wedge resection must be preferred to a Wise resection for achieving beautiful projected breasts. When this resection has been performed, most of the pendulous portion of the breast is removed (Fig. 86.2). The rest of the breast is at the level of the inframammary fold or above it. There is no need to suspend any part of the breast in a higher position. My technique does not rely on suspensions. In addition, no undermining is performed during my operation. The remaining breast is in its original configuration, which explains why the results hold for so long (Figs. 86.37 and 86.38).

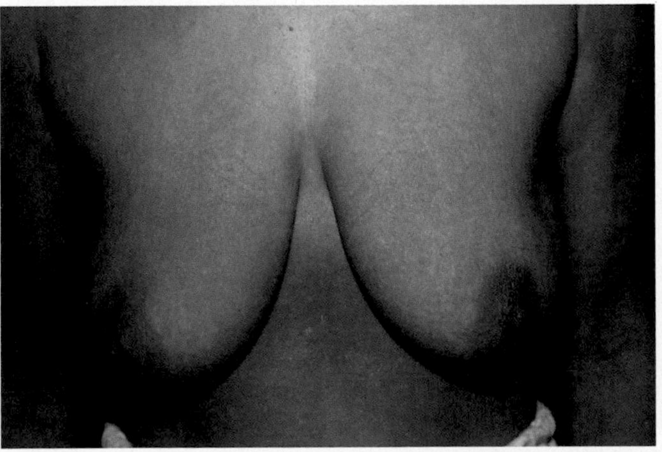

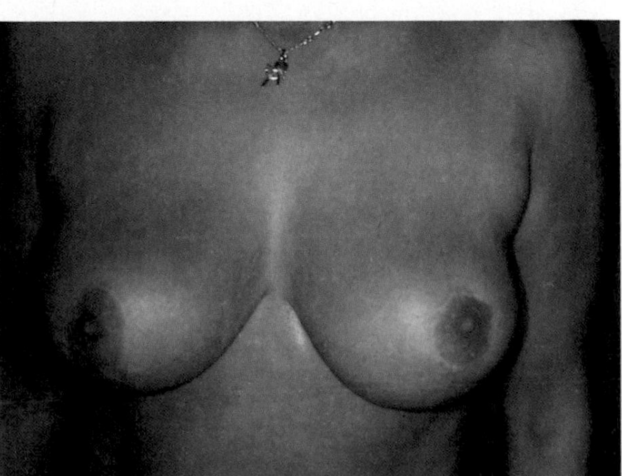

Figure 86.34. Before (**A**) and after 2 years (**B**).

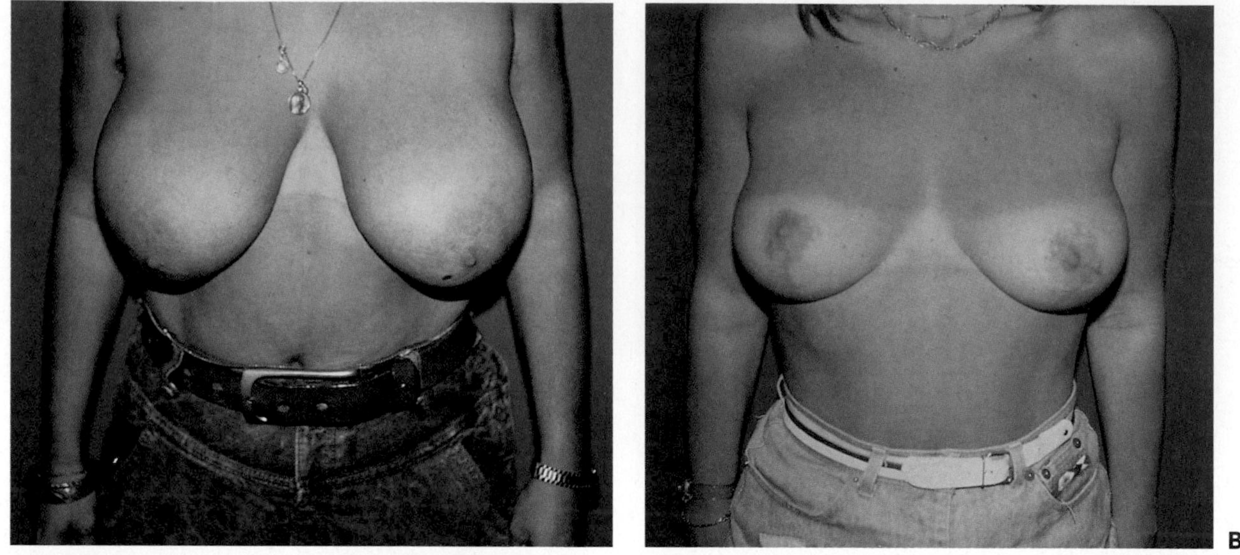

Figure 86.35. Before **(A)** and after 3 years **(B)**.

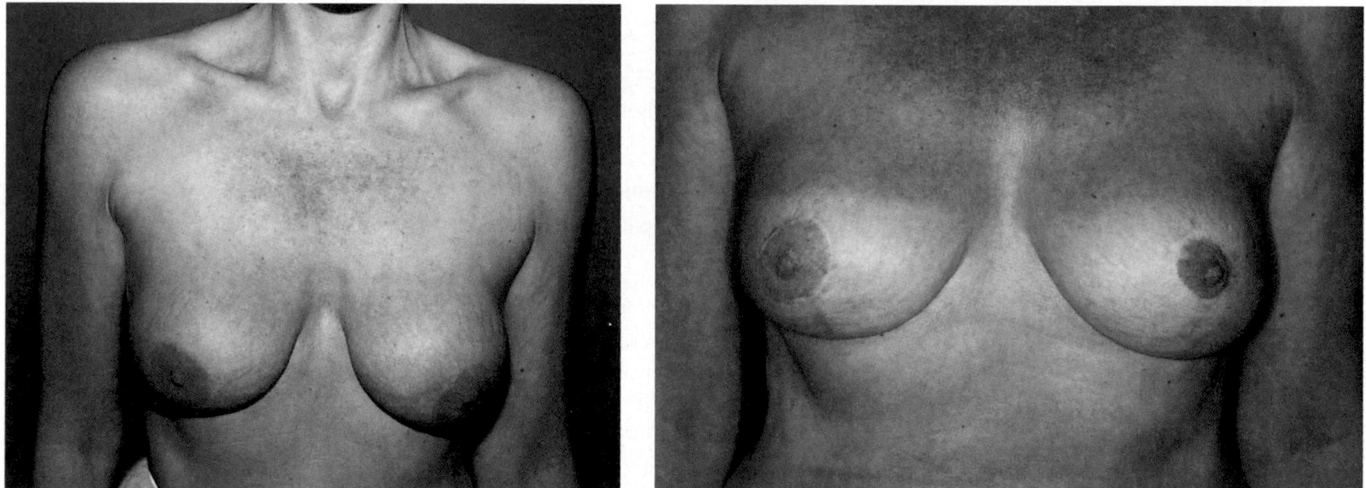

Figure 86.36. The prosthesis has been removed and the breast reshaped with vertical mammaplasty.

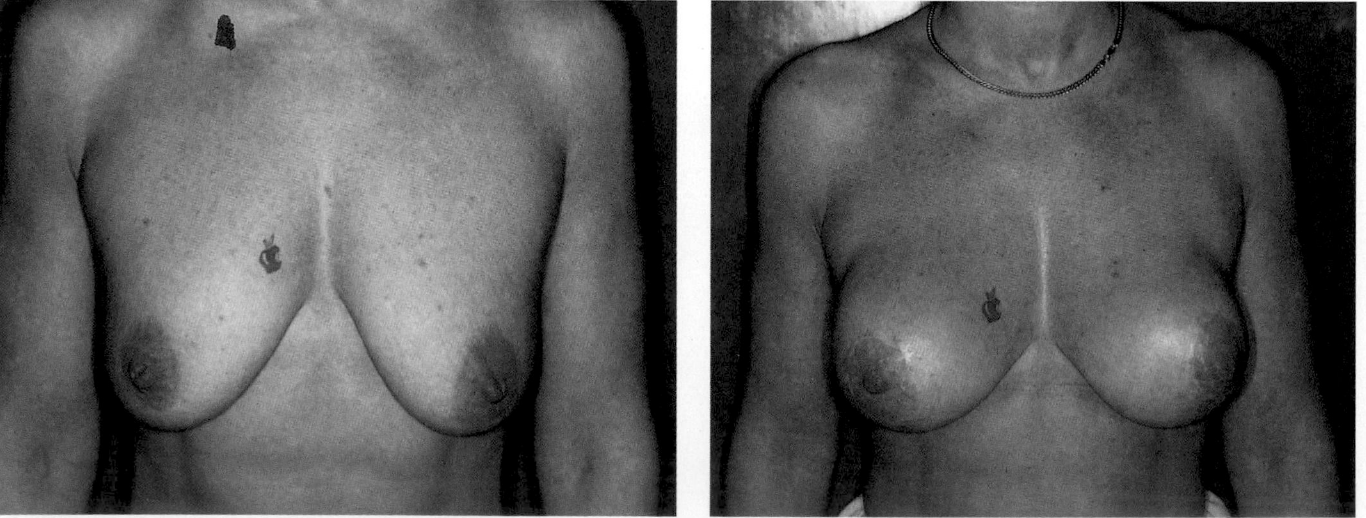

Figure 86.37. Before surgery and after breast implant plus vertical mammaplasty.

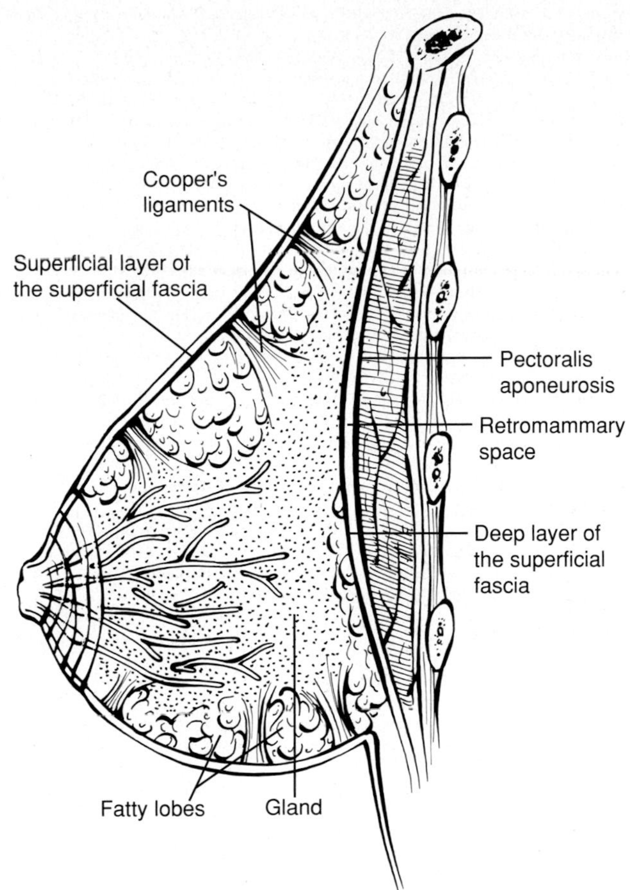

Figure 86.38. A cross section of the structure of the breast. Note the position of the Cooper's ligaments.

VERTICAL SCAR

When the central vertical wedge resection has been completed, the breast cone is reconstructed by drawing the lateral parts of the remaining breast centrally toward each other (Fig. 86.2). The two composite blocks of skin fat and gland are joined together and fit perfectly (Fig. 86.26). Healing produces a solid, fibrous band the thickness of the breast. This fibrous band plays the same role as a whale bone in a corset, which accounts for the long-lasting results. Does the length of the scar play a role in achieving excellent results? Many times I hear, "we are not allowed to compromise the shape of the breast to reduce the scars"; however, a long scar is not synonymous with an excellent result (Fig. 86.9).

EDITORIAL COMMENTS

Dr. Lassus is one of the pioneers in reduction mammaplasty and mastopexy with short scars. His vertical technique with minimal undermining is an interesting procedure for patients with mild and moderate hypertrophy or ptosis. Its application is in the modest reduction patient who is anxious to avoid the horizontal scar and is willing to endure a fair amount of prolonged healing and reshaping of the breast to obtain a vertical scar procedure without the horizontal scar component.

Clearly, patient selection is critical in this operation. It is important to select patients with only modest problems and to ensure they are prepared to deal with the vagaries of the result, as well as the prolonged period of time that must elapse before the result looks reasonable. Still, in the properly selected patient, particularly those who are anxious to avoid a transverse incision, this vertical technique with minimal undermining has its place.

S.L.S.

In this chapter, Claude Lassus, widely recognized as the originator of the vertical mammaplasty, outlines the rationale for the technique, and several points merit emphasis. First, Dr. Lassus cautions against the creation of dead space centrally. This is an important concept to keep in mind during the removal of the inferocentral segment of the breast. The space that is created must be filled in as the remainder of the breast falls into the void created by the removal of breast tissue. This filling in of the central portion of the breast is assisted by the central repair when the medial and lateral breast pillars are sutured together. Failure to adequately close down this space can lead to significant postoperative deformity with puckering and collapse of the inferocentral segment of the breast. The coning effect of the vertical pattern assists tremendously in shaping the breast, increasing projection, and narrowing the base diameter. The addition of the vertical component to the skin pattern and the description of how this maneuver helps shape the breast is one of the great achievements of vertical mammaplasty. It is a concept that has application in treating many different types of breast problems. Dr. Lassus emphasizes that no undermining is performed in his technique. In doing so, the potential for dead space creation, as well as vascular compromise to the remaining breast parenchyma, is reduced. The procedure is also performed in a semisitting position. This seemingly simple and easily overlooked technical point is of critical importance in creating a reproducible and consistent technique, and I join Dr. Lassus in emphasizing this point. One cannot accurately judge what the breast looks like when the patient is supine, and this technique requires an accurate intraoperative assessment of breast shape to be consistently successful. Dr. Lassus hypothesizes that the vertical repair creates a scar band that tends to resist the gravitational forces from above and may help limit postoperative shape change due to stretching of the lower pole skin envelope. I agree with this concept and always try to reinforce the vertical closure whenever possible in an attempt to support the lower pole of the breast. One aspect of the vertical technique that does merit further comment is the manner in which the breast settles over time. In the hands of many surgeons, an attempt is made to overcorrect the coning effect with tightening of the lower pole of the breast. Over time, these tissues relax and, in most instances, the resultant shape is excellent. However, the early postoperative appearance of the breast can be somewhat alarming. Determining how much overcorrection will be required for any given patient given the size of the reduction and the nature of the patients' tissues requires experience, and for this reason, it is best to begin using the technique on smaller breast reductions and in cases of mastopexy. With increasing experience, the technique can be used on larger breast reductions with excellent results. There is no doubt that the description of vertical mammaplasty will be remembered as one of the great advances in the field of breast surgery for years to come.

D.C.H.

SUGGESTED READINGS

Arie G. Una nueva tecnica de mastoplastia. *Rev Latinoam Cit Plast* 1957;3:23.

Balch CR. The central mound technique for reduction mammaplasty. *Plast Reconstr Surg* 1981;67:305.

Biesenberger H. *Deformation und Kosmetische Operationen der Weiblichen Brust.* Vienna: W Mandrich; 1931.

Bostwick J III. *Aesthetic and Reconstructive Breast Surgery.* St. Louis, MO: CV Mosby; 1983.

Courtiss EH, Goldwyn RM. Reduction mammaplasty by the inferior pedicle technique. An alternative to free nipple and areola grafting for severe macromastia or extreme ptosis. *Plast Reconstr Surg* 1979;59:500.

Dartigues L. Le traitement chirurgical du prolapsus mammaire. *Arch Francobelges Chir* 1925;28:313.

Durston W. Sudden and excessive swelling of a woman's breast. *Phil Trans R Soc Lond* 1731;4:78.

Georgiade NG, Georgiade GS, Riefkhol R, et al. *Essentials of Plastic, Maxillofacial and Reconstructive Surgery.* Baltimore, MD: Williams & Wilkins; 1987:694.

Georgiade NG, Serafin D, Morris R, et al. Reduction mammaplasty utilizing an inferior pedicle nipple-areolar flap. *Ann Plast Surg* 1979;3:211.

Georgiade NG, Serafin D, Riefkhol R, et al. Is there a reduction mammaplasty for "all seasons"? *Plast Reconstr Surg* 1979;63:765.

Goldwyn RM, ed. *Plastic and Reconstructive Surgery of the Breast.* Boston: Little, Brown; 1976.

Goldwyn RM, Courtiss EH. Inferior pedicle technique. In: Regnault P, Daniel RK, eds. *Aesthetic Plastic Surgery.* Boston: Little, Brown; 1986:522–526.

Hallock GG, Cusenz BJ. Salvage of the congested nipple during reduction mammaplasty. *Aesthet Plast Surg* 1986;10:143.

Hauben DJ. Experience and refinements with the supero-medial dermal pedicle for nipple-areolar transposition in reduction mammaplasty. *Aesthet Plast Surg* 1984;8:189.

Hester TR Jr, Bostwick J, Miller L, et al. Breast reduction utilizing the maximally vascularized central breast pedicle. *Plast Reconstr Surg* 1985;76:890.

Hoffman S. Recurrent deformities following reduction mammaplasty and correction of breast asymmetry. *Plast Reconstr Surg* 1986;78:55.

Lassus C. A technique for breast reduction. *Int Surg* 1970;53:69.

Lassus C. New refinements in vertical mammaplasty. Presented at the 2nd Congress, Asian Section of the International Plastic and Reconstructive Surgery Society, Tokyo, 1977.

Lassus C. Minimal scarring in mammaplasty. Presented at the Tagung der Vereinigung der Deutschen Plastischen Chirurgen, Cologne, Germany, October 18–21, 1978.

Lassus C. New refinements in vertical mammaplasty. *Chir Plast* 1981;6:81–86.

Lassus C. Treatment of impending nipple necrosis: a technical note. *Chir Plast* 1985;8:117.

Lassus C. An "all season" mammaplasty. *Aesthet Plast Surg* 1986;10:9.

Lassus C. Breast reduction: evolution of a technique. A single vertical scar. *Aesthet Plast Surg* 1987;11:107.

Lejour M. Vertical mammaplasty and liposuction of the breast. *Plast Reconstr Surg* 1994;94:100.

Lejour M. *Vertical Mammaplasty and Liposuction of the Breast.* St. Louis, MO: Quality Medical; 1994.

Lejour M, Abboud M, Declety A, et al. Réduction des cicatrices de plastie mammaire de l'ancre courte à la vertucale. *Ann Chir Plast Esthet* 1990;35:369.

Marchac D, De Olarte G. Reduction mammaplasty and correction of ptosis with a short inframammary scar. *Plast Reconstr Surg* 1982;69:45.

Marcus GH. Untersuchungen über die arterielle Blutversorgung der Mamilla. *Arch Klin Chir* 1934;179:361.

Mathes SJ, Nahai F, Hester TR. Avoiding the flat breast in reduction mammaplasty. *Plast Reconstr Surg* 1980;66:63.

Meyer R, Kesserling UK. Reduction mammaplasty with an L-shaped suture line. *Plast Reconstr Surg* 1975;55:139.

Moufarrege R, Beauregard G, Bosse JP, et al. Reduction mammaplasty by the total dermoglandular pedicle. *Aesthet Plast Surg* 1985;9:227.

Nicolle FV. The lateral pedicle technique. In: Georgiade NG, Riefkhol R, Georgiade GS, eds. *Aesthetic Surgery of the Breast.* Philadelphia, PA: WB Saunders; 1990:215.

Peixoto G. Reduction mammaplasty: a personal technique. *Plast Reconstr Surg* 1980;65:217.

Peixoto G. The infra-areolar longitudinal incision in reduction mammaplasty. *Aesthet Plast Surg* 1985;9:1.

Pitanguy I. Breast hypertrophy. In: *Transactions of the International Society of Plastic Surgeons. Second Congress, London, 1959.* Edinburgh: Livingstone; 1960:509.

Regnault P. Breast reduction: a technique. *Plast Reconstr Surg* 1980;65:840.

Reno WT. Reduction mammaplasty with a circular folded pedicle technique. *Plast Reconstr Surg* 1992;90:65.

Schwarzmann E. Uber eine neue methode der mammaplastue. *Wien Med Wochenschr* 1936;86:100.

Skoog T. A technique of breast reduction. *Acta Chir Scand* 1963;26:453.

Strombeck JO. Mammaplasty: report of a new technique based on the two-pedicle procedure. *Br J Plast Surg* 1960;13:79.

Strombeck JO. Reduction mammaplasty: some observations, and some reflections. *Aesthet Plast Surg* 1983;7:249.

CHAPTER

87

Juan Diego Mejia
Foad Nahai

Vertical Mastopexy

INTRODUCTION

The word "ptosis" is derived from the Greek vernacular and is translated as "falling" (1). "Falling" of the breast, or breast ptosis, refers to the position of the nipple relative to the inframammary crease. An aesthetically pleasing breast should have the nipple located above this crease at the most projecting part of the breast mound. The degree to which the nipple descends below the level of the crease determines the severity of the ptosis. Probably the oldest and most commonly used classification is Regnault's (2). According to Regnault, grade I ptosis is diagnosed when the nipple is at or up to 1 cm below the inframammary crease. Grade II ptosis describes the nipple at a level 1 to 3 cm below the crease but not yet at the lowest contour of the breast. Grade III ptosis describes a nipple more than 3 cm below the crease or at the lowest contour of the breast gland. A condition called pseudoptosis occurs when the lower pole of the breast falls below the inframammary crease but the nipple itself is at or above the level of the crease. It is important to recognize this entity so that the corrective plan does not result in positioning the nipple too high.

The surgical correction of breast ptosis is termed *mastopexy*. Any procedure designed to accomplish elevation of the breasts must take into account four essential elements (3): (a) elevating the nipple-areola complex (NAC) and preserving its blood supply, (b) removing redundant parenchyma if necessary, (c) removing excess skin, and (d) shaping the breast.

The preservation of the blood supply to the NAC is a top priority in any mastopexy procedure. Almost any pedicle can be fashioned to maintain the viability of the NAC. Common variations include the superior pedicle, inferior pedicle, lateral pedicle, medial pedicle, central pedicle, horizontal bipedicle, and vertical bipedicle.

The removal of excess parenchyma is more of an issue in reduction mammaplasty, but it is sometimes necessary in mastopexies to achieve the desired shape and size. The location of the pedicle will dictate the area of the breast that can be removed and in this way influence the final shape of the breast. For instance, inferior pedicle techniques imply resection of tissue parenchyma in the superior pole. This leaves a breast with lack of upper pole fullness and a potential for "bottoming out" due to the weight of the pedicle in the lower pole. Superior pedicle techniques, on the other hand, resect excess parenchyma from the central and lower pole, avoiding the bottoming-out phenomenon and leaving superior tissue for upper pole fullness.

Excess skin can be resected in different ways. The skin resection design dictates the final scar left on the breast. The most common skin resection patterns are circumareolar, vertical, lateral, and inverted T (Wise). Skin resection patterns are sometimes assumed to automatically refer to a specific type of pedicle or parenchymal resection. The inverted-T or Wise design is often associated with the use of an inferior pedicle when it can be applied with a combination of different pedicle and parenchymal resections. The same applies to the circumareolar, vertical, or lateral mammaplasty techniques. The most common vertical mammaplasty technique incorporates a superior pedicle with a central wedge resection of parenchyma. However, different combinations of pedicles (superior, inferior, lateral, medial) and glandular resection patterns have been described for vertical mastopexies (4–8).

Second only to the blood supply to the nipple-areola complex, the final shape of the breast is the most important objective in a mastopexy procedure. The surgeon cannot sacrifice shape in favor of scar length or location. Therefore, although the circumareolar technique achieves the most desirable scar, it can only be applied in small, mildly ptotic breasts with adequate breast parenchyma. Any nipple-areola elevation above 2 to 3 cm will lead to poor results with this technique (9). One of the factors that have led to the recent popularity of the vertical mammaplasty technique is that it leaves less of a scar than the Wise pattern with a better breast shape.

Vertical mastopexy is therefore a surgical procedure to correct ptosis of the breasts with a vertical skin resection pattern, leaving only a vertical scar. Even though the superior pedicle with central parenchymal resection is most common with this technique, any combination of pedicle design and parenchymal resection can be applied with a vertical scar.

EVOLUTION OF THE TECHNIQUE

Mastopexy by vertical mammaplasty was described as early as 1925 by Dartigues, but it remained nearly unknown until Arie in 1957 and then Lassus in 1969 revived the technique (4,5,10–12). In the early 1990s, Lejour introduced her vertical mammaplasty technique, which was derived from that of Lassus (4). Both Lassus and Lejour have contributed enormously to the evolution and popularization of this procedure.

Claude Lassus is considered one of the pioneers of vertical mammaplasty. In 1964, he performed a breast reduction on a patient with unilateral breast hypertrophy, and in 1969 he published this technique, which combined four principles (5,10): (a) a central vertical wedge resection to reduce the size of the breast, (b) transposition of the areola on a superiorly based pedicle, (c) no undermining, and (d) a vertical scar to finish off.

His vertical mammaplasty technique for mastopexy is similar, except that there is no removal of breast tissue (10). The central wedge of tissue, instead of being removed, is left as a superiorly based flap and is then folded back on itself and anchored to the pectoralis fascia in the upper part of the breast. This flap produces upper pole fullness and retroareolar projection. With the closing of the medial and lateral pillars, this technique achieves narrowing of the base diameter and coning of the breast.

Reapproximating the pillars in several layers extending from the chest wall anteriorly also reinforces a central column that will maintain tissue support and long-term breast shape.

The superiorly based pedicle may be a limiting feature of his operation. Superior translocation of the NAC requires folding of the pedicle and potential collapse of the venous plexus compromising the NAC. When the NAC has to be advanced more than 9 cm the risk of necrosis is high, and a medial or lateral pedicle is preferable (10). In such cases we prefer a vertical bipedicle (superior and central mound) (9). According to Lassus, since he stopped advancing the NAC more than 9 cm on a superior pedicle he has had no cases of areolar necrosis. Before that, he reported 2 cases of total areolar necrosis and 17 partial losses (10).

Lassus avoids subcutaneous or subglandular undermining, so there is less dead space and therefore less chance of hematoma or seroma. Finally, Lassus uses a vertical scar to finish off. In his original description, the postoperative vertical scar often extended vertically below the fold in large reductions and mastopexies. To avoid this, Lassus added a short horizontal incision at the crease. However, he later reverted to a vertical scar only by limiting the inferior extent of skin resection and gathering the vertical closure (8).

In 1994, Lejour introduced her vertical mammaplasty technique. It was derived from that of Lassus. It benefits from three innovative principles: (a) wider lower skin undermining to promote skin retraction and reduce the amount of scarring, (b) overcorrection of deformities to produce better late results, and (c) use of liposuction to facilitate molding of the breast and to remove unnecessary tissue prone to absorption when the patient loses weight. Lejour's vertical mastopexy also includes the elevation of the lower central portion, which is then sutured to the upper level of the retromammary dissection (4).

ANATOMY

An anatomic study of Corduff and Taylor (13) demonstrated that the major blood supply enters the NAC at a superficial level. One branch from the internal mammary artery from the second or third intercostal space supplies the NAC based on a superior pedicle. This artery passes through the subcutaneous tissue into the breast, angles obliquely downward toward the nipple, and then descends into the parenchyma. It is present at the breast meridian about 1 cm deep to the skin. This is why superiorly based pedicles can be safely thinned out up to 1 cm below the areola (5,6,10). Most arteries to the breast do not have an accompanying vein. The venous plexus is superficial and concentrated around the areola; therefore a bridge of dermis with adequate width should always be left around the NAC. Any design that necessitates folding of a long pedicle is likely to collapse the venous plexus and compromise venous return. Arterial inflow might be strong enough to overcome folding, but venous return is likely to suffer. Nipple-areola sensory innervation is provided primarily by the fourth anterolateral and anteromedial intercostal nerves; however, the third and fifth intercostal nerves, as well as nerves from the cervical plexus, also contribute to nipple-areola sensibility. This overlapping of sensory zones of the areola by multiple nerves is probably the reason most patients maintain sensory input after vertical mammaplasty (14,15).

WHY VERTICAL MASTOPEXY?

The concept of breast skin excision is three dimensional: *unidimensional* refers to perioareolar skin removal; *bidimensional* includes a periareolar and a vertical component; and *tridimensional* includes a periareolar, a vertical, and a horizontal component of skin removal. The horizontal component may include a short T, a J or L, or the long horizontal T (16).

Periareolar techniques are only indicated in small, mildly ptotic breasts where the NAC needs to be elevated less than 2 to 3 cm. Tempting as it is to confine the incision to the areola, the method leads to poor results if applied to the wrong patients. For more advanced cases of ptosis, vertical or inverted-T techniques are most commonly used. In moderate or severe ptosis, mastopexy with inverted-T skin resection is still one of the most common techniques. However, the vertical approach is becoming more and more popular as plastic surgeons are becoming aware of the advantages and pitfalls of both techniques.

The first and most obvious difference is the shorter scar, with the elimination of the inframammary scar. A survey mailed out to 94 patients who had undergone breast reduction concluded that 65% of them were dissatisfied with their scars; of these, 65% indicated that the horizontal component bothered them the most (17). The vertical scar is barely visible over the years, and it rarely becomes hypertrophic even in women with darker skin. In his 40 years of experience and 1,350 cases of vertical mammaplasty (439 mastopexies and 911 reductions) Lassus reported only 4 cases of severe hypertrophy of the vertical scar that led to a terrible result (10).

With the inverted-T technique, a horizontal ellipse of skin is resected and pulled inferiorly. The vertical arms of the T design are usually short (5 to 6 cm). These two factors limit projection and contribute to a flat breast. On the other hand, with a vertical skin pattern, the long vertical closure allows for adequate projection and coning of the breast.

Inverted-T techniques with central mound or inferior pedicles usually depend on the skin to maintain breast shape. Because skin is elastic, with time the weight of the lower pedicle or central mound parenchyma will cause the skin to stretch, and the breast tissue will migrate to the lower pole. This bottoming-out phenomenon is much less likely with vertical mammaplasty techniques because the shape of the breast does not depend on a skin brassier. The final shape of the breast is accomplished by manipulation of the breast parenchyma, and the skin is simply sutured over and allowed to adapt to this new shape. The long-lasting stable result achieved with this technique is for many its main advantage. Lassus demonstrated maintenance of shape up to 20 years following the initial procedure (5). The vertical mammaplasty leaves shorter scars, improves breast projection, narrows the wide breast, offers better long-term shape. and reduces the bottoming-out phenomenon when compared with inverted-T techniques. The vertical technique reduces breast width, while the Wise pattern maintains breast width. The vertical technique pushes up the NAC, while the Wise pattern pulls it down.

INDICATIONS FOR VERTICAL MASTOPEXY

Not all patients are suited for vertical mastopexy or the superior pedicle. In achieving excellent aesthetic results, proper

TABLE 87.1	Ideal Candidates for Vertical Mastopexy
Young patients	
Mild to moderate breast hypertrophy	
Mild to moderate breast ptosis	
Normal-quality elastic skin	

patient selection is essential. It is best to start with younger patients, with mild to moderate hypertrophy, mild to moderate cases of breast ptosis, and normal-quality, elastic skin (5,10,18,19) (Table 87.1). The technique is not suitable for women with very large breasts and/or severe ptosis. In these cases a horizontal or lateral scar will be necessary to compensate for the extra skin. The relationship between the incidence of complications and body mass index and breasts size is well demonstrated (4).The patient should be willing to accept the fact that the immediate postoperative result in breast shape and scar appearance is not aesthetically pleasing and understand that the final result may not be seen for up to 3 months (4,5,11,20–22).

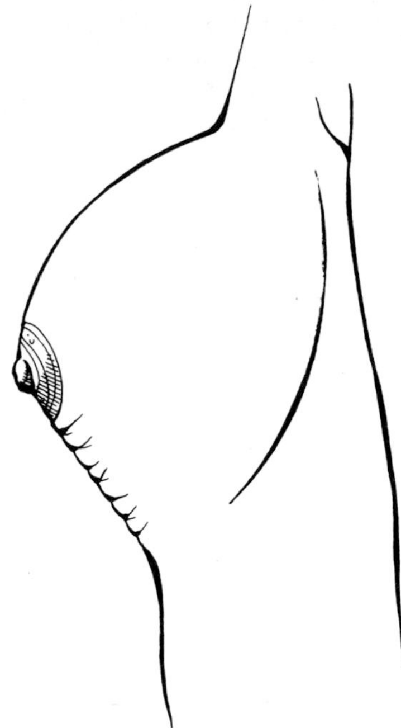

Figure 87.1. The immediate postoperative result is not aesthetically pleasing. The breast shows an excessively full upper pole, a flat lower pole, and pleats in the vertical closure compensating for skin excess. This initial appearance takes into account gravity and natural skin elasticity, which will confer some settling and rounding of the lower pole tissues in the initial postoperative months.

PREOPERATIVE PLANNING

The preoperative evaluation is essential in deciding on the best approach for the patient. The following are several key aspects to consider.

THE DEGREE OF PTOSIS

Ptosis is evaluated by assessing the position of the nipple in relation to the inframammary crease. Once the diagnosis of mammary ptosis is established, the distance from the suprasternal notch to the nipple is measured. The normal distance can average from 18 to 22 cm, depending on several factors, such as the height and build of a person, and so the use of another anatomic landmark (inframammary crease or midhumeral line) can help locate the ideal nipple position. The suprasternal notch-to-nipple distance will help to determine the distance needed to elevate the nipple to its normal position and select the safest technique and pedicle for the patient.

BREAST SIZE

Ascertaining whether the patient is content with her breast size is an important step in meeting her expectations. Asking the patient if she likes the size and shape of her breasts when wearing a bra helps to determine this. One of the advantages of the vertical mastopexy technique is the achievement of upper pole fullness. However, breasts may appear somewhat smaller following mastopexy, and the only way to add volume, particularly for upper pole fullness, is an implant. On the other hand, in patients with an excess of glandular tissue, the additional weight may actually be contributing to the ptosis, and some parenchymal resection should be considered. The technique should not be applied in women with very large breasts and/or severe ptosis. The relationship between the incidence of complications and the size of the breasts is well demonstrated (22).

SKIN QUALITY

Patients with normal elastic skin will have better and longer-lasting results. Quality elastic skin will redrape to the new breast shape faster than poor-quality skin. With this technique the vertical scar and lower breast skin may show pleats at first, but these will fade over time. The time needed for the pleats to fade is shorter (up to 2 months) if the breasts are small and the skin is elastic, or longer (5 to 6 months) in large breasts with stretched skin (4). As striae increase in size and number, it is more likely that additional skin must be excised because skin retraction in these patients is unpredictable (9).

It is important to prepare the patient about the immediate result. With this technique it takes 2 to 3 months for the breast to acquire a satisfactory appearance (8,10). We must be certain that the patient understands that the breasts will look too high for a couple of months, with excessive upper pole fullness and lower pole flattening, but will eventually take their normal place with a beautiful long-term stable result (Fig. 87.1). The vertical scar and lower skin will be pleated at first, but this will fade with time. Risks of asymmetry, altered sensation, nipple-areolar necrosis, and abnormal scarring must be explained to the patient.

OPERATIVE TECHNIQUE

The patient is marked in the standing position. The suprasternal notch-to-nipple distance is measured and recorded. A line is drawn from the suprasternal notch to the umbilicus to rep-

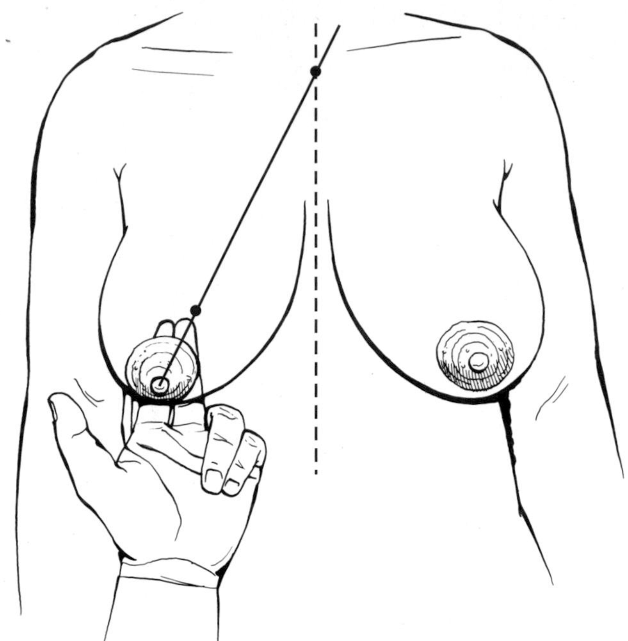

Figure 87.2. Marking the new position of the nipple-areola complex.

resent the midline. Both inframammary creases are outlined. The breast meridian is marked on each side by a line that starts at the clavicle 7 cm lateral to the suprasternal notch, extends down to the nipple, and ends at the inframammary crease below the level of the nipple, 10 to 14 cm from the anterior midline. Symmetry between these two lines is essential, as the upper part demarcates the new horizontal position of the NAC and inferiorly it will determine the limits of the medial and lateral markings and the position of the vertical scar. The new position of the nipple-areola complex (point A) is marked next by placing a finger in the inframammary crease and transposing this anteriorly along the marked breast meridian (Fig. 87.2). Anatomically and with other techniques, this point represents the new position of the nipple. However with this technique, as the pillars are brought together, the new nipple position is raised (19). This is why the new nipple position is placed a couple of centimeters lower. Therefore, point A is actually made to represent the superior aspect of the new areola. Point A is then the key to determining the medial and lateral markings. The medial marking is made by pushing the breast laterally with one hand and with the other hand drawing a straight line that joins point A with the breast meridian at the level of the inframammary crease. The lateral marking is done in the same manner but by pushing the breast medially (Fig. 87.3). This maneuver should result in a vertical ellipse design. During the surgical procedure, when this ellipse is closed into a vertical line, as explained earlier, the vertical line lengthens, bringing the inferior aspect of the vertical scar below the inframammary crease down to the abdominal skin. In addition, with this vertical mastopexy technique, the inframammary fold rises, and if the skin resection is carried close to the fold, the scar will extend downward. To keep the scar above the inframammary crease, the medial and lateral lines are joined approximately 2 cm above the crease. The bigger the breast, the higher this point should be above the crease to avoid a scar in the abdominal skin. It is very important to design the skin excision at the bottom as a U and not a V (Fig. 87.4). With the latter there will be excess skin remaining, and a "dog ear" will result that will then need to be closed with a horizontal or lateral scar. When a U is used, more skin is resected, and the closure will follow the curve of the new breast. The final step in the marking is the perimeter where the new areola will be set. At the top of the ellipse, a mosque dome shape or semicircle with variable

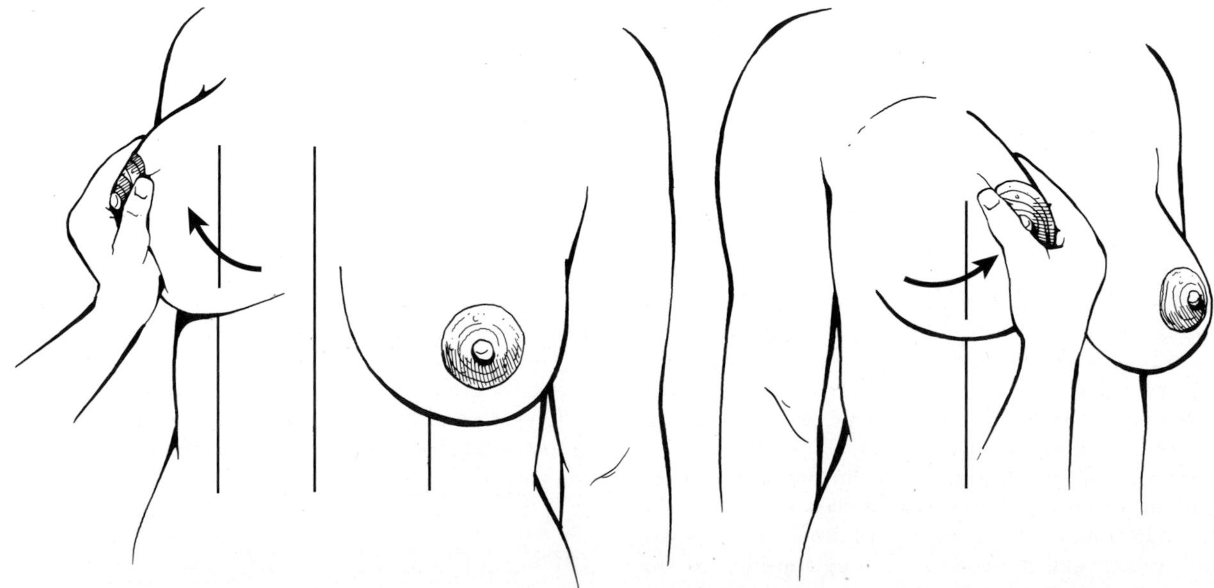

Figure 87.3. **Left:** The medial marking is made by pushing the breast laterally with one hand and with the other hand drawing a straight line that joins point A with the breast meridian at the level of the inframammary crease. **Right:** The lateral marking is done in the same manner but by pushing the breast medially.

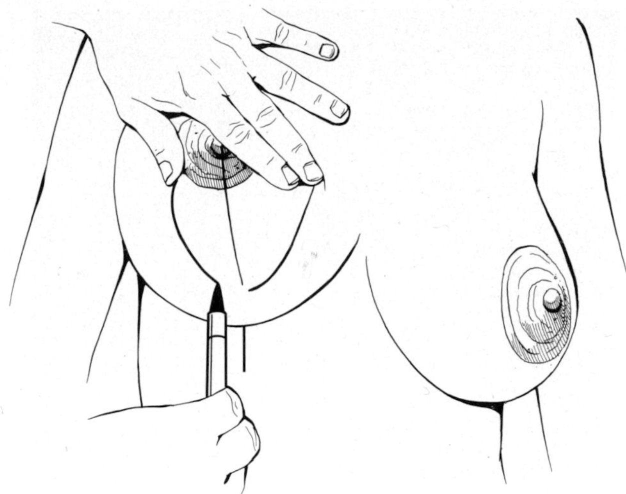

Figure 87.4. Design of the skin excision at the bottom as a U, at least 2 cm above the inframammary crease.

diameter depending on breast size joins the medial and lateral markings. Although an initial preoperative marking is a fundamental element of the vertical mastopexy procedure, it is important to keep in mind that in this technique the markings are adjustable intraoperatively as the surgeon strives to achieve the desired shape (Fig. 87.5). This is not a cookie-cutter, cut-on-the-dotted-line operation. Rather, it is more of a tailor tack technique.

Intraoperatively, the areola is marked with a 38- to 42-mm areola marker. Minimal tension is placed on the skin during the placement of the cookie cutter to avoid ending up with a small areola after the release of the skin. With the use of a Mammostat to keep the breast taut, the skin between the margins of the new areola and the lateral and medial markings is deepithelialized (Fig. 87.6A). Since this is a superiorly based

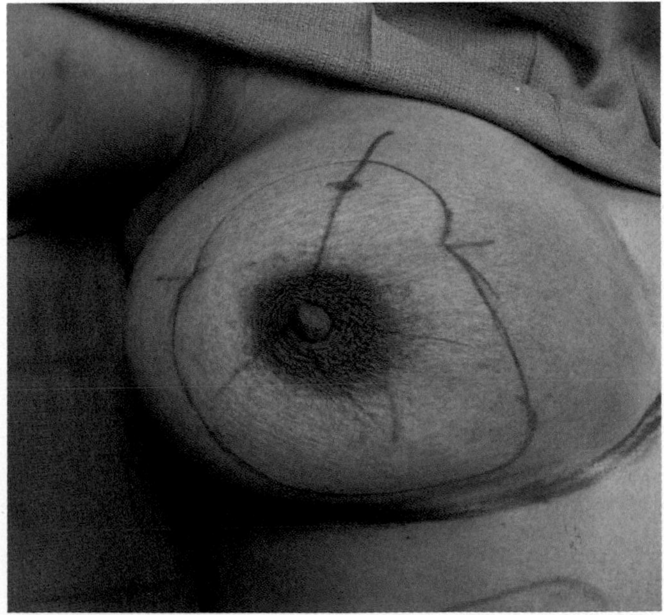

Figure 87.5. Final preoperative marking.

flap, the deepithelialized skin around the mosque dome is left intact. Below the mosque dome, the lateral and medial edges of the design are incised with electrocautery down to the pectoralis fascia (Fig. 87.6B). All of this deepithelialized lower pole breast tissue based on a superior pedicle is elevated off the pectoralis fascia (Fig. 87.6C). Continued dissection above the muscle fascia is made below the nipple-areola complex up to the level of the upper pole, creating a subglandular pocket. The superiorly based dermoglandular flap is tucked into the retroareolar pocket and sutured to the pectoralis fascia at the level of the second rib (Fig. 87.6D). This maneuver places additional parenchymal bulk behind the nipple-areolar complex and recreates the central projection. It is important to make sure that this step does not impede the advancement of the areola up to point A. After the dermoglandular flap is tucked below the breast, the areola is brought up and sutured to point A. The areolar opening is closed with a 3-0 Monocryl separating the areola from the vertical scar. At the bottom of the U, breast tissue must be resected inferiorly, medially, and laterally, making sure to leave about 1 cm of fat below the skin (Fig. 87.6E). The reason for this is that the inframammary crease rises in this technique, and it is important to have the skin hug the chest wall between the old and new inframammary folds. If this tissue is not removed inferomedially and inferolaterally, a pucker or fullness will result in the new inframammary crease. This breast resection inferiorly is similar to that of the Wise pattern; however, only the parenchyma is resected, not the skin. The extra skin medially and laterally is needed to accommodate the extra projection that results with this technique after the breast tissue is reshaped into a conical form (4,20).

The remaining pillars of underlying breast tissue are then approximated suturing the breast parenchyma together. This will cone the breast and pull in the lateral and medial fullness. Thus the breast is shaped by parenchymal tissue independent of the skin envelope (23). One of the advantages of this technique is that the shape of the breast does not rely on skin support, which, over time, may stretch and predispose to the recurrence of ptosis or pseudoptosis. Failure to suture these two pillars together may allow the superior breast tissue to push down and splay the columns, resulting in recurrent ptosis.

After approximation of the pillars the skin is reevaluated. Excess skin can make the lower pole appear ptotic. Two pickups are used to bring excess skin to the midline and stapled in place. The excess skin is marked and resected. Closure of the skin begins with multiple interrupted 3-0 Monocryl in the deep dermis. Superficial closure is achieved with an intracuticular 4-0 Monocryl. Gathering of the skin is performed to shorten the length of the vertical scar. Most of the gathering is at the inferior end of the vertical opening, where more skin retraction is desired. With the Wise pattern, it is generally accepted that the vertical scar should not exceed 6 to 7 cm in length at the end of the operation. However, when the distance from the inferior border of the areola to the inframammary fold is measured in a variety of aesthetically pleasing breasts, this distance can be up to 10 cm depending on the size of the breast (5,10). Therefore the objective is to have a final vertical scar above the inframammary crease, and focus placed on a specific measurement is not as important. In this technique it is normal for the vertical incision length to measure 8 to 10 cm (19). Lower pole length of this dimension is necessary to achieve the improved projection that vertical mammaplasty offers. If the scar is too long, a lateral skin resection of the dog ear is made along the inframammary

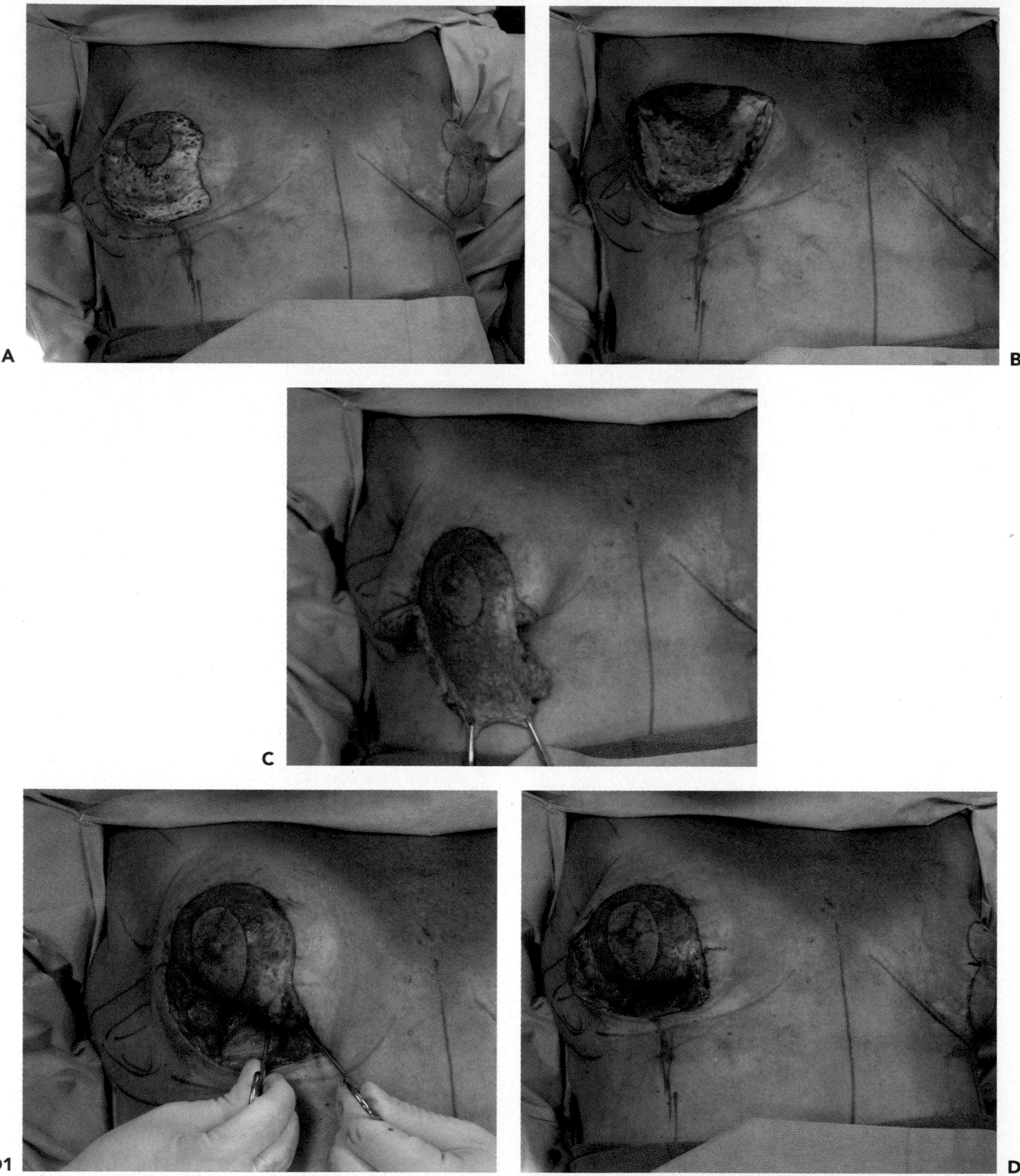

Figure 87.6. **A:** With the use of a Mammostat, the skin between the margins is deepithelialized. **B:** Below the mosque dome, the lateral and medial edges of the design are incised with electrocautery down to the pectoralis fascia. **C:** All of this deepithelialized lower pole breast tissue based on a superior pedicle is elevated off the pectoralis fascia. **D1, D2:** The superiorly based dermoglandular flap is tucked into the retroareolar pocket and sutured to the pectoralis fascia at the level of the second rib. (*continued*)

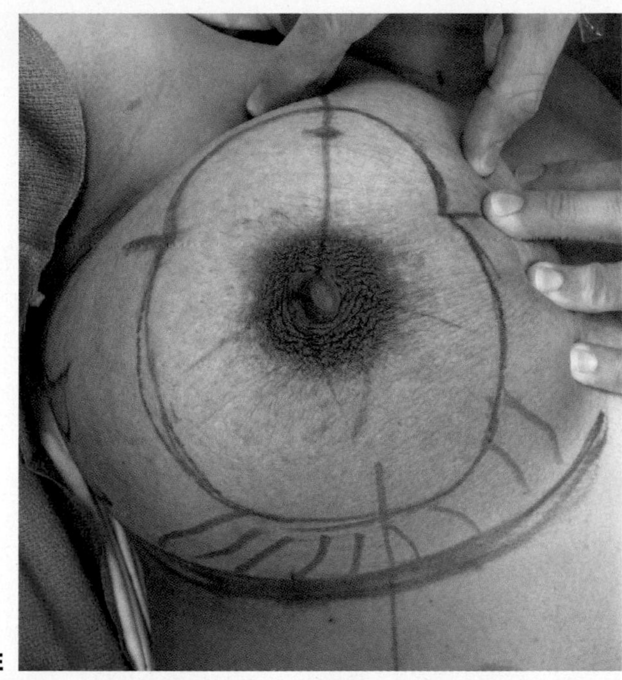

E

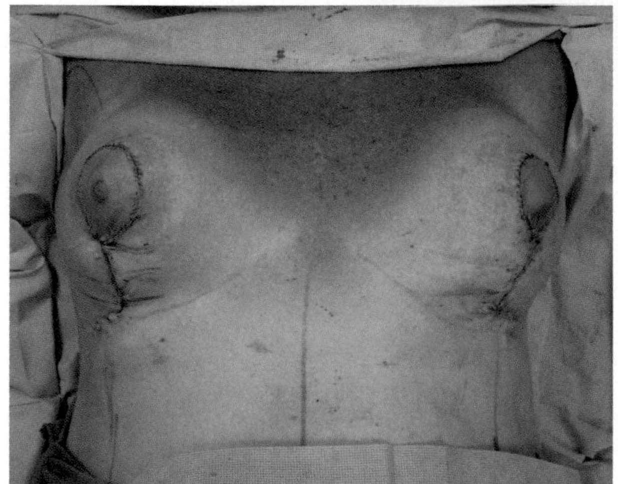

F1

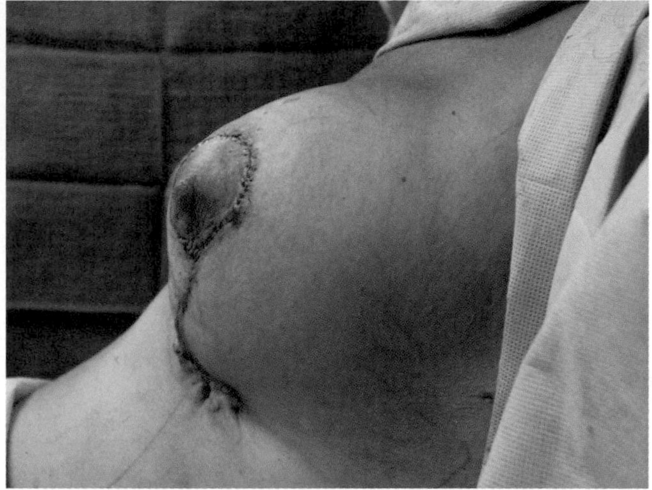

F2

Figure 87.6. (*Continued*) **E:** At the bottom of the U, breast tissue is resected inferiorly, medially, and laterally similar to the Wise parenchymal resection pattern but leaving the skin (vertical lines show area of parenchymal resection below the skin). Leaving 0.5 to 1 cm of fat below the skin is important so as not to compromise cutaneous blood supply. If this tissue is not removed, fullness will result in the new inframammary crease. **F1, F2:** At the end of the procedure the lower pole of the breast should be flat and the upper pole almost excessively full.

line to avoid placement of the scar below the crease. Placement of a drain aids in evacuation of fluid and obliteration of dead space behind the pillars.

At the end of the procedure the lower pole of the breast should be flat and the upper pole almost excessively full (Fig. 87.6F). Although this initial appearance is somewhat exaggerated, it takes into account gravity and natural skin elasticity, which will confer some settling and rounding of the lower pole tissues in the initial postoperative months (Fig. 87.7). If the lower pole is not flat initially, these same forces will result in bottoming out as opposed to a natural rounding of the lower pole.

POSTOPERATIVE CARE

The patient is given an instruction sheet containing information regarding her care at home. If a drain is placed, it is generally removed on the first postoperative day. During the first 24 hours, the color of the nipple-areola complex and skin should be checked at frequent intervals. Typically a mastopexy is associated with minor to moderate pain, so a short course of oral analgesics is usually enough. A short course of antibiotics should also be given. The patient is instructed to wear a support bra day and night for 8 weeks to help the breast heal in a

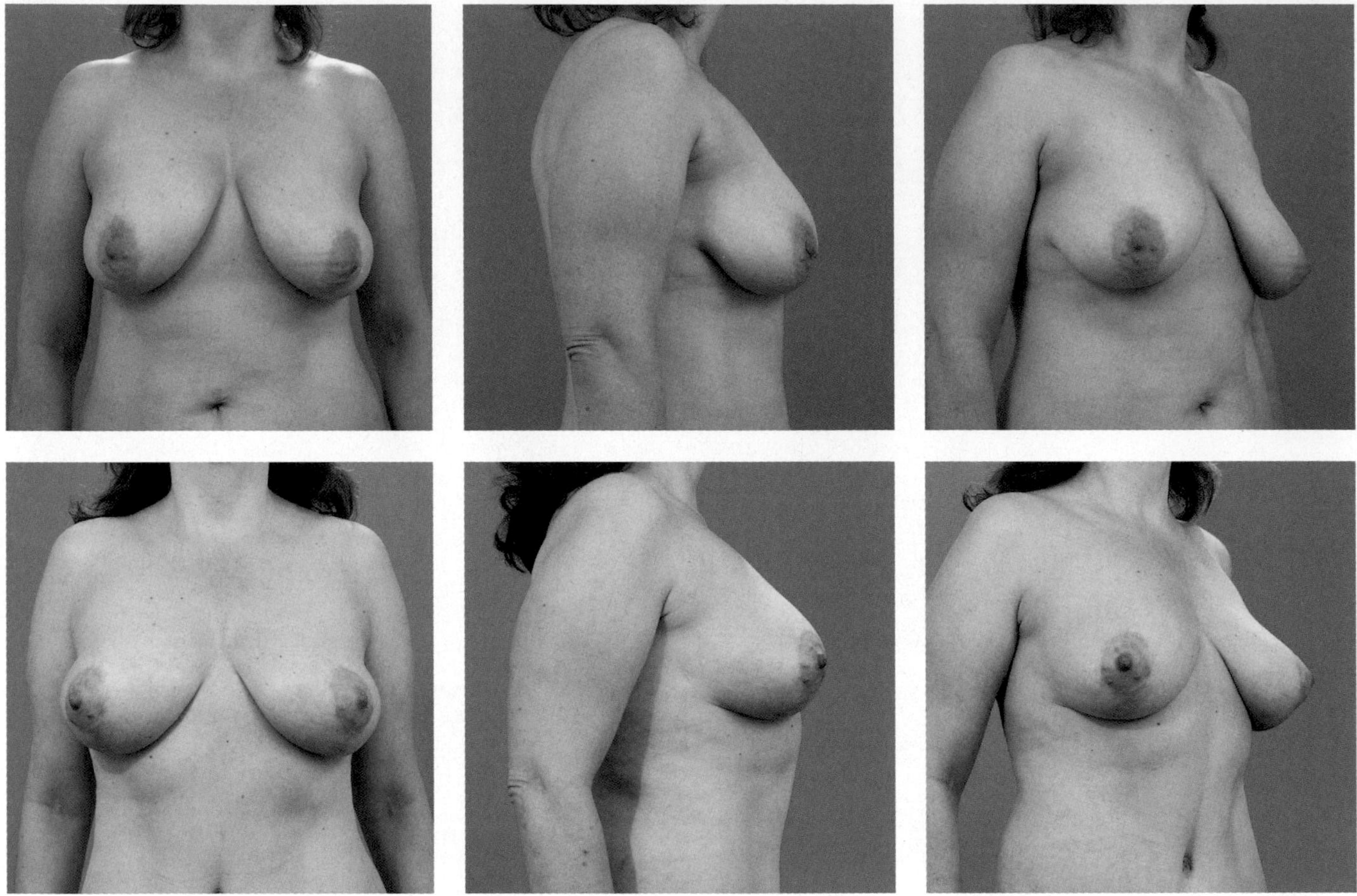

Figure 87.7. **Top:** Preoperative pictures of a 55-year-old patient with breast ptosis. **Bottom:** Postoperative images 18 months after vertical mastopexy.

high, round position. In the immediate postoperative period, the vertical scar may appear below the inframammary fold, but within 2 to 3 months, with the descent of the breasts, the scar is usually placed adequately. Since the final shape can be seen after 3 months postoperatively when the breasts descend, any surgical revisions regarding unsatisfactory breast shape or scar location should be done only after this time.

COMPLICATIONS AND OUTCOMES

The studies show that vertical mammaplasty has a low incidence of complications (4,5,19,22,24–27). The risk of complications increase with larger breasts, so in mastopexies the incidence is low. The most common early complications in vertical mastopexies are seromas, hematomas, infection, total or partial areola necrosis, and delayed healing. In Lejour's series of 476 consecutive breasts with vertical mammaplasty (reductions and mastopexies) the most frequent benign complication reported was seroma (5% of the breasts). Seromas generally appear a few days after surgery as a fluctuating swelling located under the breast. More often they remain unnoticed by the patient. Hematomas occurred in 1.2% of the cases. They appear hours after surgery and become painful if not immediately evacuated. Mastopexies are associated with lower hematoma rates because there is less dissection. Areolar necrosis was reported in two breasts (0.4%) and infection in two breasts (0.4%) (21). Lassus reported his 30-year experience using a superiorly based pedicle with no incidence of nipple necrosis in cases in which the nipple was elevated 9 cm or less (10). No healing complications occurred in Lejour's mastopexy cases as these were related to the size and fat content of the breasts (22).

Long-term complications tend to be related to scarring, breast shape, and nipple sensory changes. The scarring in vertical mammaplasty is very satisfactory. There are patients in whom the scars become virtually invisible with time. Some surgeons recommend late tanning (after 9 months) to help fade the scars (9). In his 40 years of experience and 1,350 cases of vertical mammaplasty (439 mastopexies and 911 reductions), Lassus reported only 4 cases of severe hypertrophy of the vertical scar that led to a terrible result (10).

With regard to breast shape, in her 10-year experience with 250 consecutive cases, Lejour reported that at a 1-year-follow up only 4 patients presented with recurrent ptosis (4), and this parallels our experience. Lassus demonstrated maintenance of shape for as long as 20 years following the initial procedure (5). Avoiding distorted or teardrop-shaped areolas can be achieved by gathering only the inferior aspect of the vertical scar. Wallach (28) recommended two different sutures in the closing of the vertical line. He sutures the first 2 cm of the superior aspect of the vertical incision without gathering to avoid the teardrop phenomenon. The remaining vertical incision is gathered with a different suture to obtain the desired vertical length.

Altered nipple sensation after breast procedures is a common complaint. Lejour found in her series of 170 patients with a 6-month follow-up that 7 patients reported reduced nipple sensation and 1 reported complete loss of sensation Otherwise, the overwhelming majority of patients had nipple sensitivity that was either unchanged or only temporarily reduced (4). Greuse et al. (15) in their breast sensitivity study after 80 vertical mammaplasties with Lejour's technique reported that the sensitivity on the nipple and areola was significantly decreased at 3 to 6 months postoperatively. However, at 1 year, sensitivity recovered and no NAC was insensitive. They concluded that with Lejour's technique patients recover their preoperative levels of sensitivity after an initial postoperative decline.

Breast-feeding following mastopexy is unpredictable. The thinner the dermoglandular flap that holds the areola, the less chance there will be for future breast-feeding capability. In patients who become pregnant after a mastopexy procedure, trying breast-feeding is encouraged, but they must be aware that there is a chance that they will not be able to achieve it.

CONCLUSION

Since plastic surgeons have been trained to produce the best possible results on the table, there is a reluctance of many surgeons to adopt this method because of the unusual appearance of the breasts at the end of the operation. Vertical mammaplasty results in an initial temporary shape that may be of concern to those performing the procedure for the first time. It is because of this that detractors of the vertical technique state that they would rather have a horizontal scar then a strange-looking breast. The term "short-scar" procedure is somewhat of a misnomer, however, as it implies that the shorter scar is the main benefit and the major reason the technique is performed, whereas in fact it is the concept underlying these techniques that produces a better shape with longer-lasting results (29). It is now clear that the vertical mammaplasty not only reduces scars but also improves breast projection, narrows the wide breast, offers better long-term shape, and reduces bottoming out when compared with inverted-T techniques.

EDITORIAL COMMENTS

This chapter is yet another option in performing a mastopexy in a newer way. It combines a vertical or circumvertical skin pattern with yet another variation on using parenchymal or glandular flaps to reshape the breast. The skin markings and skin excision are designed to allow access to the breast parenchyma, while the final skin excision is intended to be minimized with the skin redraping to the reshaped breast.

The authors emphasize that this technique is not for every patient and is best suited for moderate degrees of ptosis, reasonable skin quality, and breasts with more parenchyma than fat.

Similar to the technique of Barbara Hayden also described in this text, this method requires a certain amount of agility and artistry on the part of the surgeon. It is not a "cookie-cutter" technique and instead requires a significant awareness of how the breast needs to look on the table so that it looks good 6 months later.

One major concern or limitation with this technique is the repositioning of the nipple and the central parenchymal flap conflicting with each other. It is very important that the placement of the superiorly based parenchymal flap not restrict or distort the superior elevation of the nipple. The competition between these two fundamental goals of the surgery is a limitation of the technique and essentially restricts how much upper pole fullness can be achieved with this operation. For this reason, it is important that the nipple be at least tentatively fixed in place before completing the repair and recreation of the breast inferiorly.

I also agree with the authors that if there is too much excess skin at the time of redraping the skin, it is perfectly acceptable to excise the dog ear of excess skin along the inframammary fold.

M.Y.N.

REFERENCES

1. Michelow BJ, Nahai F. Mastopexy. In Guyuron B, ed. *Plastic Surgery: Indications, Operations and Outcomes.* St. Louis, MO: Mosby; 2000:2769–2781.
2. Regnault P. Breast ptosis: definition and treatment. *Clin Plast Surg* 1976;3(2):193–203.
3. Hammond D. Reduction mammaplasty and mastopexy: general considerations. In: Spear SL, ed. *Surgery of the Breast: Principles and Art.* 2nd ed. Philadelphia: Lippincott Williams & Wilkins; 2006:971–976.
4. Lejour M. Vertical mammaplasty: update and appraisal of late results. *Plast Reconstr Surg* 1999;104(3):771–781.
5. Lassus C. Update on vertical mammaplasty. *Plast Reconstr Surg* 1999;104(7):2289–2298.
6. Hall-Findlay EJ. Vertical breast reduction. *Semin Plast Surg* 2004;18(3):211–224.
7. Hall-Findlay EJ. Pedicles in breast reduction and mastopexy. *Clin Plast Surg* 2002;29:379–391.
8. Spear SL, Howard MA. Evolution of the vertical reduction mammaplasty. *Plast Reconstr Surg* 2003;112:855–868.
9. Grotting JC, Chen SM. Control and precision in mastopexy. In: Nahai F, ed. *The Art of Aesthetic Surgery.* St. Louis, MO: Quality Medical Publishing; 2005:1907–1950.
10. Lassus C. Vertical scar breast reduction and mastopexy without undermining. In: Spear SL, ed. *Surgery of the Breast: Principles and Art.* 2nd ed. Philadelphia: Lippincott Williams & Wilkins; 2006:1021–1039.
11. Graf RM, Tolazzi ARD, Ono MC. Vertical mammaplasty. In: Codner M, ed. *Techniques in Aesthetic Plastic Surgery.* Spain: Saunders Elsevier; 2009:217–227.
12. Chen CM, White C, Warren SM, et al. Simplifying the vertical reduction mammaplasty. *Plast Reconstr Surg* 2003;113(1):162–172.
13. Corduff N, Taylor GI. Subglandular breast reduction: the evolution of a minimal scar approach to breast reduction. *Plast Reconstr Surg* 2004;113:175–184.
14. Hanna MK, Nahai F. Applied anatomy of the breast. In: Nahai F, ed. *The Art of Aesthetic Surgery.* St. Louis, MO: Quality Medical Publishing; 2005:1790–1815.
15. Greuse M, Hamdi M, DeMey A. Breast sensitivity after vertical mammaplasty. *Plast Reconstr Surg* 2001;107(4):970–976.
16. Nahai F. Clinical decision-making in breast surgery. In: Nahai F, ed. *The Art of Aesthetic Surgery.* St. Louis, MO: Quality Medical Publishing; 2005:1817–1858.
17. Sprole AM, Adepoju I, Ascherman J, et al. Horizontal or vertical? An evaluation of patient preferences for reduction mammaplasty scars. *Aesthetic Surg J* 2007;27(3):257–262.
18. Hoffman A, Wuestner-Hofmann M, Basseto F, et al. Breast reduction: modified "Lejour technique" in 500 large breasts. *Plast Reconstr Surg* 2007;120:1095–1104.
19. Hidalgo DA. Vertical mammaplasty. *Plast Reconstr Surg* 2005;115(4):1179–1197.
20. Hall-Findlay EJ. A simplified vertical reduction mammaplasty: shortening the learning curve. *Plast Reconstr Surg* 1999;104(3):748–759.
21. Nahai F, Boehm K. Mastopexy. In: Evans G, Nahabedian MY, eds. *Cosmetic and Reconstructive Breast Surgery.* Philadelphia: Saunders Elsevier; 2009:109–118.
22. Lejour M. Vertical mammaplasty: early complications after 250 personal consecutive cases. *Plast Reconstr Surg* 1999;104(3):764–770.
23. De Mey A. Vertical mammaplasty for breast reduction and mastopexy. In: Spear SL, ed. *Surgery of the Breast: Principles and Art.* 2nd ed. Philadelphia: Lippincott Williams & Wilkins; 2006:1040–1047.
24. Berthe JV, Massaut J, Greuse M, et al. The vertical mammaplasty: a reappraisal of the technique and its complications. *Plast Reconstr Surg* 2003;111(7):2192–2199.
25. Lista F, Ahmad J. Vertical scar reduction mammaplasty: a 15-year experience including a review of 250 consecutive cases. *Plast Reconstr Surg* 2006;117(7):2152–2165.
26. Spector JA, Kleinerman R, Culliford AT. The vertical reduction mammaplasty: a prospective analysis of patient outcomes. *Plast Reconstr Surg* 2006;117(2):374–381.
27. Thienen CE. Areolar vertical approach (AVA) mammaplasty: Lejour's technique evolution. *Clin Plast Surg* 2002;29:365–377.
28. Wallach SG. Avoiding the teardrop-shaped nipple-areola complex in vertical mammaplasty. *Plast Reconstr Surg* 2000;106(5):1217–1218.
29. Adams WP. Reduction mammaplasty and mastopexy. *Sel Read Plast Surg* 2002;9(29):1–48.

CHAPTER

88

Albert De Mey
Diane Franck
Christophe Zirak

Vertical Mammaplasty for Breast Reduction and Mastopexy

Few operations can be considered entirely new, as one always borrows from the past to describe a surgical technique. After the description of Dartigues in 1925 (1) and Arie in 1957 (2), Lassus published a vertical scar mammaplasty in 1970 (3). The vertical mammaplasty that we will describe is derived from the technique of Lassus (4) and modified by Lejour (5) to be applicable for small breasts, as well as for large ones. The operative technique of vertical scar mammaplasty described in this chapter represents evolution based on an experience of more than 20 years of performing this technique.

Initial results obtained using the technique of Lejour (6,7) have been encouraging not only concerning the reduction of scar, but also for the achievement of a long-lasting, good-looking breast (see Fig. 88.10). The Lejour technique has been used in our department as the only technique for breast reduction since 1990. However, at the university hospital, a high rate of complications was observed when the technique was performed by multiple operators, often residents in training. This is probably due to the fact that the technique as described and performed by Lejour was based on experience in hundreds of these procedures associated with an uncommon skill. This made the outcome of that particular technique not always predictable in other hands.

In order to reduce the learning curve and make it easily applicable and teachable in a plastic surgery training center, some modifications were adopted that proved to be effective in reducing the risks of complications or unsatisfactory results (8,9) and also to be applicable even in large breasts (10).

The modified technique remains based on a superiorly based areolar pedicle with central glandular resection. Extensive wide lower skin undermining is avoided, as well as liposuction of the breast. The shape of the breast is created by suturing the gland and does not rely on the skin to maintain its form. In the majority of cases, no scar is needed in the submammary fold.

PRINCIPLES

The goals of a breast reduction are correcting the volume, improving durability of the shape and symmetry, and preserving nipple sensitivity with minimal scarring.

Volume reduction and correction of the shape can be obtained by different techniques. However, long-term results remain a concern because too often the result of surgery deteriorates with time, especially in large breasts. A high projected and narrowly based breast must be obtained and maintained. In the vertical scar mammaplasty, the reshaping is based on the suture of the glandular pillars in the medial inferior quadrant of the breast.

Scars are unavoidable but should be minimal. This, of course, must not be at the expense of the quality of breast shape. The periareolar scar is mandatory, as the nipple/areola has to be repositioned. Periareolar techniques have been described but are only applicable to small reductions and often result in a flat breast with stretched areola and irregular scars. The vertical scar allows an adequate reduction of the skin brassiere over the reduced breast volume in most cases and is the scar that fades best with time. In our technique, the horizontal submammary scar can be avoided in the majority of cases except for the reduction of more than 1,000 g per breast and inelastic skin (10). However, it can be limited in length and always well hidden in the breast fold.

DRAWINGS

The preoperative drawings are done the day before surgery, according to the description of Lejour (5), on a standing patient.

The future nipple site is positioned on a line joining the suprasternal notch with the nipple slightly lower than the inframammary sulcus as projected to the face of the breast by the index finger (Fig. 88.1). The areolar circumference is then defined by marking the upper pole on the line drawn from the nipple to the sternal notch 2 cm above the nipple site. This distance between the sternal notch and the areolar site is 18 to 22 cm. The internal limit of the areola is positioned at 9 to 10 cm from the midline, according to the width of the chest, and the external limit 7 to 8 cm externally of this point on a horizontal line drawn 3 to 4 cm below the upper marking. These three points are joined and mark the superior areolar circumference.

The submammary fold is marked, as well as the vertical axis of the breast.

The lateral markings are made by pushing the breast laterally and medially with an upward rotation movement, in continuity with the vertical axis drawn below the breast (Fig. 88.2A, B).

The lower limits of the areola are then delineated by drawing a slightly curved line between the previous areolar points and the vertical lines (Fig. 88.3).The total circumference of the areola must measure between 14 and 16 cm to match the 4.2-cm areola template.

The same markings are made on the opposite breast. To check the symmetry of the drawings, the breasts can be gently pushed together toward the midline, making the medial markings touch.

SURGICAL TECHNIQUE

Under general anesthesia, the patient is positioned in a semi-sitting position, with the hands under the buttocks. The base of the breast is constricted with an autofixed band Mammostat, and the periareolar area is deepithelialized. Two points are

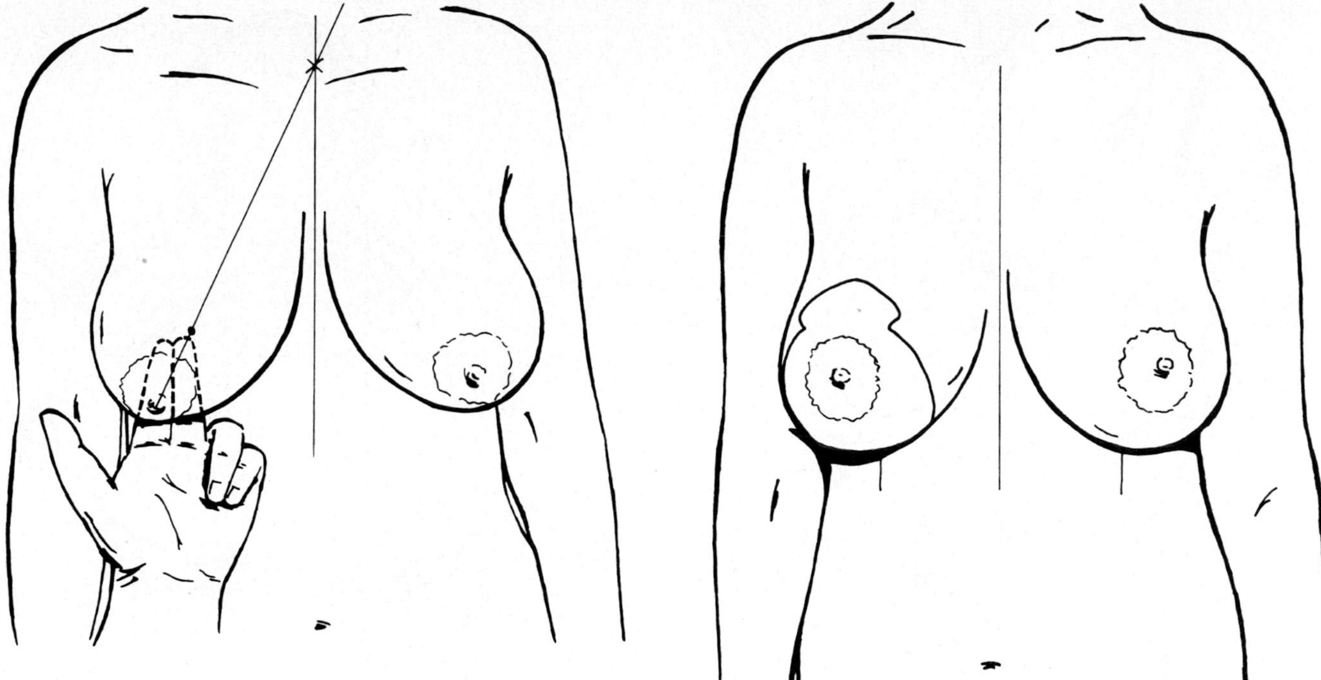

Figure 88.1. Marking of the future nipple site.

Figure 88.3. Final markings.

then marked on each vertical line 7 to 8 cm below the lower areolar point in order to determine the height of the remaining glandular pillars (Fig. 88.4).

A skin hook is placed at this point and another at the lowest part of the drawings near the submammary fold. This makes it possible to undermine the lower part of the breast subdermally, leaving not too much adipose/glandular tissue attached to the dermis down to the submammary sulcus. This dissection is performed both medially and laterally in the inferior quadrants of the breast (Fig. 88.5).

Centrally the dissection continues upward, above the pectoralis fascia, in the retromammary space, to the subclavicular

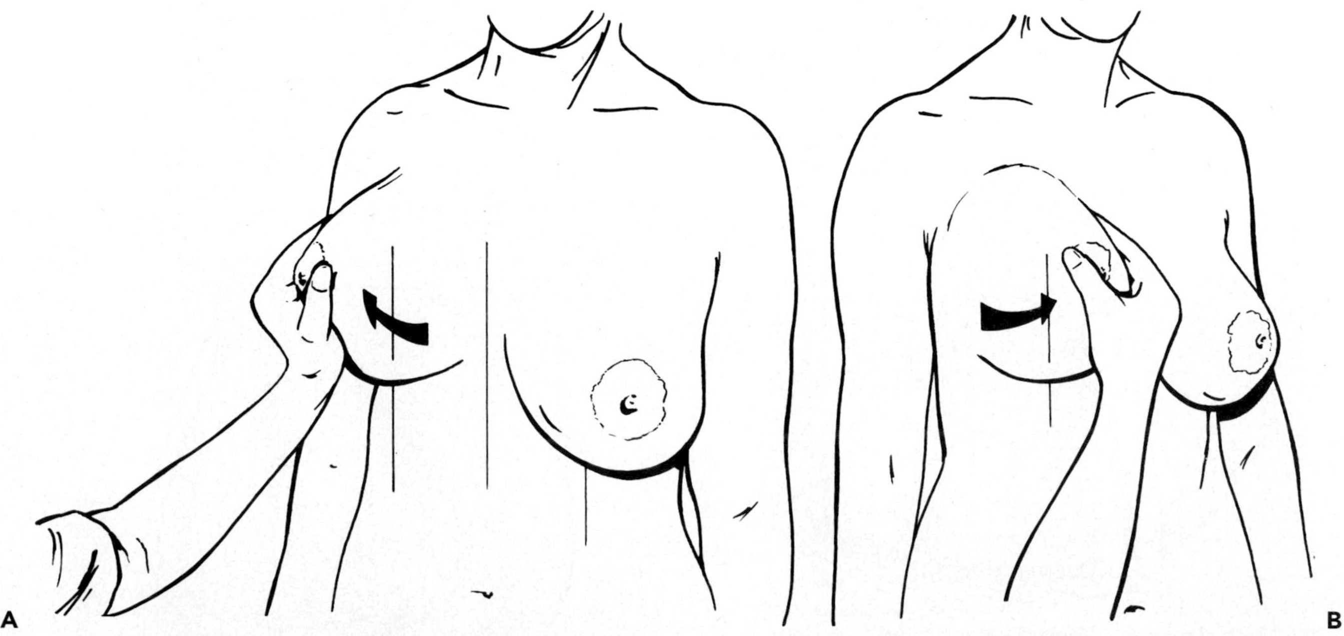

Figure 88.2. **A, B:** Vertical markings in continuity with the vertical axis of the breast drawn after pushing the breast medially, laterally, and upward.

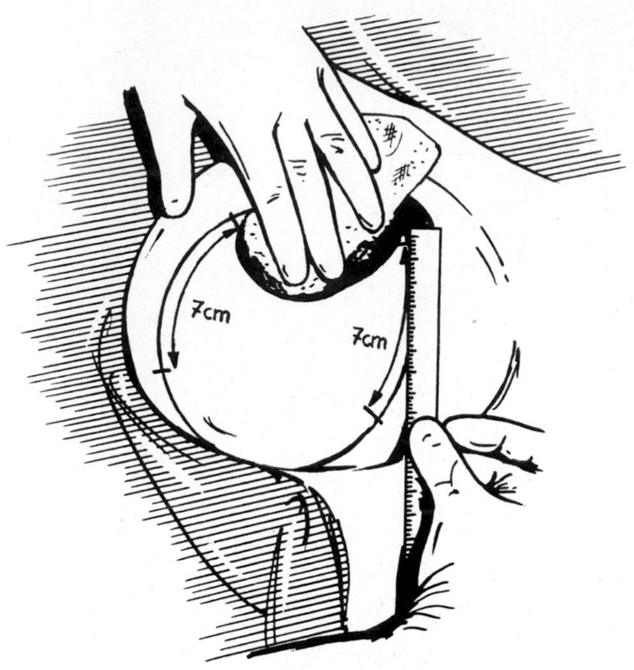

Figure 88.4. Seven-centimeter hallmark to determine the height of the medial and lateral glandular pillars.

area. This dissection must not be extended laterally, in order to preserve the blood supply and the innervation.

A hand is then placed in the retromammary space, and the breast tissue is incised vertically along the medial and lateral skin marks. By doing so, two glandular pillars are created. In the large, ptotic breast, the surgeon must be very conservative in dissecting the medial pillar but has to resect more on the lateral pillar in order to correct the inferior lateral excess of breast tissue.

A skin hook is then positioned at the lowest point of the deepithelialized area around the areola, and the central portion of breast tissue is resected in a conical fashion (Fig. 88.6).

The resected tissue is sent to the pathology department. The closure starts with the positioning of the areola by four stitches of 4.0 nylon starting at the upper pole.

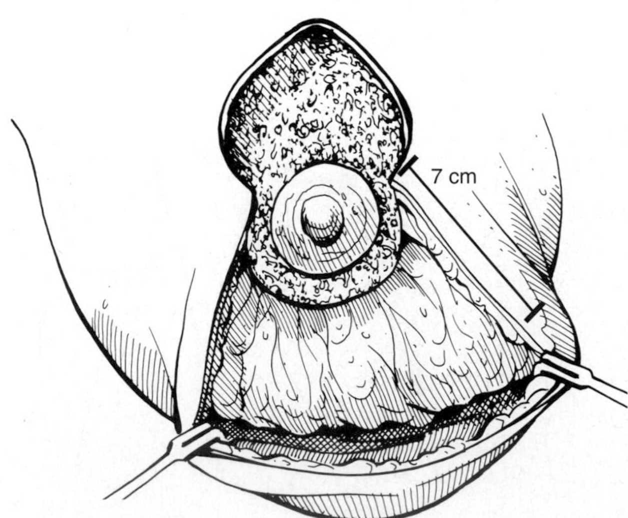

Figure 88.5. Skin undermining in the inferior part of the breast along the submammary fold.

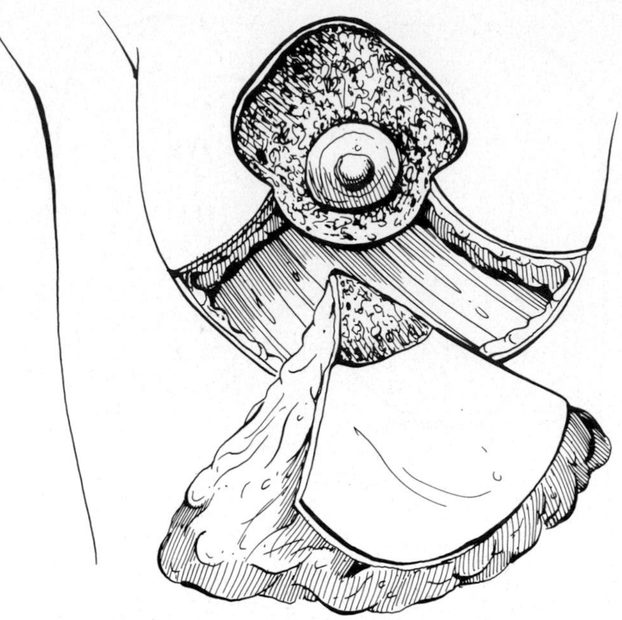

Figure 88.6. Inferomedial glandular excision.

No suture of the gland to the chest wall or pectoralis fascia is performed except in very large fatty breasts in order to facilitate the shaping of the breast by releasing some tension.

The parenchymal sutures are then performed with thick 0 resorbable suture starting at the upper part of the glandular pillars, from deep to superficial to achieve the desired conical shape of the breast (Fig. 88.7).

If necessary, some additional resection can be performed laterally and medially at the lower end of the pillars to obtain a smoothly curved submammary fold.

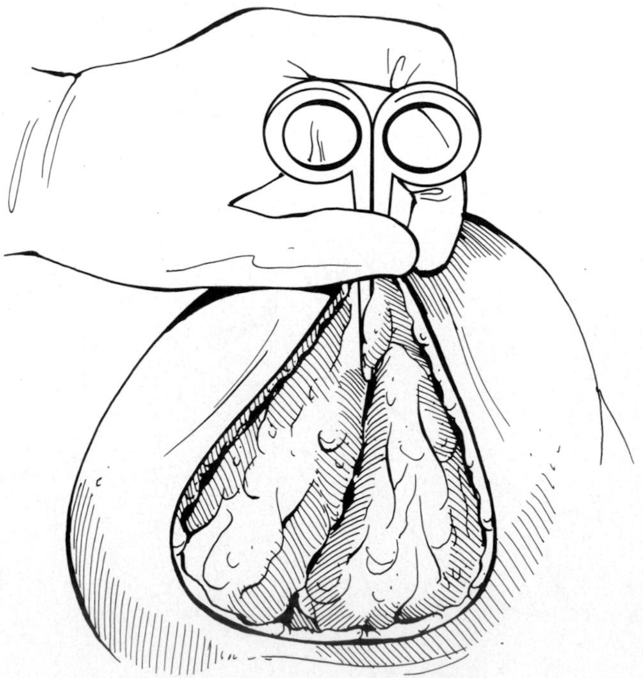

Figure 88.7. Suture of the glandular pillars.

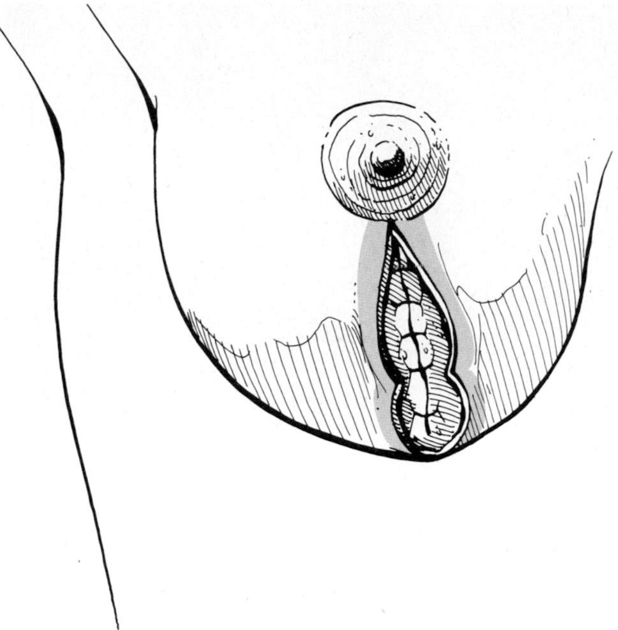

Figure 88.8. Minimal skin undermining along the vertical scar.

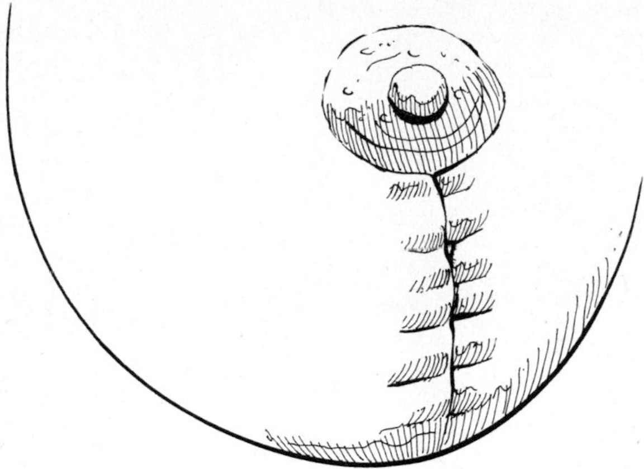

Figure 88.9. Final aspect of the skin suture with thin wrinkles evenly placed.

The last suture is then placed at the lowest part of the pillars, including the chest wall tissue.

A minimal undermining of the skin is performed along the vertical scar in a triangular fashion (Fig. 88.8) in order to avoid tension on the subdermal stitches. These are done with a 3.0 resorbable suture starting at the upper end of the vertical scar as a continuous suture, creating an evenly puckered vertical scar. The end of this suture is attached to the basis of the glandular pillars after placement of a suction drain (Fig. 88.9).

In some cases of large breast resection (1,000 g/breast), a small horizontal skin excision is performed in the submammary fold at the end of the vertical suture in order to avoid crossing the submammary fold or leaving a "dog ear." This is also recommended in patients with redundant skin and limited skin elasticity or in the presence of risk factors such as smoking and diabetes.

Finally, the skin is closed with 3.0 subcuticular nonresorbable suture. A light dressing is applied on the wounds, with an additional roll of gauze placed in the lower part of the breast to avoid a dead space in the undermined areas.

This technique is different from the original technique described by Lejour in the absence of liposuction and wide skin undermining on the glandular pillars. Moreover, skin puckering is limited, and thick skin folds or dog ears are avoided at the level of the submammary crease by performing a horizontal skin excision at that level at the end of the operation when necessary. See Figure 88.10.

RESULTS

From 2003 to 2008, 244 patients were operated at the university hospital using the vertical mammaplasty as described here (8). The average weight resected was 516 g/breast (0 to 2,015 g) and the mean body mass index (BMI) was 29.25 UI (17 to 43 UB).

Breast sensitivity was evaluated prospectively in a consecutive series of 50 patients, as superior pedicle techniques have often been criticized because of the potential damage to the nerve supply. We demonstrated that in mastopexies and

A 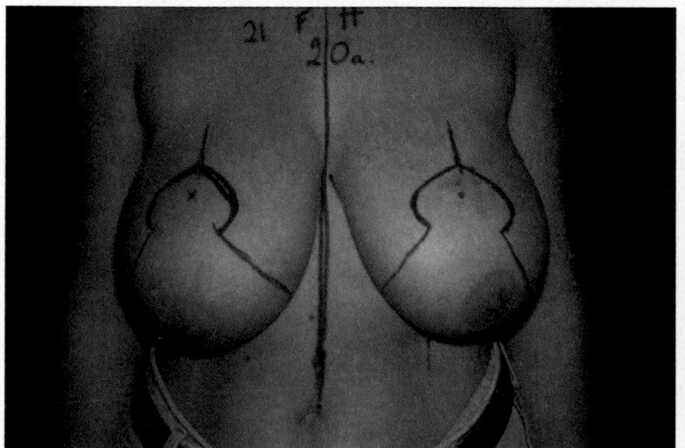

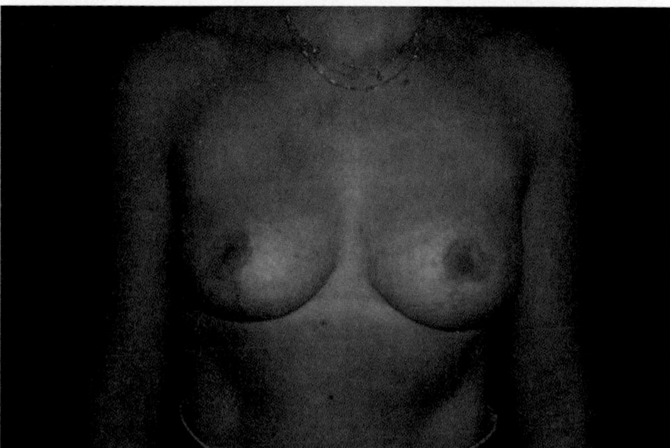 B

Figure 88.10. Reduction in a 20-year-old patient. **A:** Preoperative. **B:** At 18 months postoperative. (*continued*)

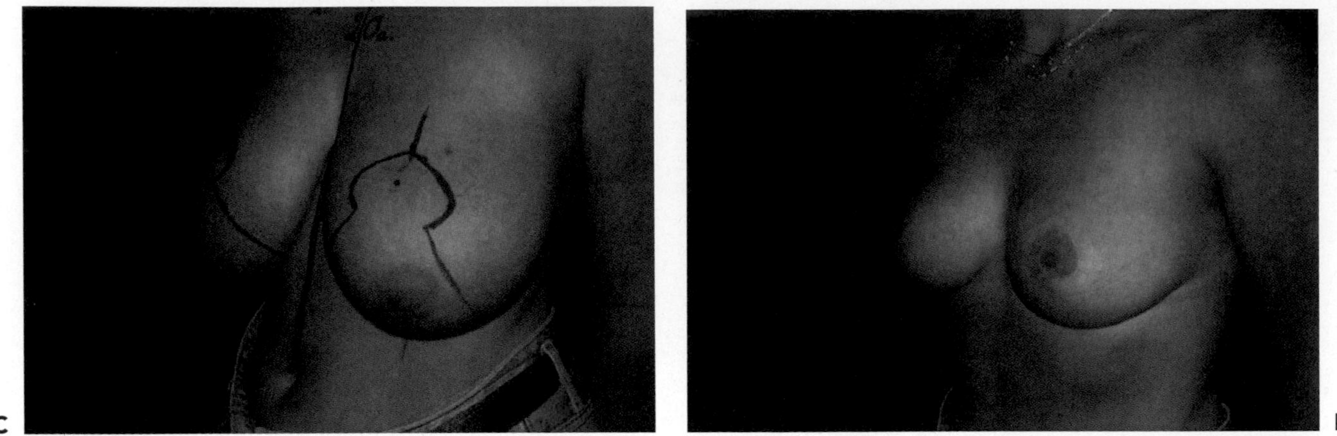

Figure 88.10. (*Continued*) **C, D:** Oblique views.

moderate hypertrophies (11) a complete recovery of the preoperative level of sensibility was observed. Although in large breast reduction (greater than 500 g/breast), pressure sensitivity recovered after 1 year, but temperature and vibration sensitivity remained decreased on the nipple and areola.

The possibility of breast-feeding was also evaluated (12) and appeared to be possible if desired in the vast majority of cases (Fig. 88.11). Finally, long-term results were evaluated and were considered to be good to excellent by the majority of patients, as well as by the surgeons (Figs. 88.12 and 88.13).

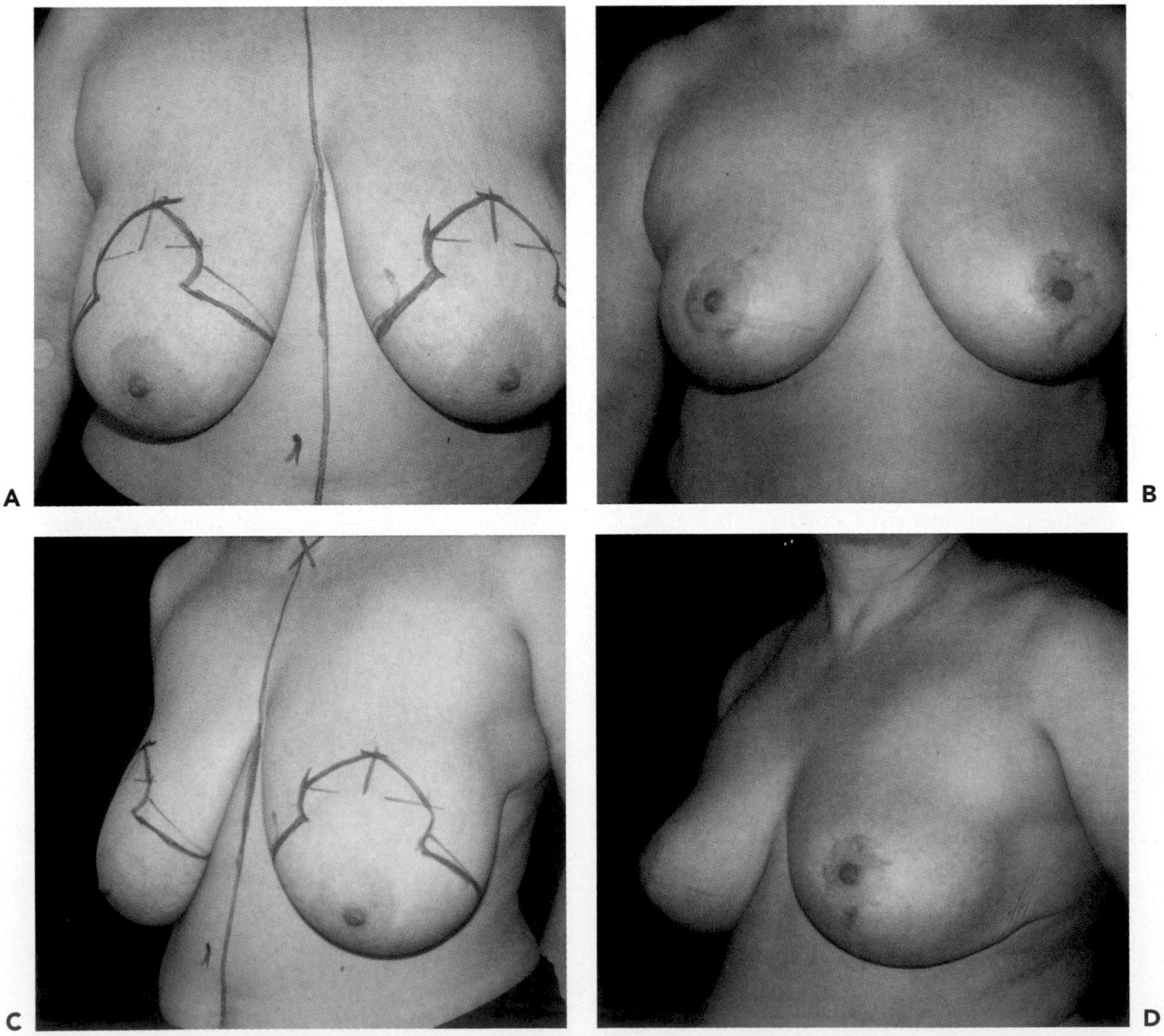

Figure 88.11. Reduction in a 23-year-old patient. **A:** Preoperative. **B:** At 3 years postoperative after 2 pregnancies and breast-feeding. **C, D:** Oblique views.

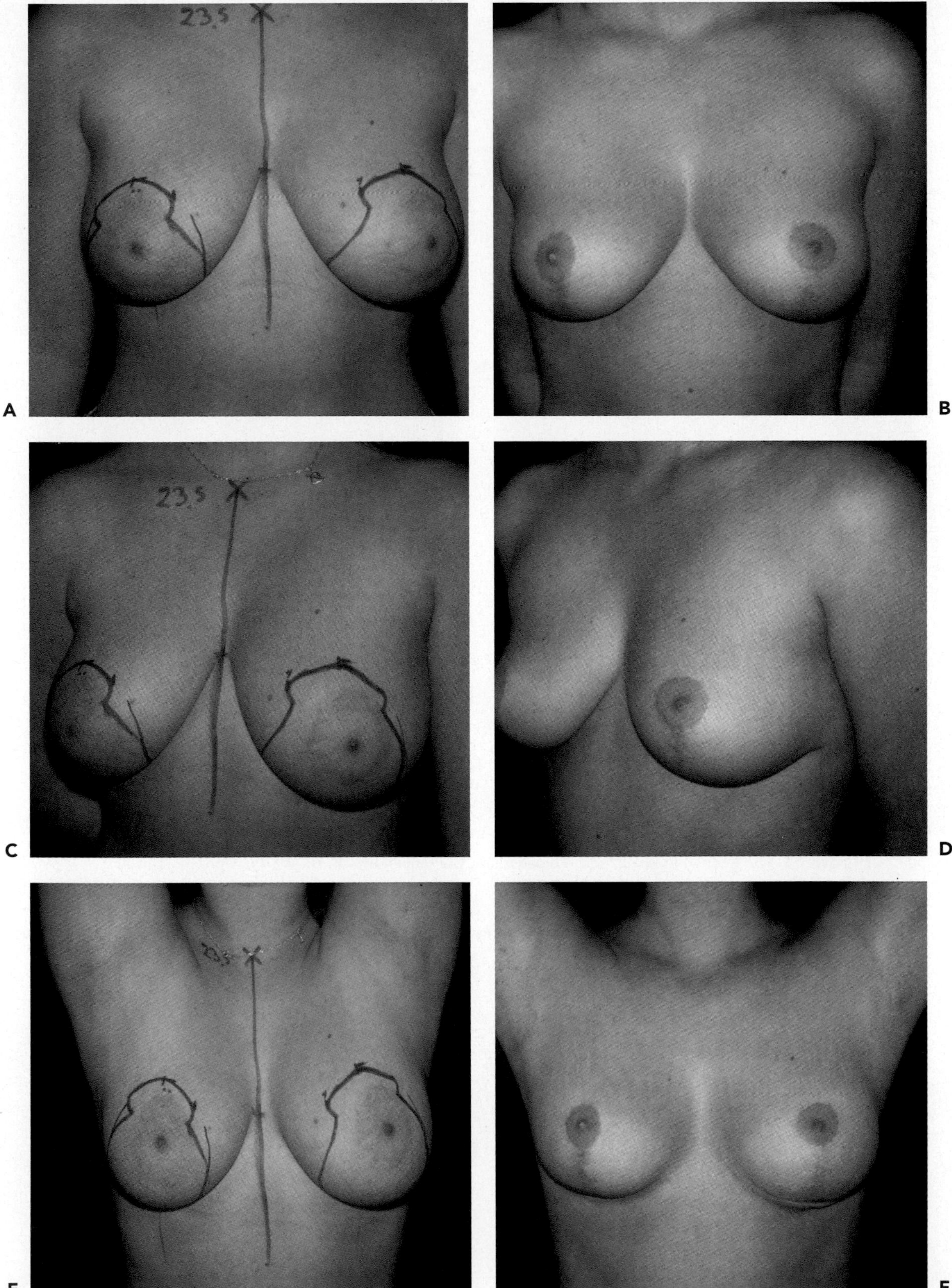

Figure 88.12. Reduction in a 44-year-old patient. **A, C, E:** Preoperative. **B, D, F:** At 5 years postoperative. **C, D:** Oblique views.

A B C D

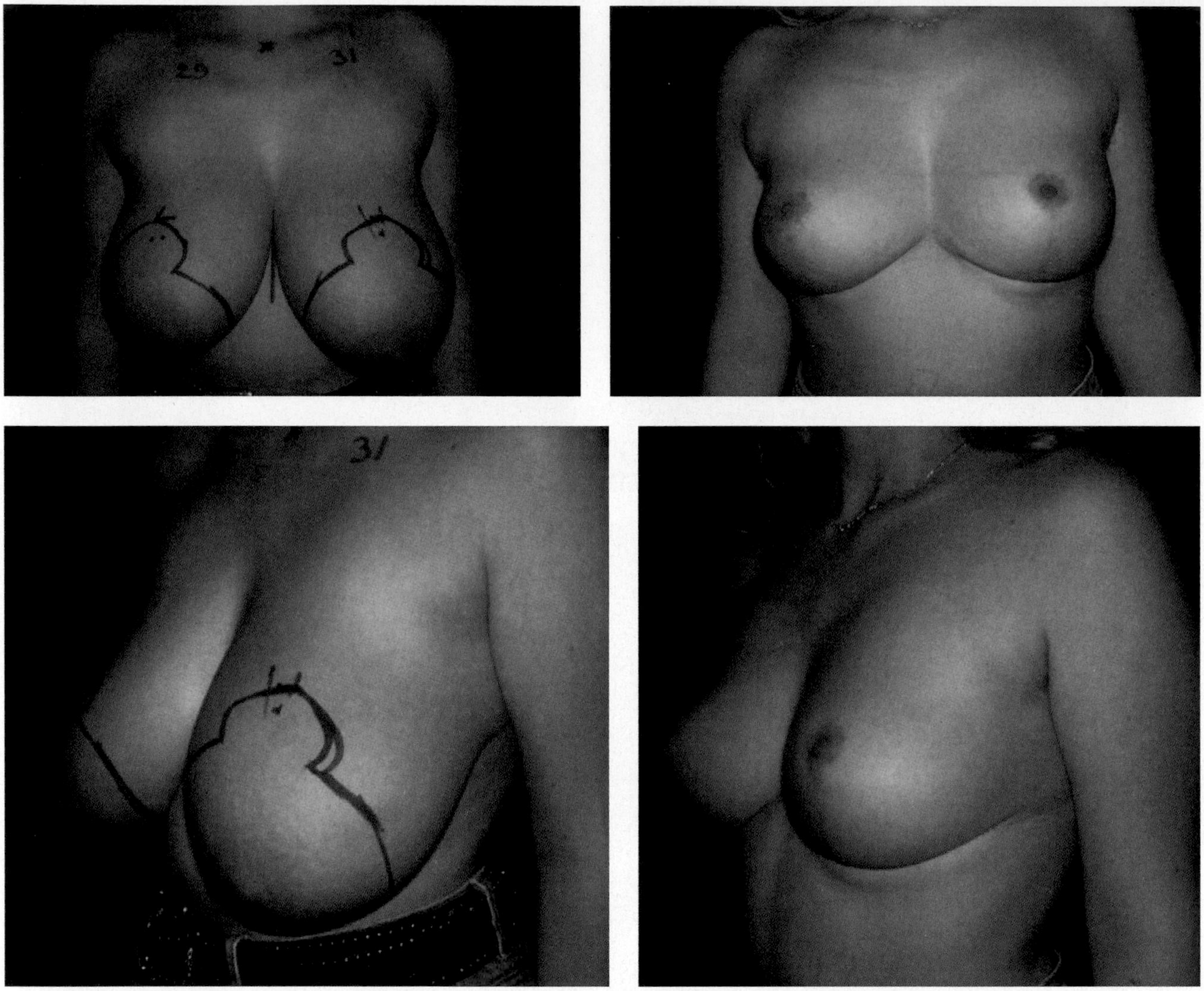

Figure 88.13. Reduction in a 22-year-old patient. **A, C:** Preoperative. **B, D:** At 8 years postoperative. **C, D:** Oblique views. **E, F:** Inferior views.

A B

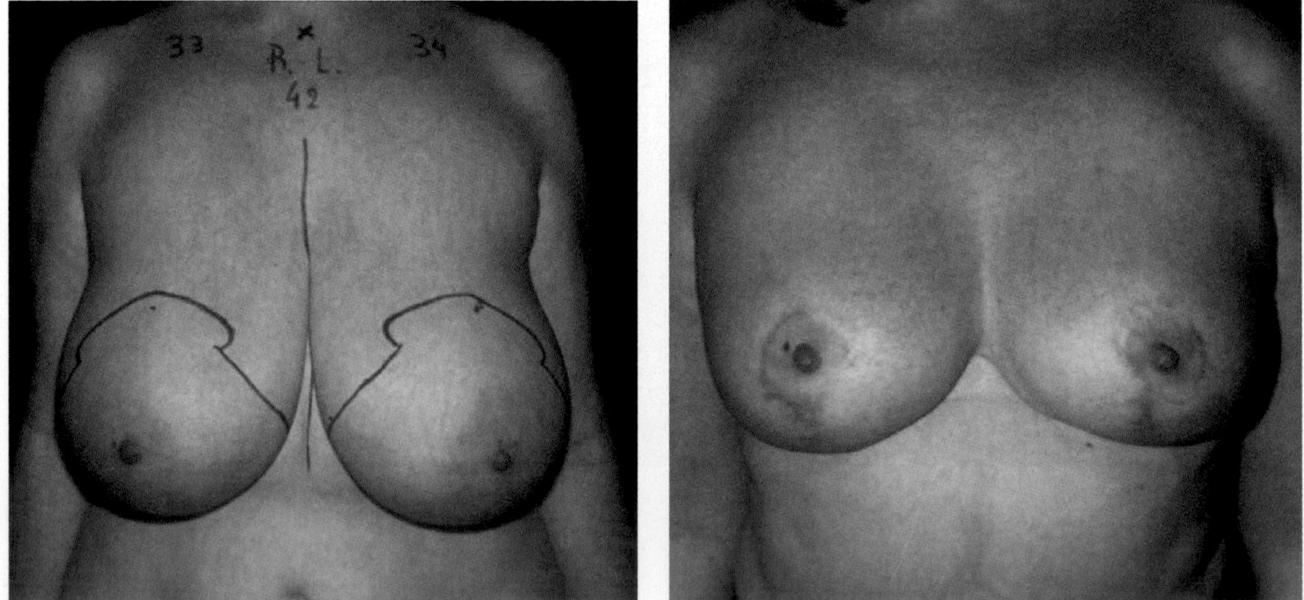

Figure 88.14. Reduction in a 42-year-old patient. **A:** Preoperative. **B:** At 13 months postoperative. (*continued*)

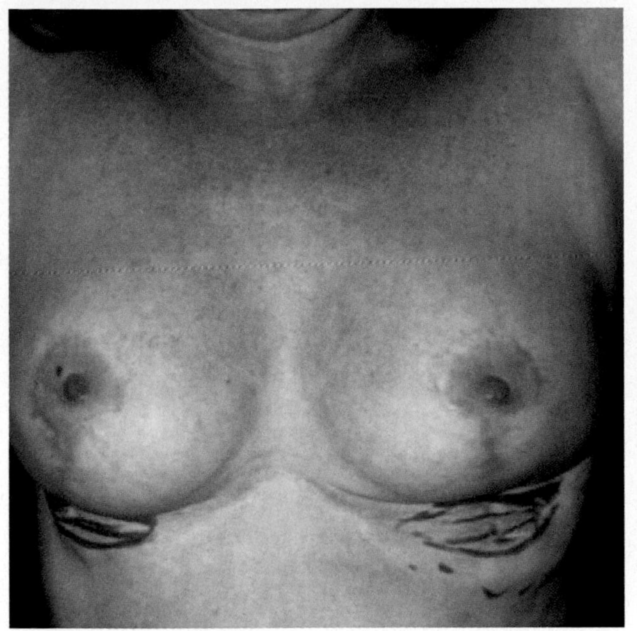

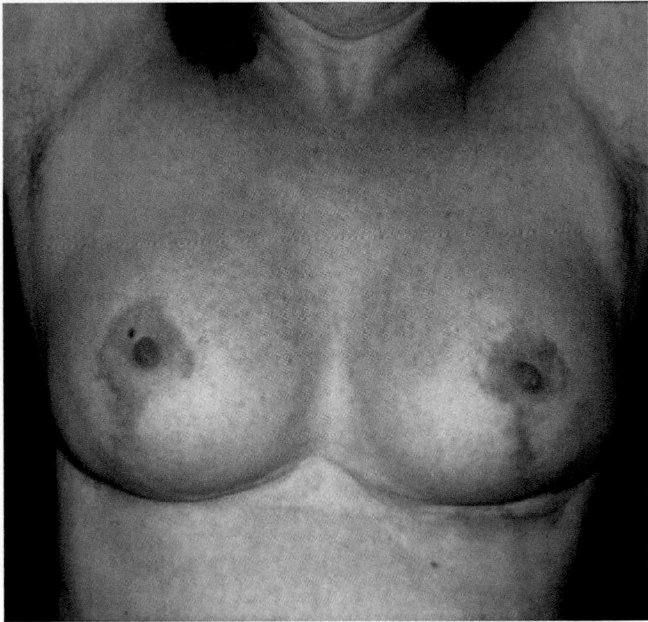

Figure 88.14. (*Continued*) **C:** Excess of skin in the submammary fold. **D:** At 6 months after small horizontal resection.

COMPLICATIONS

The complications rate decreased significantly with the technical modifications of the original technique.

We compared the results obtained at the university hospital in a series of patients operated between 1991 and 1994 with liposuction and wide skin undermining with the revised technique (13). We observed a dramatic decrease of seromas (27% vs. 4%) and hematomas (12% vs. 5%). Wound healing of the vertical scar was also improved, with less than 15% of delayed healing compared to 46%. Finally, steatonecrosis was nearly eliminated, decreasing from 22.4% to 1.3%. These figures were confirmed in the next series of 244 patients operated between 2003 and 2008 with the revised technique.

The same rate of complication was observed, with 2.4% of seromas and 2.8% of hematomas. Superficial wound-healing problems were observed in 18%. Only 2.6% developed steatonecrosis. A horizontal submammary scar was performed primarily in 47 of the heaviest cases. This scar was limited to a maximum of 12 cm and was invisible outside of the breast cone. Nevertheless, secondary corrections were still needed in 16% of the cases, mostly on the lowest part of the vertical scar to eliminate an excess of skin in the submammary fold. The need for corrections in this area was unfortunately not completely eliminated by a primary excision in the submammary fold (Fig. 88.14).

In our series, the main risk factors for complications were the BMI, the amount of resection, and the elevation of the nipple-areola complex. Eight percent of patients presented some complications after resection of less than 250 g, but 50% of complications were observed after resection of more than 1,000 g per breast, when the elevation of the nipple-areola complex was greater than 15 cm, or when the BMI was greater than 30 UI.

CONCLUSION

As we have gained experience with the vertical scar mammaplasty, refinements in our procedure have led to an increased consistency in results. The important modifications of the original Lejour technique include the avoidance of excessive skin undermining, liposuction of the breast, and the acceptance of a small submammary scar in large breasts or when the skin lacks elasticity.

Despite these very good results, many surgeons remain reluctant to use this technique as a standard. This can be due to the use of a superior pedicle for the areola with an inferomedial glandular resection (13), even though this type of glandular resection and reshaping was presented long ago by Pitanguy (14) and has proven efficacy.

The originality of the Lejour technique and its revised procedure lies in the independence of treatment of the skin and the glandular tissue. The latter is treated as with a technique following a Wise pattern, the first being redraped laterally and excised centrally only.

Understanding these factors enables surgeons to use the vertical mammaplasty successfully with more challenging cases while minimizing the scars and avoiding complications.

EDITORIAL COMMENTS

In this chapter Dr. DeMey describes several important modifications to the original Lejour technique. These modifications were adopted in an attempt to improve results while reducing the number of complications. It is interesting to note that these modifications, namely the avoidance of undermining and not using liposuction to recontour the breast, parallel the recommendations of Dr. Lassus. Internal suturing of the breast is described as a method of shaping the breast, and difficulties with the inferior portion of the vertical scar are managed with the addition of a small T-shaped resection. I agree with these modifications. In particular, the addition of a small T-shaped resection I find to be far preferable to the scalloped, irregular wound, which can sometimes result at the inferior end of the vertical incision. The scar is much shorter than the typical Wise pattern inframammary scar and is concealed within the inframammary fold. Adopting these modifications can significantly reduce the number of complications that are sometimes associated with traditional vertical mammaplasty technique.

D.C.H.

REFERENCES

1. Dartigues L. Traitement chirurgical du prolapsus mammaire. *Arch Francobelg Chir* 1925; 28:313.
2. Arie G. Una nuova tecnica de mastoplastia. *Rev Latino Am Cir Plast* 1957;3:23.
3. Lassus C. A technique for breast reduction. *Int Surg* 1970;53:69.
4. Lassus C. New refinements in vertical mammaplasty. *Chir Plast* 1981;6:81–86.
5. Lejour M. *Vertical Mammaplasty and Liposuction.* St Louis, MO: Quality Medical Publishing; 1994.
6. Lejour M. Vertical mammaplasty: update and appraisal of late results. *Plast Reconstr Surg* 1999;104:771.
7. Lejour M. Vertical mammaplasty early complications after 250 personal consecutive cases. *Plast Reconstr Surg* 1999;104:764.
8. Berthe JV, Massaut J, Greuse M, et al. The vertical mammaplasty: a reappraisal of the technique and its complications. *Plast Reconstr Surg* 2003;111:2192.
9. De Mey A, Greuse M, Azzam C. The evolution of mammaplasty. *J Plast Surg* 2005;28: 213–217.
10. Azzam C, De Mey A. Vertical scar mammaplasty in gigantomastia: retrospective study of 115 patients treated using the modified Lejour technique. *Aesthet Plast Surg* 2007;31(3): 294–298.
11. Greuse M, Hamdi M, De Mey A. Breast sensitivity after vertical mammaplasty. *Plast Reconstr Surg* 2001;107:970.
12. Cherchel A, Azzam C, De Mey A. Breastfeeding after vertical reduction mammaplasty using a superior. *J Plast Reconstr Aesthet Surg* 2007;60(5):465–470.
13. Beer GM, Spicher I, Cierpka KA, et al. Benefits and pitfalls of vertical breast reduction. *Br J Plast Surg* 2004;57:12.
14. Pitanguy I. Surgical treatment of breast hypertrophy. *Br J Plast Surg* 1967;20:78.

CHAPTER

89

Daniel A. Marchac

Vertical Mammaplasty With a Short Horizontal Scar

This chapter explains the principles and the practical realization of our technique of vertical mammaplasty with a short horizontal scar.

I devised this technique after using many different methods during my training and early experience: the lateral approach of Dufourmentel and Mouly, the Biesenberger conical remodeling with complete separation of the skin and the gland, and the Pitanguy approach with very little skin undermining and central resection. I borrowed some principles from each of these techniques, my aim being to attain natural, good-looking breasts with short scars and a stable result.

The main idea was a vertical resection of skin and glandular tissue. This created two "dog ears." The upper one corresponds to the areola and is easily adjusted by resecting periareolar skin. The lower one is the main problem. A vertical resection as proposed by Arié and Dartigues is going to show below the inframammary fold, so our idea was to limit all of our incisions to well above the inframammary fold and to make a horizontal incision at this higher level. We started doing it in this way in 1977 and published the technique in 1982. We did not know at that time that Claude Lassus had published his vertical mammaplasty approach in 1981, proposing the limitation of incisions to above the inframammary fold as well.

We also introduced the concept of upper plication and suspension to the pectoralis fascia, conical gland reconstruction, and lower support by the glandular lateral pillar sutured together.

All of these ideas have been used and modified by Madeleine Lejour in her vertical mammaplasty with skin undermining and use of skin retraction to address the lower dog ear. This is an interesting development; in principle, it is better to avoid a horizontal scar. However, we still think that a horizontal scar is a good solution in many cases to avoid the skin undermining, the extensive postoperative wrinkling, and the frequently necessary revision of a remaining dog ear by a horizontal excision. It has been said that the scar from the horizontal incision performed initially was sometimes found later higher on the breast, the inframammary fold recreating itself below. We do not think that this is a problem: The scar is not visible when the patient is standing, and the inframammary fold is completely free of scars, which is a distinct advantage when the patients are wearing a beach bra. In any event, regarding long-term results, the only really visible scar is the periareolar one.

A breast technique should meet the following requirements:

- Be safe, with no risk of areola or skin necrosis; this is achieved by a broad upper breast pedicle and limited skin undermining.
- Produce a stable result; this is achieved by glandular reconstruction of a cone with strong vertical lower pillars and suspension to the pectoralis fascia.
- Be esthetically pleasing and natural; this is achieved by the filling of the superior quadrant using the aforementioned suspension, associated with conical creation through the lower vertical resection.
- Preserve sensitivity; this is achieved by conservation of all the upper and lateral connections of the areola to the superficial sensory nerves.
- Leave nondetectable scars; this cannot, for now, be achieved 100% of the time but should be the goal.
- Scars as short and discreet as possible. This is what we are attempt to achieve with use of the vertical mammaplasty with a short horizontal scar and stitching of sutures with very limited tension on the skin.

The important goal is the final result. Scars evolve differently on the breast.

When the skin is sutured under limited tension, the vertical scar becomes hardly visible with time. The horizontal scar also becomes practically invisible, as long as it remains short. When it continues medially, it often becomes hypertrophic and, later, white. When it is prolonged laterally, spreading is common. That is why it is so important to keep the scar hidden under the breast, so that it does not show laterally or medially when the patient is standing.

The quality of the areolar scar is related to the tension applied to it. We always try to design the deepithelialized area in a way that avoids tension. A discrepancy between the edges is not a problem, but tension is. A circular nonabsorbable stitch passed around the deepidermized area can help diminish the tension.

To attain these goals, our technique relies on three main principles:

1. A vertical excision of skin and glandular tissue
2. A conical construction of the gland, associated with suspension to the pectoralis fascia
3. A short horizontal scar obtained by limiting the vertical skin resection to above the inframammary crease and converting the lower mammary strip of skin into thoracic skin

I now explain the technique step by step.

The operation is performed with the patient in the semisitting position. The head must be fixed in a central position, the arms must rest on the side of the table, with good padding, and the legs must be bent, the feet on a foot rest. Excessive pressure points must be avoided. An elastic strap is placed across the thighs to stabilize them.

We usually make our final markings while the patient is on the table, the semisitting position allowing a good evaluation of the ptosis. We nevertheless like to mark the upper limit A beforehand in the patient's room, in the standing position, to try to avoid asymmetry. For this we pinch the breast with the index

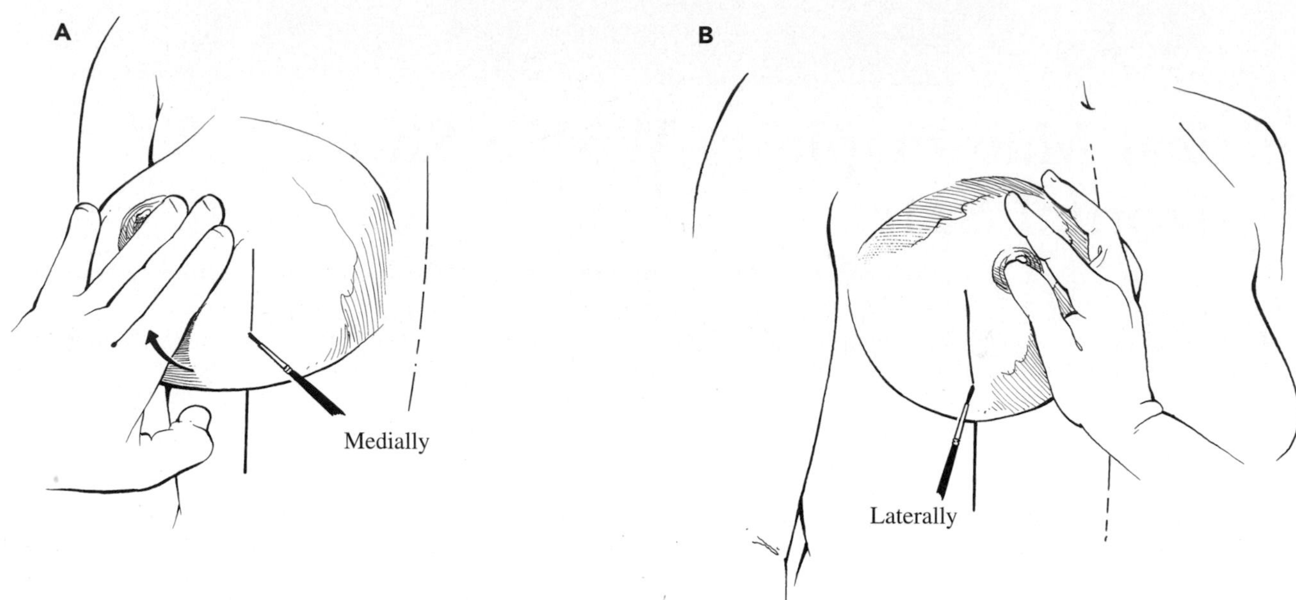

Figure 89.1. Determination of the width of the vertical excision. **A:** The axis of the breast is a vertical line drawn on the abdominal wall, below the breast, which indicates the line on which the areola should be located at the end of surgery. The breast is then pushed laterally, and a vertical line in continuity with the axis is drawn. **B:** The same maneuver is made medially. one must be sure to push the breast horizontally.

in the inframammary fold and the thumb above the areola. We mark these points A and then carefully check their symmetry on the patient standing straight. We then mark the axis of each breast. The axis of the breast is the line on which we want to have our future vertical scar and, even more important, the areola and nipple. One has to lift the breast and see in what location the areola is satisfactory. A vertical line is drawn on the thorax, usually 8 to 10 cm from the midline. Symmetry is again carefully checked.

The next step is to draw the planned vertical wedge excision. The breast is pushed gently medially and laterally, not too much, to keep some fullness, and a line is drawn on the breast in continuity with the thoracic axis. The pull on the breast should be horizontal, to end up with two vertical lines (Fig. 89.1A, B).

The horizontal lower line D–E is located by pinching the lower part of the vertical lines. One sees what level produces a nice new inframammary line, without too much tension. It is usually 3 to 4 cm above the inframammary line, according to the size of the breast and its implantation.

From points D and E one measures 4, 5, up to 6 cm, according to breast size. We thus obtain our future vertical suture. At the level of the upper markings, B and C, one marks a 0.8-cm indent to diminish the tension below the areola (Fig. 89.2A).

The periareolar line is then drawn by joining points C and B, passing through point A. A gentle, semicircular curve must be made.

The last marking is the upper limit of the pectoral undermining. The breast is lifted and pushed up, and the superior limit becomes apparent and is marked (Fig. 89.2B).

We then carefully check the symmetry of our markings. If the breasts are asymmetric, we consider the residual skin flaps on each side, which should be equal, and not the width of the resection. When in doubt, it is always better to diminish the width of the vertical resection, which can easily be adjusted at the end of the operation, because exaggerated skin tension should be avoided.

TATTOOING AND INFILTRATION

It is useful to tattoo the key points to be able to find them easily later. We tattoo points A, B, C, D, E, and G using a 30-gauge needle dipped into surgical ink or methylene blue.

The periareolar area, the vertical lines, the horizontal line, and the lower part of the breast along the inframammary crease and the retroglandular space are infiltrated with a moderate amount of lidocaine with epinephrine (0.5%).

DEEPIDERMIZATION WITH THE COSTAGLIOLA MAMMOSTAT

To provide the proper tension in the periareolar area, we use the Mammostat (Medical Z, Chambray-les-Tours, France) described by Michel Costagliola. It produces a firm stricture of the base of the breast and frees the hand of the assistant. It is adjustable to different breast sizes.

The deepidermization is then performed. We mark a circle of 7.5 cm around the areola, incise it using a no. 10 blade, and

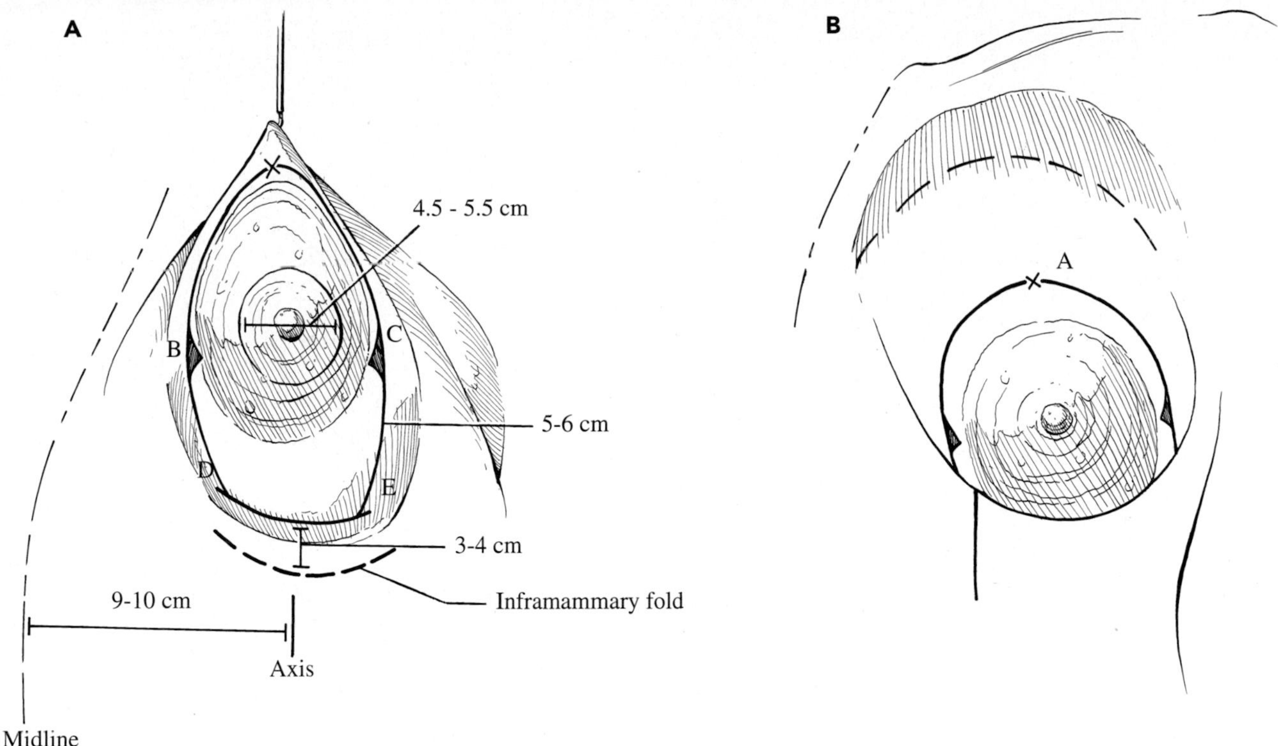

Figure 89.2. Upper and lower limits of the markings. **A:** The horizontal line D–E is located 3 to 4 cm above the inframammary fold. The upper limits of the future vertical suture, B and C, are marked at 5 cm (small breasts) to 6 cm (large breasts) from D and E. An indent is marked to diminish the tension below the areola. **B:** A gentle curve is drawn, joining B and C and passing through point A, which is usually determined by pinching the breast between the inframammary fold and the upper part of the areola. It is situated 1 to 4 cm above the areola. By pushing the breast up, one determines the upper limit of the glandular tissue, and a dotted line is traced representing the necessary undermining.

then perform the deepidermization with the mammotome manufactured by Beaver.

The lower limit of the deepidermization is about 2 cm below the areola. In case of ptosis correction in small breasts, we deepidermize the entire vertical wedge below the areola.

GLANDULAR DISSECTION AND RESECTION

From the lower horizontal line D–E, we undermine the skin down to the inframammary fold and then upward under the lower pole of the breast, to reach the pectoralis fascia (Fig. 89.3A). The posterior aspect of the breast is then freed vertically until the mark indicating the upper limit of the breast is reached (Fig. 89.3B). Laterally, the dissection is limited to avoid injuring the intercostal nerves.

The resection is then performed. An initial incision is made on each side of the drawing (B–D, C–E); the incision is made straight through the skin and the gland, creating a vertical full-thickness incision medially and laterally (Fig. 89.4A). In the upper part, one makes an incision under the central portion of the breast, to leave just 1.5 cm of thickness under the areola (Fig. 89.4B). A vertical and central resection is thus performed.

In case of large breasts with a wide base, it is often useful to associate to this vertical and central resection a circumferential excision at the base of the breast. The breast is lifted, and 2 to 4 cm of breast tissue is resected superiorly, laterally, and medially, at the base of the breast cone. We stop when the desired volume has been attained (Fig. 89.5A).

SUSPENSION BREAST REMODELING

A heavy absorbable stitch is passed through the pectoralis fascia at the upper limit of the undermining, not far from the clavicles (Fig. 89.5B), and the deep aspect of the gland, 2 cm above the areola. This stitch, carefully placed on the line of axis of the breast, plicates the upper part of the breast, filling the upper quadrant and lifting the whole breast (Fig. 89.6).

A strong lower vertical buttress is then constructed by pulling together, with several layers of heavy absorbable stitches, the two glandulous pillars (B–D, C–E) on each side of the vertical excision (Fig. 89.7A). The glandular cone is then reconstructed, the breast stands by itself, and the new, higher inframammary fold is already visible (Fig. 89.7B).

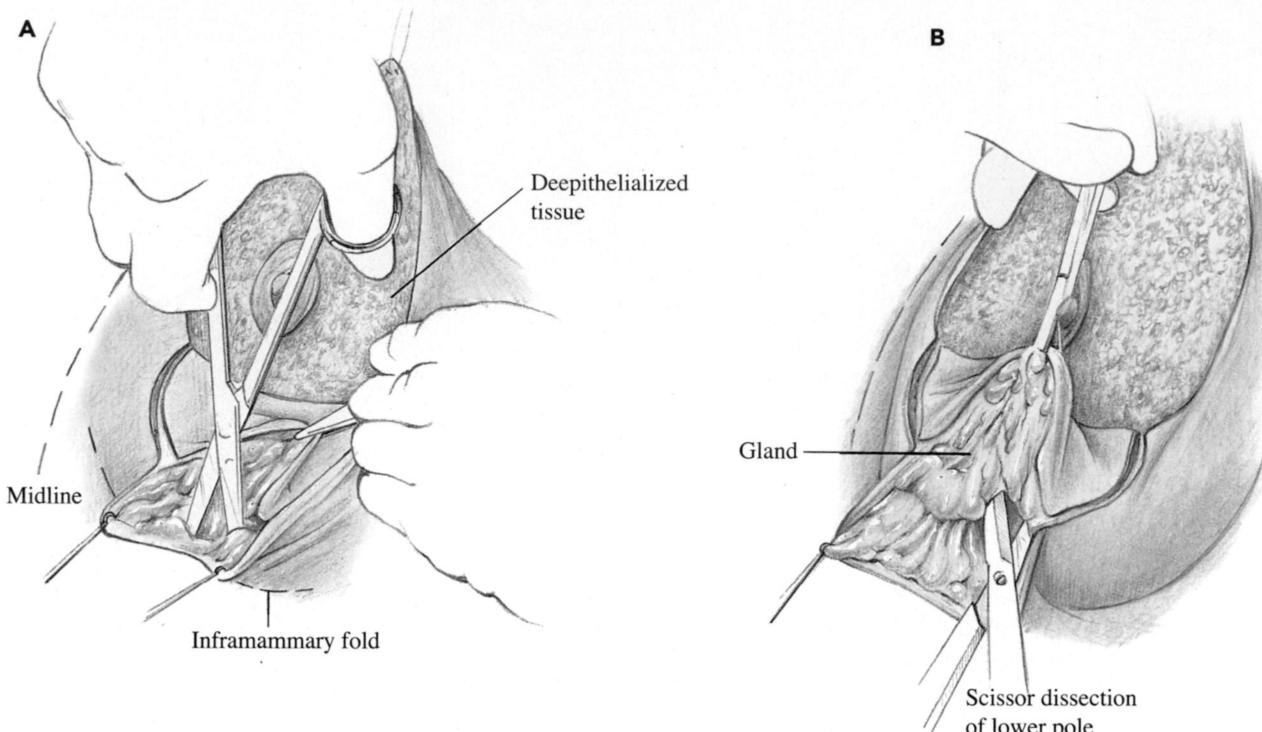

Figure 89.3. Lower and posterior dissection of the gland. **A:** From the horizontal incision, subcutaneous dissection is performed downward to the inframammary fold until the lower part of the breast has been exposed. **B:** The surgeon then dissects behind the gland, in front of the pectoralis fascia, until the dotted upper limit visible (Fig. 89.2B).

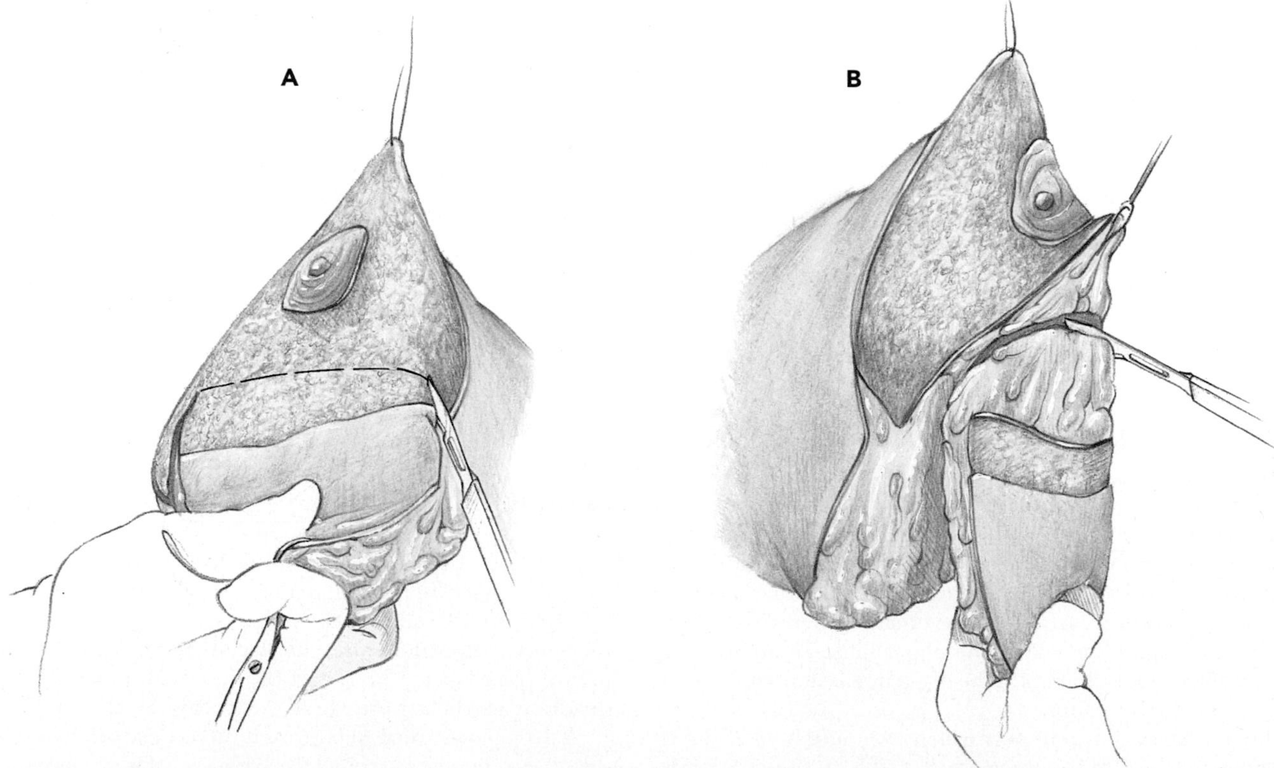

Figure 89.4. Glandular resection. **A:** With the hand introduced behind the gland, a vertical cut is made on each side along lines C–E and B–D (Fig. 89.2A), cutting through all the elements—dermis, fat, gland—in continuity, like cutting a slice of cake. **B:** While the areola complex is held horizontally by the assistant, the surgeon performs the central resection, keeping a thickness of about 1 cm under the areola.

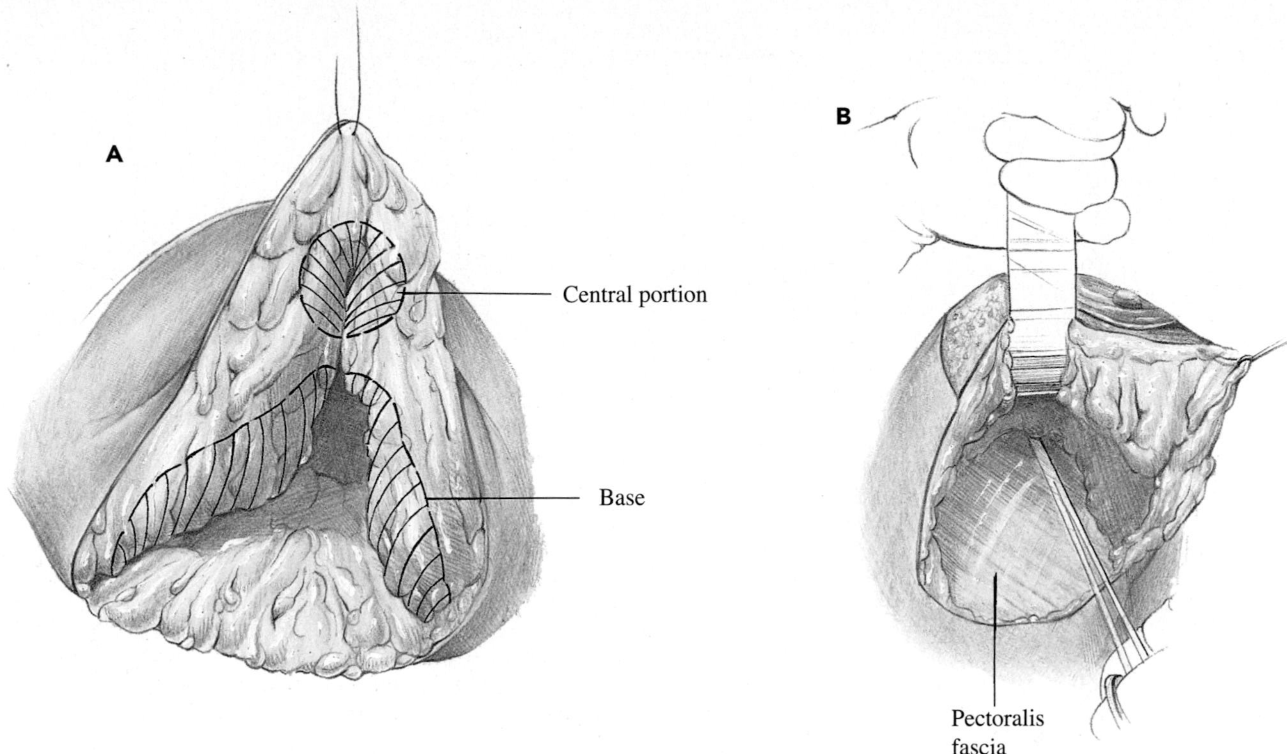

Figure 89.5. Additional resection and suspension. **A:** When the volume of the breast needs to be further reduced after the lower and central resection, more breast tissue is removed: (1) at the base of the cone, especially in large and wide breasts; (2) in the central portion. **B:** Once the desired volume has been reached, a suspension stitch is placed in the pectoralis fascia at the upper limit of the undermining.

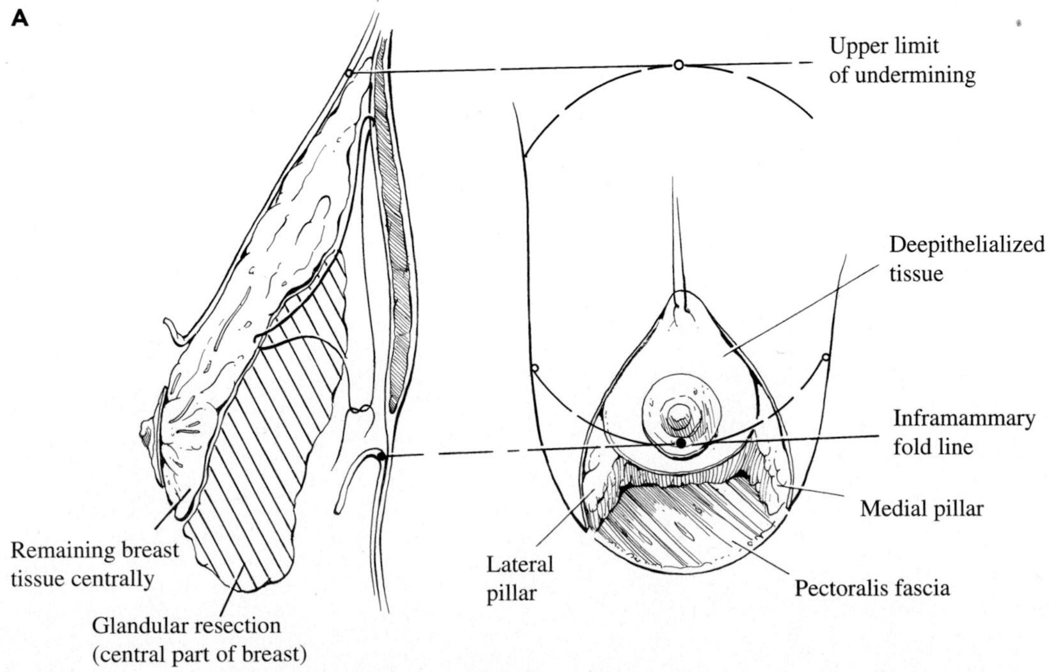

Figure 89.6. Suspension and plication of the breast. **A:** A 2-0 stitch is placed through the pectoralis fascia at the upper limit of the undermining and through the breast tissue, above the areola. (*continued*)

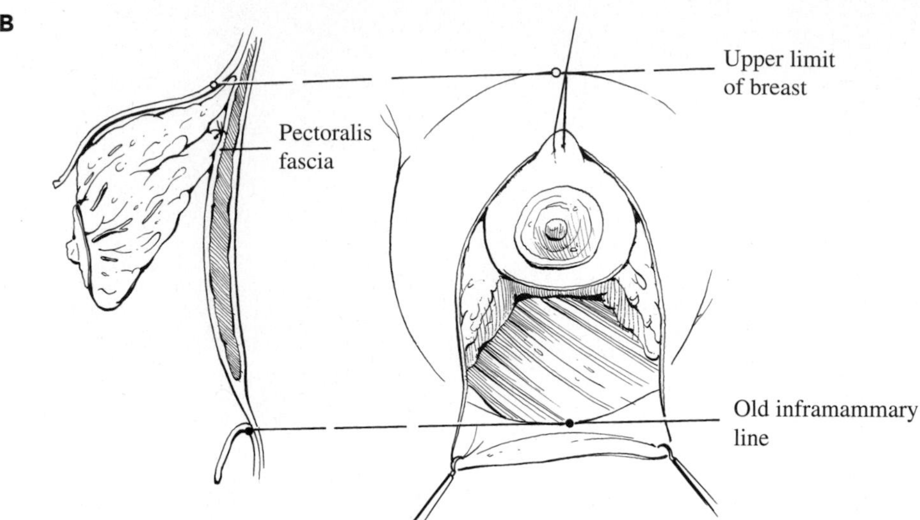

Figure 89.6. (*Continued*) **B:** The breast is plicated to fill the upper quadrant. It is lifted en bloc above the previous inframammary fold.

THE SHORT HORIZONTAL SCAR

At this stage, there is a skin dog ear at the lower end of the vertical suture. One could excise it vertically or absorb it by vertical suturing, after extensive skin undermining.

We prefer to perform a short horizontal incision (5 to 9 cm, depending on the size of the breast), lift the lower skin flap thus created, and excise it (Fig. 89.8A). There is a discrepancy between the upper and lower edges of the incision, but it is easily compensated. It is important to defat carefully on each side of the horizontal incision to help define the new inframammary fold located 1 to 1.5 cm above the original inframammary fold (Fig. 89.8B).

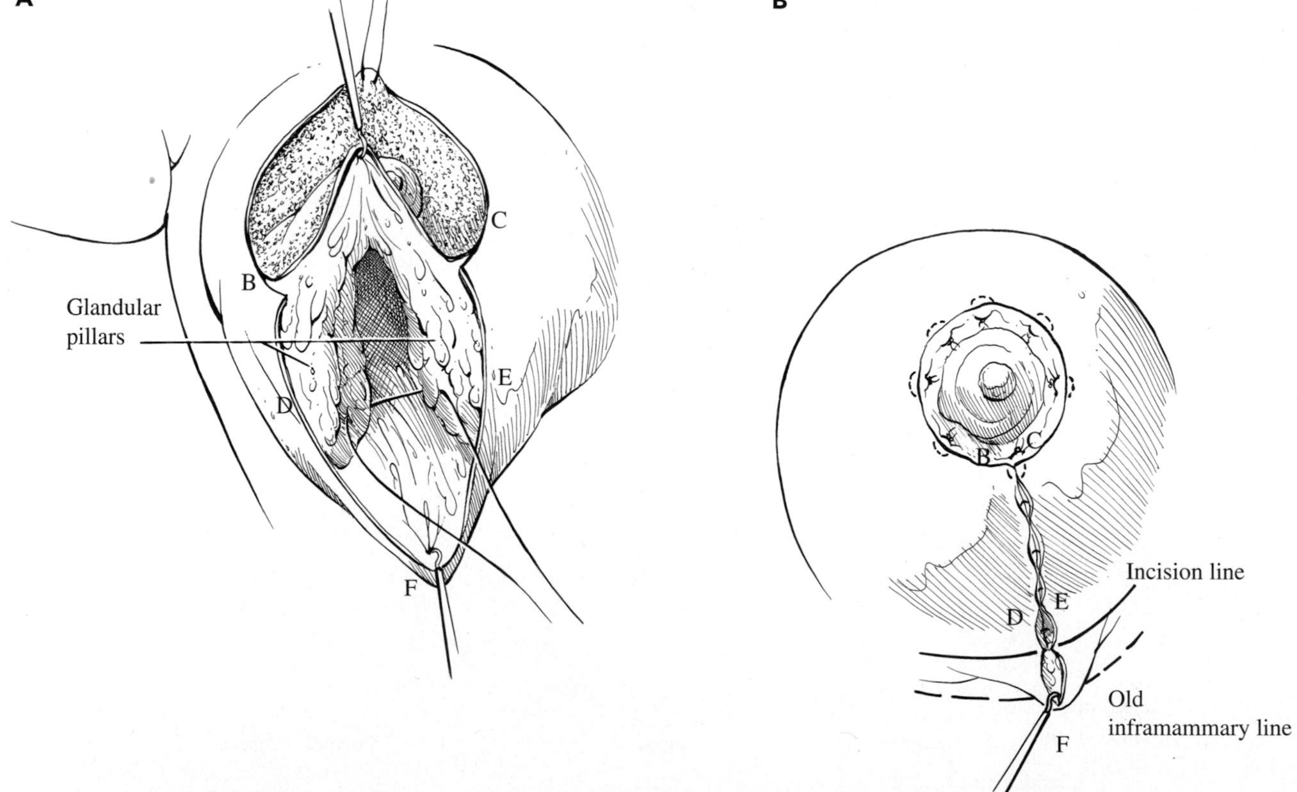

Figure 89.7. Construction of the lower pillar and vertical suture. **A:** The medial and lateral glandular pillars (usually on line with the skin incisions C–E and B–D) are sutured together in several layers. **B:** The breast now stands by itself, and new inframammary line marks itself at the level of D–E if the width of the skin and glandular excision has been well planned.

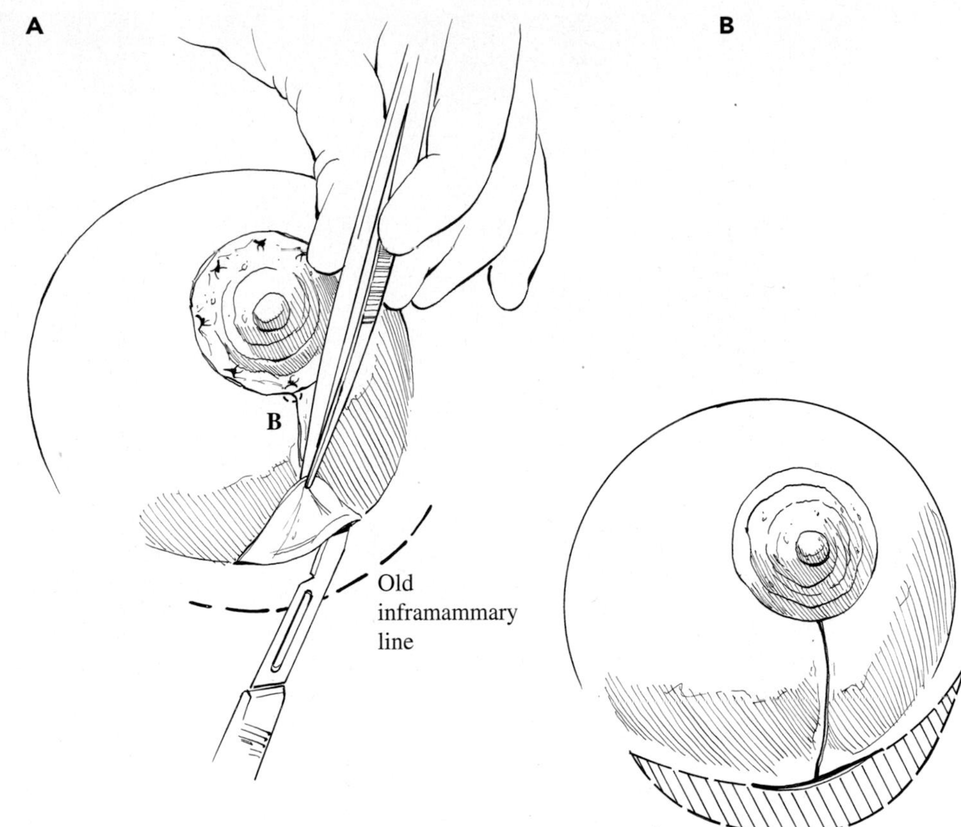

Figure 89.8. The short horizontal line. **A:** After the horizontal incision has been made at the level of D–E, the lower flap thus created is lifted and a short incision is made horizontally. **B:** The hatched area represents the area of previous mammary skin, which becomes abdominal with the elevation of the new fold. In this area, removal of residual gland and defatting must be meticulous, especially at the two extremities. In addition, one should leave a thick layer of fat to match the abdominal wall below.

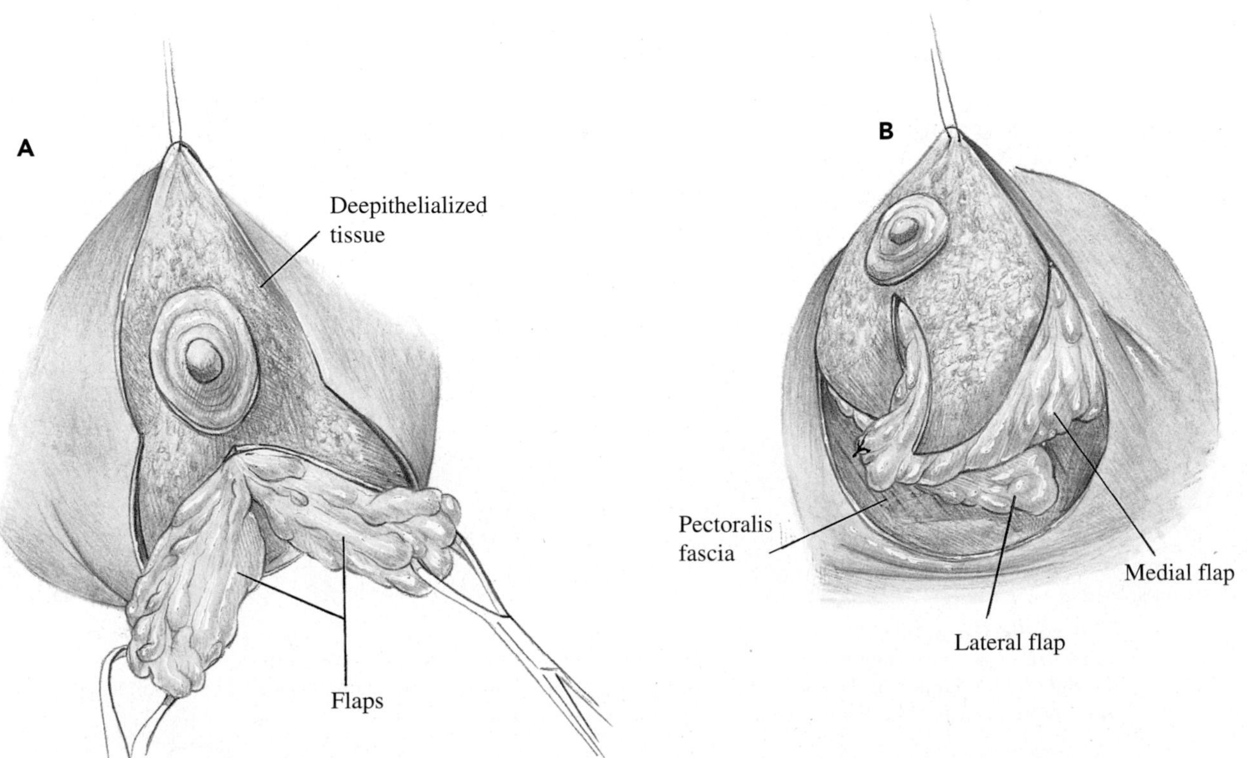

Figure 89.9. Ptosis correction. **A:** A vertical incision up to the areola is made on the lower part of the gland once it has been undermined inferiorly and posteriorly. **B:** The two flaps of gland and deepithelialized skin are overlapped: The lateral flap is first sutured medially and the medial flap sutured above it under tension.

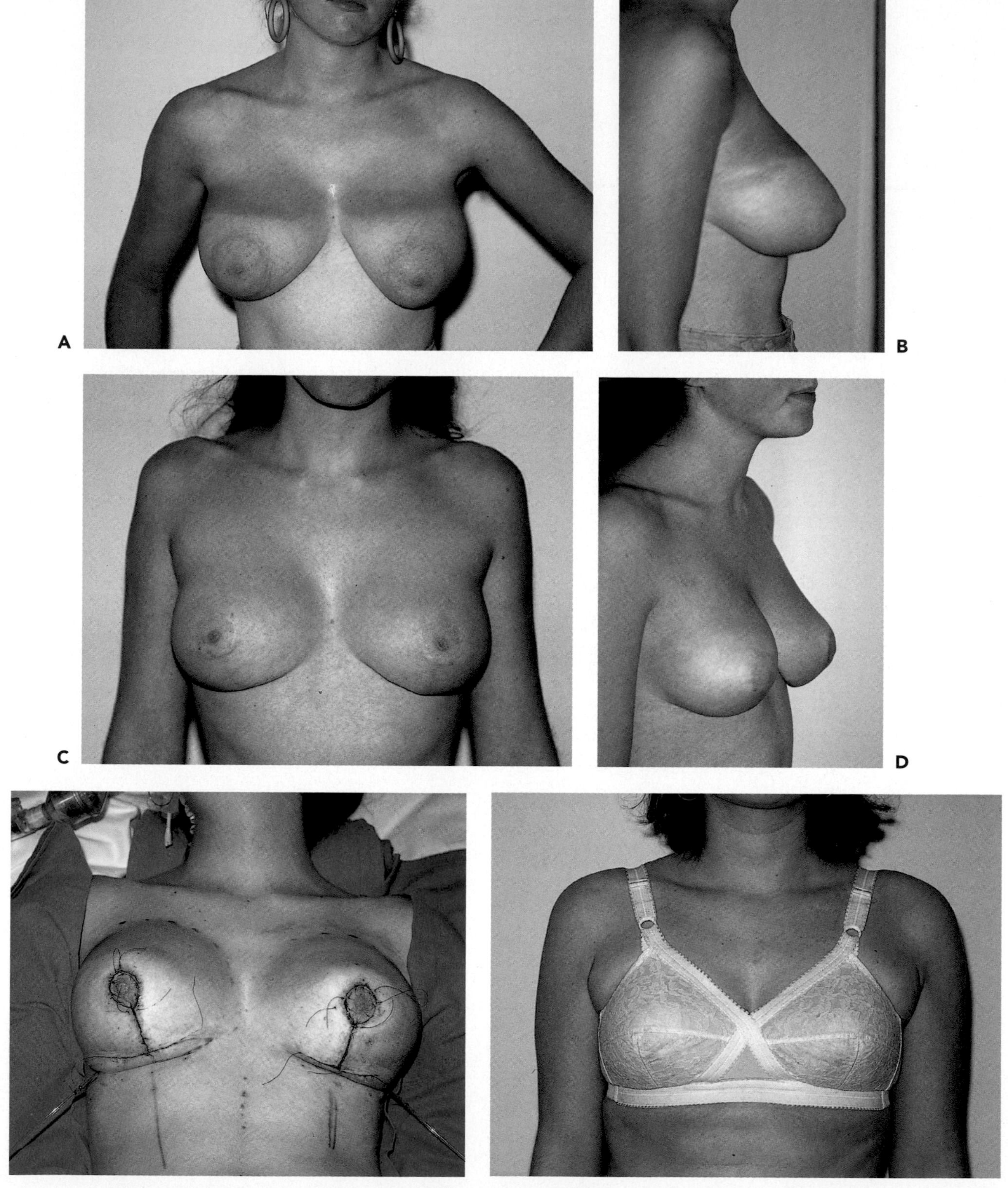

Figure 89.10. **A, B:** A 17-year-old girl presenting with an asymmetric hypertrophy and ptosis. **C, D:** One and a half years after mammaplasty, with removal of 300 g on the right side and 250 g on the left. **E:** Because the right breast was initially larger, the skin pocket located under the new inframammary scar is more visible. **F:** A bra with a wide strap is worn continuously for 2 weeks. (*continued*)

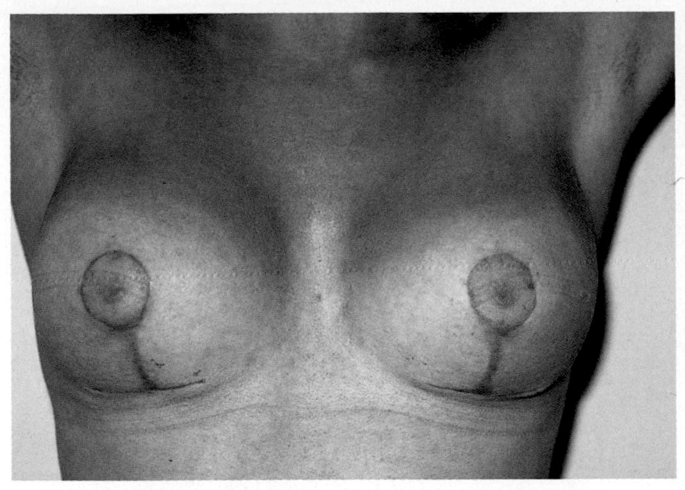

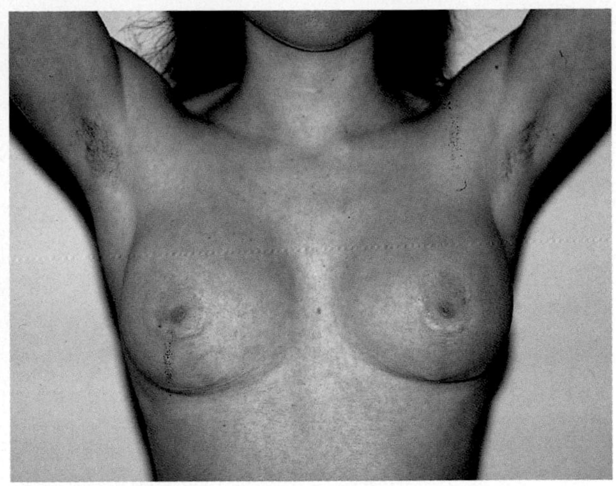

Figure 89.10. *(Continued)* **G:** Two months after surgery, the skin pocket has flattened. **H:** One and a half years after the operation, the inframammary scar is short and hardly visible.

AREOLA ADJUSTMENT

Usually the limits of the deepithelialized areas can be readily sutured to the areola. If we feel that there is still an excess of skin, we perform a purse-string–like stitch around the limits of the deepidermization and pull the stitch to obtain the desired tension. We then mark a new circle and perform an additional deepidermization.

When there is some tension on the periareolar suture, we place a slow absorbable periareolar deep suture in the dermis and pull it to obtain the desired size to fit the areola.

SPECIAL BRASSIERES

This technique produces a little horizontal skin pocket between the previous inframammary fold and the new one. It must be carefully defatted, but also must be flattened for several weeks by a brassiere with a wide lower strap. This brassiere is placed after completion of the surgery and worn day and night for 2 weeks and daily for another month.

PTOSIS CORRECTION

After deepidermization of all the marked areas and liberation of the lower pole and posterior aspect of the gland, a vertical incision is made up to the areola. The deepithelialized dermis is incised at the limit of the skin to allow mobilization of the dermis attached to the gland. The suspension is performed, and the lower epidermoglandular flaps are overlapped and sutured together (Fig. 89.9).

CLINICAL EXAMPLES

The first case (Fig. 89.10) demonstrates how the technique allows an easy correction of asymmetry and the importance of the continuous pressure provided by a brassiere with a large lower strap to flatten the skin pocket created between the old and new inframammary lines.

The second case (Fig. 89.11) demonstrates that this technique can be applied to large breasts with minimal sequelae and a stable long-term result.

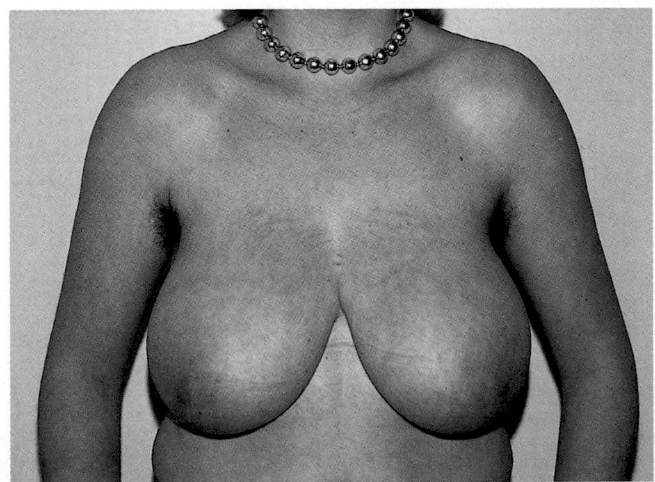

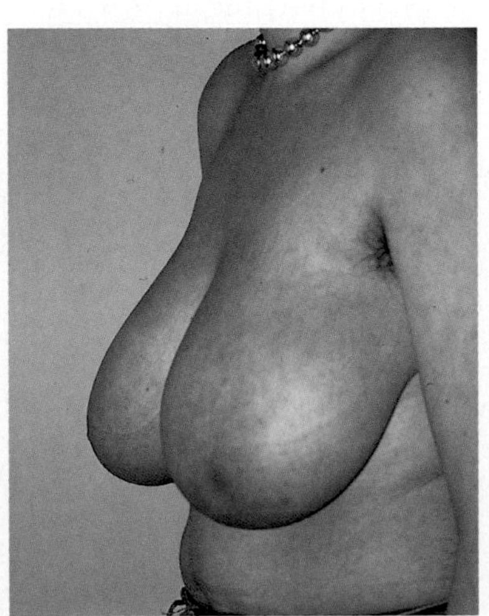

Figure 89.11. **A, B:** An 18-year-old patient with mammary hypertrophy and ptosis. *(continued)*

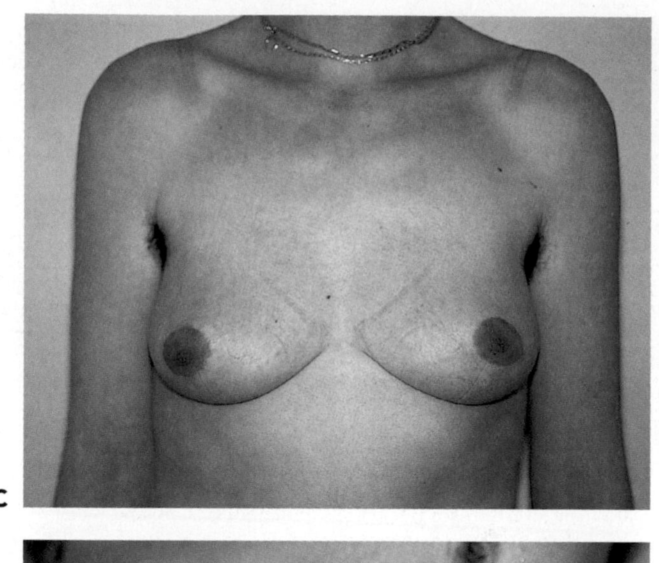

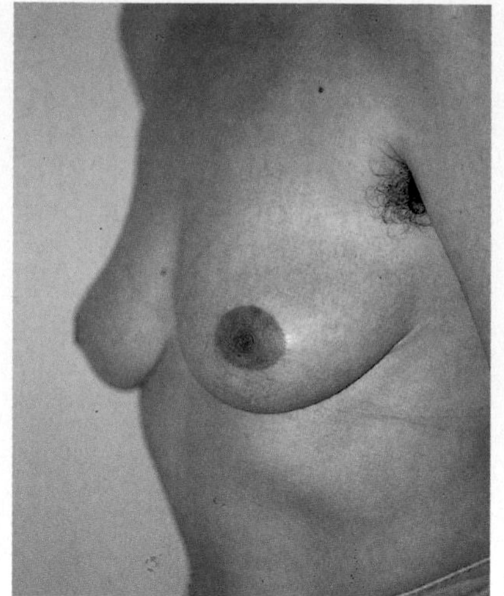

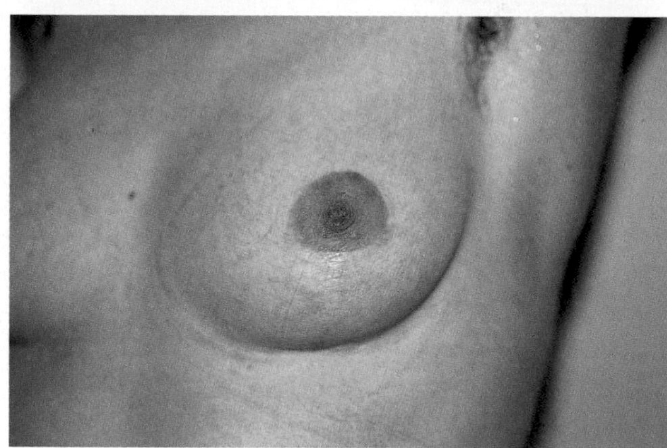

Figure 89.11. (*Continued*) **C, D:** Ten years after the mammaplasty with a 750-g resection of breast tissue on each side. In the interval, the patient lost weight and had one pregnancy but did not try to breast-feed. **E:** The close-up shows only a slightly visible scar.

EDITORIAL COMMENTS

Daniel Marchac provides an excellent review of his technique of vertical mammaplasty with a short horizontal scar. This methodology is similar to the techniques of Madeline Lejour and Claude Lassus, both of which are also described in this book. Marchac's technique varies from the other two by preferring to excise the dog ear created by the vertical mammaplasty at the time of surgery rather than waiting to see to what extent the skin will redrape and contract, thus reducing the need for excision of the dog ear.

I have used Dr. Marchac's technique on many occasions and was with him in Paris as he was developing the technique in the late 1970s. This is essentially a superior pedicle-type breast reduction, with a central or vertical glandular resection. It allows a great deal of flexibility at the time of surgery and therefore is useful in cases of asymmetry or bilateral moderate hypertrophy.

By delaying the creation of a transverse incision until the end of the operation, the creation of a short horizontal scar using the Marchac technique is unavoidable. Although cosmetically less desirable than the results of the Lejour and Lassus techniques, which do not produce a transverse scar, many American patients feel that the predictable, attractive result that is immediately visible after surgery is well worth the price of the short horizontal scar. In any case, the trade-off between the short transverse scar as described by Marchac or delayed wound healing and gratification as proposed by Lejour is one that can be discussed with the patient before making the final decision between the vertical scar–only technique or the short transverse scar technique.

For surgeons who perform a large number of breast procedures, including breast reconstruction and breast reduction, the vertical mammaplasty with a short horizontal scar as described by Marchac is a helpful tool to complement other mastopexy and reduction techniques such as the Lejour technique, the Lassus technique, and techniques associated with a vertical pedicle, such as the inferior pedicle technique or the McKissock technique.

S.L.S.

SUGGESTED READINGS

Lassus C. New refinements in vertical mammaplasty. *Chir Plast* 1981;6:81–86.

Lejour M. *Vertical Mammaplasty and Liposuction.* St. Louis, MO: Quality Medical; 1994.

Marchac D. Reduction mammaplasty with a short horizontal scar. In: Goldwyn R, ed. *Reduction Mammaplasty.* Boston: Little, Brown; 1990:317–336.

Marchac D, De Olarte G. Reduction mammaplasty and correction of ptosis with a short inframammary scar. *Plast Reconstr Surg* 1982;69:45.

CHAPTER

90

Martin Moskovitz

Breast Reduction by Liposuction Alone

INTRODUCTION

Traditional breast reduction techniques use various incisions and pedicles to form a smaller and less ptotic breast. Technically, however, a breast reduction is an operation to reduce breast size. Ptosis correction, although desirable in many cases, has been a corequisite of breast reduction surgery due to prior limitations of surgical technology that required skin incisions to accomplish reduction. Traditional breast reduction removes large blocks of skin, fat, and glandular tissue, often in contiguous pieces. Pioneering surgeons were logical in designing access incisions that maximize ptosis correction because ptosis is a common concurrent condition. Liposuction, however, has provided plastic surgeons with a method to reduce breast size without incisions. Liposuction breast reduction (LBR) is an excellent method to reduce breast size with minimal scarring and can be used in a large segment of the population. In addition, LBR provides a rapid recovery with minimal complications.

INDICATIONS

Breast hypertrophy is the obvious indication for reduction surgery. Candidates for LBR must have chief complaints directly related to their breast hypertrophy (Fig. 90.1). Pain, often in the neck, shoulder, and back, is a common complaint, and patients will often have a history of orthopedic or chiropractic care directed at these ailments. Intertrigo, poor posture, and bra-strap grooves are also common findings in breast hypertrophy patients. Difficulty with exercise and activities of daily living can also be directly attributable to hypertrophic breasts. Finally, although not necessarily medical conditions, difficulty finding proper clothing and awkwardness in social situations are common concerns for many patients with large breasts.

Candidates for LBR must also have a significant fatty component to their breasts. Patient biometrics and age are the best predictors of fat content. Patients with significant fatty deposits elsewhere on their bodies are those most likely to have fatty breasts amenable to LBR. Fatter patients tend to have fatter breasts, whereas thin patients often have predominantly glandular breast hypertrophy.

As patients age, they undergo significant glandular atrophy with replacement by fat. This process increases the success rate of LBR in older patients. Although many patients in their teens and 20s will do well with LBR, patients older than 40 years will almost universally have a successful outcome.

Asymmetry is another excellent indication for LBR. Traditional asymmetry correction relies on excisional techniques, breast implant placement, or a combination of the two procedures. These operations result in scars on the breast or possible long-term asymmetry due to implant action on one side of the chest alone. LBR removes mass without scars and does not introduce the unpredictable factor of unilateral implant placement. As long as patients will accept two breasts both of smaller proportion, LBR is an excellent alternative to traditional operations (Fig. 90.2).

Guidelines based on age, height, and weight are not universal or immutable, and there are relatively thin patients who have significant fat deposits in their breasts. Similarly, although the surgical success rate increases with age, many patients in their teens and 20s have excellent outcomes with LBR. It is important in preoperative discussions with LBR patients to give a general sense of the likelihood of successful reduction surgery based on the parameters available (Fig. 90.3).

There is currently no pragmatic preoperative test to assess fatty breast tissue volume. Mammography is unreliable in delineating the successful LBR patient because it is designed to look for calcifications and breast architectural abnormalities, not fat and glandular differences. Although radiologists often comment on glandular or fatty tissues in their official mammogram readings, in practice many patients with glandular readings have significant fatty deposits.

Some women note that their breast size increases with weight gain and decreases with weight reduction. This finding does have positive predictive value regarding LBR, and women with this situation will tend to do very well with LBR. This finding does not, however, have negative predictive value. Many patients do not lose weight in their breasts until they have achieved a state of near starvation, despite a significant fatty breast component, and they will do well with LBR surgery.

Physical examination is also limited in its ability to discern a fatty breast from a glandular one. Age and biometrics, therefore, remain the most useful predictors of success in LBR.

Concurrent medical conditions can also make LBR an intelligent alternative operation. Patients with conditions that preclude general anesthesia or a longer operating time make LBR a good option. Likewise, older patients in their 60s, 70s, and 80s may be better candidates for a faster procedure with a shorter recovery (Fig. 90.4).

CONTRAINDICATIONS

The main contraindication for the use of LBR is a chief complaint of breast ptosis. Traditional breast reduction techniques, or mastopexy alone, are much better operations for those patients who complain predominantly of ptosis-related issues.

Many patients complain of both size and ptosis issues. The majority of these patients are good candidates for LBR as long as they understand that ptosis correction will be limited to what the natural elastic recoil of their skin can supply. Patients desiring ptosis correction beyond what is possible by elastic recoil alone should be counseled to undergo traditional breast reduction surgery. Because there is no way to accurately predict how much ptosis correction can be gained through recoil, it is wise to give patients a "worst-case scenario" in which their ptosis remains unchanged. If patients think they would be satisfied

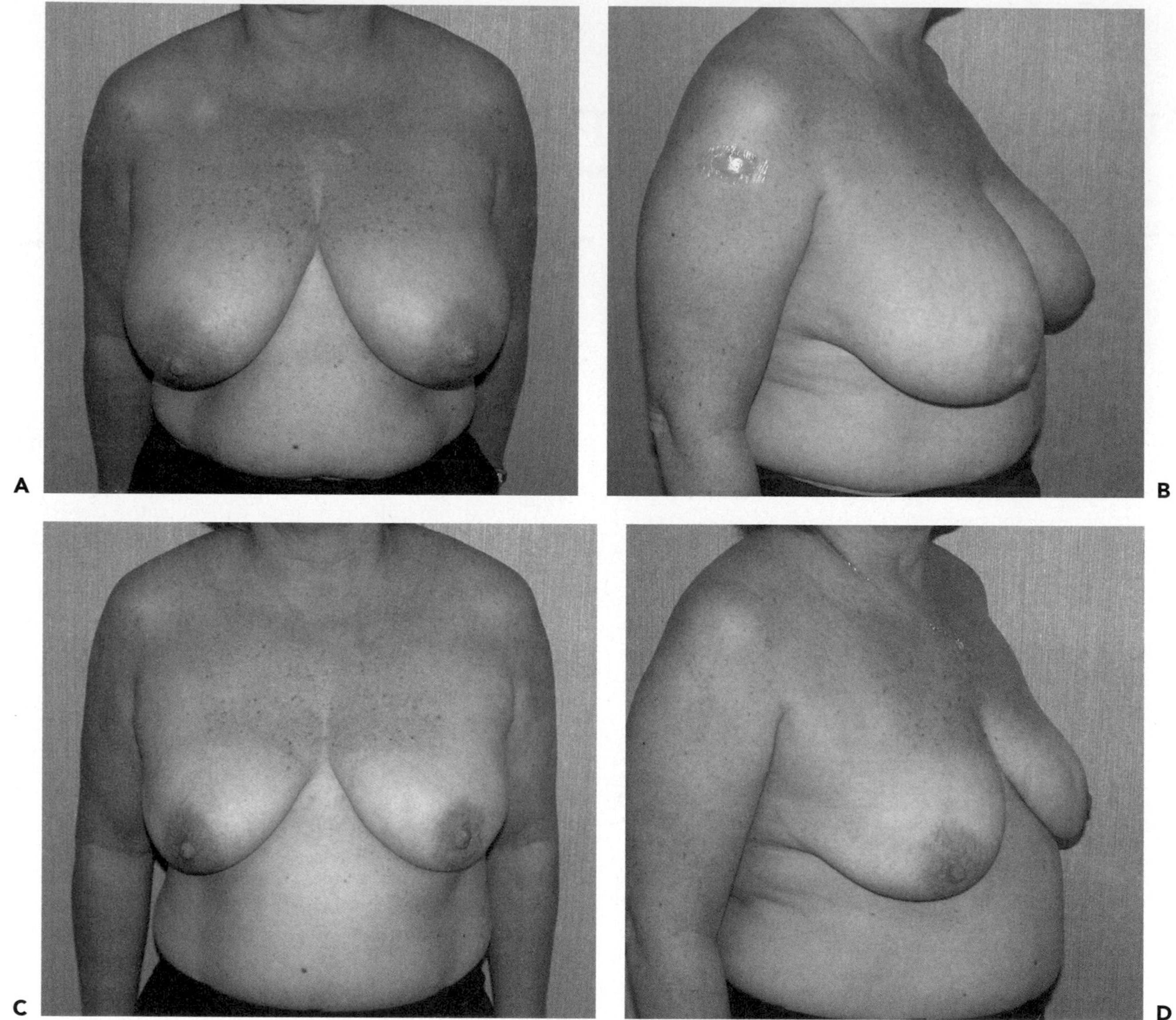

Figure 90.1. **A, B:** Preoperative views of a 46-year-old woman, 4′11″, 130 lb, DD bra cup. Patient complaints included back/neck pain and difficulty with daily activities. **C, D:** Six-month postoperative views; 650 cc fat removed from each breast. The patient now wears a C cup bra.

with smaller breasts and ptosis similar to their preoperative situation, they will usually be satisfied with the outcome of LBR. Ptosis will not increase after LBR because no new skin is created. In addition, the vast majority of patients will have a demonstrable ptosis correction, although often not of the magnitude possible with traditional mastopexy/reduction techniques.

The fact that patients with a chief complaint of ptosis are not suitable candidates for LBR does not, however, mean that patients with ptosis cannot be treated. The key is that the chief complaint be size and weight related. Previous publications (1,2) limited the role of LBR to those breasts without ptosis and, by doing so, confined the scope of this operation to a small percentage of patients. This limitation was based on the idea that breast reduction must be accompanied by ptosis correction. A broader view of patient desires, however, has shown that many patients will accept residual postoperative ptosis if they can be spared the extensive scarring of traditional reduction techniques. Large individual series (3) and outcome studies (4) have shown that LBR can be administered to a wide range of patients with good results.

The other significant contraindication to LBR is breast hypertrophy due to glandular components. Cases of virginal hypertrophy and very thin patients with large breasts and little to no body fat will probably fail LBR and should be advised to undergo traditional breast reduction surgery.

Smokers can tolerate LBR well but do run a higher risk of skin-healing complications. Smokers should stop smoking 2 weeks before surgery and refrain from smoking for 2 weeks after surgery.

Patients with fibrocystic breast disease do not pose a problem for LBR, although patients should be told that although their breasts will be smaller, the overall character of their fibrocystic breast symptoms will not likely change. Patients

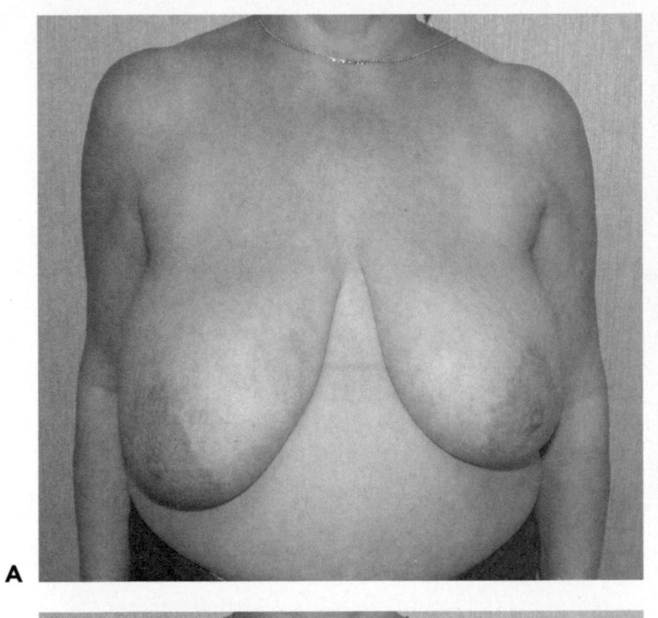

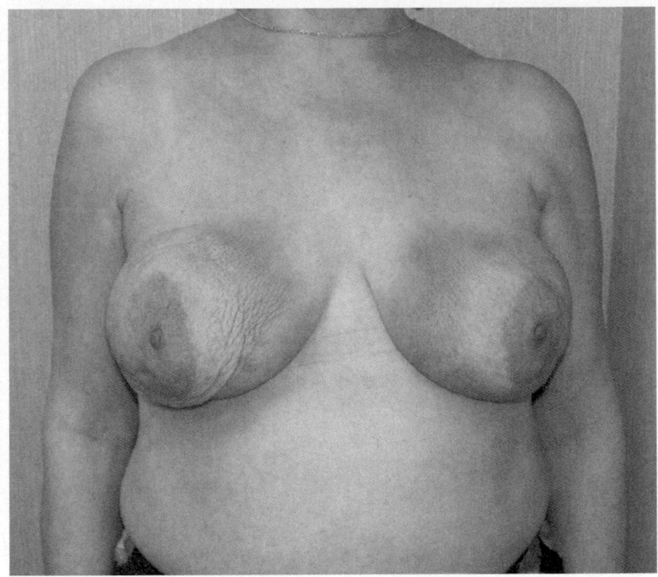

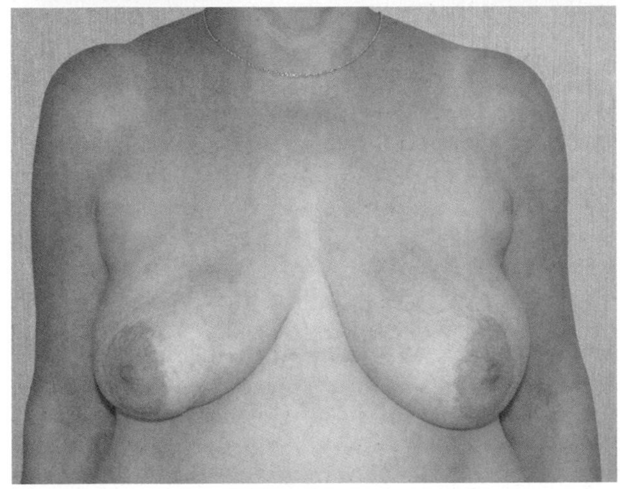

Figure 90.2. **A:** Sixty-four-year-old woman, 5′4″, 160 lb, D cup on left, DDD cup on right. **B:** One month postoperatively; 350 cc of fat removed from left, 900 cc from right. Note the significant skin retraction beginning bilaterally. **C:** Six months postoperatively. The patient now wears a C cup bilaterally.

with ongoing breast conditions, such as recurrent infections or cancer, should be counseled to seek treatment of these issues before considering any breast surgery. Postpartum patients should wait 6 to 9 months from the time they stop all lactation until surgery to avoid rare complications such as galactocele.

SURGICAL TECHNIQUE

PREOPERATIVE WORKUP

The workup for LBR begins with a physical examination, including careful breast palpation to locate any masses or nipple discharge and examination of the skin for irregularities. Blood tests should include required preoperative laboratory tests based on the patient's age and history. Mammography must be performed on all patients older than 40 years and those younger than 40 years with a significant family history of breast cancer. Studies have shown that many cases of breast cancer after traditional reduction mammoplasty take place in patients who did not have screening mammogram preoperatively (5).

SURGERY

Few markings are needed for LBR. The "danger zone" is outlined from the clavicle inferiorly, roughly one hand's-breadth (Fig. 90.5). Most hematomas will start from perforators off the lateral thoracic, acromiothoracic, and internal thoracic arteries, all of which lie high on the chest wall and far from the breast tissue to be resected. In the supine position, however, the delineation of the upper portion of the breast can be obscured, and the surgeon can inadvertently pass the cannula through this area, yielding little fat with a higher risk of hematoma. The most common site of bleeding is the acromiothoracic perforator located several centimeters inferior to the midpoint of the clavicle (6).

Markings are also made for lateral chest fat deposits, which are quite common in heavier patients and are found as a ridge extending from the lateral aspect of the breast to the back (Fig. 90.6). Treatment of these deposits dramatically helps patients in finding the proper bras and in purchasing clothing more easily.

Breast size discrepancy should be noted at this time. The larger side is clearly marked, and an estimate of the percentage asymmetry is written on the larger breast. In most cases, a visually

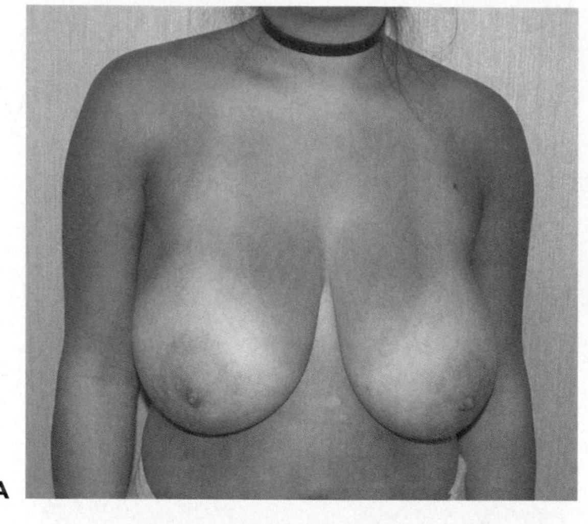

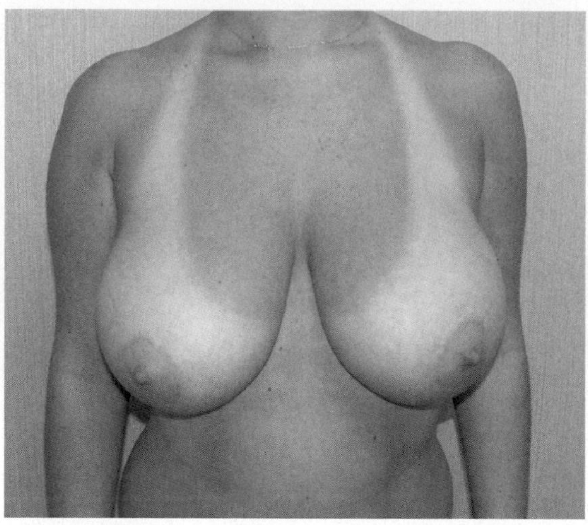

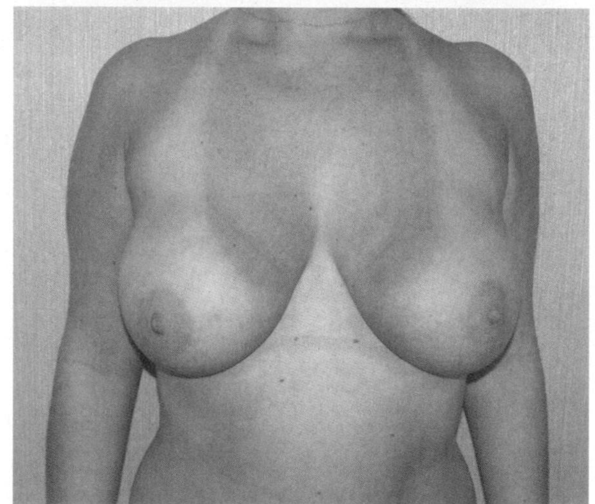

Figure 90.3. **A:** Twenty-one-year-old woman, 5′2″, 143 lb, 36DD bra. **B:** Twenty-five-year-old woman, 5′3″, 135 lb, 34DD bra. **C:** Patient B experienced a reduction from a DD to a C cup with removal of 800 cc fat from each breast. Patient A failed LBR and had no substantial change.

perceptible difference will represent at least a 20% volume difference, and many cases will have asymmetries of 20% to 40%. Surgery performed primarily for asymmetry will often have volume differences of 40% to 80% (Fig. 90.2).

The patient is brought to the operating room and placed in the supine position with arms out on armboard extensions. The incision sites for cannula insertion are marked (Fig. 90.7). One site on each breast is usually sufficient. The incision should be marked 1 to 2 cm *above* the inframammary fold in the anterior axillary line. Placement above the inframammary line prevents inadvertent jamming of the cannula handle into the abdomen and avoids the need to torque the cannula to allow safe and easy motion. Placement in the anterior axillary line allows for easy access to all fatty areas of the breast, including the lateral chest fat deposits. Very large breasts (G/H cup) may require an additional incision above the inframammary fold close to the sternum.

Anesthesia consists of intravenous sedation or inhalational anesthetic via laryngeal mask. Endotracheal intubation can be used but is not necessary. The patient is prepped and draped in standard fashion, and the incision sites are injected with local anesthetic. Stab incisions are made with a knife, and standard tumescent solution is instilled. This solution is usually 1 L of normal saline with 30 mL of 1% lidocaine and 1 mL of 1:1,000 epinephrine. The lidocaine content can be reduced if desired, but because it allows the anesthesiologist to use less medication, it does provide a marked benefit. The tumescent solution is placed throughout the breast tissue in three dimensions to allow for complete suctioning from the skin level to the pectoralis fascia.

Liposuction is then performed in standard fashion. A 4-mm cannula works well in the vast majority of patients, although a 6-mm cannula can be used to speed surgery in cases in which greater than 1,500 cc of fat are removed per breast. The cannula is directed to all areas evenly and thoroughly (Fig. 90.8). Irregularities and contour defects are not common in breast liposuction because the cannula is directed to all areas aggressively.

In cases of breast asymmetry, the surgery should always commence on the larger side. This allows maximal reduction on the larger side, which can be matched on the smaller breast. Beginning on the smaller side could result in a reduction that cannot be matched on the larger breast, and the patient would then be left with smaller, asymmetric breasts. Most women prefer a smaller reduction with breasts that are even.

The lateral chest area is far more sensitive to pain than the breast itself, and it is advantageous to suction that area first so additional boluses of medication are not given at the end of the procedure as the surgeon is preparing to finish the case and move the patient to the recovery area.

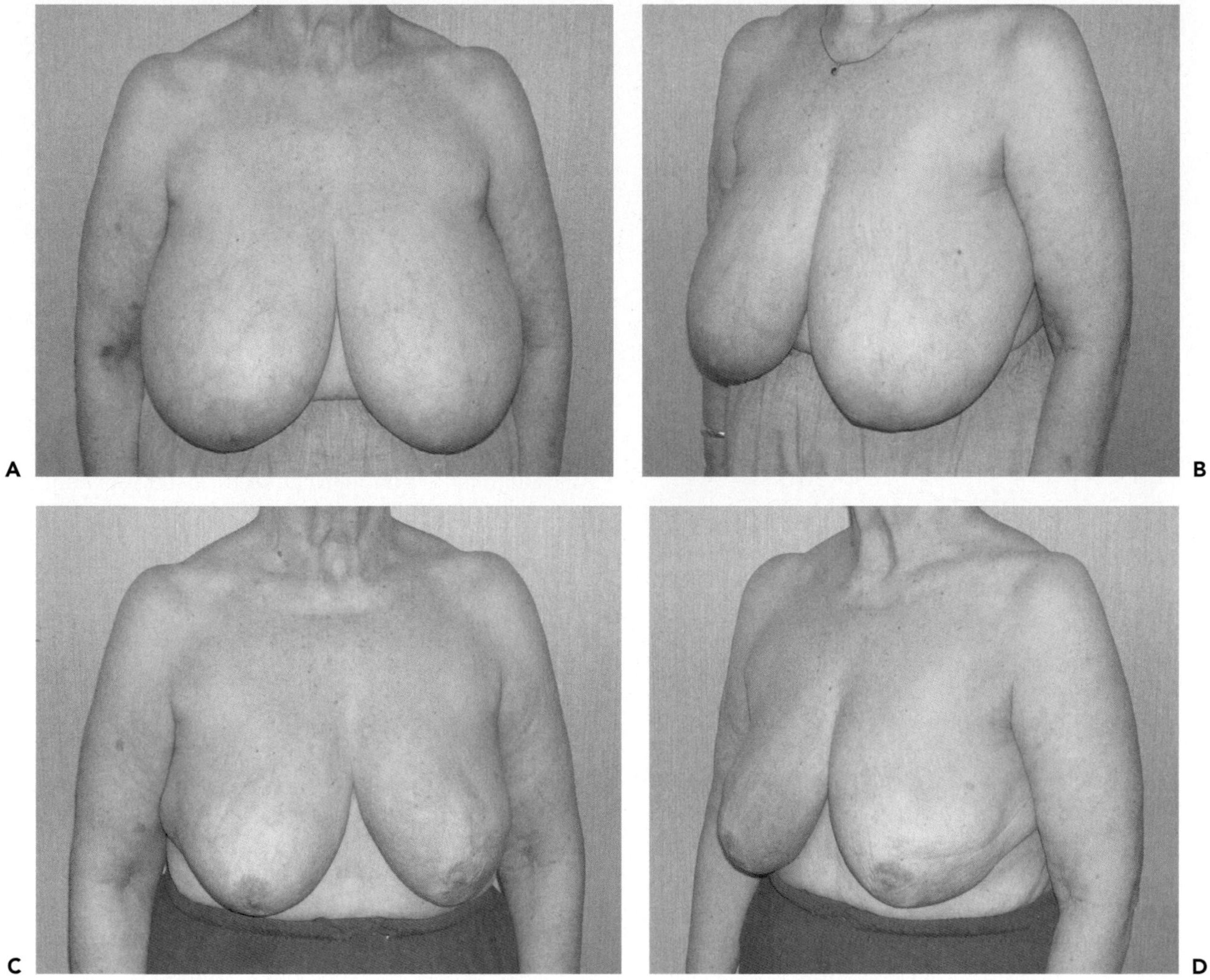

Figure 90.4. **A, B:** Preoperative views of a 70-year-old woman, 5″5′, 185 lb, DDD bra cup. **C, D:** Four months post removal of 1,700 cc of fat from each breast. The patient now wears a C cup bra.

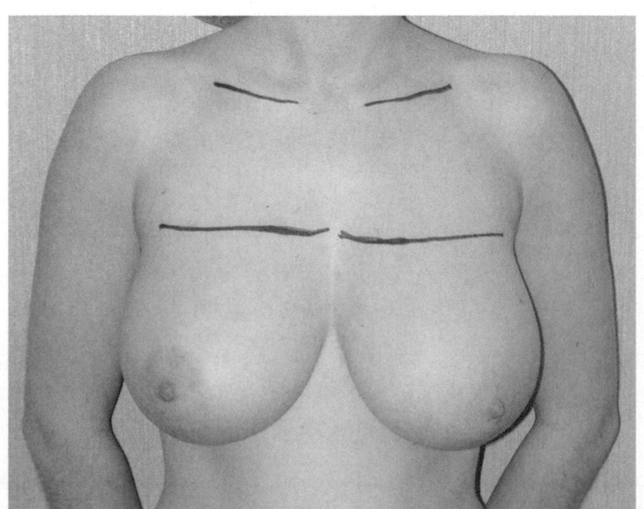

Figure 90.5. An area one hand's-breadth inferior to the clavicle is marked off to be avoided during surgery. This area contains little breast tissue but can easily be traversed during surgery and cause a hematoma.

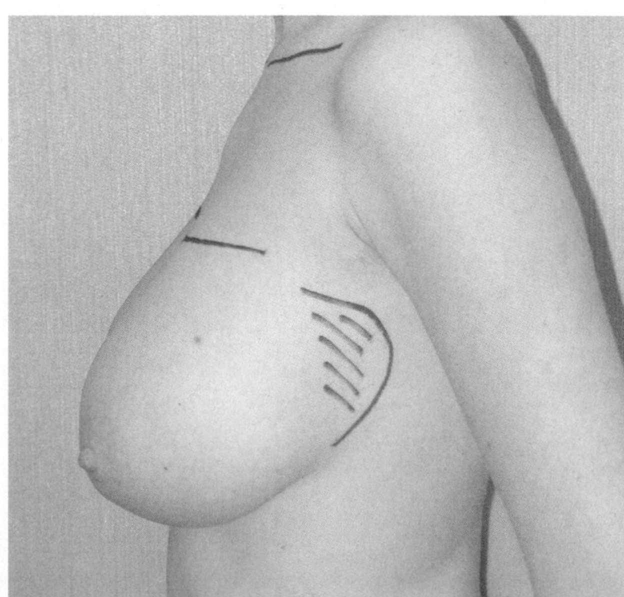

Figure 90.6. The lateral chest fat pads are marked (*hatched area*). Any asymmetry should also be marked directly on the breast to avoid confusion during surgery.

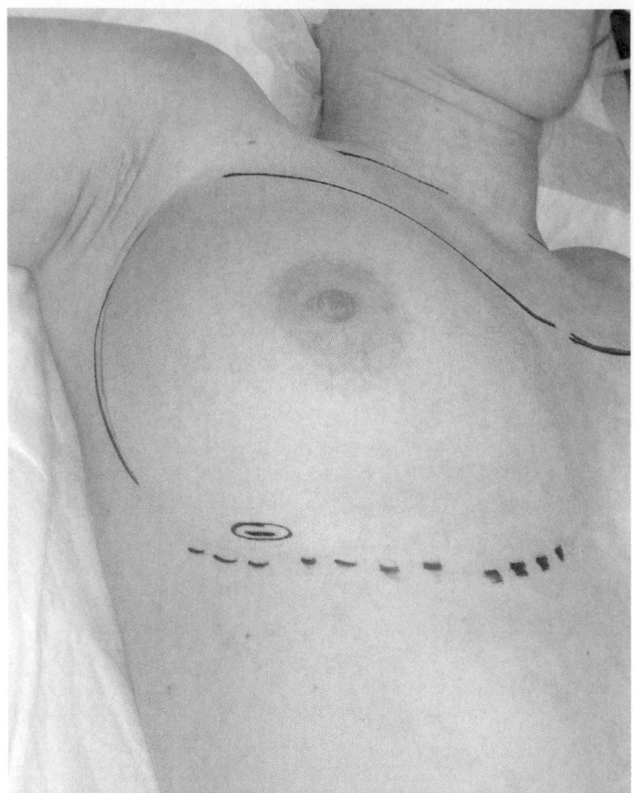

Figure 90.7. The incision site (*circled*) is marked above the inframammary crease (*dashed line*).

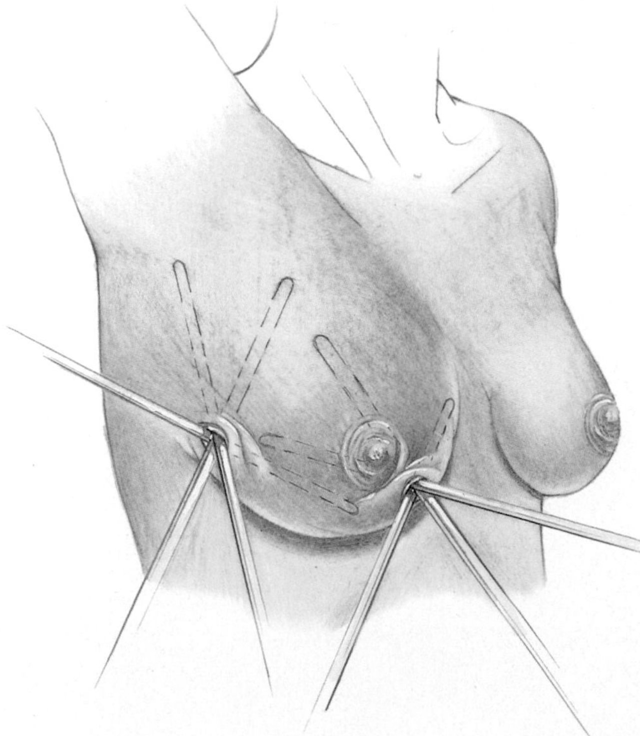

Figure 90.8. The cannula is passed throughout the breast evenly. A second insertion site can be made medially in very large breasts if needed.

The endpoint of surgery is usually reached when no further fat is returned or when the aspirate becomes bloody. Overresection of the breast using liposuction alone is nearly impossible because the skin and glandular tissue remain behind and provide substantial bulk. Individual cases in which a limited reduction is desired may require earlier termination of liposuction.

The nature of liposuction makes equal reduction of the breasts simple and provides a terrific tool in cases of asymmetry. The aspirate can be viewed easily and equal amounts removed on each side. Likewise, in asymmetry cases, a predetermined excess can be removed from the larger breast and then confirmed with physical examination. During surgery, total aspirate levels can be used as a guide because they will tend to settle to equal amounts of fat and fluid over time. The endpoint in asymmetry patients depends on whether one or both breasts are treated. If both sides are addressed, the endpoint is symmetry as seen on the operating room table. If only one breast is treated, that breast should be left slightly larger than the contralateral untreated breast at the conclusion of surgery. Swelling and tumescent solution can mask the true breast volume slightly and risk that when the treated breast is fully healed it may be slightly *smaller* than the unoperated side.

Liposuction of the breast should be more aggressive and complete than liposuction of other areas. Although aggressive liposuction of the lateral thigh, for example, would produce contour deformities and seromas in many cases, liposuction of the breast rarely, if ever, suffers from either complication. The generous lymphatics of the chest preclude seromas, and contour irregularities do not occur because the breast has been evenly suctioned throughout and is not tented tightly over a muscle base that accentuates contour deformities.

Dressings consist of an absorbent pad over the incision site and a bra followed by a tight, abdominal-type binder or Ace wraps placed around the chest.

Patients should be monitored in the recovery room for 1 to 2 hours and can be discharged as per accepted criteria. Pads should be changed as needed prior to discharge, and, to prevent blister formation, patients should not be sent home with large amounts of tape on their skin.

Histopathology of the liposuction aspirate is routinely performed to comply with the current norm of practice. Multiple aspirate specimens are examined, and reports are noted. Most samples demonstrate fatty tissue, often without demonstrable breast tissue characteristics.

RECOVERY

Patients should change the absorbent pads as needed during the evening after surgery. Feminine napkins make an excellent dressing for this purpose because they are clean and very absorbent. The dressings should be changed at least once overnight to prevent any skin creases that may have formed at the initial dressing. These creases may lead to tissue ischemia if not prevented.

Patients must be aware of the leakage they will experience so they do not become unnecessarily anxious. The leakage is light red in color and similar to that of any other liposuction procedure. Patients should understand that as long as their breasts do not swell, the drainage is normal.

Dressings should be changed at an office visit the next day, and the patient should be placed in her bra. To maximize elastic recoil, patients should be instructed to lift their breast into the bra so the nipple points upward or forward. The breast should not be flattened against the chest in a ptotic fashion; it should be lifted as much as possible.

Postoperative pain is mild to moderate and is easily controlled with oral analgesics. The lateral chest fat deposits are the most sensitive areas after surgery, and patients will note significantly more pain in those areas than in their breasts.

Ecchymosis will decrease and resolve over the first 2 to 3 weeks. Induration and a "lumpy" feeling will develop after 2 to 3 weeks and persist for 2 to 4 months. The breasts will look normal but feel irregular. Smokers will take longer to heal and may stay lumpy for 4 to 6 months.

Activity can be resumed as tolerated, with most women going back to work in 3 to 5 days and resuming full exercise in 2 weeks (4).

COMPLICATIONS

HEMATOMA

The most common complication of LBR is hematoma, with a rate of 1% to 3% (4). Nearly all hematomas are noticed in the operating room as bleeding in excess of normal. Breast swelling may or may not be present immediately due to the effect of epinephrine in the tumescent solution. Swelling will often begin 30 to 60 minutes after surgery in the recovery room as the epinephrine effect wanes. Treatment consists of expressing the blood through the incision site. If blood does not easily express, a suction device can be used at the bedside under sterile conditions to evacuate the hematoma. The patient can also be brought back to the operating room if desired. Once the blood has been removed, the patient should be redressed and the binder replaced as tightly as possible. Recurrence of bleeding is very rare; however, monitoring for hematoma is crucial because a large breast envelope can accommodate a significant amount of blood, similar to the volume of fat removed. A recurrent hematoma should be drained again and direct pressure applied to the source area with an open palm for at least 30 minutes. The patient should then be dressed tightly as noted above and monitored for recurrence for at least 2 to 3 hours.

In the weeks after surgery, the breast subject to hematoma will heal more slowly and require extra time for resolution of ecchymosis and induration. At the conclusion of the healing period, however, the two breasts will be symmetric without sequelae of the bleed. (Fig. 90.9).

SEROMA

Despite the aggressive nature of the suctioning procedure, seroma formation is very rare. This is most likely due to the multiple lymphatics of the breast area. Seromas are usually small and superficial and can easily be definitively drained with an 18-gauge needle in one treatment.

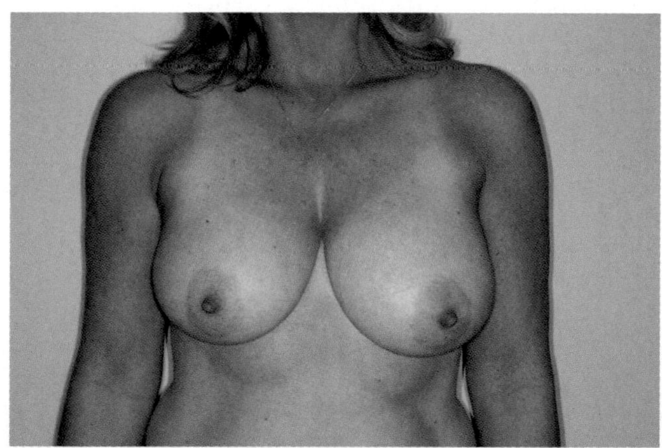
A

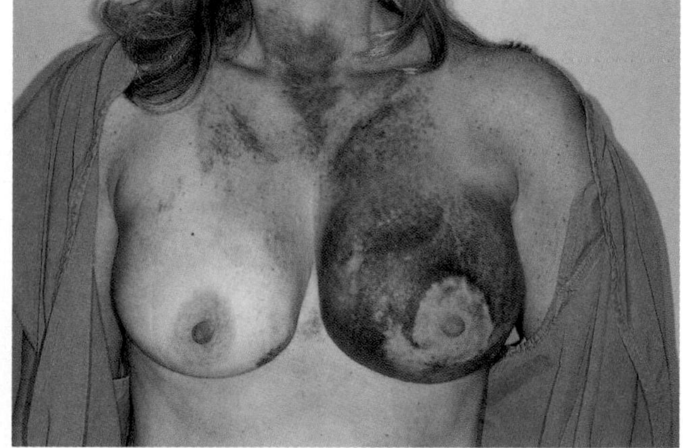
B

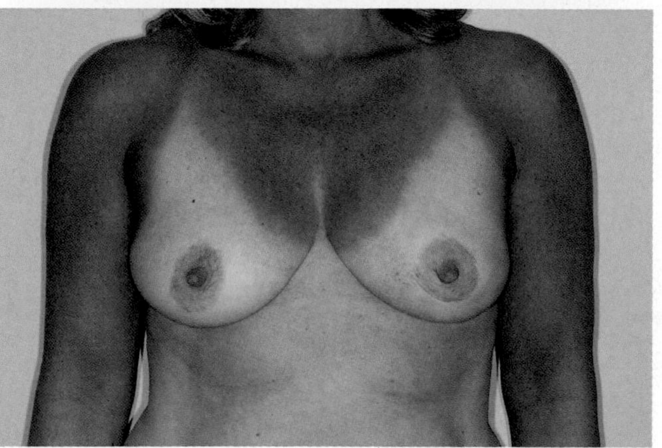
C

Figure 90.9. **A.** Preoperative view of a 41-year-old woman, 5′4″ tall, 130 lb, 36D bra cup. **B.** One week after surgery with postoperative hematoma; 600 cc fat removed from left breast, 500 cc from right breast. **C.** Six months after surgery. The patient now wears a 34C bra.

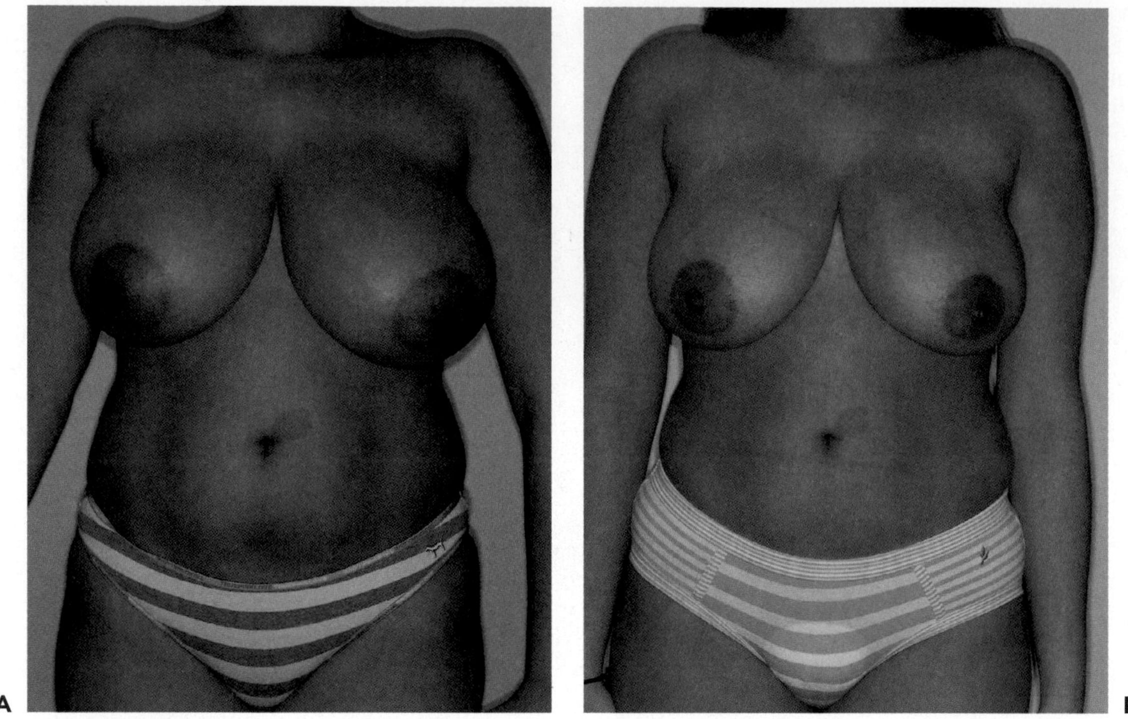

Figure 90.10. **A.** Preoperative view, 23-year-old woman, 5′5″ tall, 150 lb, 36DDD bra with asymmetry. **B.** Postoperative with 900 cc fat removed from left breast and 600 cc from right breast. She now wears a 36C cup bra.

SKIN NECROSIS

Skin necrosis is extremely rare. Smoking is the main risk factor, and necrosis has not been seen outside the smoking population. The event usually begins as an epidermal blister that proceeds to an eschar similar to those of pressure ulcers. These defects usually measure 1 to 4 cm in diameter and can occur on the skin or nipple-areolar complex. Treatment consists of thorough debridement, dressing changes, and cessation of smoking. Scarring will occur when fully healed but is usually acceptable. Scar revisions can be carried out after full maturation if desired.

INFECTION

Infection is rare in LBR, as it is in standard liposuction. Infections should be treated with antibiotics and surgical intervention as dictated by the situation.

NIPPLE INNERVATION

LBR affects nipple sensation to a limited extent. Sixty-seven percent of patients undergoing LBR noted no change in their nipple sensation, whereas 15% noted a decrease and 18%

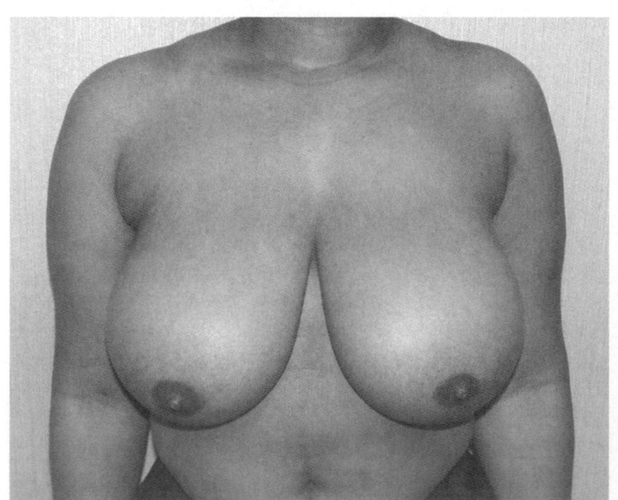

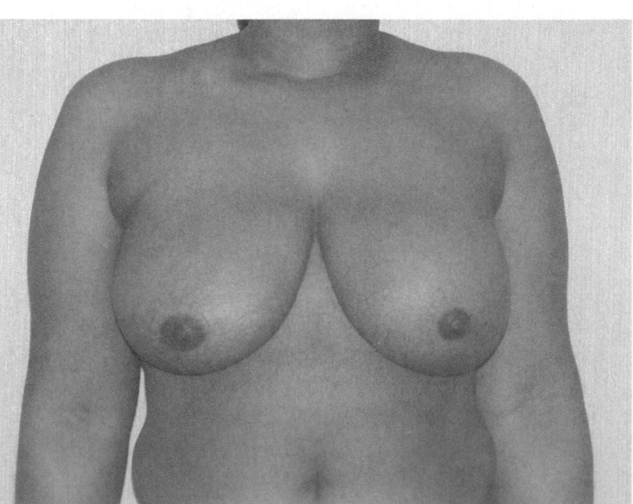

Figure 90.11. **A:** Preoperative view, 25-year-old African American woman, 5′1″, 140 lb, DD bra cup. **B:** Three-month postoperative view, 800 cc fat removed from each breast, C cup bra.

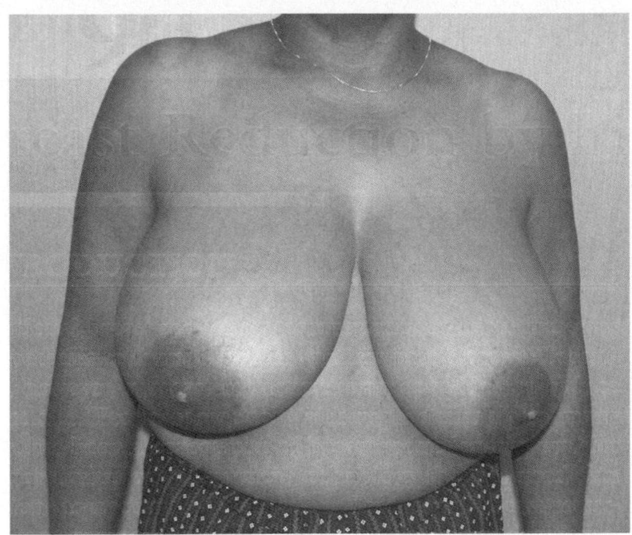
A

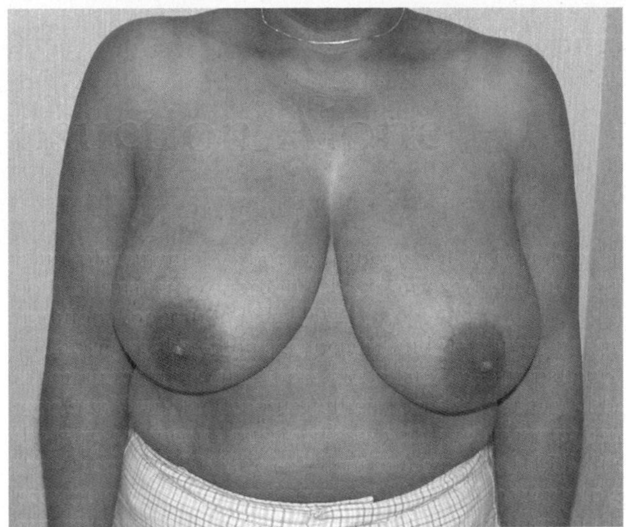
B

Figure 90.12. **A:** Preoperative view of a 46-year-old woman, 5′2″, 167 lb, DD/DDD cup bra with moderate asymmetry. **B:** Three-month postoperative view; 1,100 cc removed from left breast and 800 cc from right breast. The patient now wears a D cup bra bilaterally without difficulty.

noted an increase in sensation (4). No cases of complete sensation loss were noted.

UNDERRESECTION

Although not technically a complication, underresection of tissue is the most common complaint from LBR patients. The most crucial preventative measure for this complication is patient education and honest dialogue. Patients must understand that there is no dependable way to gauge the amount of fat in their breasts, and glandular tissue may limit the reduction. Patients who understand this concept will accept the risk in return for fewer scars and will be more comfortable with the situation should it arise. Patients who are ignorant of the possibility of underresection will feel cheated and angry. Therefore, it is important to also have a financial contingency plan for those patients who fail liposuction reduction completely or who are clearly underresected. This plan will help patients understand their situation regarding finances and surgery before the procedure.

PATIENT SATISFACTION

One of the most important measurements of surgical efficacy is patient satisfaction, and outcome studies have become a mainstay of surgical care evaluation. A more recent outcome study in LBR (4) has shown that the procedure is effective in alleviating patient complaints and providing measurable results. More than 90% of patients complaining of pain due to breast hypertrophy (shoulder, chest, back, neck) noted significant or complete symptom elimination. Ninety-six percent of patients with intertrigo noted symptom improvement, and 88% of patients reported that their shoulder bra-strap grooves were improved or eliminated. Patients noted an average reduction of two bra cup sizes after surgery, with some cases reporting a four-cup reduction. In addition, 70% of patients believed their breast ptosis was noticeably improved by LBR. On average, patients returned to work in less than 5 days and resumed exercise by 11 days. Ninety-two percent of respondents would recommend this operation to a friend, and 87% would choose LBR again. Equally important, these excellent reports were obtained with a complication rate of less than 2%.

BREAST CANCER ISSUES

The use of standard tumescent liposuction does not introduce any form of electromagnetic energy or other potential carcinogenic sources, so it does not carry a realistic risk of carcinogenesis. Although probably safe, the use of ultrasonic liposuction does involve a source of energy that could be accused of introducing some element of risk. The safety of ultrasonic liposuction in the breast is yet to be determined, and its use must be considered along with the high prevalence of breast cancer in our society.

Mammographic review has shown that LBR does not cause calcifications of the breast or other stigmata that may be confused with breast carcinoma. Some scarring of the subdermal layer is common and is similar to that found after traditional reduction. This scarring does not mask cancer nor is it easily confused with breast carcinoma.

CONCLUSION

LBR is an excellent surgical modality to treat breast hypertrophy (Figs. 90.10 to 90.12). The procedure has an above-average safety profile, and the technique is already known to plastic surgeons familiar with standard liposuction. It is, however, important to apply the technique to the proper patients, as well as to have a clear and educational dialogue with patients prior to surgery. As in many aspects of medicine, patient education, involvement, and choice have become much more important in the administration of care. LBR demands careful discussion to ascertain patient desires and to gain an insight into patient expectations. Many patients will choose LBR as an alternative to traditional breast reduction because they want a reduction in their breast size and volume and they object to some aspect of traditional breast reduction. Some patients object to the scarring, whereas others want a more rapid recovery. In any case, LBR offers a much-needed alternative to traditional breast reduction. LBR does not, however, replace traditional breast reduction. The blanket application of any one technique is a mistake, and the use of LBR in the incorrect patient is sure to yield an unsatisfactory result. The addition of LBR to the ever-growing armamentarium of plastic surgical care allows for improved patient care and increased patient satisfaction.

EDITORIAL COMMENTS

The basic goal of any breast reduction technique is to reduce the volume of the breast and relieve the upper torso complaints common to these patients. Of course, the overwhelming majority of these patients will also have some element of ptosis, and nearly every technique described for breast reduction involves some sort of ptosis correction. Dr. Moskovitz is quite right to step back and question whether ptosis correction is a required element for any given patient. As he notes, the scarring associated with standard breast reduction can be disconcerting to some patients, and persistent ptosis after breast reduction may be an acceptable outcome if these scars can be avoided. Certainly, a fatty breast is easily reduced with standard liposuction, and Dr. Moskovitz has documented the symptom relief that results after liposuction breast reduction alone. Assuming persistent ptosis is not a significant concern for the patient, the major issues that arise using this technique involve breast cancer detection. It is reasonable to conclude that liposuction of the breast should not create any more postoperative architectural distortion or scarring than standard open breast reduction, and this point is confirmed by Dr. Moskovitz. Certainly, postoperative mammography 6 months to 1 year postoperatively can easily be justified to document the postoperative appearance of the breast, just as is commonly done for standard breast reduction patients. It is unlikely that ultrasonic liposuction of the breast poses any increased risk for the development of breast cancer; however, each surgeon must assess his or her comfort level with the technique before proceeding. Given the potentially fibrous nature of the breast, ultrasonic liposuction may offer advantage over traditional liposuction in adequately reducing a patient with a more fibrofatty breast. Although the yield is likely to be low, I agree with the recommendation to send the aspirate for pathologic examination in the off chance that malignant cells might be identified. The disadvantage of a positive finding would be the inability to isolate the tumor to a specific quadrant of the breast, thus rendering lumpectomy an uncertain option. This potential outcome, in addition to the other recommendations for patient education outlined in the chapter, are best discussed with the patient preoperatively to assist in informed decision making.

D.C.H.

REFERENCES

1. Matarasso A, Courtiss EH. Suction mammoplasty: the use of suction lipectomy to reduce large breasts. *Plast Reconstr Surg* 1991;87:709–716.
2. Courtiss EH. Reduction mammoplasty by suction alone. *Plast Reconstr Surg* 1993;92(7):1276–1284; discussion, 1285–1289.
3. Gray LN. Update on experience with liposuction breast reduction. *Plast Reconstr Surg* 2001;108(4):1006–1010; discussion, 1011–1013.
4. Moskovitz MJ, Muskin E, Baxt SA. Outcome study in liposuction breast reduction. *Plast Reconstr Surg* 2004;114(1):55–60; discussion, 61.
5. Keleher AJ, Langstein HN, Ames FC, et al. Breast cancer in reduction mammoplasty specimens: case reports and guidelines. *Breast J* 2003; 9(2):120–125.
6. Corduff N, Taylor GI. Subglandular breast reduction: the evolution of a minimal scar approach to breast reduction. *Plast Reconstr Surg* 2004;113(1):175–184.

CHAPTER

91

Elizabeth J. Hall-Findlay

Vertical Breast Reduction Using the Superomedial Pedicle

HISTORY

Vertical breast reduction has been slow to achieve widespread popularity. Many surgeons are concerned about the learning curve and having to revise the pucker that can occur at the lower end of the vertical incision.

Surgeons realize that patients who are preoperatively informed are willing to accept that some time is necessary for the results to settle in most plastic surgery procedures. This is no different in breast reduction surgery than it is in rhinoplasty, facelift, or liposuction surgery.

Although most surgeons can accept that there is a certain revision rate inherent in most plastic surgery procedures, they find it more difficult to accept in breast reduction. Perhaps this is because the problems (lateral and medial dog-ears, boxy shape, and bottoming out) with the inverted-T, inferior pedicle (1,2) procedures were so difficult to correct that the revision rate remained low.

Despite the development of the vertical approach by Daniel Marchac (3) and also by Claude Lassus (4–6), not many surgeons were willing to try to reduce scarring when they had a method (inverted T, inferior pedicle) that they believed to be safe and reliable. Madeleine Lejour (7–10) popularized vertical breast reduction, but surgeons found the technique difficult and the complication rate too high.

The most common comment that I get from surgeons who try the medial pedicle vertical breast reduction is that they find it so easy and predictable. I initially had problems insetting the superior pedicle, so I tried the lateral pedicle. I assumed that the lateral pedicle would have better sensation, but I found that the medial pedicle actually gave better shape and surprisingly equal sensation. The problem with the lateral pedicle is that the base of the pedicle is the same tissue that we want to remove, and it results in a shape that has excess lateral fullness. I now almost exclusively use a medially based pedicle (11–13). The medial pedicle is easy to inset, is full thickness, has reliable circulation, and has good sensation. My results are best when I keep the pedicle full thickness, when the inferior border of the medial pedicle becomes the medial pillar, when I remove the inferior and lateral breast tissue, and when I minimize gathering of the vertical incision.

Since the mid-1990s, many of the problems with the vertical approach have been addressed, and consistency of results can be achieved. Surgeons who have adopted this approach are often surprised at how fast the learning curve can be. Those who resist the vertical approach can still be heard saying that it becomes a choice of scars over shape. However, once surgeons incorporate the vertical approach for the breast reduction and mastopexy patients, they realize that both the scars and the shape—both short and long term—are significantly improved.

Surgeons who have used the inverted-T techniques have learned to use the skin to reshape the breast. Unfortunately, over time, the skin will stretch, and some bottoming out or pseudoptosis will occur. The concepts used for "vertical" breast surgery are quite different. Instead of using the remaining skin to shape the breast, the nature of the resection and the reshaping of the breast parenchyma are used to shape the skin.

INDICATIONS

Although vertical breast reductions are best used for small to medium-sized breast reductions, the medial pedicle can be used for larger breast reductions even when an inverted T is needed to reduce the skin envelope. Very large reductions or reductions in massive-weight-loss patients are often best performed with a medial pedicle because it allows the surgeon to remove the heavy inferior breast tissue. There are times when a vertical skin excision will not be enough, and the remaining excess will need to be removed with a J, an L, or a T. Surgeons initially do not realize how well the skin redrapes to the new breast shape, and they will convert to a T far more often than is necessary.

Adding a T excision to the skin is rarely needed unless the vertical incision is longer than about 13 to 15 cm. It has been shown that adding a horizontal skin excision does not alter the revision rate (14). It may, in fact, be surprising to learn that it is difficult to know where to actually place the horizontal scar. One of the hardest things for surgeons new to this technique to accept is that a vertical incision of more than 5 cm is far from negative. A longer vertical scar is both necessary and desirable to accommodate the extra projection that occurs with the vertical techniques.

It would be ideal for a surgeon to start getting comfortable with the technique by reducing the opposite side in a breast reconstruction patient. Because reconstruction patients often require revision, there is ample opportunity to correct the inevitable problems that result over the learning curve.

CONTRAINDICATIONS

The medial pedicle vertical breast reduction is far more than just a vertical scar and a pedicle that is easy to inset. The nature of the excision (removing the inferior breast tissue) and the reshaping of the breast are what provide a good, long-lasting shape. Because of this, I will still use the same approach in very large reductions or in postbariatric patients, but I will excise the excess (poor-quality) skin that will not retract.

There are very few contraindications to performing a vertical breast reduction. The real limitations are the length of the pedicle and the amount and quality of the remaining skin.

Blood supply to the nipple may be compromised in a very long pedicle. It is impossible to give a numerical value to this. With growth, puberty, and pregnancy, the breasts become larger and more ptotic. However, as the skin and breast tissue stretch, so do the blood vessels and nerves. When the patient is lying in the supine position, it is clear that the pedicle is not as long as it appears when the patient is standing. The risk of losing blood supply results from the fact that we remove more than 75% of the tissue (and blood supply) from around the pedicle when we perform the resection.

Is the pedicle "superomedial" or "medial"? The pedicle may look as if it is "superomedial" when the patient is standing and the markings performed. However, the blood supply is actually medial, coming mainly from the internal mammary artery at the third interspace. When the pedicle appears to be excessively long, a true "superomedial" pedicle can be designed by incorporating the descending branch of the internal mammary branch that comes from the second interspace. I have "Dopplered" this vessel and transected it in most of my purely medial pedicles, and it almost always enters the areolar opening just medial to the breast meridian usually less than 1 cm deep to the surface. If the base of a long pedicle is carried up into and lateral to the 12 o'clock position of the areolar opening, the arteries from both the second and third interspaces will be included. The pedicle will now be more difficult to inset, but the artery can be preserved by resecting tissue in the deeper aspect of the pedicle, where there is a paucity of blood vessels.

An overly large pedicle may contribute to bottoming out. It may be advisable to suture the bulk of the pedicle up onto the chest wall, but it is questionable whether these sutures are actually as effective as desired. A good alternative in a very large breast is to consider free nipple grafts (15).

OPERATIVE TECHNIQUE

PREOPERATIVE PLANNING

Determination of New Nipple Position

The new nipple position is often best placed at the level of the inframammary fold. I have analyzed my results over the years and have found that there are several patients in whom the level of the inframammary fold is actually misleading, with nipples ultimately being placed too high or too low. What I have found is that the upper breast border (the junction of the top of the breast with the chest wall) is the most static and reliable landmark. The upper breast border does not change in patients in any of the postoperative photos from the preoperative photos. The surgeon can then use this landmark to visualize the result and accurately determine the new nipple position.

It is important for surgeons (and patients) to understand that some patients are "high breasted" and some are "low breasted." The actual attachment or "footprint" of the breast on the chest wall is quite variable from one patient to another. The distance from the clavicle to the upper breast border can be quite short or can be quite long. There are no surgical maneuvers of which I am aware (except implants and fat injections) that can actually raise the level of the upper breast border.

Since the upper breast border is static, it is a good landmark to determine new nipple position. The nipple is usually best located about one-third to one-half the distance up the final breast mound. This point is usually 8 to 11 cm below the upper breast border in an average C cup breast.

It is interesting to note how different both the upper breast border and inframammary fold levels can be from one patient to another. Not only are the levels very different, but also the breasts in some patients have a long vertical attachment to the chest wall (footprint), and some have a very short vertical attachment.

The new nipple position should be determined in relationship to the existing breast upper breast border and not at some arbitrary distance from the suprasternal notch (Fig. 91.1).

Marking the Upper Breast Border. The upper breast border is at the junction of the chest wall and the breast. This is very clear in some patients, with a definite demarcation line, and it is blurred in other patients, where the breast slopes gently away from the chest wall. The upper breast border is usually at the level of the upper edge of the stretch marks. The upper breast border is always below the preaxillary fullness, but in some very low-breasted patients it can be well below that level. These patients need to understand that the breast cannot be lifted on the chest wall, and if their breasts are attached at a low level, they will remain at that level.

Marking the Level of the Inframammary Fold. This level is becoming less important in determining the new nipple position, but it is important in deciding how aggressive the surgeon can be in resecting tissue at the fold in order to elevate the fold itself. Sometimes the inframammary fold can be at quite different levels on the same patient. The surgeon can thus be more aggressive with the resection of the lower fold.

Marking the Breast Meridian. The breast should be divided into halves at the level of the new nipple position. Although it does not matter where the line starts, it is easier to draw it beginning at the clavicle and then making the mark down the breast bisecting it. The nipple looks best slightly lateral to the midline and it is therefore better to err on the side of marking the meridian slightly more lateral. For surgeons who are comfortable with the inverted-T, inferior pedicle type of breast reduction, the meridian can be marked more medially because the medial pedicle vertical breast reduction is usually more effective at removing the excess lateral tissue. It is important not to draw the meridian through the existing nipple position but to draw it at the level of the desired new nipple position.

Marking the New Nipple Position. The new nipple can then be marked at the intersection of the vertical mark (8 to 11 cm from the upper breast border) and the new breast meridian (8 to 11 cm from the midline of the sternum). This position will often be at the level of the inframammary fold but not always. It is important at this stage for the surgeon to stand back and visualize the result to make sure that the nipple is designed at a good level both horizontally and vertically.

The surgeon has more flexibility with nipple position in patients with a very full upper pole, but he or she should place the nipple lower in a patient who has a ski-jump type of slope to the upper half of the breast. Nipples can always be raised if a revision is needed, but they cannot be lowered.

If there is significant asymmetry, the new nipple position should be placed up to 1 cm or so lower on the larger breast. The larger breast can be heavier, and closure of a wider vertical ellipse in the larger breast will push the nipple further up than it will on the smaller breast.

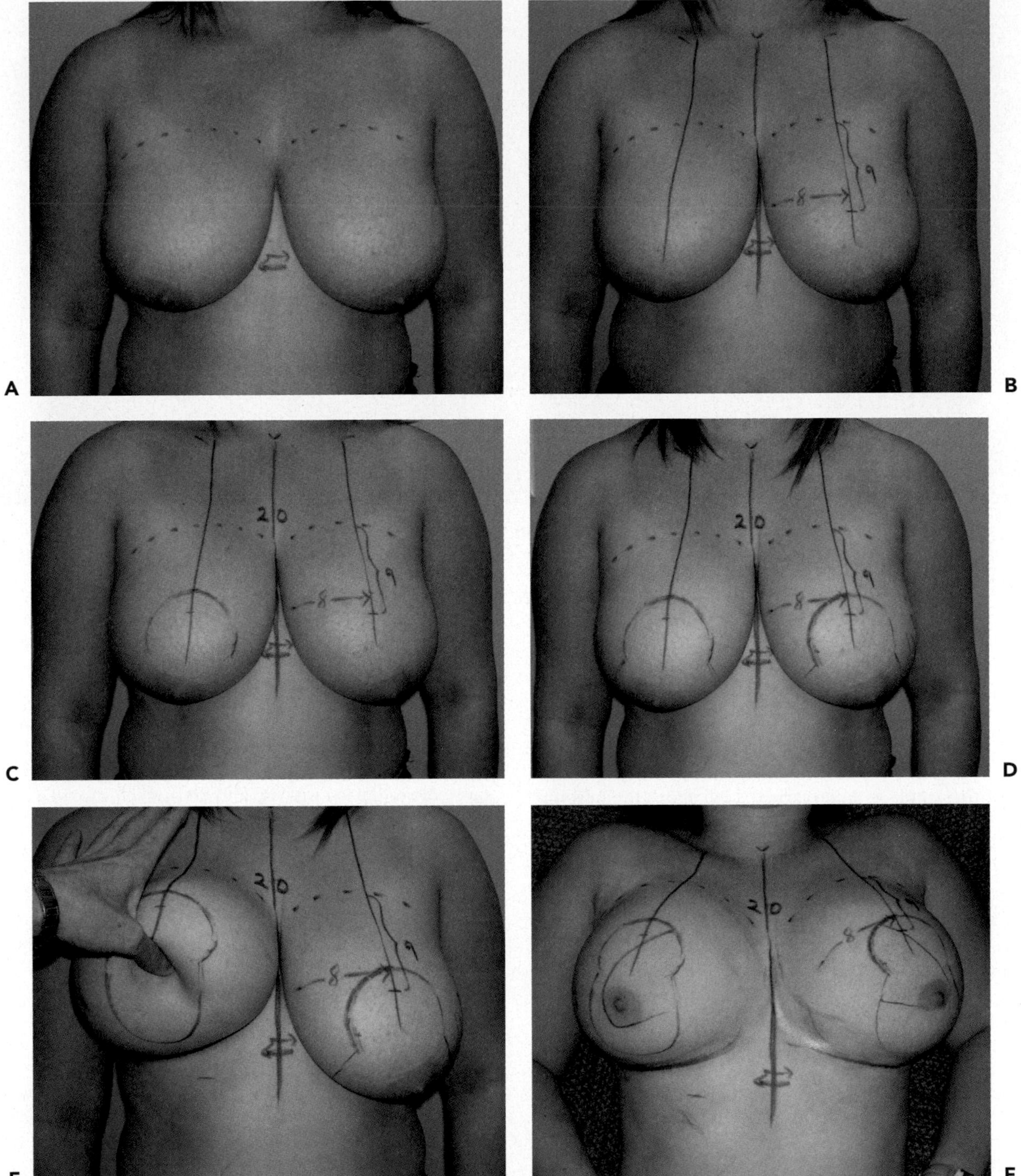

Figure 91.1. Markings. **A:** The upper breast border is marked with a dotted line at the junction of the chest wall and the breast. This patient is "high breasted," with a short distance between her clavicle and the top of her breast. Her inframammary fold level is marked between her breasts, and it is relatively low, showing that this patient has a fairly long vertical breast footprint. **B:** The breast meridian is marked. The meridian should not be drawn through the existing nipple position but through the desired nipple position. In this patient the meridian is marked at 8 cm from the chest midline (through the "air," not around the skin). The new nipple position is marked at the intersection of the breast meridian and at 9 cm from the upper breast border. **C:** The new areola is marked at 2 cm above the new nipple position. It is drawn freehand so that when closed it will complete a circle. It is drawn with a circumference of 14 to 16 cm to match a 4.5- to 5-cm-diameter areola. **D:** Then new nipple position is marked at 20 cm. This is measured from the suprasternal notch but is not determined at some arbitrary distance but as measured from the top of the upper breast border. This patient was 5′2″ tall. The vertical limbs are designed much as one would with an inverted-T approach. **E:** Instead of carrying the vertical limbs of the Wise pattern medially and laterally, they are curved around and joined about 2 to 4 cm above the inframammary fold. The surgeon can pinch the skin to make sure that not too much skin is being removed. The skin closure is not used to hold the breast, so this should be designed for a loose, tension-free closure. **F:** The patient is shown lying down with the areolar opening, the skin resection pattern, and the medial pedicle drawn. The breast slides up the chest wall when the patient is supine. (*continued*)

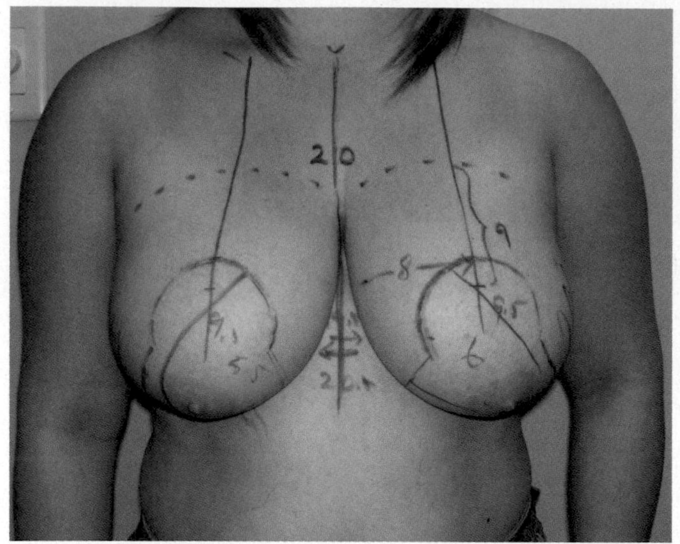

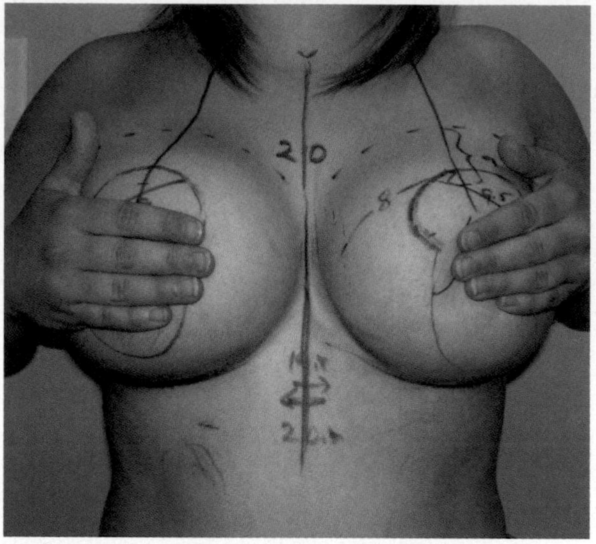

Figure 91.1. (*Continued*) **G:** The final marking with the patient standing. **H:** The final markings shown with the breasts pulled up. The skin resection pattern should be designed as a U rather than a V and it should stay well above the inframammary fold. If a V is used, the surgeon may not remove enough subcutaneous tissue just above the fold, and if the skin pattern is carried down to the fold, the scar will extend down onto the chest wall.

DESIGN OF THE SKIN RESECTION PATTERN

Areolar Opening

The top of the areola is then marked 2 cm above the new nipple position. This accommodates most areolar diameters of 4 to 5 cm. The areola is then drawn so that it will close as a circle. It does not actually need to be mosque shaped since it is probably better to take out more distance vertically than horizontally. The original Wise pattern design (16) was 14 cm in circumference, and this matches a 4.5-cm-diameter areola. A large paperclip can be used as a template because it is 16 cm in length and this matches a 5-cm-diameter areola. If the areola is not a "perfect" circle at the end of the procedure, it is quite simple to make the appropriate adjustments. It is important to make sure that there is symmetry in the design from one breast to the other.

Skin Resection Opening

The lateral and medial breast limbs are much the same as with the Wise pattern. The breast can be rotated laterally and medially to match up the breast limbs with the breast and chest wall meridians. Instead of extending these limbs at 5 cm laterally and medially, the limbs are curved down as a U and joined about 2 to 4 cm above the inframammary fold.

It is important to recognize that the medial pedicle vertical breast reduction does not rely on the skin as a brassiere, and the skin flaps can (and should) be loose enough so that there is no tension on the closure. The surgeon can pinch the skin both with the patient standing and again supine in the operating room to gauge the closure and tension.

It is tempting to bring the skin resection pattern down as a V instead of a U in order to avoid a pucker, but the surgeon will inevitably not remove enough subcutaneous tissue. Postoperative puckers are more a problem of excess subcutaneous tissue than they are a problem of excess skin. The final skin resection pattern with the areolar opening and the vertical limbs should actually resemble a snowman.

It is important to stay well above the inframammary fold because the fold itself will rise and because closure of a vertical ellipse will push down and easily cross the inframammary fold. Again it is important to match the markings on both sides to achieve symmetry.

Surgeons will initially have trouble with the idea of a vertical limb that exceeds 5 to 7 cm, but if ideal breasts are analyzed, an ideal B cup breast will have a distance of 7 cm from the bottom of the areola to the inframammary fold, an ideal C cup breast will have a distance of 9 cm from the bottom of the areola to the inframammary fold, and an ideal D cup breast will have a distance of 11 cm from the bottom of the areola to the inframammary fold.

Patients often ask for breasts that sit completely within the confines of the breast footprint, but it is important for both surgeons and patients to understand that the breast will hang like an awning off the footprint with some breast skin touching chest wall skin. An excellent shape can still be achieved, but a longer vertical distance is needed with this curved lower pole and a longer distance is needed to accommodate the increased projection that results from the vertical approach. A vertical distance of 5 cm would flatten the breast. The parenchymal pillars are best designed at approximately 7 cm, but the skin distance will be longer as it curves down over the inferior pole of a well-projecting breast.

DESIGN OF A MEDIALLY AND SUPEROMEDIALLY BASED PEDICLE

Design of a Medially Based Pedicle

The medially based pedicle will often appear to be "superomedially" based when a patient is standing up, but when a patient is lying down the true medial nature of the base can be seen. The blood supply is medial, whereas a true superomedial pedicle has both a medial and a superior blood supply. The best way to design a medially based pedicle that is easy to inset is to place half of the base of the pedicle in the areolar opening and half of the base in the vertical limb of the skin resection pattern. A base of about 8 cm is ideal, but it may extend up to 10 to 11 cm in a larger pedicle.

The veins can usually be seen just below the skin, and it would be ideal to try to include one of the visible veins within the base design. The artery to the medial pedicle comes from the internal mammary system at the level of the third interspace. It is deep as it comes around the sternum and then proceeds up in the subcutaneous tissue toward the areola. It travels separately from the veins.

The inferior border of the medial pedicle becomes the medial pillar as the pedicle is rotated up into position.

Design of a Superomedially Based Pedicle

A true superomedially based pedicle may be a good choice for the longer pedicles since it will include both the medial and superior arteries. It will, however, be more difficult to inset. Because we know that the descending branch of the artery from the second interspace almost always enters the areolar opening just medial to the breast meridian and almost always within 1 cm below the skin surface, we can create a wider base superiorly and then remove deeper tissue (that has minimal blood vessels) in order to make it easier to inset the pedicle.

OPERATIVE TECHNIQUE

Infiltration

Infiltration of the skin incisions is not recommended because it can damage some of the superficial veins, which should be preserved. Infiltration of a vasoconstrictor is usually reserved for the areas where liposuction is to be performed. If the patient is somewhat obese, then a tumescent type of infiltration is used for the lateral chest wall and preaxillary areas. In thinner patients about 40 cc of Xylocaine 1/2% with epinephrine 1/400,000 is used on each side for the lateral chest wall and preaxillary areas.

Creation of the Pedicle

The pedicle is then deepithelialized (Fig. 91.2A). Some form of compression at the base of the breast will put tension on the skin and make the deepithelialization easier. A cuff of tissue is left around the areola to help incorporate more venous drainage.

The pedicle is then carried down to the chest wall using either a scalpel or cutting cautery. A full-thickness pedicle is created by carrying the pedicle directly down to the breast meridian. Care is taken not to expose the pectoralis fascia to preserve both nerves and prevent excess bleeding (Fig. 91.2B).

The pedicle is created as a full-thickness pedicle directly down to pectoralis fascia. There is no need to make the pedicle thick laterally since there is minimal blood supply coming from that direction.

Resection of the Parenchyma

The parenchyma is then resected by beveling out medially and laterally (Fig. 91.2D). The skin is undermined but only down to the inframammary fold. The rest of the resection is accomplished by leaving about 1 cm of tissue at the skin margins and extending out laterally and more deeply as the resection progresses. It is important to resect as much tissue inferiorly and laterally as possible and to leave some tissue superiorly.

The inferior border of the medial pedicle will create the medial pillar. The surgeon should leave a lateral pillar about 7 cm long and 2 cm thick below the lateral extent of the areolar opening. Tissue can then be resected out past the pillars deep to the lateral skin flap.

It may be tempting to leave tissue superiorly and use the pedicle to try to push some tissue up to create more upper pole fullness, but it will not work. The tissue will drop down, push the bulk of the pedicle down, and create bottoming out. If the patient has a considerable amount of upper pole fullness, then some tissue can be removed to achieve an adequate resection. It is important to leave some tissue in this area as a platform for the areola (even when the pedicle is full thickness, the area under the areola itself will appear to have been thinned).

The parenchymal resection will follow the Wise pattern (16), but the skin resection pattern will look more like a snowman. If the Wise pattern is drawn on the skin, the tissue that remains is the tissue above the pattern. The 5- to 7-cm rule for the vertical limbs of the Wise pattern is good—not for the skin, but for the vertical limbs of the parenchymal pillars.

Lassus (4–6) does not remove tissue horizontally but confines his resection to a vertical ellipse. He can then chase his vertical skin excision inferiorly with less risk of the scar going onto the chest wall because the inframammary fold does not rise with his approach. When the tissue is removed inferiorly along the Wise pattern as described previously, the inframammary fold will actually rise.

Insetting of the Pedicle

It is easiest to close the base of the areola before insetting the pedicle (Fig. 91.2E, F). A single 3-0 Monocryl is used in the dermis of the pedicle and the dermis of the opposite side. No undermining is needed in the pedicle. Once this suture is in place, the pedicle is then rotated up into position.

The areola will sit easily into the new opening. The whole base of the pedicle rotates, which means that the areola sits into position with little tension or compression. The inferior border of the medial pedicle becomes the medial pillar.

Closure of the Pillars

The pillars are closed with interrupted 3-0 Monocryl. It is important to place the first pillar suture inferiorly so the pedicle is completely rotated into position. The first suture is placed right at the base of the pedicle inferiorly, but this is only about 7 cm below the areolar opening. The pillars only extend about halfway down the skin opening.

The first suture should not be deep (Fig. 91.2I). There is no point in pulling on the lateral breast tissue to try to move it medially. Tension on the breast tissue will eventually stretch, and any lateral tissue pulled inward will eventually slide back out.

Sutures do not need to be deep but should only catch enough fibrous type of breast tissue so that fibrous tissue

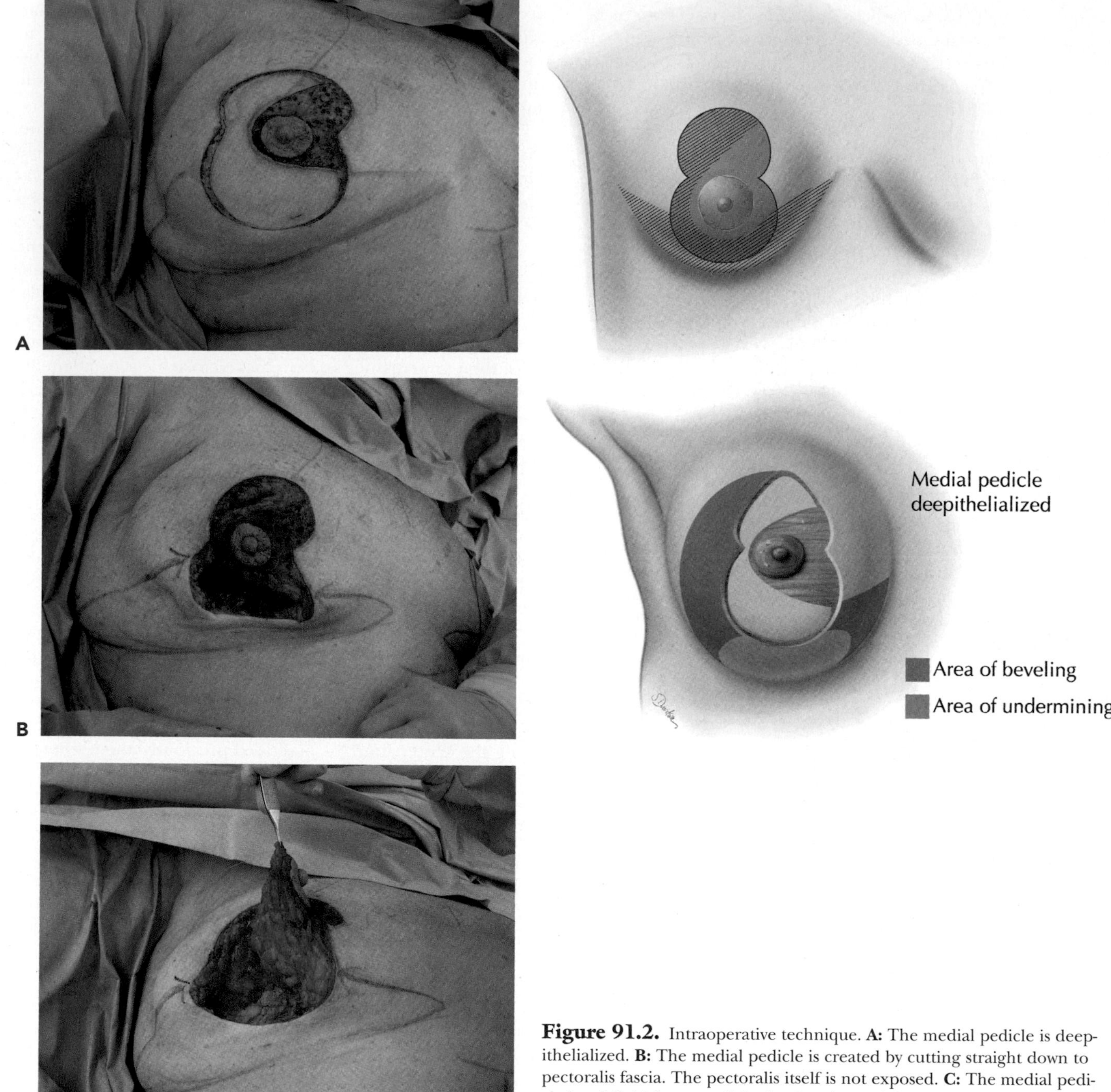

Figure 91.2. Intraoperative technique. **A:** The medial pedicle is deepithelialized. **B:** The medial pedicle is created by cutting straight down to pectoralis fascia. The pectoralis itself is not exposed. **C:** The medial pedicle is a full-thickness pedicle that is quite mobile, much like the inferior pedicle. (*continued*)

comes into contact with fibrous tissue and allows it to heal. Large constricting sutures that contain a lot of fat are not only unnecessary but are also likely to cause problems with fat necrosis.

This first suture rotates the inferior border of the medial pedicle up so that it now becomes the medial pillar. It is only necessary to coapt this suture to fibrous tissue on the lateral pillar at an equivalent position. These sutures do not need to be deep or under any tension.

Two or three more sutures are used to complete the pillar closure. More will be needed with a very bulky pedicle. Suturing the pedicle up to pectoralis fascia is not needed; however, it might be wise to suture some of the bulk of a very large pedicle up to the chest wall.

The breast parenchyma should now have good projection because closure of the vertical elliptical resection pushes the upper "dog ear" up into the areolar opening. The pillars should measure only about 7 cm in length. The area between the inferior border of the parenchyma and the original inframammary fold should be empty. It may be helpful to draw the Wise pattern on the skin to check that the parenchymal resection is adequate.

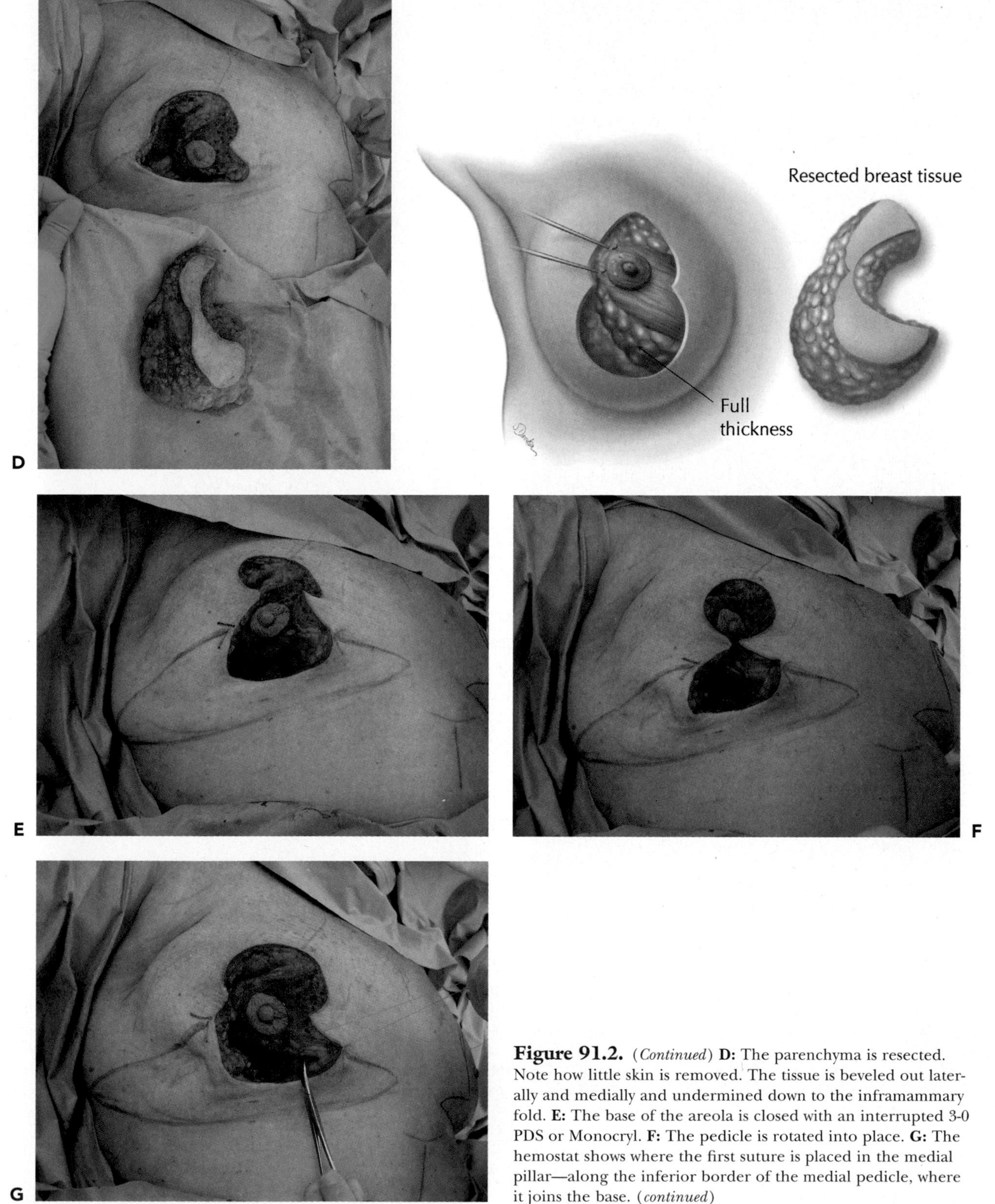

Figure 91.2. (*Continued*) **D:** The parenchyma is resected. Note how little skin is removed. The tissue is beveled out laterally and medially and undermined down to the inframammary fold. **E:** The base of the areola is closed with an interrupted 3-0 PDS or Monocryl. **F:** The pedicle is rotated into place. **G:** The hemostat shows where the first suture is placed in the medial pillar—along the inferior border of the medial pedicle, where it joins the base. (*continued*)

Closure of the Dermis

The dermis is closed with interrupted 3-0 Monocryl Plus (Fig. 91.2J). It is not necessary to suture the dermis up onto the breast parenchyma. Such sutures will actually delay resolution of the shape. Surgeons should resist the temptation to excise more skin. The skin does not contribute to the shape, and too much tension will just delay healing. The breast should have a good curve to the lower pole and not be pushed up into a concave type of shape.

Liposuction

Liposuction is then used to refine the shape (Fig. 91.2L). The subcutaneous tissue above the inframammary fold needs to be

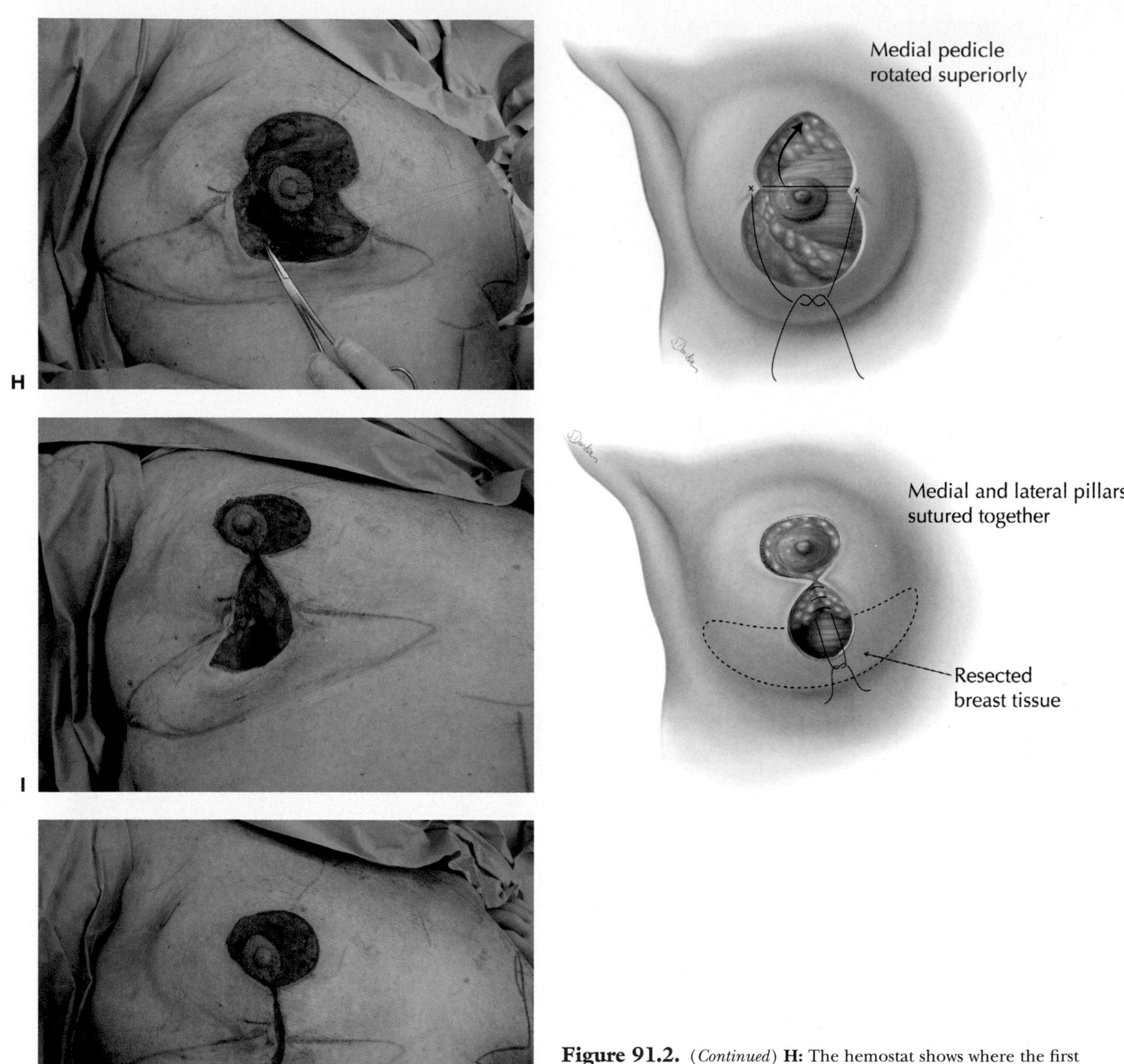

Figure 91.2. (*Continued*) **H:** The hemostat shows where the first suture is placed in the lateral pillar. **I:** The first pillar suture starts at the inferior aspect of the pillars, which is about halfway up the vertical skin opening. Note how the area below the Wise pattern has had the parenchyma removed. **J:** Closure of the dermis with deep interrupted buried 3-0 Monocryl sutures. The dermis is not sutured up onto breast parenchyma. (*continued*)

removed—all except a layer under the skin to prevent contractures or adhesions. Some of the more fibrous tissue will need to be directly excised, but the area can be easily tailored and shaped by using liposuction. It is especially important not to leave excess subcutaneous tissue just above the inframammary fold laterally; postoperative puckers are more of a problem of excess subcutaneous tissue and less of a problem of excess skin.

Liposuction is also used to reduce fullness in the preaxillary area and to reduce excess fat along the lateral chest wall.

Closure of the Skin

The skin is closed with a running subcuticular 3-0 Monocryl Plus suture. It is important not to take deep constricting bites of dermis.

Initially it was believed that gathering the skin closure would promote wound retraction; however, excessive gathering not only delays healing, but it also delays resolution of the shape. Measurements at surgery and each follow-up visit showed that the vertical distance stretched back out. A scar contracture in the skin can result, and this may need a later revision. This gathering

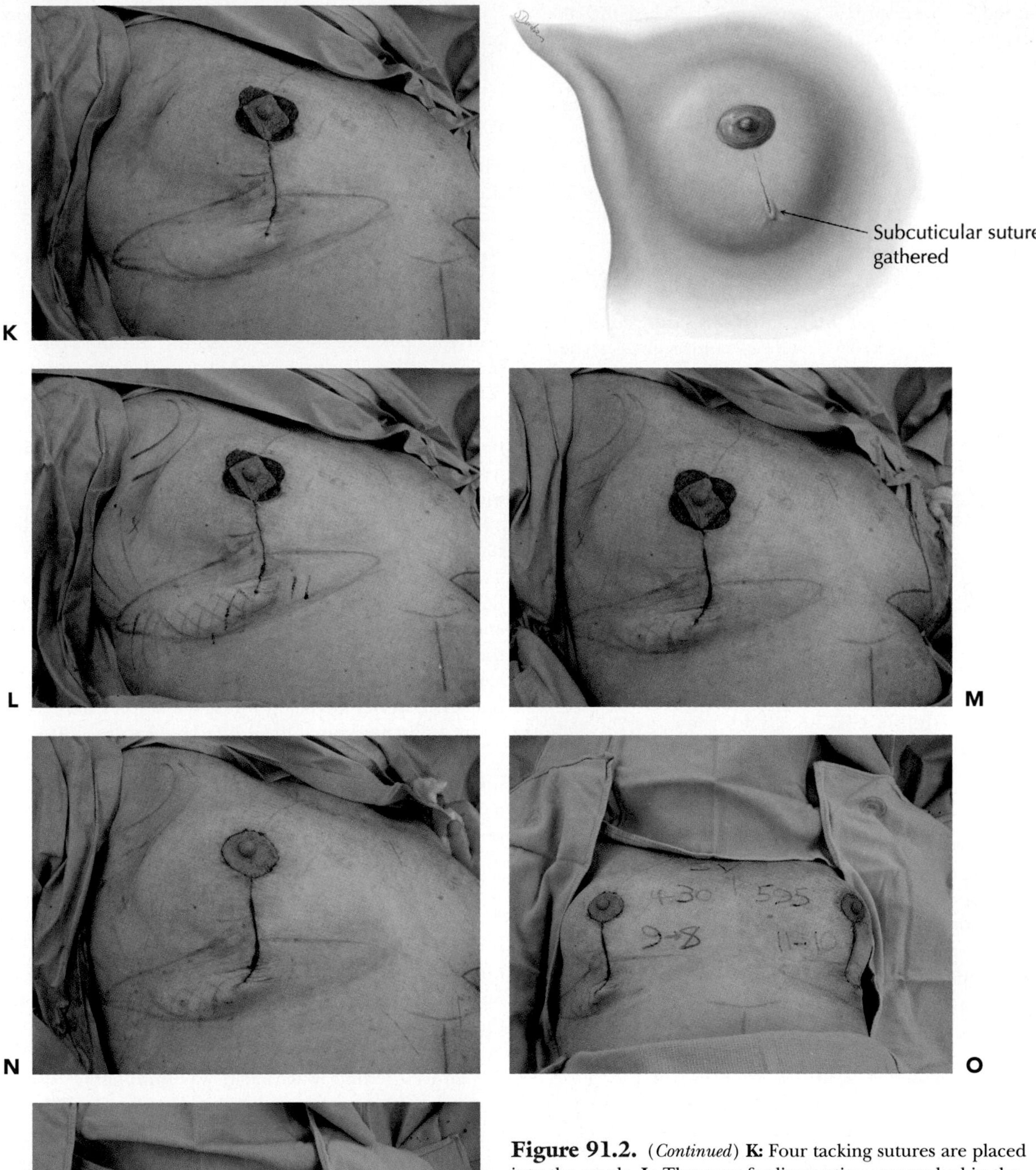

Figure 91.2. (*Continued*) **K:** Four tacking sutures are placed into the areola. **L:** The areas for liposuction are marked in the inferior breast, along the lateral chest wall and in the preaxillary areas. **M:** The liposuction has been completed. **N:** The areola suturing is completed with a running subcuticular 3-0 or 4-0 Monocryl. **O:** The dermis is closed with a running subcuticular suture. Very little gathering of this vertical incision should be done. Gathering constricts blood supply to the skin and delays resolution of the shape. **P:** Paper tape is used to cover the incisions. A couple of extra strips are placed horizontally along the inferior aspect of the breast. Drains are rarely used. The patient is allowed to shower the next day. She is told to pat the tape dry and then leave it in place for 3 weeks.

was performed because surgeons mistakenly believed that the vertical incision should be no longer than 5 to 7 cm. A longer vertical incision is actually desired to accommodate both the increased projection and the curve to the lower pole of the breast.

It may be tempting to either excise the excess skin inferiorly or even to suture it down to the chest wall. An added horizontal excision will only be necessary when the vertical incision exceeds about 12 to 14 cm or in postbariatric patients with poor-quality skin.

Closure of the Areola

The areola is closed with four interrupted stay sutures of 3-0 or 4-0 Monocryl Plus (Fig. 91.2M). The circumference is then closed with a running subcuticular Monocryl Plus suture (Fig. 91.2N).

INTRAOPERATIVE AND POSTOPERATIVE CARE

DRAINS

I rarely use drains. If there is more oozing than usual, I may leave drains in overnight (and usually through a separate stab wound). Drains do not prevent a hematoma nor do they prevent a seroma. Drains may treat a seroma, but they need to remain in place for several days. A seroma may develop that can exaggerate inferior fullness. Although a seroma may be aspirated, it can be also left alone to resolve on its own.

ANTIBIOTICS

A full week's course of intraoperative and postoperative antibiotics (cephalosporins) definitely improved problems with suture spitting and wound-healing issues. With the new guidelines, similar results have been achieved with the use of one intraoperative dose of antibiotics along with the use of an antibacterial impregnated suture.

BANDAGING AND TAPING

The incisions are covered with 3M Micropore paper tape, which is left in place for 3 to 4 weeks. Patients are allowed to shower the day after the surgery, and they are told just to pat the tape dry. It is not necessary to tape up the whole breast. The skin will settle into the new shape over time; the skin has no role in shaping the breast.

Immediately postoperatively, the breasts are covered with gauze, and a surgical (noncompressing) brassiere is then applied. The main function of the brassiere is to hold the bandages in place. After the first couple of days, patients often use panty liners inside the bra instead of gauze.

It is suggested that patients use the surgical brassiere for a couple of weeks before switching to a sports-type brassiere. They are advised to look for a bra with a wide band that extends down onto the chest wall or to find an elasticized camisole top. The bra is not used for compression but to promote a sense of support.

RECOVERY

Patients may return to desk-type work in 1 to 2 weeks. It may take 3 to 4 weeks to return to work if the job is more physical. Patients are encouraged to maintain a level of activity such as walking and to gradually increase from lower-body workouts to adding upper-body activities by 3 to 4 weeks.

CASES

The cases shown in Figures 91.3 to 91.6 are representative of the results obtained by using this technique.

RISKS

Scarring

Scarring, possible loss of sensation, and possible inability to breast-feed are the main problems with breast reduction. The vertical approaches avoid the often-unsightly horizontal scar in the inframammary fold. The vertical scar is usually good, and the periareolar scar can be slightly thicker. Proponents of the inverted-T scars say that patients do not see or complain about the inframammary scar.

After having performed inverted-T, inferior pedicle breast reductions for the first 10 years of my practice, I can say categorically that it was the inframammary scar that bothered patients the most. They were also upset with the dog-ears laterally and medially, but those puckers were difficult to correct. With the vertical approach I still see dog-ears—inferiorly—but at least now I have an effective method of correction. Most of the puckers can be corrected under local anesthesia with a small vertical skin excision and a horizontal fat resection.

Some patients would develop a slightly boxy shape with the inverted-T procedure, but they rarely complained. Patients now comment on how much they like the "perky" shape with the vertical approach.

Sensation

It is interesting that the sensation for all the pedicles is comparable. Eighty-five percent of patients recover normal to near-normal sensation. I had initially believed that sensation with the lateral pedicle would be better than the sensation with the medial pedicle, but this did not hold true. The problem with the lateral pedicle was that it was impossible to remove the excess lateral breast tissue because it comprised the base of the pedicle.

Although we often talk about the lateral branch of the fourth intercostal nerve as being the most important for nipple sensation, it is clear that there are many other sources of innervation (Fig. 91.7A). Researchers have shown that there is both a superficial and a deep branch of the fourth intercostal nerve (17). The deep branch courses just above the pectoralis fascia, and at the breast meridian it curves upward toward the nipple. By leaving the pedicle full thickness and by not exposing the pectoralis fascia, the medially based pedicle is likely to preserve this deep branch. There are also branches from the medial intercostal system and branches from the clavicular nerves that supply sensation.

Breast-Feeding

It is well known that patients with large breasts have more difficulty breast-feeding. Cruz-Korchin (18) conducted an interesting study that showed that the incidence of breast-feeding

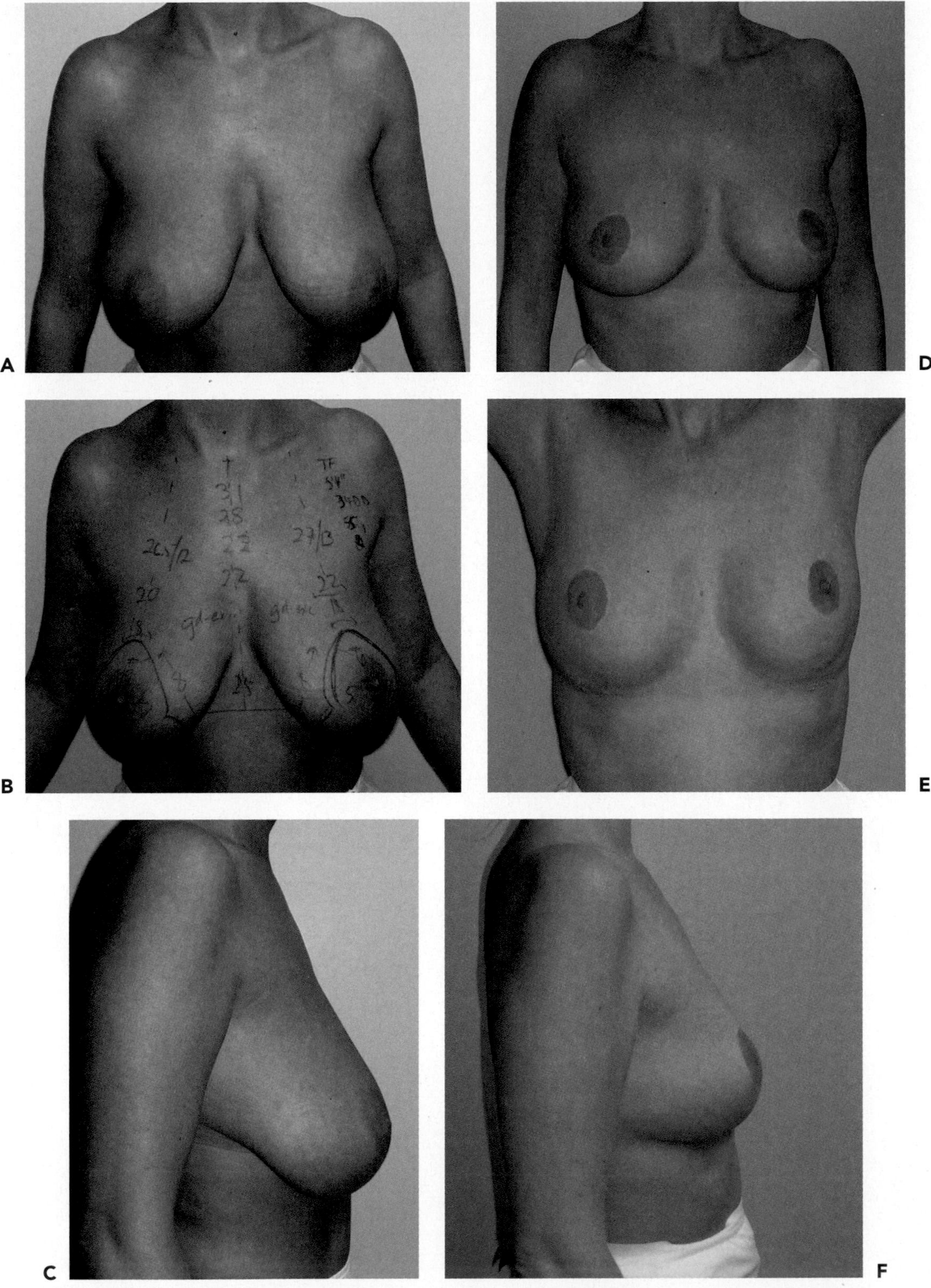

Figure 91.3. A 34-year-old woman who has a very low inframammary fold. She was 5′4″ tall, weighed 120 lb, and wore a 34DD brassiere. She had 340 g removed from the right breast and 400 g from the left breast. **A:** Preoperative frontal view. **B:** Preoperative frontal marked view. Note that the inframammary fold is actually lower than the anterior elbow crease. **C:** Preoperative lateral view. **D:** Three-year postoperative frontal view. The inframammary fold is 1.5 cm higher than it was preoperatively. **E:** Three-year postoperative arms-up view. **F:** Three-year postoperative lateral view.

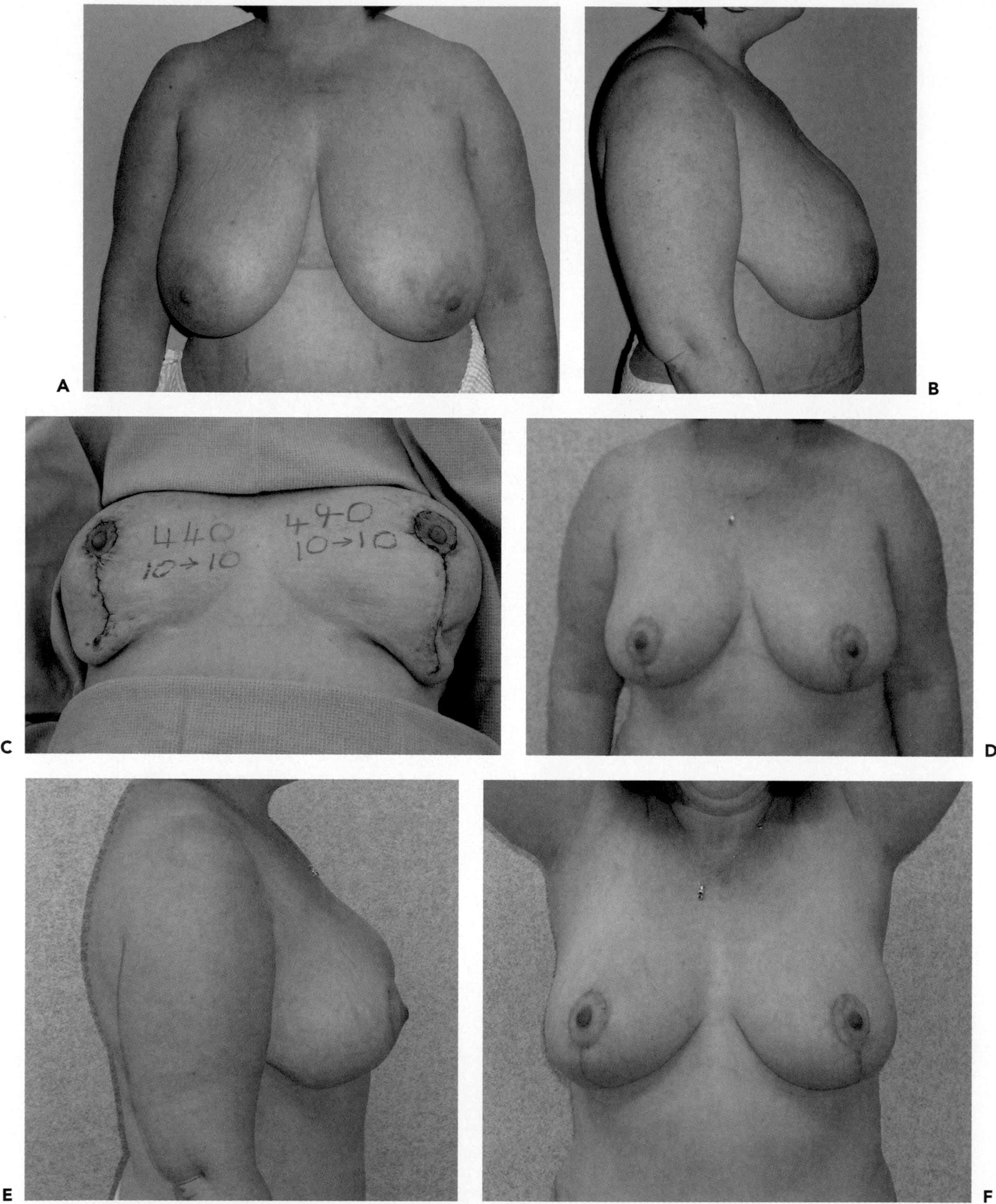

Figure 91.4. A 40-year-old patient who shows how quickly the postoperative pucker settles. She was 5′4″ tall, weighed 150 lb, and wore a 34G brassiere. She had 440 g removed from each side and another 475 cc of peripheral liposuction. **A:** Preoperative frontal view. **B:** Preoperative lateral view. **C:** Intraoperative view. Most surgeons who are unfamiliar with the vertical technique will be tempted to excise the excess skin and create a small T. This is unnecessary. **D:** Postoperative frontal view at 6 weeks. **E:** Postoperative lateral view at 6 weeks. **F:** Postoperative arms-up view at 6 weeks. Note how the inferior pucker has spontaneously tucked in. Excising the pucker and creating a short transverse scar is acceptable but far less indicated than many surgeons believe.

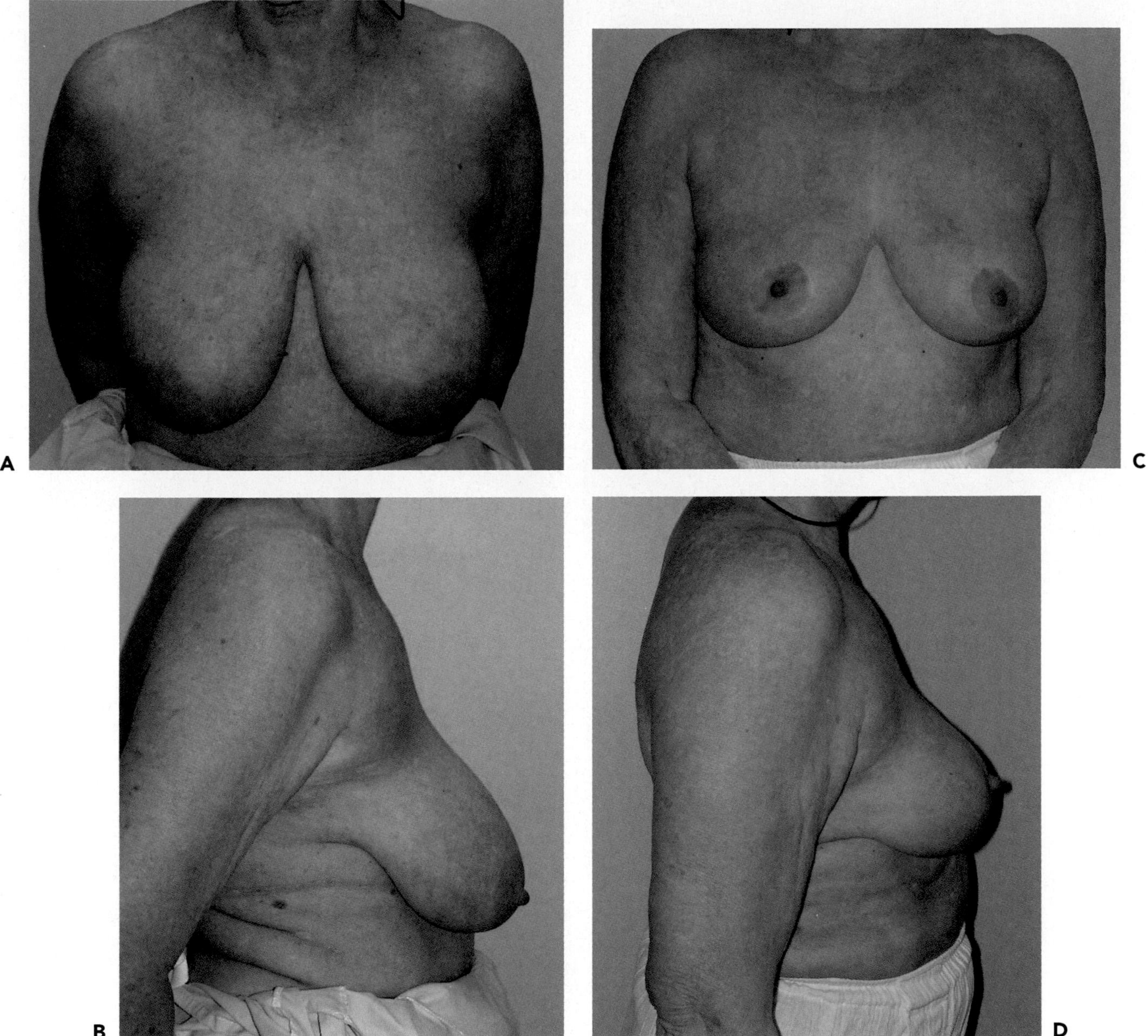

Figure 91.5. A 66-year-old patient. She was 5′6″ tall, weighed 150 lb, and wore a 36E brassiere. She had 375 g removed from the right breast and 395 g removed from the left breast. Another 375 cc of liposuction was performed peripherally. **A:** Preoperative frontal view. **B:** Preoperative lateral view. **C:** A 2 ½-year postoperative frontal view. **D:** A 2 ½-year postoperative lateral view. The vertical scar measured 10 cm on both sides. This distance is needed to accommodate the projection that results from the vertical technique. Most patients are actually quite pleased with the elegant curve that results in the lower pole of the breast.

difficulties was the same after breast reduction as it was in large-breasted women who had not had a reduction. About 60% of patients in both groups were able to breast-feed, and one fourth of those patients needed to supplement.

A full-thickness pedicle is more likely to preserve breast-feeding potential than a thinned dermal pedicle. The medially based pedicle is a full-thickness pedicle, although it often looks as if it has been thinned after it has been created. This phenomenon is common with all pedicles and has been well recognized when performing the inverted-T, inferior pedicle techniques.

The superior pedicle, in contrast, must often be thinned to allow it to be inset without too much compression or constriction. An aggressively thinned pedicle will be less likely to permit breast-feeding.

Nipple and Areolar Necrosis

Circulation to the nipple and areola complex is superficial (19,20). Taylor and coworkers showed that the arteries and veins are superficial (and actually separate from each other). This makes sense because the breast is ectodermal in origin.

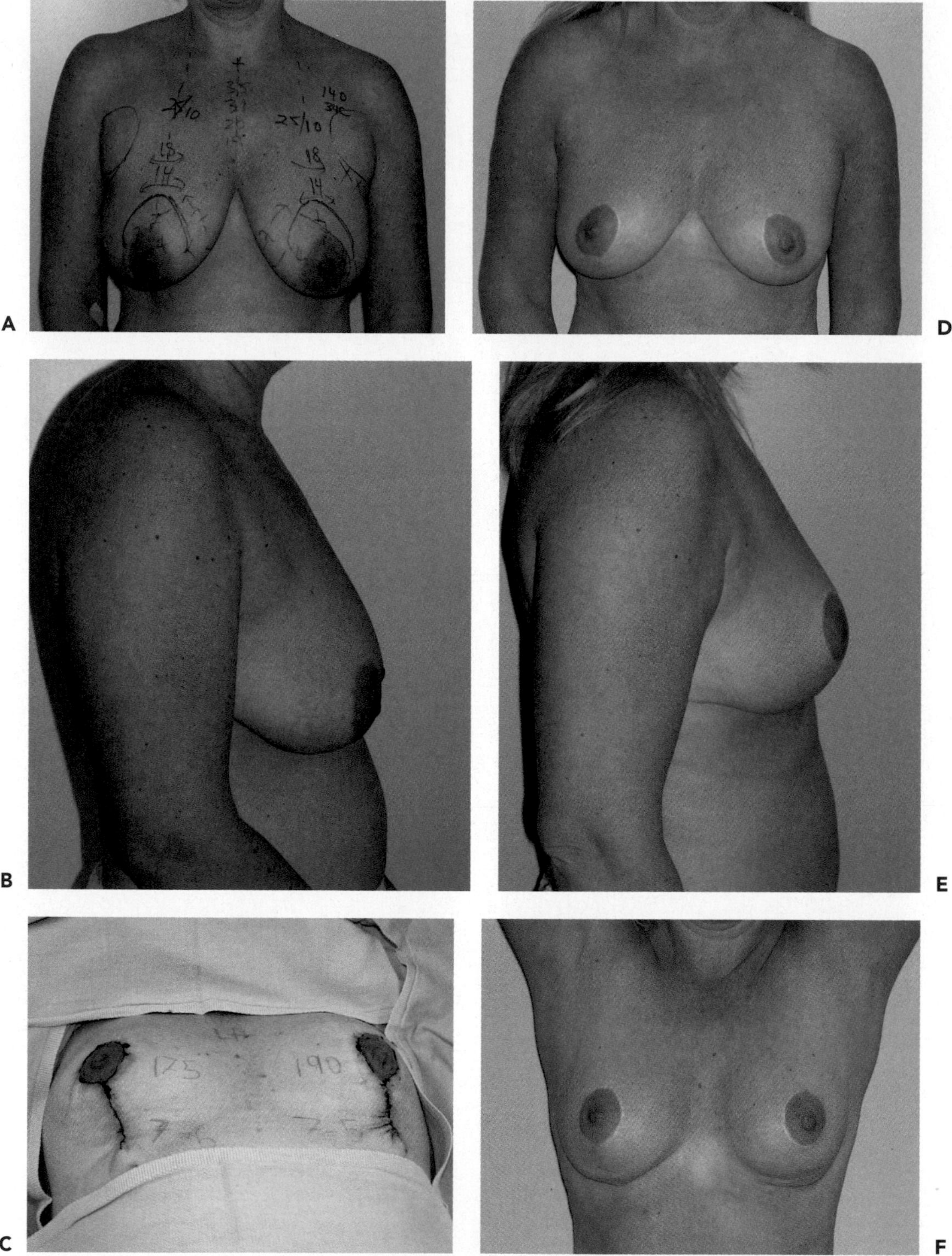

Figure 91.6. A 40-year-old patient. She was 5′4″ tall, weighed 140 lb, and wore a 34 C brassiere. She had 175 cc removed from the right breast and 190 cc from the left breast. Another 200 cc of liposuction was performed peripherally. **A:** Preoperative frontal view. Note the marking of the medial pedicle. The base of the pedicle is 7 cm. The nipple will be moved upward 5 cm. She has a high inframammary fold. Note the markings in the preaxillary area where liposuction will be performed. **B:** Preoperative lateral view. **C:** Intraoperative view. This shows more gathering of the vertical incision than I would perform now. On the right side the incision was gathered from 7 to 6 cm. On the left breast, the incision was gathered from 7 to 5 cm. **D:** A 3 ½-year postoperative frontal view. **E:** A 3 ½-year postoperative lateral view. Both vertical scars stretched out to 7 cm. The nipples were placed slightly too high. **F:** A 3 ½-year postoperative arms-up view. Note that slight puckering and irregularity remain.

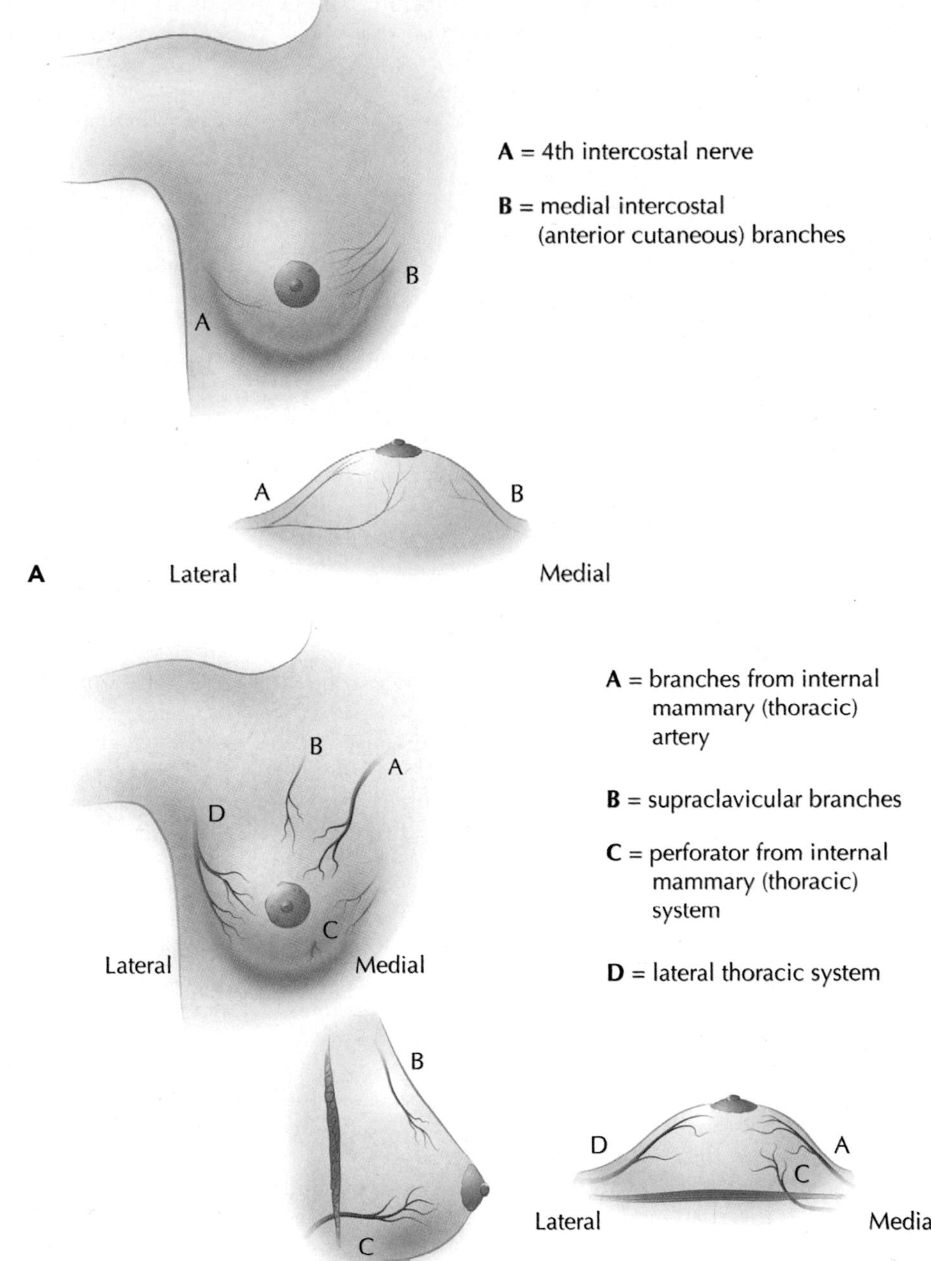

Figure 91.7. **A:** The innervation to the nipple and areola is not confined to the lateral branch of the fourth intercostal nerve. There are also medial intercostal nerve branches. The lateral branch has a superficial and a deep component. The deep branch travels just above the pectoralis fascia and turns upward toward the nipple at the level of the breast meridian. It is preserved with a medially based, full-thickness pedicle. **B:** The blood supply to the breast is superficial, except for the perforator through the pectoralis muscle, which supplies the inferior and central pedicles. There are venae comitantes accompanying this perforator. The rest of the pedicles are supplied by arterial input that enters the breast superficially. The veins do not accompany these arteries, but they are also superficial, lying just beneath the dermis. They can often be seen through the skin.

There is a main deep perforator that comes from the internal mammary system. It comes up through the pectoralis muscle just medial to the breast meridian and just above the fifth rib. It is this perforator that supplies an inferior and a central pedicle. It is the only artery that has accompanying venae comitantes.

The inferior and central pedicles need to be full thickness to incorporate these perforators. The superior, lateral, and medial pedicles can all be thinned. The superior pedicle can be safely thinned because there is a very strong vessel that originates at the second interspace and enters the breast obliquely. It is almost always about 1 cm deep to the skin surface. The lateral pedicle is supplied by the superficial branch of the lateral thoracic artery. This curves around the pectoralis muscle edge and then travels up into the subcutaneous tissue. The medial pedicle is supplied by branches of the internal mammary system mainly from the third interspace, which also travel up in the subcutaneous tissue.

The veins travel separately from the arteries, and they can be seen just deep to the skin draining mainly superomedially.

The superior pedicle often needs to be thinned to allow it to be inset without compression. In contrast, leaving the medial pedicle full thickness is more likely to incorporate the deep branch of the lateral fourth intercostal nerve and to permit some breast-feeding potential.

Breast reduction is a blood supply–reducing operation. It is inevitable that some pedicles are going to lose circulation (Fig. 91.7B). The problem is in deciding whether and when to intervene. It may be clear if there is obvious venous congestion that removing some sutures or taking the patient back to the operating room to correct any compression may be indicated.

In my experience, the problem is rarely one of venous congestion. Usually, the nipple and areola look pale and dusky. There is nothing that can be done about a lack of arterial input, except conversion to free nipple grafts. However, this is rarely a good solution because the majority of nipples will recover. Some may develop some edge necrosis or blistering, but the final result will still be better than a free nipple graft. Free nipple grafts can have healing problems of their own, especially if delayed. The nipples lack projection, do not recover sensation, preclude breast-feeding, and frequently develop patchy areas of depigmentation. I believe that it is better to reconstruct the few patients who develop complete necrosis than to subject a significant number of patients to a reoperation that has a low chance of success, with or without conversion to free nipple grafts.

Hematoma

Drains will not prevent or treat a hematoma. The best way to prevent a hematoma is to ensure that all known arteries are secured. This is especially important when vasoconstrictors are used. The vessels may not be obvious, but once the vasoconstrictor has worn off postoperatively, the artery may open up and cause a hematoma. The only treatment for a substantial hematoma is to take the patient back to surgery. Knowledge of the anatomy can help in searching for these vessels prior to closure.

Seroma

Drains do not prevent seromas either. Seromas can develop even after drains have been left in for several days. It is interesting that breast seromas behave differently from those in the abdomen. They eventually resorb.

Surgeons who are learning the vertical approach will frequently check their patients postoperatively and will find a significant number of seromas. These seromas often recur and may require repeated aspirations. They may be more common than realized but are perhaps best left alone. I have not had any long-term problems with seromas.

Infection

Although I resisted using antibiotics for years, I found that my infection rate was too high. I tried to control other factors but finally decided to put all patients on a week-long course of cephalosporins. Of interest, not only did my infection rate fall, but also patients (who had no overt evidence of infection) stopped calling my office with questions about wound-healing problems and suture-spitting issues. I had been blaming the sutures for open sores in the vertical incision.

When the infectious disease recommendations came out recommending only one intraoperative dose of antibiotics and recommending strongly against a full-week course I found that there was still a problem with open sores and suture spitting. When I switched to antibacterial sutures, the problem disappeared. I now use one intraoperative dose of cephalosporins and antibacterial (not antibiotic) sutures for closure. The Monocryl Plus suture is impregnated with triclosan.

The other key to avoiding healing problems is to avoid tension in the closure of both the parenchyma and the skin. The medial pedicle vertical breast reduction does not require skin tension to shape the breast, and the skin repair is best left fairly loose.

Wound-Healing Problems

Wound-healing problems are usually the result of poor circulation and/or infection. There is no question in my practice that wound-healing problems are more common in the larger breast reductions and more common in obese patients. The inverted T is notorious for problems in healing where skin tension is the greatest—at the T itself. As long as the vertical incision is sutured loosely and without tension, then wound healing problems are rare. I no longer gather the vertical incision, but when I did, I was careful not to backtrack and constrict the circulation to the skin margins.

Puckers

There are two puckers or dog-ears that develop with the inverted-T procedure at the lateral and medial extent of the inframammary scar. This is the expected result after closing a horizontal ellipse.

There are two puckers or dog-ears that develop with the vertical approaches to breast reduction. The excision of skin and parenchyma is performed as a vertical ellipse with both upper and lower dog-ears. The upper dog-ear is absorbed by the areola. The lower dog-ear has created a huge controversy and resistance to the vertical technique. It is the reason that there is a higher revision rate (about 5%) with the vertical approaches. However, is there is a higher revision rate because we can actually do something about the problem? There is really no good way to treat the lateral and medial dog-ears with the inverted T, and therefore the revision rate remains artificially low.

I warn all my patients that 95% of patients worry about the puckers, yet I need to fix only about 5%. They also know that I will not consider any revision for a full year because most puckers will disappear on their own.

I find it difficult to accept the argument that American patients insist on good results immediately. We seem to be able to get patients to understand that facelifts and blepharoplasties take time to settle. Rhinoplasty patients know that it will take several weeks before they feel presentable. A preoperatively informed patient is the surgeon's best ally.

Underresection and Bottoming Out

One problem I still have is that it is harder to achieve an adequate reduction with the vertical approach. It is important to adhere to the preoperative assessment of the volume that needs to be removed. The breasts look smaller on the table than with the inverted T. More tissue can be removed laterally, and occasionally some tissue will need to be removed superiorly. If a patient does not have much upper pole fullness, it is important to leave as much superior tissue as possible.

When I review my cases of bottoming out, they are invariably the result of underresection. When I tried to pull lateral tissue up and medially with a lateral pedicle, bottoming out would occur with time as the tension on the parenchyma eased. With medial pedicle vertical breast reduction the result at 1 year appears to hold out, and it is difficult to differentiate between the 1-year photos and the 6- and 10-year photos. The 1-year shape persists over time. With my inverted-T, inferior pedicle patients, the shape would deteriorate with time, and bottoming out was progressive.

I can correct the bottoming out with this vertical technique by removing inferior parenchyma without removing any skin and without any attempt to reposition the inframammary fold. The complication of bottoming out is not the fault of the procedure, but it has always been my fault in not removing enough breast tissue inferiorly.

Asymmetry

When the breasts are asymmetric, it is important to design the new nipple position lower on the larger breast. There are two reasons for this. One reason is that the skin may be stretched more on the larger breast and the marking will rise up when the extra breast weight is removed. The other reason is that closure of the vertical ellipse (both skin and breast parenchyma) on the larger side will push up the superior end even further.

The asymmetry can be sometimes better assessed in the arms-up position. It is interesting that the inframammary fold on the larger breast is not necessarily lower than on the smaller breast. Note should be made of these differences while planning the surgery. The fold can be raised to some degree by removing tissue just above the inframammary fold, either directly or with liposuction for tailoring.

Revisions in my practice are usually performed for puckers, underresection, and asymmetry. It is interesting that the patients who seem most bothered by the asymmetry are the ones who were asymmetric before surgery.

OUTCOMES

The outcomes are the same as with the inverted-T breast reduction—considerable relief of back pain, neck pain, bra-strap grooving, rashes in the skin beneath the breasts, headache, posture problems, and exercise intolerance. The vertical skin resection pattern combined with a medially based pedicle not only reduces the scars, but it also improves the shape and the longevity of the shape. The operative time, blood loss, and recovery for the patient are all less.

Most inverted-T methods use a horizontal skin and parenchymal resection. Although there is some coning of the breast tissue, the narrowing of the breast base is restricted. The skin closure is tight to try to prevent bottoming out; this unfortunately tends to flatten the breast and prevent projection. It is my belief that bottoming out is not the fault of the inverted T but is due to the fact that we remove superior tissue and then leave heavy inferior breast tissue and then use the skin to hold up the result.

Most vertical techniques use a vertical skin and parenchymal resection. Closure of the vertical ellipse of breast tissue pushes the dog-ears upward and downward. The upper dog-ear is pushed up into the areola, which actually helps with projection. With the superior, lateral, and medial pedicles, the lower dog-ear is just skin, and it tucks in underneath the breast. In vertical skin resection patterns where the inferior pedicle is used (21), the skin is used to help maintain shape much as it is with the inverted T.

It should be clear that we cannot compare apples and oranges. The inverted-T skin resection pattern with an inferior pedicle cannot be compared with a vertical skin resection pattern using a superior or medial pedicle. There are two variables—skin resection pattern and parenchymal resection pattern. The scars and the shape are separate. The shape does not depend on the type of scar that results but depends on how the parenchyma is excised and shaped.

I believe that the skin pattern is less important than the shaping of the breast tissue. Skin and dermis are elastic structures that deform with stress. Any breast tissue that is left to apply pressure with gravity on the inferior skin will cause the skin to stretch. By removing the tissue that we want to leave (superior) in an inverted-T inferior pedicle, we are likely to have progressive bottoming out. By removing the inferior breast tissue and leaving a more superiorly based pedicle, we are giving gravity less of a chance to destroy the shape.

The medial pedicle provides an elegant curve to the lower pole of the breast because the inferior border of the medial pedicle becomes the medial pillar. The breast has a good shape on the table at the end of the procedure, and it holds its shape over time. It is important to use the Wise pattern to help the surgeon decide what parenchyma should be left behind rather than what should be removed.

CONCLUSION

I switched initially to the vertical approach to reduce the scarring of breast reduction surgery. I persisted through the learning curve because of the improved shape. The vertical resection of both skin and parenchyma gave the breasts better projection. The medial pedicle simplified the procedure and gave an elegant curve to the breast. The lack of reliance on the skin brassiere then allowed the shape to hold out over time. The vertical approach using a medial pedicle has reduced the scarring and improved the shape and its longevity.

EDITORIAL COMMENTS

With the original description of the vertical breast reduction by Lassus and later by Lejour came the realization that, at times, insetting the superior pedicle was problematic. A bulky or excessively long pedicle could result in shape distortion due to tissue crowding, or more important, potential vascular compromise due to tissue tension and kinking of the pedicle. To answer these concerns, Dr. Hall-Findlay popularized the use of the superomedial pedicle. This minor alteration in pedicle orientation respected the basic tenets of the vertical mammaplasty but yet provided an easier inset of the nipple and areola. Using this technique, surgeons were able to use this modified vertical mammaplasty technique in larger breasts with less potential compromise to the vascularity of the nipple and areola. I agree that this pedicle is a safe pedicle from a blood supply standpoint. By incorporating the branches of the sizable internal mammary perforator from the second intercostal space, an axial flap is created making this pedicle one of the safest constructs used in breast reduction. Beyond this technical modification, the technique mirrors that of Lejour. All issues that tend to complicate standard vertical technique are still in play. In larger breast reductions or in patients with marked skin excess, management of the redundant skin envelope will be a challenge and, as noted, revisions will at times be required. However, with this innovative contribution to our understanding of the vertical mammaplasty, Dr. Hall-Findlay has helped bring the vertical mammaplasty concept into the mainstream, and many surgeons have successfully incorporated her technique into their own practices.

D.C.H.

REFERENCES

1. Robbins TH. A reduction mammaplasty with the areola-nipple based on an inferior pedicle. *Plast Reconstr Surg* 1977;59:64–67.
2. Courtiss EH, Goldwyn RM. Reduction mammaplasty by the inferior pedicle technique. An alternative to free nipple and areola grafting for severe macromastia or extreme ptosis. *Plast Reconstr Surg* 1977;59:500.
3. Marchac D, de Olarte G. Reduction mammaplasty and correction of ptosis with a short inframammary scar. *Plast Reconstr Surg* 1982;69:45–55.
4. Lassus C. A technique for breast reduction. *Int Surg* 1970;53:69.
5. Lassus C. Breast reduction: evolution of a technique. A single vertical scar. *Aesthetic Plast Surg* 1987;11:107–112.
6. Lassus C. A 30-year experience with vertical mammaplasty. *Plast Reconstr Surg* 1996;97:373–380.
7. Lejour M, Abboud M, Declety A, et al. Reduction des cicatrices de plastie mammaire: de l'ancre courte a la verticale. *Ann Chir Plast Esthet* 1990;35:369.
8. Lejour M. *Vertical Mammaplasty and Liposuction of the Breast*. St. Louis, MO: Quality Medical; 1993.
9. Lejour M. Vertical mammaplasty and liposuction of the breast. *Plast Reconstr Surg* 1994;94:100–114.
10. Lejour M, Abboud M. Vertical mammaplasty without inframammary scar and with breast liposuction. *Perspect Plast Surg* 1996;4:67–90.
11. Hall-Findlay EJ. A simplified vertical reduction mammaplasty: shortening the learning curve. *Plast Reconstr Surg* 1999;104:748.
12. Hall-Findlay EJ. Vertical breast reduction with a medially based pedicle. Operative strategies. *Aesthetic Surg J* 2002;22:185–195.
13. Hall-Findlay EJ. Pedicles in vertical reduction and mastopexy. *Clin Plastic Surg* 2002;20:379–391.
14. Berthe JV, Massaut J, Greuse M, et al. The vertical mammaplasty: a reappraisal of the technique and its complications. *Plast Reconstr Surg* 2003;111:2192–2199.
15. Gradinger GP. Reduction mammaplasty utilizing nipple-areola transplantation. *Clin Plast Surg* 1988;15:641–654.
16. Wise RJ. A preliminary report on a method of planning the mammaplasty. *Plast Reconstr Surg* 1956;17:367.
17. Schlenz I, Kuzbari R, Gruber H, et al. The sensitivity of the nipple-areola complex: an anatomic study. *Plast Reconstr Surg* 2000;105:905–909.
18. Cruz-Korchin N. Breast feeding after vertical reduction mammaplasty. Paper presented at the 71st Annual Meeting of the American Society of Plastic Surgeons, San Antonio, Texas, November 2–6, 2002.
19. Reid CR, Taylor GI. The vascular territory of the acromiothoracic axis. *Br J Plast Surg* 1984;37:194.
20. Corduff N, Taylor GI. Subglandular breast reduction: the evolution of a minimal scar approach to breast reduction. *Plast Reconstr Surg* 2004;113:175–184.
21. Hammond DC. Short scar periareolar inferior pedicle reduction (SPAIR) mammaplasty. *Plast Reconstr Surg* 1999;103:890.

CHAPTER

92

Dennis C. Hammond

The Short Scar Periareolar Inferior Pedicle Reduction Mammaplasty

INTRODUCTION

Since the mid-1960s, the Wise pattern inferior pedicle reduction technique has been, in one variation or another, the preferred technique for breast reduction for most surgeons across North America and around the world. However, more recent interest in reduced or "short" scar techniques has prompted plastic surgeons to more carefully evaluate other approaches. This interest stems not so much from dissatisfaction with the standard inferior pedicle approach, but rather from a desire to reduce the complications associated with the procedure. In particular, techniques to reduce the amount of cutaneous scar and provide for more aesthetic and long-lasting shapes have been actively investigated. This chapter describes one such approach called the short scar periareolar inferior pedicle reduction (SPAIR) mammaplasty (1–4).

OPERATIVE STRATEGY

In designing this approach, every effort was made to geometrically design a pattern for skin envelope reduction that would limit the scar to the central portion of the breast using a circumvertical strategy to eliminate the wide inframammary scar. Because of the general familiarity with the inferior pedicle approach, this type of pedicle is used to preserve the neurovascular supply to the breast parenchyma and nipple-areola complex (NAC). Finally, internal shaping sutures are used to more effectively reposition the remaining breast tissue to create aesthetic breast shapes that can be evaluated directly at the time of surgery, rather than waiting for time to result in breast shape change with settling. By combining these operative steps, a versatile, consistent, and reliable technique for breast reduction is developed that is applicable to a wide variety of patients.

PATIENT MARKING

The goal of the marking procedure is to estimate how much of the skin envelope must be retained around the periphery of the breast to comfortably wrap around the inferior pedicle once the excess parenchyma has been resected. With this in mind, four cardinal points are identified using existing breast landmarks. The patient is marked in the upright position. The midsternal line and the inframammary fold are identified, and the breast meridian is then drawn on each side (Figs. 92.1A and 92.1B). This meridian line bisects the breast into two equal volumetric halves and extends from the anterior portion of the breast over and around onto the chest wall. It is important to note that, in some instances, this line will not run through the nipple if the nipple is displaced off the midline of the breast either medially or laterally. The inframammary fold under each breast is joined with a line that extends across the front of the patient (Fig. 92.1C). This allows the location of the fold to be identified with the breasts in their natural orientation. The first cardinal point represents the proposed position of the superior portion of the areola. This point is based on the position of the existing fold. By measuring up from the inframammary fold in the midline 3 to 5 cm, the top portion of the pattern on each side is identified. A line parallel to the inframammary fold line is drawn across the breast (Fig. 92.1D). Where the breast meridian crosses this line represents the topmost portion of the periareolar pattern. The second cardinal point identifies the inferior portion of the pattern. This is a measured landmark based on the breast meridian. The meridian is identified at the level of the inframammary fold, and an 8-cm wide pedicle is drawn and centered on the breast meridian. On either side of the pedicle, a line is drawn up onto the breast parallel with the breast meridian. The length of this line measures 8 cm in smaller breasts, with proposed reduction amounts of 500 g or less, and 10 cm in larger breasts with proposed reduction amounts of 1,000 g or more. The tops of these two lines are then joined in a curvilinear line that parallels the inframammary fold (Fig. 92.1E). This represents the inferior segment of skin that will be preserved after parenchymal resection. The third and fourth cardinal points represent the medial and lateral portions of the periareolar pattern, respectively. These two points are identified by using the hand to elevate and slightly rotate the breast first up and out (Fig. 92.1F), then up and in (Fig. 92.1G), and then transposing visually the breast meridian onto the breast at a point level with the nipple. The goal inherent in manipulating the breast in this way is to try to mold the breast into the desired postoperative shape, and then use the breast meridian to identify the proper position of the medial and lateral resection margin to allow easy redraping of the medial and lateral skin segments around the inferior pedicle. Once these four cardinal points have been identified, they are joined in a curvilinear pattern that assumes the shape of an elongated oval (Fig. 92.1H). A proposed areolar diameter of approximately 5 cm is diagrammed and the pedicle is drawn in, skirting the top of the areolar margin by a distance of 2 to 3 cm. The segment of skin to be removed with the parenchyma is marked with horizontal lines, and the skin of the inferior pedicle that will be deepithelialized is marked with dots (Fig. 92.1I). It is helpful to measure the dimensions of the proposed periareolar pattern at this point, both in the transverse and longitudinal dimensions. Experience has shown that when either of these measurements is less than 15 cm, there is little difficulty in managing the skin envelope during the skin redraping portion of the procedure. For measurements of 15 to 20 cm, some experience in using the circumvertical concept is helpful. For

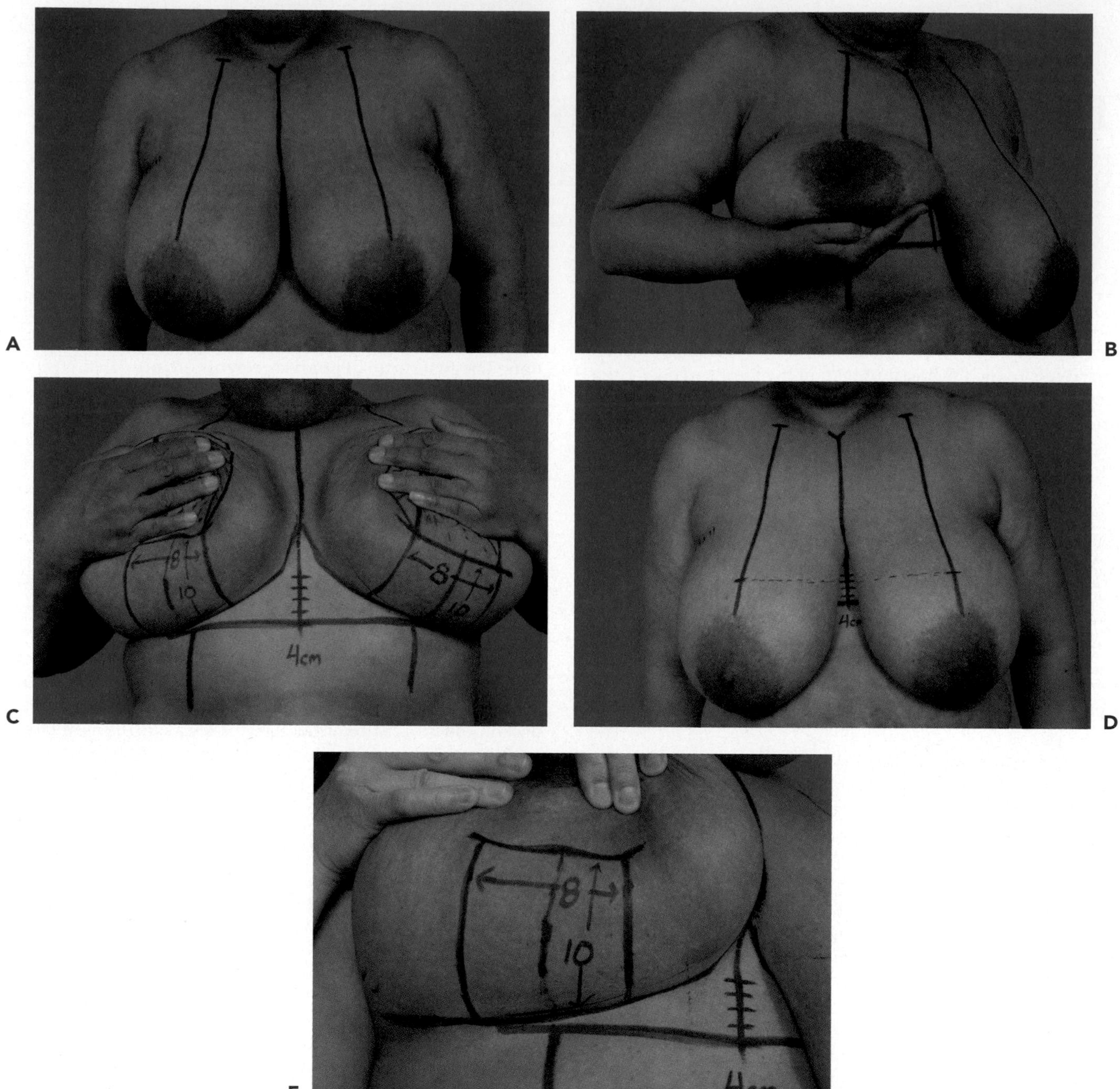

Figure 92.1. **A:** The marking for the short scar periareolar pedicle reduction mammaplasty is begun by noting the midsternal line and the breast meridian. **B:** The meridian line is carried down the central axis of the breast and is extended below the breast onto the abdomen. **C:** The midpoint of the inframammary fold is marked on each side, and these two points are connected with a line that extends across the midline of the upper abdomen. **D:** With the breasts in repose, the exact location of the inframammary fold can be seen without the need to further manipulate the breast. A transverse line is then drawn parallel to the inframammary fold across the breasts at a point 3 to 5 cm above the inframammary fold line. Where this line transects the breast meridian on each side marks the top portion of the periareolar pattern. **E:** An 8-cm pedicle width is measured along the inframammary fold, centered on the breast meridian. On either side of this pedicle, a pedicle length of 8 to 10 cm is drawn onto the breast where a line paralleling the inframammary fold line is drawn. This marks the inferior portion of the periareolar pattern. (*continued*)

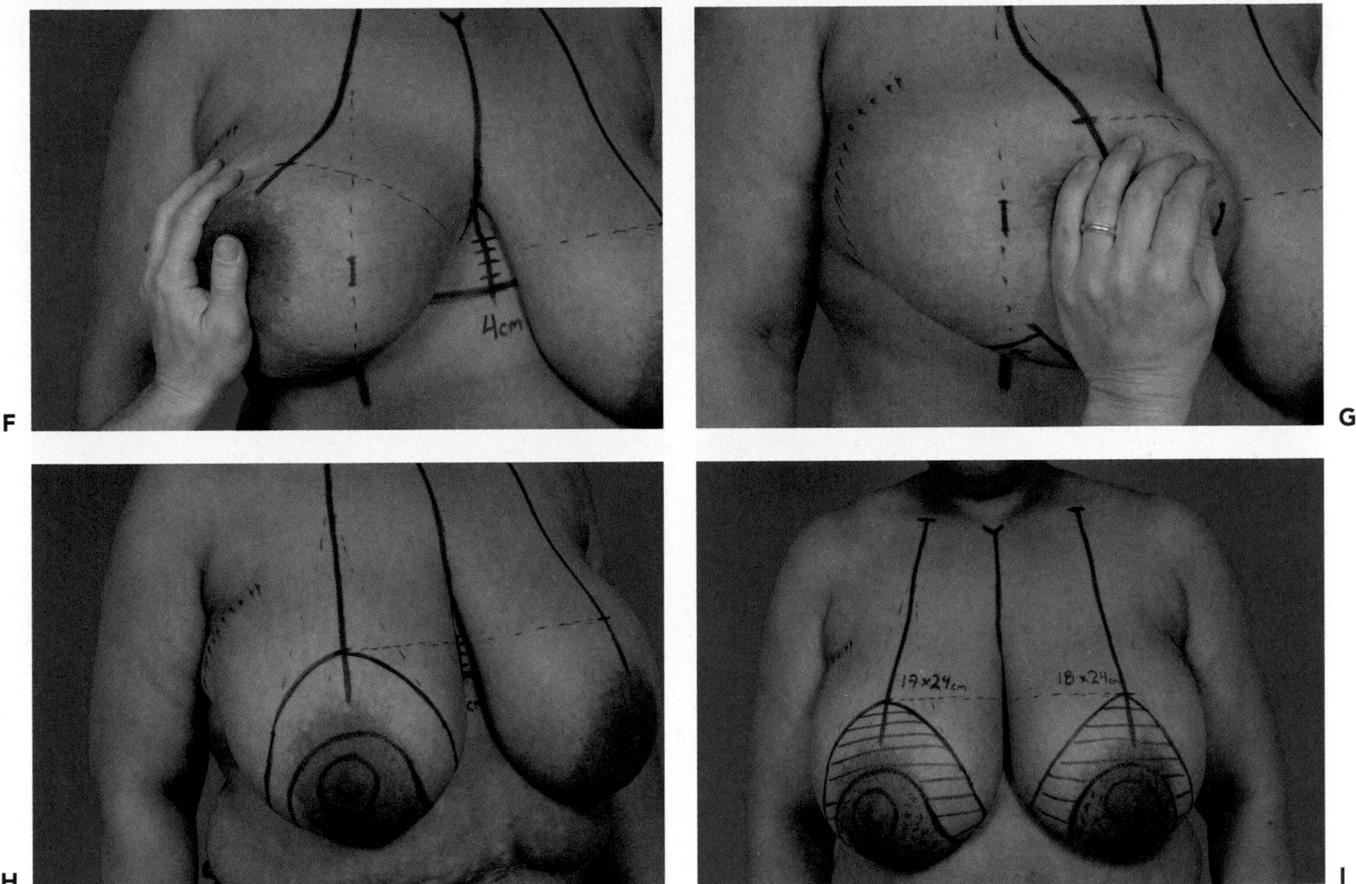

Figure 92.1. (*Continued*) **F** and **G:** The breast is then drawn first up and out, then up and in, and the breast meridian is transposed onto the breast at the level of the nipple. This sets the medial and lateral points of the periareolar pattern. **H:** The four cardinal points are smoothly connected into the shape of an elongated oval, and the upper portion of the pedicle is drawn in, skirting the top of the proposed areola by a distance of 2 to 3 cm. **I:** The final marking pattern shows symmetry in the top of the pattern, and the amount of skin destined to be left behind medially, laterally, and inferiorly after resection.

measurements of more than 20 cm, experience with the technique is recommended to achieve the best result.

OPERATIVE TECHNIQUE

At surgery, the patient must be prepared for being elevated to the sitting position during the procedure. This maneuver is mandatory to allow assessment of breast shape during skin redraping. Therefore, the arms must be secured to arm boards and the head supported on a foam headrest. Anesthesia must be informed of the need to sit the patient up during surgery to allow for adequate hydration and avoidance of postural hypotension.

All proposed incisions are infiltrated with a dilute solution of lidocaine with epinephrine. A breast tourniquet is applied, and the areola is placed under maximal stretch. A 52-mm diameter areolar mark is made with a circular template (Figs. 92.2A and 92.2B). Ultimately, the periareolar purse-string suture will be tied down to approximately 40 mm in diameter; thus, the larger areola will eventually be allowed to simply rest in the areolar opening without tension. This strategy allows a more natural-looking and tension-free areola to be created. All incisions are scored, and the inferior pedicle within the periareolar pattern is de-epithelialized, along with a rim of dermis around the periphery (Figs. 92.2C and 92.2D). This rim is de-epithelialized for a width of approximately 1 cm, and the dermis divided with Bovie cautery in such a way that a 5-mm dermal rim is created around the periareolar pattern except for the 8 cm width of the inferior pedicle. This rim of dermis will ultimately serve as a sturdy architectural dermal framework into which the periareolar purse-string suture will be placed. The dermis around the inferior pedicle is likewise divided and the tourniquet released. Medial, superior, and lateral flaps are then developed with three-dimensional sculpting of the breast in mind. The medial and superior flaps are initially dissected directly at the dermal level, with dissection then curving gently downward to create a flap that becomes progressively thicker until the chest wall is reached. At the base of the flap, the thickness of fat and parenchyma measures 4 to 6 cm. Laterally, there is a tendency for the breast to assume a "boxy" appearance if the flap is kept too thick; therefore, initial flap dissection again begins just under the dermis and then angles toward the capsule of the breast. The remainder of the lateral flap is dissected at this level down to the lateral border of the breast. Where the lateral and superior flaps merge, a smooth transition is made from the thicker base of the superior flap to the thinner base of the lateral flap. It is important to emphasize that dissection of the flaps does not violate the

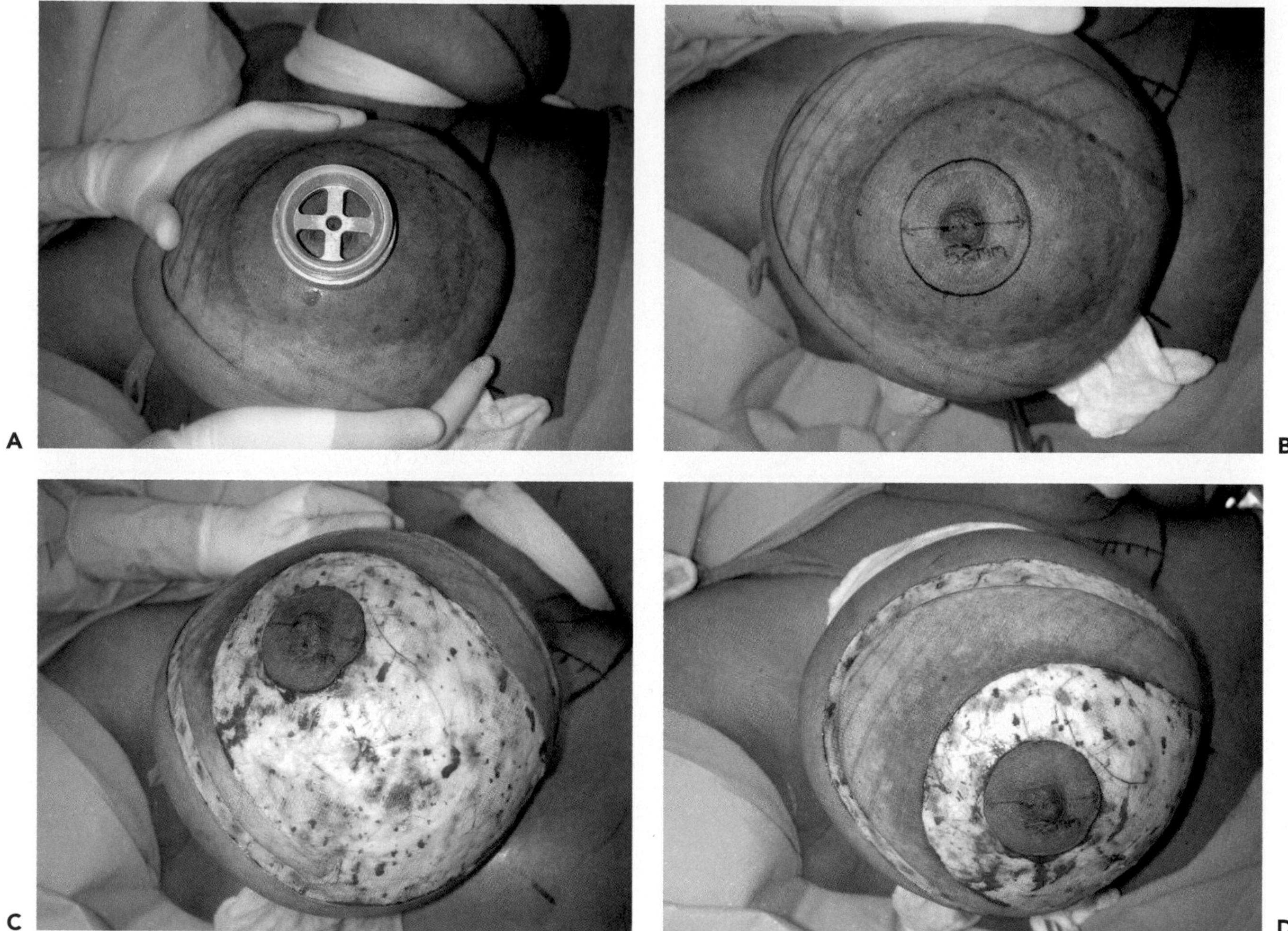

Figure 92.2. **A** and **B:** A circular areolar marker is used to diagram a perfectly round areolar incision with a diameter of 50 to 52 mm. **C** and **D:** The inferior pedicle is de-epithelialized, along with a 5-mm rim of dermis around the periareolar incision.

inframammary fold. In the medial and lateral corners of the breast flap dissection, the attachments of Scarpa's fascia to the underside of the breast are preserved. By keeping these relationships intact, the postoperative phenomenon of "bottoming out" or migration of breast parenchyma below the inframammary fold is prevented. The result is a stable breast shape postoperatively and greater control over the operative result. After the flaps have been created, the bulk of the remaining breast can be delivered from the wound, and the general contours created by the flaps can be seen (Figs. 92.3A and 92.3B). Specifically, the superior and medial contours of the breast should be smooth and full to avoid any sharp step-offs in breast shape. The pedicle is now skeletonized, making sure to avoid any undermining of the NAC (Figs. 92.3C and 92.3D). The longitudinal septum of the breast can usually be identified in the lower half of the breast during this dissection. This septum carries important perforators and should not be incised during pedicle dissection (5,6). The specimen that is removed comes off in the shape of a horseshoe with the lateral limb slightly longer than the medial limb (Fig. 92.3E). It is important to carefully create the flaps and pedicle such that, after pedicle skeletonization, the flaps and pedicle wrap around each other smoothly. This creates a pleasing breast shape and avoids any sharp or unaesthetic contours. In patients with a naturally full upper pole to the breast, no further shaping maneuvers are required, and the procedure simply continues. If, however, there is hollowness in the upper pole of the breast, reshaping with internal sutures is required. This simply involves undermining the remaining breast parenchyma in the superior pole of the breast and advancing this flap superiorly until the desired upper pole fullness is created (Figs. 92.4A–C). At this point, the underside of the flap is sutured down to the pectoralis fascia with one or two absorbable sutures to perform what is essentially an "autoaugmentation" of the upper pole of the breast (Fig. 92.4D). Usually, the leading edge of the undermined superior breast flap is relocated superiorly 4 to 6 cm. This maneuver is made possible by making the superior flap thick enough at the base during the initial flap dissection. When necessary, medial reshaping is also performed by undermining the base of the medial flap up to the level of the intercostal perforators (Fig. 92.4E) and then simply plicating the leading edge of this flap to itself to gather the medial tissues together to create a more rounded contour (Figs. 92.4F–H). Finally, the tendency for the inferior pedicle to fall off laterally into the axilla is counteracted by suturing the base of the

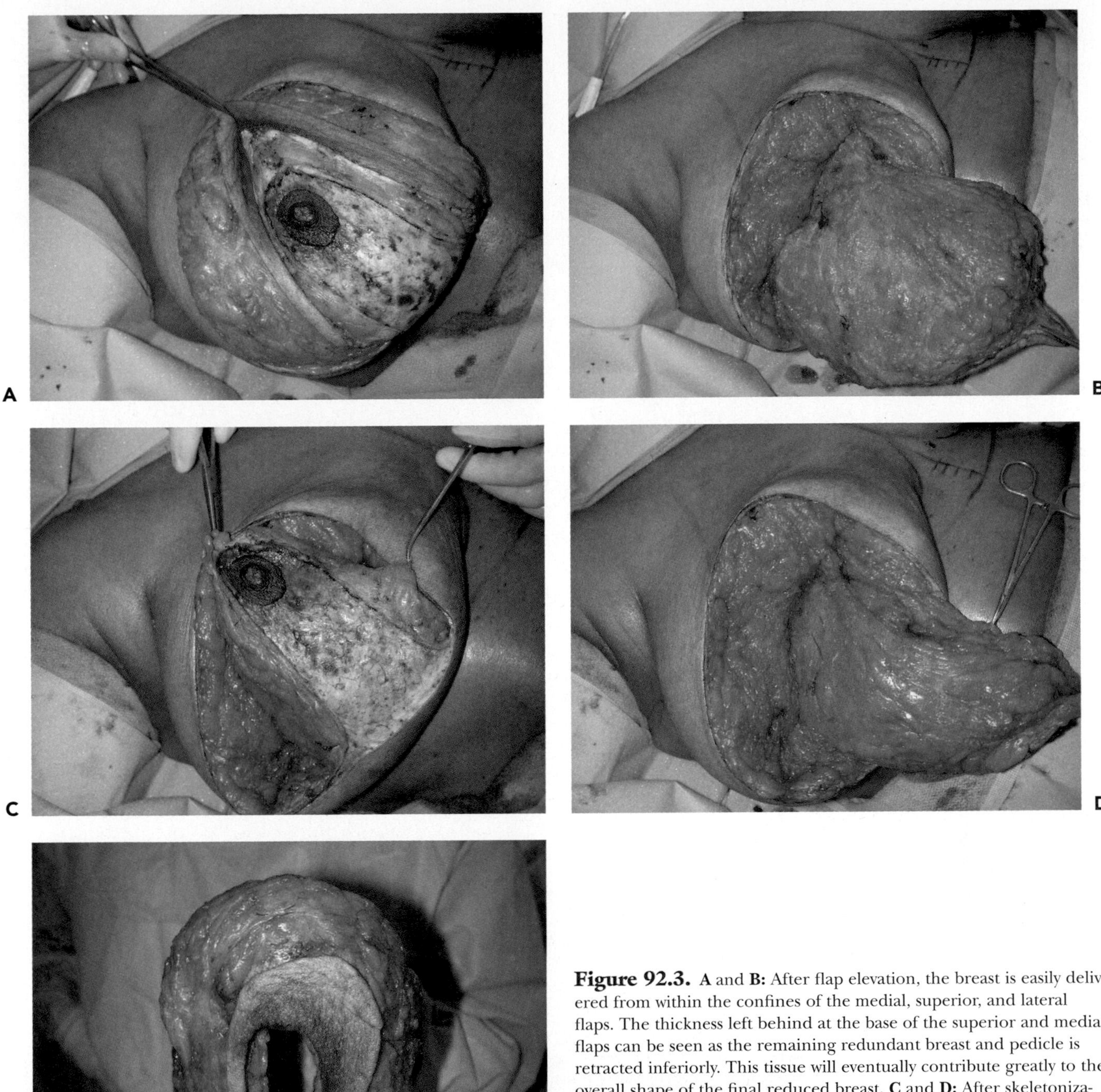

Figure 92.3. **A** and **B:** After flap elevation, the breast is easily delivered from within the confines of the medial, superior, and lateral flaps. The thickness left behind at the base of the superior and medial flaps can be seen as the remaining redundant breast and pedicle is retracted inferiorly. This tissue will eventually contribute greatly to the overall shape of the final reduced breast. **C** and **D:** After skeletonization of the pedicle, the tissue left behind for breast shaping on the flaps and the pedicle can be seen. Sculpting these two segments of tissue to fit evenly contributes greatly to the quality of the aesthetic result after skin retailoring. **E:** The specimen resembles an elongated horseshoe after removal, with the lateral limb being slightly longer than the medial limb.

pedicle down to the pectoralis fascia in the central portion of the breast (Fig. 92.4I). This centralizes the bulk of the breast tissue and assists in shaping the breast. After the breast shape has been controlled, the vertical skin incision is determined. By placing traction on the inferior pedicle, the medial and lateral breast flaps will buckle. These two buckle points are joined together with a skin stapler to position the "key staple" (Figs. 92.5A–D). This then sets the rest of the pattern. Two hemostats are used to grasp the previously de-epithelialized dermal shelf right at the key staple point, and upward traction is placed on the inferior skin envelope (Fig. 92.5E). This maneuver allows the redundant inferior skin envelope of the breast to be plicated together with staples until a smooth, rounded contour is created (Figs. 92.5F–J). The NAC is also inset with staples to complete the proposed closure (Fig. 92.5K). Adjustments are often required at this point to either tighten the skin further or loosen

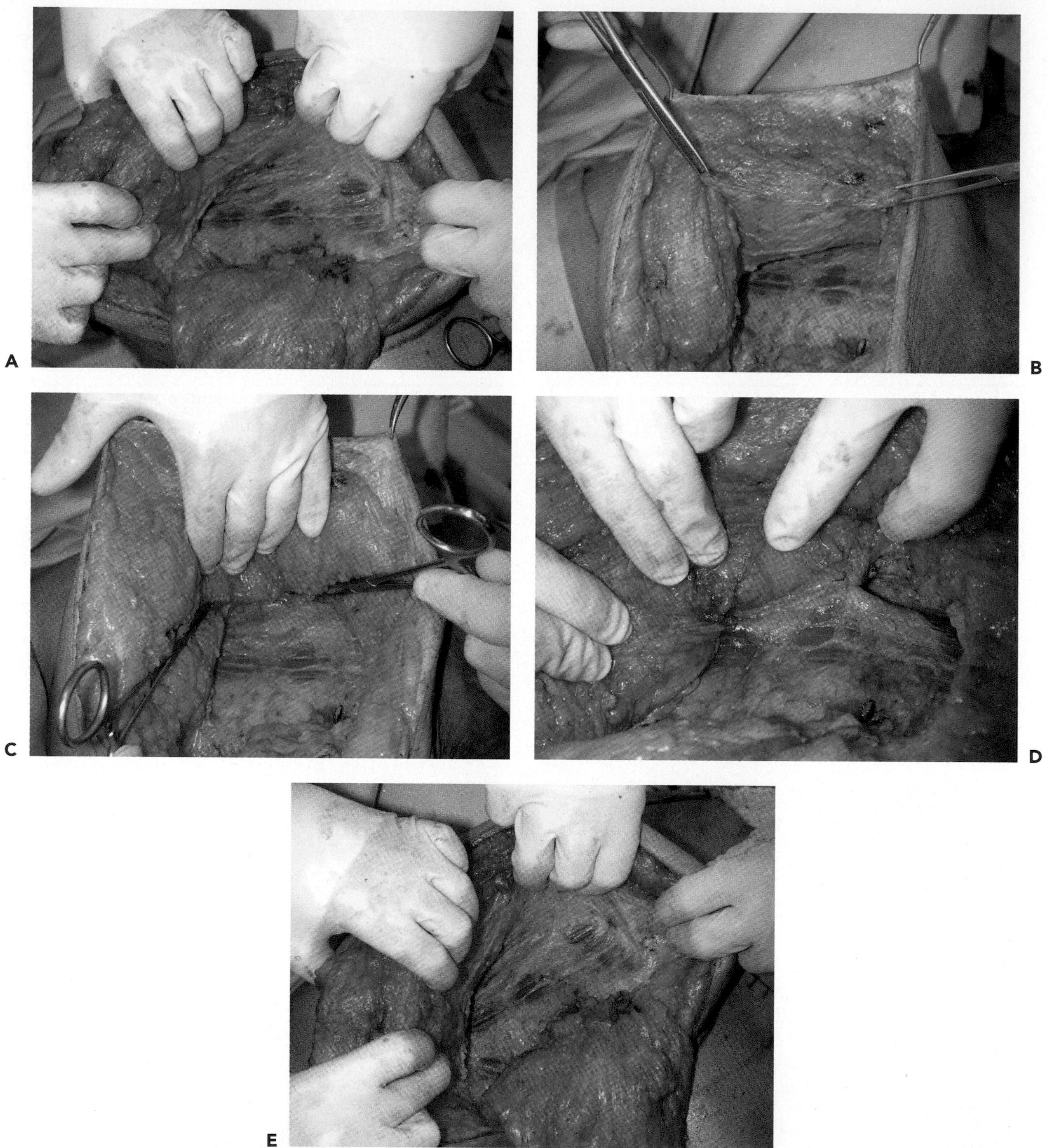

Figure 92.4. **A:** After pedicle skeletonization, the upper flap is undermined to point above and slightly beyond the superior aspect of the breast. **B** and **C:** The leading edge of this undermined flap is grasped and advanced superiorly until the mass effect of transposing this tissue under the upper pole of the breast fills the void and corrects the concavity present preoperatively. This amounts to an "autoaugmentation" of the upper pole of the breast. **D:** The leading edge of the flap is sutured to the pectoralis fascia to secure it into position with two to three evenly spaced tacking sutures. **E:** The medial flap is undermined up to the level of the intercostal perforators. (*continued*)

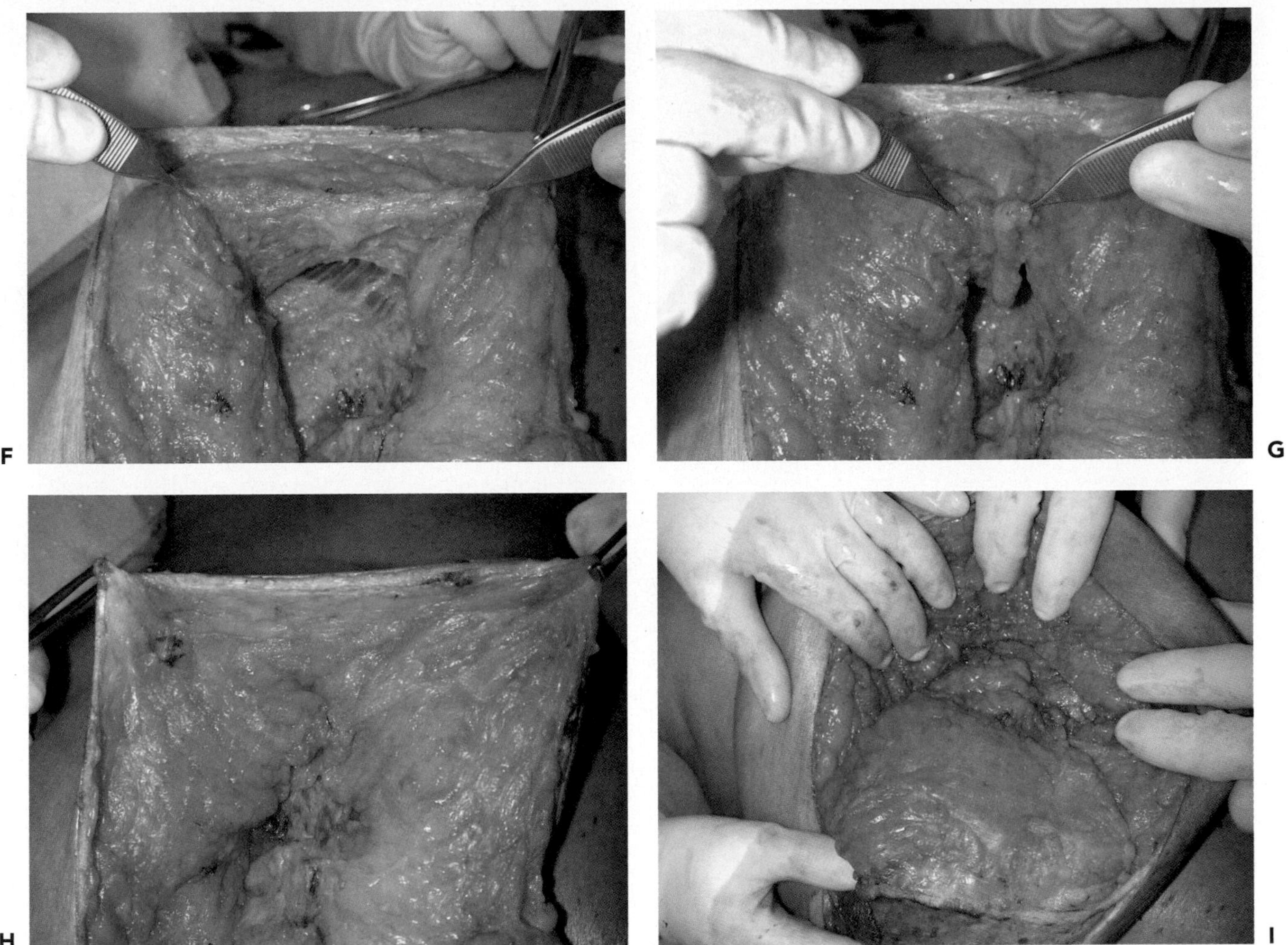

Figure 92.4. (*Continued*) **F–H:** The undermined edge of the medial flap is grasped at two points separated by 3 to 4 cm, and these two points are advanced toward each other and sutured. This has the effect of gathering the medial parenchyma together, creating a more rounded and attractive medial breast contour. **I:** Finally, the base of the inferior pedicle is secured centrally to the pectoralis major fascia to centralize the bulk of the pedicle and keep it from falling off laterally into the axilla.

the plication in selected areas to create the desired shape. It is sometimes helpful to perform this plication with the patient upright as an aid to effective shaping. After the desired shape has been created, the edges of the staple line are marked with a skin marker, and all the staples are removed (Fig. 92.5L). The area of the inferior pedicle is identified, and a small medial wedge and a larger lateral wedge of redundant skin and parenchyma are noted (Fig. 92.5M). The inferior pedicle is de-epithelialized, and the medial and lateral wedges of tissue are removed (Fig. 92.5N). In this fashion, the lateral breast flap, because it is completely incised, can be brought over to the medial breast flap on top of the de-epthelialized pedicle without tension or kinking (Fig. 92.5O). This aids in the creation of a smooth rounded inferior breast contour. Drains are placed in larger reductions of more than 700 to 800 g and are brought out laterally along the inframammary fold. The vertical incision is then closed with 4–0 absorbable monofilament, using both interrupted inverted dermal sutures and finally a running subcuticular suture (Fig. 92.5P). The dimension of the periareolar opening will be noted to be much smaller as a result of adding the vertical component to the skin pattern; however, there will still be a discrepancy between the larger diameter of the periareolar incision and the smaller diameter of the areolar incision. This discrepancy is managed by placing a purse-string suture in the periareolar dermal shelf created during the initial incision pattern (Figs. 92.6A and 92.6B). It is highly recommended that a CV-3 Gortex suture is used for this purpose. The handling characteristics of this material are ideal in that this suture material is strong, permanent, and, most important, slides easily through the dermis. This allows the purse-string suture to be closed with a great deal of control and to any desired dimension. The knot for the suture is placed so as to bury it under the edge of the dermal shelf to avoid postoperative erosion through the suture line. The suture is drawn down to create an opening of approximately 40 mm (Figs. 92.6C and 92.6D). After being secured, the patient is placed upright, and the opening is often observed to be irregular and oval shaped along an axis running from superomedial to inferolateral. By drawing a circular pattern centered on this opening and then de-epithelializing this additional skin, a perfectly circular areolar defect can be created (Figs. 92.6E–G). Care must be taken to avoid inadvertently cutting the Gortex purse string suture during this process. The areola is then inset

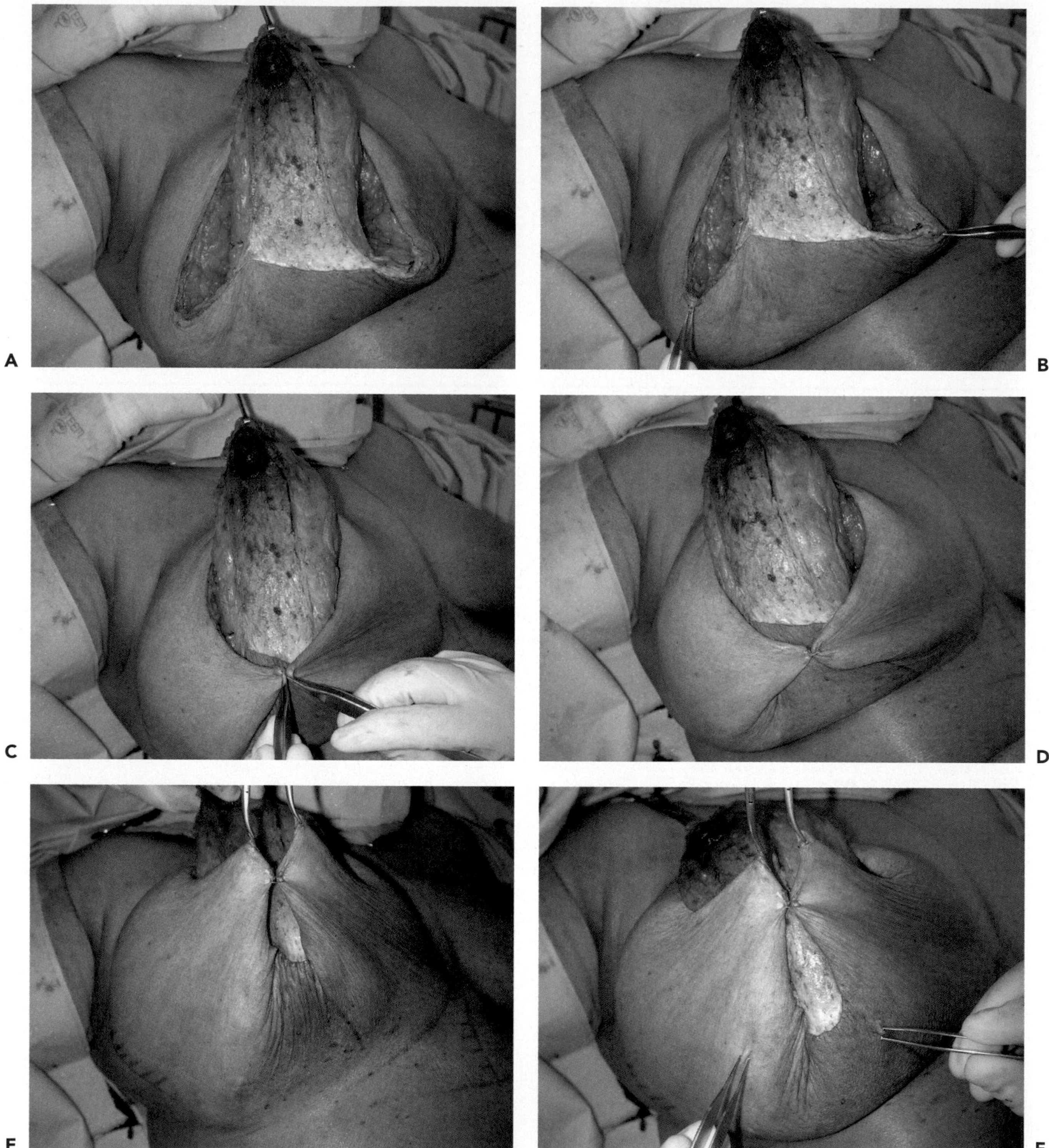

Figure 92.5. **A:** Retailoring of the inferior pole skin envelope is begun by grasping the tip of the inferior pedicle and exerting upward traction. This causes a medial and lateral buckle point to form in the skin flap on either side of the pedicle. **B–D:** These two buckle points are stapled together to identify the "key" staple. This represents the top of the vertical pattern. The remainder of the skin plication is based on the placement of this "key" staple. **E–I:** Two hemostats are used to grasp the de-epithelialized portion of the periareolar dermis near the "key" staple. By placing upward traction on these hemostats, the plication line for retailoring the inferior skin envelope can be more easily discerned. Medial and lateral skin points are sequentially brought together with temporary staples until a pleasing lower breast contour is created. (*continued*)

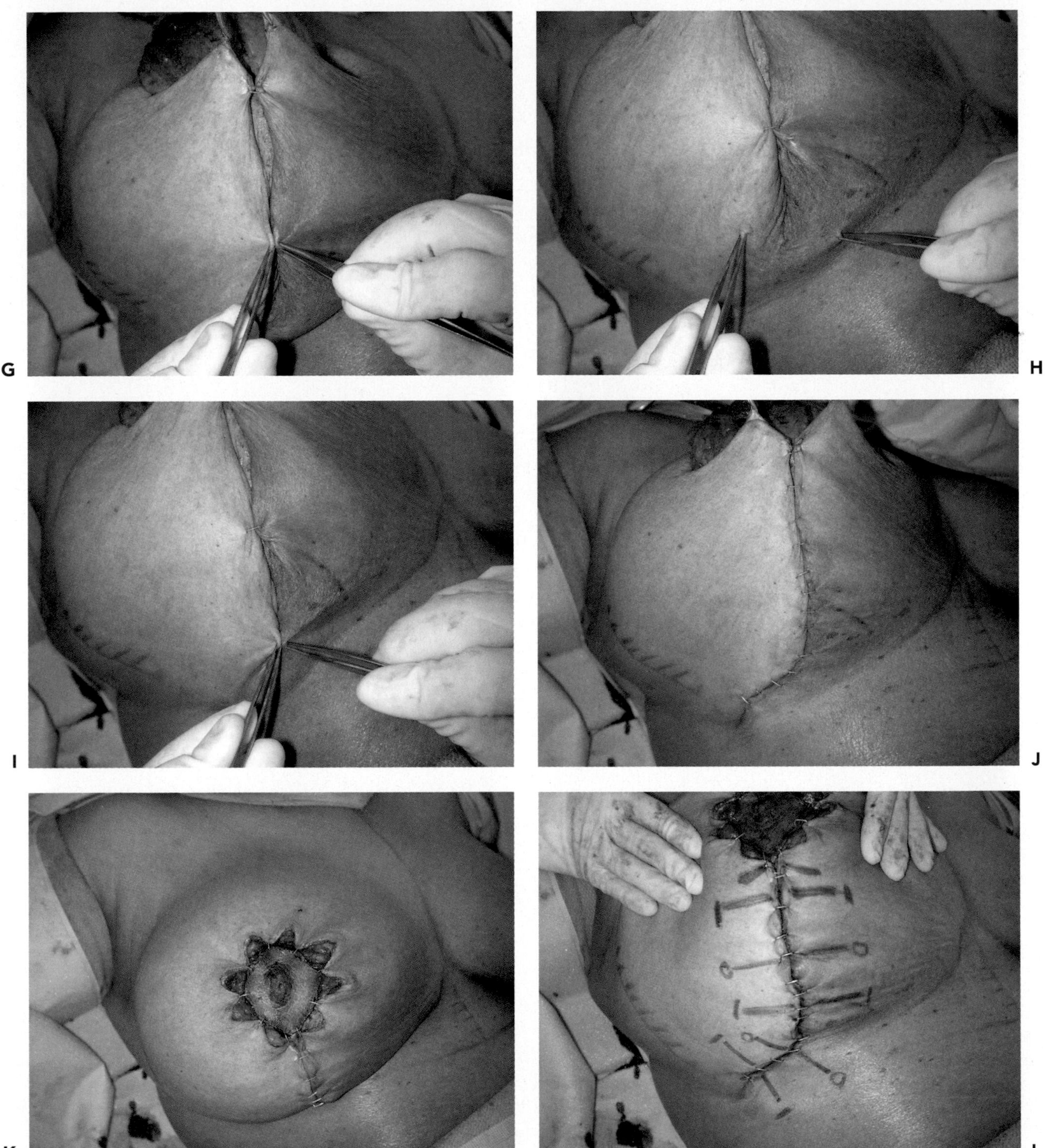

Figure 92.5. (*Continued*) **J:** Appearance of the breast after complete retailoring of the inferior skin envelope. **K:** Appearance of the breast after insetting of the nipple-areola complex. **L:** After the desired breast shape has been created, the vertical plication line is marked with a surgical marker. Orientation lines are very helpful in putting the edges back together after the redundant skin has been resected. (*continued*)

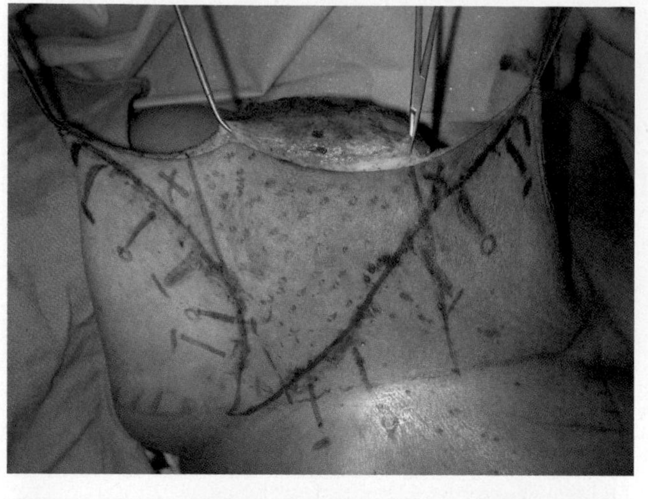
M

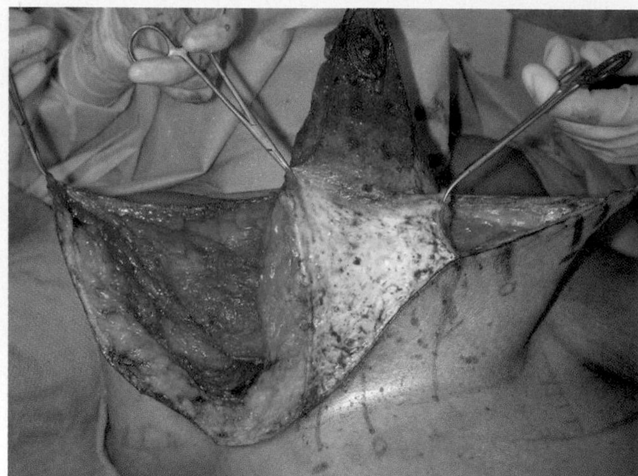
N

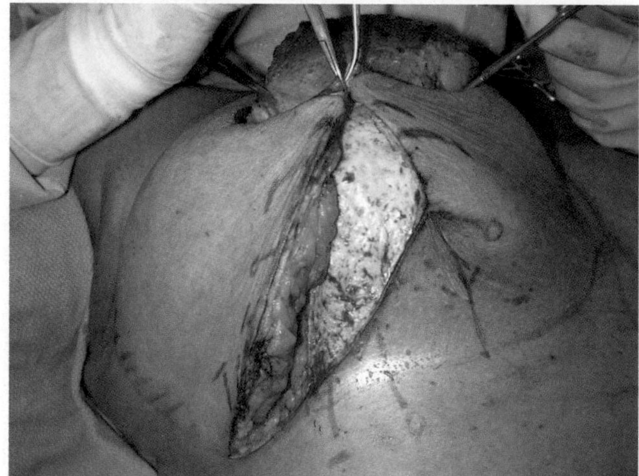
O

Figure 92.5. (*Continued*) **M:** After the staples are removed, the area of skin over the inferior pedicle that needs to be de-epithelialized can be seen. **N:** Appearance of the lower pole after de-epithelialization, and resection of the redundant medial and lateral flaps outside to the margin of the inferior pedicle. **O:** Full-thickness release of the lateral flap allows it to pass over on top of the inferior pedicle to meet the medial flap without kinking or distortion.

into the defect again with 4–0 absorbable monofilament suture (Figs. 92.6H and 92.6I). To prevent postoperative asymmetry, it is advised to perform the various steps of the operation sequentially from side to side. This gives maximum control over the volume and shape of each breast and allows proper adjustments to be made as needed. If one breast is completed first, it may become difficult to obtain absolute symmetry in the other, particularly if the second breast then ends up lacking volume compared with the first. After the procedure is fully completed, our preference is to cover the incisions with Dermabond and Opsite. A support garment is then applied.

The procedure is performed quite successfully as an outpatient procedure, although some patients are kept overnight in the hospital. A support garment is worn continuously simply for comfort and to help control swelling. Dressings and drains are removed in about 7 days and a vitamin E-containing gel is applied to the incisions and covered with paper tape every 3 to 5 days and thereafter for 6 weeks. Vigorous physical exertion is discouraged for 4 weeks after the procedure. Full maturation of the result is complete in 6 to 12 months (Figs. 92.7A–D).

RESULTS

The SPAIR mammaplasty is a versatile and predictable technique for everything from simple mastopexy up to reductions of 2,000 g per side and more. The operation is similar in every way except that as the preoperative size of the breast increases, the vertical scar extends more laterally along the inframammary fold. In cases of mastopexy, there is usually an element of upper pole breast concavity, along with a ptotic appearance to the breast. In these cases, the SPAIR technique offers considerable advantage due to the ability to directly control upper pole shape with the internal shaping sutures. Combining this feature with the reduced amount of cutaneous scar offers these patients an attractive option for operative correction of ptosis without the possibility of postoperative shape change or "bottoming out." This is an ideal combination of advantages for these patients who tend to have high expectations with regard to the aesthetics of the ultimate result.

For modest reductions up to 700 g, the technique offers the same advantages (Figs. 92.8 and 92.9). It is easily performed, the periareolar defect affords excellent exposure, allowing easy flap dissection and shaping, and skin redraping is typically not difficult. These types of patients tend to develop excellent results with few complications.

For larger reductions of 800 to 1,000 g or more, or in patients with a significant degree of ptosis with an excessive skin envelope, experience with the technique is recommended. Here, exposure is not typically a problem, but skin redraping and management of the periareolar defect can be challenging. It is not uncommon for these patients to experience

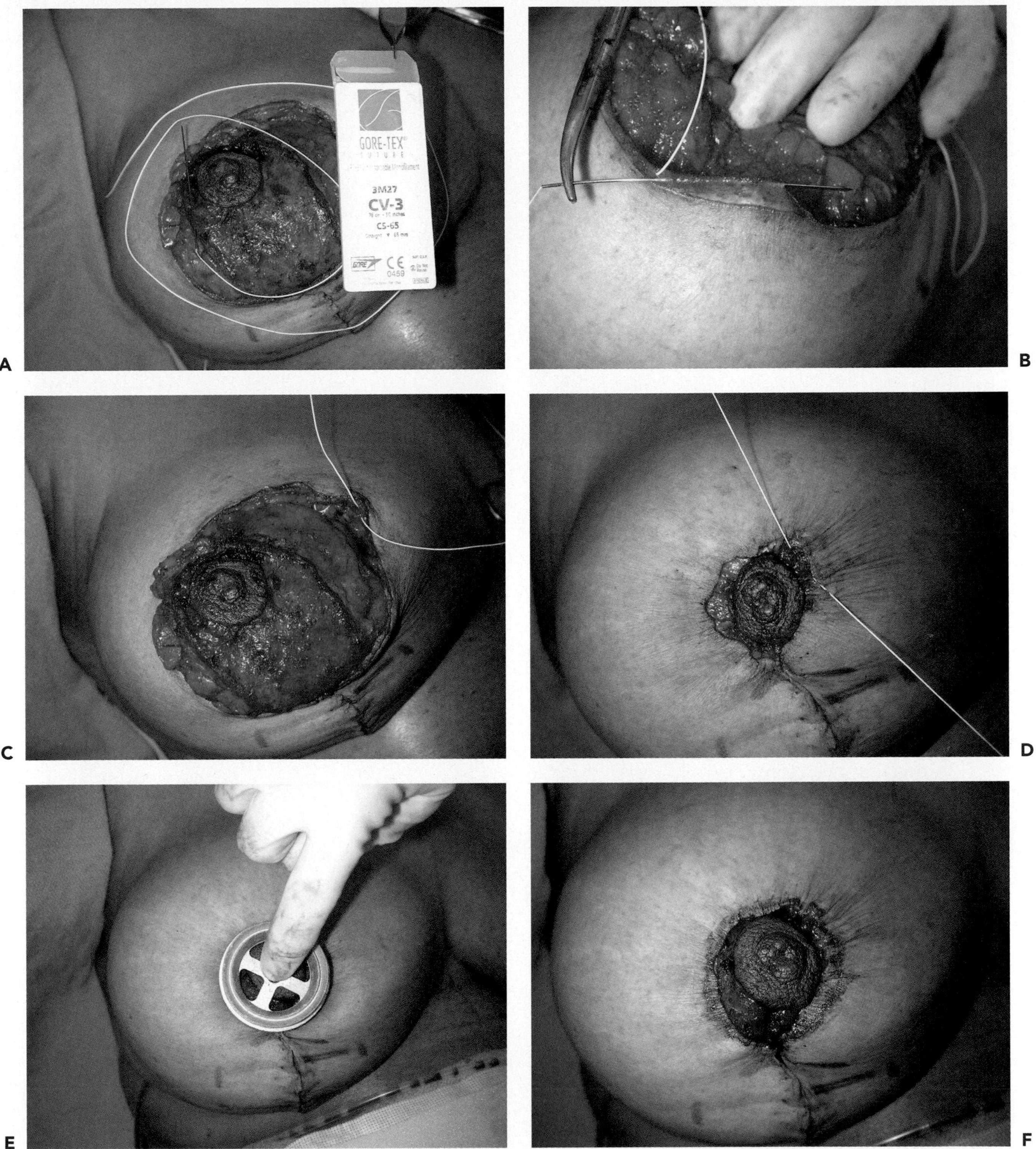

Figure 92.6. **A:** A CV-3 Gortex suture on a straight needle is used to cinch down the diameter of the periareolar incision. **B:** The needle is passed into the substance of the de-epithelialized dermal shelf created at the beginning of the procedure. **C** and **D:** By placing traction on the Gortex purse-string suture, the somewhat wide periareolar defect can be cinched down to an opening of 35 to 40 mm. The handing characteristics of this suture material make it ideal for this purpose. **E–H:** The often ovoid resulting defect is reconfigured by drawing a circular opening, often with the aid of an areolar marker, and then de-epithelializing this additional skin before final insetting of the nipple-areola complex (NAC). In this fashion, a truly round NAC can be constructed. (*continued*)

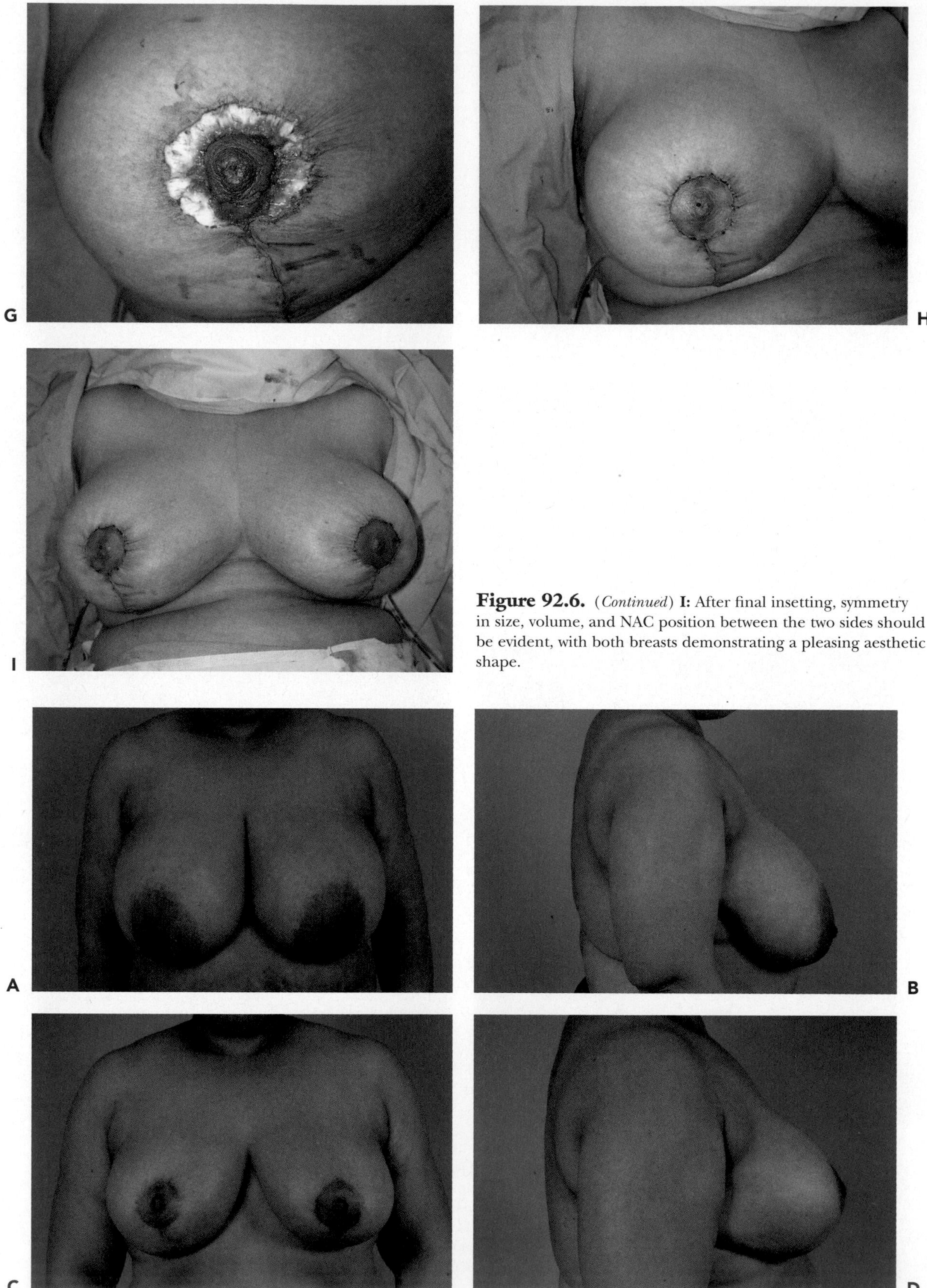

Figure 92.6. (*Continued*) **I:** After final insetting, symmetry in size, volume, and NAC position between the two sides should be evident, with both breasts demonstrating a pleasing aesthetic shape.

Figure 92.7. **A** and **B:** Preoperative appearance of a 46-year-old woman prior to breast reduction using the short scar periareolar pedicle reduction technique. This is the same patient seen in the marking and operative technique photos. **C** and **D:** Appearance 6 months after removal of 833 g of tissue from the right breast and 769 g from the left.

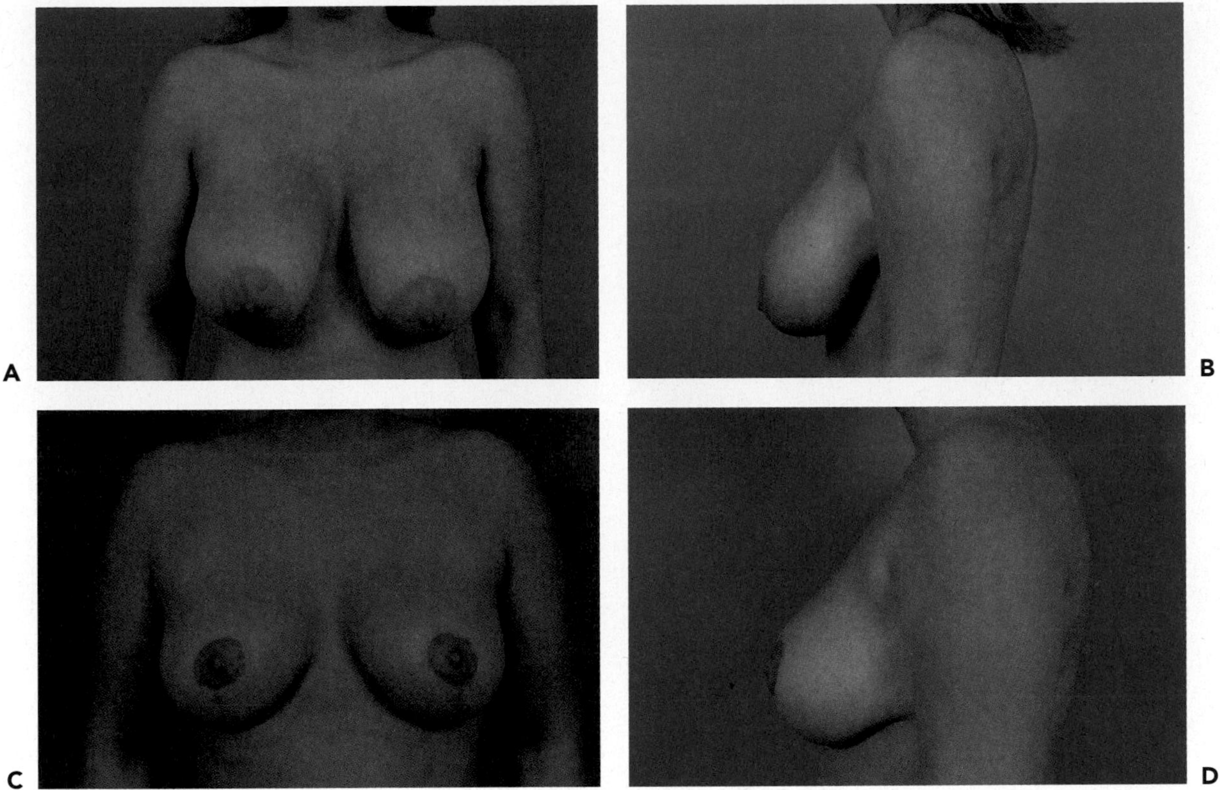

Figure 92.8. **A** and **B:** Preoperative appearance of a 17-year-old young woman prior to breast reduction with the short scar periareolar pedicle reduction technique. **C** and **D:** One year postoperative appearance after removal of 420 g of tissue from the right breast and 452 g from the left.

persistent distortion of the periareolar closure with skin pleating or irregular contours being the result. It must be remembered that the alternative for these patients would most commonly be an inverted T-type procedure, and it is my practice to educate my patients about the limitations of the SPAIR technique and accept them rather than switch to the inverted T approach. The advantage of the shorter scar, and, most important, shape stability, outweigh concerns over the periareolar scar for most patients.

COMPLICATIONS

The usual complications associated with breast reduction remain as potential complications of the SPAIR technique. Infection, bleeding, hematoma formation, wound separation, NAC or breast skin numbness, and hypertrophic scarring, while unusual, have been observed. Specific complications associated with the SPAIR technique do however merit specific comment.

SEROMA

Although unusual, several cases of seroma formation with significant capsule formation around the seroma have been observed. The cavity forms deep in the breast around the superior portion of the inferior pedicle. As the seroma fluid eventually reabsorbs, the scar capsule contracts, creating a tethering effect on the NAC. This causes the breast to appear flattened and distorted. Minor cases resolve with simple observation. Significant breast distortion, however, can persist and require operative repair. In these cases, the incision pattern is opened, and the seroma cavity is exposed and removed. Reclosure then restores an aesthetic shape to the breast without the need for further internal suturing or reshaping.

GORTEX SUTURE INFECTION

Rarely, a persistent red halo of erythema around the NAC can develop with or without small sinus tracts in the periareolar scar. This finding represents a purse-string suture infection that resolves with removal of the Gortex suture. Typically, scar has already stabilized the periareolar opening, and postoperative dilatation of the areolar diameter has not been noted after removal of the Gortex.

POSTOPERATIVE SHAPE CHANGE

True "bottoming out" of the breast with extension of breast parenchyma below the inframammary fold does not occur in the SPAIR technique because the attachments of Scarpa's fascia to the inframammary fold are not violated. However, resolution of swelling or mild skin stretch in the lower pole of the breast can detract from the overall breast shape. In addition, it is common for the areola to expand several millimeters over time. These changes are easily corrected with simple scar revision. By plicating additional skin along the vertical closure or redoing the periareolar purse-string suture, significant improvement in breast shape can usually be accomplished. However, such manipulations are only rarely required.

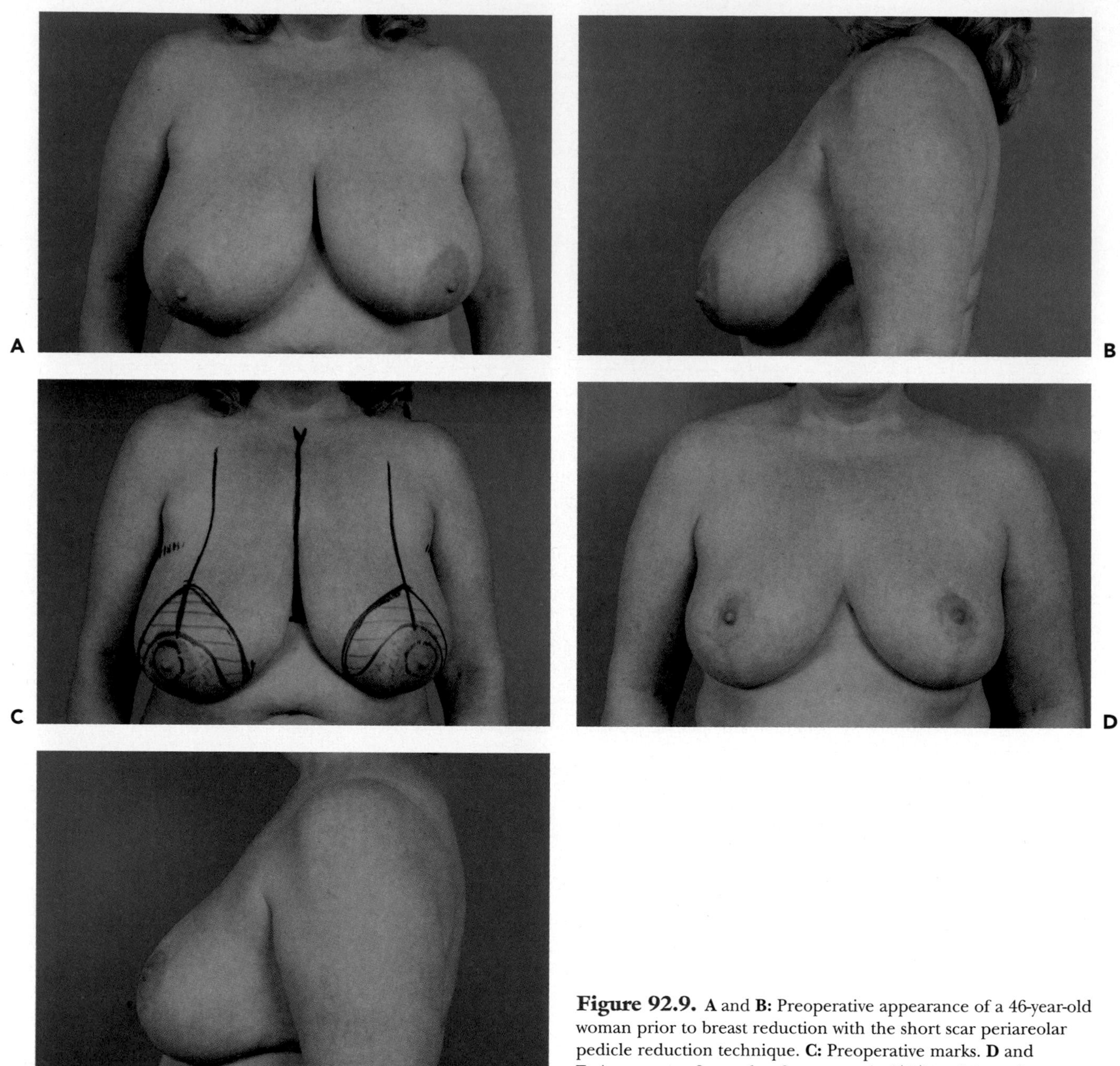

Figure 92.9. **A** and **B:** Preoperative appearance of a 46-year-old woman prior to breast reduction with the short scar periareolar pedicle reduction technique. **C:** Preoperative marks. **D** and **E:** Appearance 8 months after removal of 717 g of tissue from the right breast and 573 g from the left.

CONCLUSION

The SPAIR mammaplasty has proven to be a predictable and reliable technique for breast reduction and mastopexy. Complications are few, and surgeon and patient satisfaction are high. It is recommended as an excellent treatment option for patients interested in breast reduction and mastopexy.

EDITORIAL COMMENTS

Dr. Hammond has prepared an excellent chapter that reviews and outlines the SPAIR technique for reduction mammaplasty. I have listened to and read many of Dr. Hammonds' presentations, manuscripts, and chapters over the years, and each time I come away with more useful information. He has taken an operation that on first glance seems complex, analyzed each step, and described it in a simple and eloquent style to facilitate comprehension. Having personally been an advocate of the Wise pattern, I now frequently perform the short scar techniques much to the credit and teaching of Dr. Hammond. He clearly has an understanding of every aspect of this operation and has mastered them all to the point that he is able to obtain a consistent and predictable result in his patients. In this chapter, Dr. Hammond has described and outlined the SPAIR technique in clear and concise fashion with enough detail such that other surgeons may too be able to obtain similar results.

There are several tips and techniques advocated by Dr. Hammond that I have found particularly useful. He emphasizes that there is a learning curve associated with this operation and that surgeons should first master the smaller reductions before attempting the larger ones. The initial and perhaps most important step with this operation is to properly mark the patient in the upright position. The four cardinal points described are critical to ensure proper breast contour, position, and symmetry. Dr. Hammond describes delineating the NAC with a 5-cm pattern and then reducing it to 4 cm with a purse-string suture. I have found that enlarging the outline of the NAC has been extremely effective in eliminating the "stretched look" and maintains a natural appearance. The phenomenon of "bottoming out" has plagued many of the previous reduction mammaplasty techniques. Dr. Hammond emphasizes the importance of preserving the integrity of the inframammary fold, as well as the attachments of Scarpa's fascia, to the lateral and medial pillars to prevent the bottoming-out phenomena. I also perform the "tailor-tack" technique when closing the vertical scar to improve lower pole contour and the appearance of the incision. There are only three areas in which Dr. Hammond and I differ. These include use of the Wise pattern for severe mammary hypertrophy, use of a medial or superior pedicle on occasion, and use of suction drains for reductions that exceed 300 g. Hopefully, with time and additional personal experience using the SPAIR technique, larger reduction can be performed to meet patient expectations.

M.Y.N.

REFERENCES

1. Hammond DC. The SPAIR mammaplasty. *Clin Plast Surg* 2002;29:411.
2. Hammond DC. Short scar periareolar inferior pedicle reduction (SPAIR) mammaplasty. *Plast Reconstr Surg* 1999;103:890.
3. Hammond DC. Short scar periareolar inferior pedicle reduction (SPAIR) mammaplasty: Operative techniques. *Plast Reconstr Surg* 1999;6:106.
4. Hammond DC. Short scar periareolar inferior pedicle reduction (SPAIR) mammaplasty/mastopexy: how I do it step by step. *Perspect Plast Surg* 2001;15:61.
5. Wuringer E. Refinement of the central pedicle breast reduction by application of the ligamentous suspension. *Plast Reconstr Surg* 1999;5:103.
6. Wuringer E. Nerve and vessel supplying ligamentous suspension of the mammary gland. *Plast Reconstr Surg* 1998;6:101.

CHAPTER

93

A. Aldo Mottura

The Circumvertical Breast Reduction Technique

INTRODUCTION

Every breast reduction technique has three main parts: parenchyma removal, the choice of the pedicle for the areola, and the incision and final scar. Short-scar techniques are modern trends in surgery, to the point that in plastic surgery, Nahai (25) popularized the term "scar wars."

Twenty years ago, Benelli (3) introduced the periareolar technique, but in my hands and those of many others, the scars and final results were not always optimal. Almost at the same time, Lejour (14,15) popularized a vertical technique that was an adaptation of the original Lassus (11–13) vertical technique. Since then, in spite of the many different papers published, as well as the many hours of lectures, these two techniques and their modifications have not had universal acceptance (26). The reasons are manifold: The techniques are not easy to learn, it is not easy to obtain nice results, the indications are limited by the skin quality and large-volume breast removal, the results are not always observed at the end of the surgery, and the long vertical scars usually cross the inframammary fold (IMF) with a significant number of touch-ups (2–17).

Thirty years ago, when the idea of the purse-string suture did not exist, I started using a primitive vertical technique called at that time the Arié (1–8) technique for minor breast hypertrophies and ptosis. Fifteen years ago, in an attempt to find a way to have a shorter vertical scar, I began using a combination of the periareolar technique and a prolongation at the inferior quadrant like a vertical technique, thus developing the circumvertical reduction mastoplasty (CVRM). I found that after the inferior lateral and medial skin was undermined, a W-Wise pattern was the best means of parenchyma removal (as in the inverted-T technique) (Fig. 93.1); in most cases, no pedicle was needed for areola transposition. Initially, the areola was sutured with the purse-string suture, which was then changed for the cinching running suture. As I observed that the skin retracted during surgery, I resected less skin and obtained an acceptable result at the end of the surgery. As happens with every new technique, with time and experience, refinements improved the initial technique (18–24).

CHOICE OF THE PATIENT AND MARKING

In general, for small-volume breast removals (200 to 300 g) I use the periareolar or the vertical Lassus technique (11–13); when the areola is too low, I plan a medial or lateral pedicle (7); and for huge breasts (gigantomastia) I use the inverted-T technique or the Yousif–Lalonde (9,10,28) techniques. CVRM is selected when the breast removal is between 300 and 1,000 g.

In order to select CVRM, the skin has to have a good tone and the areola should not be located more than 10 cm away from its ideal anatomic placement. I move the areola with my fingers, and if I foresee that it will be difficult to move, I consider a pedicle. In cases of more than 10 cm of areola ascension, I also select a pedicle for its transposition.

Before surgery, with the patient standing, I mark the IMF on both sides and the ideal future location of the areola (i.e., the whole areola over the IMF). If the areolas are going to be moved upward, I follow a vertical line coming from the middle part of the clavicle. In case the areolas are place laterally and need to be moved medially, I follow a line that unites the sternal notch to the areola (Figs. 93.2 and 93.3). Then, at 4 to 6 cm lateral and medial of the nipple, I mark the lateral limit of the periareolar. The superior future areola border mark is continued with curved lines, with the lateral marks forming the superior part of the CVRM. From these points two curvilinear lines are drawn downward converging at a point located 2 to 4 cm above the IMF (Fig. 93.4).

Because women have different breast shapes and volumes, the volume to be removed on each side is penciled on the skin. As a guideline, I imagine breast implant volumes. The shape of each breast is studied, and the areas of breast resection are marked. The breast projection is also analyzed, as are how to preserve the good projected breast and how to project a flat one. What I mark is what I am going to do at surgery.

THE SURGICAL TECHNIQUE

Every surgery is performed using local anesthesia and deep sedation controlled by an anesthesiologist (18). When the patient is asleep, before beginning the surgery, each breast is thoroughly infiltrated with 250 to 300 cc of anesthetic solution, at the subcutaneous inferior half of the breast skin and under the areola and at the subglandular layer. The anesthetic solution is prepared with 25 mL of 2% lidocaine, 25 mL of 0.5% bupivacaine, and 1 mL of 1/1,000 epinephrine diluted in 450 to 550 cc of saline solution or Ringer lactate solution.

Once the whole periareolar skin is deepithelialized (Fig. 93.5), the skin is undermined at the inferior half of the breast medially and laterally, leaving 1-cm-thick subcutaneous to preserve its blood supply. The inferior half of the breast is also detached from the pectoralis major muscle up to the fourth intercostal space, where the perforant of the fourth intercostal nerve usually emerges. As a consequence of this dissection, the breast comes out, and with the parenchyma in my hands, holding up the breast with a hook on the areola, I mark a W-Wise pattern resection at the inferior quadrant and at the inferior part of the medial and lateral quadrants, marking 10 cm of what will be the future areola–submammary fold (SMF) distance (Fig. 93.6). After the resection, the lateral and medial glandular edges are sutured medially in two to three layers using 3/0 Vicryl suture (Fig. 93.7). In case I want to obtain a central projection of the breast, both pillars can be imbricated. To have a more projected

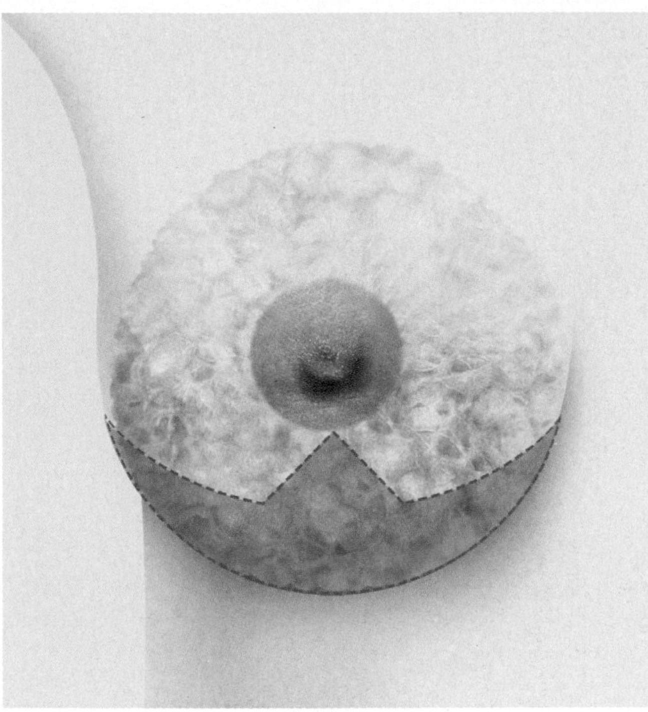

Figure 93.1. The W pattern of the parenchyma removal.

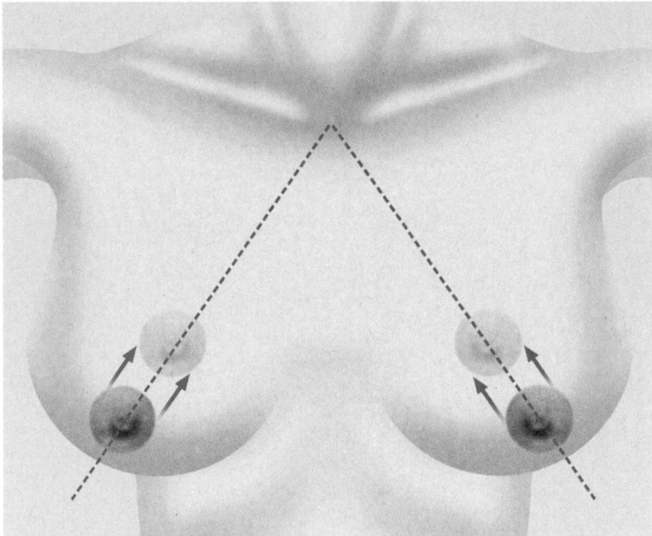

Figure 93.3. Areolas are going to be moved up and medially following the sternal notch line.

breast, two or three stitches are placed at the base of the cone in order to keep the pillars together. Once I have obtained a conic-shaped breast (Fig. 93.8), the inferior edge of the parenchyma is sutured to the pectoralis fascia where it now sits, using five to seven 3/0 Vicryl separate stitches placed all along what will be the future SMF (Fig. 93.9). In this moment, some defatting could be done to have an even rounder breast shape. Then I move the areola to the superior border of the skin, and I fix it with two or three subdermal 3/0 Vicryl sutures.

To begin skin closure, a stitch is placed at 8 to 10 cm from the inferior part of the skin angle, dividing the wound into two figures: the superior round periareolar and the inferior vertical ellipse (Fig. 93.10). Then another stitch moves up this vertical wound to the areola (Fig. 93.11). The inferior wound is sutured in a vertical fashion with a 3/0 Vicryl subdermal running suture. The periareolar skin is sutured to the areolar border with another subdermal cinching running suture. This running suture takes large 10- to 20-mm horizontal bites at the skin dermis and 2- to 3-mm vertical bites at the areola dermis. In this way,

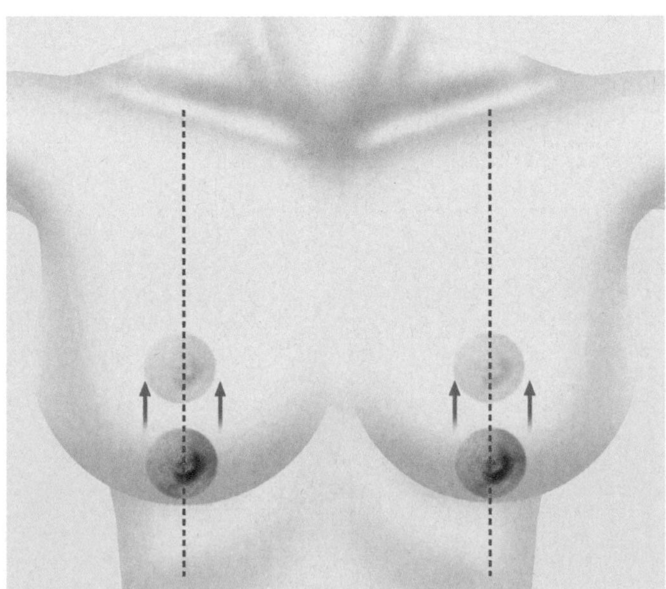

Figure 93.2. The areolas are going to be moved upward following the vertical middle clavicular line.

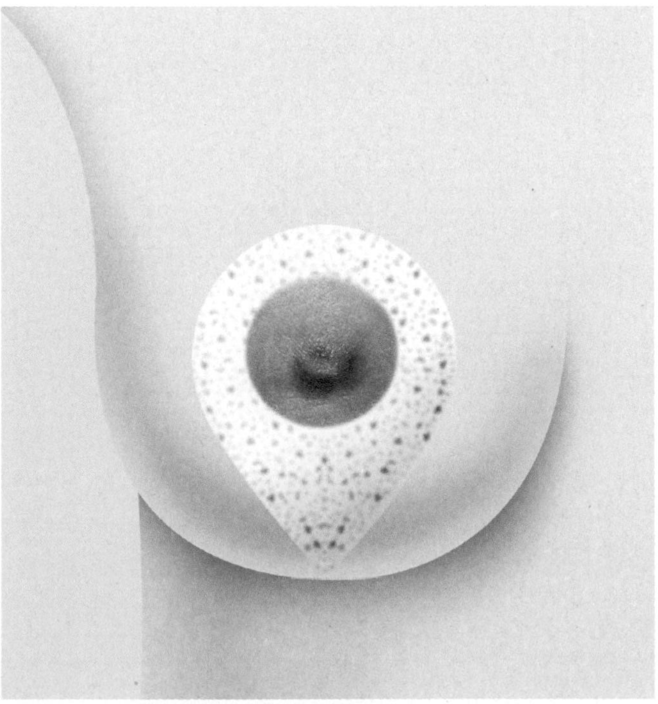

Figure 93.4. Circumvertical design.

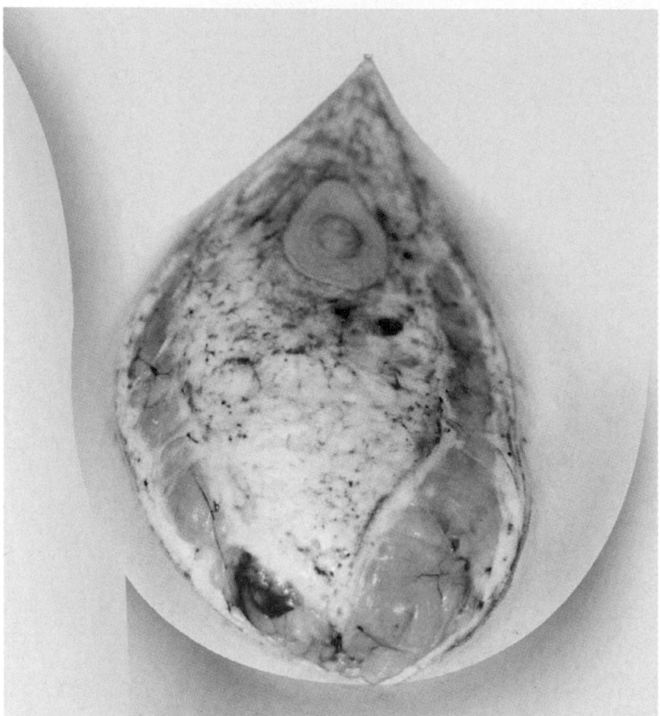

Figure 93.5. The periareolar and vertical area deepidermized.

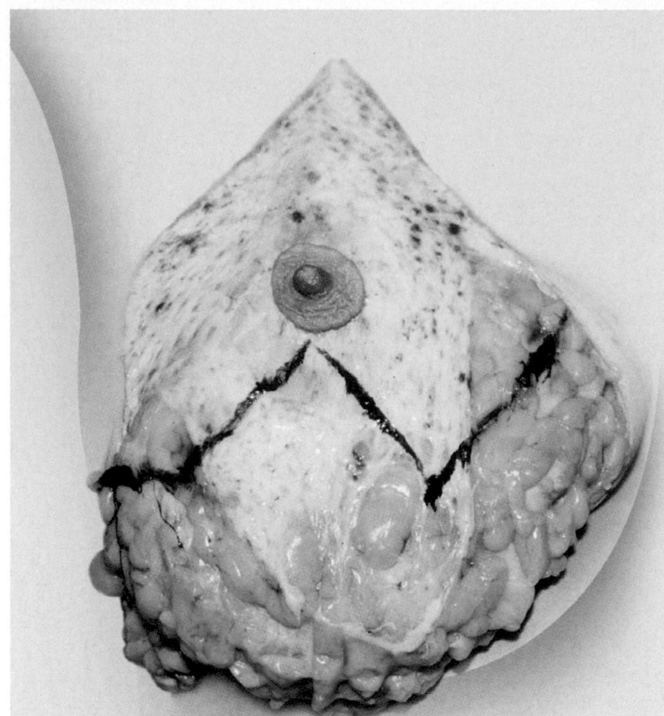

Figure 93.6. Once the parenchyma comes out, the W pattern is marked.

after three passes, the thread is strongly pulled and the skin is gathered toward the areola. Then I continue the suturing all along the areola to have a harmonious distribution of the wrinkles all along the areola in order to avoid leaving dead spaces (Fig. 93.12). To finish the surgery, all the wounds are closed with intradermal 5/0 Vicryl suture. Aspiration drains are placed laterally, and the wounds are covered by paper tape. To keep the flap attached to the parenchyma, strong aspirative drainage is used. After the suturing is finished, a 3-mm cannula can be introduced from the lower part of the vertical wound

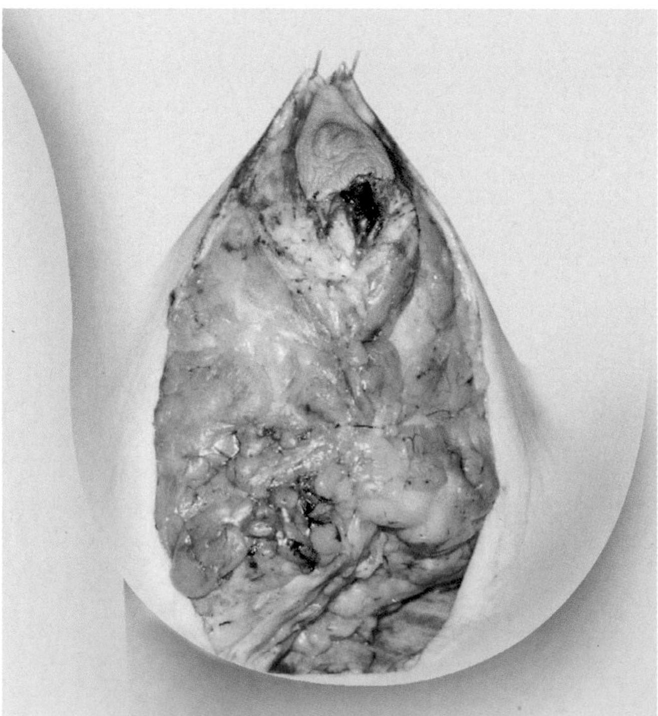

Figure 93.7. After parenchyma removal, pillars are sutured.

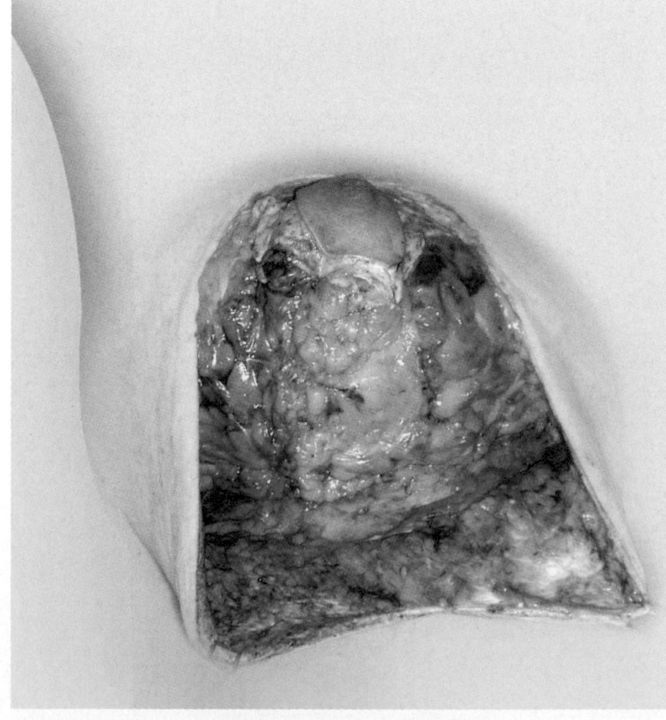

Figure 93.8. A round-shaped breast can be built.

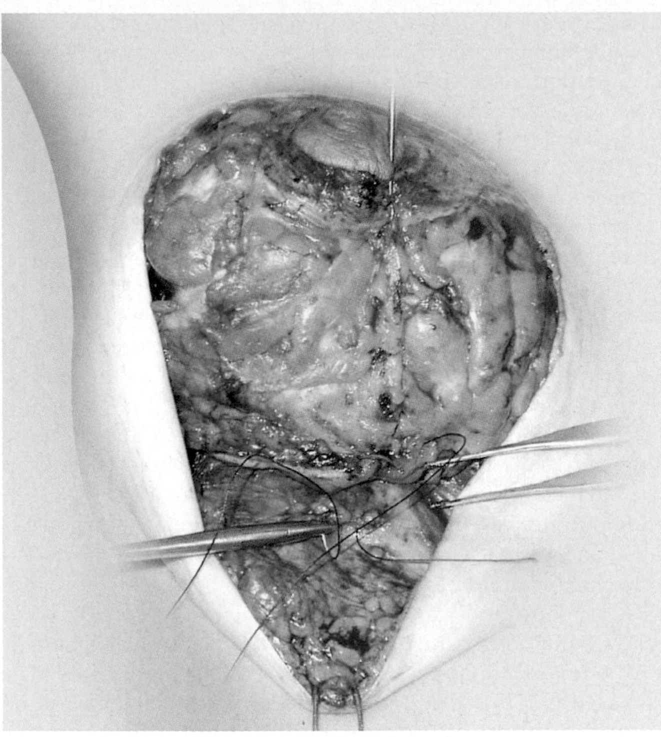

Figure 93.9. The inferior parenchyma wedge is sutured to the pectoralis fascia.

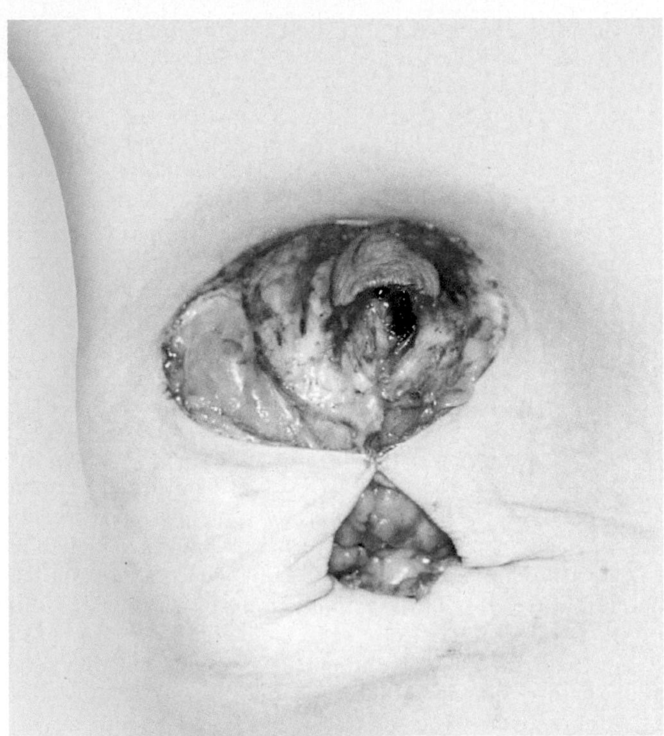

Figure 93.10. A stitch divides the wound into circumvertical and vertical ones.

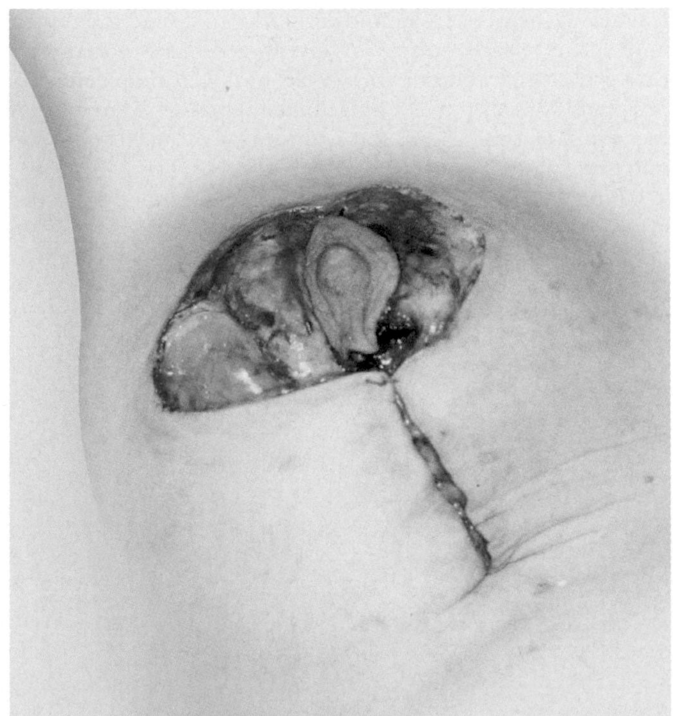

Figure 93.11. The vertical ascends by suturing to the areola.

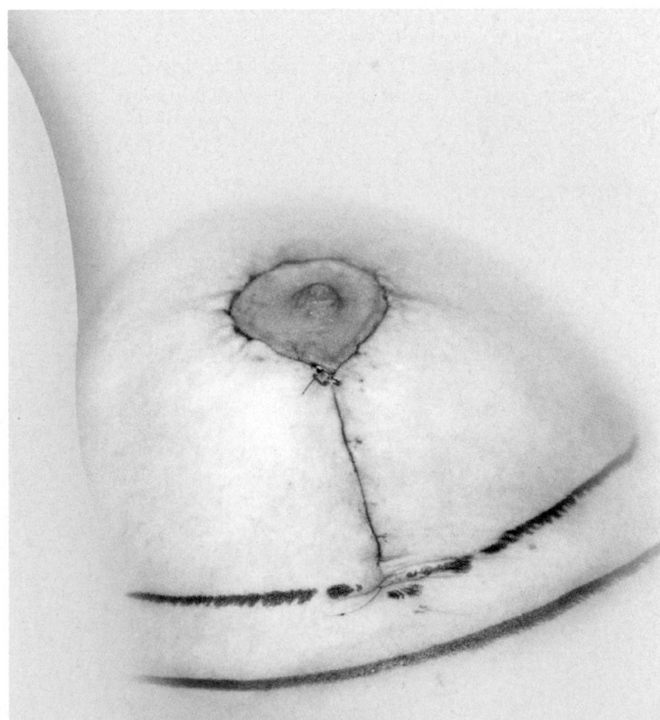

Figure 93.12. Around the areola, a harmonious distribution of the wrinkles is observed. The vertical wound does not cross the new inframammary fold. A round-shaped breast is observed at the end of the surgery.

and used as a complementary tool for minor asymmetries of the shape of the breast or to remove the lateral quadrant of the parenchyma.

When the inferior part of the breast is removed, the skin that previously covered the breast will now attach to the thoracic wall. As the pleats are harmonically distributed at the periareolar and vertical wounds and the undermined skin retracts during surgery, an acceptably good result can be observed at the end of the surgery.

RESULTS

In the ideal case—a moderate breast removal (prospective 400 to 700 g), with a good skin tone and areolas not too low—the results are nice. I have used CVRM for removing more than 1,200 g, but even when the scars are vertical, the results are suboptimal. The main complication I had was the skin slough at the periareolar vertical junction, but since a very limited amount of skin is removed without compressing the flaps, this problem is very seldom observed. Hematomas are present in 4% of the cases, and since wounds are washed out with cefazolin before suturing, there are no infections to report. Because no pedicle is used and the blood supply of the areola is preserved, no areolar necrosis was observed.

Because this is not the only technique of breast reduction I use, in 16 years I have dealt with more than 400 cases. At the beginning, when it was the fashion to have small breasts, I had to revise around 10% of my cases because women wanted to have smaller breasts. In those cases, I used a vertical parenchyma removal without moving the areola. Now, when larger breasts are fashionable, these revisions are rare.

I never have to revise a long vertical scar crossing down the IMF because when I see that this will probably happen, I plan and use a small inverted-T technique (16–27).

DISCUSSION

Good selection of cases, meticulous planning, and marking are the keys to good results.

In surgery I follow the penciled line and the estimation of the glandular removal I planned before surgery. This is especially important when there are asymmetries. Because there is a great variety of breast hypertrophies, I also plan, before surgery, from which part of the breast I have to remove more tissue. When there are difficult asymmetries I usually draw a draft of the future areas to be removed as a surgical guide.

I do not use liposuction to reduce the volume because I can better reshape a firm conic breast with scalpel and sutures. Suturing the breast pillars vertically and at the base of the breast, I can project a flat breast, obtaining a conic shape. By suturing the new inferior border of the breast to the pectoralis fascia, a clear IMF is defined and the gland is fixed to the muscle, thus avoiding the possible bottoming out of the breast.

In case of flat breasts, to project them, I prefer two to three stitches that are placed at the base of the cone in order to keep the pillars together (4) rather than an inferior pedicle (5,6). In the opposite case of overprojected round breast, no suture is used, and then at the base of the breasts, pillars can move out, reducing the breast projection (Fig. 93.13A, B). The suture that divides the wound can be regulated during surgery. If it the stitch is placed in a higher position, the periareolar diameter will be reduced and the vertical wound will be longer, while if it is placed in a lower position, the periareolar diameter will be wider and the vertical shorter (Fig. 93.14A, B). The possibility of such variations is important when a harmonic distribution of the pleats has to be determined.

I began by using the purse-string suture and then changed to the cinching running suture. The subdermal running periareolar cinching suture approximates the skin to the areola, thus avoiding dead spaces. As the pleats are harmoniously distributed at the periareolar and vertical wounds and the undermined skin retracts during surgery, an acceptably good result can be observed when the surgery is finished. Complementary postoperative skin retraction will complete the tightening of the skin. For this reason, the selection of patients with good skin tone is important.

Once the areola is moved and fixed to the superior border of the skin, all the skin moves toward the areola. Then the superior part of the vertical is sutured to the 6 o'clock areolar dermis, raising the vertical wound and avoiding crossing the

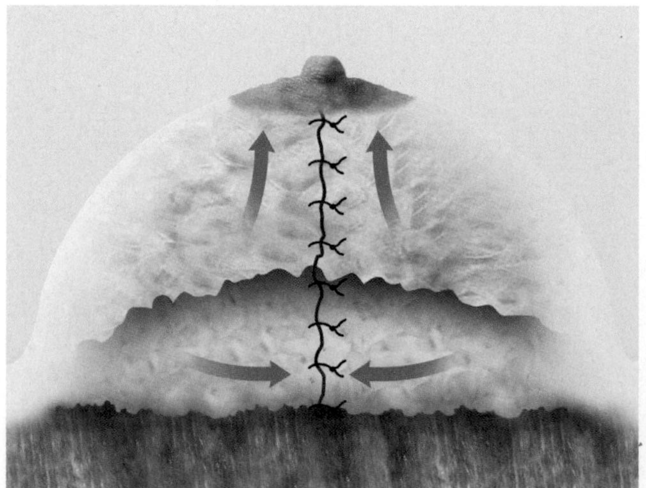

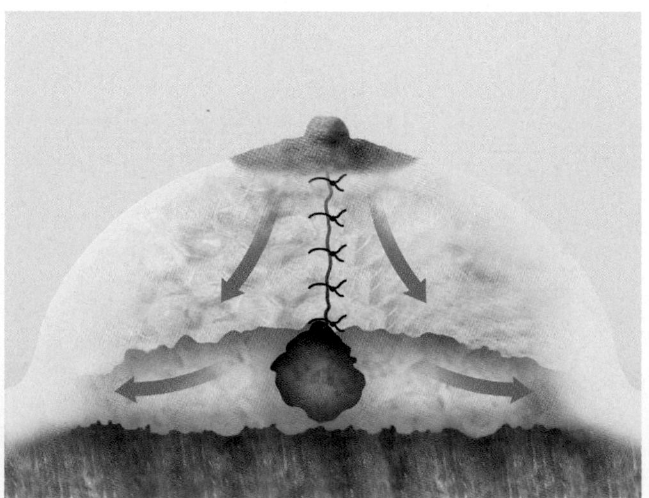

Figure 93.13. **A:** Pillars sutured at its base project the breast. **B:** When unsutured, the breast remains flat.

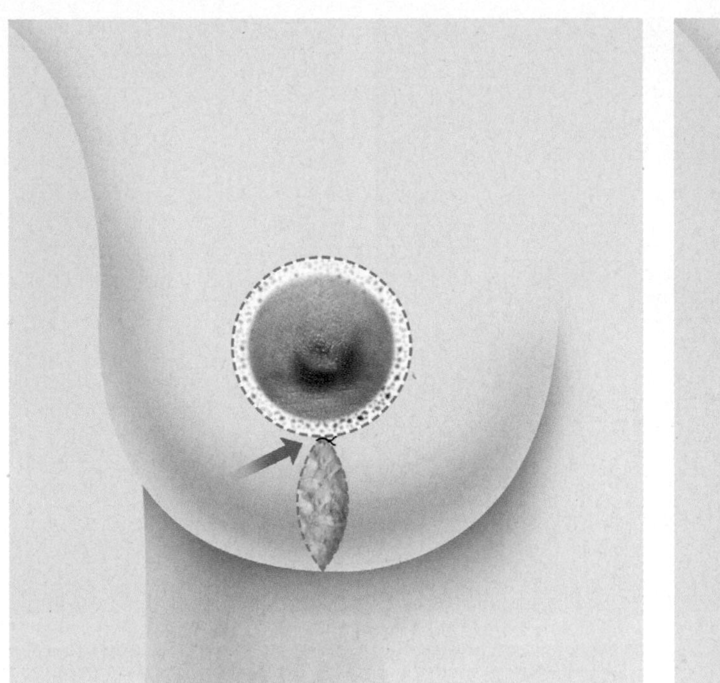

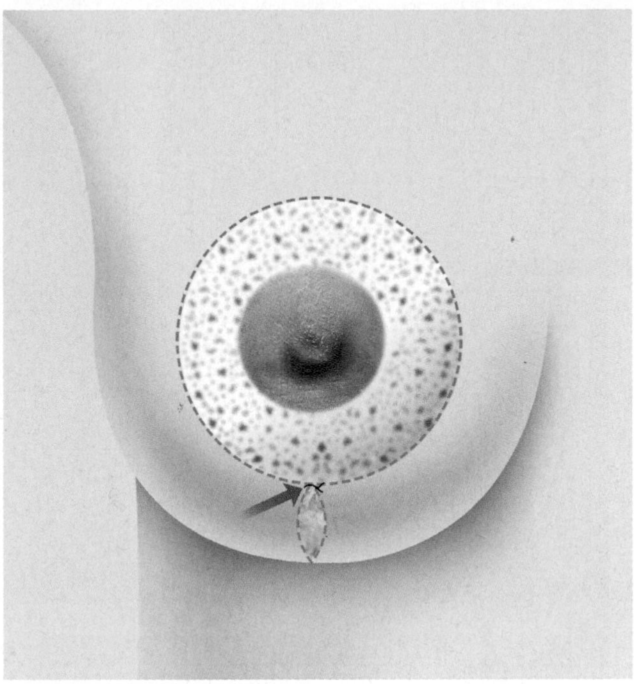

Figure 93.14. **A:** If the stitch is placed in a higher position, the periareolar diameter will be reduced and the vertical wound will be longer. **B:** If it is placed in a lower position, the periareolar diameter will be wider and the vertical shorter.

IMF (Fig. 93.15). Therefore, I never have to turn a vertical into an inverted T at the end of the surgery.

If the areola is moved without any pedicle, its blood supply and the venous flow are not altered. As the lactiferous ducts are not transected either, the lactation function is not disturbed. When the glandular removal is at the inferior part of the breast and the areola transposition moves upward without a pedicle, the normal anatomy is almost unaltered, an important factor in controlling the breast with mammograms over the years.

When the inferior part of the breast is removed, the skin that previously covered the breast will attach to the thoracic wall. This skin is what is routinely removed with the inverted-T technique, leaving the horizontal scar.

When large amounts of diluted anesthetic solution are infiltrated, the bleeding decreases, the hydraulic dissection facilitates the surgery, and the use of bupivacaine gives some hours of postoperative pain relief.

The periareolar skin resection is very conservative because, as happens after superficial liposuction, the undermined skin retracts during surgery. Retraction after surgery will contribute even further to the skin retraction. In order to avoid skin slough at the periareolar vertical junction, conservative skin resection has to be done and no compression in undermined skin areas is used. A strong aspirative drainage keeps the flaps attached to the parenchyma (Figs. 93.16 and 93.17).

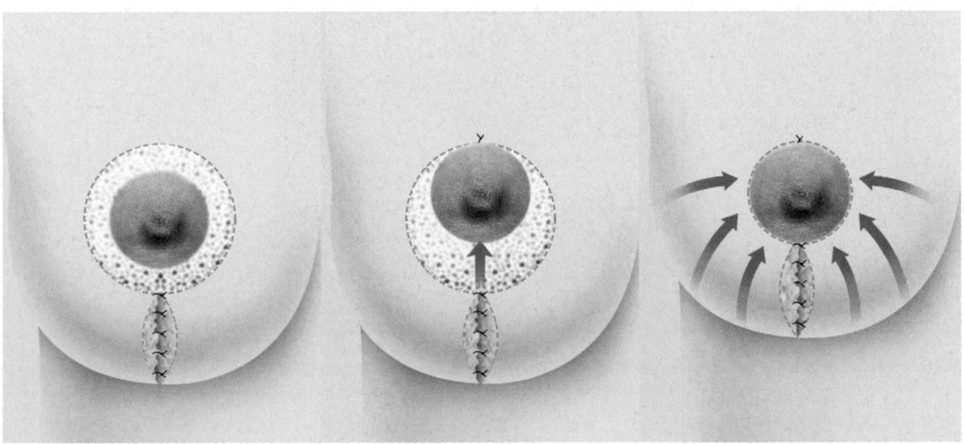

Figure 93.15. Once all the skin moves toward the areola, the vertical wound ascends, avoiding crossing the inframammary fold.

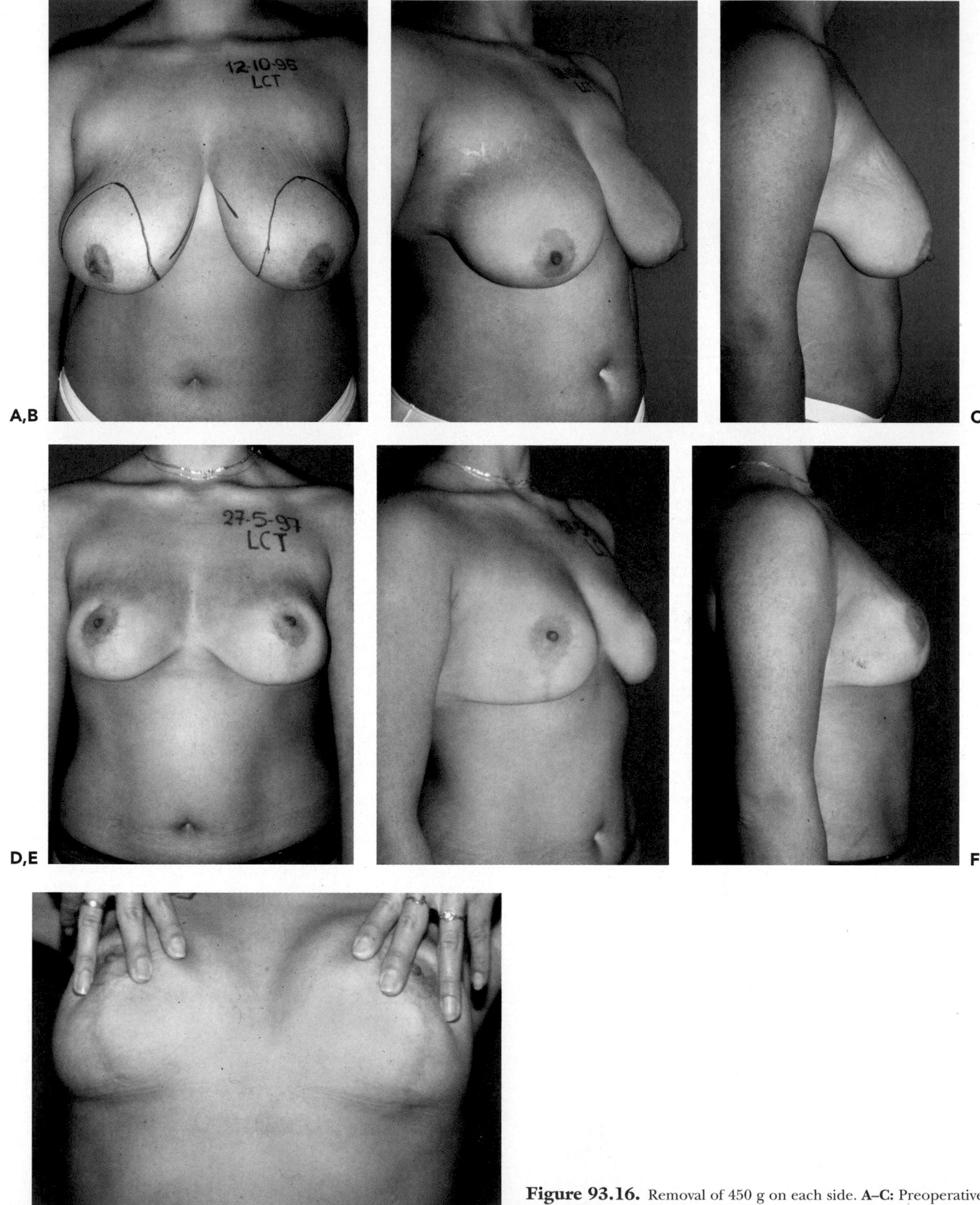

Figure 93.16. Removal of 450 g on each side. **A–C:** Preoperative views. **D–G:** At 19 months postoperatively.

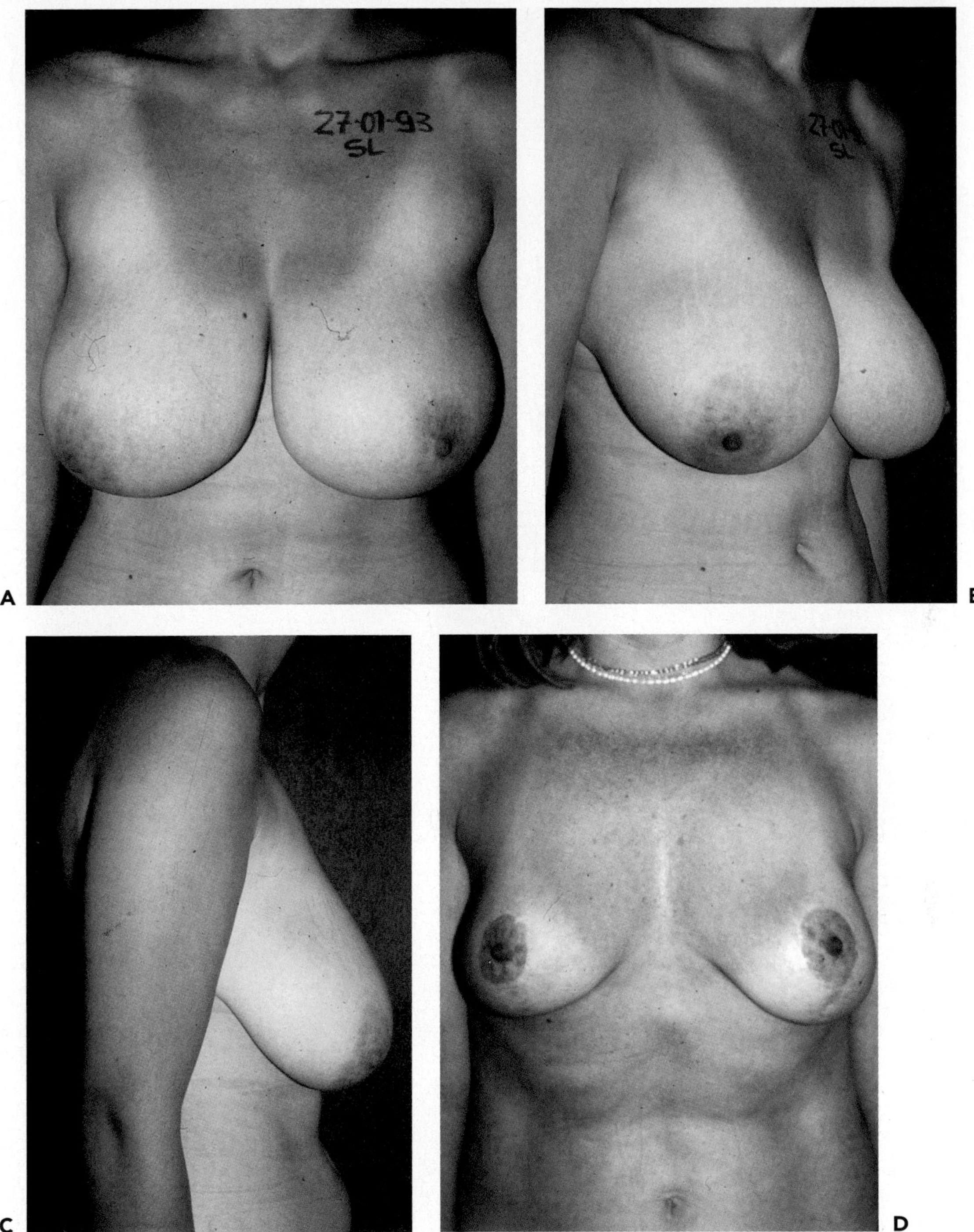

Figure 93.17. Removal of 700 g on each side. **A–C:** Preoperative views. **D–F:** At 8 years postoperatively. (*continued*)

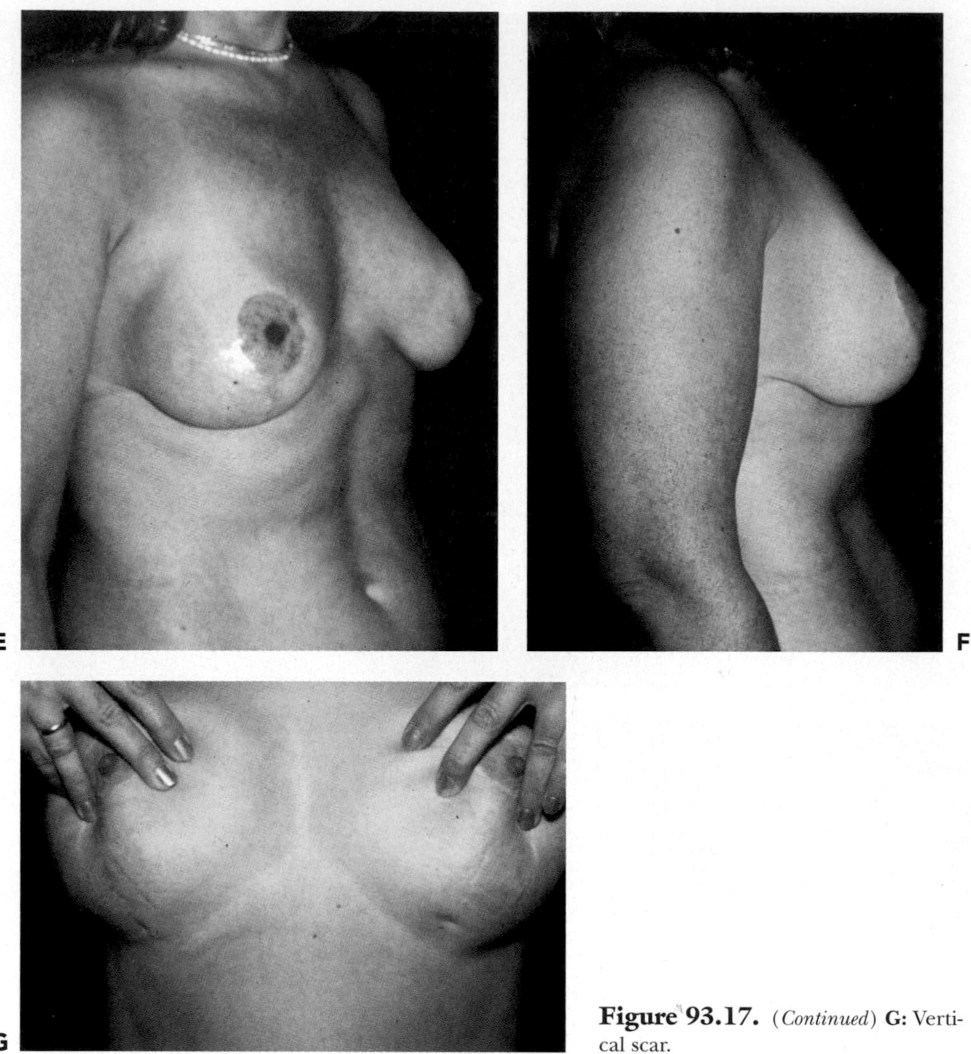

Figure 93.17. (*Continued*) **G:** Vertical scar.

CONCLUSION

CVRM is a combination of the periareolar and the vertical techniques on the skin. The parenchyma is removed according to the W-Wise pattern, the parenchyma can be projected during surgery, and the periareolar skin is sutured using a cinching running suture. Once the breast is removed using CVRM, there is a conic breast reshaping, a new IMF is defined, and the parenchyma is fixed to the pectoral fascia. Most of the skin is gathered around the areola, there is a harmonic distribution of the pleats all along the periareolar wounds, and the vertical wound never crosses the IMF. Without any pedicle for areola transposition, its blood supply and breast-feeding function remain unaltered. An acceptable result can be observed at the end of the surgery.

EDITORIAL COMMENTS

In this chapter, the significant advantage of combining the periareolar incision pattern with a vertical takeout is highlighted. This strategy has been utilized in many breast reduction and mastopexy techniques including the SPAIR mammaplasty, a technique I have been using for the past 14 years. Utilizing the periareolar skin removal accomplishes a lifting of the position of the areola while the addition of a vertical segment is a powerful shaping maneuver that can reduce the dimensions of the skin envelope, and narrow the base diameter of the breast. Both techniques also complement each other very well as the vertical resection effectively reduces the dimensions of the periareolar defect, resulting in less stress being placed on the periareolar closure. Despite this synergy of technique, occasionally the results can be compromised by unwanted spreading of the areola postoperatively, particularly in larger reductions. For this reason, rather the using cinching sutures, it can be helpful to utilize the interlocking technique described elsewhere in this book. Incorporating this technique with a combined periareolar and vertical skin pattern can allow such maneuvers to be used in even the largest of breast reduction. Using these modifications allows the breast to be reduced or lifted in nearly any circumstance making the need for an inverted T pattern an uncommon circumstance.

S.L.S.

In this chapter, the significant advantage of combining the periareolar incision pattern with a vertical takeout is highlighted. This strategy has been utilized in many breast reduction and mastopexy techniques including the SPAIR mammaplasty, a technique I have been using for the past 14 years. Utilizing the periareolar skin removal accomplishes a lifting of the position of the areola while the addition of a vertical segment is a powerful shaping maneuver that can reduce the dimensions of the skin envelope, and narrow the base diameter of the breast. Both techniques also complement each other very well as the vertical resection effectively reduces the dimensions of the periareolar defect, resulting in less stress being placed on the periareolar closure. Despite this synergy of technique, occasionally the results can be compromised by unwanted spreading of the areola postoperatively, particularly in larger reductions. For this reason, rather the using cinching sutures, it can be helpful to utilize the interlocking technique described elsewhere in this book. Incorporating this technique with a combined periareolar and vertical skin pattern can allow such maneuvers to be used in even the largest of breast reduction. Using these modifications allows the breast to be reduced or lifted in nearly any circumstance making the need for an inverted T pattern an uncommon circumstance.

D.C.H.

REFERENCES

1. Arié G. Una nueva técnica de mastoplastia. *Rev Latinoam Cir Plast* 1957;3:23.
2. Azzam C, De Mey A. Vertical scar mammaplasty in gigantomastia: retrospective study of 115 patients treated using the modified Lejour technique. *Aesthet Plast Surg* 2007;31(3):294–298.
3. Benelli L. A new periareolar mammaplasty: the "round block" technique. *Aesthet Plast Surg* 1990;14:93–100.
4. Berrino P, Galli A, Rainero ML, et al. Unilateral reduction mammaplasty: sculpturing the breast from the undersurface. *Plast Reconstr Surg* 1988;82(1):88–98.
5. Graf R. In search of better shape in mastopexy and reduction mammoplasty. *Plast Reconstr Surg* 2002;110:309.
6. Graf R. Breast shape: a technique for better upper pole fullness. *Aesthet Plast Surg* 2000;24:348.
7. Hall-Findlay E. A simplified vertical reduction mammaplasty: shortening the learning curve. *Plast Reconstr Surg* 1999;104:748.
8. Juri J, Juri C, Cutini J, et al. Vertical mammaplasty. *Ann Plast Surg* 1982;9(4):298–305.
9. Lalonde DH, Lalonde J, French R. The no vertical scar breast reduction: how to delete the vertical scar of the standard T scar breast reduction and produce an excellent breast shape. *Perspect Plast Surg* 2001;15:103.
10. Lalonde DH, Lalonde J, French R. The no vertical scar breast reduction: a minor variation that allows to remove vertical scar portion of the inferior pedicle wise pattern T scar. *Aesthet Plast Surg* 2003;27(5):335–344.
11. Lassus C. New refinements in vertical mammaplasty. *Chir Plast* 1981;6:81–86.
12. Lassus C. Breast reduction: evolution of a technique—a single vertical scar. *Aesthet Plast Surg* 1987;11:107–112.
13. Lassus C. Update on vertical mammaplasty. *Plast Reconstr Surg* 1999;104:7.
14. Lejour M. Suction mammaplasty. Correspondence. *Plast Reconstr Surg* 1992;89:161.
15. Lejour M. Vertical mammaplasty and liposuction of the breast. *Plast Reconstr Surg* 1994;94:1.
16. Marchac D, de Olarte G. Reduction mammaplasty and correction of ptosis with a short inframammary scar. *Plast Reconstr Surg* 1982;69(1):45–55.
17. Menke H, Restel B, Olbrisch RR. Vertical scar reduction mammaplasty as a standard procedure. Experiences in the introduction and validation of a modified reduction technique. *Eur J Plast Surg* 1999;22:74–79.
18. Mottura AA. Local anesthesia in reduction mastoplasty for out-patient surgery. *Aesthet Plast Surg* 1992;16:309–315.
19. Mottura AA. Mastoplastia reductiva periareolar. *Rev Arg Cir Plast* 1996;2:25.
20. Mottura AA. Zirkumverticale mammareduktionplastik. In: Lemperle G, ed. *Aesthetische Chirurghie.* 1st ed. Landsberg, Germany: Ecomed, Grand Werk; 1998:1–5.
21. Mottura AA. Circumvertical reduction mastoplasty. *Aesthet Surg* 2000;20:199–204.
22. Mottura AA. Circumvertical reduction mastoplasty. *Clin Plast Surg* 2002;29:393–400.
23. Mottura AA. Circumvertical reduction mastoplasty: new considerations. *Aesthet Plast Surg J* 2003;27:85.
24. Mottura AA. Mastoplastia reductiva circumvertical: nueva alternatica. In: Coiffman F, ed. *Cirugía Plastica Reconstructiva y Estética.* Bogota, Colombia: Amolca; 2008:Chapter 303.
25. Nahai F. Scar wars. *Aesthet Surg* 2000;24:461.
26. Rohrich RJ, Gosman AA, Brown SA, et al. Current preferences for breast reduction techniques: a survey of board-certified plastic surgeons. *Plast Reconstr Surg* 2002;114(7):1724–1733; discussion, 1734–1736.
27. Spear SL, Howard MA. Evolution of the vertical reduction mammaplasty. *Plast Reconstr Surg* 2003;112(3):855–868; quiz, 869.
28. Yousif NJ, Larson DL, Sanger JR, et al. Elimination of the vertical scar in reduction mammaplasty. *Plast Reconstr Surg* 1992;89(3):459–467.

CHAPTER

94

Navin K. Singh
Marwan R. Khalifeh

Inferior Pedicle Technique in Breast Reduction: Basic Concepts

INDICATIONS

Indications for breast reduction, regardless of the technique is used, include (a) self-identification of problems, (b) referral from another health care provider, and (c) issues of symmetry related to a lumpectomy or mastectomy for contralateral breast cancer.

Because of the wide dissemination of knowledge facilitated by the proliferation of health-related websites, prospective patients are often able to self-diagnose the cause of the stereotypical symptom cluster of macromastia. By surfing plastic surgeons' websites, a woman seeking breast reduction will often have gained a reasonable fund of knowledge regarding the benefits that breast reduction may offer. She is likely to become well educated about the range of techniques being offered, the likely functional and cosmetic outcomes, and the expected aesthetic shape. It is, of course, the in-person surgical consultation with an appropriately trained and credentialed plastic surgeon that can help to confirm the diagnosis, clarify the patient's do-it-yourself understanding, and correct any misinformation that the woman may have received. Some women are free of physical symptoms and seek breast reduction solely for aesthetic purposes, yet all women want an aesthetically proportioned breast shape delivered along with volumetric reduction.

Other women are referred for a plastic surgery consultation from their primary care physician, gynecologist, chiropractor, or spine specialist for conditions such as symptoms of back pain, neck pain, shoulder grooves, breast pain, intertrigo in the inframammary folds (IMFs), inability to exercise or participate in sports, or inability to fit into clothes. Most have failed some attempt at conservative management, such as physical therapy, exercise, weight loss, massage, or nonsteroidal anti-inflammatory drugs (NSAIDs). Attempts at weight loss are a "catch-22": Inability to exercise because of neck, back, and shoulder pain impedes their ability to lose weight, and thus the macromastia persists. Since the underlying problem of large, pendulous breasts remains uncorrected, it does seem illogical that conservative measures would suffice: Such women would have to undergo lifelong physical therapy or lifelong NSAIDs and be at risk for their adverse renal and gastric effects (1,2).

Given the high incidence of breast cancer in North American women, many patients undergo a lumpectomy followed by radiation therapy. This leads to fibrosis, breast volume loss, and contraction of the breast. Alternatively, if a woman has had a unilateral mastectomy followed by reconstruction (autologous or prosthetic based) that tends to have less ptosis and is smaller because of limitations in donor-site availability, the normal, unoperated breast will continue to age and have more ptosis and be larger. Hence, women may seek a unilateral breast reduction to match a side that has been treated for cancer.

CONSULTATION

A detailed history is obtained to ensure that the patient is suitable for surgery from medico-surgico-psychosocial perspective. A notable family history of breast cancer should be worked up for genetic susceptibility (BRCA testing). This may precipitate bilateral mastectomy and immediate reconstruction instead of bilateral breast reduction. Mammograms are obtained as necessary to bring them up to date with current guidelines for baseline mammography and screening for breast cancer. American Cancer Society guidelines recommend a baseline mammogram at age 40 years and annually thereafter for women of average risk. Any detected anomalies should be referred to a breast oncologic surgeon to ascertain need for biopsy, imaging, or deferring of surgery to observe any suspicious radiographic abnormalities over time.

During the consultation process, measurements are undertaken for both the medical record and for third-party payer coverage criteria documentation. Typically, height, weight, sternal notch-to-nipple distance, and nipple-to-IMF distance are recorded bilaterally, and discrepancies in IMF and nipple-areolar complex (NAC) positions are pointed out to the patient. The degree of ptosis (none, mild, moderate, or severe) is assessed. During the focused breast exam, the breasts are screened for masses or nodules, axillary lymphadenopathy is checked, and the skin is examined for ulcerations, erosions, or postinflammatory hyperpigmentation. Nipple discharge is ruled out, and NAC size is noted (small, average, or dilated). Standard-view photography of the patient is done.

Lalonde breast sizers or a water displacement technique can be used to estimate the volume in each breast (3). With newer digital imaging technologies, it may be possible to estimate the volume from stereophotography.

Current bra size is elicited, and the desired cup size is discussed with the patient. Patients do not always understand the bra sizing system, and some request going from a 38DD to a 32B, for instance. The band size usually will not change (unless axillary liposuction is also done) since this reflects the underbust chest circumference. Ranges for volume resection that correlate with each one-cup-size reduction are from 200 to 350 cc, with little consensus. Some heavy-set women request a small breast cup size and should be counseled about choosing a cup size that is proportional to their overall body habitus. Lastly, cup size serves as a lay parlance discussion tool only. Cup sizes vary significantly by bra manufacturer, and these are not medical measurements. They serve as general guideposts to facilitate dialogue about a woman's desired target size.

The volume to be resected in each side, which may be different based on preexisting asymmetries, is estimated. Broad generalizations suggest that approximately 200 to 350 g is required for each one-cup-size change, and that each 1 cm of asymmetry in NAC position between the breasts accounts for 100 g of breast volume asymmetry. Most insurance companies establish volume requirements of breast tissue to be resected to reimburse for the procedure. While there are many variations, some third-party payers require 500 g of resection at least. Other companies use a nomogram based on height and weight to determine how much breast tissue needs to be removed to be eligible for reimbursement.

INSURANCE SYSTEMS

Preauthorization from insurance companies is sought with a copy of the consultation and the foregoing measurements, photographs of the torso in frontal and lateral views, and International Statistical Classification of Diseases and Related Health Problems-9 (ICD-9) and Current Procedural Terminology (CPT) codes. The ICD-9 codes frequently used in conjunction with breast reduction symptomatology are 611.1 (breast hypertrophy), 611.71 (breast pain), 692.9 (intertrigo), 724.8 (symptoms referable to back), 724.1 (back pain), 723.1 (neck pain), 723.9 (shoulder pain), 738.3 (shoulder grooves), and 709.0 (dyschromia). The CPT code is 19318-50. (Breast reduction preformed unilaterally to correct asymmetry with a reconstructed postmastectomy breast is covered by insurance without regard to size and volume criteria, as mandated by the Women's Health and Cancer Rights Act of 1998.)

When coverage for breast reduction is denied, an appeal letter may be considered, reminding the payer that recent scientific literature and evidence-based studies published in peer-reviewed journals strongly support the position that women undergoing reduction mammaplasty for symptomatic breast hypertrophy experience significant improvement in their preoperative signs and symptoms. Managed care organizations rate outcome or cost-effectiveness analyses as the most important factor in determining reduction mammaplasty coverage policies (4).

The plastic surgeon's office can often facilitate the appeal process, but the ultimate responsibility rests with the patient. The objective, ethical, and honest account of the patient's health care problem is captured in the office consultation note prepared by the physician, and a copy may be provided directly to the patient, supplemented with photographs. The patient may be encouraged to contact her payer or employer directly about her dissatisfaction. Some women will pay for services out of pocket in the face of denial and/or use their flexible health savings accounts to fund the surgery.

PREOPERATIVE DISCUSSION

After a thorough medical history and physical exam, the patient is screened for outpatient surgery. Smoking or secondhand smoke exposure must be stopped for 6 to 8 weeks prior to surgery. Nicotine exposure via gum or patch is also eliminated. A newer, non–nicotine-containing medication, varenicline, may be initiated. Patients should additionally remain free of tobacco smoke and nicotine for the postoperative healing period of at least 6 weeks. Weight loss, if indicated, is desirable to get closer to ideal body weight, but this is frequently unrealistic, as discussed earlier.

Preoperative testing is directed by medical history, physical findings, and age per anesthesia criteria. Young, healthy women may not need any testing except for a history and physical examination. Those with medical illnesses may need a complete blood count, electrolytes, liver function tests, pulmonary function tests, chest x-ray, and/or electrocardiogram. Those with a significant cardiopulmonary history should be cleared by their internist or cardiologist.

The patient is instructed to stop medications that predispose to a bleeding diathesis, such as NSAIDs, aspirin, salicylic acids, and over-the-counter medications that may contain these ingredients. Herbal medications and vitamin supplements, especially in large doses, are also eliminated. In particular, vitamin E, gingko biloba, St. John's wort, and garlic are to be discontinued.

Estrogenic medications such as oral contraceptive pills (OCPs) and postmenopausal hormone replacement therapy should be discontinued to lower the risk of deep vein thromboses (DVTs) and venous thromboembolism (VTE) associated with surgery. Patients on OCPs should practice an alternate form of contraception in the preoperative and postoperative interval because OCPs (even when not discontinued) may have decreased effectiveness due to metabolism of other medications during the episode of surgical care.

During the consultation, the patient and her significant others are educated regarding the risks and benefits of breast reduction surgery, as well as the alternative techniques available such as (a) no surgery and attempt at weight loss, (b) breast liposuction, (c) periareolar incision, (d) a vertical pattern or short-scar procedure, (e) a transverse scar (Passot) procedure, or (f) Wise-pattern breast reduction.

Having no surgery and seeking reduction in breast size through exercise and weight loss is also a possibility, especially if the patient can achieve a weight loss to get to a normal body mass index (BMI). She may then be reevaluated at some future date to see whether she still needs a breast reduction or only a mastopexy. Breast liposuction may be successful in decreasing one or two cup sizes for some women with moderate hypertrophy without mild to moderate ptosis and should be considered. Liposuction does not address NAC ptosis and may worsen it. Periareolar techniques may have a role in mild hypertrophy but remain technically challenging and unpredictable. Vertical or short-scar reduction has the advantage of eliminating the transverse IMF scar; however, this has a 15% to 20% revision rate with possible future or intraoperative conversion to a Wise pattern or J or L scar. These breast reductions do not achieve their optimal shape right away and do so over time. This is less likely to have bottoming out or parenchymal maldistribution (pseudoptosis). The transverse scar technique is typically used with a superomedial or superior pedicle and/or with free nipple graft. However, the inferior pedicle reduction technique can be used with the transverse scar.

The Wise skin pattern is most commonly associated with the inferior pedicle breast reduction technique. This incision pattern can be used, however, with superior or superomedial pedicle techniques, as well as with free nipple grafts. Nevertheless, the Wise or inverted-T scar technique is most commonly associated with the inferior pedicle technique. The inferior pedicle breast reduction in combination with the anchor T incision remains the most popular method of breast reduction and is the most predictable (5). Approximately 75% of plastic surgeons in the United States use this technique, and approximately 50% of surgeons use this technique exclusively. It is the most versatile and has a straightforward learning curve. It bears emphasizing that pedicle and skin pattern can be chosen independently of each other in most, but not all, scenarios.

CONSENT

The written informed consent is a supplement to the patient education process that occurs during the consultation. It should cover the risks including, but not limited to, infection, bleeding, hematoma, seroma, wound dehiscence, delayed healing, poor healing, and swelling. The patient is told about the potential for scarring, such as keloids, hypertrophic scar, hypopigmentation or hyperpigmentation, and dark or pink, itchy, or tender scars, which may be visible outside or through garments. Adverse sequelae include asymmetry, numbness, stiffness, pain, chronic pain, or anxiety and/or depression related to changes in body image. The patient is informed of the chance for further unplanned surgery with its additional risks, financial responsibilities, and time required for surgery and recuperation. Potential hospitalization may not be covered by insurance, since most reduction mammaplasties are done as outpatient cases at ambulatory surgery centers.

Urine pregnancy tests are recommended. If the woman is pregnant, she could be exposed to medications and anesthetics that cause birth defects or miscarriages.

There is the potential, but fortunately extremely rarely, for blood transfusion with major surgery and the accompanying risks including bacterial and viral infection (e.g., HIV, hepatitis) and transfusion reaction. There may be partial or total flap and tissue loss, fat necrosis, and loss of skin or of the NAC. Incomplete relief or no relief of the symptoms (e.g., back pain, neck pain) may occur, or the patient may be dissatisfied with the results of the surgery. No guarantee can be made of fitting into a particular clothes size or bra cup size or to match a digital simulation. Any surgery of the breasts leads to scars, both internal and external, and hence may hinder cancer surveillance and detection efforts. Magnetic resonance imaging may be required instead of mammograms for follow-up of calcifications from surgery.

Those patients who travel a great distance to a particularly well regarded surgeon may incur higher risks associated with traveling soon after surgery (e.g., flying, driving) such as DVTs or pulmonary embolisms from immobility in a confined car or airplane.

Comorbidities must be addressed in the informed-consent process as well. For instance, obesity and diabetes (controlled or uncontrolled) may contribute to poor healing and raise the rates of infection. After discussing best-case, worst-case, and average outcomes and scenarios and looking at representative photographs/diagrams, the patient and her family should feel comfortable that they grasp the likely benefits and potential for untoward events. They must understand the diagnosis, medical necessity versus elective nature of the surgery, goals of the procedure, pain management, expected time course of recovery and management of complications should they arise, and warning signs and symptoms of complications. Patients are provided sufficient time to consider the procedure in depth and should demonstrate their comprehension by being able to relate the information back to the surgeon and voice their understanding of the procedure in plain, lay language.

CAUTIONS AND CONTRAINDICATIONS

One contraindication is recent postpartum state in which breast size is still changing and has not reached an equilibrium plateau from involution. Active lactation is similarly a contraindication to breast reduction.

Age must be considered as well. With earlier and earlier age of thelarche and menarche in Western women, teen-aged girls are encountered with greater frequency with symptoms of macromastia, some of which is related to higher obesity rates in teens. The decision must be tailored to the physical findings, expected future growth, maturity level, and willingness to accept the potential for a repeat reduction mammaplasty in the future. There are no absolute age-related criteria, and the decision to operate is multifactorial.

Prior irradiation for breast conservation therapy (BCT) after lumpectomy is not a contraindication but should be given due consideration, as it may precipitate the need to alter the surgical plans. If an inferocentral lumpectomy has been performed, then the vascularity for an inferior pedicle reduction may not exist, and the plan should be changed in favor of an alternate pedicle. Radiation, independent of the lumpectomy site, will lead to slight modification of the surgical plans. For instance, the skin brassiere is not undermined widely, and, in general, more conservative markings are used.

Similarly, a prior breast reduction may be a contraindication to an inferior pedicle technique. Previous operative notes should be obtained when practical, since the inferior pedicle may have been resected during the surgery. Even if the prior reduction was an inferior pedicle procedure, the risks of injury to the pedicle and consequent loss of the NAC are nonetheless possible (6).

Diabetes, as a disease that compromises microvascular circulation, poses a challenge in breast reduction surgery. In this situation, as for radiation, the skin brassiere is not undermined as widely, pedicle width is enlarged, and longer distances for NAC are not transposed. Failure to modify the markings and extent of the reduction can contribute to higher rates of fat necrosis, NAC necrosis, and skin necrosis, particularly at the T junction.

Active smoking is a contraindication. Patients are insisted to be tobacco and nicotine free for a period of several weeks prior to surgery. This includes abstinence from nicotine gum or patch and from second-hand-smoke exposure. Urine cotinine tests may be indicated to encourage compliance. Urine cotinine tests are reported to detect tobacco use as recent as 2 to 10 days. Rarely, a carboxyhemoglobin test is indicated from an arterial blood gas sample in the preoperative holding area. Despite efforts to persuade and educate patients into smoking cessation for their own benefits, noncompliance is often encountered. Even with compliance, higher rates of complications are expected because of the aggregate toll that smoking has taken on their tissues.

A high BMI is not an absolute contraindication but may contribute to an overall anesthesia or surgical contraindication. The goal of getting patients into a 10% to 15% range of a normal BMI is not realistic. These patients find it impossible to exercise and thus difficult to lose weight precisely because the symptomatic macromastia makes them unable to exercise.

Very large reductions or those with dramatic ptosis and long sternal notch-to-nipple distance risk devascularizing the NAC and should be handled with a free nipple graft technique rather than an inferior pedicle procedure.

When several of these cautionary findings are found in conjunction, such as a diabetic patient who smokes or a previously radiated patient who also smokes, the surgeon must consider delaying the surgery until one or several factors can be optimized or mitigated.

MARKINGS

Markings, which determine the entire operation except for some minor intraoperative adjustments, are done with the patient standing upright with arms adducted. Shoulders are placed squarely, and a midline reference line is drawn from the sternal notch to the umbilicus. Existing scoliosis and kyphosis of the spine and asymmetries are demonstrated to the patient. The IMFs bilaterally are drawn with an indelible surgical site marker. The IMFs are typically 21 to 25 cm from the sternal notch and about the level of the midhumeral point.

The midbreast lines are drawn vertically through the nipple to the IMF with the breast weight gently supported to decrease stretch traction on the supra-areolar skin. Obstetric calipers may be used to transpose the level of the IMF onto the anterior supported breast skin, or this can be done through bimanual palpation. The new nipple position is determined by placing a finger in the IMF and marking the anterior projection on the vertical midbreast line. This mark is confirmed against several landmarks, including the midhumeral point, or within a range of 18 to 24 cm from the sternal notch, and in comparison to the contralateral side.

Once the provisional neo-NAC position is chosen, two oblique lines (which, when closed, will be the vertical limb of the T incision) are dropped to make an inverted V. The vertical limbs are set to 4.5 to 7 cm to allow for future bottoming out. The limbs may be drawn with the assistance of an NAC template such as a McKissock keyhole pattern. The angle of divergence of the vertical limbs (which form an inverted V) is determined by the skin excess, as judged by pinching the excess skin. The greater the amount of skin, the wider the V will open. At a first approximation, the limbs of the V should be tangent to the NAC since the dilation of the NAC is typically proportionate to the degree of hypertrophy. When in doubt, one should make the V narrow since more skin can be excised during the tailor-tack phase. If too much skin is resected, then primary closure may not be possible—a mistake to be avoided.

Finally, a horizontal line is drawn from the inferior end point of the vertical lines to the IMF. They need not extend all the way to the medial extent or the lateral extent of the breast—a pearl gleaned from experience with the vertical-only approach. The horizontal lines meet the IMF at 1 to 4 cm from the lateral sternal border and roughly at the lateral limit of the breast crease (Fig. 94.1).

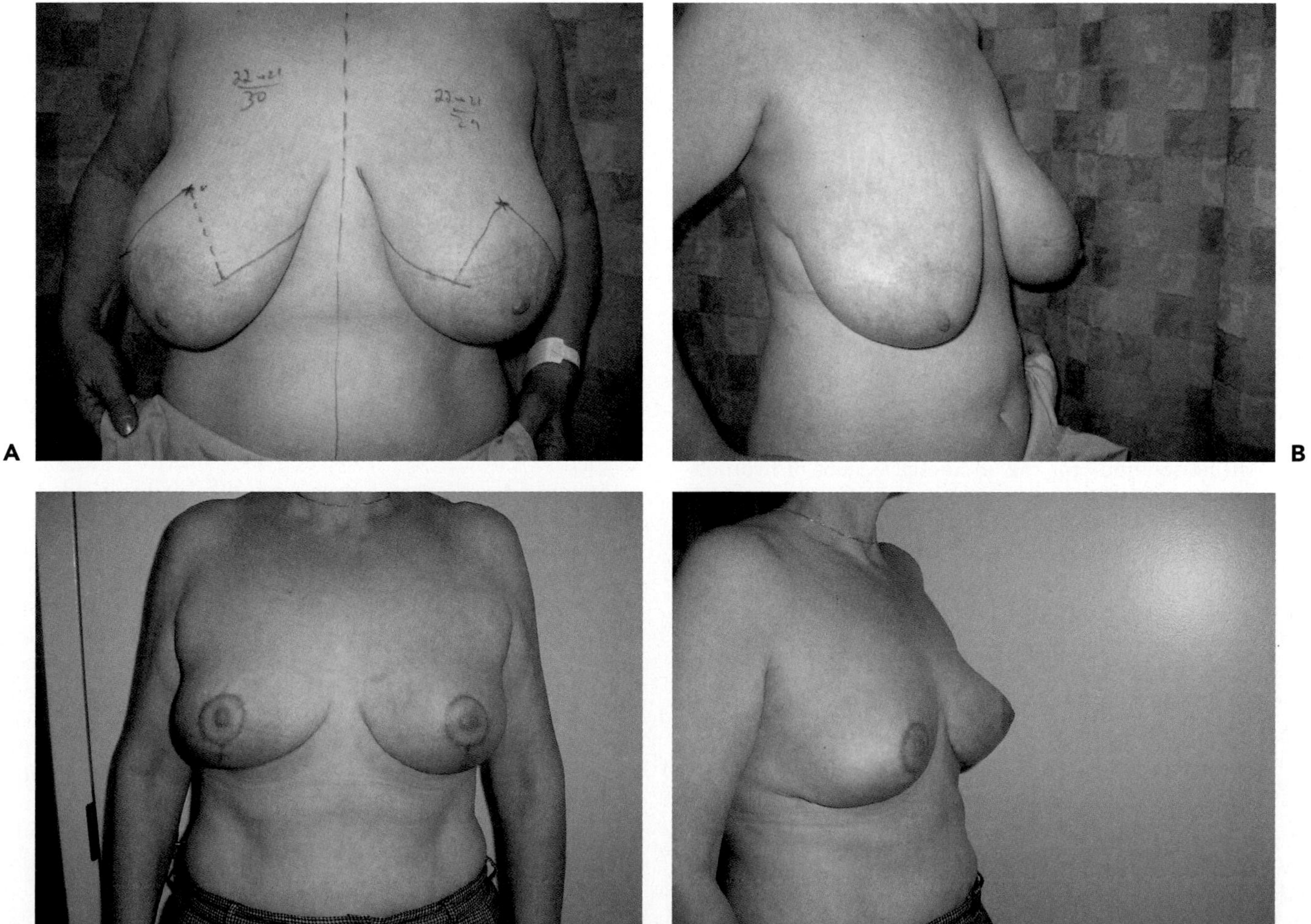

Figure 94.1. **A:** Preoperative sternal notch-to-nipple distance is 30 cm on the right and 29 cm on the left. The inframammary fold is at 22 cm bilaterally and the neo–nipple-areolar complex will be sited at 21 cm bilaterally. **B:** Oblique view. **C:** Postoperative result at 3 months, frontal view. **D:** Postoperative result at 3 months, oblique view.

OPERATIVE DETAILS

The patient is scheduled as an outpatient procedure for 2 to 3 hours and admitted to the hospital only if necessary. Criteria for conversion to in-patient or 23-hour observation unit include presence of medical comorbidities, high blood loss, long surgical duration, uncontrolled postoperative pain, and intractable postoperative nausea and vomiting.

In accordance with the Joint Commission on the Accreditation of Healthcare Organizations guidelines for surgical infection prevention, preoperative antibiotics targeted at skin flora for a clean case are administered intravenously within 60 minutes prior to incision. They are discontinued 24 hours after surgery. First-generation cephalosporins are most commonly indicated in the non–penicillin-allergic patient to minimize surgical site infections.

Venodynes should be applied and activated prior to the induction of anesthesia. Chemoprophylaxis for VTE is administered when the patient is considered at elevated risk for DVT. Unfractionated heparin, low-molecular-weight heparins such as enoxaparin or dalteparin, or synthetic antithrombotics such as fondaparinux may be administered preoperatively and continued postoperatively for chemical prophylaxis of thrombotic events (7).

The patient is positioned supine with arms abducted to approximately 90 deg in a well-padded and cushioned fashion. A lower-body warmer is used to maintain normothermia during the operation.

General anesthesia is commonly used via an endotracheal tube, a laryngeal mask airway, or total intravenous anesthesia with agents such as propofol, midazolam, and fentanyl. Alternate techniques include spinal anesthesia or intravenous sedation with local anesthetics. When intravenous sedation is used as for anesthesia, infiltration of local anesthetics as a field block is requisite (8). However, even when general anesthesia is employed, a local field block or intercostal blocks with the addition of tumescent anesthesia may help to provide long-lasting postoperative pain relief and thus minimize use of postoperative narcotics. Some surgeons place indwelling catheters with pain pumps for postoperative pain management. Some surgeons use tumescent infiltration (dilute lidocaine and dilute epinephrine solution) for the additional benefit of hydrodissection and local hemostasis.

Assistants at surgery are used to help retract, suction, and expedite wound closure, thus minimizing the operative time and anesthetic experience. A smoke evacuator may be used during the surgery to minimize the smoke plume associated with the electrocautery.

The planned pedicle is an 8-cm-wide area centered about the breast meridian originating at the IMF and continuing to the level of the NAC. For larger reductions, the width should be increased to 10 cm. The pedicle is deepithelialized except for the NAC, which is left intact as a 42- or 45-mm-diameter circle. The NAC can be cut as a perfect circle using a Freeman cookie cutter, or small undulations and imperfections (like a running W-plasty) are tolerated to mimic a more natural NAC. The superior skin flap is elevated to reveal the underlying breast parenchyma. An omega- or horseshoe-shaped excision of parenchyma is performed, leaving a broadly attached, 8-cm-wide pedicle originating at the IMF and continuing to the level of the NAC. The pedicle that remains is vascularized by branches from the lateral thoracic, internal mammary, and intercostals vessels.

This excises tissue from the medial, superior, and lateral quadrants of the breast. Some prefer to resect tissue from each area separately, which is not as efficient as an en bloc excision but affords the opportunity to compare and shape each region more selectively. Medially, the tissue must not be overresected, so as to optimize cleavage. A layer of loose areolar tissue should be left on the pectoralis fascia to preserve the nerves traveling in this plane. The specimen from each side is separately labeled and weighed.

Finally, a tailor-tack method is used to shape the breast. The surgeon shapes the breast by transposing the pedicle cephalad and supporting it with medial and lateral breast flaps. Skin staples or provisional sutures are used to create guidelines for closure. Then the patient is sat up intraoperatively, and size, shape, and symmetry are assessed. If the desired target size is not reached, additional piecemeal tissue may be excised from the pedicle or from the surrounding flaps. Differential resection is undertaken from each breast to account for preexisting asymmetries in size. Symmetry must be assessed, and if asymmetry exists, additional tissue may be excised unilaterally. Sterile Lalonde sizers may be used intraoperatively to judge symmetry of retained volumes. Once the desired volume of resection to achieve the requested bra cup size is achieved, the specimen may be sent to pathology, individually labeled for left and right sides. A request to use intraoperative weights is sent with the specimens to pathology since there may be some volume loss related to specimen desiccation postoperatively.

The remaining pedicle and flaps are finally assessed for adequacy of vascularity. Healthy uniform punctuate arterialized bleeding should be confirmed from the deepithelialized pedicle and its edges. The NAC should have good turgor and demonstrate contractile areolae. If there is a question, it may be pin pricked with a 25-gauge needle to assess pink bright bleeding. Rapid, dark congested blood suggests venous insufficiency. Another technique is to administer intravenous fluorescein and inspect the surgical site with a Wood ultraviolet lamp and to visualize fluorescence along all concerning areas to assure viability and vascularity.

All areas are irrigated with warm saline, and hemostasis is meticulously confirmed. Electrocautery is typically used for the smaller vessels, but suture ligation of larger vessels may be needed.

Shapes are optimized by advancing the medial and lateral skin flaps to help shape the breast parenchyma. In addition, the flap is advanced superiorly, and shaping sutures may be used to create a fuller central mound that is less dependent on skin support. This shaping technique is less effective in the setting of fatty breasts and has better outcomes with breasts with a greater glandular component that can hold suture. The patient is sat up again, and the positions for the neo-NAC are chosen. They should be placed at the point of maximal breast projection at a distance of 5 to 7 cm from the IMF. In larger breasts, one must be careful not to let the NAC fall too laterally or too high. If skin quality is poor, one can anticipate some future "bottoming out" or pseudoptosis and place the NAC a little lower. Once the neo-NAC is marked with a cookie cutter, the 38- to 45-mm-diameter circle of skin is excised, and the NAC is exteriorized and anchored with 3-0 inverted Vicryl suture. See Figure 94.2.

NAC viability should be assessed at this point. If there is good 2-second capillary refill with neither sluggish nor brisk refill, then closure is continued with 4-0 monofilament

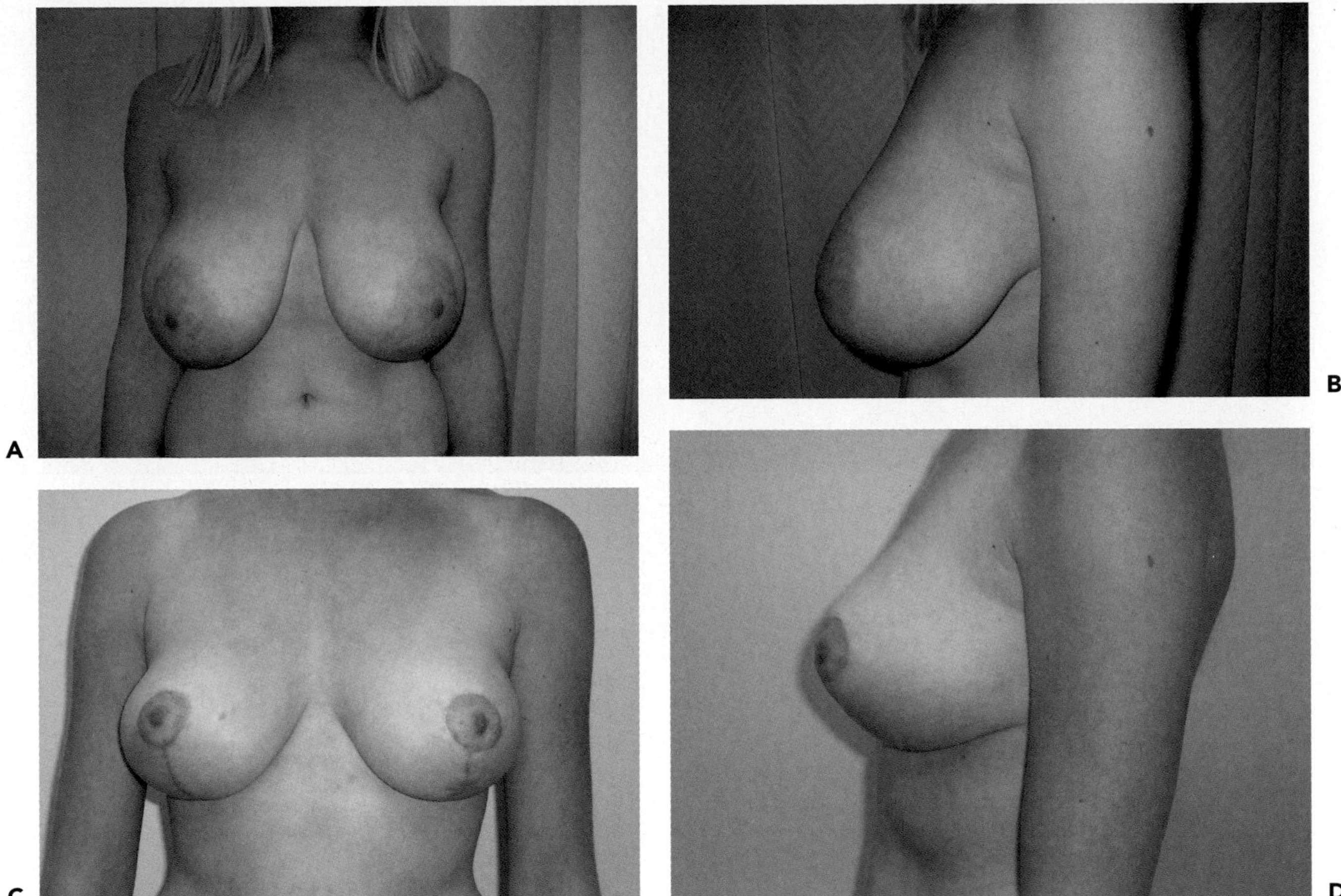

Figure 94.2. **A:** Frontal view, preoperative. **B:** Lateral view, preoperative. **C:** Frontal view, 6 months postoperative, glandular shaping sutures used to avoid bottoming out. **D:** Lateral view, postoperative.

absorbable suture. If there is a question of viability at this point, the sutures should be realized, and the wounds inspected for hematoma causing pressure on the flap, kinking of the pedicle, or undue tension from a tight skin closure. If correcting these potential causes of vascular insufficiency to the NAC does not restore vascularity, the NAC should be harvested as a full-thickness skin graft. After defatting, it can be grafted onto a deepithelialized circle on healthy breast skin flaps.

Drain use varies widely. Some surgeons use no drains, others us them only overnight, and some use them for a week or until drainage is lower than approximately 30 cc per 24-hour period. There is no difference in hematoma, seroma, or overall complication rates with or without drain use (9).

Concomitant axillary liposuction may be undertaken during breast reduction as an adjunct technique. This may not be covered by insurance, and prior arrangements should be made by the patient to address any fees for the surgeon, facility, or anesthesia associated with this. Liposuction may decrease the chest wall diameter by several inches, allow for better contouring of the lateral breast, and help prevent dog-ears in the incisions. It permits better-fitting brassieres postoperatively and can address unsightly bulges toward the lateral chest wall. Superwet technique employs infusion of tumescent solution in a proportion of approximately 1:1 or 2:1 with the anticipated volume of aspirate. A traditional or power-assisted cannula in the 2- to 4-mm range is used to aspirate fat in a smooth, graduated, and tapered fashion to contour the lateral chest. Ultrasonic or laser energy is typically not needed in this soft fat. The portal for liposuction may be placed through a separate stab incision that might be repurposed for a drain exit site (if one is used), or the cannulas may be placed from within the breast reduction incisions, thus minimizing additional scars.

Final closure of all incisions is typically with 3-0 Monocryl deep-dermal and 4-0 Monocryl subcuticulars. The NAC may be closed with running 6-0 fast-gut. Incisions may be dressed with surgical adhesive glue or Steri-Strips. After dry, sterile dressings are applied, the patient is then placed into an appropriate-sized surgical bra for support.

POSTOPERATIVE CARE

Antibiotics are stopped 24 hours after surgery. Oral narcotic analgesics are continued as necessary—typically 1 week—and then NSAIDs can be initiated for both analgesia and as an anti-inflammatory. Postoperative nausea and vomiting are managed

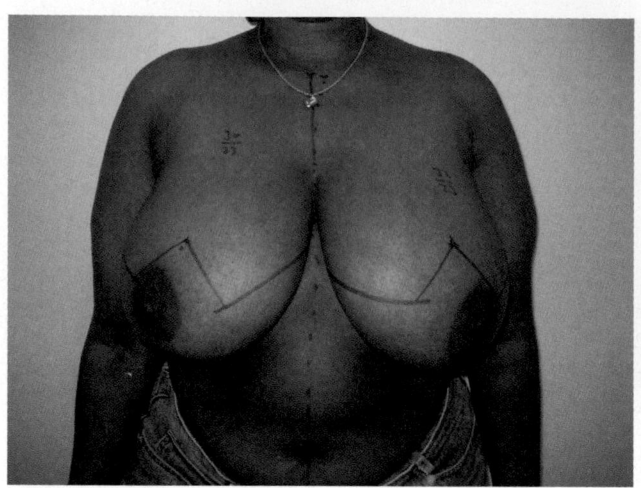

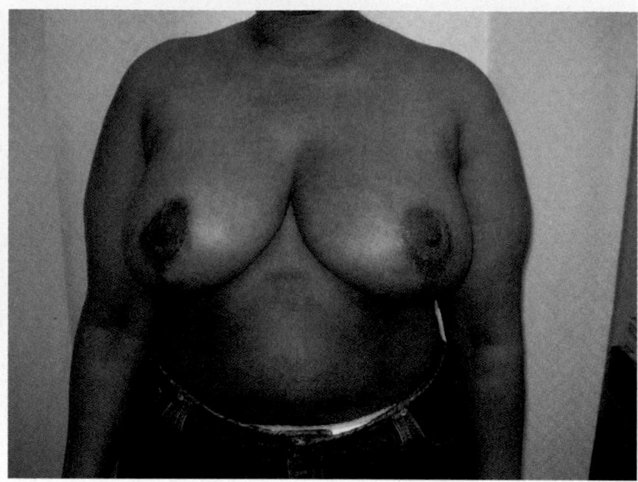

Figure 94.3. **A:** Preoperative view with markings. Note the deep shoulder grooves. In larger breasts, the nipple must be moved more medially. **B:** Postoperative view with hypertrophic scars.

with antiemetics as needed. Hydration and stool softeners can mitigate the constipative effects of narcotics.

Patients are allowed to shower after 48 hours, with or without drains. Steri-Strips may fall off by themselves at this stage.

Patients should be active and ambulating on the night of surgery and may increase to brisk walking in 3 to 5 days postoperatively. Running and other jarring motions should be avoided for 4 to 6 weeks postoperatively, but elliptical machines or stationary bicycle work can be started in 2 weeks. Patients are dissuaded for lifting objects greater than 10 lb for 2 to 4 weeks. After 6 weeks they may resume more strenuous aerobic work and lifting activities as tolerated.

Scar management and optimization is begun at about 4 weeks after surgery. Silicone gel sheets can afford better scars, as can scar massage with creams or vitamin E oils. See Figure 94.3. Gentle massage of scars and breasts is encouraged at 3 to 4 weeks to help scars mature, as well as to desensitize scars and encourage return of skin sensibility. Areas of prolonged numbness (such as the lateral chest after liposuction) tend to be perceived by patients as "fat," much as a numb lip after a dental block tends to feel fat. Warm compresses may be applied, with the caveat that an insensate area can suffer a burn if compresses are too warm or applied for too long an interval. Patients return to the use of a normal bra or camisole at 4 weeks.

COMPLICATIONS

While major complications are unusual, minor complications are frequent. Small areas of delayed healing are frequently identified at the T junction at the level of the IMF, and these heal with local wound care such as antibiotic ointment (e.g., bacitracin) and a Band-Aid. For larger areas of skin loss, wet to dry gauze dressings may be prescribed. If a dry eschar forms, it may be treated with silver sulfadiazine 1% topical ointment twice daily until it separates. Rarely, larger areas of full-thickness skin loss may need operative debridement and closure with a negative-pressure device (vacuum-assisted closure) or, rarer still, with a skin graft.

If a hematoma occurs, it may observed if it is small, noninfected, and not compromising the skin. The risk of developing calcifications around the hemorrhage exists. A hematoma may be needle aspirated—a liposuction cannula is particularly effective. For larger hematomas, operative evacuation and hemostasis are indicated. Seromas should be needle aspirated (10).

Superficial infection can be treated with oral antibiotics, but if significant or if the patient becomes systemically ill, intravenous antibiotics are recommended in an inpatient setting. The need to debride is unusual.

Dog-ears may develop in the lateral breast area and are touched up under local anesthesia with elliptical excision. Hypertrophic or keloid scars may need revision once the inciting etiology (tension during closure) is removed. They may also be treated with injections of triamcinolone. Lasers may be used. Off-label intralesional injections of antineoplastic agents such as 5-fluorouracil have also been reported. See Figure 94.4.

Occasionally the patient will report that she is still too large after reduction. A period of observation to allow edema to subside and for the patient to now attempt weight loss to get closer to a normal BMI (if she was overweight to start) should be undertaken.

An undesirable yet consistent long-term outcome of inferior pedicle and Wise-pattern breast reduction is "bottoming out" and developing a high NAC. A vertical skin excision may address the pseudoptosis sufficiently. Many techniques exist to lower the NAC, including excising excess skin in the IMF, but sometimes a scar above the NAC becomes necessary.

Fat necrosis should be treated conservatively initially since much of it will soften and improve. However, if after 6 to 9 months of massage and observation the fat necrosis is persistent, it should be excised through existing scars.

Nipple necrosis is managed conservatively until healed. Then, the nipple is reconstructed using the techniques for breast reconstruction (e.g., C-V flap, keyhole flap) and then tattooed. See Figure 94.5.

Malignancy is an uncommon finding in the breast specimen, but if found, it is discussed with the patient, pathologist, and a breast oncologic surgeon. If the malignancy is surrounded by a healthy margin of normal tissue, it can be considered an

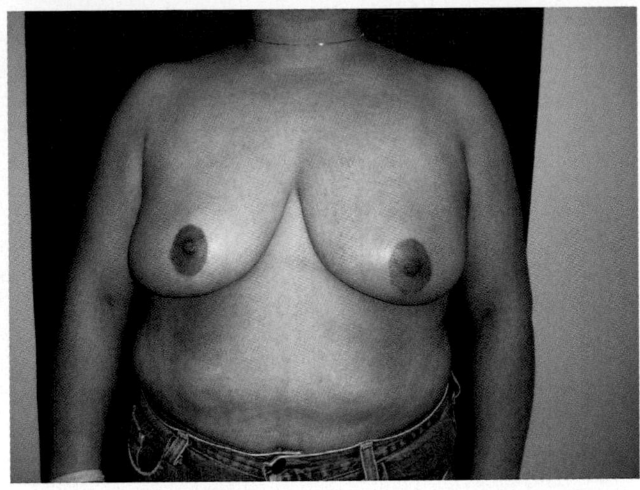

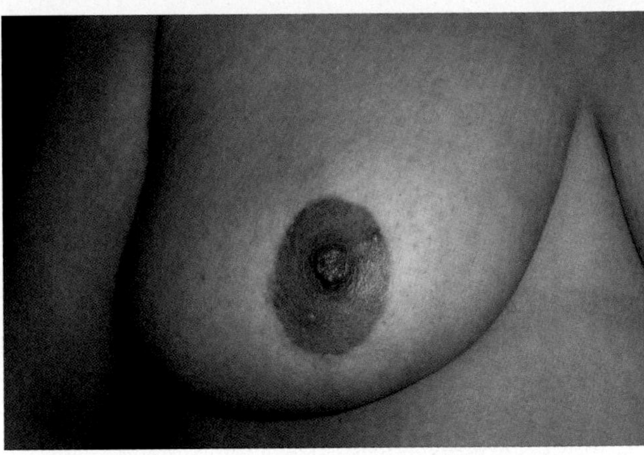

Figure 94.4. **A:** Long-term shape. Notice the fading of scars in this African American patient. **B:** Close-up view of incisions.

adequate lumpectomy. If not, then a mastectomy is indicated. Axillary lymph node sampling may be done via a sentinel lymph node technique. Radiation therapy would be indicated for this method of BCT.

OUTCOMES

Numerous meta-analyses and prospective cohort studies provide level I and level II evidence that breast reduction is effective in addressing the symptoms associated with macromastia and that there is generally high patient and physician satisfaction (11). In breast reduction, the inferior pedicle technique takes center stage, as it is the most commonly subscribed to technique in the United States, has a low rate of complications, is versatile yet predictable, and preserves vascularity and sensation to the nipple (12).

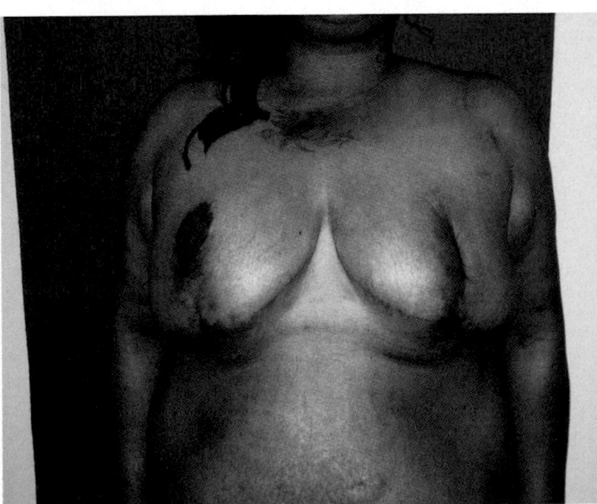

Figure 94.5. Unilateral loss of nipple-areolar complex in a patient with fat necrosis throughout both breasts.

EDITORIAL COMMENTS

The authors provide a very comprehensive guide for the management of the breast reduction patient. We must interpret this as their personal approach and not necessarily accept their comments as indicating anything approaching a standard of care. As I read this chapter prior to discussing it, I wished that they had spent more time describing the technique and less time on the more peripheral issues like insurance coverage, bra sizes, and so on. However, this chapter does provide an interesting overview regarding many aspects of managing the breast reduction patient.

There are many examples of where I might differ from the authors. For example, I do not measure the distance from the nipple to the IMF and prefer instead to measure how much the breast gland overhangs the fold, which is also much easier to measure than N-IMF. Similarly, I do not measure the size of the areola but refer to the preoperative pictures instead.

I find the discussion about bra sizes ambiguous. Although patients speak in terms of bra sizes, surgeons do not. We speak in terms of grams, and our concern is estimating as accurately as possible how much breast tissue we can safely remove. I often find that the bra sizes that patients report vary widely even for breasts of similar size. My experience is that for women with very large breasts who report DD, DDD, F, and G baseline bra cup sizes, the final postoperative bra size is often still a D or larger, but now it at least fits. The comment regarding nipple asymmetry corresponding to weight discrepancy in a ratio of 1 cm to 100 g is interesting but probably highly unreliable. My experience is often the opposite, with the more ptotic nipple sitting on the smaller more pendulous breast.

The authors' description of the informed-consent process is very personal and comprehensive. Mine is somewhat different, and I rely heavily on staff, printed materials, and commercially available information to round out the informed-consent process.

Regarding smoking, we strongly recommend that patients stop smoking for at least 2 weeks either side of surgery. We recognize that some patients cheat, and so we try to operate on previous smokers with more conservative technique than on nonsmokers.

The authors mention using obstetric calipers to transpose the IMF to the breast surface. I would like to think that using such calipers is pretty much a historical footnote.

All in all, this chapter is a thorough overview of the breast reduction experience particularly as it relates to reduction using the inferior pedicle.

S.L.S.

This chapter highlights the advantages associated with the use of an inferior pedicle in breast reduction. Several points are worthy of further emphasis. The authors rightly point out that the inverted-T skin pattern can be used with a number of different pedicles. However, using the inverted T with an inferior pedicle offers a strategic advantage due to the fact that the skin envelope and the pedicle with the attached NAC are managed separately. This allows the NAC to be lifted with no restriction, as opposed to a traditional vertical or superomedial technique, in which the pedicle base is part of the surrounding skin pattern and can therefore limit NAC transposition in cases of a short pedicle. The reader is also directed to the literature regarding the internal breast septum. This internal septum has profound influence on the vascularity of an inferior pedicle, and maintenance of the septal perforators is critical to the successful use of an inferior pedicle in cases of larger breast reductions with longer pedicles (13,14). Another aspect of the technique described in this chapter that is of particular importance is the practice of defining the final location of the NAC until the end of the case after the resection and skin tailoring have been performed. By sighting in the NAC position in this fashion as opposed to committing to the position of the NAC in the initial markings, inadvertent asymmetries or, perhaps more important, unwitting superior malpositions of the NAC can be prevented. As for complications, it stands to reason that the very tip of the inferior pedicle would be the area most at risk for ischemia, and it is in this location that fat necrosis is generally found in cases in which the length of the pedicle outstrips the ability of the vascular supply to nourish the tissues. Therefore, when firmness or an outright mass is noted just above the NAC postoperatively, the etiology is nearly always fat necrosis at the tip of the pedicle. Observation over months will generally result in gradual resolution of the mass, leaving behind only a mild thickening. At one year postoperatively, if there is any persistence of a mass, it is advisable to remove the affected area to prevent any confusion with or masking of any underlying breast malignancy. As for bottoming out, if the attachments of Scarpa's fascia are left intact during the parenchymal resection along the inframammary fold, postoperative change in the shape of the breast will be greatly minimized, as the overlying breast parenchyma will be prevented from slipping inferiorly into the loose subscarpal space. By combining these concepts with the principles outlined in the chapter, the inferior pedicle will continue to serve as the gold standard for breast reduction surgery, now and into the future.

D.C.H.

REFERENCES

1. Kerrigan CL, Collins ED, Striplin DT, et al. The health burden of breast hypertrophy. *Plast Reconstr Surg* 2001;108:1591–1599.
2. Collins ED, Kerrigan CL, Striplin DT, et al. The effectiveness of surgical and nonsurgical interventions in relieving the symptoms of macromastia. *Plast Reconstr Surg* 2002;109:1556–1566.
3. Sigurdson LJ, Kirkland SA. Breast volume determination in breast hypertrophy: an accurate method using two anthropomorphic measurements. *Plast Reconstr Surg* 2006;118(2):313–320.
4. Krieger LM, Lesavoy MA. Managed care's methods for determining coverage of plastic surgery procedures: the example of reduction mammaplasty. *Plast Reconstr Surg* 2002;107:1234–1240.
5. Rohrich RJ, Gosman AA, Brown SA, et al. Current preferences for breast reduction techniques: a survey of board-certified plastic surgeons 2002. *Plast Reconstr Surg* 2004;114(7):1724–1733.
6. Matarasso A, Klatsky SA, Nahai F, et al. Secondary breast reduction. *Aesthet Surg J* 2006;26(4):447–455.
7. Khalifeh M, Redett R, The management of patients on anticoagulants prior to cutaneous surgery: case report of a thromboembolic complication, review of the literature, and evidence-based recommendations. *Plast Reconstr Surg* 2006;118(5):110e–117e.
8. Singh NK, Bluebond-Langner R, Nahabedian MY. Impact of anesthesia technique on breast reduction outcome: review of 200 patients with case-controls. *Aust N Z J Surg* 2003;73:A153–A330.
9. Wrye SW, Banducci DR, Mackay D, et al. Routine drainage is not required in reduction mammaplasty. *Plast Reconstr Surg* 2003;111(1):113–117.
10. Nahai FR, Nahai F. MOC-PSSM CME article: breast reduction. *Plast Reconstr Surg* 2008;121(1 suppl):1–13.
11. Chadbourne EB, et al. Clinical outcomes in reduction mammaplasty: a systematic review and meta-analysis of published studies. *Mayo Clin Proc* 2001;76:503–510.
12. Schreiber JE, Girotto JA, Mofid MM, et al. Comparison study of nipple-areolar sensation after reduction mammaplasty. *Aesthet Surg J* 2004;24(4):320–323.
13. Würinger E, Mader N, Posch E, et al. Nerve and vessel supplying ligamentous suspension of the mammary gland. *Plast Reconstr Surg* 1998;101(6):1486–1493.
14. Würinger E. Refinement of the central pedicle breast reduction by application of the ligamentous suspension. *Plast Reconstr Surg* 1999;103(5):1400–1410.

CHAPTER

95

Saul Hoffman

Inferior Pedicle Technique in Breast Reduction: Practical Steps

In 1975, Ribeiro described a new technique for reduction mammaplasty in which the nipple is based on an inferior dermal flap (1). Two years later, Robbins (2) and then Courtiss and Goldwyn (3) reported a similar procedure. Soon thereafter, Reich (4), then Georgiade and et al. (5), published their experience with the same method. Since then, the inferior pedicle technique has become one of the most common methods of breast reduction in use today. In 1987 a survey of the members of the American Society of Plastic and Reconstructive Surgery found that 36% preferred this method (6). This may have changed with the introduction of newer techniques, such as the short-scar technique of Marchac (7), the Lejour vertical mammaplasty (8), and the round block operation of Benelli (9).

The operation is versatile and safe and can be used for most cases of breast hypertrophy. There are virtually no contraindications, except perhaps in cases of gigantomastia. The pedicle in these cases will be large, and adequate reduction may not be possible. Free nipple grafting for this group of patients is preferred. An inferior flap consisting of dermis and glandular tissue with free nipple grafting will prevent overresection and maintain an aesthetic contour.

The term "inferior pedicle" is descriptive but misleading because it implies that the blood supply comes through an inferiorly based pedicle. A more accurate description, as given by Labanter et al. (10), is the inferior segment technique. The main blood supply of the breast is from the lateral thoracic, internal mammary, and intercostal vessels. It is therefore possible to resect the inferior segment without compromising the blood supply (Fig. 95.1). A procedure using this principle was described by Hester et al. (11) in an operation using a central breast pedicle. An understanding of the anatomy is essential if one is to maintain circulation and sensation to the nipple. A layer of tissue over the fascia must be preserved to protect the vessels as they enter the pedicle. The pedicle can be sculpted to the appropriate size and the flaps thinned when further reduction is required. (Patients often complain of lateral fullness after a reduction mammaplasty if adequate resection has not been performed in this area.) On the other hand, care must be taken to preserve enough tissue medially for adequate cleavage. Before closure, the pedicles and the thickness of the flaps should be compared in order to obtain the best possible symmetry. Suction-assisted lipectomy can be added for further refinement.

PREOPERATIVE PLANNING

Precise planning is essential if one is to achieve a good result. Patients are now being admitted on the day of surgery, so it is more efficient to mark them in the office within a few days before the operation. The markings are made in the routine fashion with a marking pen and reinforced with a sharpened applicator stick that is dipped into a 20% solution of silver nitrate. The silver nitrate leaves a brown stain on the skin that lasts for 7 to 10 days. The patient can shower preoperatively without disturbing the markings.

Marking is begun with the patient in the standing position. The vertical axis of each breast is marked (Fig. 95.2). This line extends through the nipple to the inframammary fold—in some patients the nipple is located medial or lateral to the vertical axis. Next the nipple position is determined by placing a finger in the inframammary fold and marking the anterior projection on the vertical axis (Fig. 95.3). This position is checked by measurement to the clavicle and to the midline and with the contralateral nipple to ensure symmetry. In large breasts, the nipple position may need to be lower or more medial in order to avoid positioning it too high or too lateral. The amount of skin to be resected is then determined by pinching the breast between the thumb and index finger (Fig. 95.4). These points are marked.

An inverted V-shaped incision is then outlined from the new nipple site to these two points. A distance of 7 cm is measured along the limbs of the inverted V from the apex (Fig. 95.5). The inframammary fold is marked and the medial and lateral skin excision outlined so that the upper and lower limbs are approximately the same length (Fig. 95.6). With experience, one will determine a range for these measurements. In order to keep the incision from extending too far medially and laterally, the lower incision can be moved above the fold onto the skin of the breast.

OPERATIVE PROCEDURE

After preparation and draping, the incision lines and areas to be deepithelialized are infiltrated with a mixture of local anesthetic with epinephrine. Marcaine will relieve the postoperative discomfort for several hours. The nipple is circumscribed with an areola marker of the appropriate size (usually 42 mm). An inverted U-shaped incision is made around the areola based on the inframammary fold, creating the so-called inferior pedicle. The skin over the pedicle is deepithelialized. The incision is then deepened, beveling outward to avoid undercutting the pedicle. A layer of tissue should be left over the pectoral fascia to protect the underlying vessels and nerves to the pedicle (Fig. 95.7). Incising along the inframammary fold will facilitate this dissection, which is extended peripherally to the upper markings. The inverted V-shaped incision is then made and connected medially and laterally to the inframammary fold incision. The specimen is removed (Fig. 95.8). Additional tissue can be resected from under the

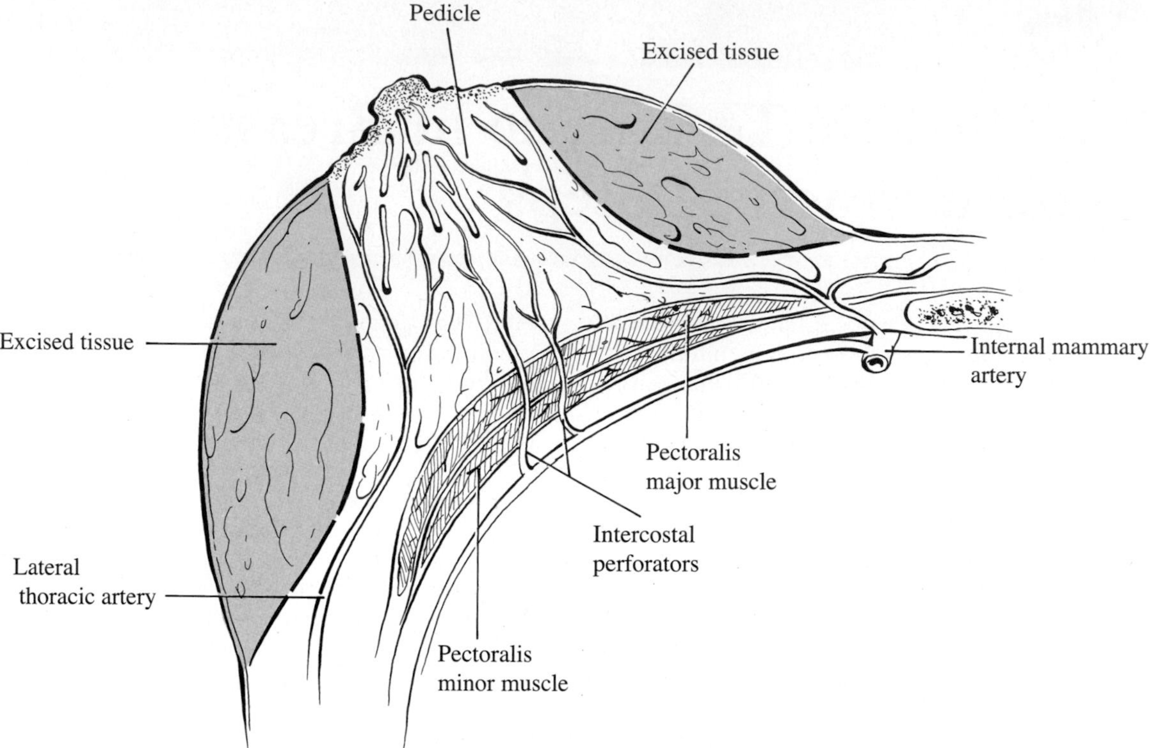

Figure 95.1. Anatomic basis for the "inferior pedicle" technique.

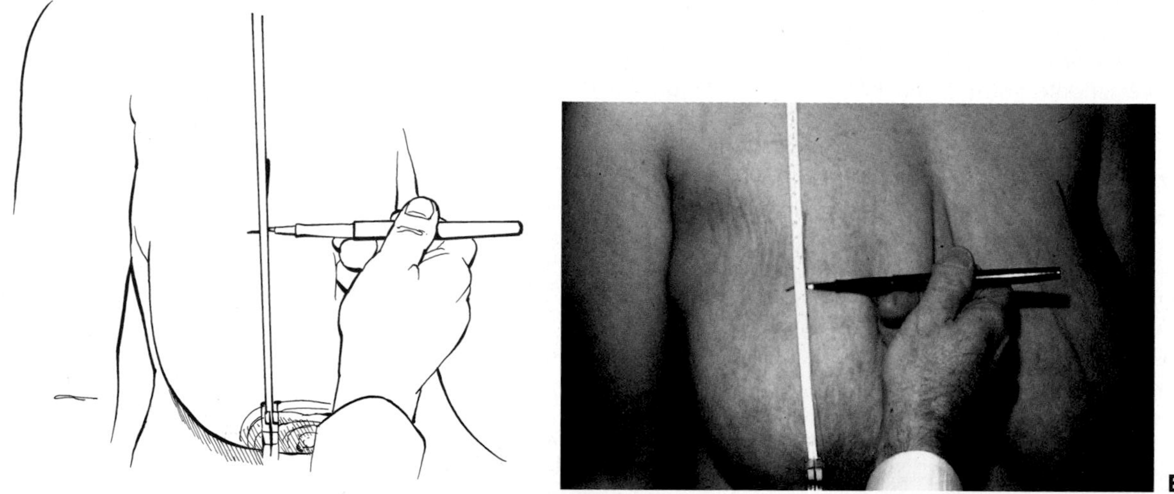

Figure 95.2. The vertical axis of the breast.

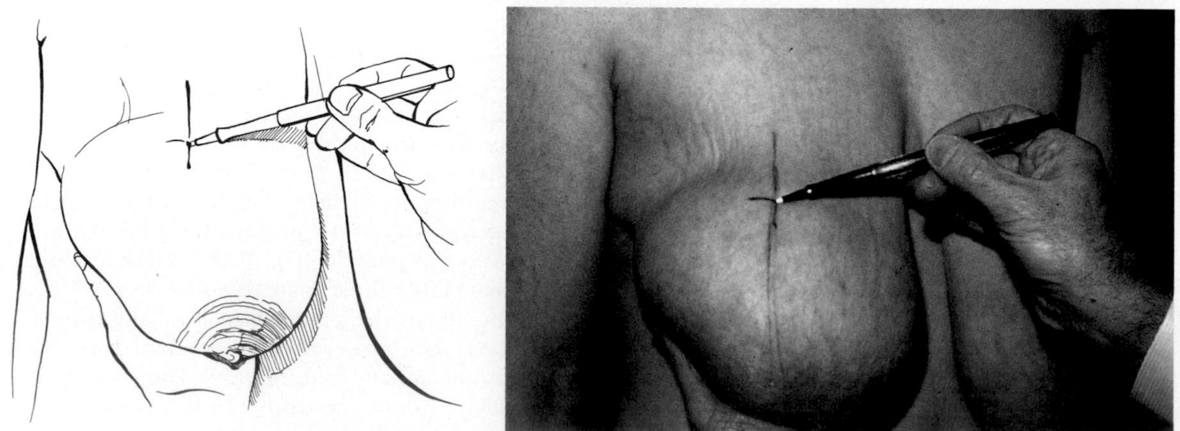

Figure 95.3. The nipple position is determined and marked.

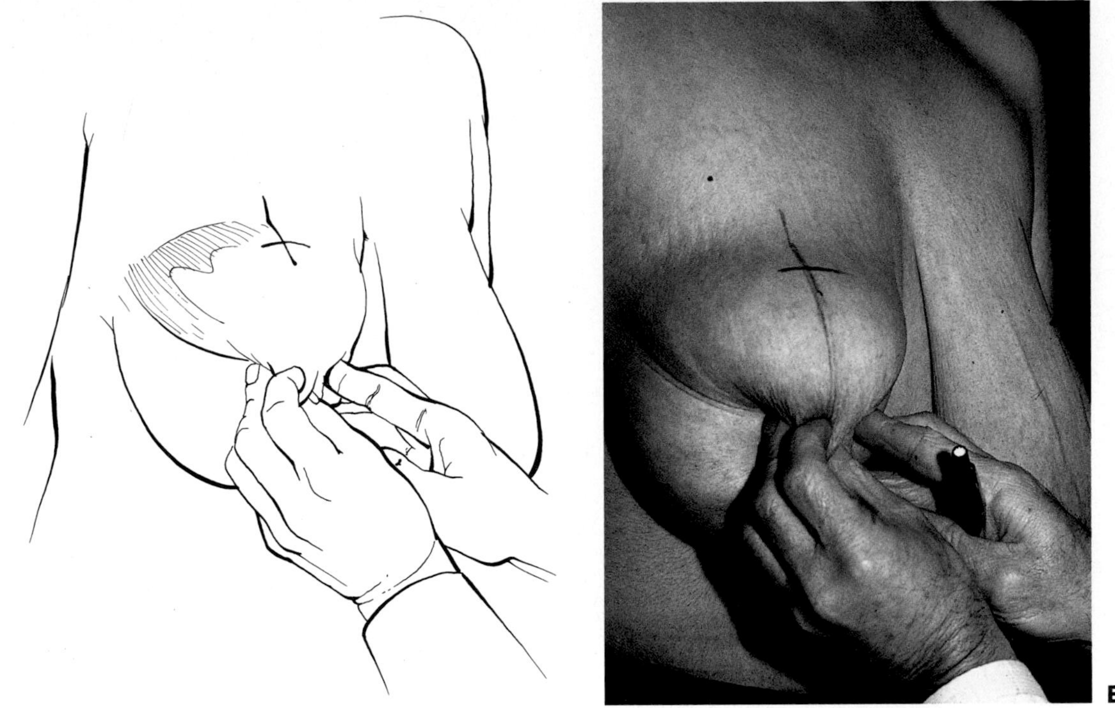

Figure 95.4. Determining the amount of skin resection.

flaps, carefully assessing the thickness of the flaps as one proceeds. Usually more tissue is taken from the lateral flap to avoid postoperative fullness in this area. When hemostasis has been secured, a key suture of 3-0 nylon is placed slightly above the corners of the flaps through the apex of the inferior triangle (Fig. 95.9). The corners of the flaps are trimmed to avoid breakdown at this point of maximum tension. The flaps are sutured in two layers beginning at the corners to avoid "dog-ears." Additional fat removed from the angles will also prevent medial and lateral dog-ears. Despite careful suturing, however, dog-ears occasionally remain and can be removed at a later date. (It is a good idea to warn the patient that this might be necessary.) The skin is closed with a continuous intradermal suture and Steri-Strips. An absorbable suture such as polydioxanone will eliminate the need for suture removal and results in a scar free of suture marks. The flaps are sutured together temporarily, burying the pedicle. The final nipple position is then determined (Fig. 95.10), and a circle of skin of the same diameter as that of the areola is deepithelialized. The nipple is then delivered and examined to be certain that the circulation is adequate. If one is in doubt, the nipple can be removed and applied as a full-thickness

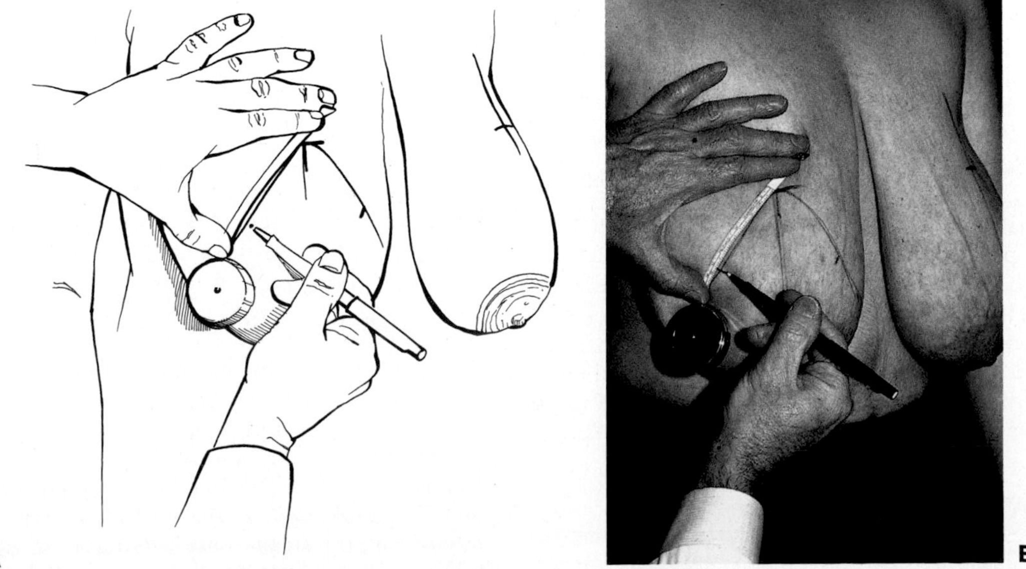

Figure 95.5. The inverted-V incision. Each limb measures 7 cm in length.

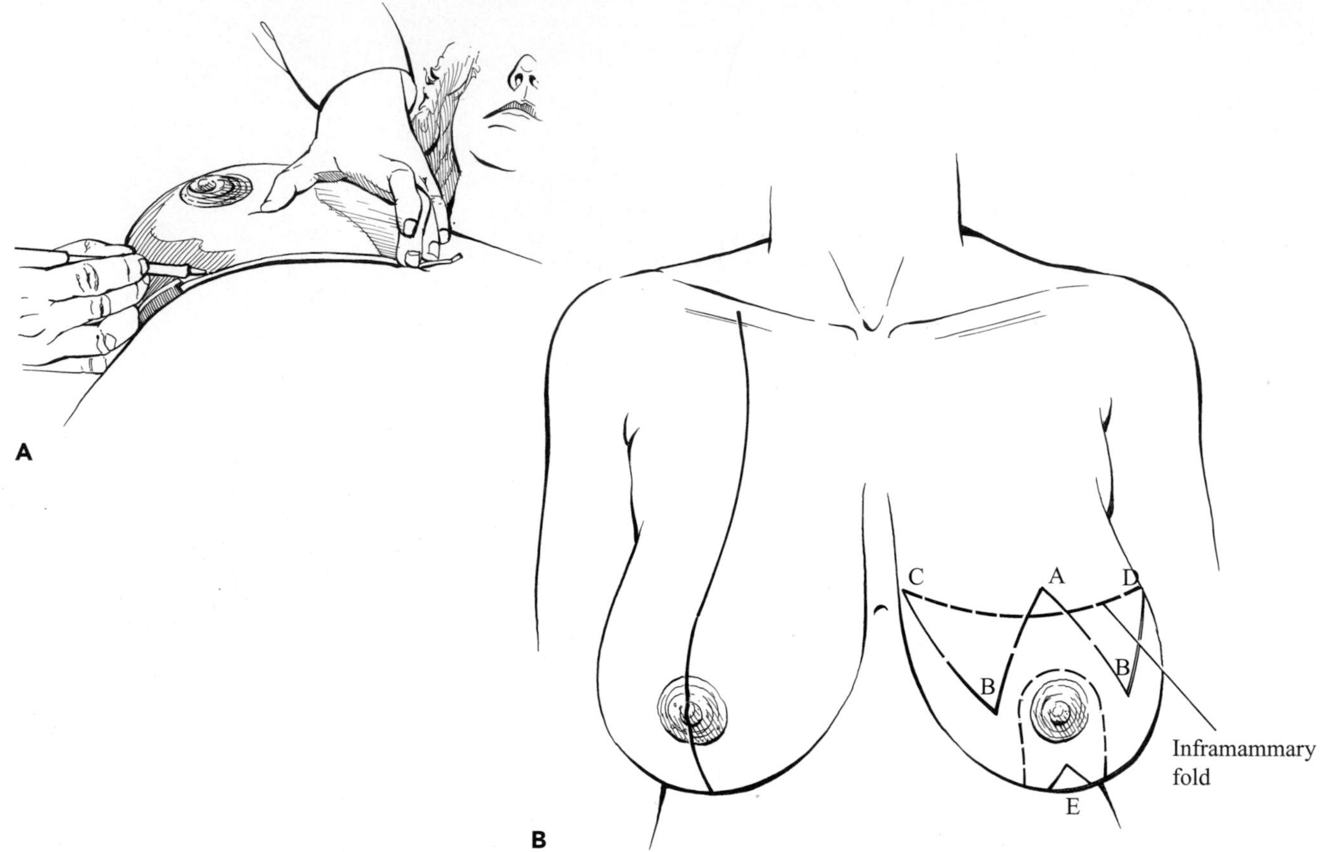

Figure 95.6. The V incision is extended medially and laterally to connect with the inframammary fold incision. Distance B–C should equal distance C–E, and B–D should equal D–E. Note the triangle of skin at E.

graft and the pedicle trimmed to remove any devascularized tissue. When it has been determined that the circulation is adequate, the deepithelialized circle of skin is removed, leaving a peripheral shelf of dermis approximately 8 mm in width to support the nipple. This prevents the tendency to inversion. The nipple is sutured into place. Drains are brought out through the lateral end of the inframammary fold incision. After removal of the drains (usually 24 hours), the intradermal suture can be pulled tight to close the drain site for better healing of this area.

POSTOPERATIVE CARE

A circumferential mild compression dressing is applied. After several days the patient can shower and apply a composite pad to the wounds, held in place by one of her old brassieres. The tapes can be left in place until they come off by themselves, usually in 10 to 14 days. Mild exercise such as walking, using a stationary bike, and so on is allowed after the first week, but more vigorous exercises such as jogging, playing tennis, and using the upper arms are not allowed for approximately 6 weeks.

COMPLICATIONS

Complications should be rare in a properly planned and executed reduction mammaplasty, but no operation is entirely immune (Figs. 95.11 and 95.12).

AVASCULAR NECROSIS

Because a certain amount of tension is necessary to maintain the skin brassiere in this procedure, occasional loss of tissue will result at the junction of the vertical and transverse incisions. The use of the interposing triangle has helped to prevent ischemia at the corners of the flaps. When this occurs, however, it usually can be managed conservatively and will heal with careful wound care. Fat necrosis also may result when areas of fat become devascularized. Temperature elevation, tenderness, and induration with occasional mottling of the overlying skin are manifestations of fat necrosis. This may lead to areas of induration that can continue for several days or weeks but usually disappear in time. Infection can accompany tissue necrosis, necessitating removal of the necrotic tissue. Prophylactic antibiotics are not used routinely in this operation.

HYPERTROPHIC SCARRING

The patient should be informed about the nature of the scars after reduction mammaplasty. Most women with severe breast hypertrophy are willing to accept the resultant scars, but severe hypertrophy can have a disturbing effect in an otherwise satisfactory result. The inframammary fold scar tends to become more hypertrophic than the vertical or circumareolar scar. For this reason, the shorter-scar techniques of Lejour and others have been developed. My indications for these operations are in younger women with minimal to moderate hypertrophy and good tissue elasticity. Lejour extended her indications to

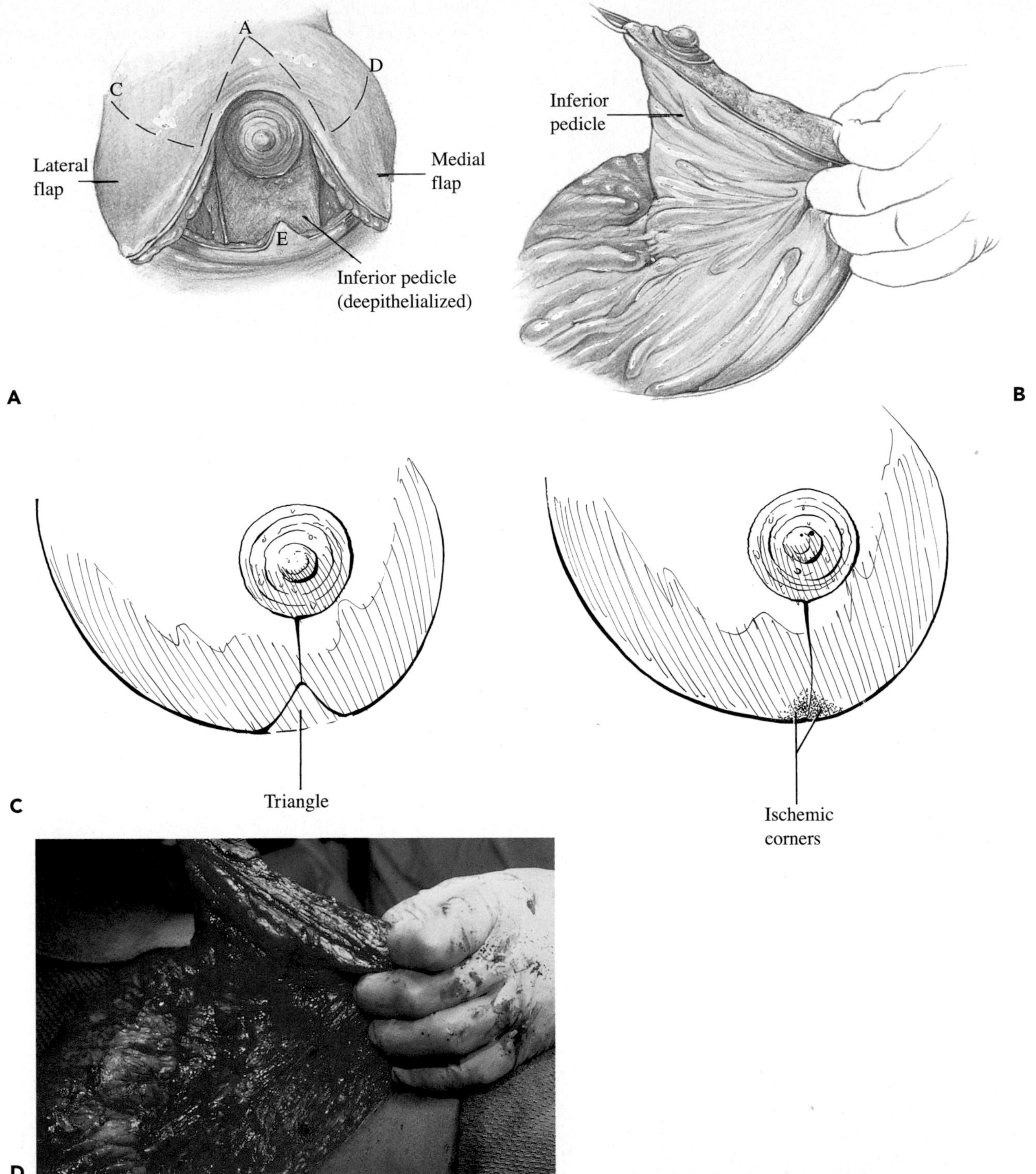

Figure 95.7. **A:** Inferior pedicle deepithelialized and medial and lateral flap developed. **B:** Pedicle dissected; note that the pectoral fascia is not exposed, so blood vessels and nerves are preserved. **C:** Note the interdigitation of a triangle of skin and the excision of flap corners to facilitate healing and avoid necrosis at the junction of the two incisions.

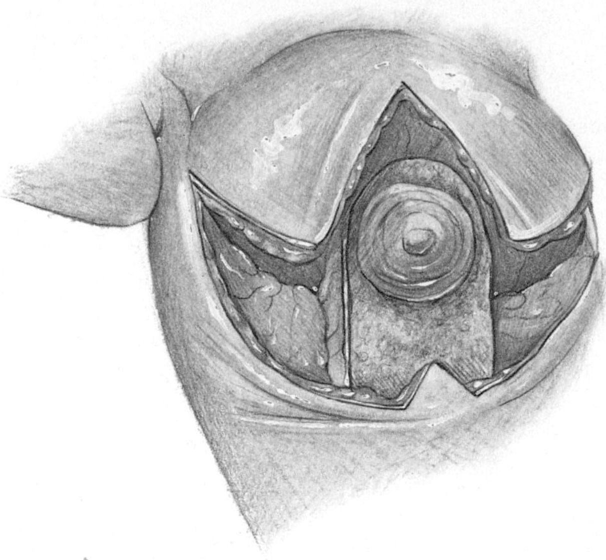

Figure 95.8. Specimen has been removed; ready for closure.

include almost all hypertrophies, with satisfactory results. The occasional addition of a transverse component results in a much shorter inframammary fold scar than is usual with the inverted-T incision.

Hypertrophic scars will eventually subside but may require treatment such as application of silicone sheeting and/or injections of steroids.

LOSS OF SENSATION

The patient should be warned that loss of nipple sensation of variable degree may occur after a reduction mammaplasty. In some cases the reduction is temporary, but in approximately 20% of cases using the transposition technique, permanent loss of sensation can be expected.

AESTHETIC COMPLICATIONS

With careful preoperative planning, aesthetic complications such as overresection or inadequate resection and asymmetry should be avoided. Occasional revisional surgery is sometimes

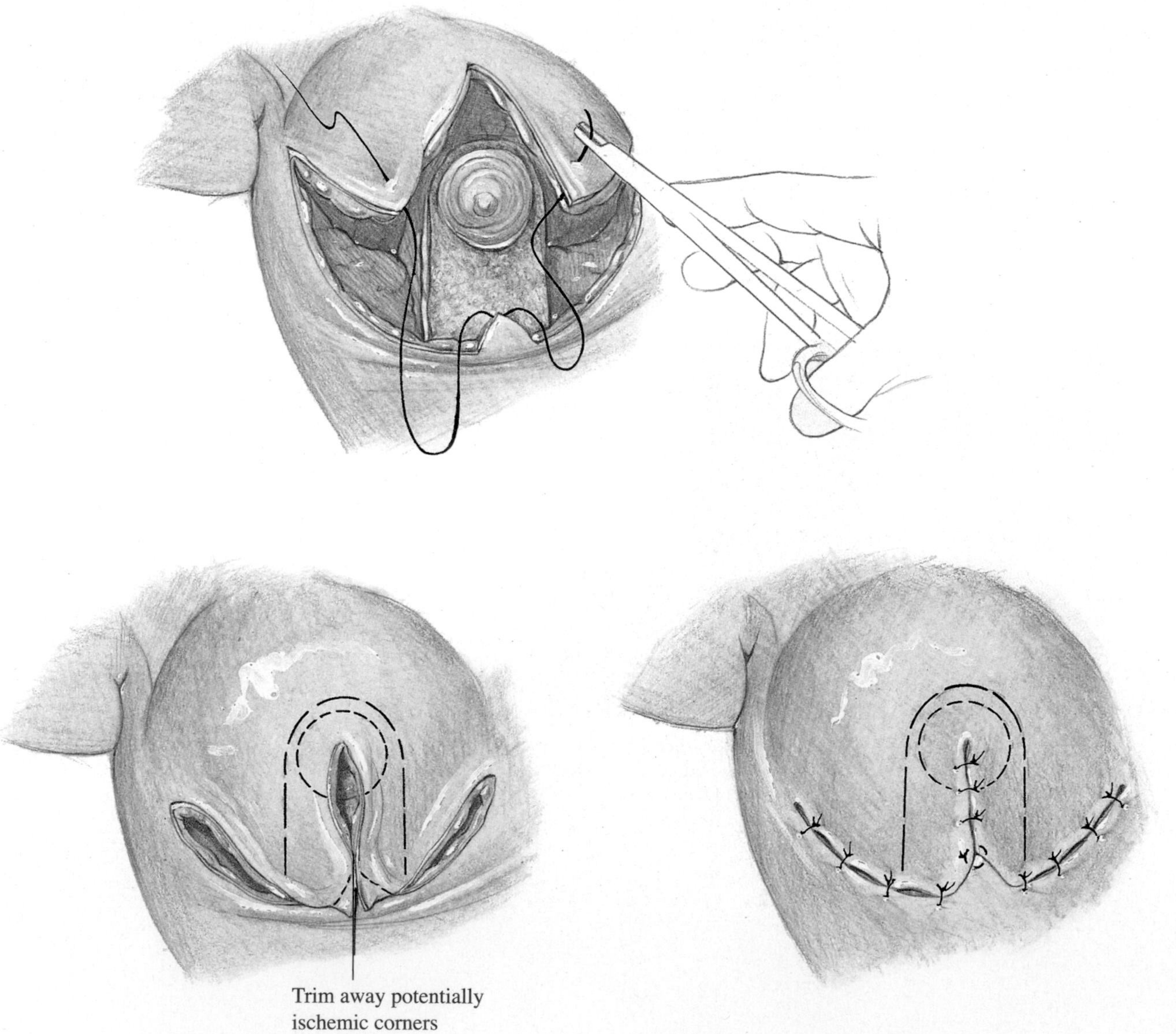

Trim away potentially
ischemic corners

Figure 95.9. Temporary closure. Three-corner suture through skin and dermis.

A

B

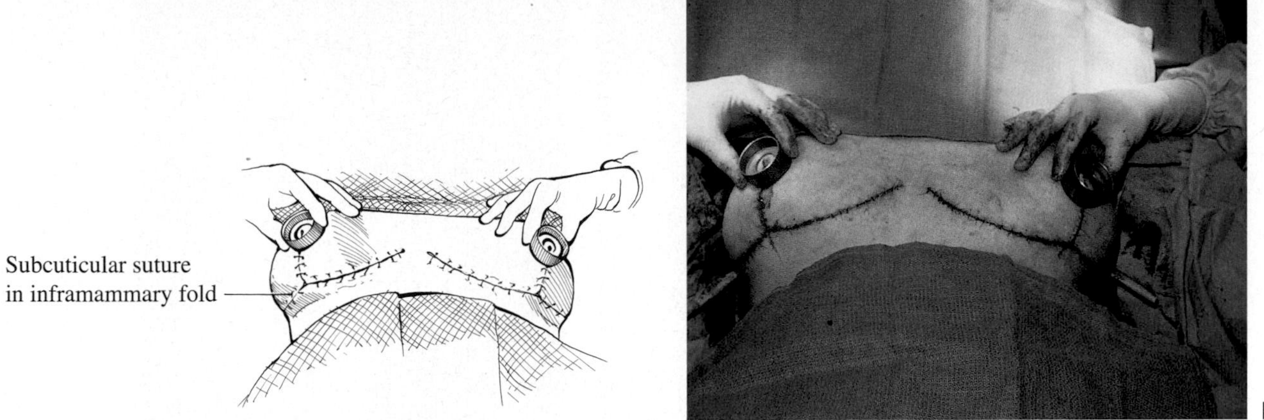

Figure 95.10. Determining nipple position with patient sitting.

A

B

C

D

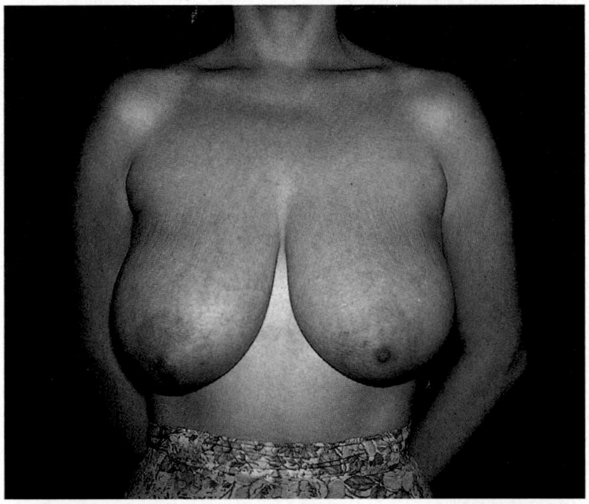

Figure 95.11. In the absence of complications, good results should be the routine. **A–C:** Preoperative 30-year-old woman with large, pendulous symptomatic breasts. Note asymmetry. (*continued*)

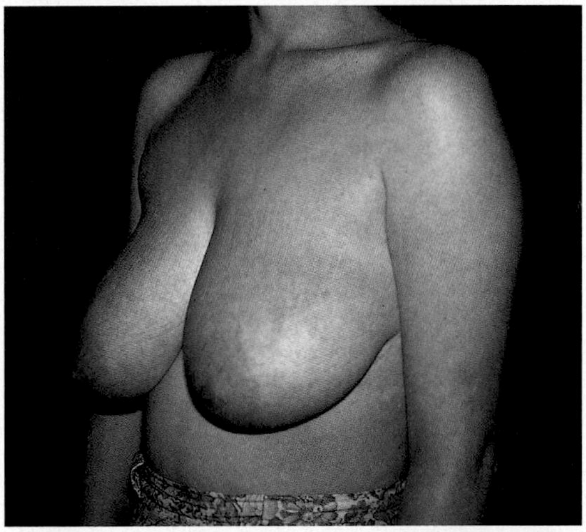

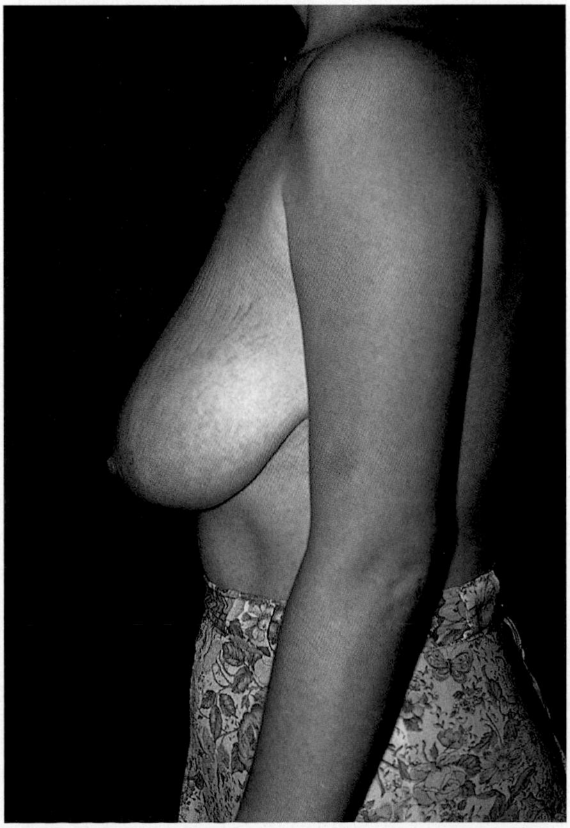

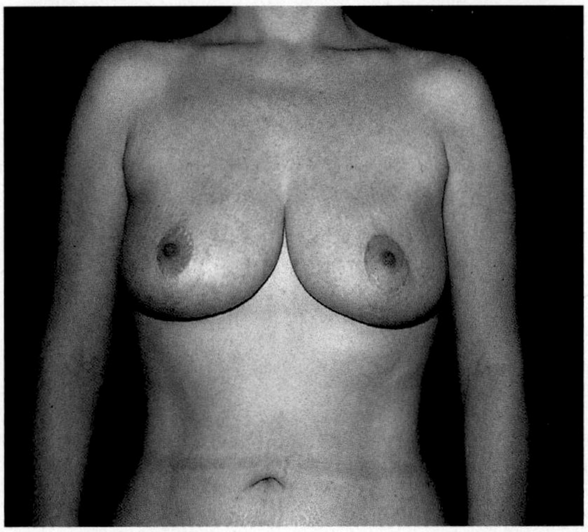

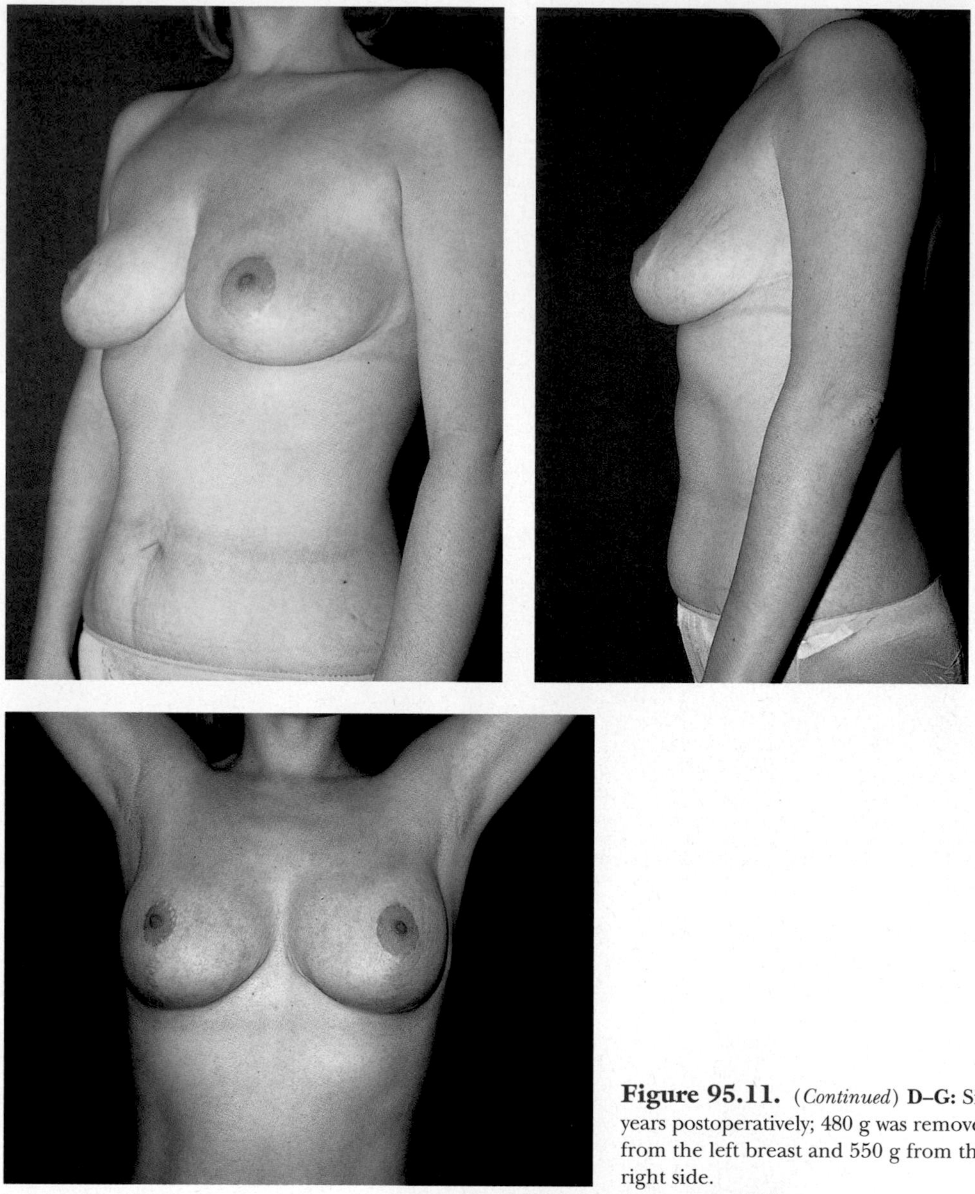

E

F

G

Figure 95.11. (*Continued*) **D–G:** Six years postoperatively; 480 g was removed from the left breast and 550 g from the right side.

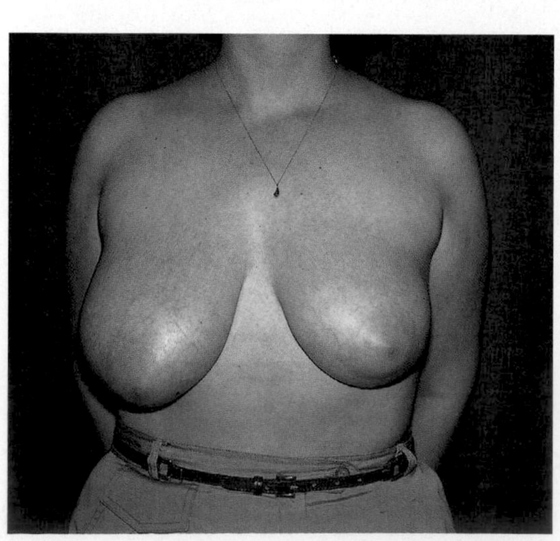

A

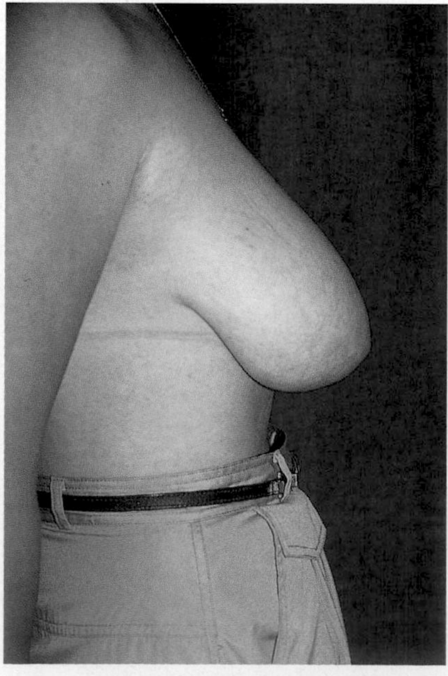

B

Figure 95.12. Another typical good result. **A–D:** Preoperative 26-year-old woman with breast hypertrophy and asymmetry. (*continued*)

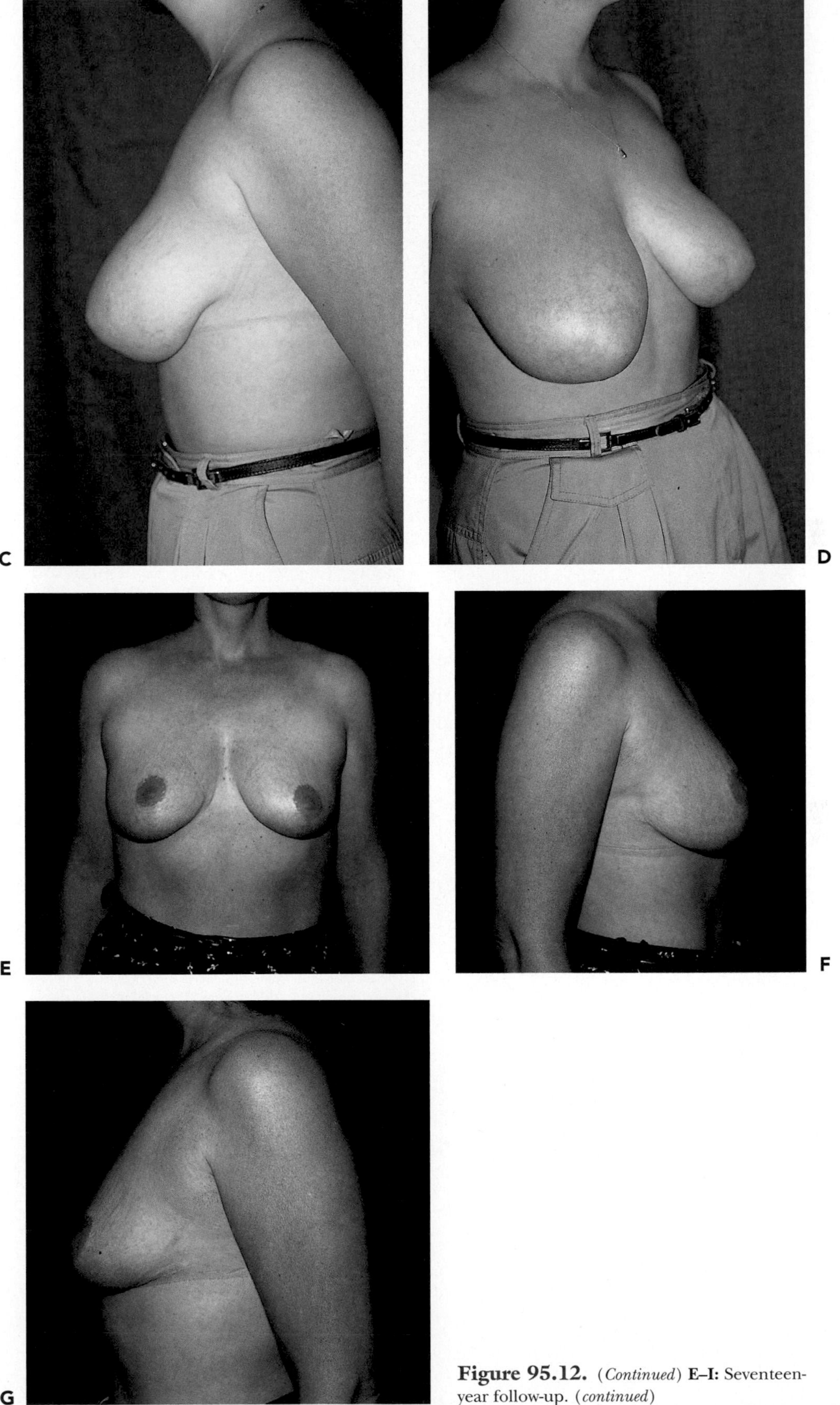

Figure 95.12. (*Continued*) **E–I:** Seventeen-year follow-up. (*continued*)

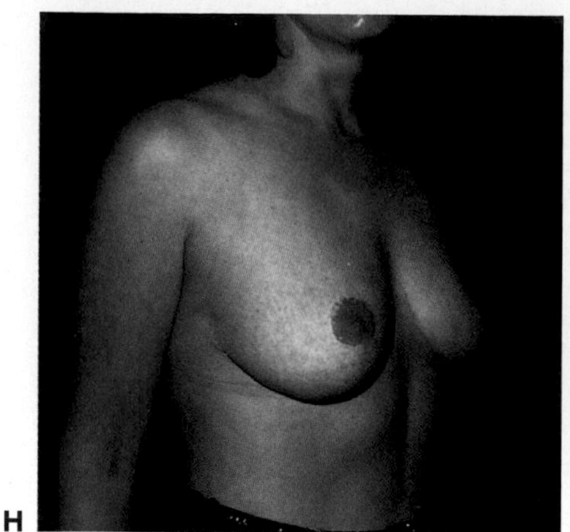

H

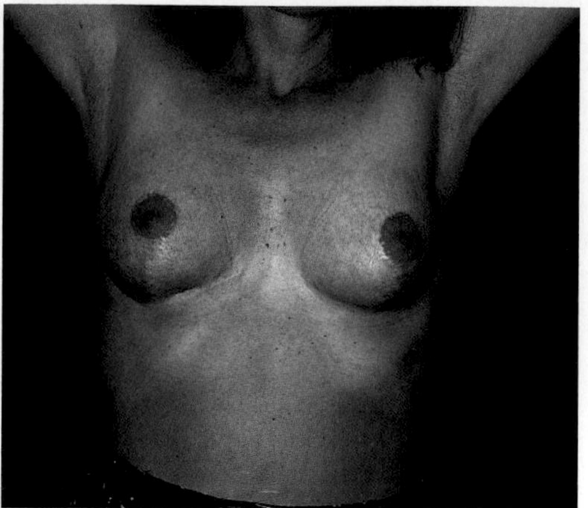

I

Figure 95.12. (*Continued*)

necessary. For a more detailed discussion of complications, the reader is referred to Chapter 27 and Hoffman (12).

EDITORIAL COMMENTS

The interior pedicle method of breast reduction as described by Dr. Hoffman has become the real workhorse of breast reduction surgery in the United States. Most surveys of American plastic surgeons show that this is by far their preferred breast reduction method. As Dr. Hoffman implies, the description of the pedicle or the name is somewhat misleading because the blood supply really comes not just inferiorly but also from the inferior–posterior region of the nipple-areola. In fact, it is really as much a posterior pedicle as it is an inferior pedicle. Its popularity is primarily due to its simplicity of design and execution and its consistently good results with relatively few complications. Episodes or instances of nipple necrosis or breast skin flap necrosis are relatively uncommon with this operation and have been reported in the neighborhood of 1% to 2%. Nipple sensitivity and the ability to lactate are also most likely optimized with this procedure, which leaves adequate breast tissue immediately subjacent to the nipple without removing the nipple.

The most common drawback of this operation has been the final breast shape, often described as being somewhat flattened. In addition, this operation is considered by many to be prone to bottoming out or to result in a nipple that rotates superiorly with a gland that descends inferiorly over time.

Still, because of its reliability and simplicity, this operation remains the most commonly performed in the United States despite the possible limitations of breast shape both short and long term. Although I tend to prefer the McKissock procedure over the inferior pedicle, I feel that the inferior pedicle technique is a safe and predictable option for most patients.

S.L.S.

REFERENCES

1. Ribeiro L. A new technique for reduction mammaplasty. *Plast Reconstr Surg* 1975;55:330.
2. Robbins TH. A reduction mammaplasty with the areola-nipple based on an inferior dermal pedicle. *Plast Reconstr Surg* 1977;59:64.
3. Courtiss EH, Goldwyn RH. Reduction mammaplasty by the inferior pedicle technique. *Plast Reconstr Surg* 1977;59:500.
4. Reich J. The advantage of a lower central breast segment in reduction mammaplasty. *Aesthet Plast Surg* 1979;3:47.
5. Georgiade NG, Serafin D, Morris R, et al. Reduction mammaplasty utilizing an inferior pedicle nipple areola flap. *Ann Plast Surg* 1979;3:211.
6. Hoffman S. Reduction mammaplasty: a medicolegal hazard? *Aesthet Plast Surg* 1987;11:113.
7. Marchac D, DeOlarte G. Reduction mammaplasty and correction of ptosis with a short inframammary scar. *Plast Reconstr Surg* 1982;69:45.
8. Lejour M, Abboud M. Vertical mammaplasty without inframammary scar and with liposuction. *Perspect Plast Surg* 1990;4:67.
9. Benelli L. Technique de plastie mammaire: le "round bloc." *Rev Fr Chir Esthet* 1988;50:7.
10. Labanter HP, Dowden RV, Dinner MI. The inferior segment technique for breast reduction. *Ann Plast Surg* 1982;8:493.
11. Hester TR, Bostwick J, Miller L, et al. Breast reduction utilizing the maximally vascularized central breast pedicle. *Plast Reconstr Surg* 1985;76:890.
12. Hoffman S. Complications of reduction mammaplasty. In: Noone RB, ed. *Plastic and Reconstructive Surgery of the Breast.* Philadelphia: BC Decker; 1991:285.

CHAPTER

96

Daniel P. Luppens
Mark A. Codner

Reduction Mammaplasty Using the Central Mound Technique

INTRODUCTION

The central mound technique differs fundamentally from most popular techniques of breast reduction in that it relies predominately on a broad-based glandular blood supply to the nipple. The central mound technique involves separating the skin from the gland of the breast, resecting the desired portion of gland, and resecting a customized pattern of skin to achieve the desired result. Rather than rely on the skin resection only or gland resection only for the final breast shape, the central mound technique relies on the interaction of the gland with the remaining skin envelope. Additional advantages to the central mound reduction include simple preoperative markings, no limitations due to breast size or ptosis, preservation of nipple sensitivity and the potential to breast-feed, and excellent aesthetic results with a minimal secondary revisions.

The central mound approach to breast reduction surgery was introduced by Hester in 1985 (1,2). Hester's technique is a modification of earlier methods of achieving breast reduction by separating the skin from the gland. In 1921, Biesenberger described a technique of separation of the skin from the gland, leaving the nipple and areola attached, followed by resection of the lateral half of the breast. The remaining gland was then sutured to create a cone and the skin redraped over the new breast contour. Biesenberger's technique threatened the blood supply to the nipple because of extensive lateral dissection and the 180-deg glandular rotation performed during shaping (3,4). In order to better preserve blood supply to the nipple, early modifications to the technique were made by a number of surgeons, including Schwarzmann, Gillies, and McIndoe (5–9).

Unlike some previous modifications, the central mound technique has a firm anatomic basis explaining the adequate blood supply to both skin flaps and the gland of the breast. The principles of this reliable technique depend on the blood supply from the lateral thoracic artery, intercostal perforators, and internal mammary perforators through the pectoralis major muscle. The skin and subcutaneous flaps are elevated off the gland, which allows the breast mound to be reduced and shaped according to the surgeon's desire. The nipple remains at the apex of the gland, which can be reduced and sculpted like a breast implant, preserving a broad blood supply from the chest wall. After the desired breast volume is obtained by sculpting the gland, the skin and subcutaneous flaps are then closed around the reduced gland as a well-fitting "brassiere" to support and further refine the final size and shape of the breast. Breast projection can be customized independent of preoperative patterns and glandular resection. The technique has proven in clinical experience to be reliable and versatile and can be used similarly as a technique for mastopexy. The central mound technique has been used for nearly 20 years with reliable and reproducible results.

ANATOMY

Consideration of the blood supply to the breast is important to maximize blood supply to both the gland and the skin flaps. The blood supply to the breast includes branches from the lateral thoracic and thoracoacromial arteries, as well as pectoralis major perforators supplied by the anterolateral intercostal perforators, anteromedial intercostal perforators, and the internal mammary perforators (Fig. 96.1). The central mound technique exposes the breast gland following elevation of thick skin and subcutaneous dermoglandular flaps. The lateral and medial skin flaps also have a robust blood supply from the lateral thoracic and internal mammary perforators, respectively (Fig. 96.2). The skin flaps should not be too thin or elevated down to the chest wall in order to preserve blood supply at the base of the glandular pedicle. Instead, a layer of breast and adipose tissue measuring a thickness of 3 to 4 cm is preserved over the thoracic fascia to prevent division of the vessels and sensory nerves. The primary sensory nerve to the nipple is the lateral cutaneous branch of the fourth thoracic nerve, which enters the breast along the lateral border. Once the breast mound is exposed, the excess gland is resected in a tangential fashion (10).

TECHNIQUE

Compared to the markings of some other techniques of breast reduction that often commit the surgeon to a pattern that can result in a shortage of skin during closure, the markings for the central mound reduction are quite simple. With the patient in the upright position, the initial mark should be made at the sternal notch. The second point is marked at the approximate level of the inframammary fold transposed to the anterior aspect of the breast in the central meridian. Although a number of techniques have been described to localize this point, it is approximately 21 cm from the sternal notch, with the excess weight taken off the breast. If the breast is not supported to reduce the excess weight, this point will retract superiorly once reduction has taken place, resulting in a nipple that is too superiorly positioned. This mark will approximate the new level of the superior aspect of the areola, which will place the nipple at 23 cm from the sternal notch. Anticipated changes in breast shape following all reduction techniques include "bottoming out" or glandular ptosis. As ptosis recurs, the distance from the inferior aspect of the areola to the inframammary fold increases. Placing the nipple slightly lower on the breast mound has been found to maintain a better aesthetic appearance as changes occur after surgery.

The inframammary fold is then marked, as well as a vertical line at the meridian of the breast at the lowest point of the

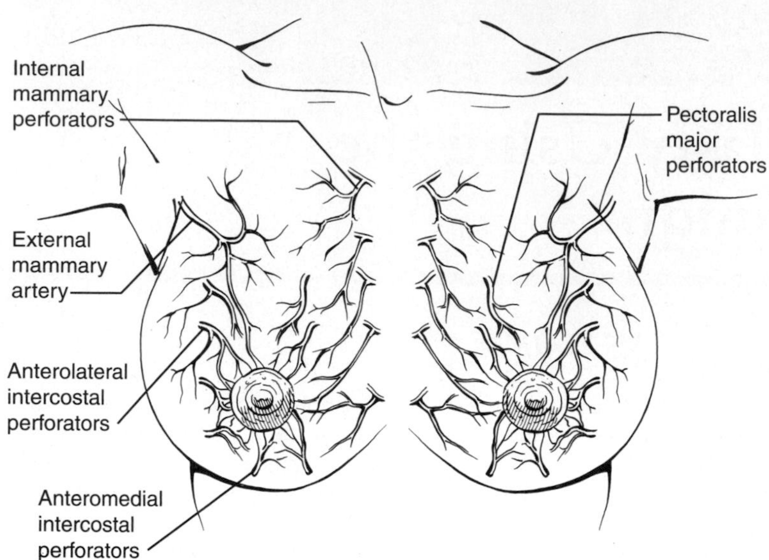

Figure 96.1. Blood supply to the breast, demonstrating medial and lateral perforators.

inframammary fold, which is approximately 11 cm from the midline. Excess adipose tissue at the axillary tail of Spence is circled to indicate the areas that require liposuction during the reduction. An inverted V is drawn from the mark at the apex of the new nipple-areola complex position to the width of the existing areola (Fig. 96.3). At this point, two parallel lines are drawn from the medial and lateral aspect of the areola inferiorly to the inframammary fold. Although this area represents the skin to be deepithelialized, the dermal pedicle does not contribute significantly to the blood supply of the nipple. Furthermore, some patients with a wide areola and minimal skin excess may have the maximal skin tension during closure just below the existing areola. Therefore, a modification of the marking may include a single incision from the inferior aspect of the areola to the inframammary fold to preserve skin for closure (Fig. 96.4).

The patient should be prepped and draped with the arms properly secured to arm boards extended at right angles from the operating table. A nipple marker with a 42-mm diameter is used to mark the nipple while the assistant places the areola on a gentle stretch. Vigorous stretching of the areola during marking can result in tension on the areola during closure and can compromise the blood supply, resulting in peripheral areolar necrosis. A circular incision is made around the areola. Then the skin is deepithelialized above and below the areola within the preoperative markings down to the level of the inframammary fold (Fig. 96.5A).

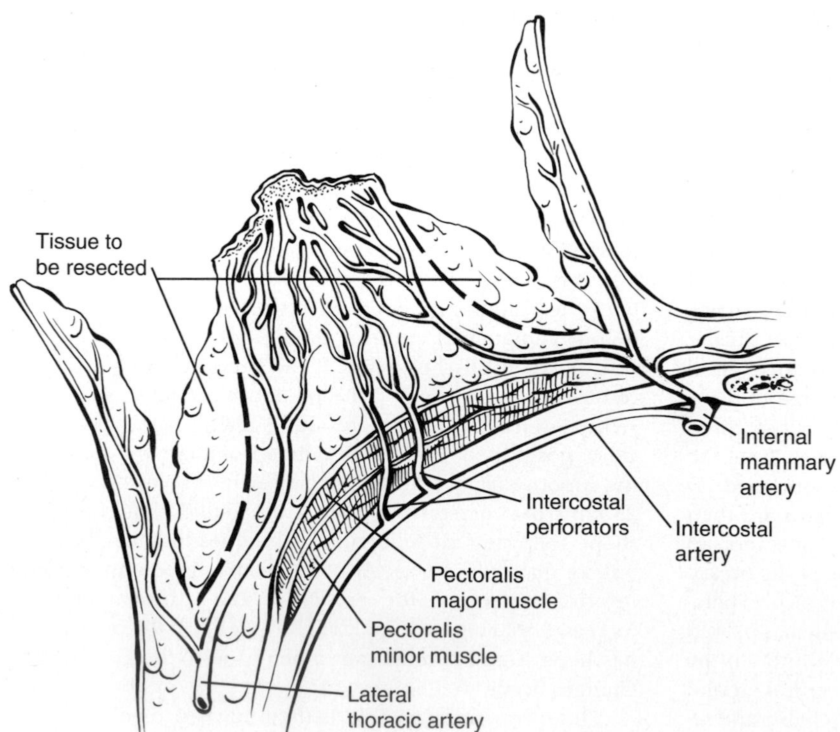

Figure 96.2. Cross-sectional anatomy of the blood supply to the breast and dermoglandular flaps.

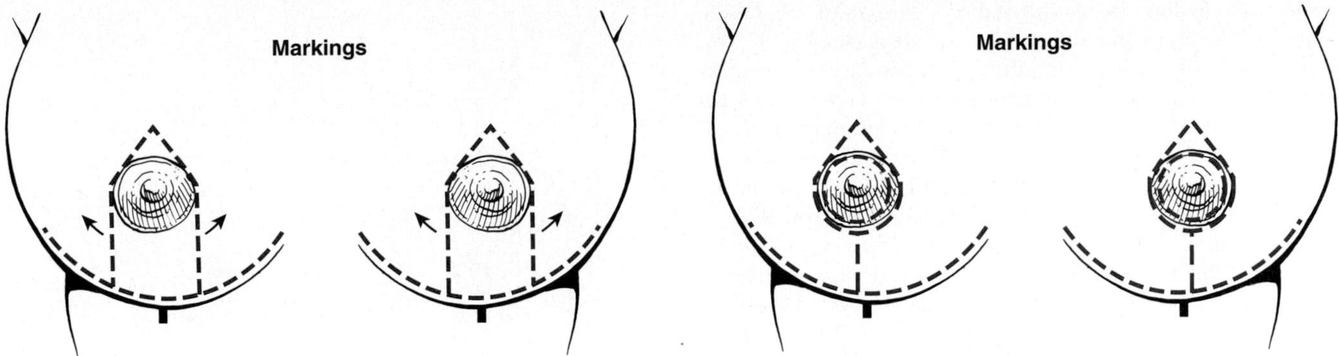

Figure 96.3. Preoperative markings of the inverted V and inframammary fold.

Figure 96.4. Modification of the markings for anticipated skin shortage below the areola.

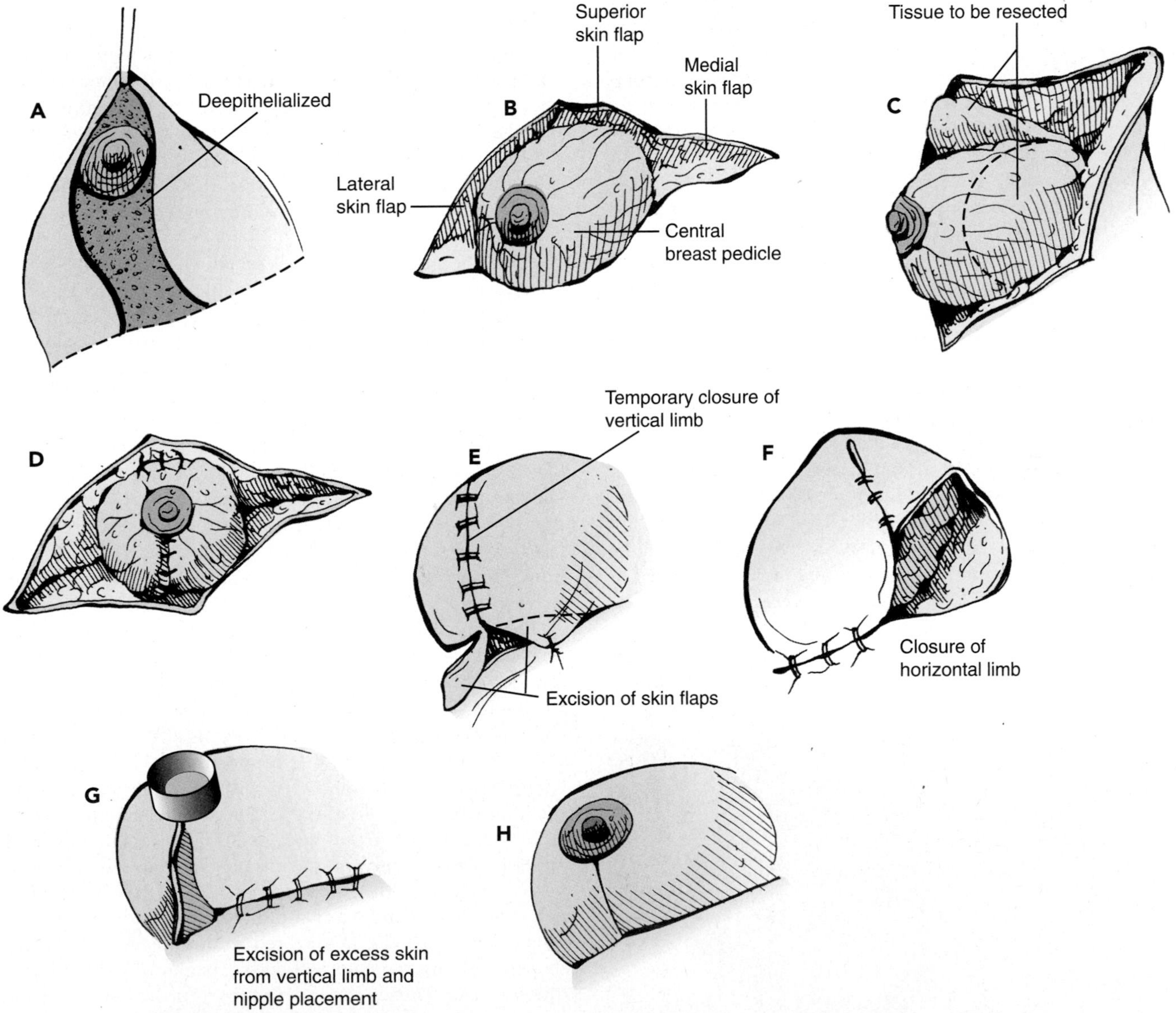

Figure 96.5. Key steps in central mound reduction. **A:** The pedicle is marked for deepithelialization. **B:** Skin flaps are raised, and central breast pedicle is exposed. **C:** Tangential resection of tissue from central breast pedicle is performed. **D:** Central breast pedicle is shaped with sutures and sutured to the chest wall. **E:** Vertical limb is temporarily closed, and medial and lateral skin flaps are excised. **F:** Horizontal limb is closed temporarily with staples with advancement toward the central to eliminate lateral and medial dog-ears. **G:** After tailor tacking to determine extent of excision, excess skin is excised from the vertical limb. **H:** Vertical and horizontal limbs closed with nipple inset.

After the pedicle is deepithelialized, skin flaps are raised, separating the breast gland from the skin flaps (see Fig. 96.5B). An incision is then made along the inframammary fold, excluding the area that was deepithelialized to preserve the dermal pedicle. The incision is then extended vertically along the markings, and electrocautery is used to elevate the skin flaps. The undermining used in these dermoglandular flaps should be thicker than the technique used in mastectomy flaps. We recommend flap thickness of approximately 2 to 3 cm. Dense breast tissue that is often present in younger patients defines the plane of dissection. The medial flap is initially elevated while the assistant retracts the flap with double hooks and the surgeon retracts the entire breast laterally. Dissection should proceed, leaving 3 to 4 cm of tissue overlying the internal mammary perforators above the chest wall. Overdissection will expose the pectoralis major muscle fascia. Once medial dissection is complete, the assistant retracts the breast mound medially and the lateral flap is similarly elevated. The lateral chest wall should not be exposed, to preserve the neurovascular supply to the breast. Once the medial and lateral flaps have been elevated, the superior flap is dissected to the level of the clavicle to create a superior pocket for the reduced breast mound. The flaps should be of uniform thickness to reduce contour irregularities from the underlying glandular resection, particularly for dense breast tissue. Following completion of the flap elevation, the flaps are retracted, exposing the entire breast mound (Fig. 96.5B). Liposuction of the lateral aspect of the breast can be performed through the lateral incision with minimal risk to the blood supply of the central mound.

The breast tissue is marked, centering the nipple-areola complex on the desired breast size (Fig. 96.6). The gland can be resected in a conical shape with the nipple at the apex of the cone (Fig. 96.5C). The gland is reduced, followed by numerous circumferential tangential excisions (Figs. 96.5D and 96.7). The breast can be elevated with two Kocher clamps, while care is taken not to undermine the base of the breast, which is preserved to maximize blood supply. The tissue surrounding the areola is also preserved. The majority of the breast tissue is removed from the lateral quadrant, followed by the superior quadrant. Although tissue is resected from the inferior quadrant, the dermal pedicle is preserved if possible. Conservative resection from the medial quadrant should be performed to maintain postoperative medial projection for

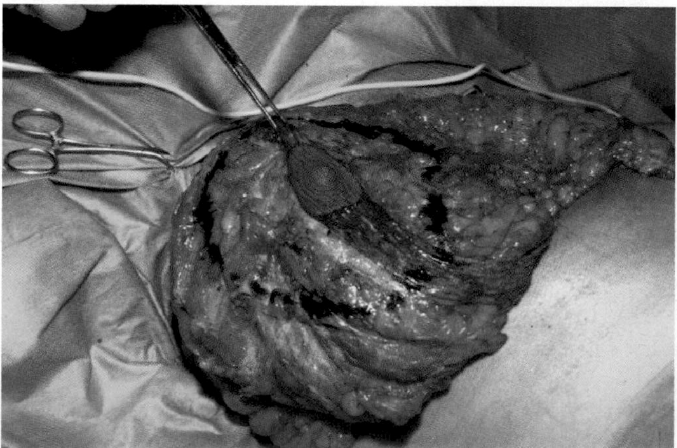

Figure 96.6. Outline of the breast mound to be preserved prior to tangential resection.

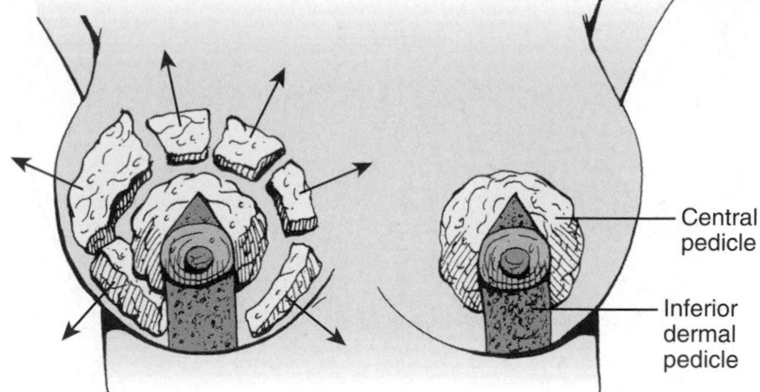

Figure 96.7. Tangential resection of the central breast mound with the majority of the resection from the superior and lateral quadrants.

cleavage. Glandular resection continues in a stepwise fashion until the desired size is obtained. The limitation on the amount of breast tissue that can be safely removed is determined by the preserved tissue centered under the nipple-areola complex to the chest wall. Although patients with very large breasts are good candidates for this technique, achieving a small B cup may be difficult, and alternate reduction techniques should be considered.

After the gland has been resected to achieve the desired size, the gland is further shaped by suturing the gland to itself as well as to the chest wall (Fig. 96.5D). The projection of the gland can be increased by plicating the glandular tissue inferiorly. The gland can be anchored to the chest wall superiorly in the desired position. Glandular sutures are designed to increase projection and minimize the risk of bottoming out. The principle of glandular sutures is to include techniques similar to vertical breast reduction by using lower pole pillars to maintain inferior glandular support. The upper pole sutures suspend the superior part of the breast mound to the prepectoral fascia. Vicryl 2-0 sutures are used for internal glandular plication (Fig. 96.8). This technique places less emphasis on the skin envelope to shape and support the central breast mound.

Following tangential resection and shaping of the gland, final shaping of the breast is performed using a freehand technique to tailor the skin flaps. The skin envelope is closed using temporary staples in a manner that produces the desired breast contour (see Fig. 96.5E). Closure begins at the apex of the inverted V and proceeds to the inframammary fold. The desired length of the vertical limb is determined by minimal tension on the inframammary fold at the intersection of the inverted-T incision. The distance from the apex to the inframammary fold is approximately 10 cm, and the distance from the inferior aspect of the areola should be approximately 6 cm. The excess tissue below the medial and lateral inframammary fold is marked and resected (Fig. 96.5E). During reduction, the excess triangular shaped flaps are resected and beveled superiorly to remove additional tissue. During mastopexy procedures, these flaps can be deepithelialized and folded inward to add volume to the breast.

Following resection of the excess tissue, the final projection is refined by advancing the medial and lateral breast skin toward the meridian incision beginning at the areola and continuing to the inframammary fold (Fig. 96.5G). As the skin is tightened below the areola, projection of the breast can be increased (Fig. 96.9). In addition, any "dog-ears" can be reduced

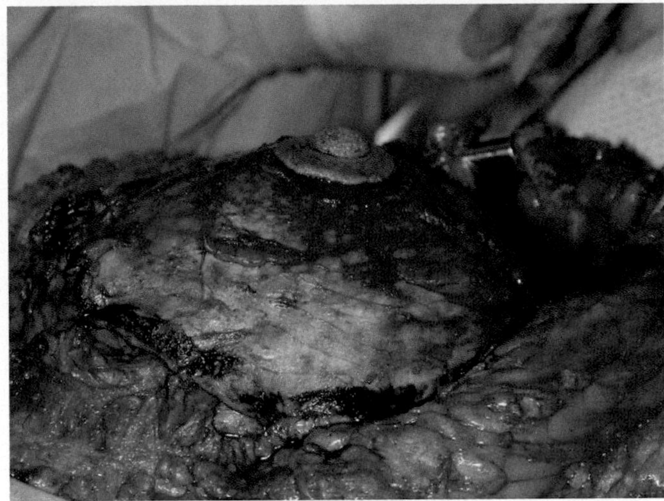

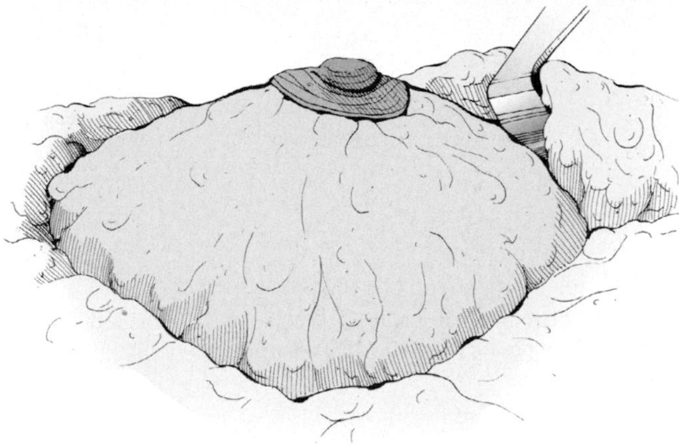

Figure 96.8. Shaping of the gland by suturing the gland to itself and to the chest wall.

by advancing the lateral and medial flaps toward the breast meridian and trimming the excess skin. Methylene blue is used to mark the final skin resection. The position of the nipple is planned with the superior aspect of the areola at the apex of the incision rather than the nipple at the apex. The staples should be removed from the apex for approximately 4 cm inferiorly so that when the 38-mm-diameter nipple marker is used to mark the areola, there is no horizontal tension on the skin. Horizontal tension on the skin at the site of the new areola will cause the circular excision to widen into an oval-shaped areola. The excision of excess skin from the vertical limb is performed such that when the nipple-areola complex is brought through the incision, minimal tension is placed on the areola during closure (Fig. 96.5G). If excess tension is present, a purse-string closure of the new areola site can be used prior to insetting the areola. Similar technique is performed on the opposite side, and breast symmetry is confirmed in the semisitting position. Preoperative determination of the amount of tissue to be removed from each breast, as well as the amount of asymmetry present, can be useful to achieve a symmetric result. A preliminary weight following glandular tangential resection and a final weight following removal of the excess flaps can be helpful to balance the amount of resection from side to side. Final skin closure is performed in two layers with absorbable sutures to produce a shape and skin closure that are satisfactory immediately postoperatively (Figs. 96.5H and 96.10). Drains have not been used routinely. Steri-Strips and a Tegaderm dressing are used, so the patient can shower the evening of surgery.

RESULTS

We have used this technique in more than 200 reductions during a 10-year period. The range of reduction was from 200 to 1,100 g, with an average of 500 g. The technique has been

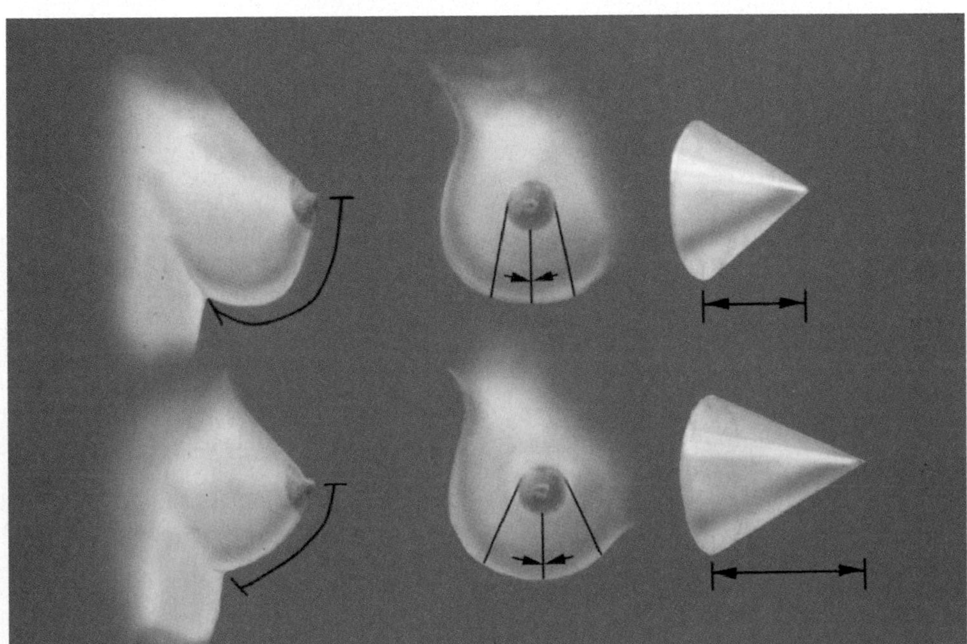

Figure 96.9. Projection of the breast is determined by shaping of the cone by shortening the distance from the nipple to the inframammary fold and tightening the skin below the areola.

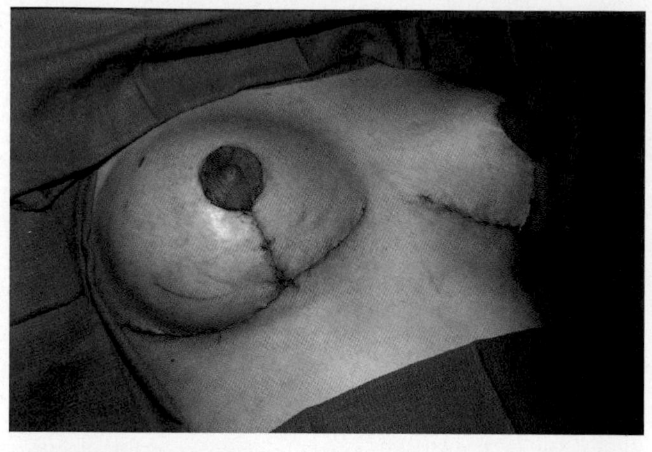

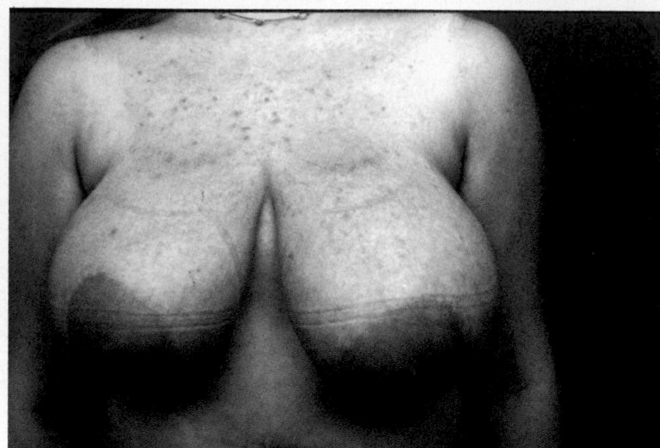

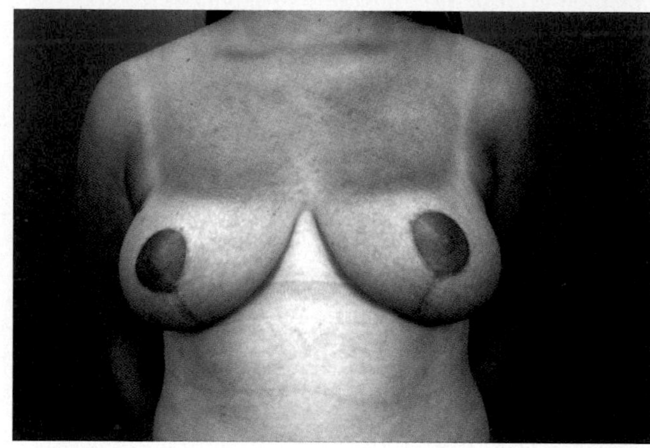

Figure 96.10. **A:** Final shape at the completion of the reduction. **B:** Preoperative photograph. **C:** Early postoperative result 3 months after reduction.

versatile, with minimal limitations based on preoperative size. No conversions to free nipple grafts have been required. Most patients are observed in the hospital for 23 hours and are treated with postoperative patient-controlled analgesia and intravenous antibiotics. Complications have been minimal. Unilateral partial areolar necrosis of the perimeter of the areola occurred in 2 patients (Fig. 96.11). Conservative management resulted in a viable nipple, and no surgical revision of the areola was required. Cellulitis occurred in 2.5% of patients, and hematoma occurred in less than 1% of patients. Delayed healing or dehiscence of the inverted-T scar occurred in 2% of patients. Surgical revision was performed in 7% of patients for correction of lower pole fullness, asymmetry, or revision of the inframammary scar. The patient satisfaction has been high, with good aesthetic results (Figs. 96.12 and 96.13). The breast shape has adequate projection, and nipple sensation is preserved.

DISCUSSION

The described central mound approach to reduction mammaplasty has several inherent advantages. Commonly used inverted-T Wise pattern techniques rely primarily on the pattern of skin resection to determine breast shape, whereas techniques such as Hall-Findlay's vertical approach rely primarily on the pattern of gland resection to affect final breast shape. The central mound technique separates the gland from the skin flaps. Because of this, the gland and skin can be modified independently, and the final breast shape is determined by the interaction between the remaining skin and gland, making this an artistic and highly versatile technique. No predetermined markings or patterns are required. This flexibility provides the surgeon with a high level of control over tailoring the desired breast shape and allows control of the amount of tension on the skin flaps. The robust blood supply that uses a broad glandular pedicle helps to minimize the risk of nipple-areola necrosis. Furthermore, there is no limitation to the amount of nipple-areola repositioning that can be achieved. Patients who may be poor candidates for other techniques due to a large distance from the sternal notch to the nipple or who may need free nipple grafts are candidates for the central mound reduction. The shape and projection of the breast are apparent at the time of surgery with minimal postoperative time for the shape to settle. Complication and revision rates have been low. In addition to preserving the appearance of the breast, the central mound reduction maintains nipple sensibility and the ability to breastfeed after surgery.

Although the central mound reduction mammaplasty requires a horizontal scar, the length can be kept to a minimum, often less than 10 cm. Other disadvantages include wide skin glandular separation that may contribute to delayed healing of the flaps. The tailor-tacking technique of the skin brassiere slightly increases the operative time, with average times of 3 to 4 hours. Although all techniques of breast reduction are associated with long-term ptosis or bottoming out, simple secondary correction can be performed by wedge excision of the inframammary fold with reestablishment of the distance to the areola. Overall, the patient and surgeon satisfaction rates have been high.

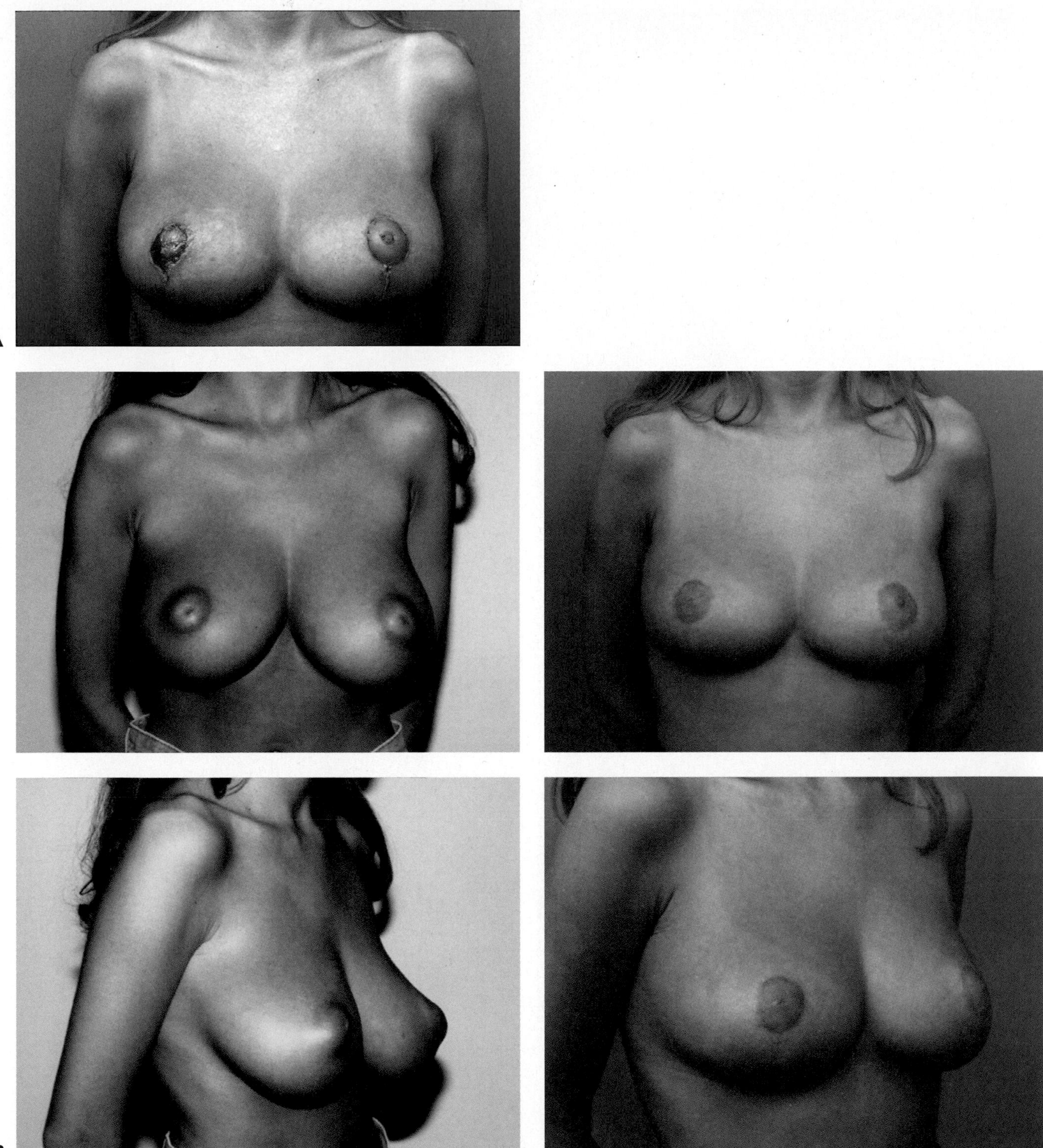

Figure 96.11. **A:** Complication demonstrating right partial areolar necrosis. **B:** Conservative management with results before and after central mound reduction.

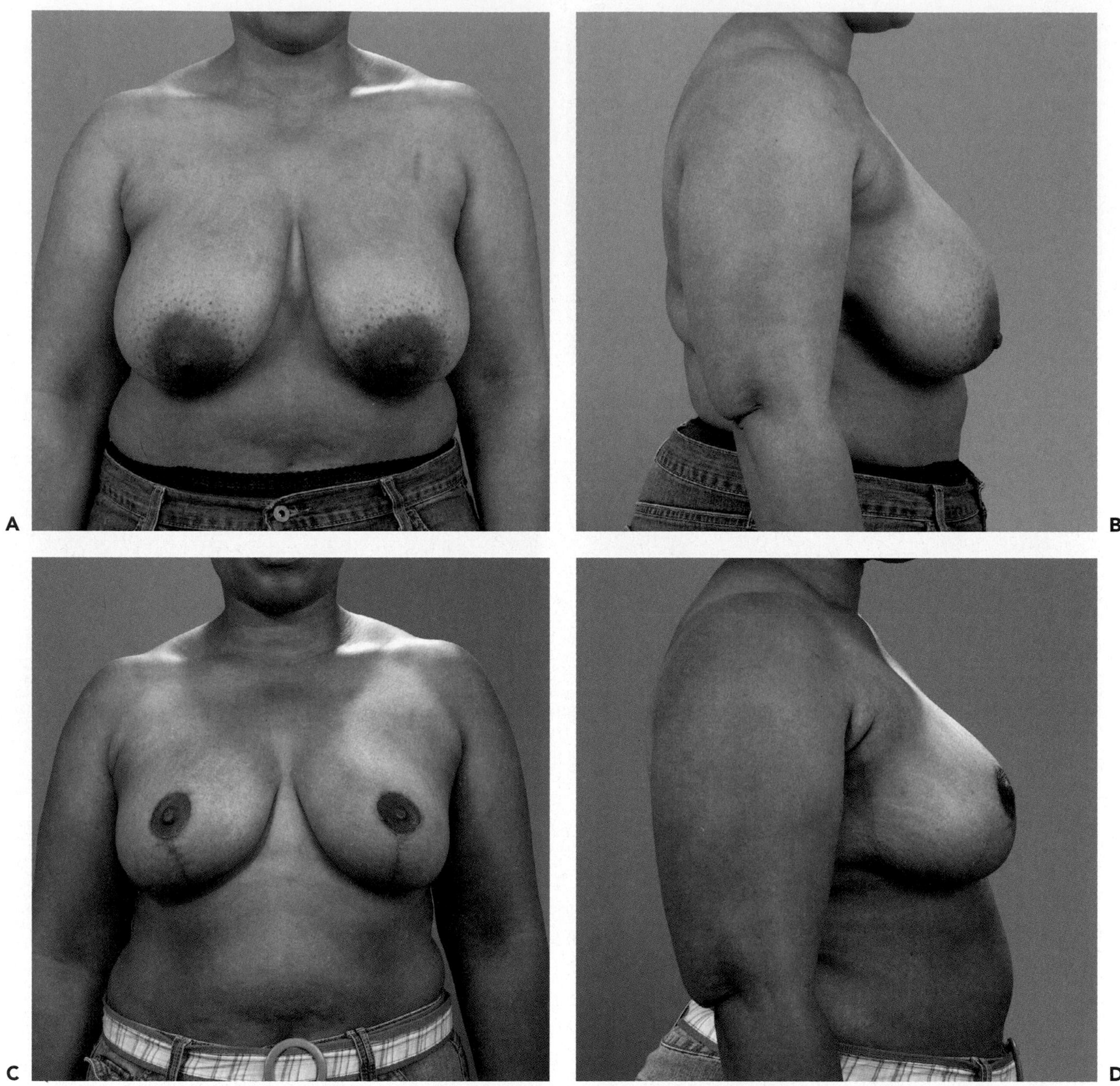

Figure 96.12. **A:** Preoperative frontal view. **B:** Preoperative lateral view. **C:** Postoperative frontal view. **D:** Postoperative lateral view.

EDITORIAL COMMENTS

The authors describe a technique for breast reduction that follows the philosophy of many South American surgeons, that being separation of the skin from the gland, reducing or reshaping the gland directly, and then retailoring the skin. It is a very artistic approach that is quite versatile and produces excellent results. The vascular supply to the nipple and areola is well preserved, and complications are few. Several points merit emphasis. In this technique, it is important that the flaps are constructed to complement the volume and shape of the central mound. For this reason, the three-dimensional sculpting of the flaps as described becomes quite important. How well the flaps and the central mound interact will go a long way toward determining the ultimate shape of the breast. The tangential resection of breast tissue reduces the breast, and suturing the remaining parenchyma can help cone the breast as well. With the breast shape directly controlled, skin retailoring is then performed based on the new size and shape of the breast. Although somewhat labor intensive, this skin resection can be customized for each individual patient to provide the best aesthetic result possible. These maneuvers, either in

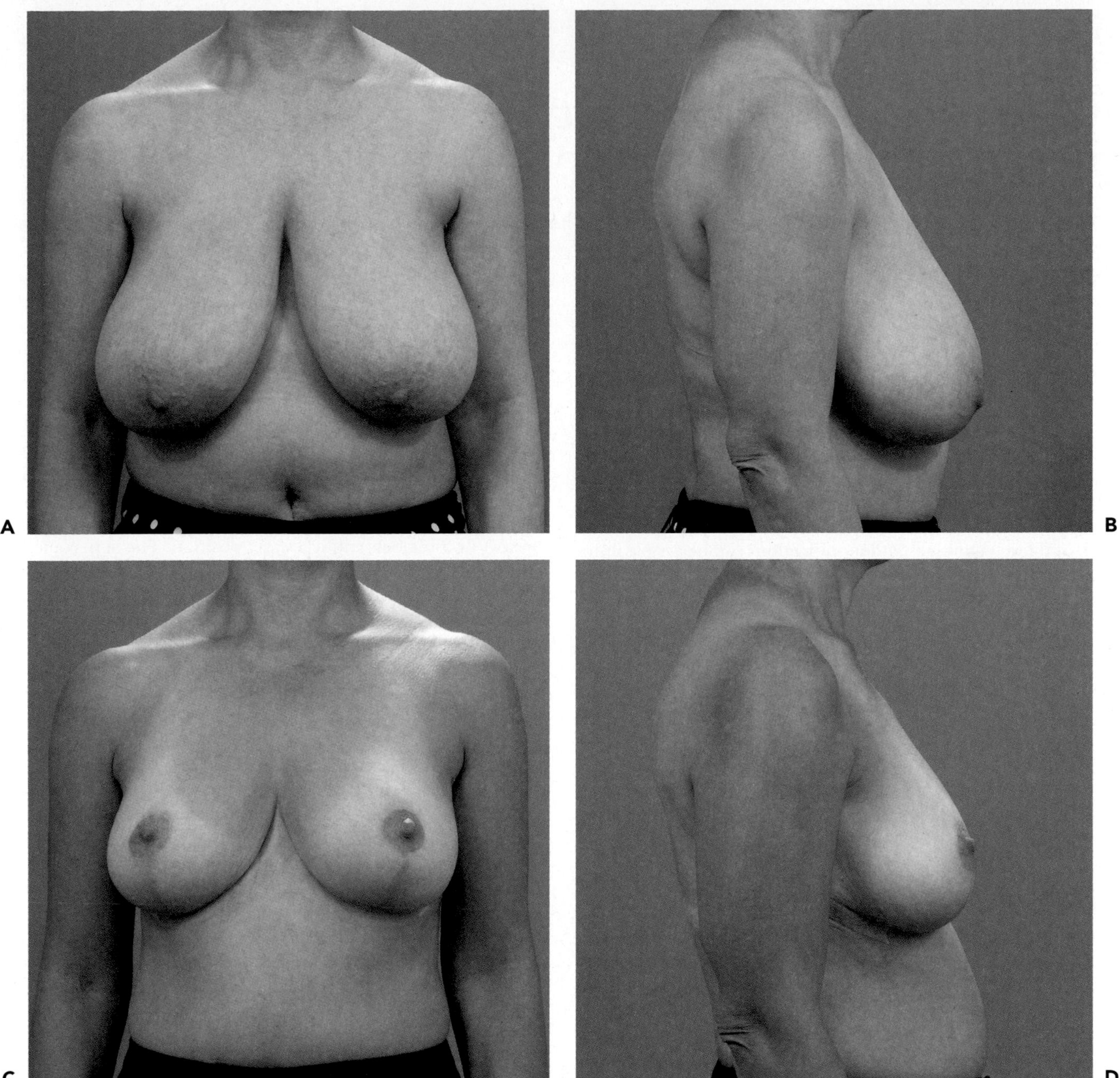

Figure 96.13. **A:** Preoperative frontal view. **B:** Preoperative lateral view. **C:** Postoperative frontal view. **D:** Postoperative lateral view.

whole or in part, can easily be incorporated into the existing technique of many surgeons, with improved aesthetic results likely being the ultimate result.

D.C.H.

REFERENCES

1. Hester TR, Bostwick J, Miller L, et al. Breast reduction utilizing the maximally vascularized central breast pedicle. *Plast Reconstr Surg* 1985;76:890.
2. Hester TR, Cukic J. Central breast pedicle and "free-hand" technique for alteration of volume and skin envelope of the breast. *Clin Plast Surg* 1988;15:613.
3. Biesenberger H. *Deformitaten und kosmetische operationen der Weiblichen brust.* Vienna: Wilheim Mauderich; 1921.
4. Biesenberger H. Eine neue methode der mammaplastik. *Zentrabl Chir* 1928;55:2382.
5. Carlsen L, Tirshakowec MG. A variation of the Biesenberger technique of reduction mammaplasty. *Plast Reconstr Surg* 1975;55:658.
6. Courtiss EH, Goldwyn RM. Reduction mammaplasty by the inferior pedicle technique: an alteration to free nipple and areolar grafting for severe macromastia or extreme ptosis. *Plast Reconstr Surg* 1977;59:500.
7. Schwarzmann E. Die technik der mammaplastik. *Chirurg* 1930;2:932.
8. Gillies H, McIndoe AH. The technique of mammaplasty in conditions of hypertrophy of the breast. *Surg Gynecol Obstet* 1939;68:658.
9. McIndoe A, Rees TD. Mammoplasty: indications, technique and complications. *Br J Plast Surg* 1958;10:307.
10. Codner MA, Ford DT, Hester TR. Reduction mammaplasty using the central mound technique. In: Spear SL, ed. *Surgery of the Breast: Principles and Art.* 2nd ed. Philadelphia: Lippincott Williams & Wilkins; 2006; 1145–1154.

CHAPTER

97

Ethan E. Larson
Maurice Y. Nahabedian

Reduction Mammaplasty Using Medial Pedicles and Inverted-T Incisions

INTRODUCTION

The evolution of reduction mammaplasty has been witness to a variety of techniques, principles, and concepts. Many of these have related to skin pattern design, parenchymal reshaping, and pedicle orientation. Skin pattern designs can include short-scar techniques such as the vertical and horizontal incisions as well as the inverted-T or Wise pattern. Parenchymal reshaping can be achieved using internal sutures or reliance of the skin envelope. Pedicle orientation can essentially be in any direction and includes inferior, superior, lateral, or medial. Each of these techniques and modifications can be a topic unto itself based on the subtleties associated with each. This chapter, however, focuses specifically on Wise pattern reduction mammaplasty using a medial or superomedial pedicle.

ANATOMY

The anatomy of the breast is complex but relatively constant. The borders of the breast typically extend vertically from the second to the sixth rib and horizontally between the lateral sternal border and the anterior to midaxillary line. The breast is composed of numerous lobules and ductules that lead to the nipple-areolar complex. There is a layer of investing fascia surrounding the breast that provides shape and contour.

When considering a reduction mammaplasty, a thorough knowledge of the vascularity and innervation of the breast and nipple-areolar complex (NAC) is important. The vascularity of the breast is derived from various sources that include the perforating branches of the internal mammary, the lateral thoracic artery, perforating branches from the pectoral vessels, and the intercostal vessels (Fig. 97.1). The innervation to the breast and NAC includes the medial and lateral division of the intercostal nerves between the second and sixth vertebrae. Studies on the vascular territories of the breast and NAC have demonstrated the internal mammary artery to be the dominant blood supply in 70% of patients (1). Studies on the innervation of the NAC have demonstrated fine branches from both the anterior (medial) and lateral fourth, fifth, and sixth intercostal nerves (2,3).

HISTORY OF THE MEDIAL AND SUPEROMEDIAL PEDICLES

Preserving the vascularity to the NAC during a reduction mammaplasty is accomplished by designing a pedicle of tissue that includes the NAC at its distal aspect (Fig. 97.2). The number of potential pedicles is large, and the indications for use are described in other chapters. There are two medially based pedicles that include the superomedial pedicle and the medial pedicle. The superomedial pedicle was introduced by Orlando and Guthrie in 1975 (Fig. 97.3) (4). Its design was intended to shorten pedicle length while broadening the pedicle as a means to enhance blood flow and maintain innervation of the NAC. Subsequent reports by Hauben and Finger et al. verified the safety, reliability, and speed of this procedure (5–7). The medial pedicle was introduced several years later by Hall-Findlay in 1999 using vertical scar techniques and by Nahabedian et al. in 2000 using Wise pattern techniques (8,9). The medial pedicle differed from the superomedial pedicle in that the medial edge of the pedicle was oriented at 10 o'clock (left breast) or 2 o'clock (right breast) position. The superomedial pedicle is oriented such that the medial edge is at the 12 o'clock position. The advantage of medial pedicle was to facilitate the arc of rotation and to prevent kinking of the pedicle. In 2005, Abramson et al. confirmed the durability of medial pedicle reduction mammaplasty (10). As with all pedicles, there was lengthening of the distance between the inframammary fold (IMF) and nipple that increased by 11% after 1 year when the resection volume was between 500 and 1,200 g per breast and by 34% when the resection volume exceeded 1,200 g per breast. The complication rate in this series was 6.8%. Davison et al. in 2007 reported on the benefits of the superomedial pedicle for breast reduction in a series of 279 patients and reported no cases of nipple loss and an overall complications rate of 18% with a time savings of 41 minutes over the inferior pedicle technique (11). Landau et al. in 2008 reported a series of 122 women following superomedial reduction mammaplasty and demonstrated no cases of nipple loss in women who had a resection volume that averaged 1,379 g per breast (12).

INDICATIONS FOR USING A MEDIALLY BASED PEDICLE

The indications for using the superomedial or medial pedicle are several. In general, a superomedial pedicle is used when the distance of nipple areolar elevation ranges from 4 to 6 cm (Fig. 97.4). The medical pedicle is used when the distance is greater than 6 cm (Fig. 97.5). The reason for this is based on the arch of rotation of each pedicle. When the distance of nipple elevation is less than 6 cm, the NAC will not rotate easily when based on a medial pedicle. However, it will advance easily when based on a superomedial pedicle. In some cases, a small back-cut will be necessary at the origin or base of the pedicle to facilitate rotation and advancement. In contrast, when the distance of NAC elevation exceeds 6 cm, the medial pedicle will rotate easily without kinking or twisting. When the distance of NAC elevation is less than 4 cm, it is our preference to use a central cone technique in which the vascularity of the NAC is based on

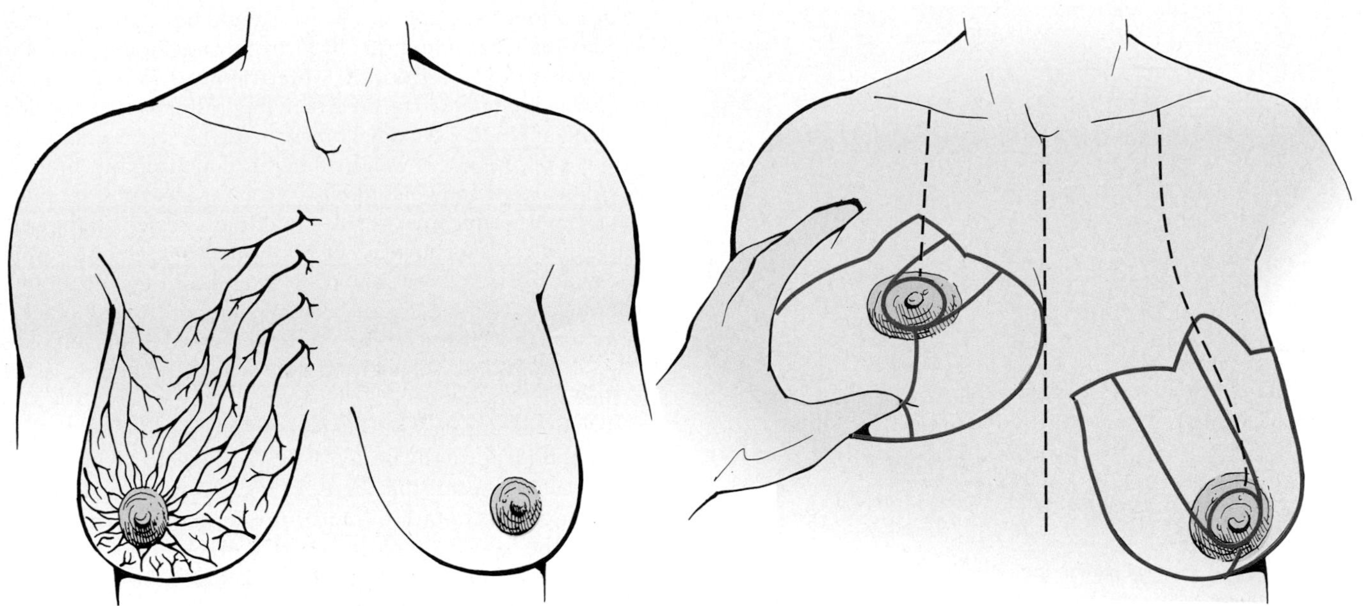

Figure 97.1. The general vascularity and the markings for the medial pedicle of the breast. The principal blood supply to the breast includes perforating branches from the internal mammary and lateral thoracic systems.

the perforating branches emanating off of the pectoralis major muscle. The NAC is easily advanced using this technique.

In addition to the anatomic indications, the medial pedicle offers other advantages. By conserving breast tissue medially and resecting tissue inferiorly and laterally, this technique tends to augment the medial portion of the breast, providing fullness where it is most desired and eliminating tissue where it is not. Although medial pedicles will have some degree of "bottoming out" over time, it is generally less than that associated with inferiorly based pedicles. The risk of "boxy"-appearing breasts, particularly in the immediately postoperative period, is also diminished. Medial pedicles permit ample lateral parenchymal excision and can be designed with a limited horizontal incision to improve shape and contour. With several reduction techniques, internal suturing techniques are recommended for shape and contour; however, with the medial pedicle approach, internal suturing is rarely necessary. Because the majority of skin excision is inferior, the upper cutaneous envelope is usually sufficient to support the retained parenchyma on the skin envelope alone.

In cases of severe mammary hypertrophy, defined as resection volume exceeding 1,200 g per breast, the medial pedicle is an excellent option (9). The NAC is often well vascularized based on the internal mammary and chest wall perforating

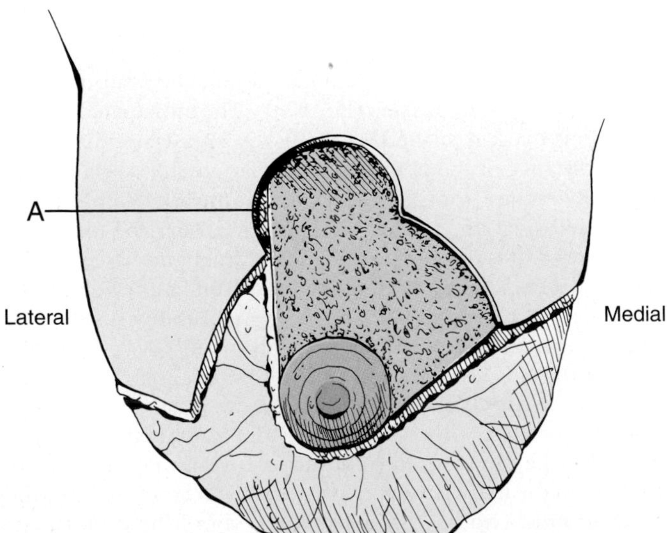

Figure 97.2. The general outline of the superomedial pedicle. Note that the central arm of the pedicle is oriented vertically.

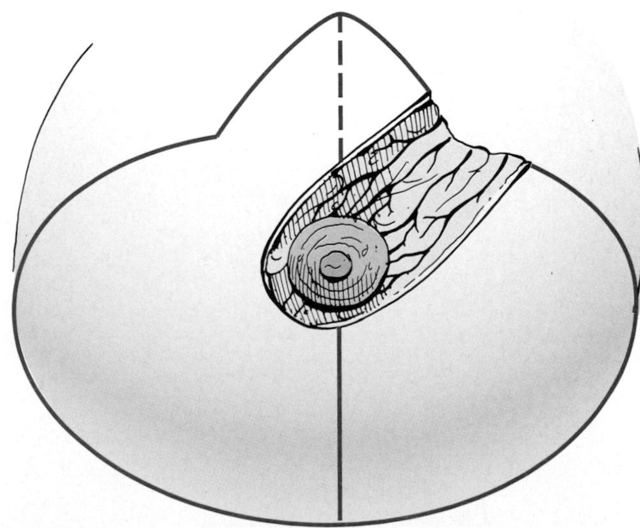

Figure 97.3. The general outline of the medial pedicle. Note that the central arm is oriented obliquely.

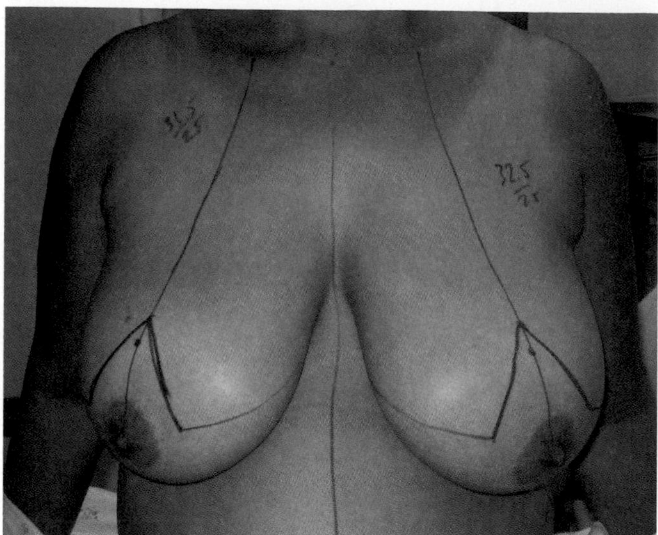

Figure 97.4. A typical patient for a superomedial pedicle. The distance of nipple-areolar complex elevation usually ranges from 4 to 6 cm.

vessels. This is frequently an alternative to amputation and free nipple graft. Resection volumes in excess of 2 g per breast are frequently amenable to a medial pedicle reduction mammaplasty. In order to minimize the incidence of partial or total NAC necrosis, the distal edges of the pedicle are evaluated for arterial and venous bleeding. When absent, it can be assumed that perfusion will be compromised, and the operation is converted into an amputation technique with free nipple graft.

PREOPERATIVE CONSIDERATIONS

As with all breast reductions, a standard medical history and examination of the pertinent systems should be performed (13). Special attention should be given to any history of bleeding diathesis. Similarly, conditions affecting wound healing, including tobacco use and diabetes, should be addressed. Problems arising from mammary hypertrophy, including back and neck pain, shoulder "grooving," intertrigo, and skin ulceration, should be documented. A breast-feeding history should be documented, including maximal breast size achieved. Similarly the patient's preoperative weight, height, cup size, and bra size should be noted and goals discussed for her ideal postoperative size. Deep vein thrombosis risk should be assessed, along with a history of contraceptive use or hormone replacement. Family history of breast cancer should be sought and a preoperative mammogram obtained in any woman younger than 40 years of age with a family history of breast cancer or older than 40 years of age without one. Subjective nipple sensitivity should also be documented and recorded.

A set of measurements can also be useful as guidelines in selecting the ideal candidate for a medial pedicle breast reduction as well as to assess the degree of breast symmetry. These include the nipple-to-IMF distance, the nipple-to-sternal notch distance, the base width of the breast, and the proposed length of the pedicle (measured from the medial skin flap to the nipple). Body mass index (BMI) should also be calculated and an estimate of the final resection volume made.

There are several breast-related parameters that should be noted and considered before considering a medial pedicle reduction mammaplasty. The ideal candidate should have a pedicle length that does not exceed 16 cm. Pedicles exceeding 16 cm sometimes necessitate a free nipple graft (10,11). Previous breast incisions that could compromise vascularity should be noted, and the pedicle design should be adjusted accordingly. The medial pedicle can safely be employed in reductions of up to 2,500 g per side and has been reported in reductions of up to 4,100 g (6,9). Women of a larger body habitus should be counseled preoperatively regarding the additional possible problems with wound healing, the possibility of conversion to a free nipple graft, and the likely emergence of their lateral axillary fat roll and large abdomens as possible aesthetic problems in the future.

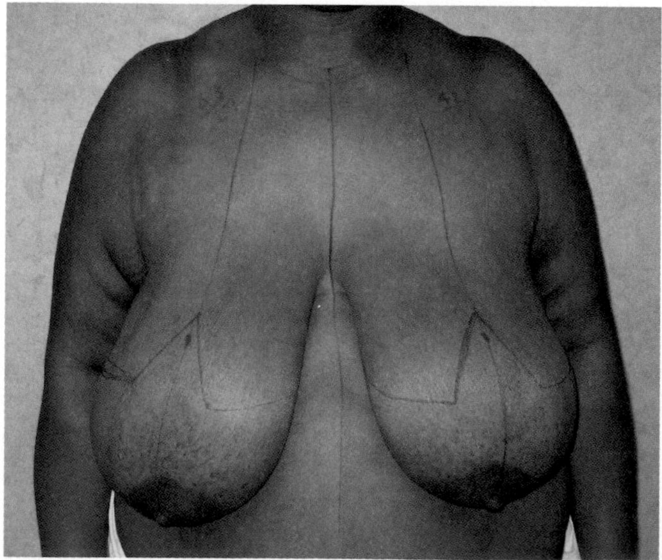

Figure 97.5. A typical patient for a medial pedicle. The distance of nipple-areolar complex elevation usually ranges from 6 to 16 cm.

PATIENT MARKINGS: MEDIAL PEDICLE

The patient is always marked in the standing position. Standard breast landmarks include the sternal midline, IMF, suprasternal notch, and breast meridians (Fig. 97.6). The anticipated nipple position is marked at the IMF along the breast meridian. The actual distance of the NAC to the sternal notch is variable and is usually ranges from 22 to 26 cm. The inverted-T pattern is delineated (Fig. 97.7). This can be drawn using the templates or freehand. It is our practice to draw it freehand based on the standard breast landmarks. The vertical limbs of the pattern are usually 8 to 9 cm. The apical angle of the vertical limbs ranges from 50 to 70 deg but is usually 60 deg. A keyhole pattern for the NAC can be delineated if desired, but it is our preference to excise the keyhole following the parenchymal resection rather than prior to it. The horizontal limbs of the inverted-T pattern extend from the inferior point on the vertical limb to the lateral point along the IMF. In larger breasts, the surgeon must choose a point laterally where the breast ends and the axillary adipose tissue begins. These marking are typically drawn outside of the operating room. The remaining markings are made in the operating room.

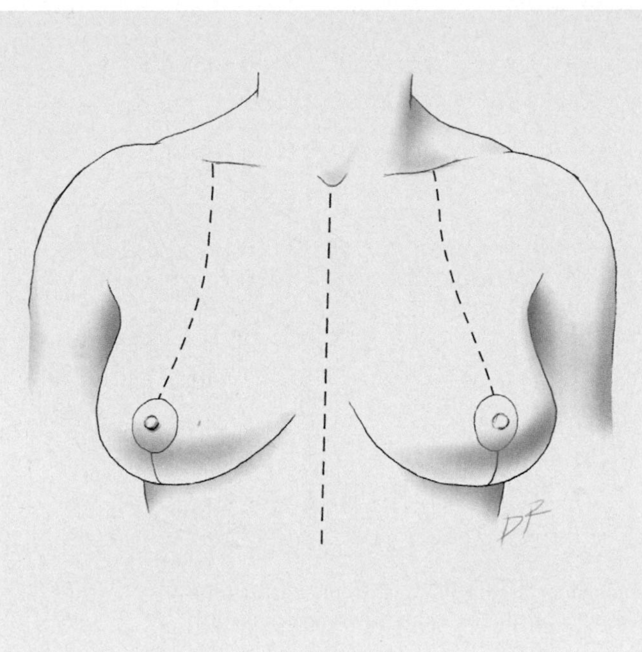

Figure 97.6. Standard preoperative markings include the sternal midline, breast meridians, and the inframammary folds.

In the operating room, the patient is placed in the supine position. The medial pedicle is designed with a base width that ranges from 5 to 10 cm and a pedicle length that ranges from 8 to 16 cm (Fig. 97.7). The superior arm of the medial pedicle is based at the midpoint of the 8-cm vertical limb of the inverted-T pattern. This point will allow for the NAC (with a diameter of 4 cm) to rotate into the apex of the vertical limbs following the parenchymal resection.

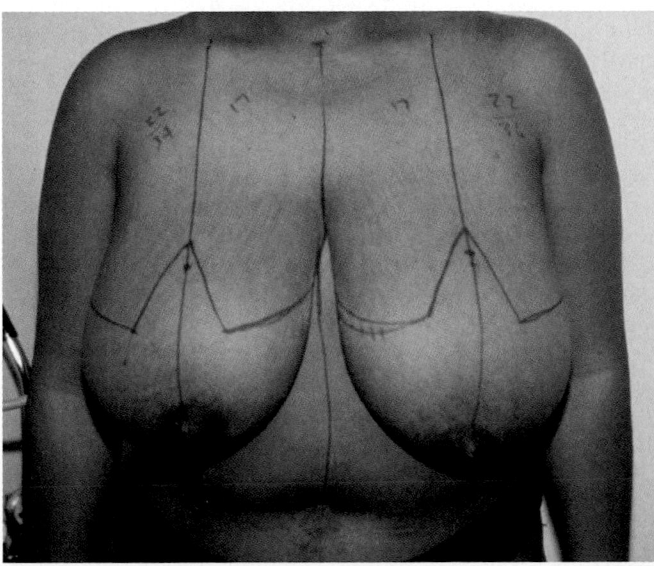

Figure 97.7. Standard inverted-T markings. The new nipple-areolar complex position is located at the level of the inframammary fold. The horizontal limbs extend to the apices of the inframammary fold.

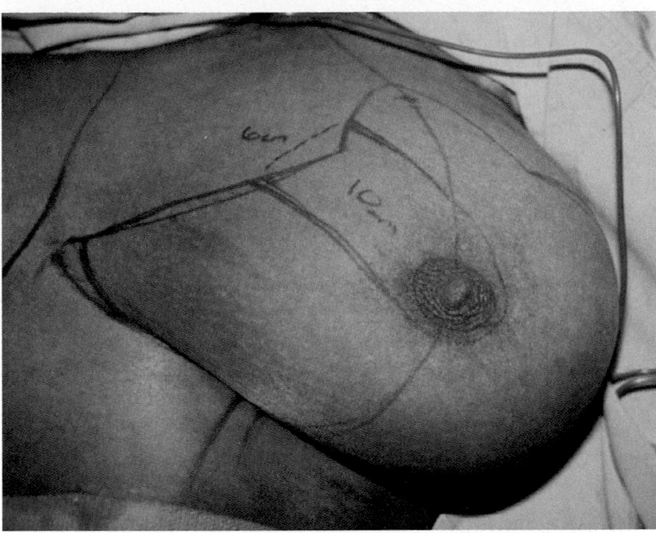

Figure 97.8. The typical markings for a relatively short medial pedicle. The base and length of the pedicle are 6 and 10 cm, respectively.

PATIENT MARKINGS: SUPEROMEDIAL PEDICLE

The inverted-T markings and the breast landmarks are identical to those of the medial pedicle technique. The superomedial pedicle differs in that the superior arm on the pedicle extends vertically in to the apex of the vertical limbs (Fig. 97.2).

OPERATIVE TECHNIQUE: MEDIAL PEDICLE

Following the markings, the patient is placed in the supine position under general anesthesia. We do not use local, regional, or sedative anesthesia techniques. The patients' arms are usually extended at about 75 deg from the operating table to allow for access to the soft tissues along the anterior and midaxillary line. Betadine prep is typically used, although a variety of agents are effective. The markings are redelineated and adjustments made (Figs. 97.8 and 97.9). Local anesthesia

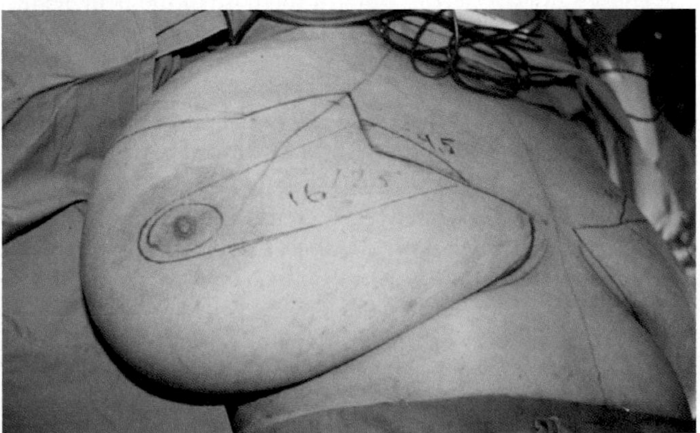

Figure 97.9. The typical markings for a long medial pedicle. The base and length are 9.5 and 16 cm, respectively.

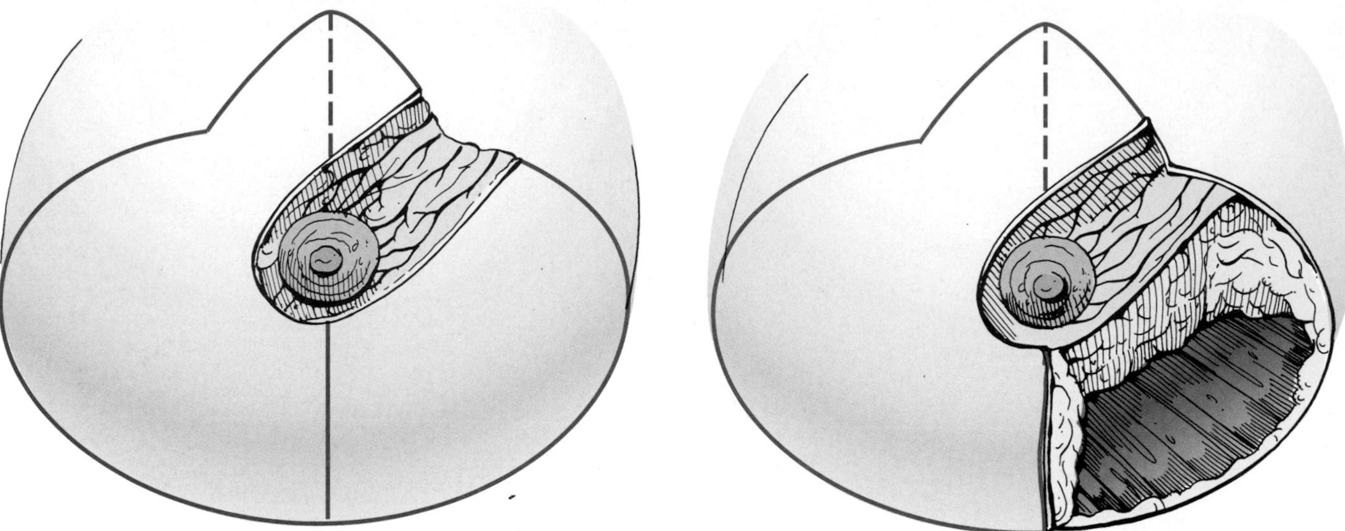

Figure 97.10. The sequence for medial pedicle reduction mammaplasty. Following deepithelialization, inferior, medial, and lateral dermoglandular wedge excision is performed. The dermoparenchymal medial pedicle is preserved.

consisting of diluted lidocaine and epinephrine may be used to minimize bleeding from the initial incisions. Tumescent solution may be infiltrated, sparing the pedicle, to further reduce operative blood loss, particularly if the majority of the resection is to be done sharply. Figures 97.10 and 97.11 are schematic illustrations highlighting the key steps of the medial pedicle reduction mammaplasty .

The specific operative details will be described and illustrated. The areola is marked with an appropriate nipple sizer and sharply incised to the level of the dermis. This is done bilaterally at the start of the case to minimize size change over the course of the procedure. The medial pedicle is then incised and deepithelialized either with a sharp blade or with curved scissors, leaving the nipple and incised areola intact (Fig. 97.12). It is recommended to maintain the dermal layer as much as possible to avoid injury to the underlying subdermal plexus (14). The pedicle is then defined with extra attention paid to avoiding undermining and maintaining medial attachments to the chest wall (Fig. 97.13). Toward the base of the pedicle, dissection should be flared out to maximize blood supply. Dermoglandular wedge excisions are performed, with the majority of tissue coming from the inferior and lateral compartments. The medial component is partially excised, leaving a thin layer of fat on the pectoralis fascia throughout. The lateral resection is aggressive and may extend into the mid to posterior axillary line. Care must be taken in the lateral excision not to pull too hard when separating the tissues from the chest wall. This can traumatize the pectoralis or serratus fascia and possibly compromise nerve supply. These excisions can be performed en bloc or segmentally, depending on the size of the breast and the volume of resection. Following the resection, the medial pedicle is assessed for bleeding at the distal aspects to ensure perfusion (Fig. 97.14). Absence of bleeding may indicate a need for conversion to a free nipple graft, particularly if the pedicle length is long.

Following irrigation and hemostasis, the medial pedicle is rotated superiorly into position toward the apex of the vertical limbs (Fig. 97.11). Twisting or kinking of the pedicle is avoided. A small back-cut may be safely made in the dermis along the inferior junction of the pedicle with the medial vertical limb if more mobility is needed in the rotation. A temporary trifurcation suture is placed at the caudal portion of the vertical limbs and at the meridian of the breast (Fig. 97.15). The skin edges are temporarily stapled, and the patient is sat upright to assess volume, symmetry, and nipple position. The patient is then returned to the supine position, and minor adjustments are made. The NAC is exteriorized by excising the apical skin and fat from the apex of the vertical limbs. This is designed such that the inferior aspect of the areola is approximately 5 cm to the IMF.

All sutures and staples are then removed, and final hemostasis is achieved. One drain is placed in each breast and can be brought out either through the lateral apex of the horizontal incision or via a separate stab incision. The skin is closed in two layers that include an absorbable interrupted dermal layer and a running continuous subcuticular layer. Lateral dog-ears are managed immediately by direct excision following the course of the lateral mammary fold. If there is a full lateral roll, additional liposuction can be employed either using a dilation and curettage cannula or standard liposuction cannula once appropriate tumescence has been infiltrated. A typical final appearance is depicted in Figures 97.16 and 97.17. Sterile dressings are then applied with a supportive, non-underwire postoperative bra selected to provide mild compression without being tight enough to compromise vascular supply. Typically, the patient is ready to return home on the day of the procedure. Drains are typically removed at 24 hours but may remain longer if necessary. Figures 97.18 and 97.19 illustrate preoperative and postoperative views following reduction mammaplasty using a medial pedicle.

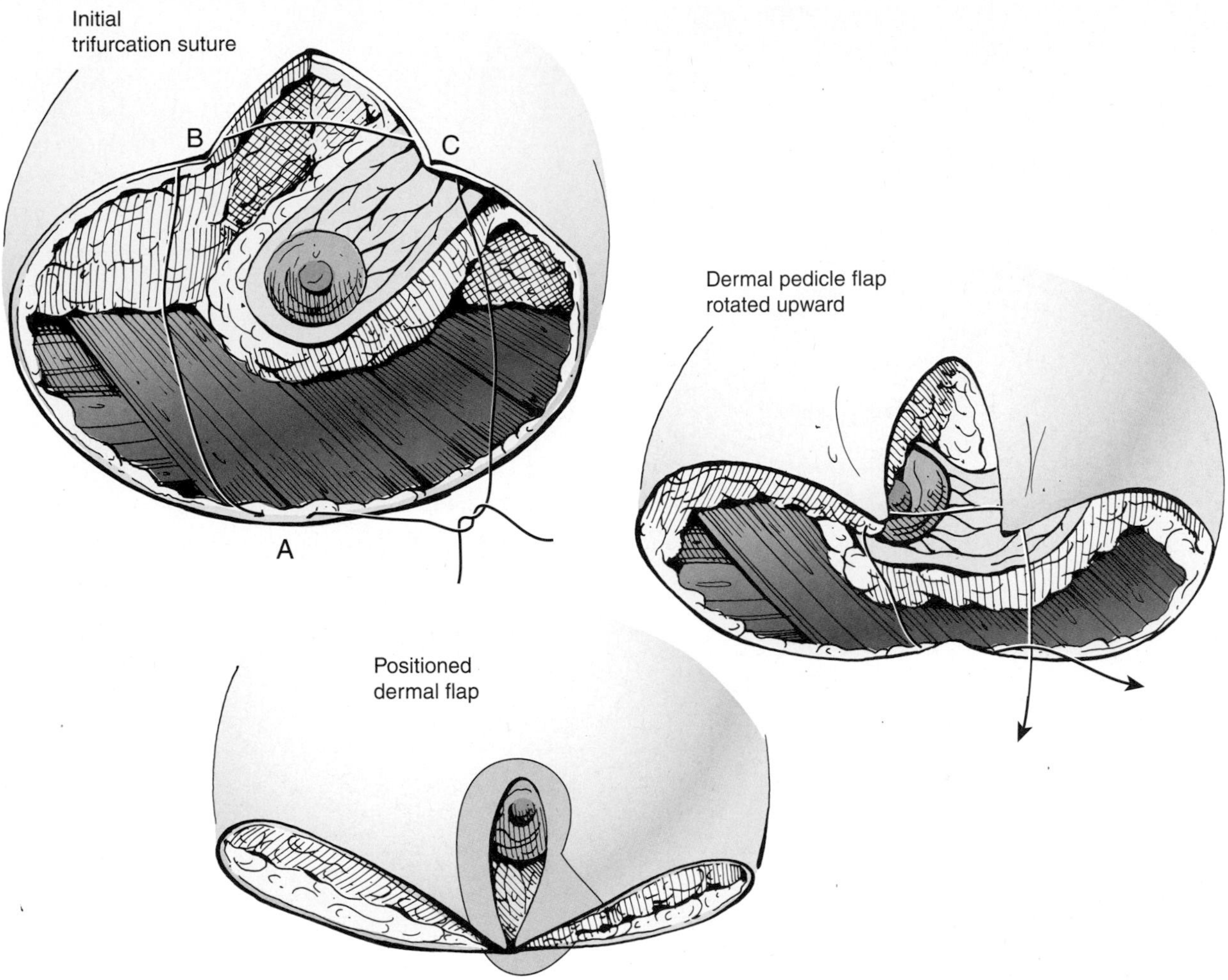

Figure 97.11. Following the excision, a trifurcation suture is placed at the two upper limb apices and to the central portion of the inframammary incision.

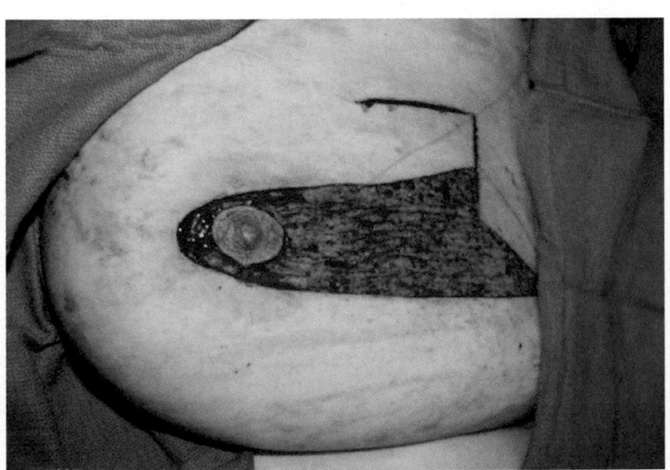

Figure 97.12. The initial step in the process is to incise around the nipple-areolar complex and deepithelialize the medial pedicle.

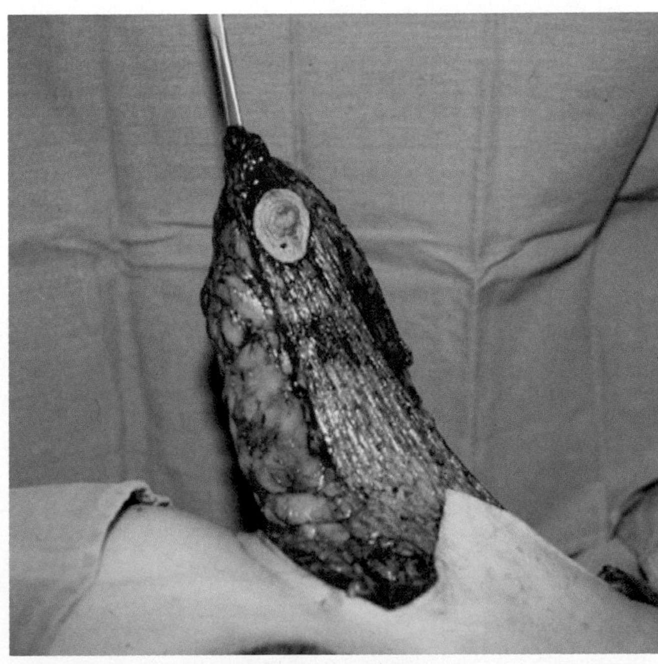

Figure 97.13. The medial pedicle is elevated.

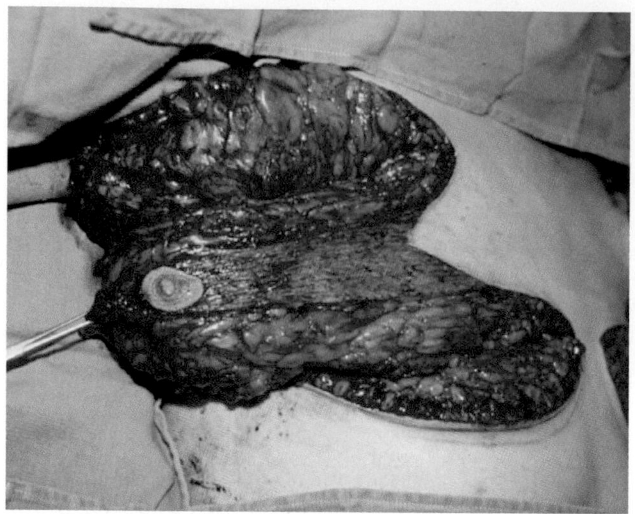

Figure 97.14. The medial pedicle is being prepared to rotate into the apex of the vertical limbs.

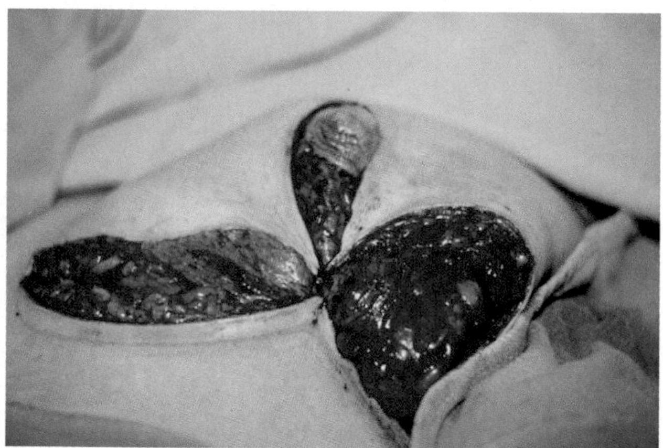

Figure 97.15. The medial pedicle has been rotated into the vertical apex, and the temporary trifurcation suture has been placed.

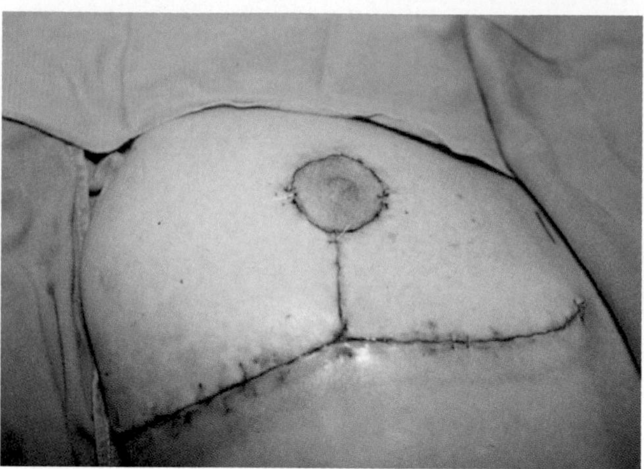

Figure 97.16. The final appearance of the breast following permanent closure.

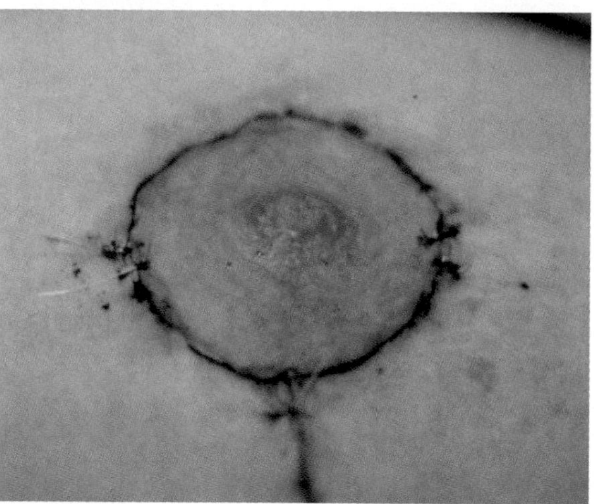

Figure 97.17. A close-up of the nipple-areolar complex demonstrating normal color and viability.

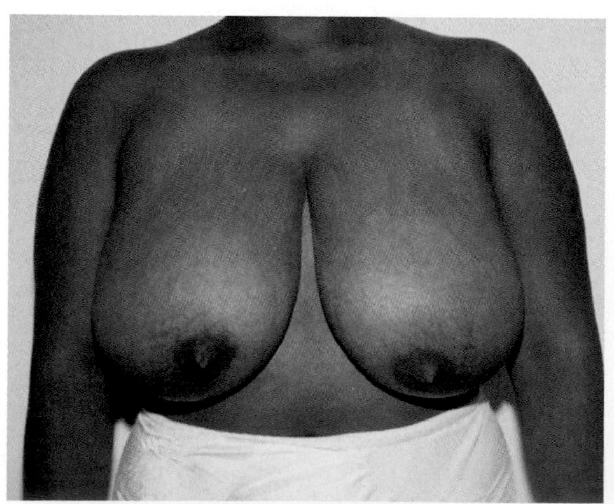

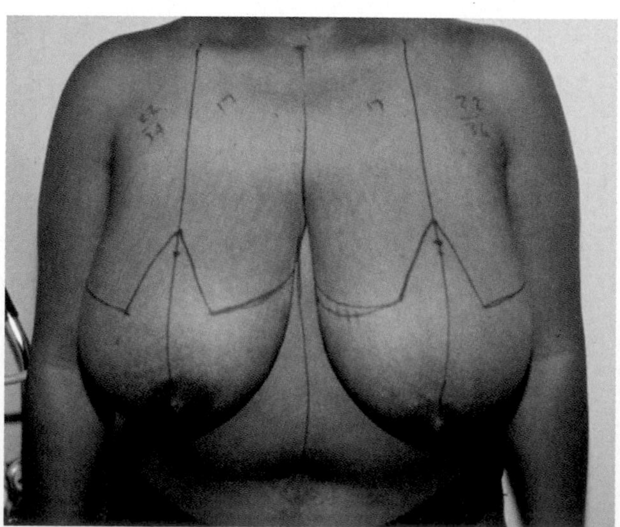

Figure 97.18. **A:** A preoperative view of a woman with moderate to severe mammary hypertrophy. **B:** The inverted-T pattern. The distance of the sternal notch to the nipple-areolar complex was 36 cm on the left and 34 cm on the right. The new nipple position is 22 cm from the sternal notch bilaterally. (*continued*)

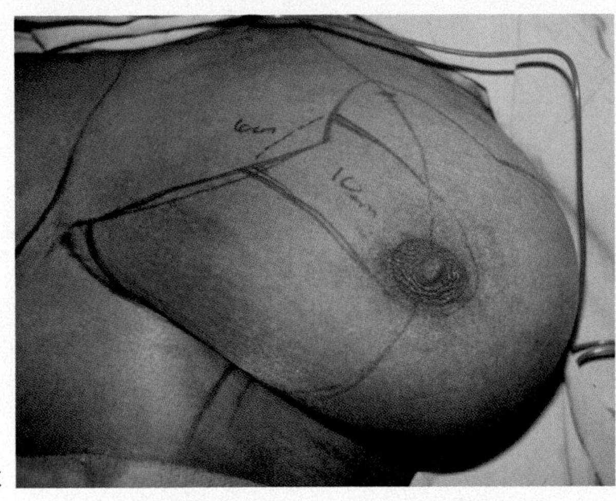

C

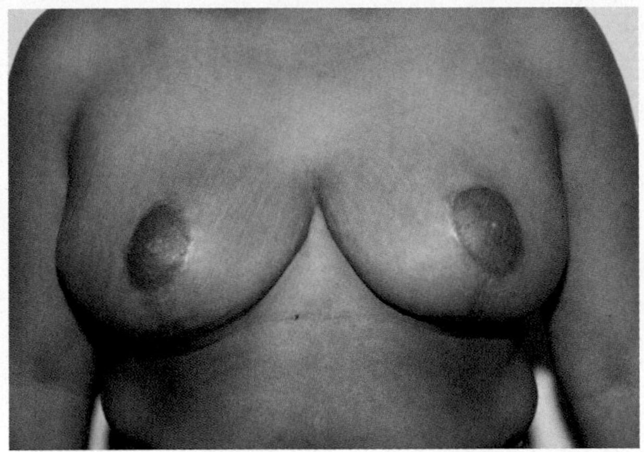

D

Figure 97.18. (*Continued*) **C:** The medial pedicle is delineated and measures 6 by 10 cm. **D:** The final appearance following medial pedicle reduction mammaplasty at 1-year follow-up. The resection was approximately 1,300 g per breast.

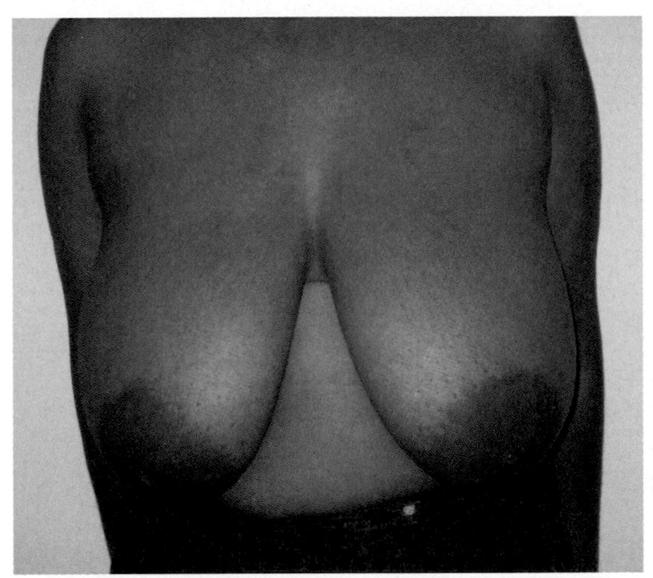

A

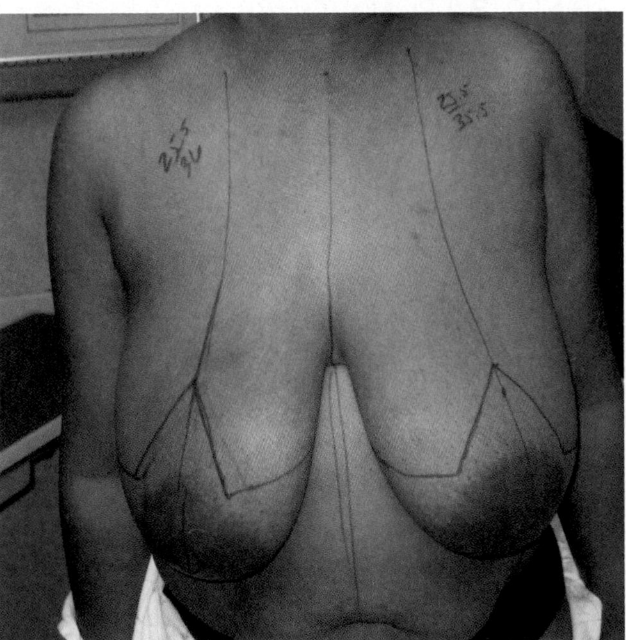

B

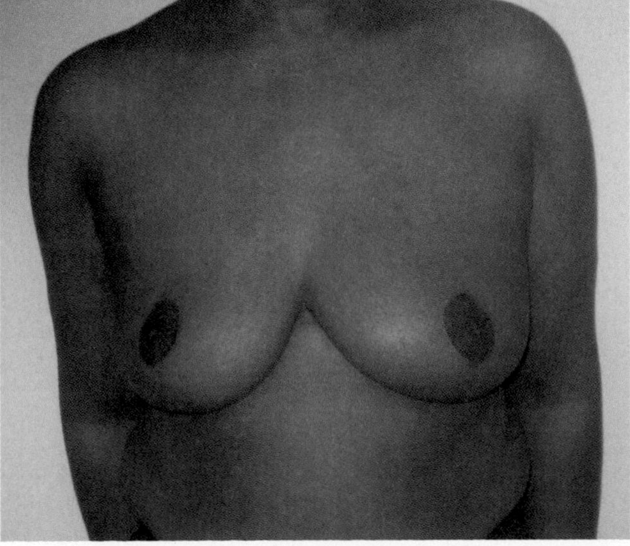

C

Figure 97.19. **A:** A preoperative view of a woman with moderate mammary hypertrophy. **B:** The inverted-T pattern. The distance of nipple-areolar complex elevation is approximately 10 cm. **C:** The final appearance following medial pedicle reduction mammaplasty at 1-year follow-up. The resection volume was approximately 700 g per breast.

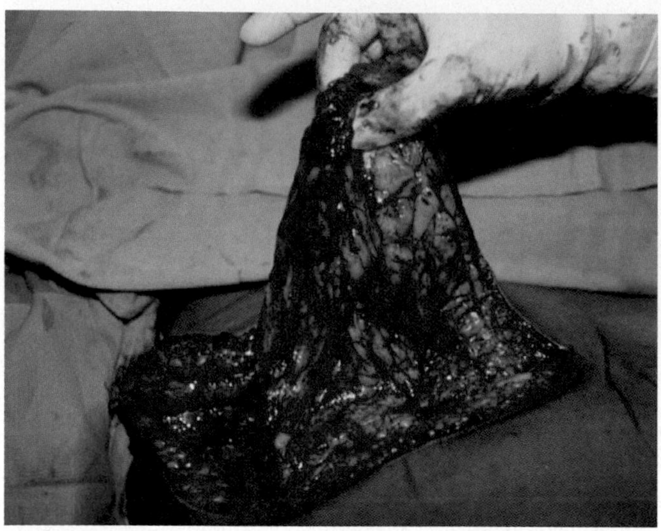

Figure 97.20. The superomedial pedicle is elevated.

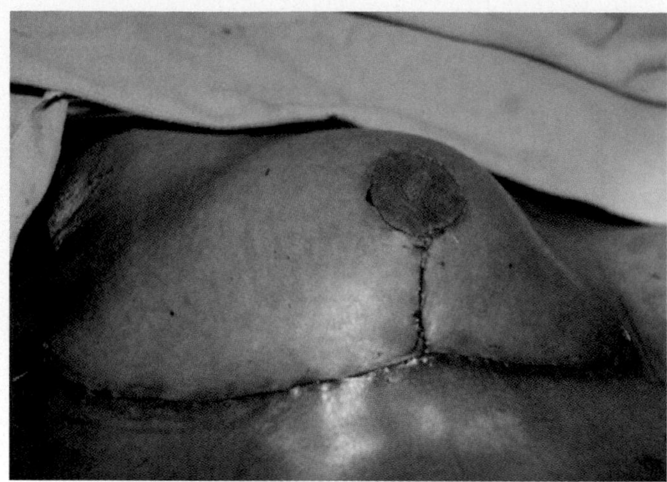

Figure 97.22. A typical immediate postoperative appearance following superomedial pedicle reduction mammaplasty.

OPERATIVE TECHNIQUE: SUPEROMEDIAL PEDICLE

The superomedial technique is almost identical to the medial pedicle technique except for a few minor details. The superomedial pedicle is elevated with the superior arm of the pedicle oriented vertically (Fig. 97.20). The superomedial pedicle is rotated or advanced into the apex of the vertical limbs (Fig. 97.21). A back-cut of the inferior arm at the cutaneous junction may be necessary to facilitate movement. The closure is identical to that of the medial pedicle. The typical immediate appearance is depicted (Fig. 97.22). Figures 97.23 and 97.24 illustrate preoperative and postoperative views following reduction mammaplasty using a superomedial pedicle.

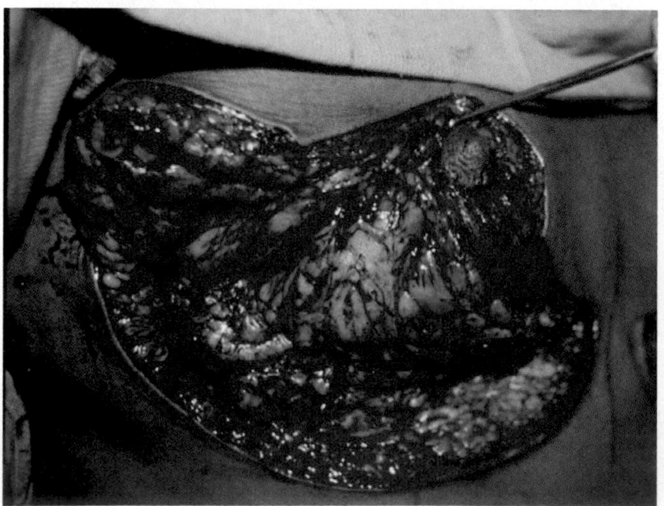

Figure 97.21. The superomedial pedicle is routed into the vertical apex.

DISCUSSION

The medial or superomedial pedicle can be employed either with a vertical skin resection pattern or with an inverted-T pattern, depending on the experience of the surgeon and desires of the patient. These pedicles are versatile and well perfused, and they can provide aesthetic benefits that are more difficult to achieve with other pedicles. Combining the medial or superomedial pedicle with an inverted-T pattern has the potential to provide a predictable and reproducible outcome for the patient and relatively quick operation for the surgeon.

The safety and efficacy of this procedure have been examined in numerous publications (5–7,9,11,12,15). Hauben stated that this procedure provides a technique that is “safe, simple, and speedy,” preserving “sensation and symmetry and producing suitably shaped and ‘sexy’ breasts” in a “sine sanguine (bloodless) operation” (5,7). The techniques of reduction mammaplasty have evolved based on earlier reports (5–7). Historically, the NAC was based on a true dermal pedicle without a parenchymal attachment to the chest wall. Most current pedicles are dermoparenchymal in nature with a direct attachment to the chest wall that provides amply blood supply. Previous reports demonstrated the incidence of total NAC necrosis at 0.8% and sensory changes at 14.8% (6). Utilizing current techniques, minor and infrequent complications include T-junction breakdown, hypertrophic scarring, and dog-ear excision, with reports of hematoma being rare. Most wound complications can be managed conservatively with dressing changes or with a minor scar revision in the office.

The vascular supply of the medial pedicle has been shown to be advantageous over other pedicles in anatomic studies (16). The medial pedicle is principally perfused via the perforating branches from the internal mammary artery and vein. These vessels are considered by some to provide the dominant blood supply to the breast. A single dominant arterial vessel tends to be present within the pedicle, while the venous drainage is via an extensive branching network (14). Both vascular patterns traverse the pedicle in a superficial plane. Similarly, the innervation of the NAC was found to be provided by intercostal

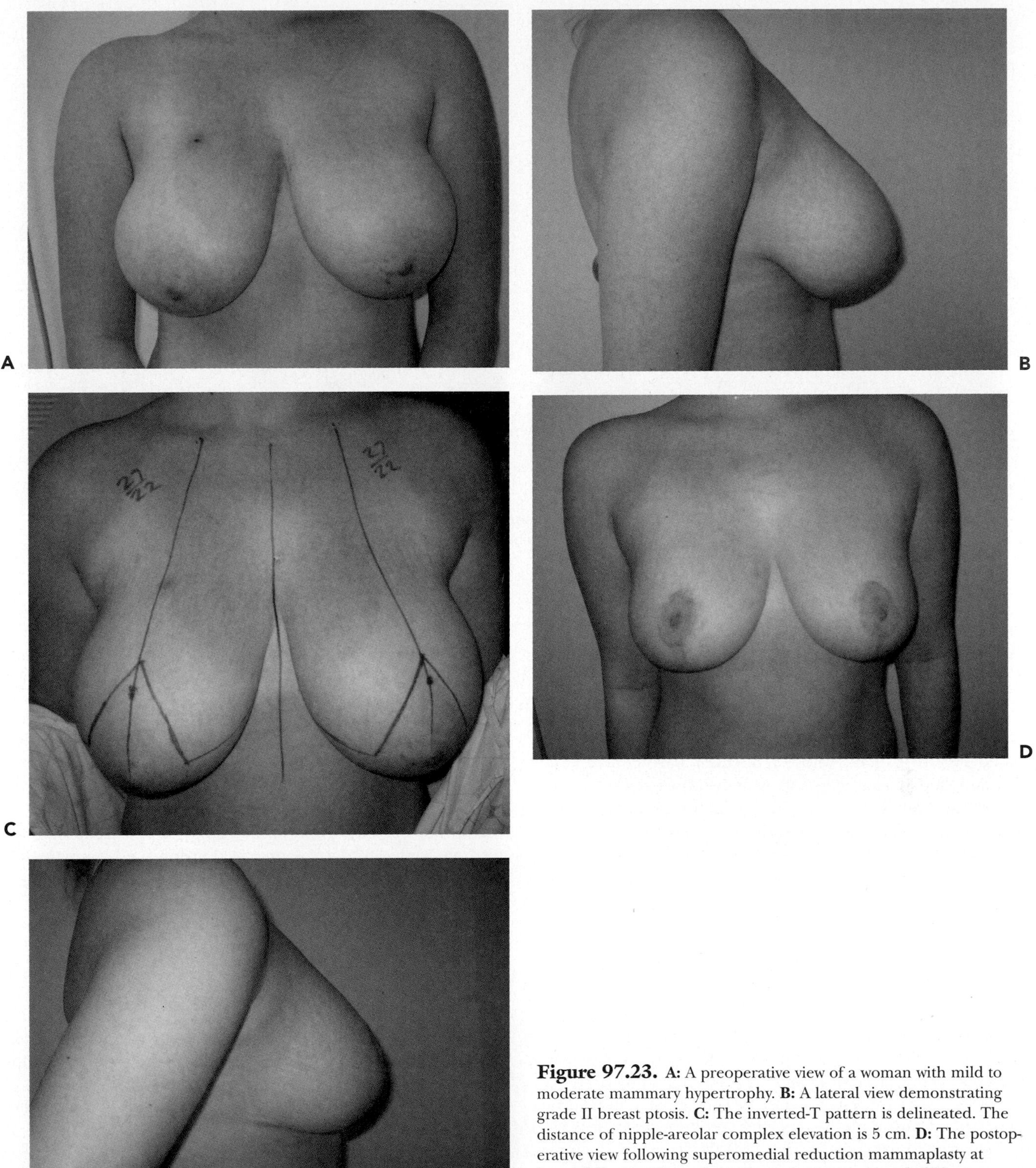

Figure 97.23. **A:** A preoperative view of a woman with mild to moderate mammary hypertrophy. **B:** A lateral view demonstrating grade II breast ptosis. **C:** The inverted-T pattern is delineated. The distance of nipple-areolar complex elevation is 5 cm. **D:** The postoperative view following superomedial reduction mammaplasty at 1-year follow-up. Resection volume was approximately 350 g per breast. **E:** The lateral postoperative view of the breast demonstrating correction of the ptosis.

nerve branches that course extremely superficially within the pedicle (17).

With regard to the safety and complication rate of this operation, there are several studies of note. In a 2007 study of 279 superomedial breast reductions in a variety of resection volumes, Davison et al. demonstrated no cases of nipple loss and an overall complication rate of 18% (11). Of these, 74% of the complications occurred in patients with a BMI greater than 30, and 29% of the complications occurred in smokers. This rate was significantly lower than in other reports of patients with a BMI larger than 30. In this same report, only 0.91% of patients had subjective complaints of hypesthesia. In another study,

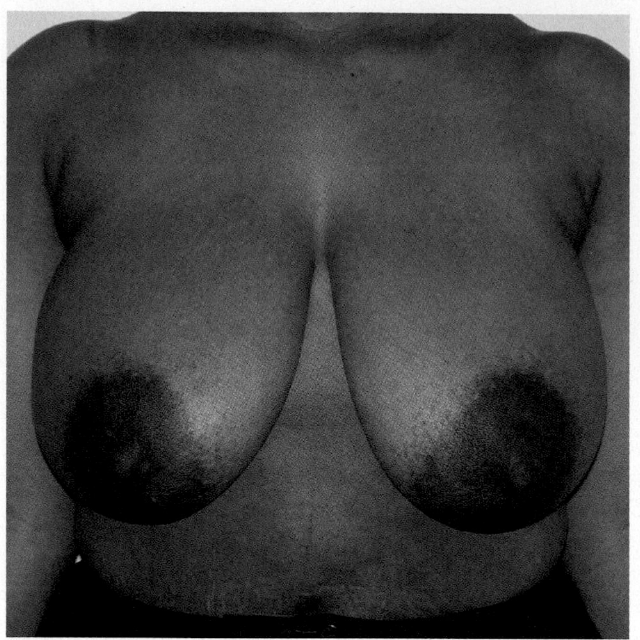

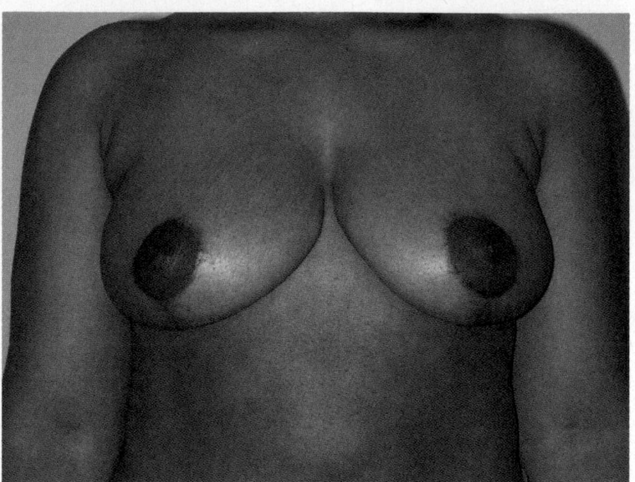

Figure 97.24. **A:** A preoperative view of a woman with moderate mammary hypertrophy. **B:** The postoperative view following superomedial pedicle reduction mammaplasty at 1-year follow-up. The resection volume was approximately 650 g per breast.

Abramson et al. examined 88 women with an average resection volume of 1,814 g per side and demonstrated that the average operative time was 104.5 minutes (10). The complication rate found in this series was found to be 6.8%, with one partial nipple loss. At 1-year follow-up, the nipple-to-IMF distance increased 11% in patients whose reductions were between 500 and 1,200 g per side and 34% in patients whose reduction was greater than 1,200 g per side. This is in comparison to an average of a 48% to 72% increase in this same distance in inferior pedicle breast reduction.

The medial pedicle technique has also been successful in managing cases of gigantomastia or severe mammary hypertrophy (9,12). Vascularity based on viability and innervation based on sensation have been preserved in the majority of cases. In a study of 45 breasts with an average resection of 1,604 g, Nahabedian et al. demonstrated that transposition of the NAC on a medial pedicle successfully transposed the nipple in 98% of patients, with preservation of sensation in 98% of NACs (9). Hypopigmentation was not observed, and central breast projection was restored in all patients. In another study of 61 patients with an average resection of 1,379 g, Landau and Hudson demonstrated no nipple loss, partial areola necrosis in 6.5%, and T-junction breakdown in 18% (12). With regard to nipple sensitivity following a medial pedicle reduction, it was objectively measured in several studies (18,19). One study demonstrated an inverse relationship between preoperative breast size and sensitivity and significant interpatient variability (18). It was found that when comparing inferior with medial pedicle reduction mammaplasty techniques, there was no significant difference in postoperative sensory outcomes, despite larger (1.7 vs. 1.1 kg) reductions in the medial pedicle group. All patients did, however, exhibit some degree of postoperative objective sensation loss. This result was supported by the results of another study of 25 patients undergoing superomedial breast reduction; however, of interest, most patients did not complain about this decreased sensation (19).

Lactational performance has also been studied in the medial pedicle breast reduction (20,21). When compared with 151 unoperated controls with macromastia, the 59 women who underwent medial pedicle reduction demonstrated equivalent breast-feeding success, 62% versus 65%, respectively. This was equivalent with the other breast reduction techniques studies. Thirty-four percent of the control group supplemented breast-feeding, while 38% of the operated group used supplementation. Successful breast-feeding was defined as breast-feeding of 2 weeks or more.

The superomedial pedicle has been employed with some modification in the management of the post–massive-weight-loss breast (22). In these patients, gland resection is limited and the Wise pattern is used as a guide primarily for skin excision. To achieve projection, the medial and lateral pillars of the breast are plicated. The superomedial pedicle may also be employed in oncoplastic breast reconstruction and may be particularly suited to tumors located in the lower pole of the breast (23).

In summary, reduction mammaplasty based on a medial or superomedial offers several key advantages:

- This is a safe operation in which nipple preservation rates approach 100% with high rates of nipple sensation and a relatively low risk of morbidity.
- The vascularity to the medial and superomedial pedicles is principally based off the perforating branches from the internal mammary artery and vein. These are considered to be the dominant vascular supply to the breast and nipple-areolar complex.
- The medial and superomedial pedicles allow for relatively rapid deepithelialization with a predictable and rapid resection pattern to minimize operative time.

- The shape of the reduced breast can be consistently created with aesthetically desirable superior and medial fullness while minimizing the risk of "bottoming out" over time.
- This is a versatile operation that can be consistently applied to a variety of breast sizes and shapes.

EDITORIAL COMMENTS

While the inferior pedicle breast reduction technique has been and remains the most popular technique in the United States, medial and superomedial techniques are increasing in popularity for reasons made apparent in this chapter.

The medial pedicle is shorter and more efficient than the inferior. Resecting inferior breast and retaining superior or medial breast makes inherently more sense than the opposite.

The superomedial and medial pedicles are my preferred technique and I use one or the other depending on the planning preoperatively. There are a few areas where I do things somewhat differently than the authors. I plan the inverted V for the resection such that it may be drawn with a wider angle and with limbs wider apart in cases where appropriate such as patients with very large and wide breasts. My preference in breast reduction and mastopexy is to narrow the breast more aggressively in certain cases and narrowing is facilitated by making the angle of the pattern more obtuse. I have also learned to keep sufficient breast on the lateral flap such that the breast can be coned with parenchymal sutures between the lateral flap and the pedicle and medial flaps.

While I was taught to plan the entire lower incision in the inframammary fold, I have learned that the fold can be altered by removing the underlying breast tissue. In many patients, I now gently angle the ends of the lower incision superiorly both medially and laterally. This does 3 things: First, it helps to minimize the common discrepancy in length between the lower and upper incisions where the lower incision is much shorter than the upper incision requiring a great deal of gathering of the skin of the breast flaps. Second, it also helps reduce the likelihood of a dog ear because the skin lengths are more equal and the incision can be blended into the commonly present lateral fat roll. And finally, it facilitates shortening the incisions because the lower incision no longer has to mindlessly extend the full length of the fold particularly in patients where the fold seems to run on forever as it joins a lateral back roll.

REFERENCES

1. Palmer JH, Taylor GI. The vascular territories of the anterior chest wall. *Br J Plast Surg* 1986;39:287.
2. Jaspars JJ, Posma AN, van Immerseel AA, et al. The cutaneous innervation of the female breast and nipple-areola complex: implications for surgery. *Br J Plast Surg* 1997;50:249.
3. Sarhadi NS, Dunn JS, Lee FD, et al. An anatomical study of the nerve supply of the breast, including the nipple and areola. *Br J Plast Surg* 1996;49:156.
4. Orlando JC, Guthrie RH. The superomedial dermal pedicle for nipple transposition. *Br J Plast Surg* 1975;28:42.
5. Hauben DJ. Experience and refinements with the supero-medial dermal pedicle for nipple-areola transposition in reduction mammaplasty. *Aesthet Plast Surg* 1984;8:189.
6. Finger RE, Vasquez B, Drew GS, et al. Superomedial pedicle technique of reduction mammaplasty. *Plast Reconstr Surg* 1989;83:471.
7. Hauben DJ. Superomedial pedicle technique of reduction mammaplasty. *Plast Reconstr Surg* 1989;83:479.
8. Hall-Findlay EJ. A simplified vertical reduction mammaplasty: shortening the learning curve. *Plast Reconstr Surg* 1999;104:748.
9. Nahabedian MY, McGibbon BM, Manson PN. Medial pedicle reduction mammaplasty for severe mammary hypertrophy. *Plast Reconstr Surg* 2000;105:896.
10. Abramson DL, Pap S, Shifteh S, et al. Improving Long-term breast shape with the medial pedicle Wise pattern breast reduction. *Plast Reconstr Surg* 2005;115:1937.
11. Davison SP, Mesbahi AN, Ducic I, et al. The versatility of the superomedial pedicle with various skin reduction patterns. *Plast Reconstr Surg* 2007;120:1466.
12. Landau AG, Hudson DA. Choosing the superomedial pedicle for reduction mammaplasty in gigantomastia. *Plast Reconstr Surg* 2008;121:735.
13. Nahai FR, Nahai F. MOC-PS CME article: breast reduction. *Plast Reconstr Surg* 2008;121:1.
14. Michelle Le Roux C, Kiil BJ, Pan WR, et al. Preserving the neurovascular supply in the Hall-Findlay superomedial pedicle breast reduction: an anatomical study. *J Plast Reconstr Aesthet Surg* 2010;63(4):655–662.
15. van der Meulen JC. Superomedial pedicle technique of reduction mammaplasty. *Plast Reconstr Surg* 1989;84:1005.
16. O'Dey DM, Prescher A, Pallua N. Vascular reliability of the nipple-areola complex-bearing pedicles: an anatomical microdissection study. *Plast Reconstr Surg* 2007;119:1167.
17. Schlenz I, Sandra Rigel S, Schemper M, et al. Alteration of nipple and areola sensitivity by reduction mammaplasty: a prospective comparison of five techniques. *Plast Reconstr Surg* 2005;115:743.
18. Mofid MM, Dellon AL, Elias JJ, et al. Quantitation of breast sensibility following reduction mammaplasty: a comparison of inferior and medial pedicle techniques. *Plast Reconstr Surg* 2002;109:2283.
19. Ferreira MC, Costa MP, Cunha MS, et al. Sensibility of the breast after reduction mammaplasty. *Ann Plast Surg* 2003;51:1.
20. Cruz NI, Korchin L. Lactational performance after breast reduction with different pedicles. *Plast Reconstr Surg* 2007;120:35.
21. Cruz N, Korchin L. Breast feeding after vertical mammaplasty with medial pedicle. *Plast Reconstr Surg* 2004;114:890.
22. Losken A, Holtz DJ. Versatility of the superomedial pedicle in managing the massive weight loss breast: the rotation advancement technique. *Plast Reconstr Surg* 2007;120:1060.
23. Munhoz AM, Montag E, Arruda EG, et al. Superior-medial pedicle dermoglandular pedicle reduction mammaplasty for immediate conservative breast surgery reconstruction: technical aspects and outcome. *Ann Plast Surg* 2006;57:502.

CHAPTER

98

Armando Chiari, Jr.
James C. Grotting

The L Short-scar Mammaplasty

INTRODUCTION

Breast reduction has consistently resulted in a high degree of patient satisfaction, despite the various techniques employed. However, the extensive incisions required with standard or so-called "inverted-T" reduction patterns have led plastic surgeons to seek short-scar techniques. These involve shortening or eliminating a portion of the vertical or horizontal incision while still attaining adequate reduction with good projection, shape, and symmetry.

Although these goals have proven to be elusive in very large breasts, we have found that the "L short-scar" or Chiari reduction mammaplasty yields excellent results in properly selected patients. The guiding principle of this technique is "that which remains is much more important than that which is removed." The surgical procedure consists of resection of skin and breast tissue from the inferior and deep central portions of the breast with preservation of the main ductal system. In almost all cases of reduction, the breast base is amputated while the third, fourth, and fifth lateral intercostal nerves are preserved.

INDICATIONS AND PATIENT SELECTION

Breast hypertrophy is classified as mild (resections up to 300 g), moderate (300 to 600 g), large (600 to 900 g), and very large (900 to 1,200 g or more). The Chiari reduction is best suited for women with mild to moderate mammary hypertrophy, with a resultant L short scar. Since 1999, the vertical variant of the technique has been emphasized, but now the vertical resultant scar and the mini-L scar are used for mild hypertrophies and ptosis (Figs. 98.1 and 98.2) and especially for mastopexies with associated silicone prosthesis. Patients undergoing large resections often require a secondary revision using the same technique, depending on the grade of ptosis and elasticity of the skin. Variations of the technique may be employed to avoid such revisions (see discussion). However, very large reductions, severe ptosis (grades III to IV), and insufficient skin elasticity contribute to less-than-ideal postoperative aesthetics, and such patients should be considered for an alternative reduction technique.

Because the technique is based on what will remain and not on what will be resected, we believe that one of the most important indications is the correction of asymmetry (Figs. 98.3 to 98.5). It is much easier to conceptualize reduction in the case of asymmetric breasts if one is not concerned about comparing the amounts resected from each side.

PREOPERATIVE MARKINGS

To the surgeon unfamiliar with the Chiari reduction, the preoperative markings will appear somewhat daunting. The following description sets them down in a stepwise fashion. Since 1999, the original (1) mathematical delineation has been used only for the amount of skin necessary for reshaping the medial portion of the breast and not for the lateral portion.

Markings are based on the chest width, the vertical meridian of the chest, and the inframammary fold, rather than on a predetermined pattern. Again, the focus is on what will remain, not on what will be resected.

With the patient standing, the midmammary and midsternal lines are marked. The chest width, defined as the distance between the axillary folds, is divided by four to yield the key measurement, *X*. The examiner's hand is then placed behind and under the breast, gently supporting it, to determine point A. This is the projection of the inframammary fold onto the anterior breast skin along the midmammary line above the nipple. Point A′ is now marked 2 cm above point A along the midmammary line (Fig. 98.6). The patient is now placed supine, and all subsequent marks are made with the skin under tension (Figs. 98.6B and 98.7B).

Point C is marked at a distance *X* cm (average 8 cm) from the midsternal line and 1 cm above the inframammary fold (Fig. 96.6). Point B is placed *X* + 2 cm (average 10 cm) from the midsternal line and 8 cm above point C (Figs. 96.6B and 98.7B). For larger breasts, line BC can be up to 16 cm. Point B′ is placed at one level between point A and the nipple, determined by trial and error (Figs. 98.6 and 97.7). Opposing point B to point B′ with bidigital maneuvers (Fig. 98.7A), we show the new breast cone, which must have good projection without tension (Fig. 98.7A). Point C′ is marked 7 cm from point B′, originating line B′C′C, with the skin of the lateral portion of the breast stretched in a superior and medial direction (Fig. 98.7B). Finally, point D is placed laterally, 1.5 cm above the inframammary fold along the end of the skin fold formed when line BC and B′C′ are opposed (Fig. 98.6B). The final markings form a distorted trapezoidal shape with the line B′C′ always positioned above BC. When united, lines BC (longer) and B′C′ (shorter) form the vertical reduction scar. The arching line C′D is opposed along CD to form the lateral horizontal limb (Figs. 98.6 to 98.8).

SURGICAL TECHNIQUE

The periareolar skin bounded by points A, B, and B′ and by a vertical line extending inferiorly from B′ and by a horizontal line at the level of B is now deepithelialized. The line CD (Fig. 98.6B) is incised, and the breast tissue is dissected superiorly in the direction of the pectoralis major muscle, nearly 1 cm above the inferior border of this muscle. The breast is then extensively undermined at the level just above the pectoralis fascia, from the inferior margin of the pectoralis major to the superior breast border. Laterally, the dissection continues to the third, fourth, and fifth intercostal nerves and medially to the level of the anterior cutaneous branches of the same intercostal nerves.

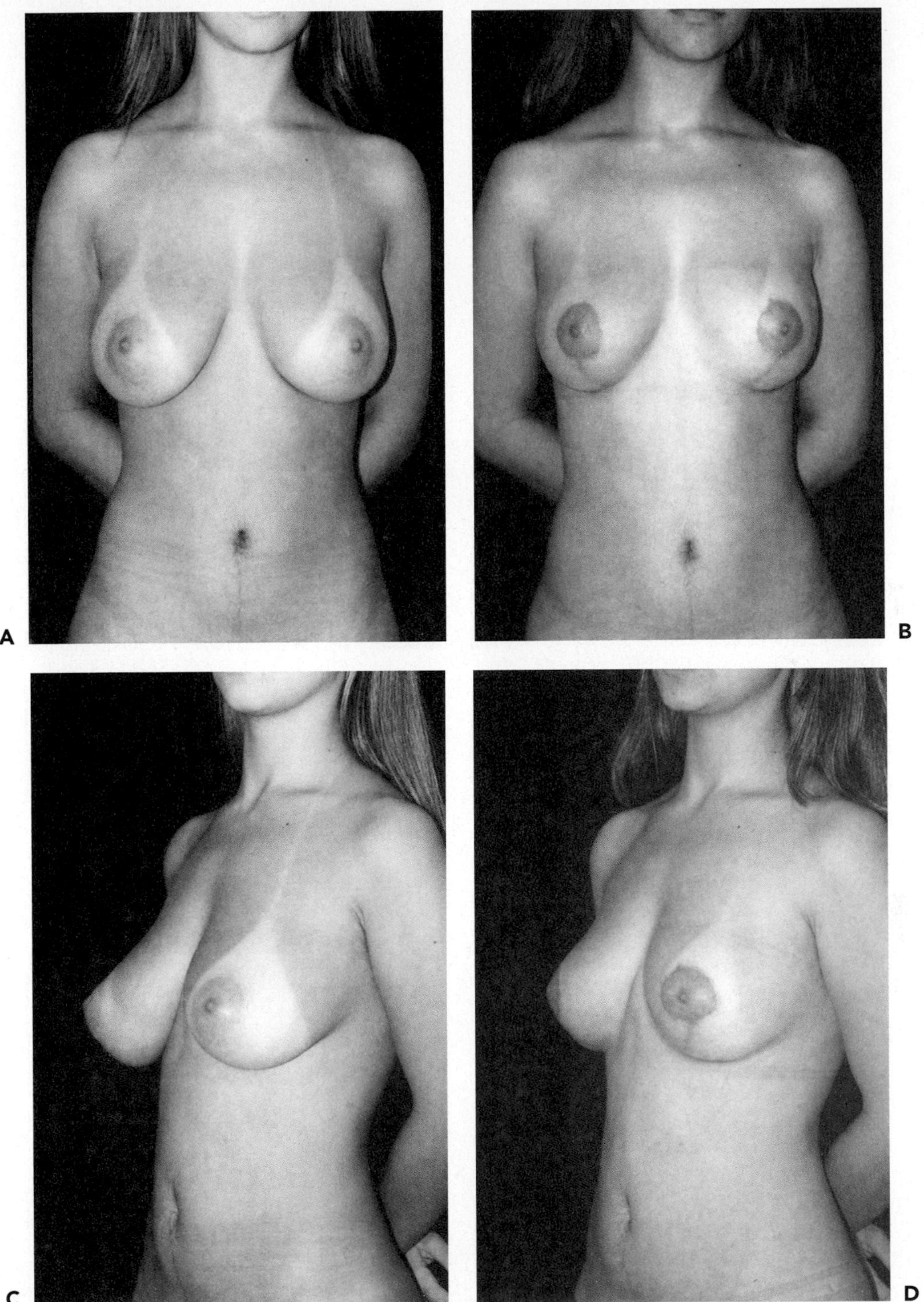

Figure 98.1. A 20-year-old patient before **(A, C)** and 1 year after **(B, D)** resection of 155 g from the left breast and 180 g from the right breast, with a "mini-L" resultant scar.

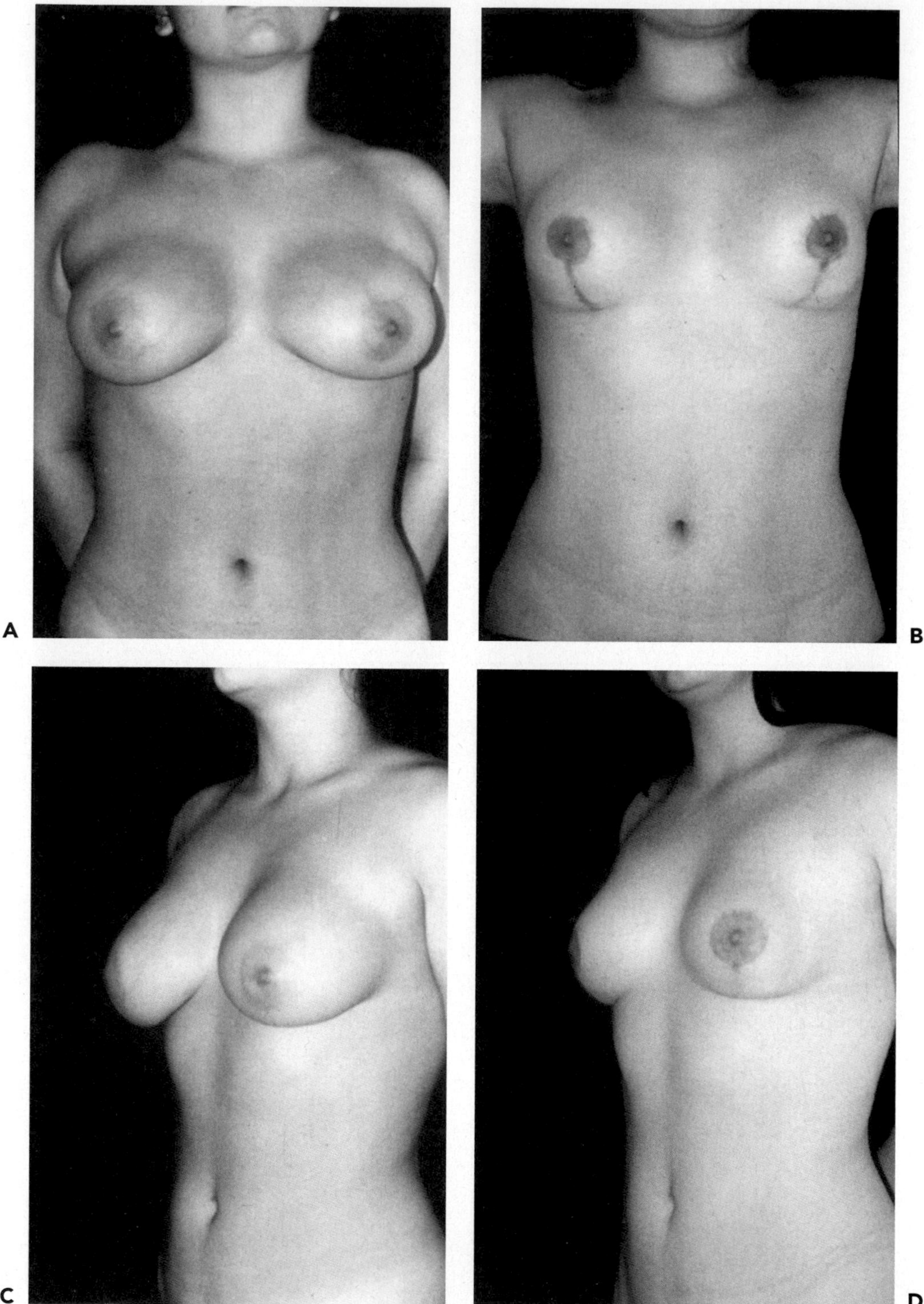

Figure 98.2. An 18-year-old patient before **(A, C)** and 1 year after **(B, D)** resection of 230 g from the left breast and 200 g from the right breast, with a vertical resultant scar.

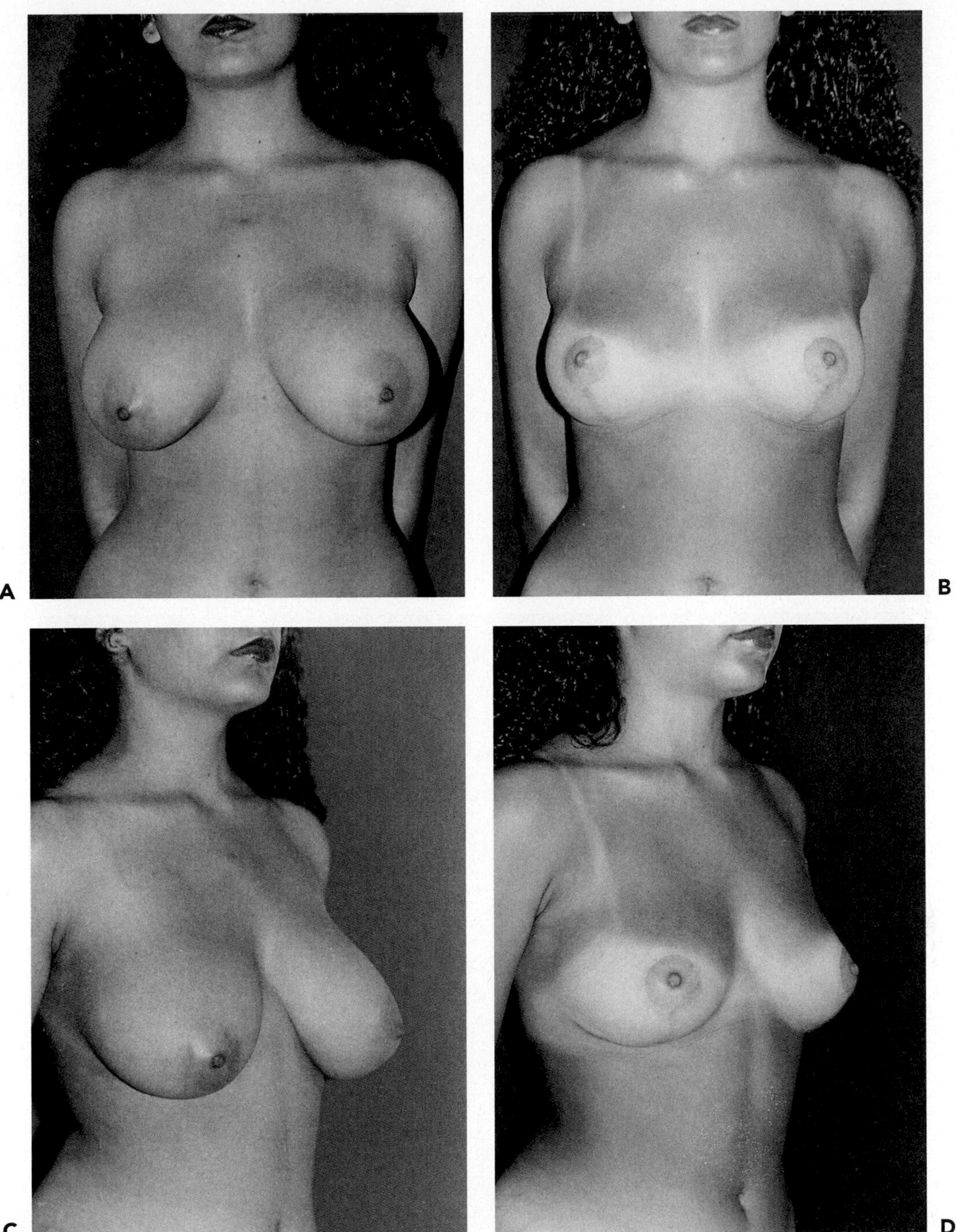

Figure 98.3. A 16-year-old patient before **(A, C)** and 14 months after **(B, D)** resection of 340 g from the left breast and 260 g from the right breast.

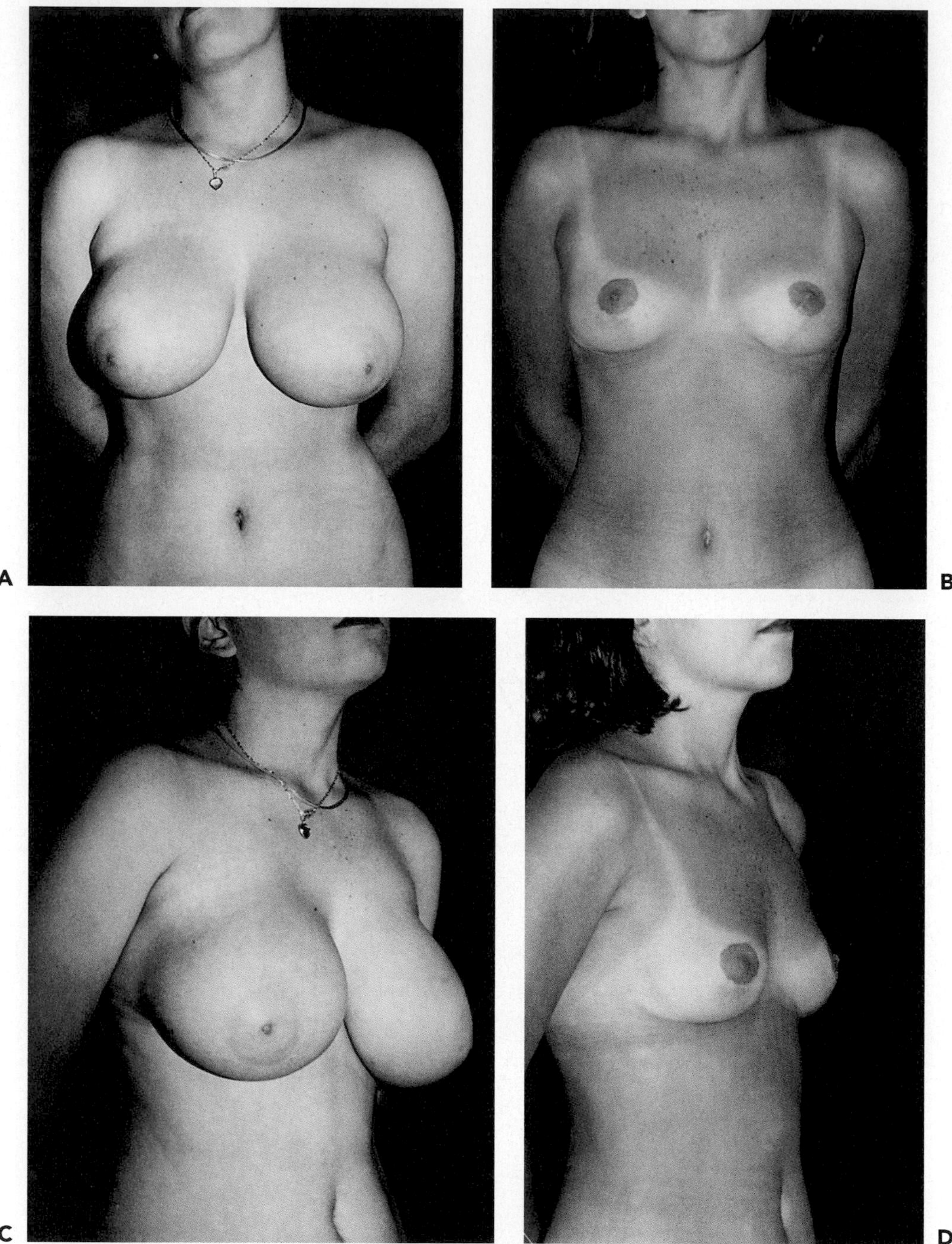

Figure 98.4. An 18-year-old patient before **(A, C)** and 8 years after **(B, D)** surgery and 1 year after the birth of her child, who she successfully breast-fed for 1 month. Resection of 710 g from the left breast and 580 g from the right.

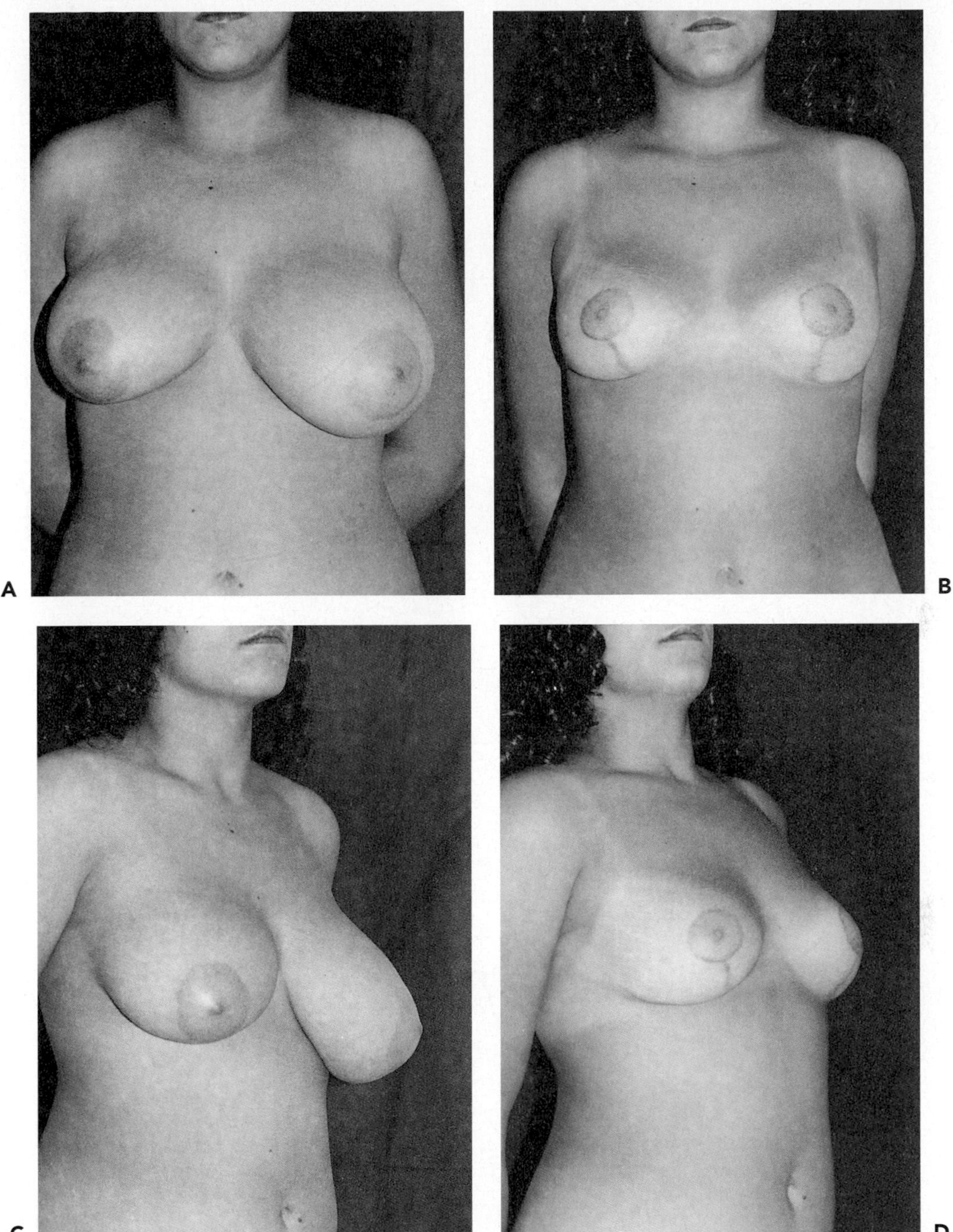

Figure 98.5. A 16-year-old patient before **(A, C)** and 8 months after **(B, D)** resection of 730 g from the left breast and 350 g from the right breast. Note the asymmetry on preoperative photos.

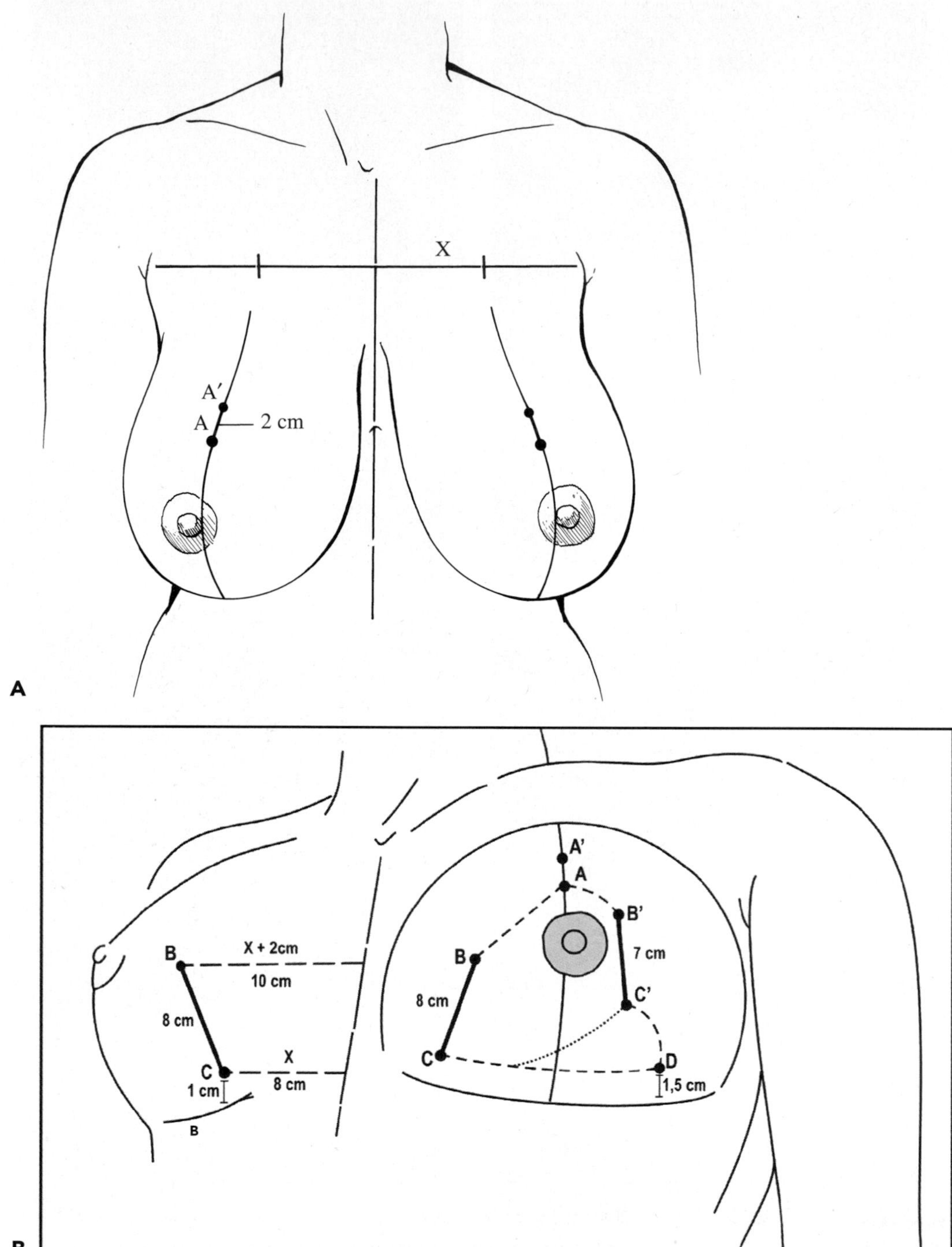

Figure 98.6. **A:** With the patient standing, the chest width is divided by 4 to yield the key measurement, *X*. Point A is the projection of the inframammary fold onto the anterior surface of the breast. All the subsequent marks are made with the patient in a supine position and the skin under tension. **B:** The medial marks are made with reference to the key measurement (*X*) and the inframammary and midsternal lines.

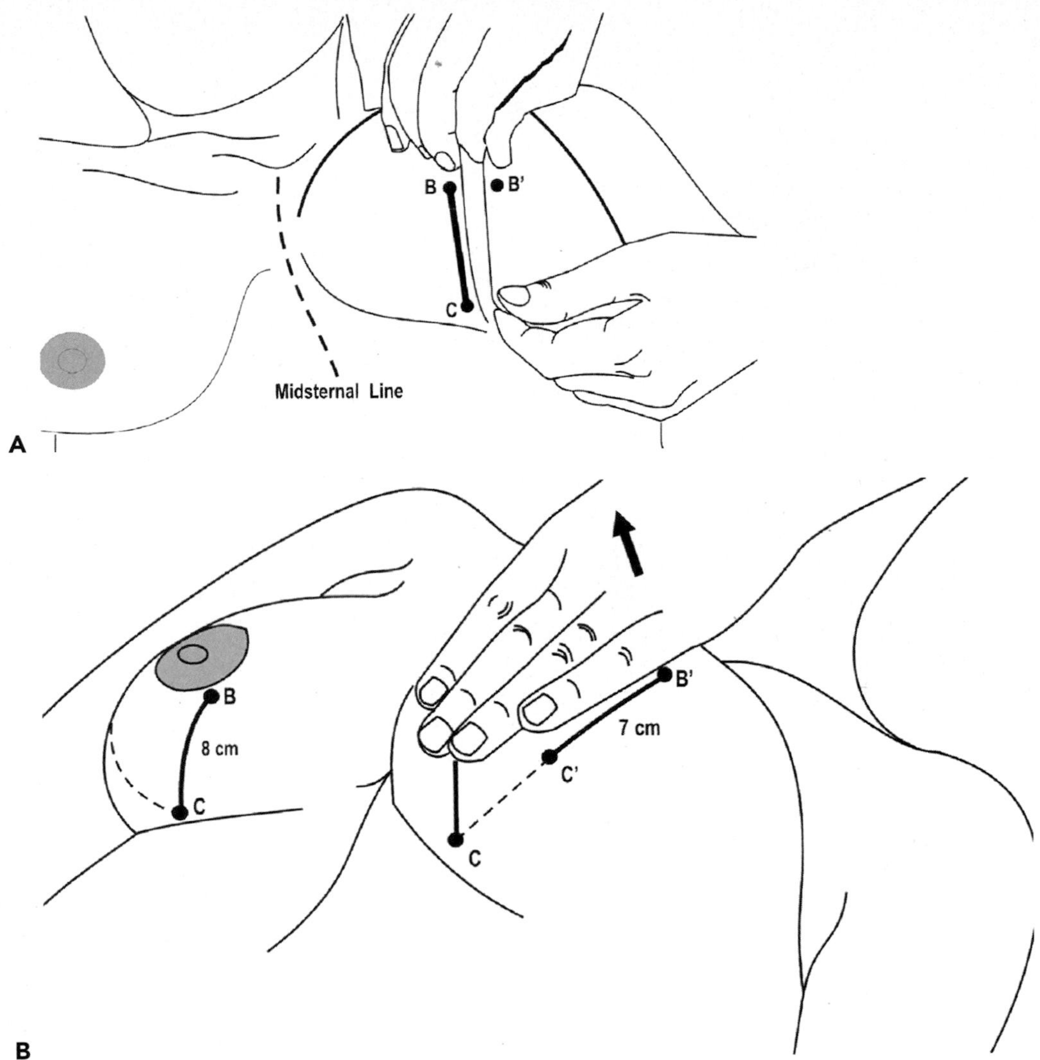

Figure 98.7. **A:** Opposing point B to point B′ with bidigital maneuvers, we show the new breast cone, which must have good projection without tension. **B:** Line B′C′ has a length of 7.0 cm and is marked in direction of point C, with the breast skin stretched in a superior and medial direction.

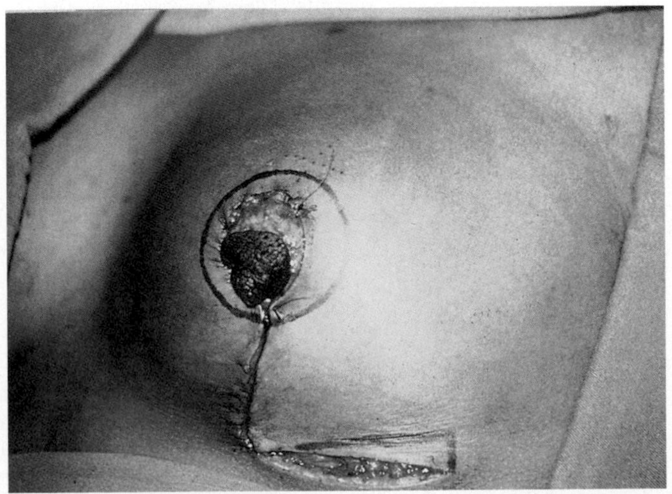

Figure 98.8. The site of the new areola is created with an eccentric skin excision designed with a compensation pouch to remove as much surplus skin medially as possible.

The patient is placed in the semisitting position for the parenchymal resection. The breast is retracted upward at point A. The parenchyma is divided along C′D perpendicular to the skin. Incisions are made along BC and B′C′, converge at an angle of 60 deg (Fig. 98.9), and meet at the pectoralis fascia along the midmammary line. This wedge of tissue is removed, except with mastopexies when it can be preserved as a superiorly based flap used to fill out the upper pole (Figs. 98.10 to 98.12). Gland remains in the upper pole, centrally below the nipple and medially and laterally as two pillars (Fig. 98.13). A final incision dividing parenchyma only is directed along a line from B′ (Fig. 98.9) toward the ipsilateral axilla lateral to the ductal system. For breasts with soft parenchyma this maneuver is not necessary, but for breasts with very firm tissue this incision or resection of some breast tissue could be important. This detaches the lateral pillar from the remaining breast and allows it to swing into position along with the overlying skin. The bases of both pillars are now resected, leaving a pillar height of 7 cm (Fig. 98.13). Again, care is taken to preserve the lateral intercostal nerve branches.

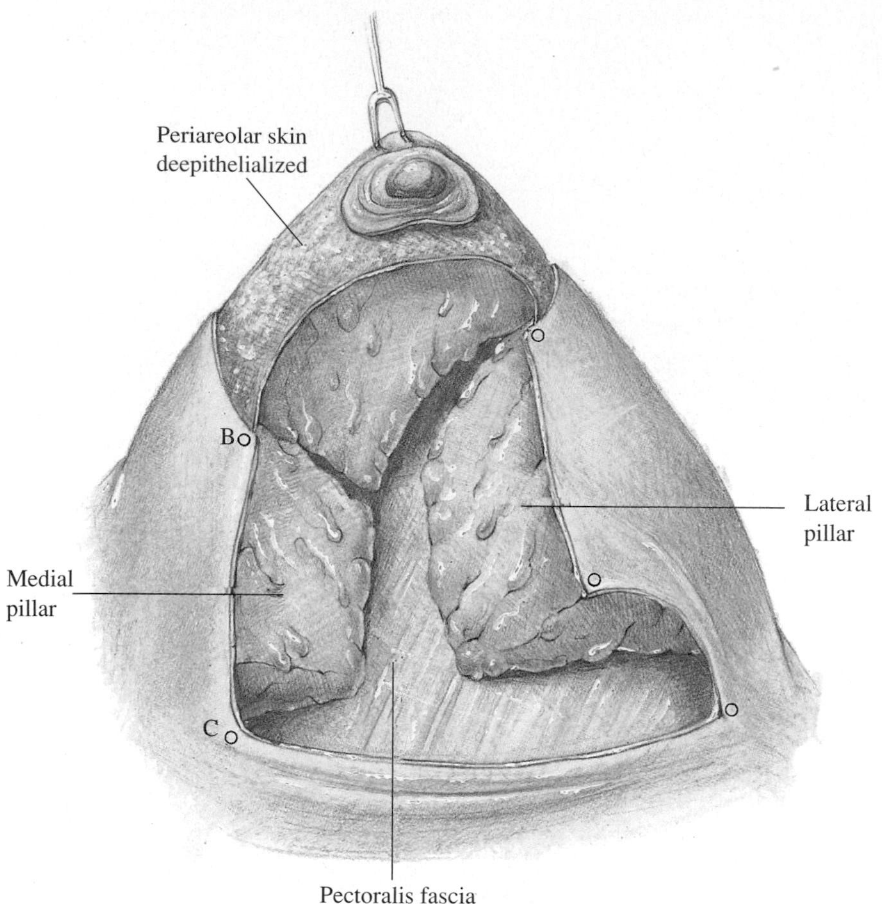

Figure 98.9. Incisions along BC and B′C′ converge at an angle of 60 deg to the chest wall.

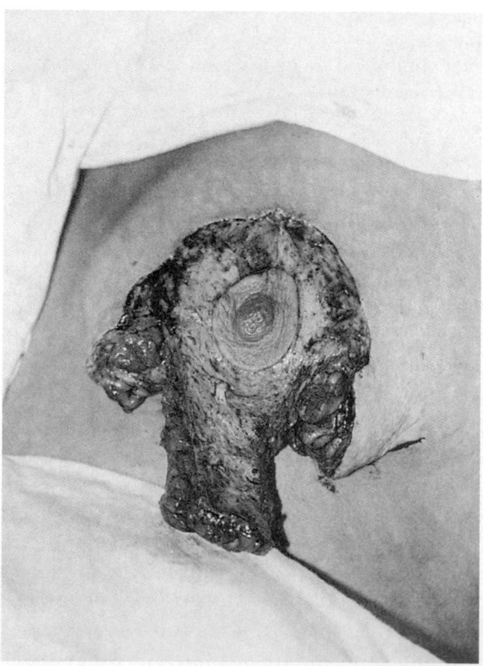

Figure 98.10. For mastopexies, the wedge of tissue between lines BC and B′C′ is preserved as a superiorly based flap and used to fill the upper pole.

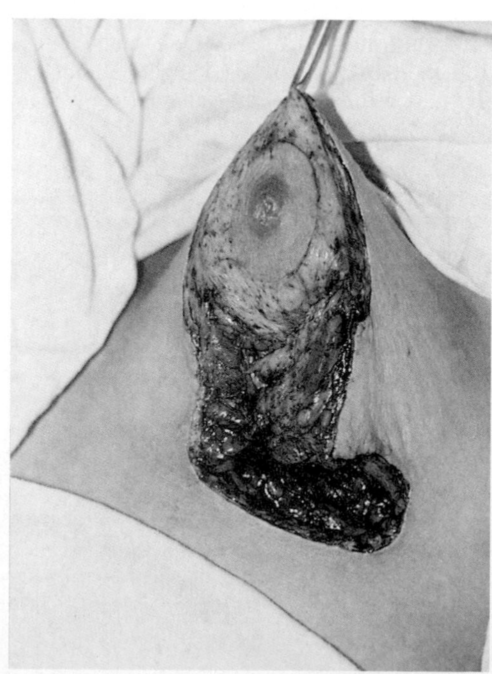

Figure 98.11. The superiorly based flap is placed in the upper pole when the medial and lateral pillars are sutured together.

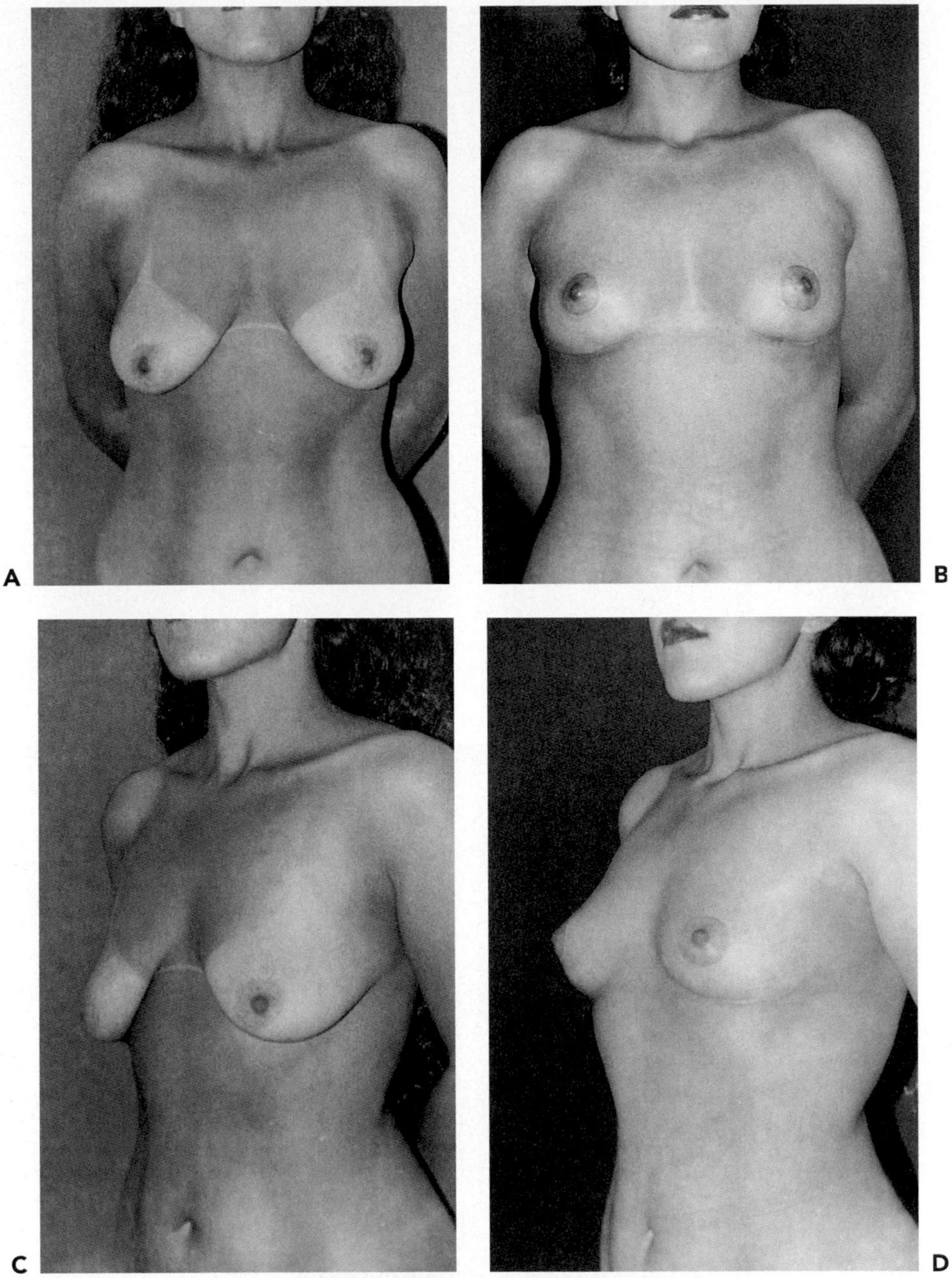

A B C D

Figure 98.12. An 18-year-old patient before **(A, C)** and 12 months after surgery **(B, D)**. No parenchyma was resected. All tissue was used as a superiorly based flap to fill the upper pole.

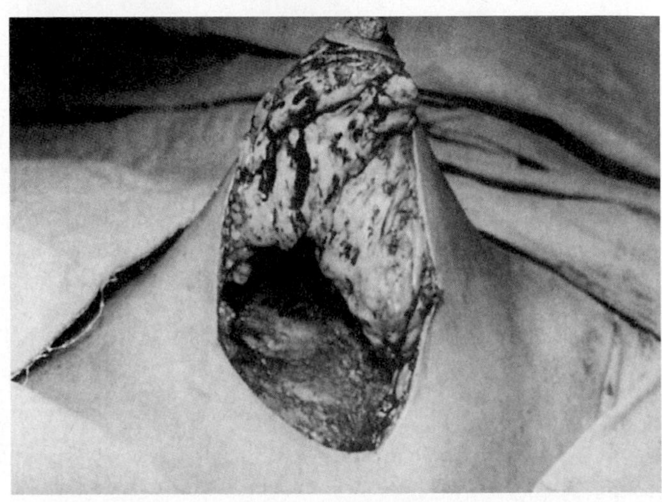

Figure 98.13. The resection preserves glandular tissue in the upper pole, centrally below the nipple, and laterally and medially as two pillars.

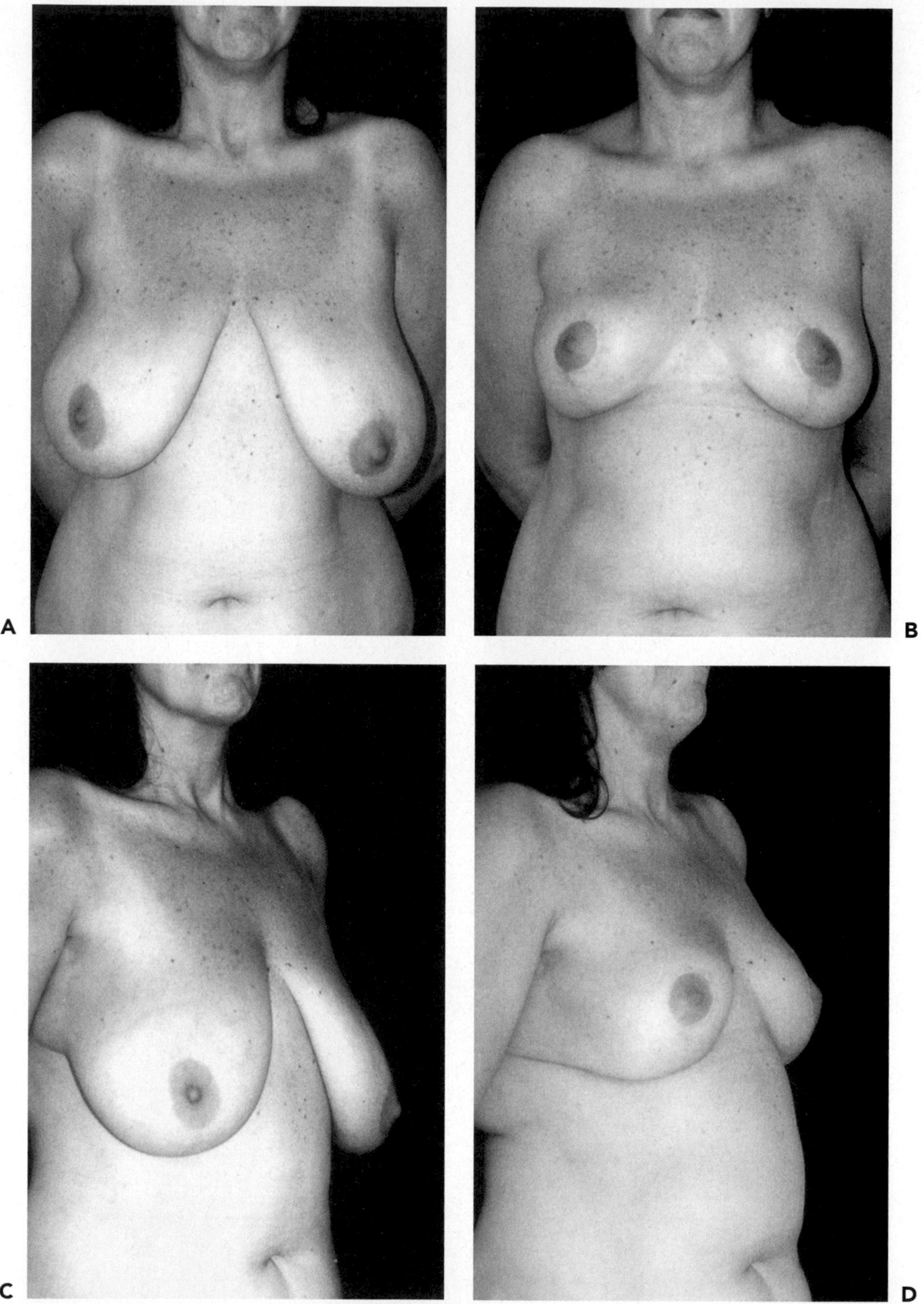

Figure 98.14. A 37-year-old patient before **(A, C)** and 1 year after **(B, D)** resection of 415 g from the left breast and 400 g from the right breast.

Beginning at the bases, the medial and lateral pillars are sutured together (Figs. 98.13 and 98.11). This effectively opposes BC to B′C′ and CD to C′D. Any surplus skin located above BAB′ is resected (Fig. 98.8). The new areolar position is marked and deepithelialized with A′ as the vertex. In all cases, we have made a circular intradermal continuous suture, with a colorless 4-0 Monocryl, like the "round block" of Benelli (2) (Fig. 98.14), to avoid areolar enlargements. The vertical scar should measure from 3.5 to 6.0 cm. It may be necessary to adjust the horizontal scar superiorly by resection of a small, laterally based skin triangle (Fig. 98.8).

RESULTS

The procedure has been uniformly safe, with few complications. There was minor loss of areola in 6 of 1,822 operated breasts (911 patients). Six patients underwent unilateral reduction only. Four patients required secondary liposuction below the site of the new inframammary fold. Nipple-areola sensory preservation has been excellent. Although the lactiferous ducts are preserved, especially in mild hypertrophies, the success rate of postoperative breast-feeding is unknown.

For women with mild to moderate mammary hypertrophy, lines BC and B′C′ are traced on distended skin with a length of 8.0 and 7.0 cm, respectively (Figs. 98.6 and 98.7). For moderate to large hypertrophy, line BC can be up to 16 cm. With the breast remodeled and without skin distention, the vertical stem of the L-shaped scar (originated by the union and compensation of these lines) has an average length of 5.0 to 6.0 cm (Fig. 98.8).

PROBLEMS, PITFALLS, AND COMPLICATIONS

The Chiari reduction has attained uniformly good results, especially in patients with a considerable degree of skin elasticity and moderate ptosis (Figs. 98.1 to 98.3 and 98.15) and even in patients with hypertrophy requiring resections of 600 to 900 g

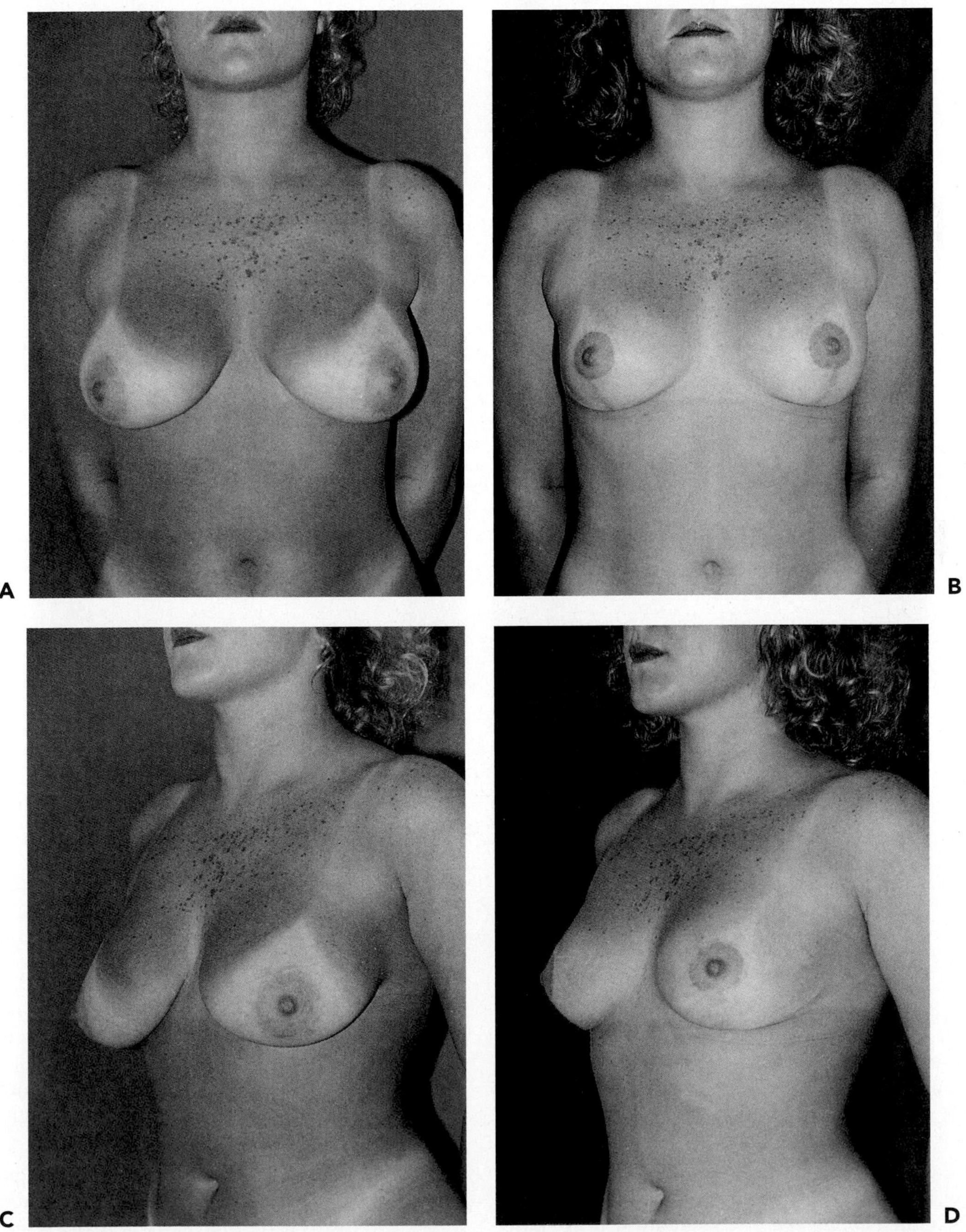

Figure 98.15. A 22-year-old patient before **(A, C)** and 1 year after **(B, D)** resection of 230 g from the left breast and 240 g from the right breast.

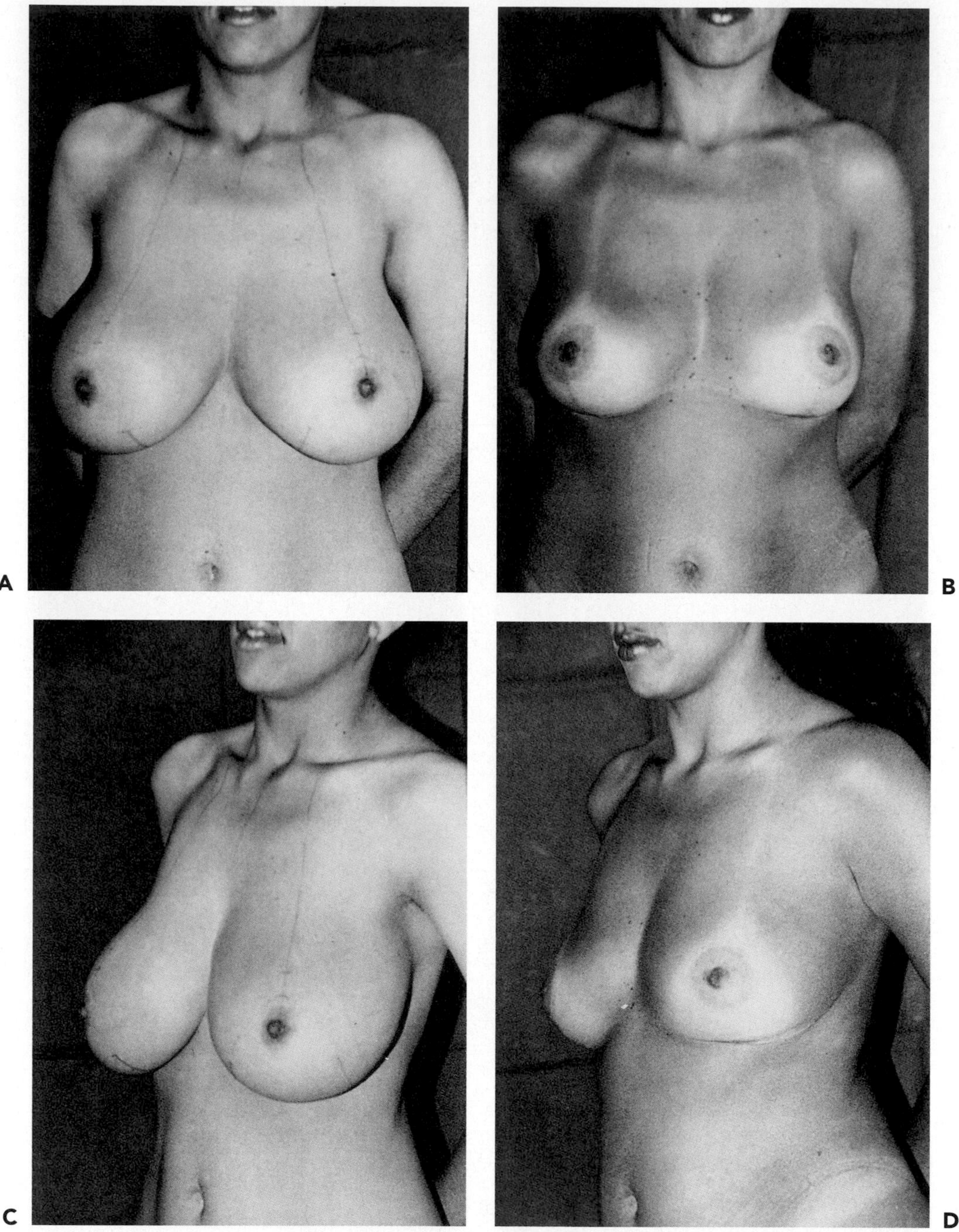

Figure 98.16. A 27-year-old patient before **(A, C)** and 3 years after **(B, D)** resection of 580 g from each breast.

(Figs. 98.4, 98.5, 98.16, and 98.17). Patients with significant hypertrophy, insufficient skin elasticity, and severe ptosis (Fig. 98.18) often require a secondary revision if this technique is chosen. To avoid this second operation, one can draw line BC longer than the 8.0 cm (the minimum distance). The resulting surplus skin in the inferomedial pole is removed by the opposition of the skin in BC with the shorter segment B′C′, as well as by resection of a medial dog ear. The resultant scar will have an "L-T" shape, always smaller than a classic inverted-T scar (Fig. 98.18).

Between 1999 and 2003, the vertical and the "mini-L" variants of the technique were emphasized (Figs. 98.1, 98.2, and 98.14) and shown in two publications in 2001 (3) and 2002 (4). However, some patients with poor skin elasticity and greater ptosis had areolar enlargement and early return of the ptosis. Since 2003, the vertical and the "mini-L" resultant scars have only been used for patients with mild hypertrophies and ptosis with good skin elasticity (Figs. 98.1 and 98.2) and especially for mastopexies with associated silicone prosthesis.

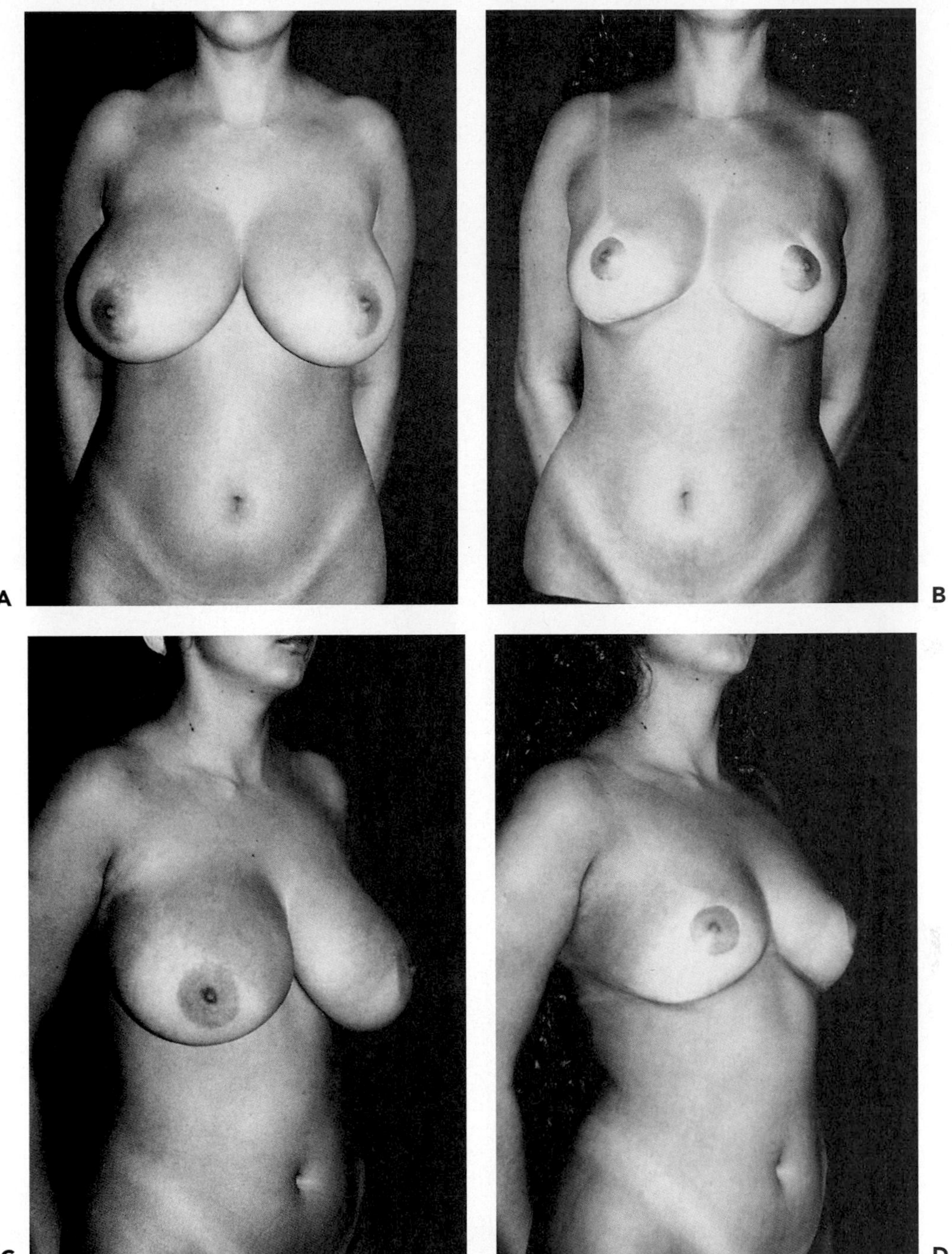

Figure 98.17. A 20-year-old patient before **(A, C)** and 2 years after **(B, D)** resection of 530 g from the left breast and 610 g from the right breast.

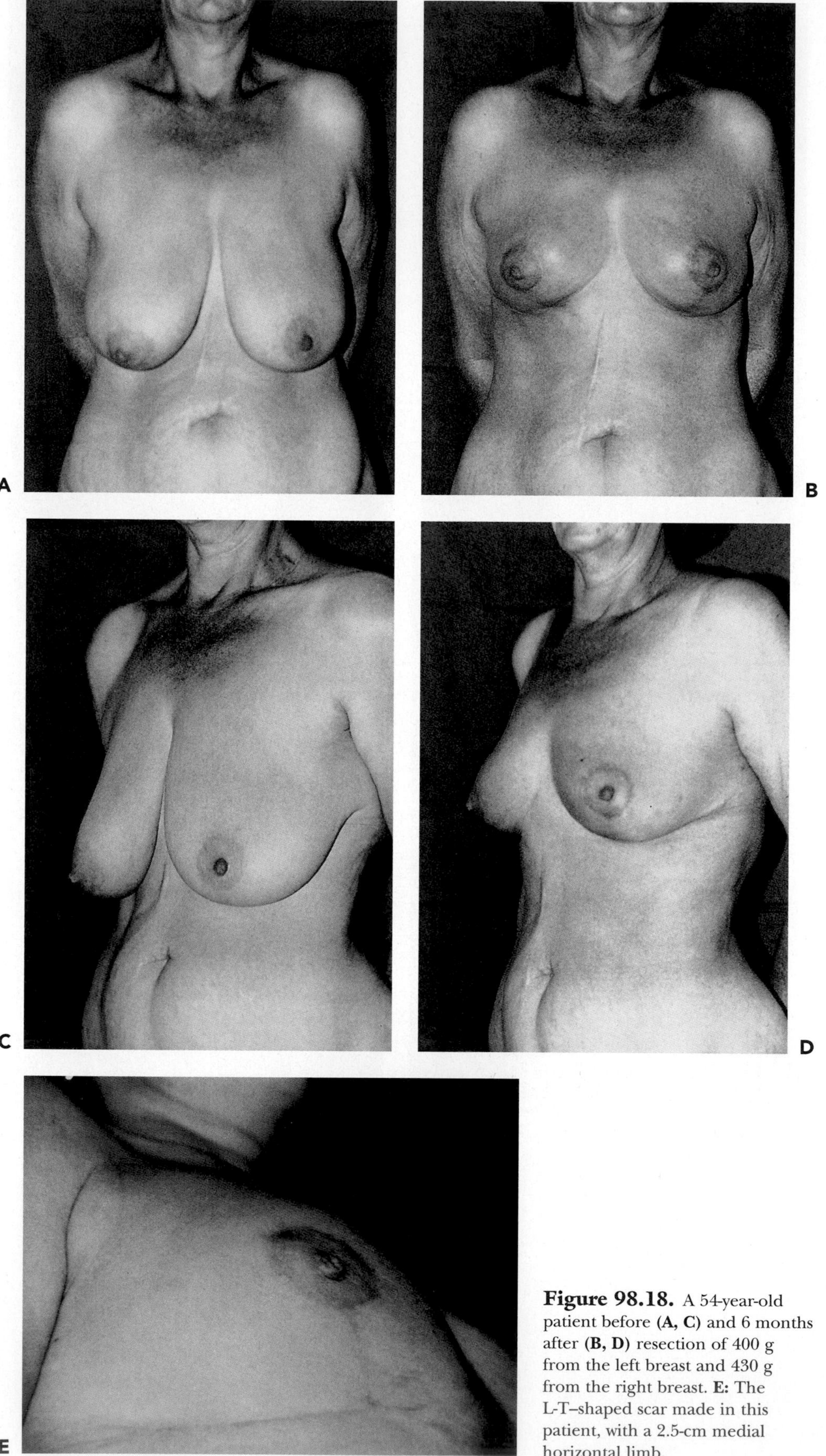

Figure 98.18. A 54-year-old patient before **(A, C)** and 6 months after **(B, D)** resection of 400 g from the left breast and 430 g from the right breast. **E:** The L-T–shaped scar made in this patient, with a 2.5-cm medial horizontal limb.

CONCLUSION

The Chiari or "L short-scar" breast reduction is an effective technique that should be considered when small to moderate reductions are indicated. Its major advantages relate to the scars, which are well positioned and have a good quality. In addition, they are short, with elimination of the medial limb, a shortened lateral limb, and preservation of an undistorted areola. As supported by a large series, breast shape, projection, and innervation are preserved. The Chiari reduction should be part of the armamentarium of every aesthetic breast surgeon.

EDITORIAL COMMENTS

Drs. Chiari and Grotting present lovely results after breast reduction using the L short-scar technique. This operation is reminiscent of similar techniques that involve geometric planning and specific breast shaping performed according to an architectural plan in order to achieve nice results. It bears some resemblance to the Regnault-B technique and the Dufourmentel reduction technique with a lateralized scar. Several other European and South American authors have described and written about similar procedures.

The authors are quite correct that the drawing and planning of this operation can be daunting to the uninitiated. I recommend, therefore, that anyone who is interested in using the L short-scar mammoplasty technique spend some time with another surgeon who is familiar with it and can achieve consistent, good results. Although the McKissock, inferior pedicle, and free nipple graft techniques benefit from simplicity and ease of revision, the L-shaped short-scar mammoplasty technique and similar techniques achieve attractive results at the price of some complexity and the risk of occasional disappointing and difficult-to-revise results.

S.L.S.

REFERENCES

1. Chiari A Jr. The L short-scar mammaplasty: a new approach. *Plast Reconstr Surg* 1992;90: 233–246.
2. Benelli L. A new periareolar mammaplasty: the "round block" technique. *Aesthet Plast Surg* 1990;14:93–100.
3. Chiari A Jr. The L short-scar mammaplasty: 12 years later. *Plast Reconstr Surg* 2001;108:489–495.
4. Chiari A Jr. The L short-scar mammaplasty. *Clin Plast Surg* 2002;29:401–409.

CHAPTER

99

Simon G. Talbot
Julian J. Pribaz

The No-vertical-scar Breast Reduction

INTRODUCTION

Reduction mammaplasty is one of the most commonly performed breast operations in the United States. In 2007, over 106,000 breast reductions were reported by the American Society of Plastic Surgeons (a 167% increase since 1992) ranking it among the top five reconstructive procedures performed in the United States (1). Reduction mammaplasty is consistently associated with high patient satisfaction and improved quality of life (2,3).

The primary goal of all methods of breast reduction is to remove and reshape excess and redundant parenchyma and skin while preserving nipple-areola complex vascularity (4). The ideal breast reduction technique would produce the "perfect" breast size and shape with minimal scarring, intact nipple vascularity and sensation, good projection, a stable inframammary fold, preservation of the ability to lactate, and structural stability over time (5). In addition, an ideal method should be easy to perform, reproducible by other surgeons, easy to teach, expeditious, and free from complications. However, as evidenced by the number of operations available, no one procedure is ideal "for all seasons," and good patient selection is key to obtaining the optimal result for any individual. Breast reduction without a vertical scar is no exception.

A wide variety of breast reduction techniques exist, resulting in combinations of vertical, horizontal, and periareolar scars. In addition, nipple-areolar blood supply may be based on inferior, lateral, superomedial, central, vertical, and horizontal pedicles or bipedicles. While countless variations and combinations of incisions, scars, and pedicles have been developed, the most popular technique currently remains one of the various forms of inverted-T scar methods (4,6). In a subset of patients with significant ptosis requiring large-volume reductions, a technique using only periareolar and inferior horizontal incisions can produce excellent results, with good shape, less scarring, a well-vascularized and innervated nipple-areola complex, the ability to lactate, and stability of the inframammary fold. The technique detailed here is relatively fast and simple, reliable, reproducible, expeditious, easy to teach, and relatively free from complications.

Several arguments can be made for methods without a *vertical* scar in breast reduction surgery. First, extensive scarring due to inverted-T pattern reductions can be unaesthetic, wound complications may occur, especially at the "T-intersection" of the incisions, and this region is prone to hypertrophic scarring (5,7). In addition, while surgeon evaluations suggest similar hypertrophy and color matching for periareolar, vertical, and inframammary scars, vertical scars do have a tendency to widen in time (3). Second, methods that significantly interfere with the inframammary fold may results in loss of shape through pseudoptosis or "bottoming out," resulting in an unfavorable change in breast shape in the long term. Third, in cases of very large breast reductions, the length of a typical narrow, inverted-T-style inferior pedicle may be too long to reliably support the nipple-areola complex, with some authors advocating free nipple grafting when transpositions of greater than 10 cm are required (8). Many methods of breast reduction are well suited to small reductions, and their translation to larger reductions may compromise nipple vascularity and sensation (7). Fourth, wound healing and contraction of the vertical scar may distort the periareolar scar, causing an ovoid and unnatural shape to the areola (6). With these points in mind, periareolar scars have been shown to be most popular with patients, and a well-placed scar located at the lower aspect of the breast and hidden by the breast mound when viewed from in front is very acceptable (3,6,9). Thus, avoiding a vertical scar may have significant benefits in some patients.

HISTORY OF THE PROCEDURE

Breast reduction surgery dates to 1669, with a procedure performed by William Durston from England (10). After studies of subdermal plexus blood supply to the nipple in the 1930s many newer techniques involving deepithelialized pedicles were developed (11). It was from this basis that Wise published a paper in 1956 on the geometry of the breast, giving rise to the now popular "Wise-pattern" breast reduction, based on an inferior deepithelialized pedicle and inverted-T scar with excisions of "wedges of gland from one or more quadrants" (12). Since the 1960s, surgeons such as Arié, Pitanguy, Strömbeck, McKissock, and Skoog have used a variety of deepithelialized pedicles beneath an inverted-T scar to expand the array of breast reduction techniques and options (13–15).

A further evolution in breast reduction has been the minimization of scarring. Despite high patient satisfaction with breast reduction surgery, scarring remains a significant concern for many patients (3). Surgeons such as Benelli (4,16) (periareolar reduction), Lassus (13) (vertical reduction), Lejour (17,18) (modification of the vertical reduction), and Hall-Findlay (19) (simplified vertical reduction) have developed techniques based on periareolar scars, vertical scars, or reduction of the horizontal/inframammary fold scars (20).

Passot (6,21) is frequently credited with developing the first breast reduction technique in the 1920s that avoided a vertical scar. Excess tissue was removed as a wedge from only the inferior pole of the breast. This technique was used in cases with minimal hypertrophy and moderate ptosis (22).

The original Robertson technique of breast reduction, published in 1967, removes a central wedge of breast tissue through the horizontal mid-axis of the breast (23). Central breast tissue underlying the nipple is resected, an inferior, bell-shaped flap is advanced superiorly, and the nipple-areola complex is resited by free grafting. The steep, bell-shaped inferior incision and straight superior incision eliminate the discrepancy between incision lengths but result in a bell-shaped, curved scar through the mid-axis of the breast and new nipple-areola complex.

Ribeiro (22,24) repopularized Passot's technique in 1975 with modifications based on techniques used by Thorek, Maliniac (25), and Conway (26), all of whom frequently used free nipple grafts. Ribeiro's technique is marked by sutures producing a conical breast mound and no free nipple grafting with a postoperative plaster dressing to support breast shape while healing. Notably, Ribeiro places the inferior incision 2 cm *below* in the inframammary fold and, in contrast to other authors, refers to this dropping to the "proper position" after healing. Ribeiro's later publications discuss dissatisfaction with breast flattening and long horizontal scars, encouraging reversion to an inferior glandular dermolipo pedicle in modified inverted-T, vertical scar, and periareolar techniques (27).

In a paper by Hurst et al. (28) from 1983, the first modification of the Robertson technique uses a broad, bell-shaped *inferior* pedicle 10 cm in height, with a deepithelialized flap above this containing the nipple-areola complex. There is adequate vascularity to the nipple-areola complex, so that a free nipple graft is not required, but the end result is still with a bell-shaped scar crossing the mid-axis of the breast, as in the original Robertson technique (28).

In the early 1990s, Yousif et al. (9) published a paper explaining their use of a no-vertical-scar technique for cases of very large and/or ptotic breasts. Their "apron technique" was developed to reduce unsightly scars in cases in which the nipple-areola complex is greater than 7.1 cm from the center of the planned new nipple location (29). This allows draping of a superiorly based flap over the pedicle, which forms the lower pole after the remaining breast tissue is tacked together in an axial plane. Emphasis is placed on "internal mound contouring" into a conical shape to produce a stable form rather than relying on a shaped skin envelope. In addition, excess inferior skin is gathered to the center of the incision, creating several small cones to help maintain projection.

Our no-vertical-scar breast reduction (also called the Boston modification of the Robertson technique) has evolved from the modified Robertson technique and includes further modification and several refinements. It is fundamentally different from Passot's technique, which removed a wedge of breast tissue inferiorly and was used only for small reductions. It is also different from the original Robertson (23) and Hurst (28) (modified Robertson) techniques, which have a scar visible from the front and through the horizontal mid-axis of the breast. There are additional shaping maneuvers to narrow the transverse diameter of the breast and improve projection. Incision placement and the siting of the nipple-areola complex differentiate it from a technique described by Keskin et al. (30). The no-vertical-scar breast reduction places the flat, bell-shaped inframammary scar 1.5 to 2 cm above the inframammary fold so that it is still hidden in the shadow of the breast and is not irritated by the bra, thus making it far less visible while maintaining the advantage of a large and broad pyramidal nipple-areola complex pedicle (5). This broad pedicle allows avoidance of a free nipple graft even in very large reductions.

INDICATIONS

The no-vertical-scar breast reduction has provided us with an effective and reliable reduction mammaplasty operation for large, ptotic breasts. It requires 6 to 7 cm (but a minimum of 5 cm) of nonpigmented skin between the position of the inferior edge of the new areola and the superior edge of the existing pigmented areolar skin (5,6). This allows adequate coverage of the lower pole without a visible scar through the center of the breast. A lack of ptosis or a very large areola can preclude this. This technique is not effective for mastopexy alone.

Several key points underscore the benefits of this technique for these large reductions. First, it eliminates a vertical scar, and hides a transverse scar in inferior breast shadow. Second, it removes the need for free nipple grafting due to the wide inferior and central pyramidal pedicle. Third, pseudoptosis is minimized by an undisturbed inferior and central pyramidal pedicle and intact inframammary fold. Fourth, the superiorly based "apron" flap overlying the pedicle acts to support the breast tissue like an intrinsic brassiere, thus eliminating stretch typically seen in inverted-T scar breast reductions and avoiding problems with dehiscence of the T-incision. Fifth, this technique is reliable, is easy to learn and teach, and can be performed safely in obese patients.

This reliability of this technique in extreme ptosis is underscored by considering the pathophysiology of breast changes with progressive hypertrophy. Typically, as the breast enlarges and becomes ptotic, the nipple-areola complex descends; the distance from the sternal notch to nipple progressively increases and may get to 50+ cm. However, the distance from the nipple-areola complex to the inframammary fold increases to a much lesser degree, rarely to more than 20 cm (31). The result is that the nipple-areola complex may descend so that it is not visible from frontal view. Why this happens is not entirely clear. It may be related to Cooper ligaments. Thus, resection of skin and breast parenchyma, which contributes to the upper pole lengthening, makes sense in cases with very large mammary hypertrophy and ptosis. In addition, an inferior and central pyramidal pedicle is optimal at maintaining nipple vascularity and sensibility.

A final key indication for this method of breast reduction is in those patients requiring contralateral symmetry operations after mastectomy and transverse rectus abdominis myocutaneous (TRAM) flap breast reconstruction. A reconstructed breast may be significantly smaller, less ptotic, and flatter, and this method allows better symmetry with the contralateral reconstructed side (9).

CONTRAINDICATIONS

As for other methods of breast reduction, there are a few contraindications to this operation.

This method of breast reduction is contraindicated in patients without significant ptosis. If less than 5 cm of skin exists between the new areola position and planned inframammary fold, a sufficient apron of tissue cannot be draped over the pedicle, and either the inferior scar will be visible or the nipple will be too high. In addition, there is a subgroup of patients with marked ptosis but who have very large areolae. In these cases there may not be a sufficient skin bridge between the lower border of the new nipple-areola complex site and the top of the areola to perform this operation without leaving pigmented tissue in the incision or raising the scar.

A history of a prior reduction may be a contraindication to this technique if a different pedicle was used. Nipple-areola vascularity from a prior pedicle should not be violated with new incisions and resections. This method of reduction can, however, be modified to incorporate an alternate pedicle (the same as for a prior breast reduction) while still avoiding a vertical scar and hence maintain viability of the nipple-areola complex.

Of course, patients may not be candidates for this surgery if they have severe underlying systemic disease that would make the anesthetic risk or ability to recover from surgery unsafe.

PREOPERATIVE PLANNING AND OPERATIVE TECHNIQUE: THE NO-VERTICAL-SCAR BREAST REDUCTION

The no-vertical-scar breast reduction (or Boston modification of the Robertson technique) involves a central inverted, U-shaped tissue resection and a broad deepithelialized, steep, bell-shaped pyramidal pedicle (including both a central and inferior pedicle) with a low and flat, bell-shaped scar just superior to the inframammary fold. This technique is best suited to large reductions in patients with significant ptosis.

Preoperative evaluation consists of the following:

- A full history, including breast disease and family history
- Examination of breast size and extent (including the size of the lateral roll), the degree of ptosis, breast consistency (fatty, fibrous, or glandular), skin quality (striae, turgor, thickness, rashes), and the size and sensibility of the nipple-areola complex
- A recent mammogram to rule out breast pathology
- Informed consent, including the risks detailed in what follows
- Routine preoperative anesthesia evaluation

In breast hypertrophy and reduction, several important issues must be taken into consideration. First, breast hypertrophy occurs in all dimensions. A breast reduction technique must be able to manage both the vertical and transverse dimensions in order to obtain the ideal breast shape and to manage ptosis and width, respectively. Reducing a breast in the vertical dimension alone results in a "boxy" appearance. Second, as a breast hypertrophies, the nipple-areola complex descends, increasing the grade of ptosis. Thus, the sternal-notch (SN) to nipple (N) distance increases disproportionately to the inframammary fold (IMF) to nipple distance. This increase in SN-N to IMF-N ratio make nipple-areola vascularity stable when based on an inferior pedicle technique since even with a large transposition of nipple location, the inferior pedicle may remain relatively short. Third, the use of a pyramidal (central *and* inferior) pedicle ensures maximum support of breast tissue under the nipple-areola complex. This ensures good vascularity in breasts of all sizes, shapes, and degrees of ptosis. Fourth, avoiding undermining of the pyramidal pedicle and superior to the new nipple location (i.e., removing solely a wedge of tissue) ensures adequate vascularity of overlying skin flaps. Fifth, by excising a wedge up to, but not including, the pectoral fascia and with no undermining at this level, nerve supple to the overlying breast is minimally disturbed, helping with skin and nipple-areola sensation. Sixth, in very large breast reductions, particularly in the obese, the roll of tissue lateral to the breast must be addressed since it appears to become part of the reduced breast when the previously larger breast is no longer able to hide this region. We manage this by using a moderate excision of tissue from the breast laterally, liposuction of this lateral roll, and quilting of the lateral tissue to the chest wall to prevent fullness here or movement of the breast pedicle into this area.

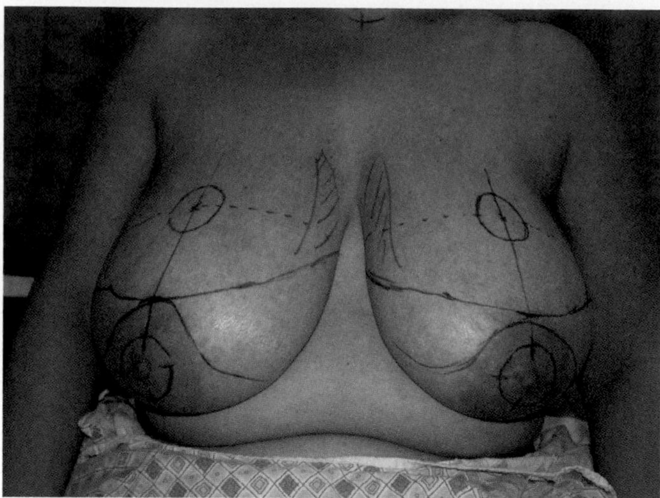

Figure 99.1. Preoperative markings, frontal view, in a 34-year-old woman with bilateral mammary hypertrophy.

Reliable preoperative markings in this technique are important to the outcome, and by making all markings entirely preoperatively, the operation is predictable and expeditious. Initial markings include the vertical and transverse mid-axial lines. The site of the new nipple is drawn on the anterior aspect of the breast at the level of the inframammary fold (*not* a preset distance) along the vertical axis of the breast. A 42-mm cookie cutter is used to size the areola. The superior incision of the wedge resection (creating a 6- to 7-cm flap below the inferior border of the new areola) is drawn. This allows sufficient apron to drape over the new inferior breast pole to hide the horizontal scar. The inferior incision of the wedge resection is drawn below this in a flattened bell-shaped curve just above the inframammary fold (Figs. 99.1 to 99.3). It is important to keep this above the inframammary fold to avoid irritation from brassieres

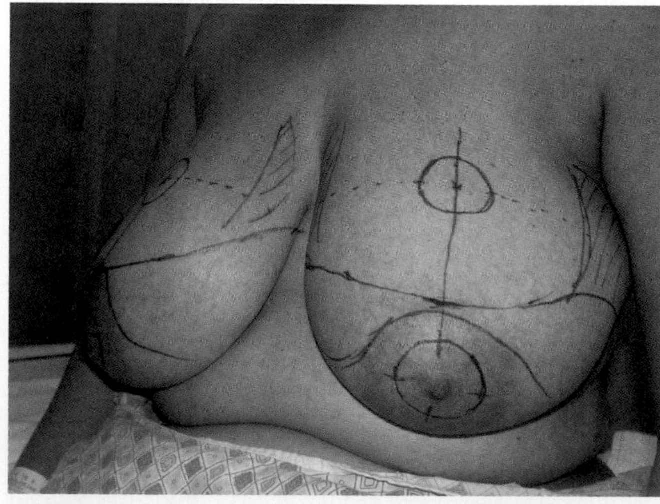

Figure 99.2. Preoperative markings, oblique view.

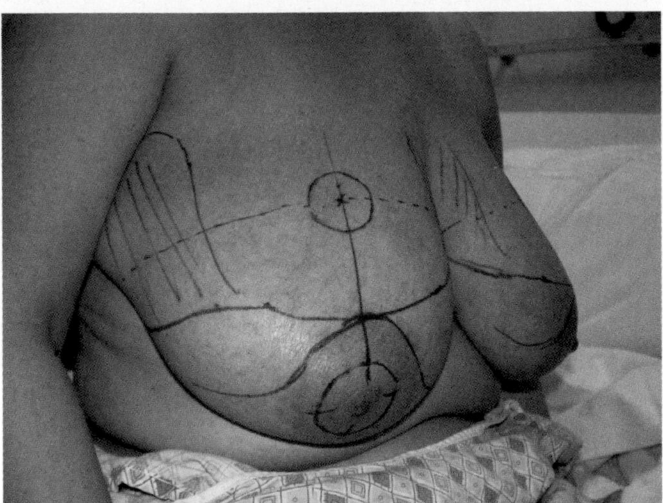

Figure 99.3. Preoperative markings, oblique view.

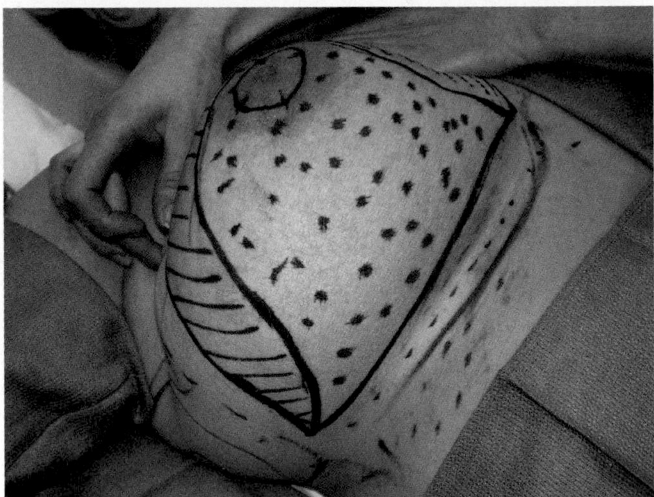

Figure 99.5. The inferior incision is marked above the inframammary fold.

and consequent scar hypertrophy. Neither the inframammary fold nor any ligaments are disturbed, to ensure that "bottoming out" cannot occur. The steep, bell-shaped curve of deepithelialized inferior and central pedicle helps to create a pyramidal pedicle that projects well. A wide deepithelialized pyramidal pedicle with the nipple-areola complex and an additional rim of breast tissue at the apex of bell curve incorporating the full width of the breast are marked. The areola is marked using a 42-mm cookie cutter, to be left intact. Medial and lateral debulking markings are made, and the lateral roll may be marked for liposuction (Figs. 99.4–99.6).

Tumescent solution is injected medially and laterally into regions being resected to reduce blood loss and to firm otherwise redundant tissue, making resection easier. The steep, bell-shaped pyramidal pedicle and new nipple-areola site are deepithelialized, leaving the inframammary fold and 42-mm-diameter nipple-areola complex intact. Marks are scratched in the epidermis of the areola at 12 and 6 o'clock to aid with later positioning. The dermis of the new areola site is incised in a cruciate fashion leaving dermis for later suturing and to maintain a "cushion" for the new areola (Fig. 99.7). Corresponding marks are made in the epidermis at 12 and 6 o'clock to help with inset of the areolae later. The superior incision is made, and the flap is undermined, leaving a 1.5-cm-thick flap up to the horizontal mid-axis of the breast (Fig. 99.8). From this new nipple location, a cut is made straight down to pectoral fascia with no further superior undermining. Avoidance of undermining ensures good skin perfusion and prevents dead space, which can predispose to seroma or hematoma formation. The main breast excision is made en bloc in a transverse inverted-U shape from the lateral, superior, and medial aspects, leaving behind a broad-based pyramidal deepithelialized pedicle (Fig. 99.9). If needed, prior to wedge resections, lateral fold liposuction is performed beyond the edges of the breast tissue to thin the lateral roll, which otherwise becomes more pronounced with the breast reduced. Following this, a larger

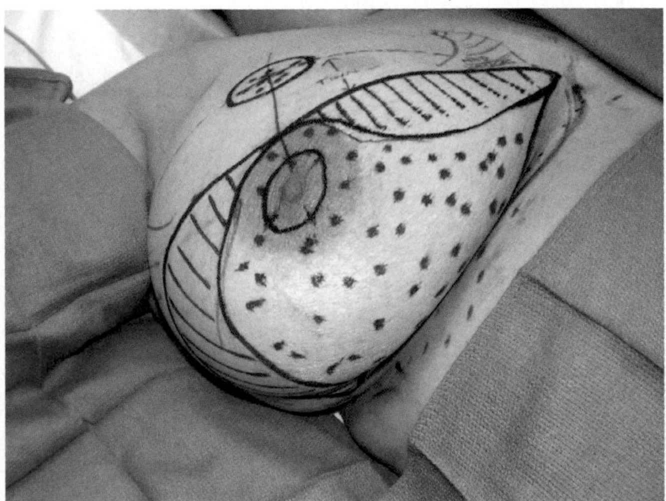

Figure 99.4. The inferior pedicle, excision, and areolae are marked.

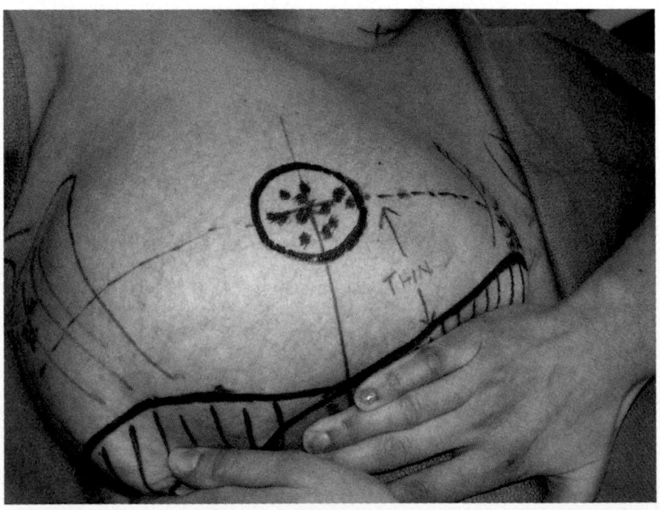

Figure 99.6. A lateral and medial wedge of tissue is marked for direct excision, and the central apron is marked for thinning, as this will overlie the pedicle.

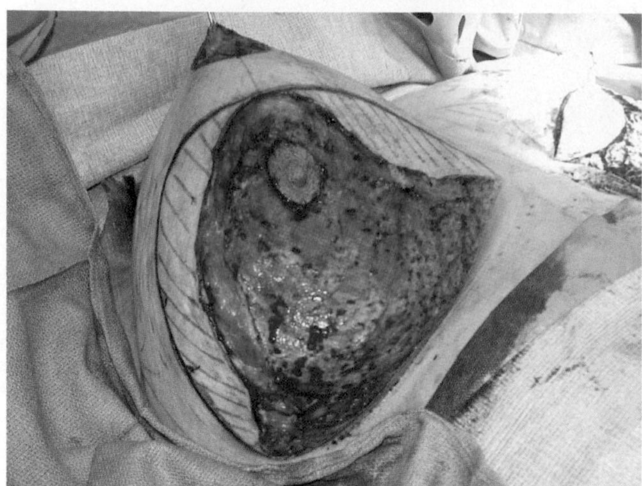

Figure 99.7. The marked incisions made through the dermis, the inferior pedicle, and new nipple-areola complex site are deepithelialized, and a cruciate incision is made at the site of the new areola.

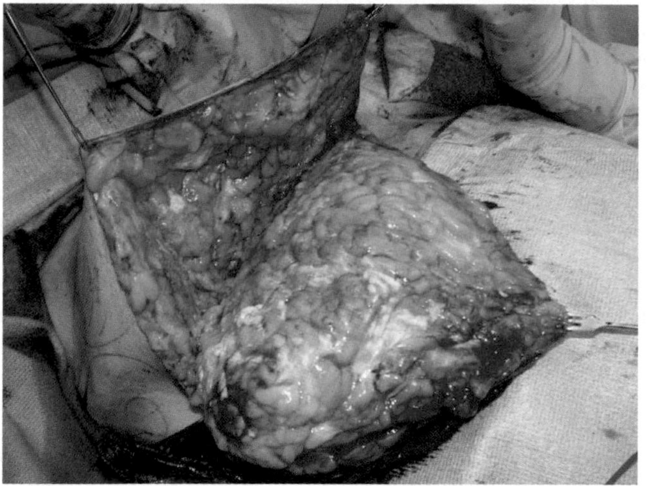

Figure 99.8. The apron of the breast is developed up to the site of the new nipple-areola complex, thinning this flap to cover the inferior pedicle.

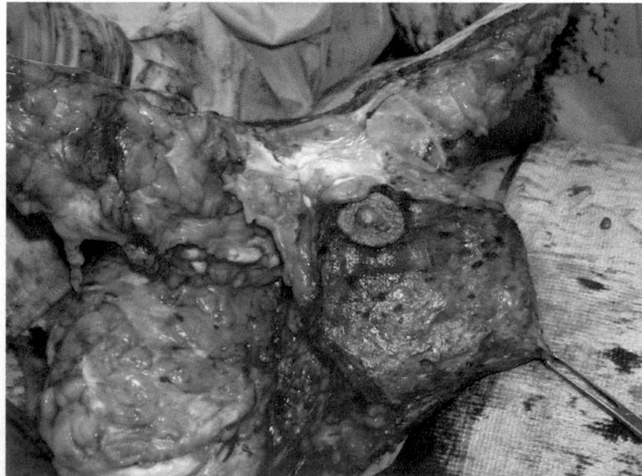

Figure 99.9. An inverted-U transverse breast excision is performed by sharply excising tissue in a plane directly down from the new nipple-areola complex to the chest wall.

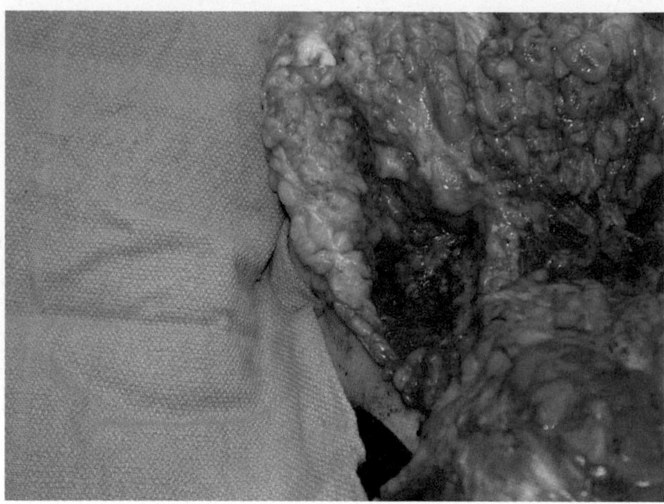

Figure 99.10. A larger lateral wedge excision with liposuction of the roll lateral to breast parenchyma is performed to reduce the horizontal dimension of the breast and minimize the lateral roll of the breast; lateral quilting sutures may be placed.

lateral wedge (Fig. 99.10) and a smaller medial wedge (Fig. 99.11) are then excised from the remaining breast. This helps to reduce the transverse diameter of the breast. Now, there remain thinned flap with a hole for the new nipple-areola complex, a superior flap narrowed in the transverse dimension, and a deepithelialized, broad, pyramidal (central and inferior) pedicle based along the entire inframammary fold. All tissue is now sent to pathology (Fig. 99.12). Lateral quilting sutures are used to obliterate dead space and further narrow the transverse diameter of the breast. Complete separation between the new, smaller breast mound and any residual excess tissue in the lateral roll area prevents the lateral roll tissue from appearing to be part of the breast, which causes an aesthetic broad, boxy appearance. No special manipulation of the central breast parenchyma containing the nipple-areolar complex is done,

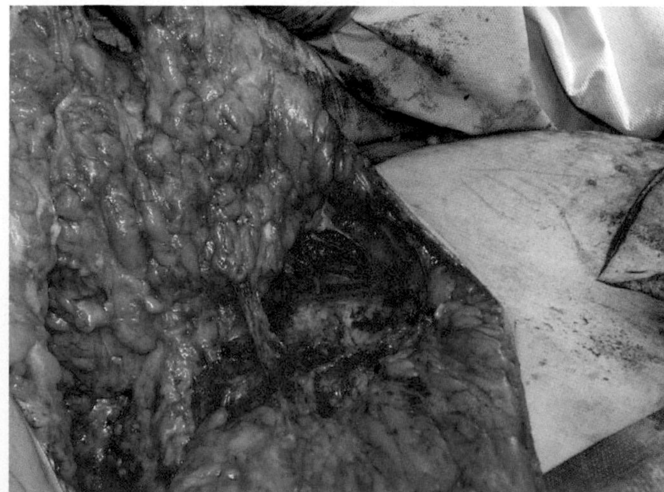

Figure 99.11. A small medial wedge excision is performed to reduce the horizontal dimension of the breast without flattening the medial pole, reducing the "boxy" appearance.

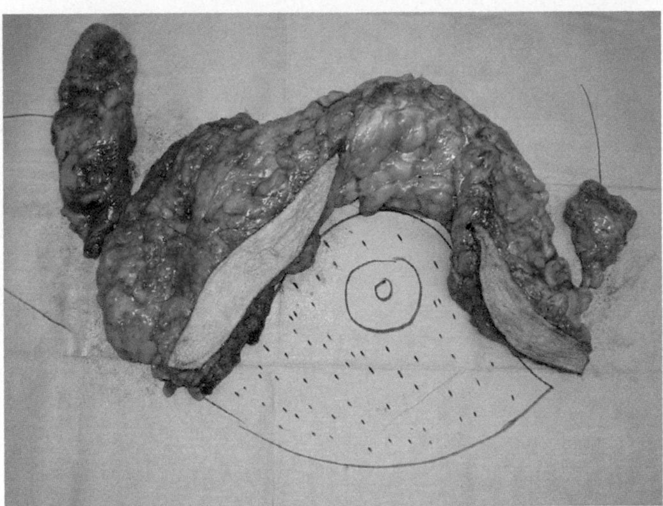

Figure 99.12. Excised inverted U of tissue from the right breast (1,290 g).

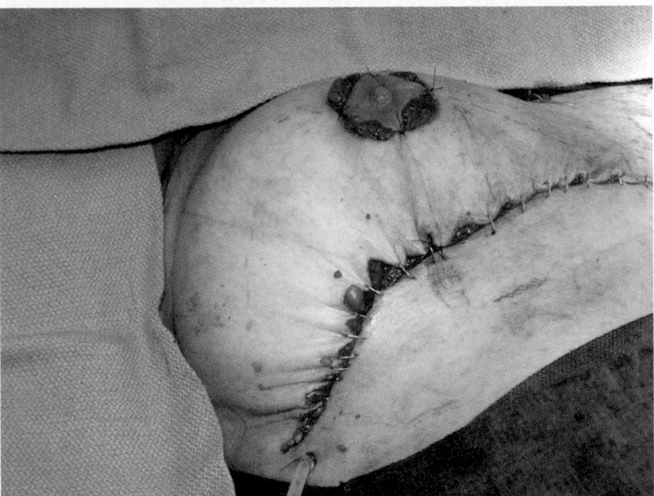

Figure 99.14. A drain is brought out laterally, and tacking staples are placed to minimize dog-ears prior to final closure.

and no breast tissue is resected superior to the site of the new nipple-areolar complex within the apron flap (in contrast to the procedure of Ribeiro, who reshapes the remaining breast). A suction drain is placed laterally from each breast.

The superior apron flap is then brought down over the inferior pedicle and preliminarily stapled while the nipple-areola complex is sutured in place with interrupted and then running absorbable sutures (Figs. 99.13 and 99.14). The redundancy of the longer superior flap is worked centrally to minimize "dog-ears," and a running suture is placed along this pleating, which resolves as healing and contraction occur (Fig. 99.15). The postoperative appearance is shown in Figures 99.16 to 99.19.

This technique causes minimal distortion to the remaining breast tissue as there is no internal rearrangement, shaping, or deep suturing. It also minimally disturbs the neurovascular supply though the pedicle, thereby alleviating any need for a free nipple graft. A free nipple graft has never been required even with very large reductions of greater than 3 kg per side. In addition, the broad pyramidal (central and inferior) pedicle allows for lactation. The undisturbed inframammary fold, intact ligaments and ducts, and broad central/pyramidal pedicle prevent "bottoming out" of the remaining breast tissue. This tends to occur if a narrow, thin, inferior dermal pedicle is used in which most of the normal ligaments and ducts are removed, thus weakening the support of the breast so that the weight of the remaining superior breast eventually descends.

A number of authors describe similar techniques of breast reduction to avoid vertical scars.

Savaci (32) describes a central pedicle technique that avoids a vertical scar, similar to the procedure of Passot. Savaci describes a resection that "will resemble a slice of melon" being taken from between a superior incision and the inframammary sulcus. This technique also necessitates a 6-cm distance between the new and old areola sites. In contrast to the aforementioned technique, however, this method skeletonizes the breast tissue in a conical shape, basing nipple-areola complex vascularity and innervation on pectoral perforators.

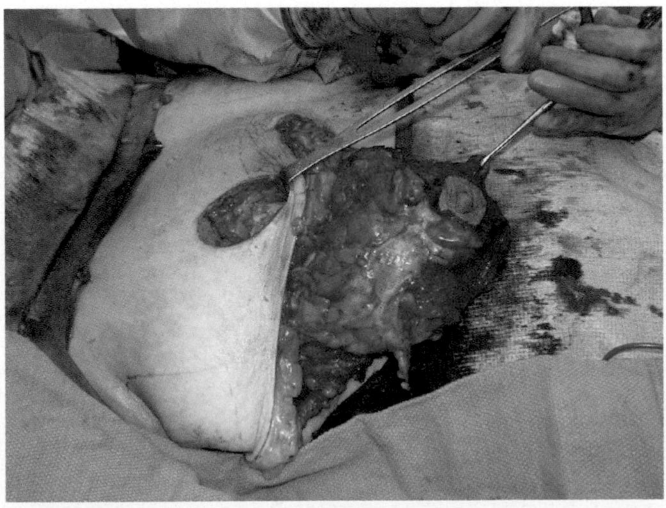

Figure 99.13. The pedicle is placed beneath the apron flap.

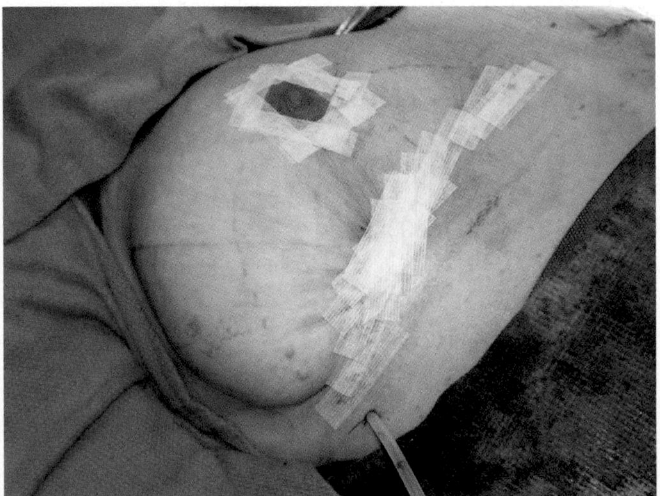

Figure 99.15. The skin is closed with interrupted, then running intradermal sutures, and Steri-Strips are placed on the incisions.

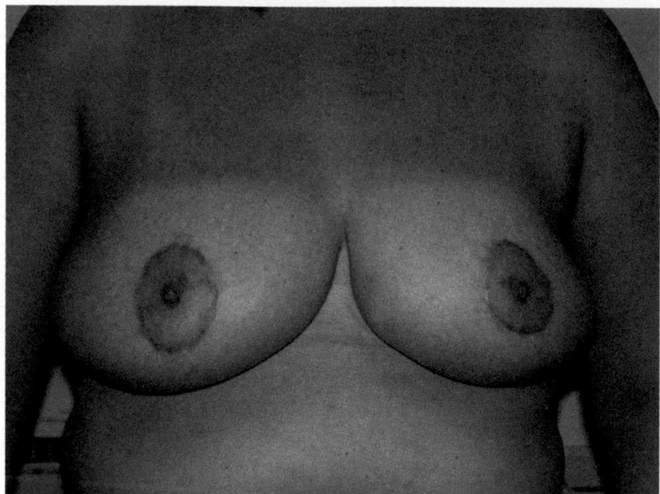

Figure 99.16. Postoperative appearance at 8 months (excision right 1,290 g; excision left 1,095 g; with additional bilateral 450-g lateral liposuction) (frontal view).

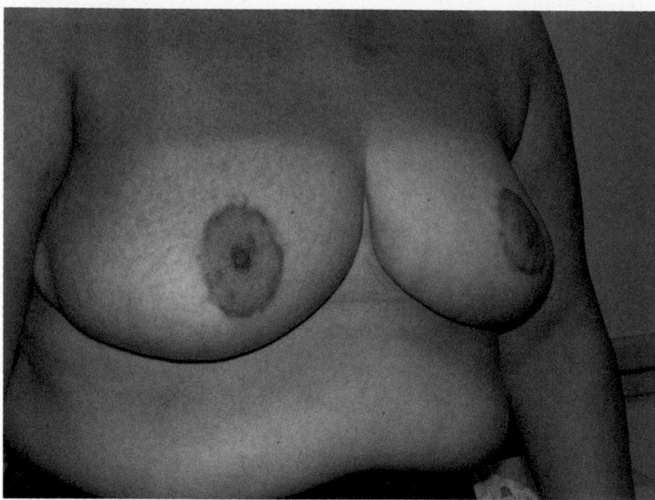

Figure 99.18. Postoperative appearance at 8 months, oblique view.

Lalonde et al. (6,33) explain their breast reduction using an inferior pedicle for large, ptotic breasts. They refer to the ideal candidate as having considerable ptosis and 5 cm between the lower edge of the new areola and the upper edge of the pigmented areola skin. In patients with less distance below the new areola site, they elevate the scar and deepithelialize less tissue inferiorly, hide the pale areola skin in the inframammary fold, or wedge out the residual areola skin in a short vertical scar. Key differences from the method given here include a 17-cm inferiorly directed curved incision directly in the inframammary fold to minimize its visibility; internal shaping with "pillar sutures" to improve projection; and emphasis on minimization of tension in the periareolar incision by cutting a smaller hole in the breast flap than the cut-out areola.

Thomas et al. (7) describe their experience with very large and very ptotic breasts using a "design-enhanced breast reduction" involving no vertical scar. This technique was developed due to problems with prior procedures, including fat necrosis, skin and nipple necrosis, shaping difficulties, decreased nipple sensation, and bleeding. They describe a technique similar to our no-vertical-scar breast reduction, in which they use a wide-based glandular deepithelialized pedicle, preservation of the fourth intercostal nerves, mesial advancement of thick skin flaps, and the use of tumescence. Similar to Lalonde's method, the design-enhanced reduction utilizes an inferior incision in the inframammary fold.

Keskin et al. (30) recently published their experience with breast reductions avoiding a vertical scar in 145 patients. Their central pedicle technique pre-sites the nipple and inframammary folds at 19 to 21 cm and 6 cm below this, respectively. In addition, they conically shape the pedicle. Their results demonstrate good results despite large reductions (average, 1,073 g excised bilaterally) and excellent maintenance of a circular areola.

Other authors (34,35) have modified the long-standing amputation with free nipple-areola grafting technique of breast reduction in order to eliminate the vertical scar. This has the merit of being a rapid operation with little blood loss. By use of a backfolded dermoglandular flap deepithelialized from the edge of the superior flap, projection can be maintained.

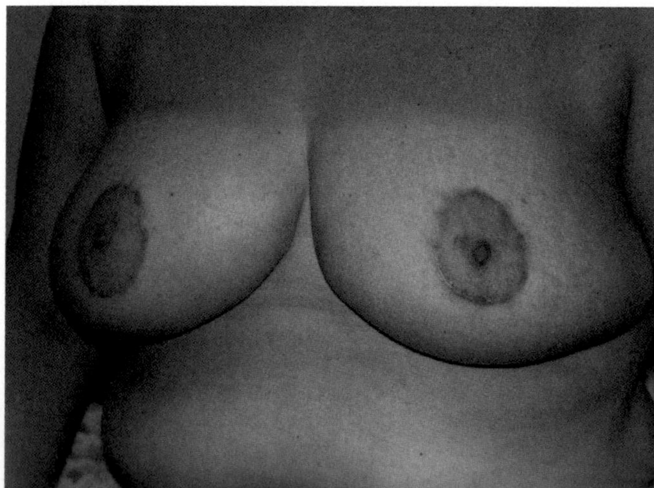

Figure 99.17. Postoperative appearance at 8 months, oblique view.

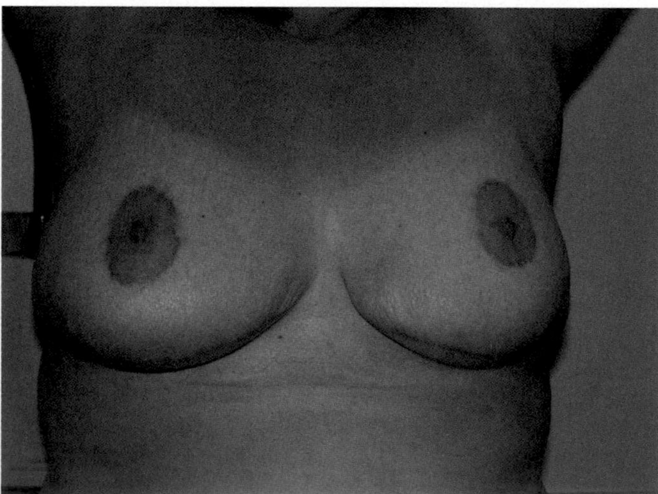

Figure 99.19. Postoperative appearance at 8 months, arms lifted.

However, in general, ideal cosmetic outcomes remain difficult to achieve in this operation.

INTRAOPERATIVE AND POSTOPERATIVE CARE

Intraoperative care and precautions are similar to those for other breast operations. Patients are positioned supine with arms extended on arm boards. Patients are intubated and receive cephalosporin prophylactic antibiotics, pneumatic compression boots, and padding of prominent pressure areas. The procedure takes approximately 2 hours.

Postoperatively, patients are admitted to a routine surgical floor overnight, diet advanced, and transitioned from intravenous to oral pain medications. Bilateral drains are removed on postoperative day 1, and patients are typically discharged that morning.

Patients are allowed to shower at 24 hours. They continue to wear a firm bra (without an underwire) at all times for several weeks. Routine follow-up is at 1 to 2 weeks post-surgery. Heavy lifting and exercise are allowed to resume at 2 weeks.

CASES

We favor the no-vertical-scar breast reduction technique in a number of specific situations. First, it is a safe and reliable technique for very large breast reductions. Due to the pyramidal nature of the pedicle in which the inferior nipple-areola complex pedicle is not undermined, vascular supply to the nipple is maintained, alleviating the need for free nipple grafting, which may be required in large reductions using other methods (Fig. 99.20). Second, this technique is most useful in those patients with significant ptosis. In these patients the majority of tissue resection is required in the vertical dimension, making them ideally suited to a horizontal incision method. Furthermore, the lack of disturbance of the support structures of the inframammary fold makes this method less apt to "bottom out" in these patients (Fig. 99.21). Third, we like this technique of breast reduction for patients requiring symmetry procedures after a contralateral TRAM breast reconstruction. Patients must still qualify with significant ptotic hypertrophy. Autologously reconstructed breasts are often flatter and broader than the unreconstructed counterpart, and the no-vertical-scar technique tends to produce a slightly flatter breast that better matches the reconstructed side (Fig. 99.22).

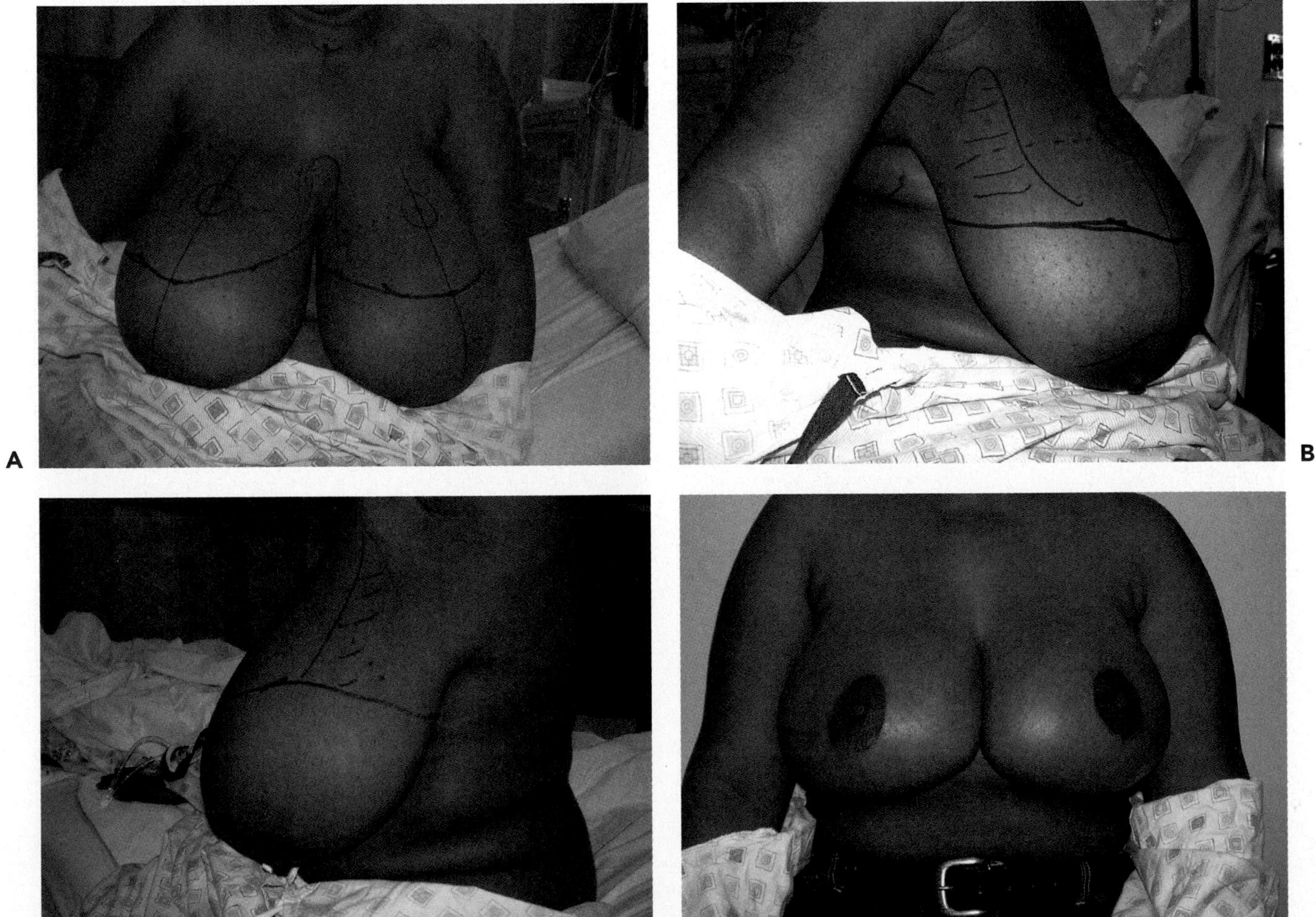

Figure 99.20. The no-vertical-scar breast reduction is useful for very large breast reductions. **A–C:** Preoperative appearance of a 40-year-old woman; sternal notch-to-nipple distance is 47 cm bilaterally. **D–F:** Postoperative appearance at 3 months, with breast reduction of 2,165 g on the right and 2,370 g on the left. (*continued*)

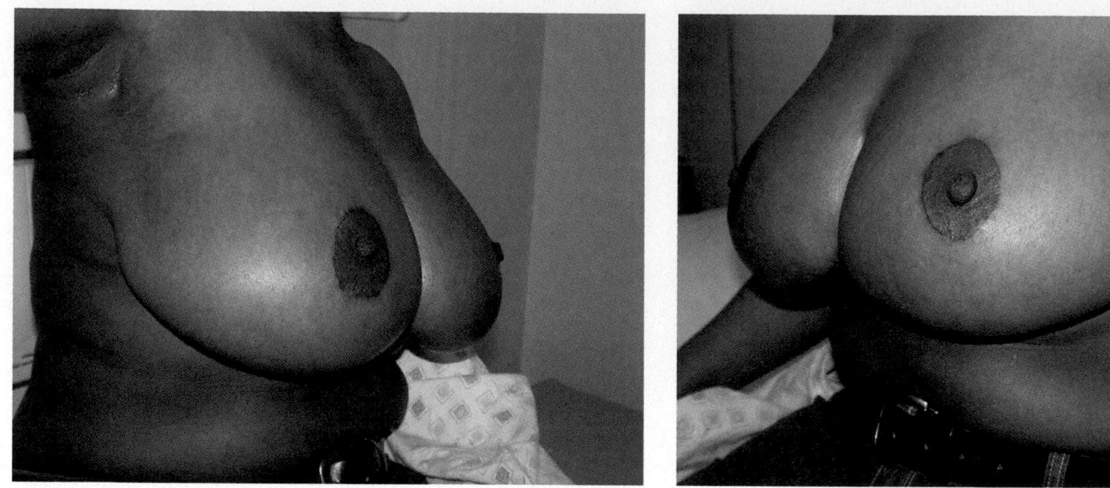

Figure 99.20. (*Continued*)

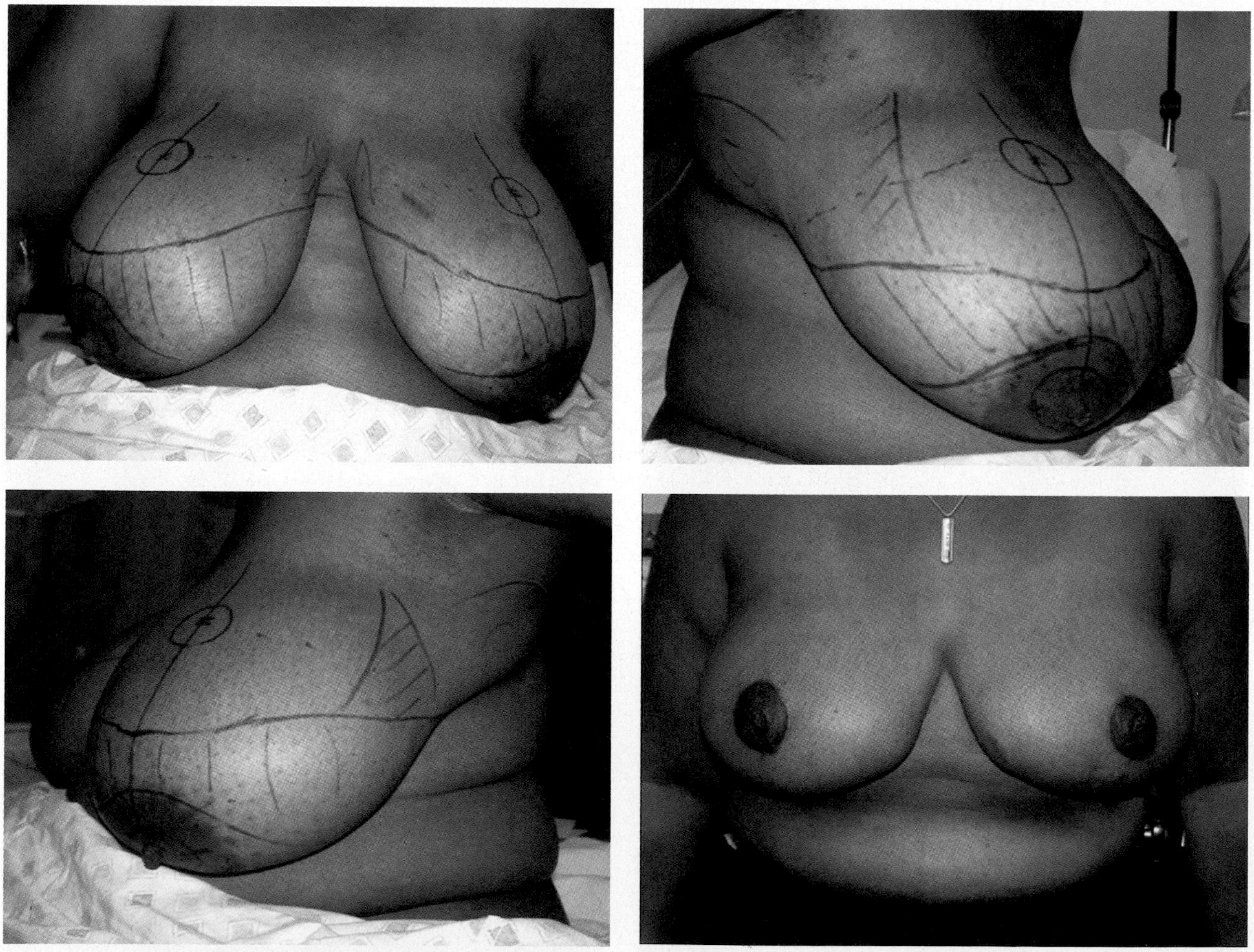

Figure 99.21. The no-vertical-scar breast reduction is especially useful and only possible in cases with significant breast ptosis. **A–C:** Preoperative appearance of a 38-year-old woman with grade 3 ptosis. **D–F:** Postoperative appearance at 6 weeks, with breast reduction of 1,600 g on the right and 1,590 g on the left with 250-g liposuction. (*continued*)

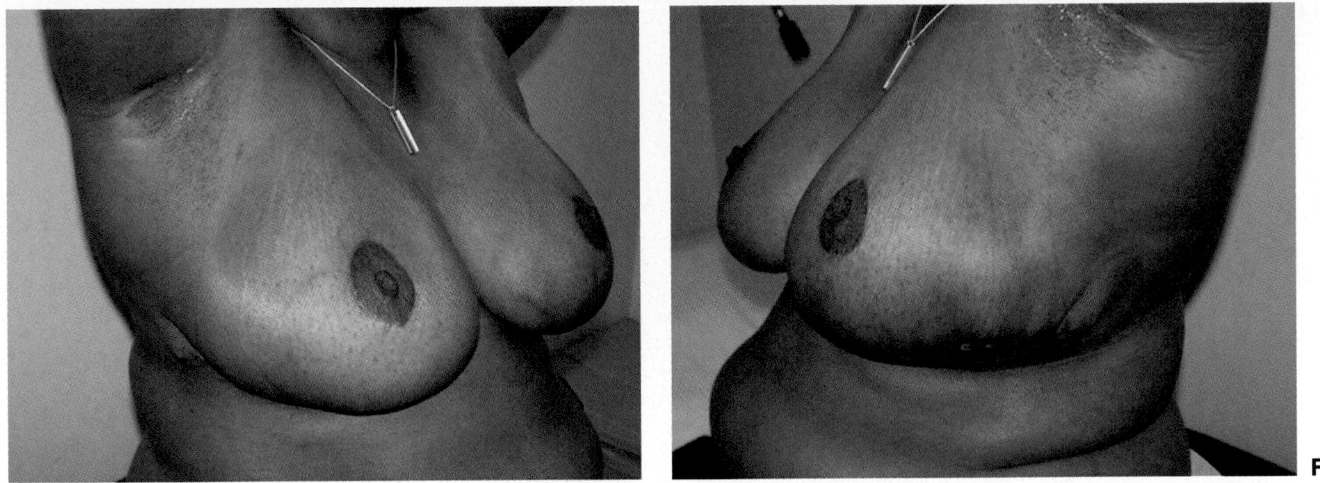

Figure 99.21. (*Continued*)

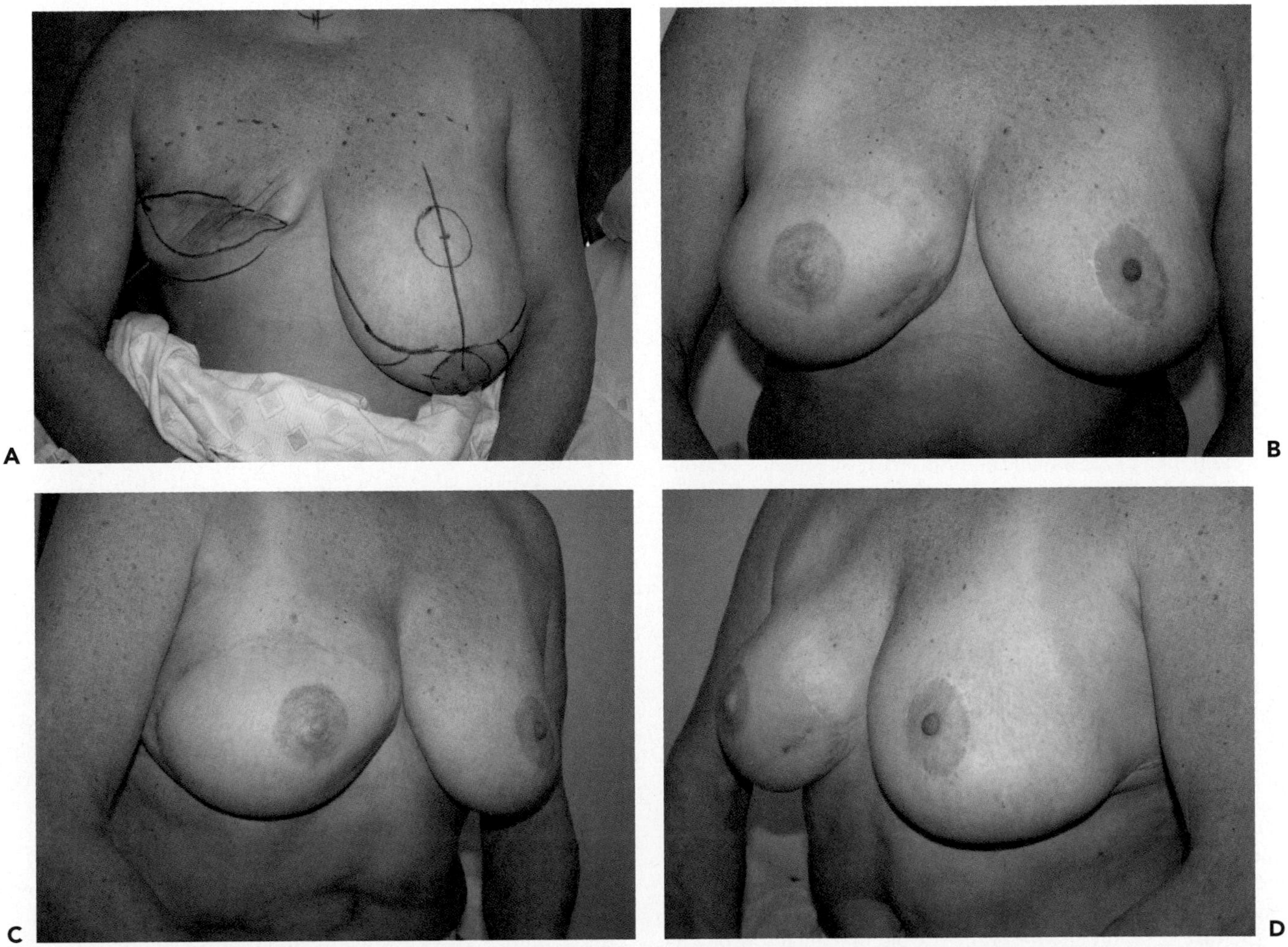

Figure 99.22. The no-vertical-scar breast reduction may be used to gain excellent symmetry when matching a contralateral autologous breast reconstruction. **A:** Preoperative appearance of a 49-year-old woman. **B–D**: Postoperative appearance at 2 years.

RISKS

Risks for breast reductions without a vertical scar are comparable to those for other common methods of breast reduction. Perioperative and intraoperative risks include anesthetic risks, significant bleeding, hematoma, seroma, infection, fat or skin necrosis, areolar pigment changes, nipple-areola necrosis, changes in sensation, and wound-healing problems. As with any bilateral and soft tissue operation, postoperative risks of asymmetry, dissatisfaction with breast size, scarring, and keloid formation exist.

Overall, the lack of a vertical scar is favorable in reducing several risks common to other methods of breast reduction. Damage to the vascularity and nerve supply of the nipple-areola complex is rare, given the pyramidal pedicle, which does not violate the pectoral fascia or neurovascular structures entering the complex from deep. Due to the lack of a vertical incision bearing tension from the breast parenchyma, wound dehiscence (which is relatively common at the T-junction of a Wise-pattern breast reduction) is rare. In addition, due to the hidden location of the scars, unsightly scarring is less obvious and obtrusive.

OUTCOME DATA

Although nonrandomized, we have found a lower rate of routine complications; including significantly less hematoma formation, and trends toward less wound dehiscence and scar hypertrophy. This is in spite of patient selection bias making this technique more popular for patients who were more obese and more ptotic and required larger resections (5).

Pseudoptosis or "bottoming out," which is frequently written about in forms of inverted-T scar breast reductions, is rarely seen in the no-vertical-scar methods, even after extended follow-up (36). Furthermore, the bell-shaped incision *superior* to the inframammary fold allows operative versatility and good nipple projection and reduces pseudoptosis by keeping the inframammary fold intact. Our long-term results have consistently demonstrated stable long-term outcomes. However, in spite of breast reduction surgery, the breast will continue to age, and the natural progression of ongoing ptosis will still occur.

One key paper directly compares patient satisfaction in 29 patients who underwent reduction with a no-vertical -scar technique against 2 patients with an inverted-T scar technique. They state a significantly higher satisfaction with scars and a higher postoperative activity level in the no-vertical-scar group. However, the inverted-T-scar patients rated nipple position as better. Groups rated their overall aesthetic satisfaction similarly (14).

Some authors mention that the transverse scar can end up too lateral on the chest wall (6). This is especially true in obese patients with fat rolls extending onto the back (5). Lalonde minimizes this occurrence by marking the medial edge of this incision below the visible cleavage crease and keeping the incision length to 17 cm along an inferiorly curved incision similar to the wire in an underwire bra. We avoid making a scar far laterally by managing this lateral tissue with liposuction and quilting of the lateral tissues.

Other authors have criticized the no-vertical-scar techniques as leading to a "boxy" appearance. This is especially true when medial and lateral resections are insufficient to narrow the base of the breast. Adequately resecting medial and lateral tissue, liposuctioning, and quilting lateral tissue narrows the transverse diameter of the breast, thereby minimizing this problem.

Medial and lateral dog-ears can be a problem (6). This is best dealt with by gathering the vertical pleating in the transverse incision toward the center of the incisions (5,7). This problem is unique to methods in which the horizontal scar remains low on the chest wall causing a discrepancy between superior and inferior incision lengths. We find that these pleated incisions "even out" rapidly during healing and that dog-ears and pleating rarely become a significant problem. Furthermore, dog-ears can be easily revised under local anesthetic in the office if necessary.

Horizontal scar hypertrophy is reduced by placing the incision above the line of the inframammary fold, avoiding irritation from clothing and brassieres.

One paper describes two cases of skin loss on the infra-areola skin. The authors ascribe this to thinning the skin apron flap too much and do not report a case after their first year of experience (6). We maximize perfusion to the nipple-areolar complex and skin by avoiding undermining, ensuring thick skin flaps, and using a central and inferior pyramidal pedicle based on the entire inframammary fold.

CONCLUSION

Over the last 90 years, various methods of breast reduction have been developed and modified to eliminate the need for a vertical scar. We have found the no-vertical-scar breast reduction to be particularly useful in *large ptotic breasts*, allowing excellent breast size and shape with minimized scarring, normal nipple vascularity and sensation, good projection, a stable inframammary fold, the ability to lactate, and structural stability over time. It is easy to perform, reproducible, simple to teach, and expeditious and has an acceptable rate of complications.

ACKNOWLEDGMENTS

We thank Anne Fladger and Meaghan Muir for their invaluable help in obtaining articles.

EDITORIAL COMMENTS

Conspicuous in the last edition of this text was the absence of a chapter on breast reduction without a vertical scar. Over the last few decades, as described by the authors, several surgeons have independently reported similar concepts of reducing the breast primarily through an inframammary incision, bringing the nipple-areola out through a buttonhole at some prescribed distance from the fold on a superiorly based skin flap. I think that is fair to say that these different techniques have never achieved much of a following or otherwise caught on widely. That is particularly surprising in light of the compelling arguments made in this chapter by Talbot and Pribaz.

The technique described here is appropriate for particularly large breasts where there is sufficient skin available below the new nipple site and above the old areola to provide at least 5 cm and preferably 7 to 8 cm of unpigmented skin. Inherent to the design is the tendency to create a short, wide, and somewhat boxy-looking breast. Hence the authors emphasize contouring and shaping the inferior/central pedicle, which is inherent to the technique.

The irony with this technique is that it runs pretty much contrary to current trends. Those trends include superior, medial, and/or central pedicles. In addition, the move toward vertical scars in lieu of inframammary scars, and finally the emphasis on narrowing, shaping, and even coning the breast using glandular pillars and parenchymal sutures.

The group that would seem the most appropriate for this approach is made up of women with very large breasts often with an obese body habitus. This approach would be an alternative to a free-nipple graft or risky long pedicle of one design or another. The trade-off using this method seems to be creating a wide, short, and somewhat flat-appearing breast but avoiding nipple-areola hypopigmentation or possible total loss.

The argument as to scars versus shape continues. There are those who seek to avoid a scar in the fold and evidently those who want to avoid a vertical scar.

From my perspective, having followed these discussions for many years, I would argue the following points. First and foremost, shape, consistency/predictability, and safety trump all other considerations. Second, the most important scar is the one around the areola. The scar around the areola is the one that is the most visible and most important. Third, surgeons have made the inframammary scar excessively and unnecessarily long. The proponents of the vertical techniques have shown us that the breast can be reduced without the need for such long inframammary fold scars. Fourth, in the vast majority of cases, the vertical scar is not objectionable or even important. Fifth, many breast reduction techniques continue to produce unattractive results with breasts that are excessively wide and short.

Thus, the best argument for the "no-vertical-scar" technique is not avoiding the vertical scar, but creating a better circumareolar scar and reducing the risk of nipple loss or hypopigmentation in the high-risk patient who otherwise might be a candidate for a free-nipple graft technique.

S.L.S.

REFERENCES

1. National Clearinghouse of Plastic Surgery Statistics. *2008 Report of the 2007 Statistics.* Arlington Heights, IL: American Society of Plastic Surgeons; 2008.
2. Thoma A, Sprague S, Veltri K, et al. A prospective study of patients undergoing breast reduction surgery: health-related quality of life and clinical outcomes. *Plast Reconstr Surg* 2007;120:13–26.
3. Celebiler O, Sonmez A, Erdim M, et al. Patients" and surgeons" perspectives on the scar components after inferior pedicle breast reduction surgery. *Plast Reconstr Surg* 2005;116: 459–464.
4. Spear SL, ed. *Surgery of the Breast: Principles and Art.* 2nd ed. Philadelphia: Lippincott Williams & Wilkins; 2006.
5. Movassaghi K, Liao EC, Ting V, et al. Eliminating the vertical scar in breast reduction: Boston modification of the Robertson technique. *Aesthet Surg J* 2006;26:687–696.
6. Lalonde DH, Lalonde J, French R. The no vertical scar breast reduction: a minor variation that allows to remove vertical scar portion of the inferior pedicle Wise pattern T scar. *Aesthet Plast Surg* 2003;27:335–344.
7. Thomas WO, Moline S, Harris CN. Design-enhanced breast reduction: an approach for very large, very ptotic breasts without a vertical incision. *Ann Plast Surg* 1998;40:229–234.
8. Giovanoli P, Meuli-Simmen C, Meyer VE, et al. Which technique for which breast? A prospective study of different techniques of reduction mammaplasty. *Br J Plast Surg* 1999;52:52–59.
9. Yousif NJ, Larson DL, Sanger JR, et al. Elimination of the vertical scar in reduction mammaplasty. *Plast Reconstr Surg* 1992;89:459–467.
10. Thorne C, Grabb WC, Smith JW. *Grabb and Smith's Plastic Surgery.* 6th ed. Philadelphia: Wolters Kluwer Health/Lippincott Williams & Wilkins; 2007.
11. Schwarzman E, Goldan S, Wilflingseder P. The classic reprint. Die Technik der Mammaplastik (the technique of mammaplasty). *Plast Reconstr Surg* 1977;59:107–112.
12. Wise RJ. A preliminary report on a method of planning the mammaplasty. *Plast Reconstr Surg* 1956;17:367–375.
13. Lassus C. A 30-year experience with vertical mammaplasty. *Plast Reconstr Surg* 1996;97: 373–380.
14. Hosnuter M, Tosun Z, Kargi E, et al. No vertical scar technique versus inverted T-scar technique in reduction mammoplasty: a two-centre comparative study. *Aesthet Surg J* 2005;29: 496–502.
15. Greer SE. *Handbook of Plastic Surgery.* New York: Marcel Dekker; 2004.
16. Benelli L. A new periareolar mammaplasty: the "round block" technique. *Aesthet Surg J* 1990;14:93–100.
17. Lejour M, Abboud M, Declety A, et al. Reduction of mammaplasty scars: from a short inframammary scar to a vertical scar. *Ann Chir Plast Esthet* 1990;35:369–379.
18. Lejour M. Pedicle modification of the Lejour vertical scar reduction mammaplasty. *Plast Reconstr Surg* 1998;101:1149–1150.
19. Hall-Findlay EJ. A simplified vertical reduction mammaplasty: shortening the learning curve. *Plast Reconstr Surg* 1999;104:748–759.
20. Ramirez OM. Reduction mammaplasty with the "owl" incision and no undermining. *Plast Reconstr Surg* 2002;109:512–522.
21. Passot R. La correction esthetique du prolapsus mammarie par le procede de la transposition du mamelon. *Presse Med* 1925;33:317.
22. Ribeiro L. A new technique for reduction mammaplasty. *Plast Reconstr Surg* 1975;55: 330–334.
23. Robertson DC. The technique of inferior flap mammaplasty. *Plast Reconstr Surg* 1967;40: 372–377.
24. Smith GA, Schmidt GH. Experience with the Ribeiro reduction mammaplasty technique. *Ann Plast Surg* 1979;3:260–263.
25. Maliniac J. Evaluation of principal mamma-plastic procedures. *Plast Reconstr Surg* (1946) 1949;4:359–373.
26. Conway H. Mammaplasty; analysis of 110 consecutive cases with end-results. *Plast Reconstr Surg* (1946) 1952;10:303–315.
27. Ribeiro L, Accorsi A Jr, Buss A, et al. Creation and evolution of 30 years of the inferior pedicle in reduction mammaplasties. *Plast Reconstr Surg* 2002;110:960–970.
28. Hurst LN, Evans HB, Murray KA. Inferior flap reduction mammaplasty with pedicled nipple. *Ann Plast Surg* 1983;10:483–485.
29. Yousif NJ, Larson DL. The apron technique of reduction mammaplasty: elimination of the vertical scar. *Perspect Plast Surg* 1994;8:137–144.
30. Keskin M, Tosun Z, Savaci N. Seventeen years of experience with reduction mammaplasty avoiding a vertical scar. *Aesthet Plast Surg* 2008;32:653–659.
31. Jackson IT, Bayramicli M, Gupta M, et al. Importance of the pedicle length measurement in reduction mammaplasty. *Plast Reconstr Surg* 1999;104:398–400.
32. Savaci N. Reduction mammaplasty by the central pedicle, avoiding the vertical scar. *Aesthet Plast Surg* 1996;20:171–175.
33. Nahai F. Breast reduction with no vertical scar. *Aesthet Plast Surg* 2004;28:354.
34. Manstein ME, Manstein CH, Manstein G. Obtaining projection in the amputation free nipple/areolar graft breast reduction without a vertical scar: using breast parenchyma to create a new mound. *Ann Plast Surg* 1997;38:421–424.
35. Aydin H, Bilgin-Karabulut A, Tumerdem B. Free nipple reduction mammaplasty with a horizontal scar in high-risk patients. *Aesthet Plast Surg* 2002;26:457–460.
36. Chalekson CP, Neumeister MW, Zook EG, et al. Outcome analysis of reduction mammaplasty using the modified Robertson technique. *Plast Reconstr Surg* 2002;110:71–79.

CHAPTER

100

Scott L. Spear
M. Renee Jespersen

Breast Reduction With the Free Nipple Graft Technique

HISTORY

Breast reduction with free nipple graft is a powerful technique ideally suited to a specific patient population. Patients who require a large-volume reduction, present a high risk for adverse outcome from a pedicle reduction, and exhibit certain physiologic changes associated with gigantomastia can benefit from this technique.

Adams first presented the free nipple breast reduction for gigantomastia in 1944 (1). The drawbacks of the free nipple technique include the loss of lactation, the short-term loss and variable return of nipple sensation and contractility, common changes in pigmentation, and potential graft failure (2–7). Patients who are ideally suited for this technique therefore are often at increased risk for nipple loss after pedicle reduction, do not have highly sensate and contractile nipples, and are willing to forego breast-feeding. In fact, patients with gigantomastia frequently have poor nipple sensation and contractility, which may improve following free nipple breast reduction (5–7).

Pedicle reduction places the nipple at risk in gigantomastia. In general, nipple necrosis is more common in patients with severe macromastia requiring resections of 1,000 g or more, patients with longer preoperative suprasternal notch-to-nipple distance, obese patients, smokers, and otherwise unhealthy individuals (6,8–11). In gigantomastia, the folding of an excessively long pedicle can compromise circulation and lead to nipple necrosis (11). In pedicle reductions, the distance of the nipple-areola complex (NAC) transposition may be as important in increasing the risk of developing postoperative complications as the volume resected (12). This risk of nipple ischemia and necrosis can be mitigated by the free nipple technique. Blood flow to the areola measured 2 weeks after pedicle reduction is decreased below baseline, while after free nipple graft reduction it is increased (13).

Opponents of the free nipple technique claim the inferior pedicle blood supply is reliable and that nipple-to-inframammary fold (IMF) distance is consistent, regardless of the degree of gigantomastia (14). This statement fails to account for the increased risk of nipple loss in the severely macromastic patient and is counterintuitive because as the sternal notch-to-nipple distance increases, the nipple descends and the skin stretches. It would seem that the greater the descent, the greater is the distance from the IMF. Detractors also criticize the free nipple technique for leaving a flat, boxy-appearing breast due to the loss of central volume, as will any procedure that fails to create a conical breast shape. Simply amputating the inferior breast tissue leaves medial and lateral flaps with thin fat only, as in a large, severely ptotic breast most of the breast parenchyma has descended into the inferior amputated portion (11). Because of this problem, modifications of the free nipple breast reduction technique have been designed to retain parenchymal volume and create projection. Gradinger retains breast tissue in the vicinity of the inferior pole to avoid a boxy, flat appearance in the lower portion of the breast (Fig. 100.1A). He provides breast projection by suturing medial and lateral pillars together when parenchyma is adequate, or by retaining parenchyma between the medial and lateral flaps and imbricating it when there is inadequate parenchyma (15,16). Casas et al. increase the length of the vertical limbs, deepithelialize the additional length, and fold it under the inferior pole (17). Casas et al. also close the vertical limb with a cone deformity at the nipple site to improve nipple projection and suction the lateral breast to enhance contour.

We prefer to retain the parenchymal tissue and dermis between the vertical limbs to create central volume projection (Fig. 100.2). Proponents of the free nipple graft technique argue that over the long term, the breast bottoms out less and maintains shape better than with the pedicle reduction technique because there is no pedicle that can shift or change shape with the passage of time (15,16).

INDICATIONS

The free nipple breast reduction is ideally suited for ptotic gigantomastia when more than 1,000 g is planned on being removed in postmenopausal women with no pleasurable nipple sensation (Fig. 100.3). The procedure plays a role in treating gigantomastia patients with obesity, poor health, or tobacco use, where the NAC has increased risk of necrosis. Some systemic diseases, such as diabetes mellitus, collagen vascular disease, peripheral vascular disease, and rheumatoid arthritis, might affect vascularity and increase risk of nipple loss (9). The free nipple breast reduction can be performed faster than the pedicle reduction, which may be useful in patients at higher risk of anesthetic complications. Breast reduction with free nipple graft is also applicable in special situations, such as repeat reduction mammaplasty with an unknown original pedicle (18) or prior breast biopsy in the vicinity of a proposed pedicle.

In addition to those patients who have medical problems that warrant a free nipple graft reduction, we find that there is a population of patients who may prefer the results offered by this technique. As previously mentioned, patients with gigantomastia may have little to no pleasurable nipple sensation. In this group of patients who are also past childbearing age and desire the most aggressive reduction possible, the free nipple technique offers a distinct advantage. The pedicled technique of breast reduction requires that structural elements of the breast be retained in addition to the tissue supporting the vascular pedicle. Because the free nipple technique allows the

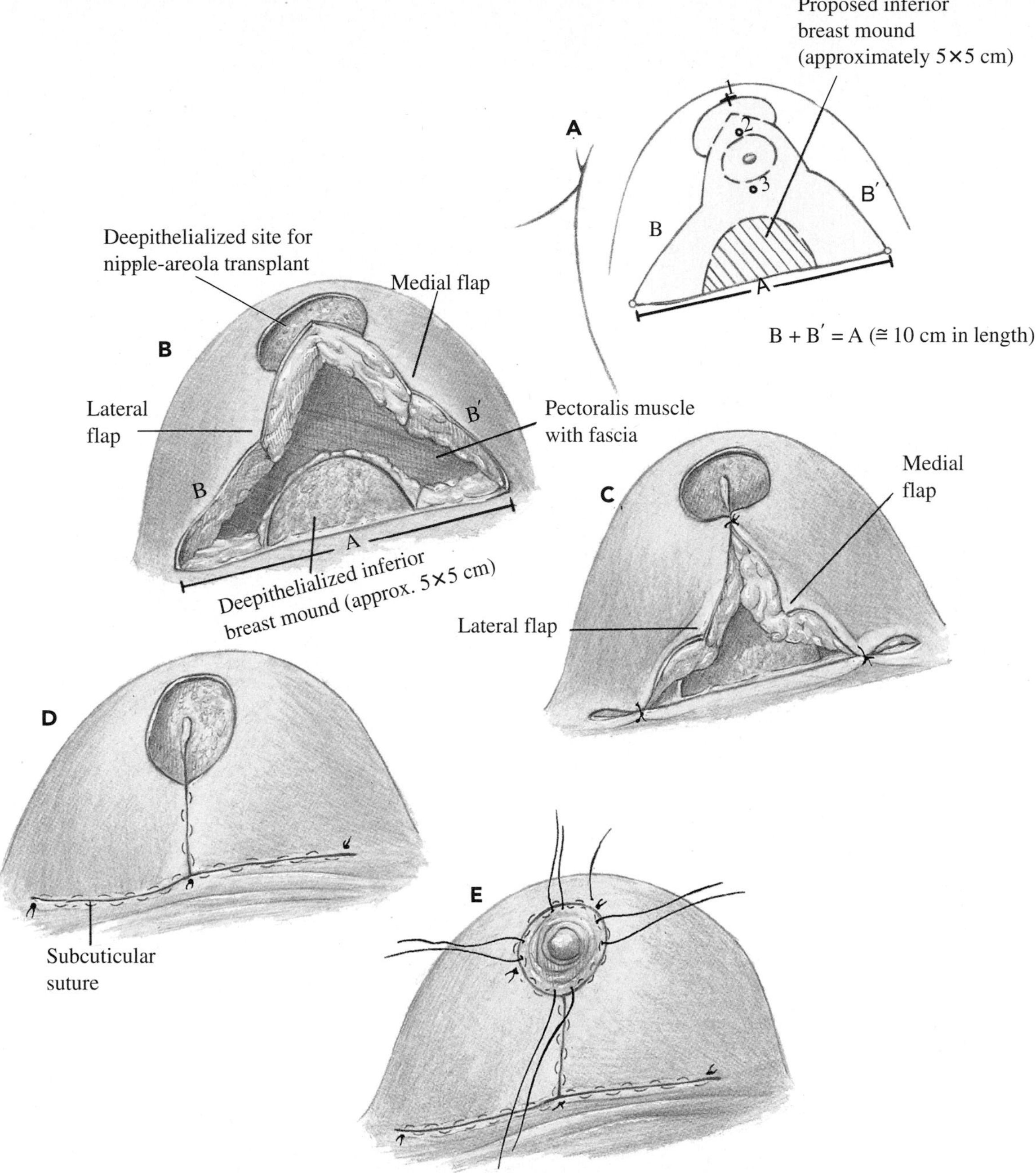

Figure 100.1. Retained inferior breast mound technique. **A:** View of the markings from underneath. Points 1, 2, and 3 correspond to the top of the areola, bottom of the areola, and inferior point of the vertical closure, respectively. Note that B + B′ = A. The lengths B and B′ were determined by how widely the Wise pattern had to be opened so that, when added together, they would be the same length as A. The other point to note on this series of markings is the proposed inferior breast mound, which will act as a buttress. **B:** Resection of the breast tissue in a perpendicular fashion with relation to the flaps and their medial margins and retention of the deepithelialized breast mound. **C:** The initial sutures are shown, and the inferior closure is started at the medial and lateral ends rather than in the middle so any differences can be adjusted without extending the incision. **D, E:** Closure before and after suturing the graft.

surgeon to remove all tissue not contributing to the desired shape and size of the final breast, a greater amount of bulk can be removed than in the pedicled technique. This gives the surgeon more control over the final shape and size of the breast, as well as the ability to cone the parenchyma aggressively without distorting nipple position or compromising pedicle vascularity.

Patients who are offered a free nipple graft reduction as a treatment alternative must understand, however, that return of nipple sensation and contractility is not guaranteed and that no chance of breast-feeding remains. In addition, they must understand that the grafting procedure can also fail, and that color and texture changes are still possible drawbacks even when it is successful.

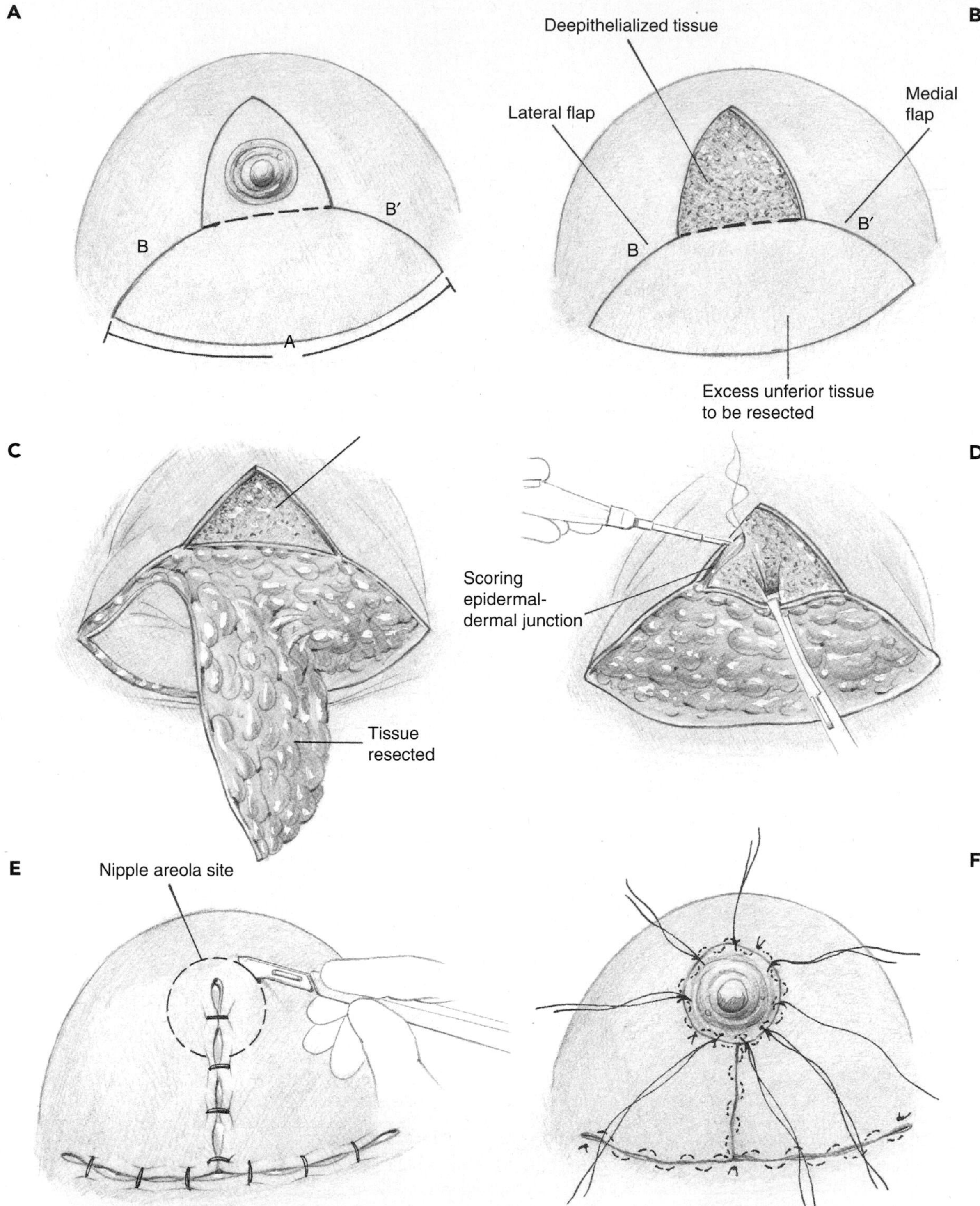

Figure 100.2. Infolding tissue between vertical limbs technique. **A:** The length of the horizontal limbs should equal the length of the incision along the inframammary fold. Note that B + B′ = A. **B:** The area between the vertical limbs is deepithelialized after the nipple-areola complex (NAC) graft is removed and saved. **C:** The excess tissue below the horizontal limbs is resected, leaving ample tissue between the vertical limbs. **D:** The epidermal–dermal junction is scored along the vertical limbs with the electrocautery unit. **E:** The NAC site is deepithelialized after marking with a 42-mm cookie cutter while the patient is upright, and then it is bilaterally reduced and temporarily closed with staples. **F:** The 4-0 silk tie is sutured through the graft and the breast skin edge to anchor the graft to the dermal platform. The vertical and horizontal skin edges are closed with a deep, interrupted 3-0 Monocryl and a running, subcuticular 3-0 Monocryl.

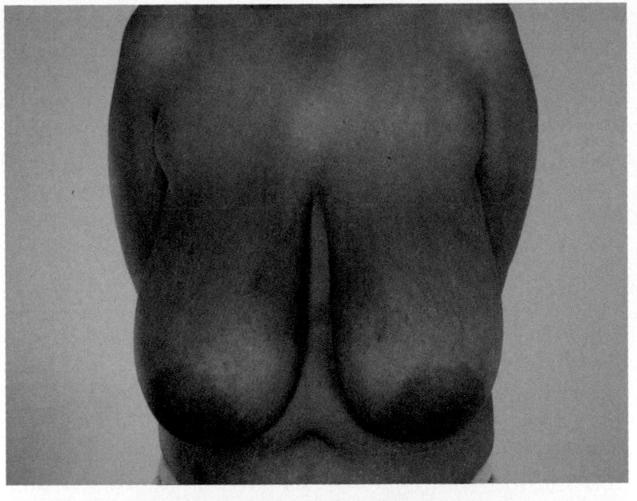

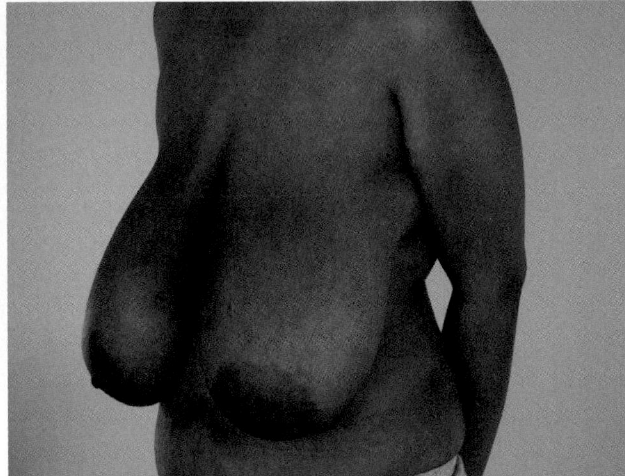

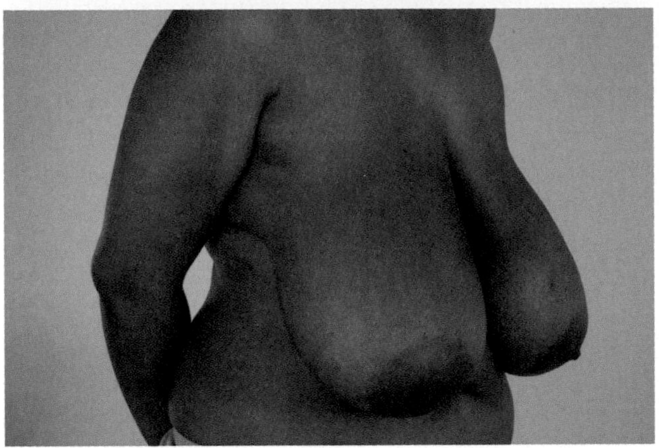

Figure 100.3. The patient is an obese 34-year-old woman with a 42F bra size, an appropriate candidate for the free nipple graft technique.

CONTRAINDICATIONS

The free nipple graft breast reduction is contraindicated in women of childbearing age who hope to breast-feed and in women who want to preserve existing erotic nipple sensation and erectility. Darker-skinned women should be counseled about hypopigmentation of the nipple after free nipple graft, although microinjection of pigment (tattoo) may improve areas of hypopigmentation. Punch grafts from the areola to the nipple have also been shown to be effective at correcting hypopigmentation.

PREOPERATIVE PLANNING

The preoperative consultation includes obtaining a medical history with emphasis on the patient's desires and goals related to breast reduction. The physical examination includes measuring height, weight, breast size, ptosis, nipple-to-fold distance, symmetry, upper pole volume, fold height, body habitus, skin quality, nipple projection, and sensation. Patient expectations and risks should be reviewed with the patient as part of the informed-consent process. The patient should expect smaller breasts with scars and altered nipples/areolas. Loss of the ability to breast-feed, change in nipple sensation, loss of nipple erection, possible hypopigmentation, and possible nipple loss should be discussed.

During surgical marking, the patient should be upright. The landmarks are identified and marked, including the midline from the suprasternal notch toward the umbilicus, the IMF continuously across the midline, and the breast meridian from the clavicle to the IMF, then extended inferiorly onto the upper abdomen.

The nipple position is not based on a predetermined distance from the suprasternal notch or supraclavicular line. Instead, the new nipple position is determined by transposing the IMF to the anterior breast and intersecting it with the breast meridian. The intersection of the transposed IMF and breast meridian becomes the approximate site of the proposed top of the areola, 2 cm above the new nipple site. To make the proposed site more accurate, the surgeon may need to mark the NAC slightly lower or gently support the breast to account for skin recoil after the heavy breast weight is removed. A nipple too high relative to the chest wall and the prominence of the breast mound is unnatural. The final nipple position should be at the most prominent portion of the breast on profile. Aesthetics of the surgery hinge on the nipple being at the breast apex supported by an elevated breast shape that resists settling. The breast shape is formed by joining the medial and lateral breast parenchymal pillars in a conical manner. This takes the tension off the skin closure as the skin advances with the parenchymal closure.

The Wise pattern is marked on the breast with the keyhole centered on the new nipple position and the vertical limbs 5 to

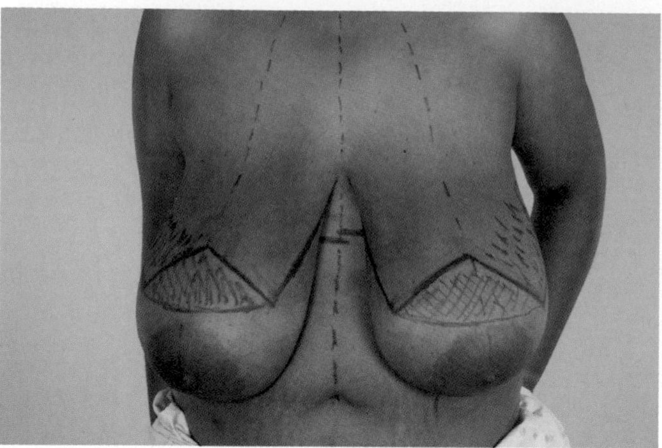

Figure 100.4. Using a Wise pattern centered at the new nipple position, an inverted V is drawn by joining the vertical limbs. The blue dashes indicate the proposed lateral undermining, and the red and black hatches indicate the deepithelialized central portion.

7 cm in length (19,20). As an alternative to drawing the keyhole, accurate nipple positioning can also be achieved by extending the medial and lateral limbs superiorly to create an inverted V (Fig. 100.4).

This method allows for adjusting the final nipple position at the time of surgery. However, the top of the areola cannot be lower than the top of the inverted V without resulting in a visible supra-areolar scar. Elongating the vertical closure length therefore displaces the NAC superiorly.

The width of the inverted V is determined by the size of the preoperative areola, width of the breast, volume distribution, skin quality, and desired size and aesthetics. The vertical limbs have to be drawn far enough apart to avoid incorporating the pigmented, areolar skin into the new inferior breast. A wider pattern will result in a more conical, projecting breast and a tighter skin envelope. If the breasts are asymmetric, the wider breast should have a wider inverted V. On the broad, flat, ptotic breast of gigantomastia, the procedure will have a more aesthetically pleasing outcome if a wider pattern is used. The greater the tension created by suturing the medial and lateral breast pillars, the greater is the breast projection. Next, lines are drawn freehand, starting at a right angle from the end of the vertical limbs of the pattern to the medial and lateral IMF. The medial limb joins the IMF discreetly away from the midline. The junction of the lateral freehand line and the IMF should be adjusted so the lateral line is approximately equal to the distance to the IMF lateral to the breast meridian. Moving the point of intersection superiorly off of the current IMF will lengthen the IMF portion and shorten the lateral upper incision. The reverse is true if the junction is moved inferiorly. The lateral limb incision should not extend beyond the lateral border of the breast, keeping the inframammary scar as short as possible and using care to avoid extending the incision into the roll of tissue that frequently extends onto the back. When this technique is used, the resultant horizontal scar will not be visible with the patient in the upright position unless the arms are raised above the head. Lateral fat rolls should be suctioned to smooth the lateral breast and thoracic contour and avoid dog-ear deformities. The surgeon may shorten the horizontal scar somewhat by pleating the excess skin or otherwise reconfiguring the pattern.

INTRAOPERATIVE TECHNIQUE

In the operating room, the nipple graft is marked with a 42-mm cookie cutter centered on the nipple (Fig. 100.5A). The graft is taken as a full-thickness graft. It is, in fact, a composite graft because it contains smooth muscle fibers deep to the nipples. Revascularization of the muscle provides postoperative nipple erection without direct innervation (Fig. 100.5B). Because the nipple portion of the graft is relatively thick, the superficial portion may undergo necrosis and delayed healing, which is why there may be loss of pigment in the nipple. Thinning of the areola and the deep portion of the nipple is crucial to graft survival and has in our experience shortened healing time (Fig. 100.5A, B).

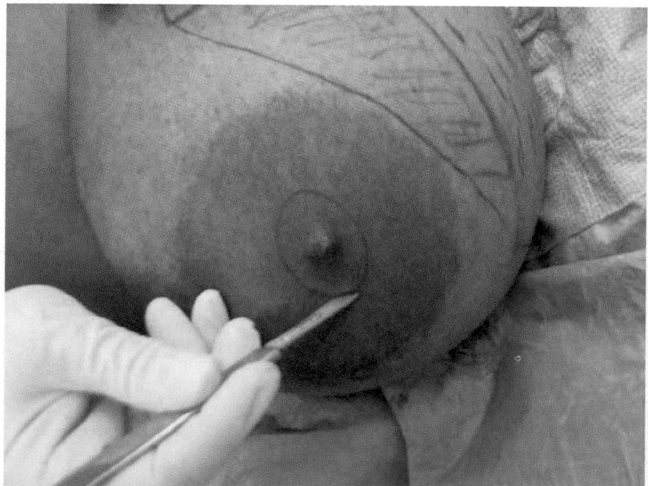

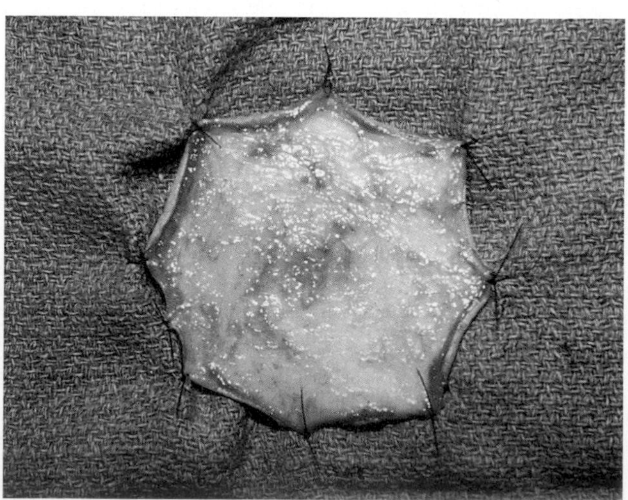

Figure 100.5. Intraoperative photographs of the free nipple breast reduction. **A:** The nipple graft is marked with a 42-mm cookie cutter centered on the nipple. **B:** Breast tissue and fat have been removed from the deep surface of this composite graft (*continued*)

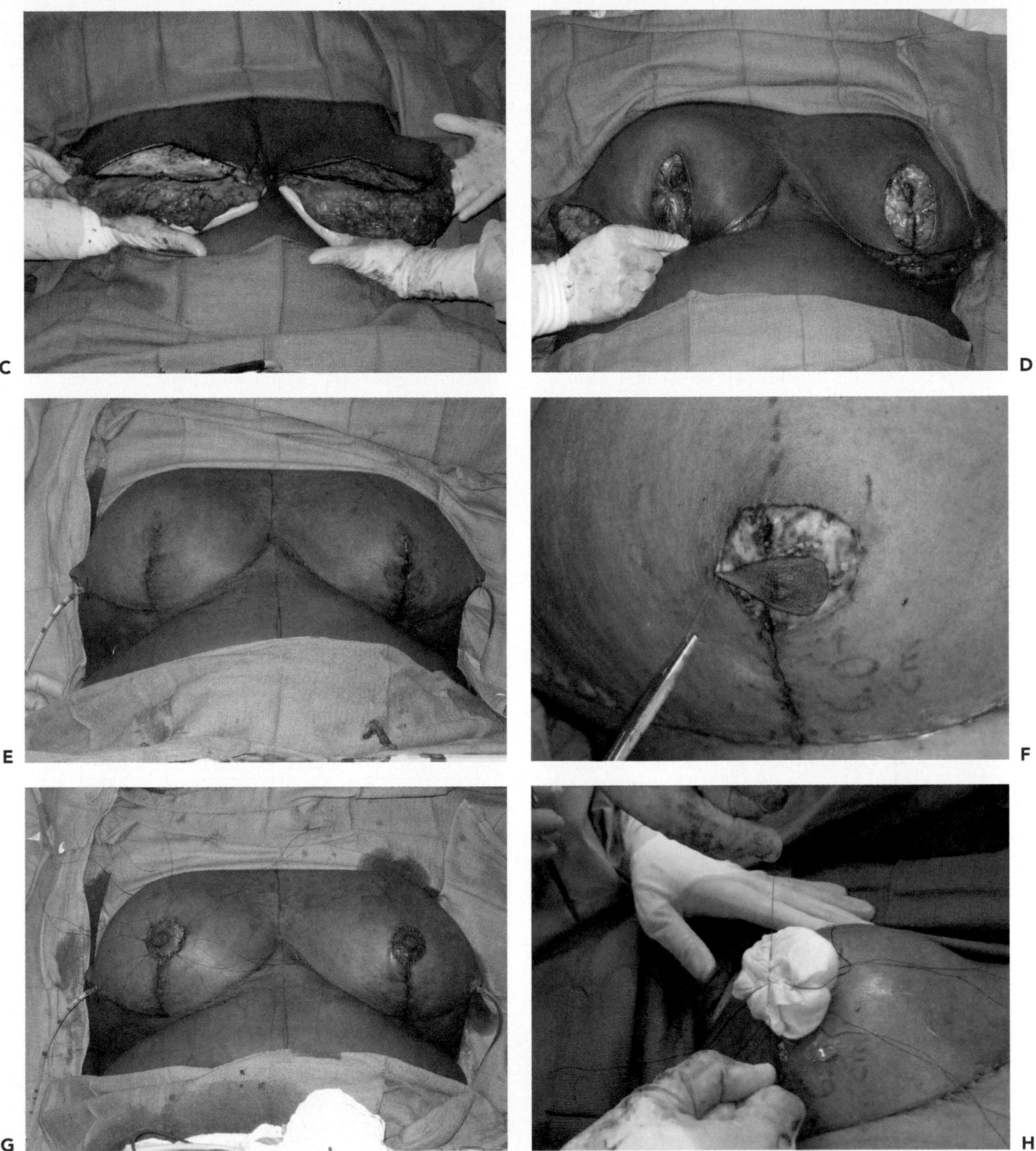

Figure 100.5. (*Continued*) **C:** The area between the vertical limbs is deepithelialized and the inferior breast is resected. **D:** The retained soft tissue in the central portion of the breast is incised through the dermis and imbricated to give the reduced breast projection. **E:** The incisions are closed and the patient sat upright to position the nipples. **F:** The free nipple graft is sutured to the deepithelialized NAC site. **G:** The patient with nipples in place before bolster dressings are added (ties for the right nipple bolster are in place). **H:** The bolster of petroleum-impregnated gauze with cotton soaked in mineral oil is secured with the 4-0 silk bolster ties.

The tissue between the vertical limbs is deepithelialized, and the horizontal limbs are incised. The inferior portion of the breast is then amputated (Fig. 100.5C). The medial and lateral flaps are undermined along the vertical limbs to allow for rotation advancement closure of the pattern and to create space for the imbricated central portion. The medial flap tissue is retained for cleavage. The lateral flap is thinned to minimize lateral breast bulk and create a pleasing breast contour. The deepithelialized central portion is separated from the vertical limbs by incising the dermis with electrocautery. The process is repeated on the contralateral side, and the breast is closed temporarily with staples to check for symmetry. Most breasts are asymmetric, resulting in different resection weights. When a satisfactory symmetry is achieved, the breast is opened, hemostasis is achieved, and 7-mm Jackson-Pratt drains are placed either through small axillary incisions or through the lateral aspect of the inframammary incision.

The medial and lateral breast pillars are then sutured over the folded retained central parenchyma to create the breast shape (Fig. 100.4D). This is done with 2-0 PDS suture and is the most important step in determining breast shape. Without "re-coning" the breast, the operation is a simple amputation and will leave a flat mound. By securing the parenchymal pillars together, the surgeon builds breast projection. The skin is then closed, and the patient is placed in the sitting upright position (Fig. 100.5E). Because the parenchymal suturing is such a powerful determinant of breast shape and projection, symmetry must be reassessed after this step. In addition, the nipple position should not be determined before this step is complete, as the nipple should sit at the apex of the new breast mound.

Once the mounds have been created, the nipple positions are marked at the apex of each mound. The breasts frequently appear quite conical at this step, which is in fact the desired result. As edema subsides, the breast shape will lose some of the "pointy" appearance; however, the coning of the tissue that creates it is critical to create an aesthetically pleasing mound (Fig. 100.6). Any bulk creating a dog-ear deformity of the lateral breast is then liposuctioned to contour the overall result. The skin is closed with interrupted deep dermal and running subcuticular 3-0 Monocryl sutures. The NAC site is deepithelialized, and the free nipple graft is sutured to the site with interrupted circumareolar, fast-absorbing sutures (Fig. 100.5F). A tie-over bolster of petroleum-impregnated gauze with mineral oil soaked cotton is secured with 4-0 silk sutured through both the graft and the skin edge at eight circumferential points (Fig. 100.5G, H). The remaining wounds are dressed with Dermabond, and a surgical bra is placed on the patient.

RETAINED INFERIOR BREAST MOUND TECHNIQUE

Alternatively, the free nipple breast reduction can be designed to retain an inferior breast mound for projection (Fig. 100.1). The Wise pattern is drawn with the keyhole. The inferior breast mound is marked 5 cm wide and long in the vicinity of the typical inferior pedicle. After the nipple-areola composite graft has been excised, the nipple-areola recipient site is deepithelialized, and the skin is removed from the inferior breast mound buttress. The leading edges of the medial and lateral flaps are left with full-thickness breast tissue beneath them. The full thickness of skin and breast tissue outside the markings of planned retained tissue is excised without skeletonizing the lateral pectoralis fascia. The lateral flap is usually thinned posteriorly. Except for skin incisions, all resection is performed with the electrocautery unit. After saline irrigation and drain placement, the medial and lateral parenchymal flaps are brought together with 3-0 Monocryl sutures. The skin is closed in two layers, the nipple-areola composite graft is sutured to the recipient site, and the tie-over bolster is secured.

POSTOPERATIVE CARE

The nipple graft bolster is removed at postoperative days 5 to 7. Typically, the areola shows signs of neovascularization, whereas the nipple appears partially necrotic. Eschar at the nipple is not uncommon and may last as long as 4 to 6 weeks. Patient expectations should be managed accordingly. If no partial necrosis exists at the nipple site, the graft may have been thinned too much, and the nipple projection and erectility may be decreased. Prominent nipples will lose some projection with the free nipple graft technique. By the same token, inverted nipples will be released from tethering breast tissue and gain some projection. The NAC should be dressed carefully with antibacterial ointment, petroleum-impregnated gauze, layers of gauze with an aperture to prevent nipple compression, and a surgical bra until the NAC is completely reepithelialized. The drains are removed per the surgeon's preference.

RESULTS OF THE SURGERY

Hypopigmentation is common and especially noticeable in African American patients. The patient in Figure 100.6 received an aesthetic and much improved breast mound shape, albeit with prominent hypopigmentation 2 months after surgery. This may resolve with time or require tattoo. Hypopigmentation did not occur in a 26-year-old, obese, African American smoker with 40DD bra size and greater than 15 cm distance from the nipple to the IMF (Fig. 100.7). She received an excellent result and comparable postoperative nipple projection in the absence of eschar and hypopigmentation. The free nipple breast reduction was successfully used in a 63-year old, obese, white patient with 40DD bra size, hypertension, and von Willebrand disease (Fig. 100.8). She received a satisfactory shape. The NAC has minimal if any pigment change. The weight loss patient in Figure 100.9 underwent free nipple graft breast reduction and abdominoplasty with marked improvement. The senior author performed 20 free nipple breast reductions between 2002 and 2009. The procedure is not performed unless the patient meets the criteria discussed in the indications section. He achieved satisfactory to excellent results, no loss of NAC, and no major complications requiring return to the operating room. Gradinger performed 156 free nipple grafts between 1979 and 1982, and only 1 failed to "take" successfully (15). Gradinger found that the free nipple graft breast reduction sometimes enhanced nipple projection (Fig. 100.10) and reliably maintained shape and nipple position (Fig. 100.11).

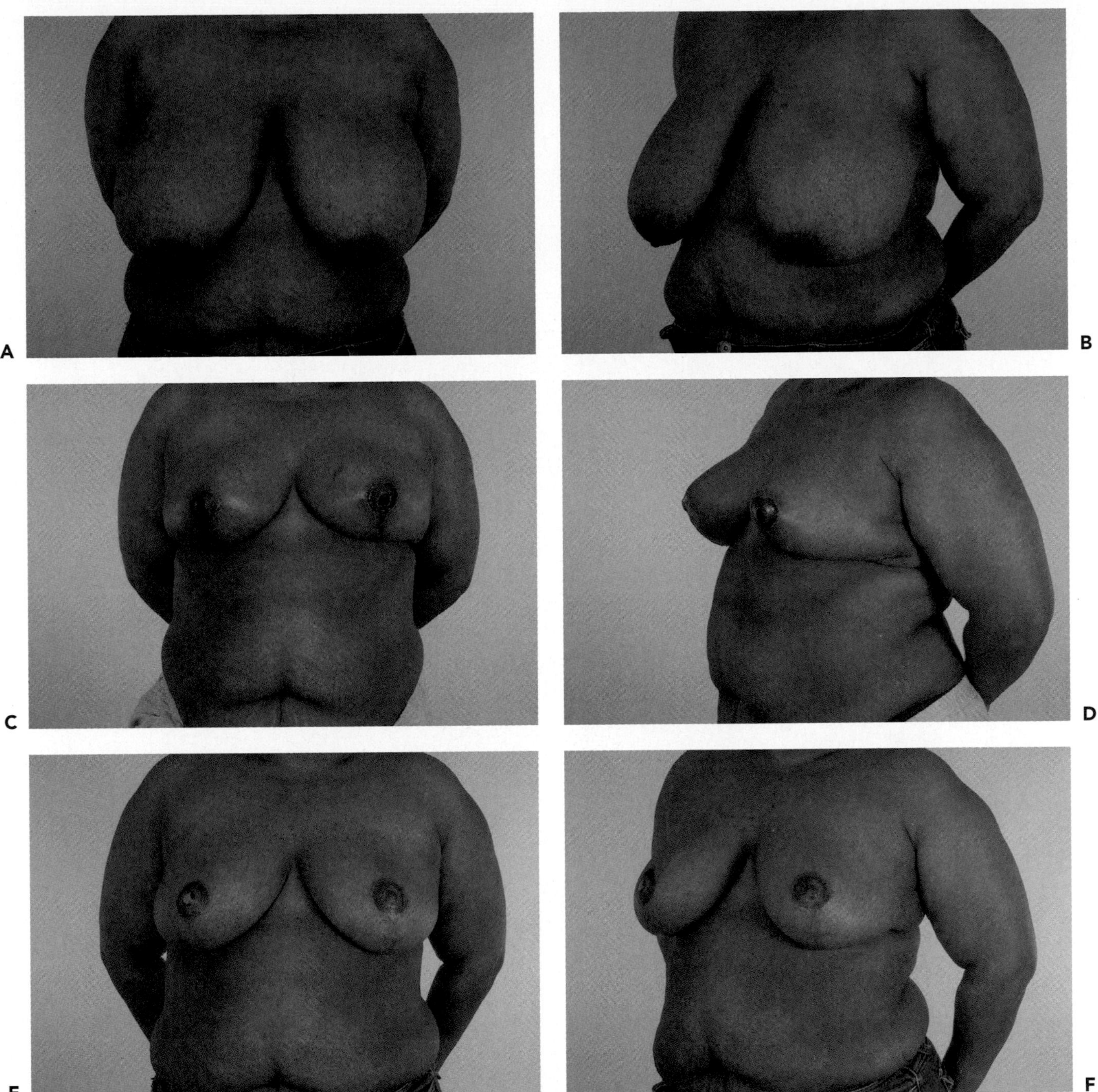

Figure 100.6. This 39-year-old patient with a 46DD bra size, a body mass index of 41, and a history of hypertension underwent free nipple breast reduction. **A, B:** Preoperative. **C, D:** Two weeks postoperatively (note the very conical shape of her breasts on the lateral view). **E, F:** Six months postoperatively. Note that the conical shape has relaxed, but the breast has retained projection. Note also the mild depigmentation common in these patients.

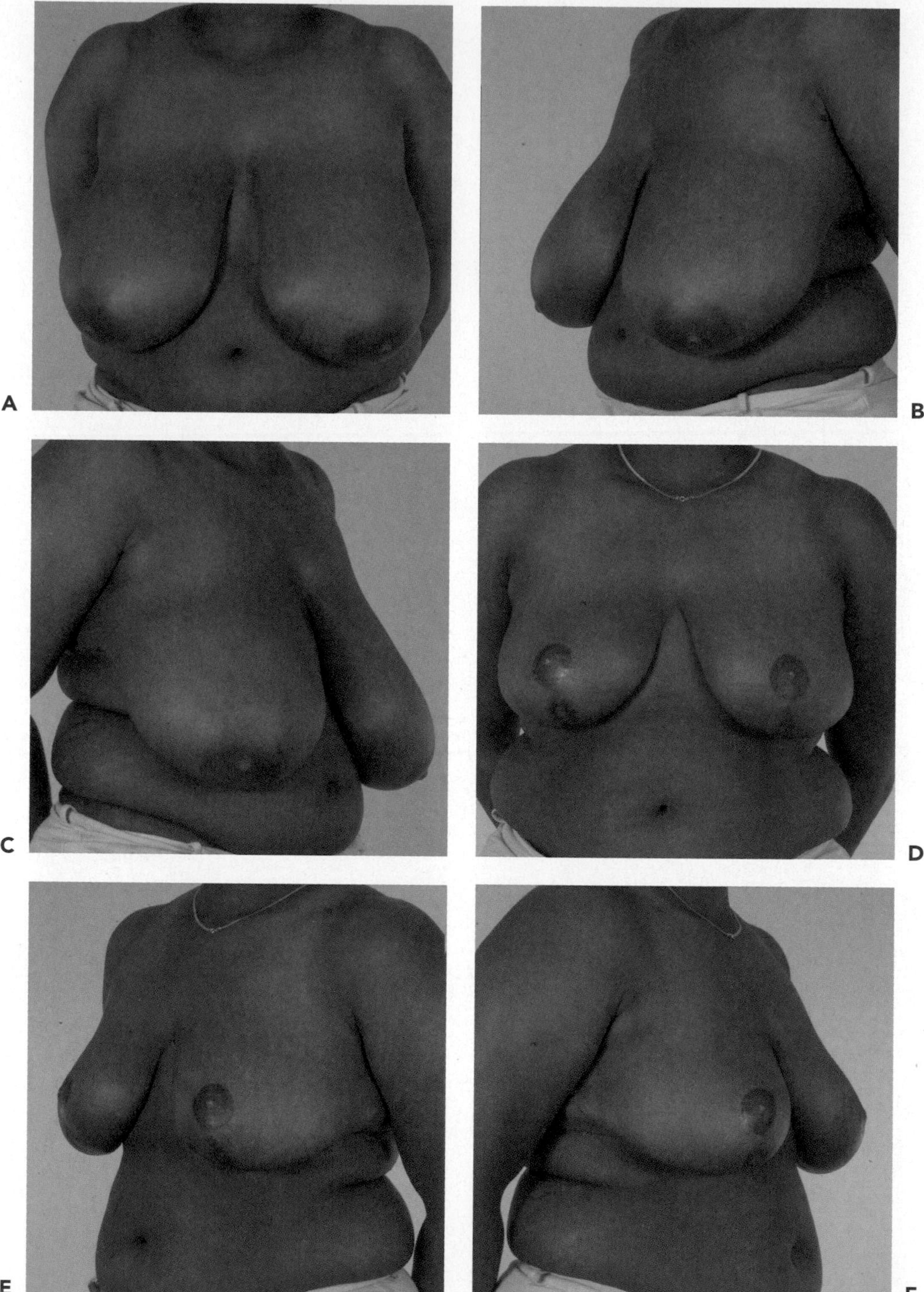

Figure 100.7. This obese 26-year-old patient with 40DD bra size and history of smoking underwent free nipple breast reduction. **A–C:** Preoperative. **D–F:** Nine months postoperative. She received an excellent result, and retained the pigmentation of the nipple-areola complex.

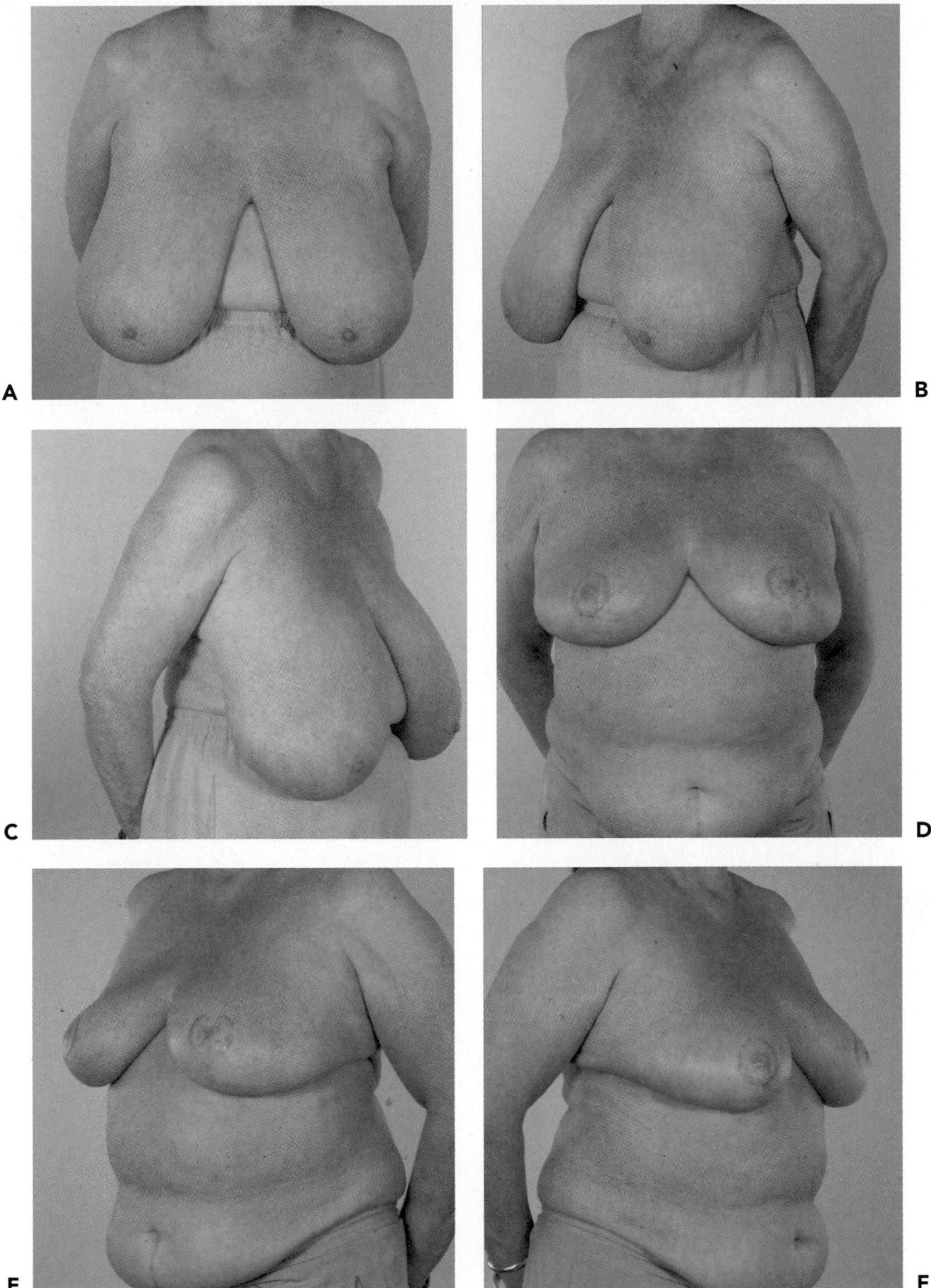

Figure 100.8. This 63-year-old obese patient with 42DD bra size and history of hypertension and von Willebrand disease underwent free nipple breast reduction. **A–C:** Preoperative; 2,290 g were removed from the right breast and 2,235 g from the left. **D–F:** One year postoperative. She has a satisfactory result.

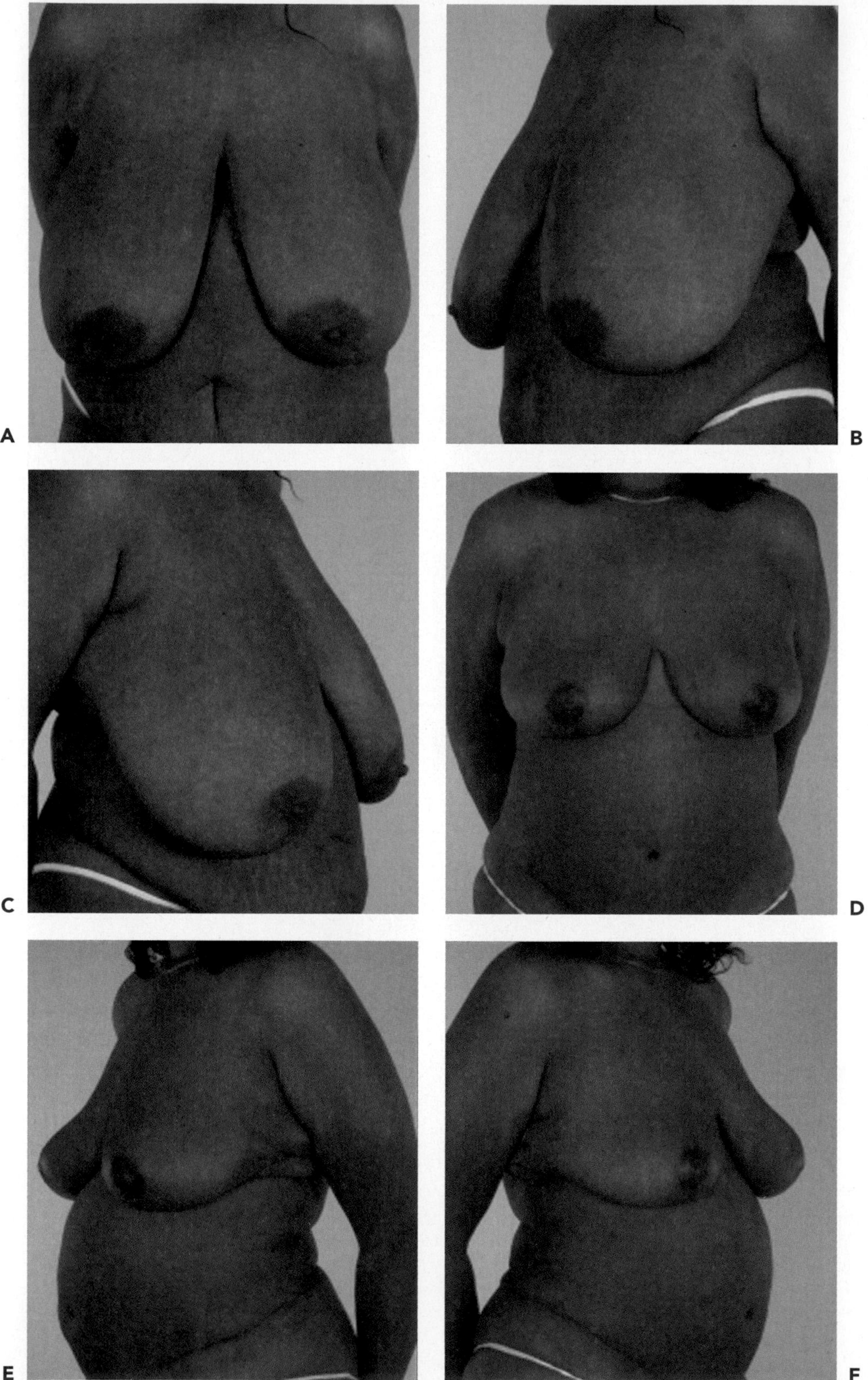

Figure 100.9. This 40-year-old obese patient with 40DD bra size after 80-lb weight loss underwent free nipple graft breast reduction and abdominoplasty with marked improvement at 2 months. **A–C:** Preoperative; 1,710 g were removed from the right and 1,940 g from the left. **D–F:** Three months postoperative. She has marked improvement.

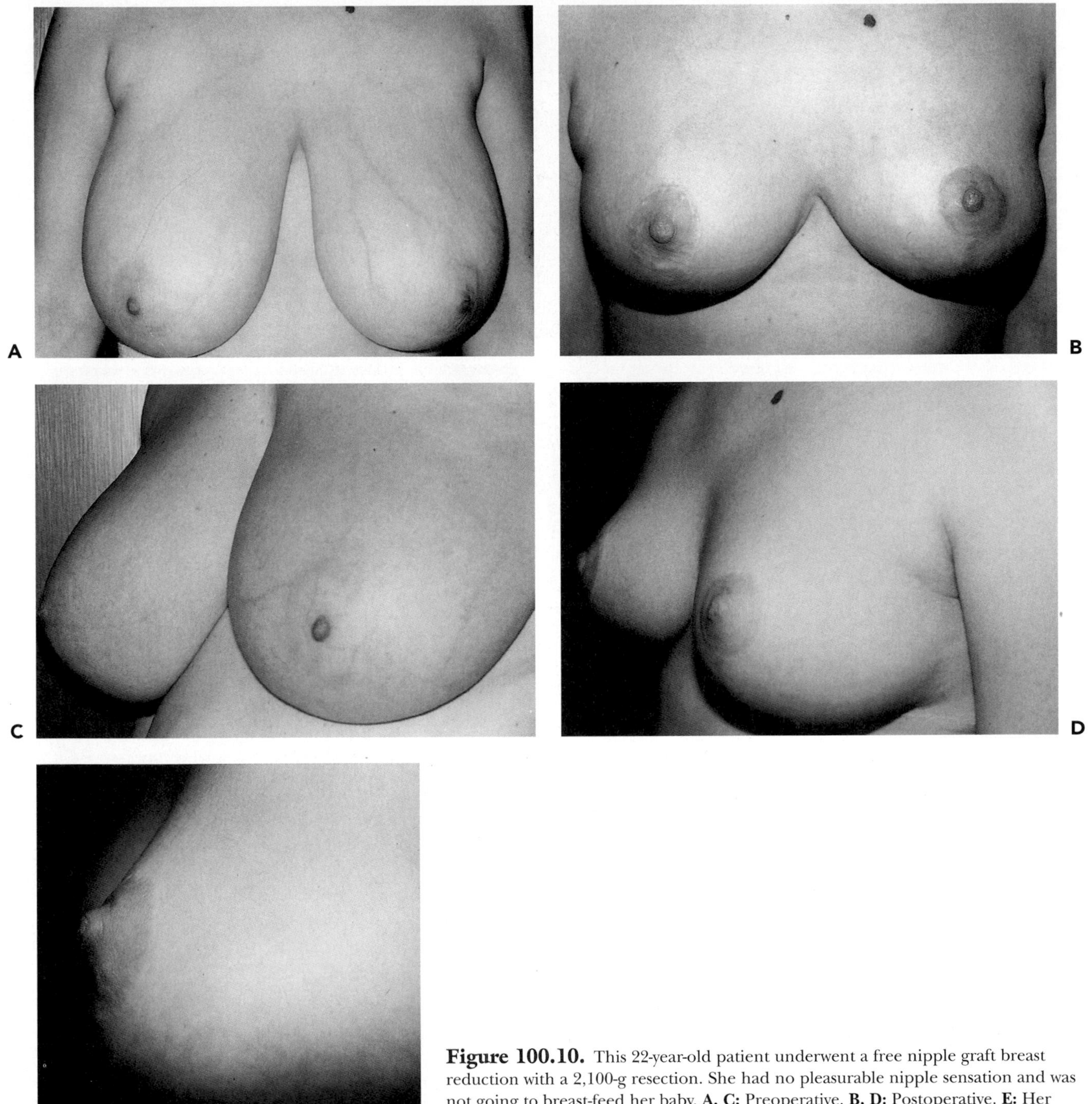

Figure 100.10. This 22-year-old patient underwent a free nipple graft breast reduction with a 2,100-g resection. She had no pleasurable nipple sensation and was not going to breast-feed her baby. **A, C:** Preoperative. **B, D:** Postoperative. **E:** Her nipple projection has been enhanced by surgery.

RISKS

The risks of free nipple graft breast reduction include unfavorable scars, nipple malposition, NAC hypopigmentation, nipple loss, sensation loss, erectability loss, fat necrosis, and other general complications. The quality of the scars is more a product of the patient than the technique. The circumareolar and vertical suture lines tend to form good-quality scars, whereas the horizontal suture line sometimes hypertrophies. The tendency for the breast tissue to fill dependent areas and the nipple to be too high for the breast mound is greatly reduced in the free nipple technique with proper parenchymal suturing, as there is no parenchymal pedicle to descend. Pigment loss is common with skin grafts and more noticeable in patients with darker complexions. Hypopigmentation can be corrected with tattooing or areola grafting. Complete nipple graft slough is a rare complication that is treated with local flap nipple reconstruction and a full-thickness graft from the groin or tattooing for the areola. Minor hematoma, cellulitis, or fat necrosis may occur but generally do not require subsequent operations or intravenous antibiotics.

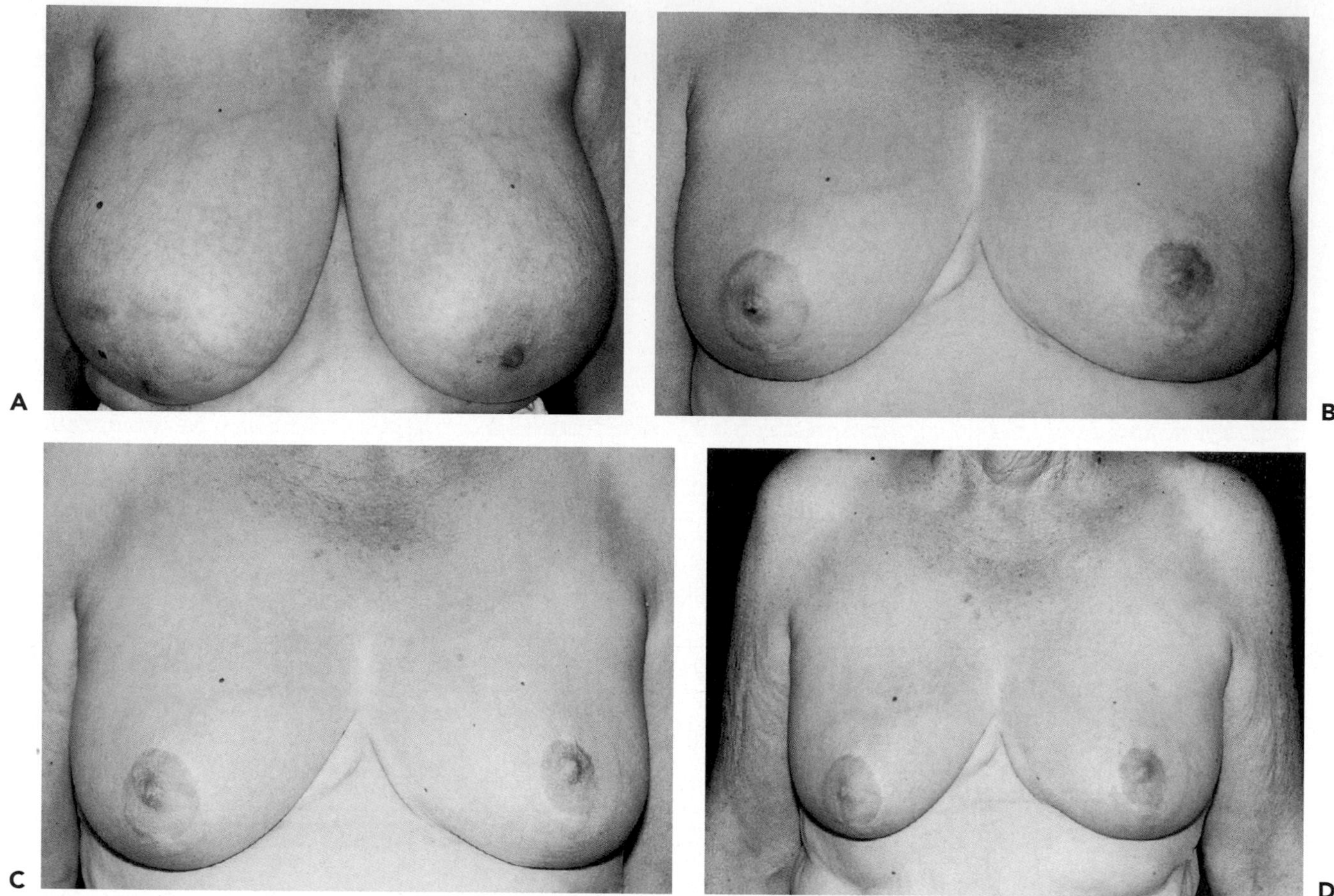

Figure 100.11. This 60-year-old patient had a total of 1,900 g resected. Note that she had minimal preoperative nipple projection. **A:** Preoperative view. **B:** One year postsurgery. **C:** Seven years postsurgery. **D:** Twelve years postsurgery. Other than minor ptosis, little change occurred during the 12-year period.

CONCLUSION

The free nipple breast reduction is appropriate for select patients with breast hypertrophy and consistently produces an aesthetic breast mound without complications due to an excessively long, folded pedicle. The preoperative planning is precise and the procedure simple due to minimal intraoperative adjustments. The free nipple breast reduction maintains the shape of the breast over the long term and facilitates the postoperative breast examination without the irregularities caused by bulky or folded pedicles. It is a powerful technique for creating an aesthetically coned breast that is ideal for certain patients with gigantomastia.

EDITORIAL COMMENTS

At first glance, it would seem that managing the NAC as a full-thickness graft in breast reduction would be an unusually risky operative strategy. If compromise of the graft occurs, the final result will be less than ideal. Such compromise can manifest as either partial or complete graft loss, loss of nipple projection, or, more subtly, loss of areolar pigmentation. Certainly, NAC innervation is assuredly disrupted, with reinnervation being incomplete even under the best of conditions. For these reasons, the technique should only be employed in the most tenuous of circumstances as far as potential disruption of the blood supply to the NAC in pedicled breast reduction is concerned. As pointed out by the authors, obese patients, patients with profound macromastia, patients with preexisting medical conditions such as hypertension, and patients who smoke are all at risk for diminished blood flow to the NAC after pedicled breast reduction. It then becomes a judgment call for the plastic surgeon to assess the risk of performing a pedicled reduction versus the risk of compromise to the vascularity of the NAC.

In any breast reduction, the best of all circumstances would be to be able to perform the procedure successfully in a pedicled fashion. In this manner, both innervation and vascularity would be preserved; parenchyma would remain attached to the NAC, theoretically preserving the ability to breast-feed; and shape would be enhanced by preserving volume under the NAC. When any of the previously noted risk factors come into play, I employ a "reconstructive technique ladder" to guide my eventual method of preserving the viability of the NAC. The simplest maneuver is to simply be less aggressive with the dissection, make the pedicle wider, and avoid extensive undermining. Alternatively, augmentation of the unipedicle into a bipedicle can provide additional vascular support to the NAC. Here, instead of using only an inferior pedicle, a combination superior/inferior pedicle as described by McKissock can be useful. When the possibility of needing a free NAC graft is anticipated, I prefer to proceed with the pedicled procedure and then assess the viability of the NAC before final insetting. If there is any question as to the vascularity of the NAC at that point, then the NAC is removed as described by the authors, the pedicle trimmed back to viable tissue, and the graft applied to the well-vascularized dermal bed of the pedicle. It should be emphasized that in patients with profound macromastia, the pedicle, even if well vascularized, can be of such dimension that blood supply can be compromised due to kinking when the pedicle is folded into the breast. In these cases, the free nipple graft technique has an advantage because the shaping of the breast can be done with the flaps, which is much more straightforward than when the pedicle must be relied on to supply the NAC.

Finally, when the free nipple graft technique is employed, it is critical that the surgeon obtain detailed informed consent for the procedure. In my experience of reviewing cases, the medicolegal risk for this procedure is high, and sufficient documentation to protect the surgeon and patient must be present to avoid not only patient disappointment, but also protracted legal proceedings.

M.Y.N.

REFERENCES

1. Adams WM. Free transplantation of the nipples and areolae. *Surgery* 1944;5:186.
2. Courtiss EH, Goldwyn RM. Breast sensation before and after plastic surgery. *Plast Reconstr Surg* 1976;58:1.
3. O'Conor CM. Glandular excision with immediate mammary reconstruction. *Plast Reconstr Surg* 1964;33:57.
4. Craig DP, Sykes PA. Nipple sensitivity following reduction mammaplasty. *Br J Plast Surg* 1970;23:165–172.
5. Townsend PLG. Nipple sensation following breast reduction and free nipple transplantation. *Br J Plast Surg* 1974;27:308.
6. Ahmed OA, Kolhe PS. Comparison of nipple and areolar sensation after breast reduction by free nipple graft and inferior pedicle techniques. *Br J Plast Surg* 2000;53:126.
7. Slezak S, Dellon AL. Quantitation of sensibility in gigantomastia and alteration following reduction mammaplasty. *Plast Reconstr Surg* 1993;91:1265.
8. Hawtof DB, Levine M, Kapetansky DI, et al. Complications of reduction mammaplasty: comparison of nipple-areolar graft and pedicle. *Ann Plast Surg* 1989;23:3.
9. Oneal RM, Goldstein JA, Rohrich R, et al. Reduction mammoplasty with free-nipple transplantation: indications and technical refinements. *Ann Plast Surg* 1991;26:117.
10. Romano JJ, Francel TJ, Hoopes JE. Free nipple graft reduction mammoplasty. *Ann Plast Surg* 1992;28:271.
11. Koger KE, Sunde D, Press BHJ, et al. Reduction mammaplasty for gigantomastia using inferiorly based pedicle and free nipple transplantation. *Ann Plast Surg* 1994;33:561.
12. Wray RC, Luce EA. Treatment of impending nipple necrosis following reduction mammaplasty. *Plast Reconstr Surg* 1981;65:242.
13. Tracy CA, Pool R, Gellis M, et al. Blood flow of the areola and breast skin flaps during reduction mammaplasty as measured by laser Doppler flowmetry. *Ann Plast Surg* 1992;28:160.
14. Jackson IT. Importance of the pedicle length measurement in reduction mammaplasty. *Plast Reconstr Surg* 1999;104:398.
15. Gradinger GP. Reduction mammoplasty utilizing nipple-areola transplantation. *Clin Plast Surg* 1988;15:641.
16. Gradinger GP. Breast reduction with the free nipple graft technique. In: Spear SL, ed. *Surgery of the Breast: Principles and Art.* Philadelphia: Lippincott-Raven, 1998;807–821.
17. Casas LA, Byun MY, Depoli PA. Maximizing breast projection after free-nipple-graft reduction mammaplasty. *Plast Reconstr Surg* 2001;107:955.
18. Hudson DA, Skoll PJ. Repeat reduction mammaplasty. *Plast Reconstr Surg* 1999;104:401.
19. Wise RJ. Preliminary report on a method of planning the mammaplasty. *Plast Reconstr Surg* 1956;17:367.
20. Wise RJ, Gannon JP, Hill JR. Further experience with reduction mammaplasty. *Plast Reconstr Surg* 1963;32:12.

CHAPTER

101

Scott L. Spear
Amer Saba

Reduction Mammoplasty in the Irradiated Breast

INTRODUCTION

More breast cancer patients are treated with conservation therapy (lumpectomy, axillary lymph node dissection, and whole breast irradiation) than with mastectomy. Historically, patients with very large breasts were considered to be poor candidates for such conservative therapy because they often obtained cosmetically less acceptable results; however, more recent radiotherapeutic techniques have led to increased cases of women with macromastia and breast cancer receiving radiation therapy (1,2). Thus, we have seen and will continue to see patients with symptomatic breast enlargement who have already been treated for breast cancer with lumpectomy, axillary dissection, and radiation therapy.

BACKGROUND

Impairment of wound healing in irradiated tissue by fibroblast inhibition and microvascular disease is supported in numerous studies (3). There is an increased rate of infections, fat necrosis, and seromas in irradiated patients. Overweight women or women with large pendulous breasts tend to have more fibrosis of the breast, leading to poorer cosmetic outcome. However, the increased fat content in large breasts, or the greater dose inhomogeneities due to the greater tangent separation, could also explain the poorer results in these women (1).

Although there has been little data in the literature on breast reduction in the irradiated patient, it is clear from the data on breast reconstruction in patients after breast irradiation that reconstructive surgery on a radiated breast is more prone to complications and yields cosmetically suboptimal results (3,4).

This chapter addresses the nature of breast reduction in the previous irradiated patient and the safety of performing such a procedure. It also addresses the preferable methods and evaluates the cosmetic results. Finally, the question of the effect of breast reduction on cancer surveillance is discussed.

TECHNIQUES

Reduction of the radiated breast could be performed safely using a variety of techniques. The method of reduction alone does not seem critical as long as the pedicle is wider and shorter than normal to avoid nipple necrosis or loss. Flaps must be designed to avoid complications such as seroma or flap necrosis (5). This includes less or no undermining or elevation of the flaps. For that reason, the Lejour technique, as well as other reduction mammoplasty techniques, which requires extensive undermining and redraping of significant amounts of remaining breast skin, would not seem safe for the irradiated breast.

TIMING

Reduction mammoplasty for the irradiated breast should be delayed until the acute postradiation response has subsided. At 1 year postoperatively, breast edema has significantly subsided, with very few patients displaying edema at longer follow-up. Telangiectasia is essentially nonexistent at 1 year, and skin thickening after 1 year is no different in patients with macromastia compared with the average patients. One advantage of delaying the reduction for 1 year is that the procedure can be performed with a more accurate estimate of how much tissue should be removed to obtain symmetry. It is unclear whether there is any advantage or disadvantage to postponing the procedure for longer intervals. From the psychological point of view, most patients are unlikely to seek reduction mammoplasty immediately after radiation therapy because they are still preoccupied with the issues surrounding their breast cancer, including the possible need for adjuvant chemotherapy. To avoid any delay in cancer treatment, the breast reduction procedure should not be performed until the cancer treatment is complete.

Although lumpectomy combined with reduction and followed by radiation therapy is the subject of another chapter in this book, there are several related issues to be raised. Simultaneous lumpectomy and reduction might create the awkward situation of residual positive margins, which could be difficult to locate in the patient if the reduction has already been performed. Does reduction after lumpectomy complicate the delivery of radiation therapy? Should the site of lumpectomy be somehow marked with surgical clips during the reduction process so the site can be subsequently identified for radiation planning and long-term follow-up? In patients with clean margins after lumpectomy, there would not appear in principle to be any adverse effect of reduction prior to radiation. The surgical margins would be greater; there would be less breast tissue left to examine and follow; the patient would be relieved of the breast enlargement; and by performing the reduction prior to radiation, the risks of operating on a radiated breast would be avoided (5).

COSMETIC RESULTS

Although the cosmetic results in irradiated patients are acceptable, the radiated breast are generally less attractive. The healing process is also delayed with more and longer induration and swelling (6).

CANCER SURVEILLANCE

The architecture of the breast is changed by the breast conservation, and there is resulting scar tissue seen on the mammogram films. Those postoperative changes become the patient's new baseline for future mammographic surveillance. This is no different than dealing with scars created by other procedures such as biopsies and lumpectomies, not to mention breast reduction procedures in nonradiated patients.

CASE REPORTS

CASE 1

A 45-year-old woman seeking consultation for a reduction mammoplasty was diagnosed with left breast cancer 8 months ago. The patient had been treated with lumpectomy and axillary dissection, followed by chemotherapy for 1 of 38 positive nodes. Chemotherapy was followed by radiation therapy consisting of 6,100 cGy. At the time of plastic surgery evaluation, her breasts were 34DD with moderate ptosis and a nipple-to-fold distance of 8 cm. Although there was no evidence of recurrence, she was asymmetric, and there was persistent thickening of the left breast at the lumpectomy site (Fig. 101.1).

Three months after completing her radiation therapy, she underwent bilateral reduction mammaplasty using the McKissock bipedicle technique. She healed uneventfully but did have a minor scar revision in the office for an inframammary dog ear 9 months later. At the time of the reduction, 505 g were removed from the normal (right) side, and 510 g were removed from the treated breast side. Liposuction of approximately 100 cc was performed on each side.

The McKissock technique used in this procedure was modified from our usual technique. The inferior base of the pedicle was designed to be 8 cm instead of our usual 6 cm, and the dissection was more gradually tapered to the chest wall to broaden the pedicle attachment. The medial and lateral breast flaps were minimally undermined and were thinned as necessary with liposuction rather than excision. The superior pedicle bridge was left 3 cm thick instead of our usual 2 cm. The pathology from both sides showed fibrous mastopathy. Mammograms performed at 3 and 18 months postoperatively showed only minor postoperative changes.

CASE 2

A 46-year-old woman seeking consultation for bilateral breast reduction to correct her underlying breast hypertrophy and distortion secondary to recent breast conservation therapy for breast cancer. Patient was diagnosed 6 months ago with ductal carcinoma in situ of the left breast and underwent lumpectomy and postoperative radiation therapy of 5,000 cGy to the breast, with a boost of 1,000 cGy to the tumor bed. On examination, she had a 38DDD size breast with 10 cm of nipple ptosis on the right but only 1 cm of nipple ptosis on the radiated left side. The surgical site on the left breast located across the upper hemisphere remained indurated (Fig. 101.2).

Approximately 8 months after completion of her radiation therapy, she underwent bilateral reduction mammaplasty. The nonradiated right side was reduced using a standard McKissock vertical bipedicle technique. On the left side, a superior pedicle procedure was performed with only a few centimeters of nipple elevation on that side. From the right breast, 905 g were removed, and from the left breast, 450 g were removed. The patient's postoperative course was uneventful, and the final outcome in terms of size and symmetry was good. The pathology on both sides showed fibrocystic changes and apocrine metaplasia.

CASE 3

A 48-year-old woman sought plastic surgery consultation for bilateral reduction mammaplasty 16 months after right

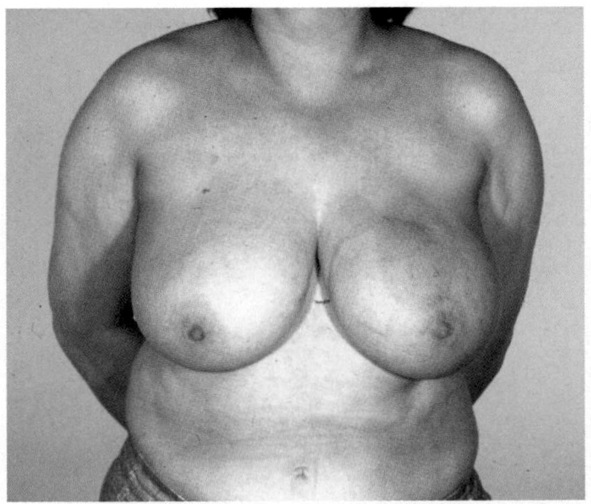

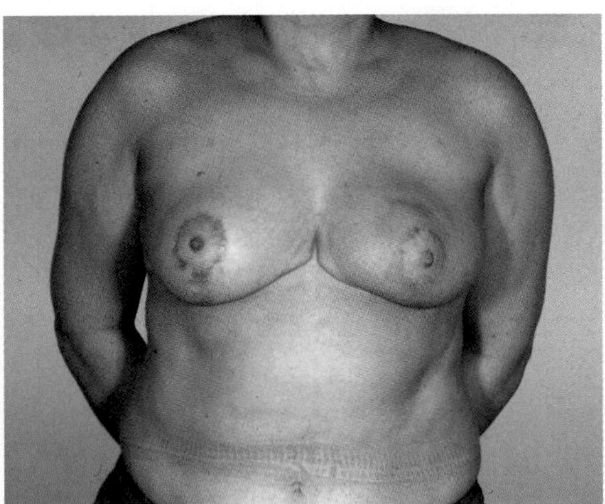

Figure 101.1. (*Left*) Preoperative view of a 45-year-old woman (case 1) previously treated with left breast lumpectomy and postoperative radiation therapy. (*Right*) Postoperative view after bilateral McKissock reduction mammoplasty, removing 505 g from the right breast and 510 g from the left breast. (Reprinted from Spear SL, Burke JB, Forman D, et al. Experience with reduction mammoplasty following breast conservation surgery and radiation therapy. Plast Reconstr Surg 1998; 102: 1913, with permission.)

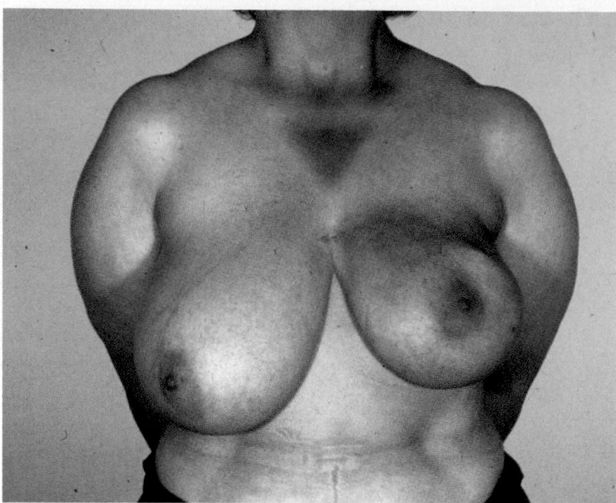
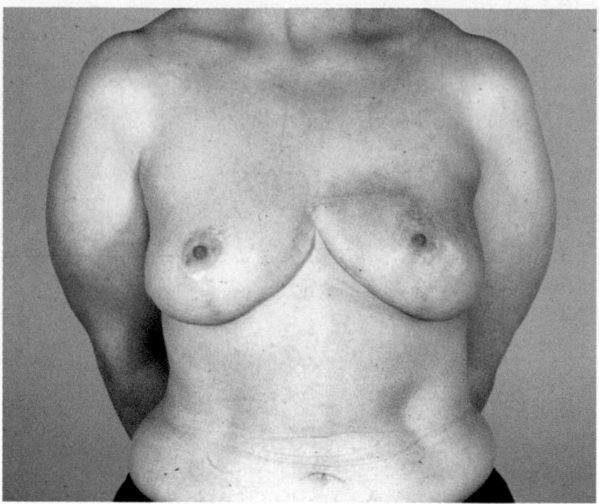

Figure 101.2. (*Left*) Preoperative view of a 46-year-old woman (case 2) previously treated with left breast lumpectomy and postoperative radiation therapy. (*Right*) Postoperative view after right McKissock reduction and left superior pedicle reduction mammoplasty, removing 905 g from the right breast and 450 g from the left breast. (Reprinted from Spear SL, Burke JB, Forman D, et al. Experience with reduction mammoplasty following breast conservation surgery and radiation therapy. Plast Reconstr Surg 1998; 102: 1913, with permission.)

lumpectomy and radiation therapy for ductal carcinoma. Her radiation treatment included 5,040 cGy to the right breast, with an additional 1,000 cGy to the tumor bed. At the time of examination, she had 38DD breasts with severe ptosis and a nipple that overhung the inframammary crease by 11 cm. The unoperated left breast was larger and more ptotic than the radiated right side. The lumpectomy scar was above the right areola. Twenty-four months after her lumpectomy, she underwent bilateral inferior pedicle breast reductions, with special attention given to avoid undermining the flaps, particularly of the right breast (Fig. 101.3).

In total, 1,070 g were removed from the left breast, and 830 g were removed from the right breast. The patient healed uneventfully, although the right breast remained edematous for several months. The pathology of the left breast revealed fibrocystic changes with stromal fibrosis and apocrine metaplasia, whereas the radiated right side showed stromal fibrosis.

CONCLUSION

Reduction of the radiated breast can be done safely in a variety of ways, including using the McKissock, inferior, and superior pedicle techniques (5). Special care is recommended in designing the pedicle to keep it wider and shorter than normal. Extensive breast flap elevation and undermining is, in all likelihood, risky. The cosmetic results, although not as good as on nonradiated breasts, are still acceptable. Follow-up of these patients and mammographic surveillance for recurrent breast cancer does not seem to be impeded by the reduction procedure.

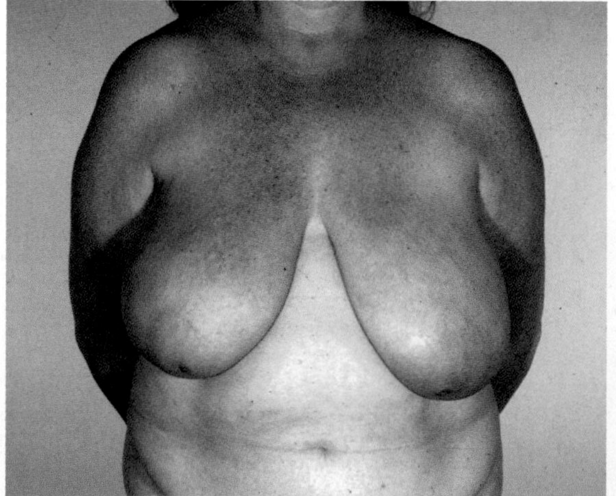
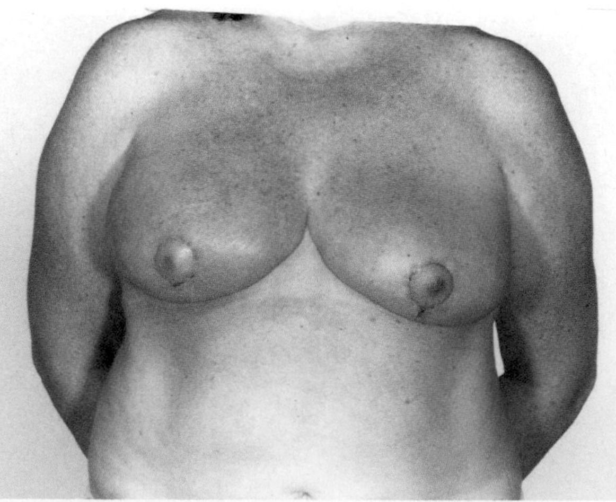

Figure 101.3. (*Left*) Preoperative view of a 48-year-old woman (case 3) previously treated with right breast lumpectomy and postoperative radiation therapy. (*Right*) Postoperative view after bilateral inferior pedicle reduction mammaplasty, removing 1,070 g from the left breast and 830 g from the right breast. (Reprinted from Spear SL, Burke JB, Forman D, et al. Experience with reduction mammoplasty following breast conservation surgery and radiation therapy. Plast Reconstr Surg 1998; 102: 1913, with permission.)

EDITORIAL COMMENTS

Since the mid-1990s, radiation therapy has become more commonly used as an adjunct in the treatment of breast cancer than ever before. As a result, plastic surgeons are seeing more patients who require breast procedures where the involved tissues have been previously irradiated. As the authors point out, extreme caution must be exercised when contemplating surgical procedures on these previously irradiated breasts. It cannot be emphasized enough that the ability of these tissues to withstand surgically induced ischemia is significantly reduced. As a result, delayed wound healing, prolonged edema, and potential tissue necrosis are all a significant concern in these patients, particularly if the breast has been operated on previously. As noted by the authors, it is best to be conservative when designing an operative plan for these patients. Prudent technical modifications, including wide pedicles, limited resections, and avoidance of wide undermining, can all serve to head off potential complications. By heeding these recommendations, safe and complication free procedures can be offered to these patients to hasten their recovery from breast cancer.

D.C.H.

REFERENCES

1. Gray JR, McCormick B, Cox L, et al. Primary breast irradiation in large-breasted or heavy women: analysis of cosmetic outcome. *Int J Radiat Oncol Biol Phys* 1991;21:347.
2. Cross MA, Elson HR, Aron RS. Breast conservation radiation therapy technique for women with large breasts. *Int J Radiat Oncol Biol Phys* 1989;17:199.
3. Williams JK, Bostwick J III, Bried JT, et al. TRAM flap breast reconstruction after radiation treatment. *Ann Surg* 1995;21:756.
4. Kroll SS, Schusterman MA, Reece GP, et al. Breast reconstruction with myocutaneous flaps in previously irradiated patients. *Plast Reconstr Surg* 1994;93:460.
5. Spear SL, Burke JB, Forman D, et al. Experience with reduction mammoplasty following breast conservation surgery and radiation therapy. *Plast Reconstr Surg* 1998;102:1913.
6. Handel N, Lewinsky B, Waisman JR. Reduction mammoplasty following radiation therapy for breast cancer. *Plast Reconstr Surg* 1992;89:953.

CHAPTER

102

J. Peter Rubin
Joseph Michaels V

Breast Reduction and Mastopexy After Massive Weight Loss

INTRODUCTION

The prevalence of morbid obesity continues to grow at an alarming rate. The implications of morbid obesity have been well documented throughout the literature. To reduce the rate of obesity-related complications, many people seek to lose weight through either bariatric surgery or diet and exercise. Following weight loss, patients are often left with redundant skin and excess subcutaneous tissue; however, significant fat deposits may remain. We frequently see patients presenting for postbariatric body contouring procedures after they have undergone massive weight loss (MWL), defined as weight loss greater than 50 pounds.

Correction of breast deformities remains a high priority for woman presenting for body contouring, but there is a wide variation in the presentation of these deformities. Although most women previously had full breasts prior to weight loss, the majority of women are left with deflated and asymmetric loss of breast volume. Common findings on examination include breast ptosis, medialization of the nipple-areolar complex, poor skin tone, and a lateral skin fold that blends into the breast (1).

INDICATIONS

Given the wide variety of breast deformities seen in MWL patients, each consultation must be individualized. There have been many descriptions for breast contouring following MWL (2–9). Several factors will determine which procedure is appropriate for each patient: (a) the severity of the aforementioned breast deformities, (b) the desired breast size of the patient, and (c) the surgeon's experience. Irregardless of which procedure is chosen, it must deliver the size and shape that the patient desires.

INADEQUATE BREAST VOLUME

Patients who have undergone significant breast involution or who do not have sufficient lateral skin folds to provide sufficient tissue for autoaugmentation of the breast will require breast implants if they desire larger breasts. Most of the patients that fall into this category are young women with good skin tone. These patients can be considered for an isolated breast augmentation if there is minimal ptosis and skin redundancy. Our preferred approach to breast augmentation is with an inframammary fold (IMF) incision. Patients falling into this category represent less than 2% of the breast deformities we have corrected. Description of this technique can be found in the chapters of this text dealing with augmentation mammaplasty.

Patients with inadequate volume associated with grade 2 or 3 ptosis, significant skin redundancy, an enlarged nipple-areolar complex (NAC), and/or an inadequate lateral skin fold on physical examination will require a mastopexy in addition to augmentation mammaplasty. In select patients we perform a mastopexy-augmentation through a vertical access incision made beneath the NAC. After submuscular placement of the implant, we tailor-tack the skin envelope to the correct nipple position and control the redundant skin envelope. It is not uncommon to require a significant inframammary extension to control the redundant skin. The patient must be made aware of this potential scar burden preoperatively. In complicated cases in which there is significant asymmetry or a loose IMF, we prefer to perform a staged mastopexy-augmentation to optimize the aesthetic outcome. In some cases, the patients have been satisfied with their breast size following the mastopexy, obviating the need for later augmentation.

EXCESSIVE BREAST VOLUME

Approximately 20% of patients presenting for breast surgery have excessive breast volume necessitating a breast reduction. Our preferred technique is a Wise-pattern reduction mammaplasty using either a medial or inferior pedicle. The decision as to which pedicle is used will depend in part on the nipple-to-fold distance and on the experience of the surgeon. These techniques are described in detail in chapters dealing with reduction mammaplasty and mastopexy. Although the procedure is performed in a similar manner as for non-MWL patients, there are special preoperative considerations and modification to the markings that may need to be addressed. Some patients have significant medialization of the NAC. In these patients, it may be difficult to adequately rotate the pedicle to its new position on the breast meridian. If we believe that this might be an issue, then we choose an inferior pedicle. Since these patients may also have a considerable lateral skin fold, the posterior extension and width of the lateral excision can be significantly larger than for non-MWL patients. It is important to come out of the breast crease laterally when performing the markings to prevent a "boxy" appearance to the breast. The width of the lateral excision can be estimated with a pinch test. Liposuction of the lateral skin fold may be useful to further contour the lateral fold of the breast. This is best performed after the skin resection has been performed and the skin has been temporarily closed with staples.

Short-scar techniques in the MWL may result in a large inferior dog-ear due to the excessive skin redundancy and poor skin tone. This dog-ear will require a horizontal excision to remove the redundancy. A pitfall of the short-scar technique would be to chase the dog-ear inferiorly, which would leave an unsightly scar below the IMF. In addition, short-scar techniques will have minimal impact on the lateral skin fold that is present in the majority of MWL patients.

ADEQUATE BREAST VOLUME

Although many of the women presenting after MWL feel that they need a breast reduction, the majority of these woman have adequate volume to give them the size and shape they desire. Careful examination of the breast parenchyma will determine whether there is sufficient parenchymal volume. The lateral skin fold is also evaluated to assess how much tissue can be recruited into the breast for autoaugmentation. In patients who have adequate parenchymal volume, severe ptosis, and an adequate lateral skin fold, our preferred technique is dermal suspension with total parenchymal reshaping and autologous augmentation from the lateral chest wall (2–4). This technique provides reliable results with the ability to intraoperatively individualize the size and shape of the breast. Since the parenchymal reshaping and the amount of tissue recruited for autologous augmentation can be customized for each breast, this technique allows for the correction of difficult breast asymmetries often encountered in these patients.

As with all of our MWL patients desiring body contouring procedures, a thorough history and physical examination is performed (10). Specific questions about a personal and family history of breast cancer are asked, and all patients undergo mammography in accordance with the American Cancer Society guidelines (11). A nutritional assessment is also performed to ensure that the patient is optimized prior to surgery.

There are relatively few contraindications to this procedure. The only true contraindication to this procedure is previous breast surgery that may compromise the undermined tissue. We defer surgery in all active tobacco users due to the degree of undermining required to perform this procedure. Patients with a positive smoking history are screened with a cotinine urine test prior to surgery. We also defer patients that have active severe intertrigo or other active dermatologic conditions.

SURGICAL TECHNIQUE

MARKINGS

The procedure is based on an extended Wise pattern with preservation of both a central and an inferior pedicle (Fig. 102.1). A new breast meridian in marked in the center of the breast mound that ignores the medial position of the nipple. The new nipple position is referenced to the IMF along the breast meridian. The top of the NAC is marked 2 cm above the new nipple position. A keyhole pattern with 5-cm vertical limbs is drawn. The lateral portion of the Wise pattern extends posteriorly to encompass the lateral skin roll. The robust blood supply through the lateral thoracic perforators allows for sufficient tissue to be rotated into the breast for autologous augmentation. This lateral extension can be used in its entirety or can be trimmed, depending on the desired size and degree of asymmetry.

TECHNIQUE

The areola is marked using a 42-mm cookie cutter. The skin within the entire Wise pattern is then deepithelialized. The dermis is completely incised except for a pedicle base width of approximately 10 cm inferiorly along the IMF. The lateral and

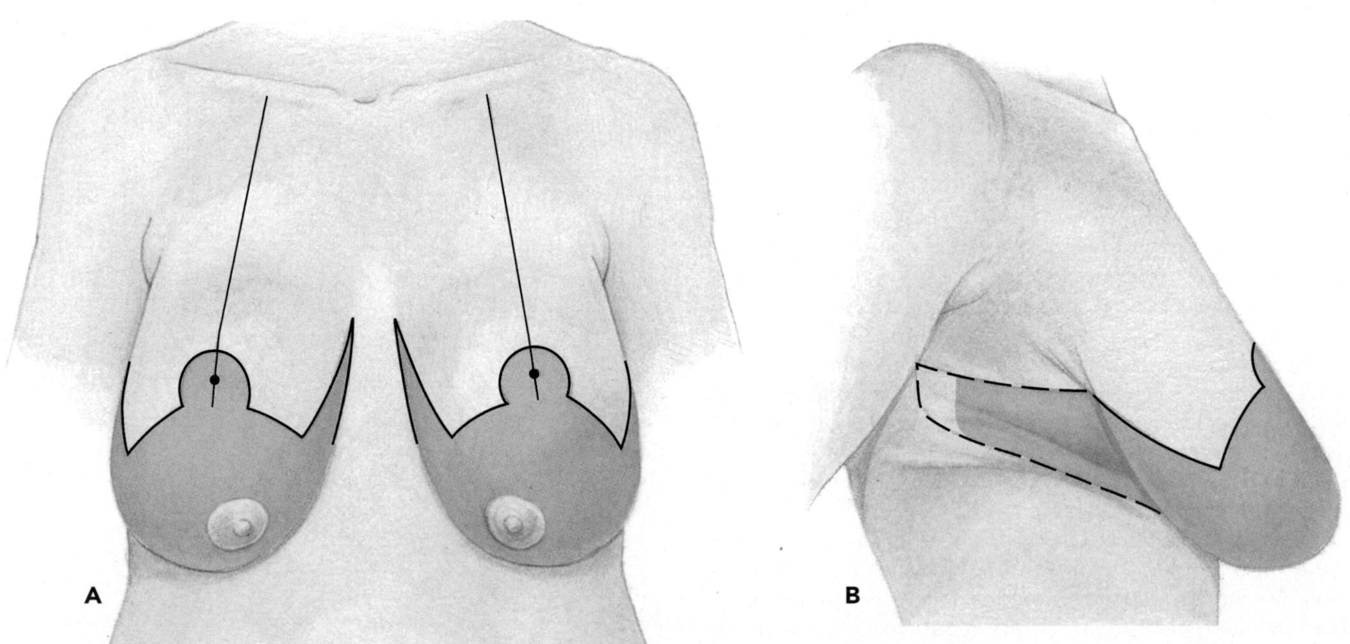

Figure 102.1. **A:** A diagrammatic representation of the extended Wise pattern. The new breast meridian is drawn to correct the medialized nipple position. The total area within the Wise pattern will be deepithelialized. **B:** The lateral extension will be designed to encompass the lateral skin fold. The amount of lateral skin deepithelialized will depend on the autologous volume needed to achieve the desired breast size. Any remaining portion of the lateral roll is discarded.

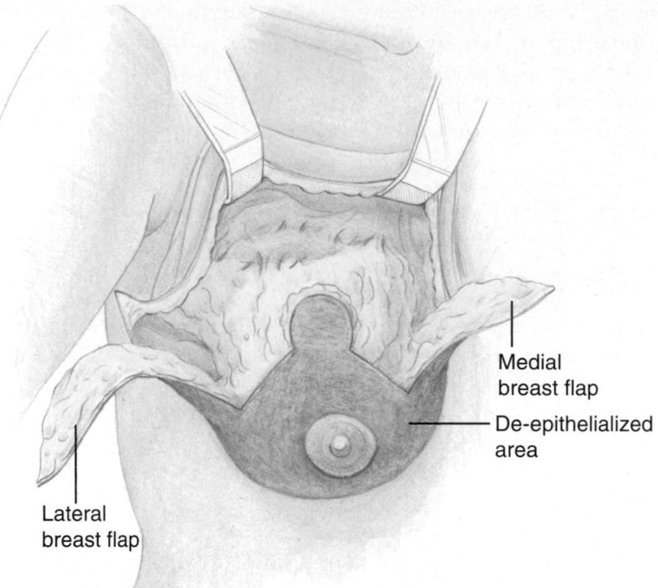

Figure 102.2. The breast parenchyma is degloved to the level of the clavicle by raising 1-cm-thick flaps. Medial and lateral parenchymal flaps are elevated off the chest wall.

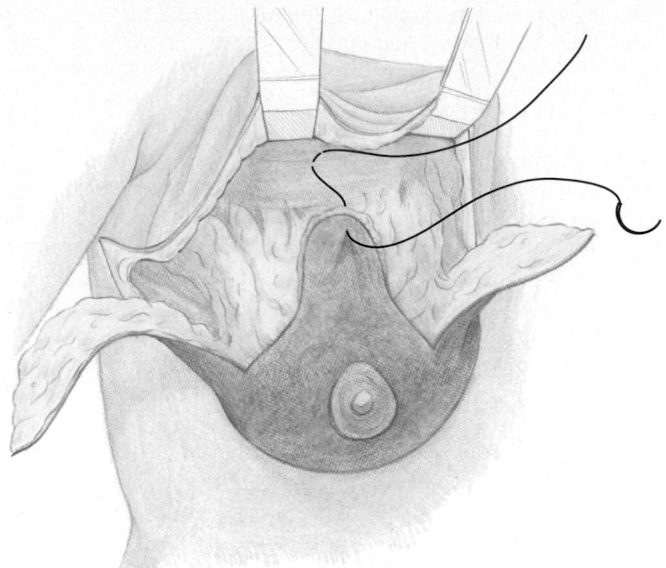

Figure 102.3. The central dermal extension is fixated to the second or third rib in the plane of the new breast meridian using braided nylon sutures. The rib utilized is determined by which position suspends the nipple to the desired final position.

medial extent of this pedicle will correspond to the approximated pivot points for the medial and lateral parenchymal flaps. The entire breast is then degloved by raising skin flaps with a thickness of 1 to 1.5 cm. This dissection is carried down to the pectoralis fascia and then extends in a cephalad direction to the level of the inferior border of the clavicle. The nipple will survive on a healthy central pedicle. Preservation of the attachments to the sternum is essential during medial dissection or symmastia may result. The medial and lateral flaps are then elevated down to the level of the chest wall fascia taking care to preserve any perforating vessels at the flap base (Fig. 102.2). Dissection should be limited to the minimal amount necessary to rotate the flaps to obtain the desired shape. The extent of the lateral flap will vary depending on the amount of volume needed to obtain the desired size, as well as on the degree of asymmetry that needs to be corrected. When dealing with large lateral extended flaps, the flap margins should be checked for healthy bleeding prior to rotation.

Once the breast has been degloved, the next step is to suspend the breast parenchyma to the chest wall. The central dermal extension is suspended to the periosteum of either the second or third rib along the new breast meridian. To safely perform this maneuver, the fingers of the nondominant hand are used to palpate the rib and guide the needle pass. The level of suspension will depend on which rib allows the nipple to lie in the intended final position. Braided 1-0 braided nylon is used (Fig. 102.3).

The lateral breast flap is then rotated and fixated most often to the third rib periosteum. The level of fixation should be where the suspension provides good lateral curvature to the breast parenchyma. The size of the lateral flap can be adjusted prior to this maneuver to obtain the desired volume of autologous augmentation. The medial flap is then rotated superiorly, most commonly to the fourth rib, and fixated to the periostrum in a similar manner (Fig. 102.4). During suspension of the parenchymal flaps, it is helpful to continuously redrape the skin flaps to assess the shape and volume of the breast. If the suspension does not provide the desired nipple position or breast shape, it should be removed and repeated.

Following the dermal suspension, the parenchyma is plicated into its final shape. The dermis of the lateral flap is plicated to the central pedicle dermis using 2-0 absorbable polyglactin

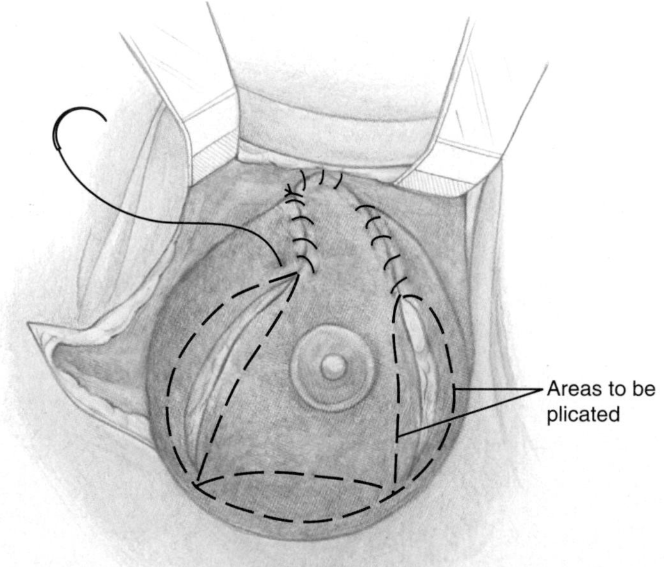

Figure 102.4. The lateral breast flap is then medially rotated to recreate the lateral curvature of the breast. The size of this flap is determined by the amount of tissue required for autologous augmentation. This flap is often sutured adjacent to the first fixation point. The dermis of the medial flap is then fixated to the chest wall, most commonly to the fourth rib periosteum. The dermis of the medial and lateral flaps is sutured to the central dermal extension using a running suture.

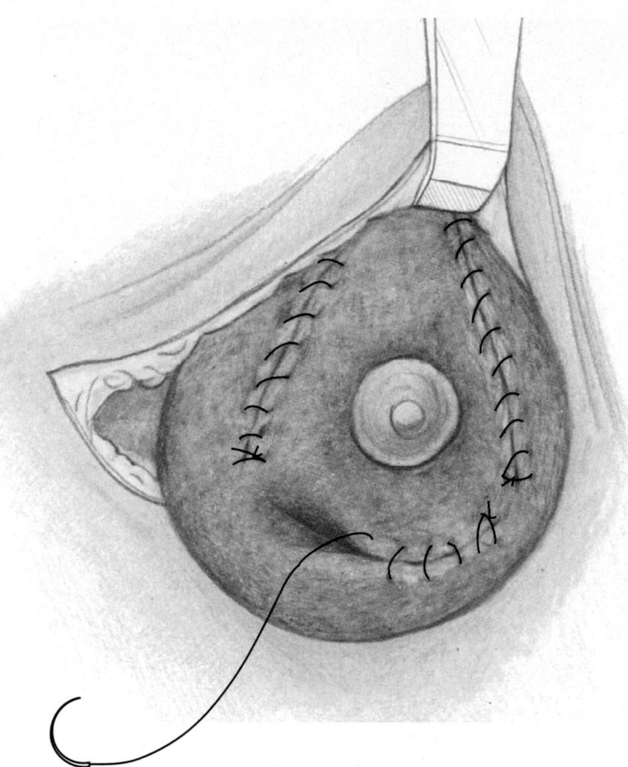

Figure 102.5. The dermis of the inferior pole is then plicated to shorten the nipple to inframammary fold distance. Additional plication sutures can be placed to optimize the breast shape.

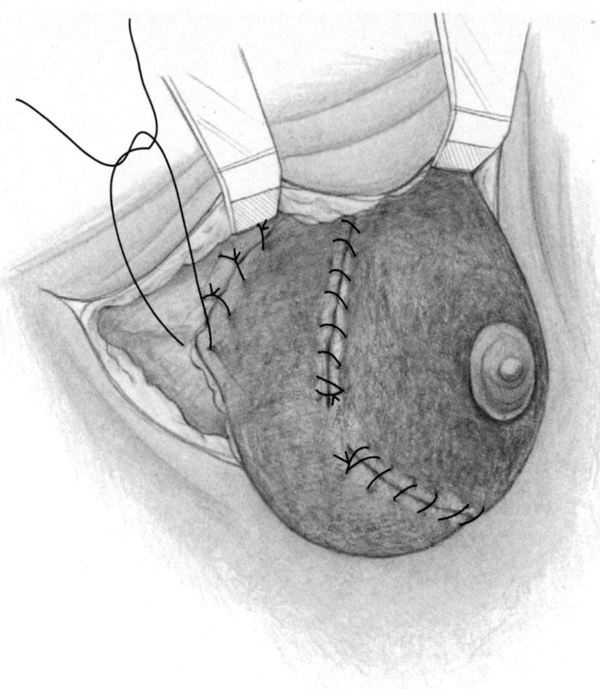

Figure 102.6. The lateral aspect of lateral breast flap is sutured to the chest wall to prevent the breast parenchyma from "herniating" laterally. This maneuver will also increase nipple projection.

sutures. This is performed with the medial flap in similar fashion (Fig. 102.5). If suturing the dermis of the medial and central flaps distorts the medial breast contour, we simply approximate the deep breast parenchyma of these two flaps. The final plication is inferiorly. The desired distance from the IMF to the NAC is 5 cm. Plication is performed inferiorly to achieve this distance, which also helps to increase nipple projection.

The sequence of dermal suspension and parenchymal reshaping is best performed simultaneously on both breasts while the patient is in the sitting position. As the patterns of suspension and plication cannot be predicted preoperatively, it is easier to achieve symmetry if each step is performed synchronously. In addition to the three main rows of dermal plication, additional individual sutures or rows can be added to contour the final parenchymal shape. Constant redraping of the skin flaps will assist in any minor adjustments. To further improve nipple projection and add definition to the lateral sweep of the breast, the lateral dermal edge from the lateral parenchymal flap is sutured to the chest wall fascia (Fig. 102.6). This will also prevent lateral herniation of the parenchyma. The lateral flap is not sutured to the periosteum in this position to minimize the risk of injury to the long thoracic nerve and the thoracodorsal nerve and pedicle.

Prior to closure, the skin flaps are redraped for a final time to ensure that the desired breast shape has been achieved and to assess final symmetry. Closure begins with a 0-polypropylene half-buried stitch tied over a Xeroform bolster to secure the medial and lateral skin flaps to the IMF. A single drain is placed laterally that wraps around the pedicle. The vertical and horizontal skin incisions are closed with a combination of absorbable buried interrupted and running sutures in the dermis.

It may be necessary to release the dermis around the NAC to bring it into its final desired position (Fig. 102.7). It is safe to release the dermis over one half of the circumference of the NAC, given the robust central pedicle blood supply. If the dermis is not released in these cases, the nipple may have a retracted appearance postoperatively. The NAC is secured to the skin flaps with absorbable buried dermal sutures. Cyanoacrylate glue is used along all incisions.

For preoperative and postoperative photographs, see Figures 102.8 to 102.12.

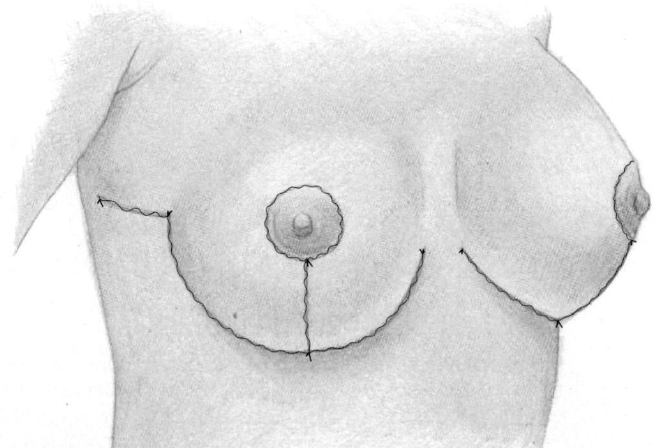

Figure 102.7. The skin flaps are redraped and reapproximated. The dermis around the nipple can be scored around half of its circumference to prevent a tethered appearance of the nipple.

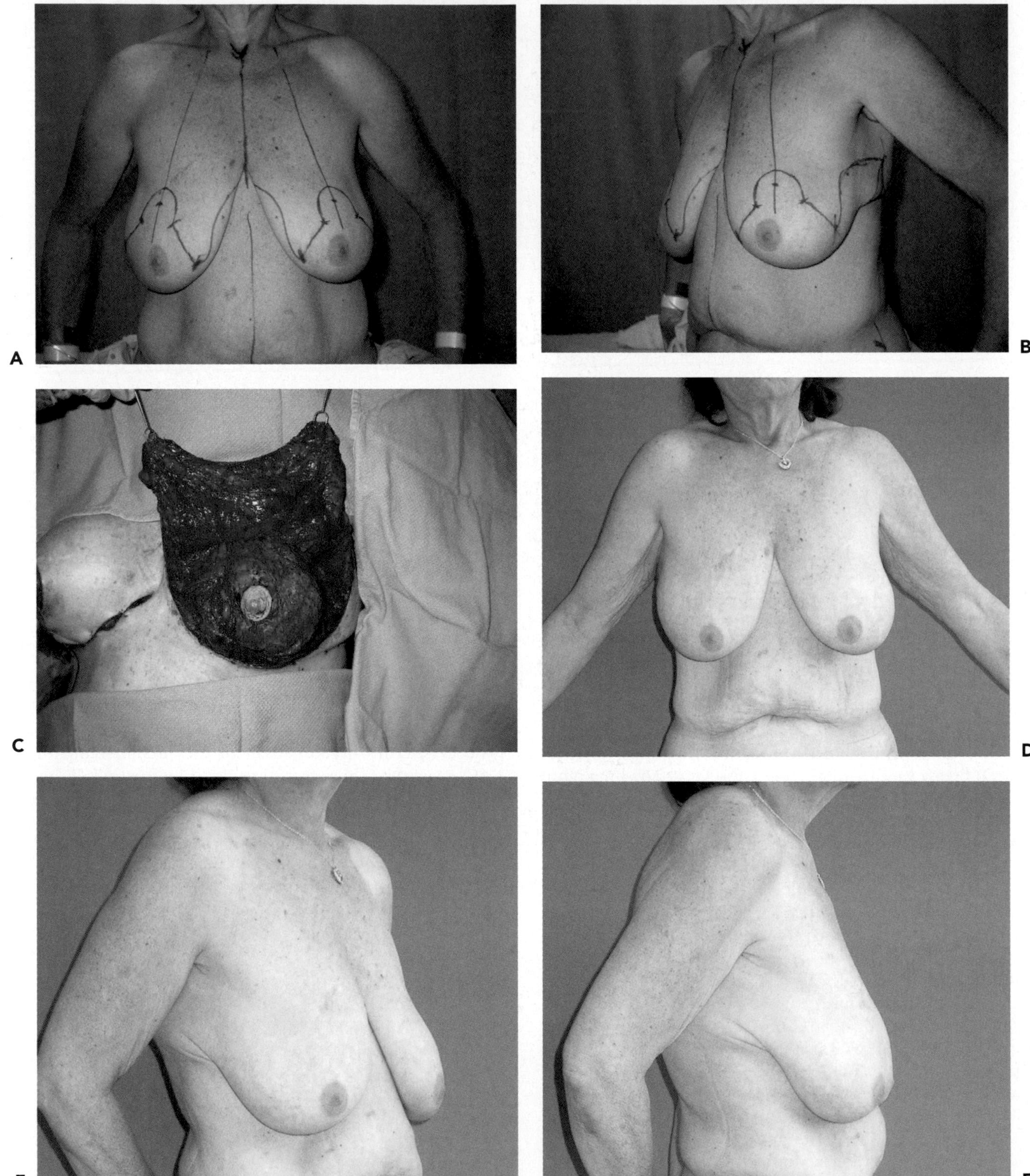

Figure 102.8. **A, B:** A 57-year-old woman after a 130-pound weight loss. The markings demonstrate the extended Wise pattern that encompasses the lateral skin fold and moves the nipple to a more medial position along the new breast meridian. **C:** Intraoperative view demonstrating the suspension and breast shape control achieved with parenchymal reshaping. **D–F:** Preoperative views. (*continued*)

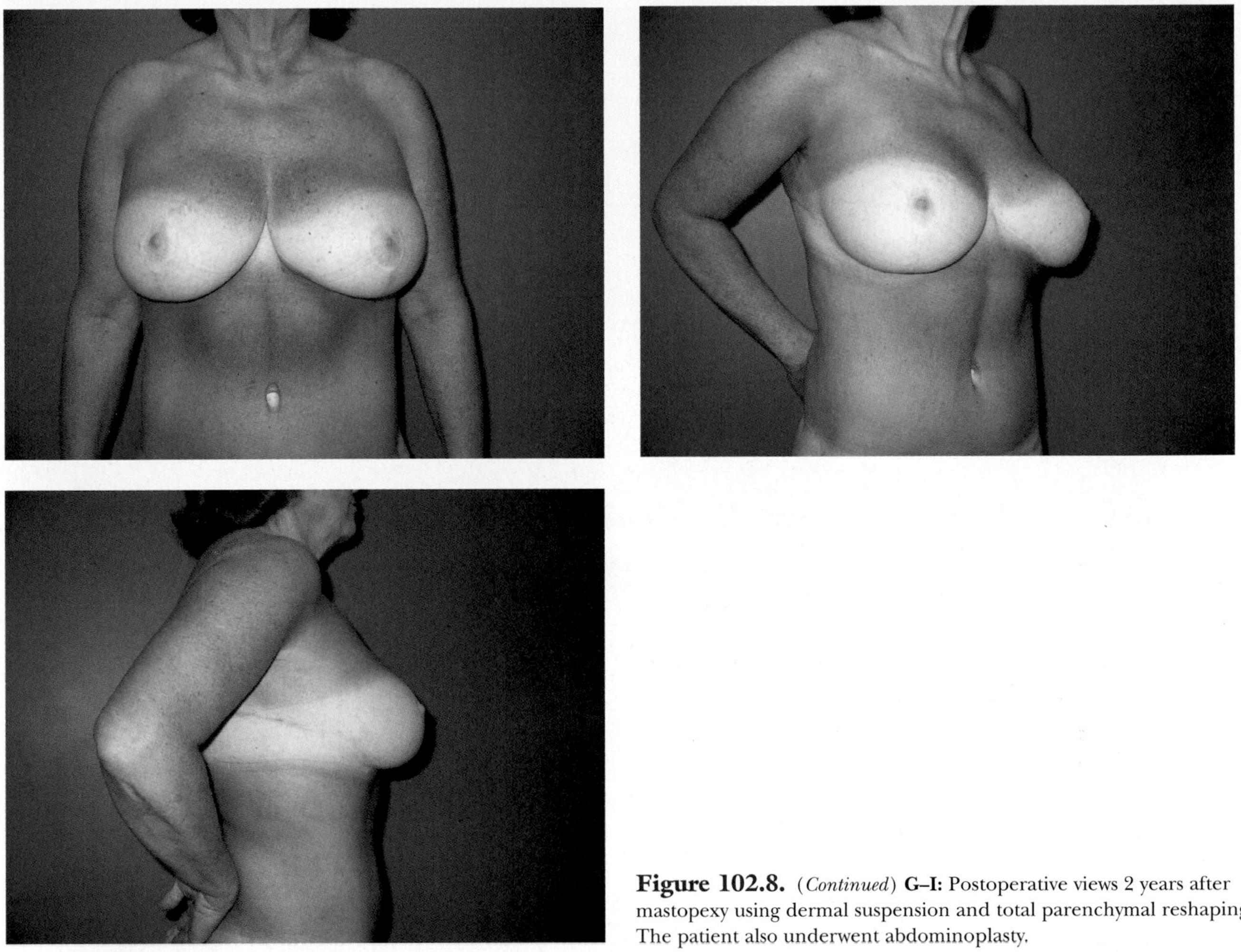

Figure 102.8. (*Continued*) **G–I:** Postoperative views 2 years after mastopexy using dermal suspension and total parenchymal reshaping. The patient also underwent abdominoplasty.

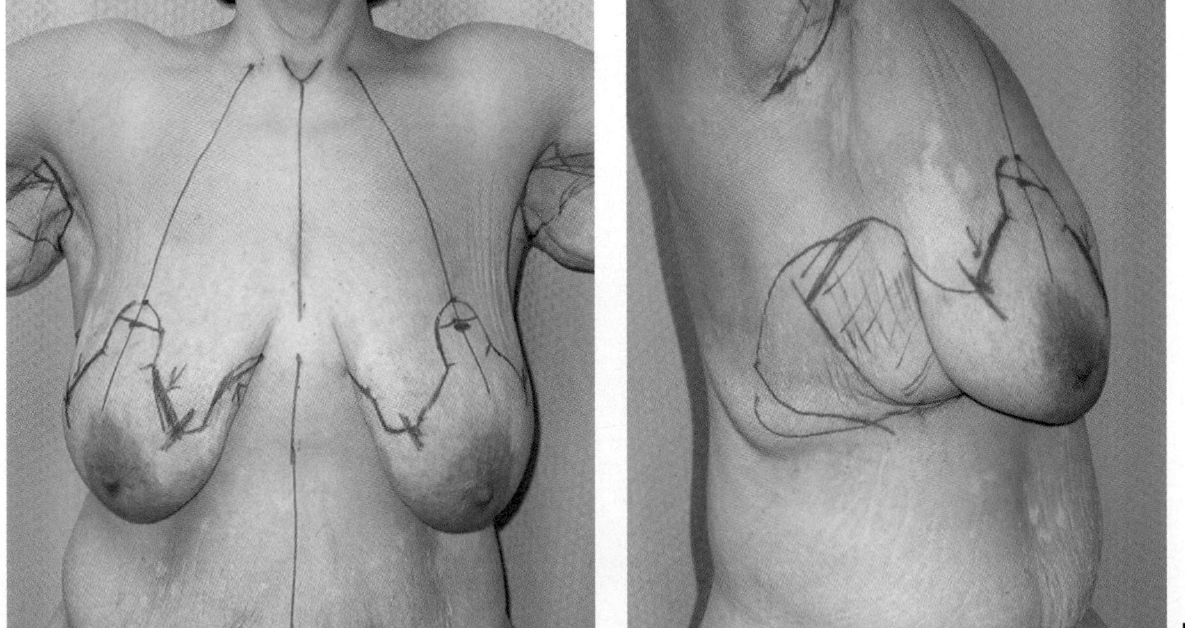

Figure 102.9. **A, B:** A 40–year-old woman following a 135-pound weight loss. The lateral markings demonstrate how varying amount of tissue from the lateral skin fold can be used for volume augmentation and the remaining skin fold tissue is discarded. (*continued*)

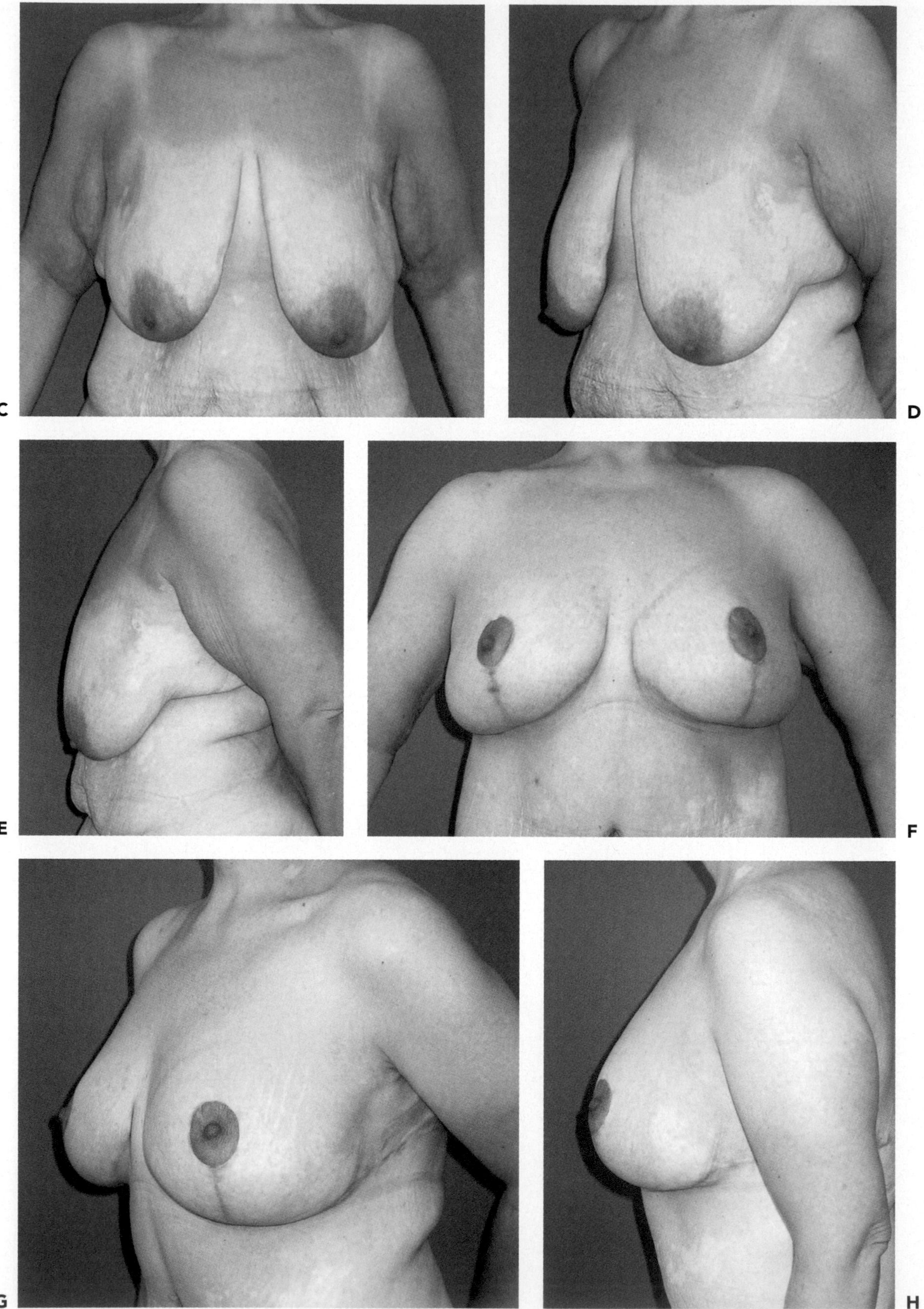

Figure 102.9. (*Continued*) **C–E:** Preoperative views. **F–H:** Postoperative views 6 months after surgery. The patient also underwent abdominoplasty.

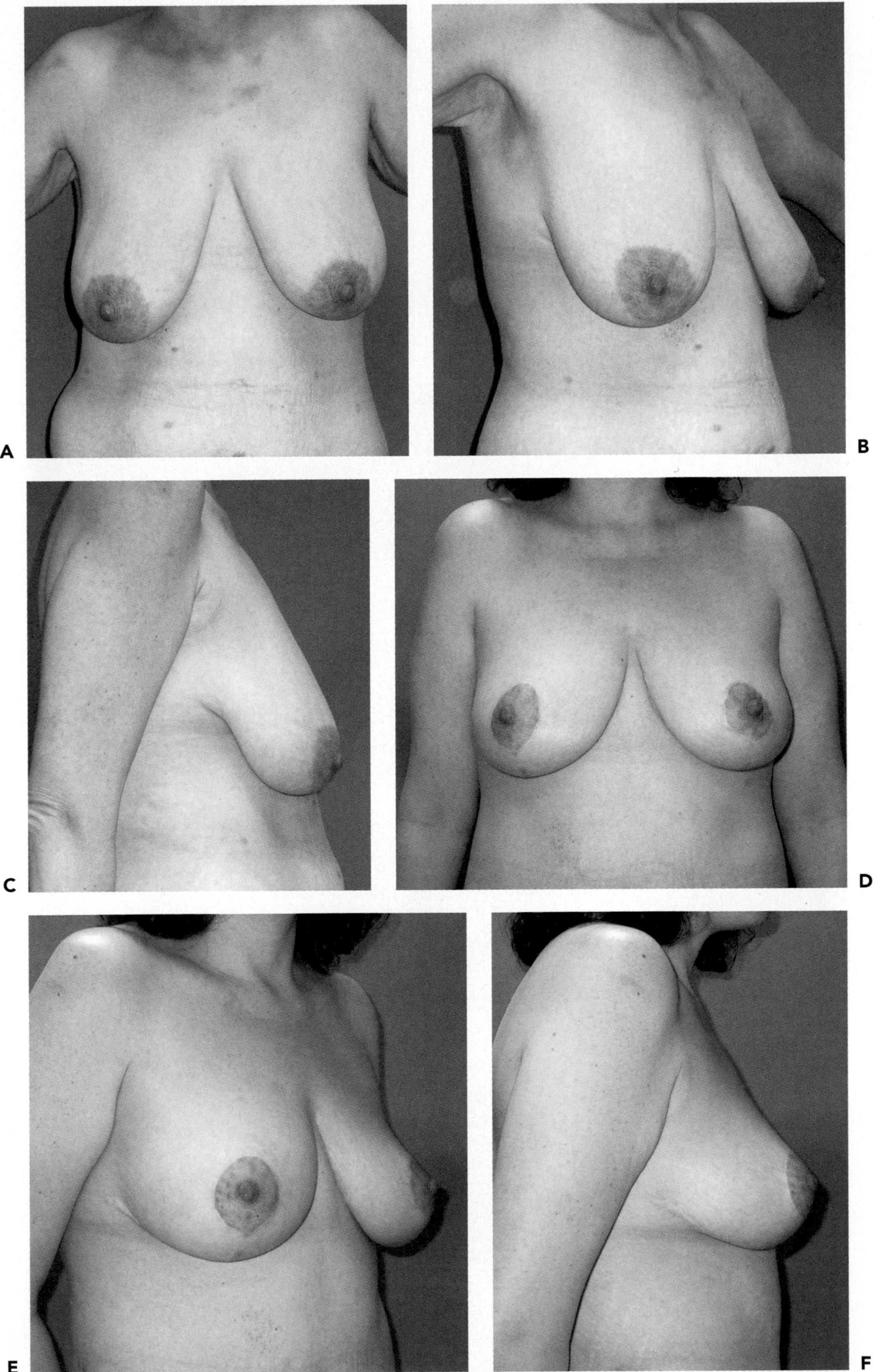

Figure 102.10. A 43-year-old woman 18 months after a Roux-en-Y gastric bypass with a weight loss of 110 pounds. Her preoperative body mass index was 26 kg/m^2. **A–C:** Preoperative views. **D–F:** Postoperative views 2 years following mastopexy with dermal suspension and total parenchymal reshaping. This patient had a small lateral fold allowing the lateral scar to be shorter. The patient also had a concurrent abdominoplasty.

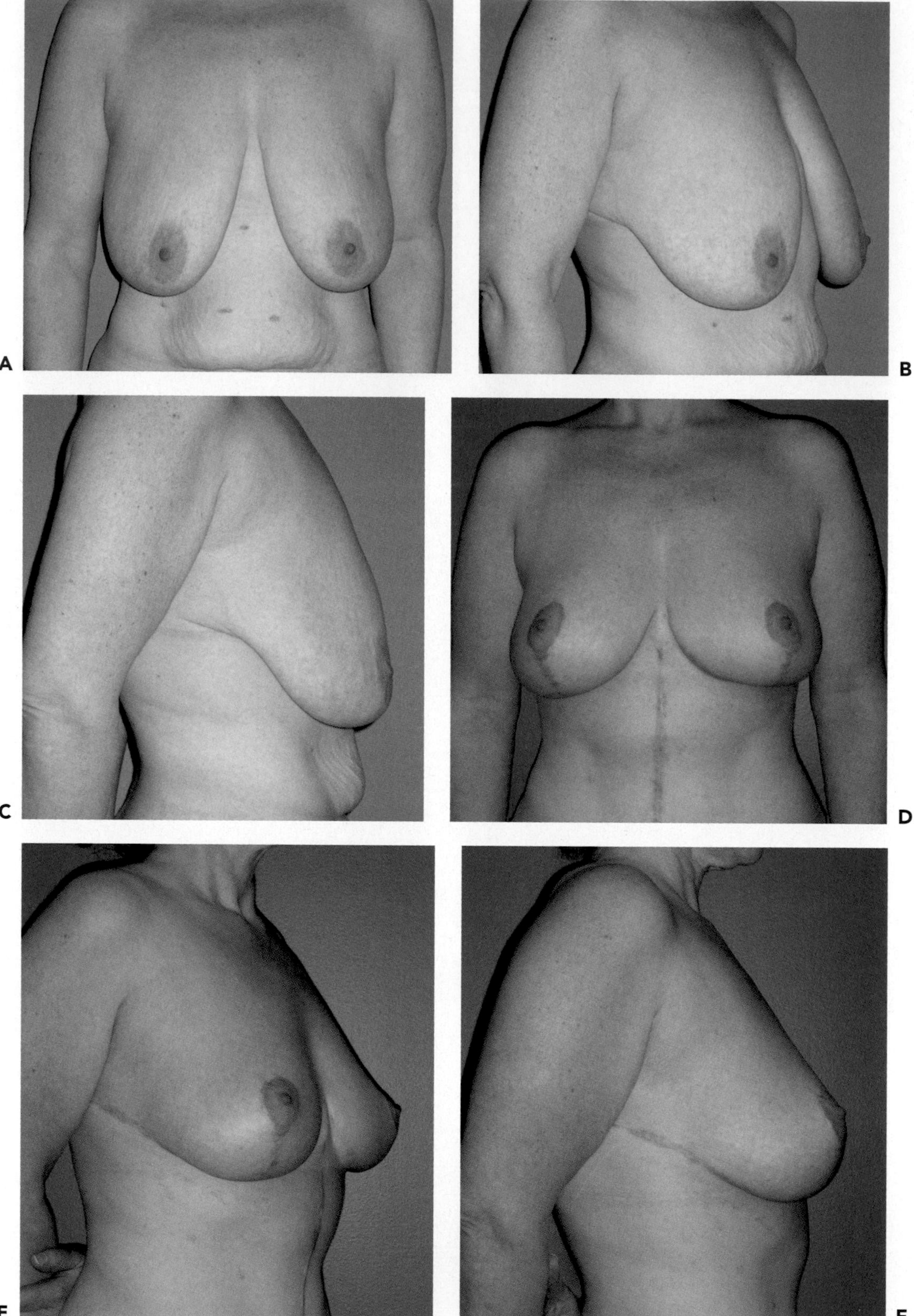

Figure 102.11. **A–C:** Preoperative views of a 46-year-old woman after a 150-pound weight loss. **D–F:** Postoperative views 21 months after mastopexy using dermal suspension and total parenchymal reshaping. A vertical abdominoplasty was also performed.

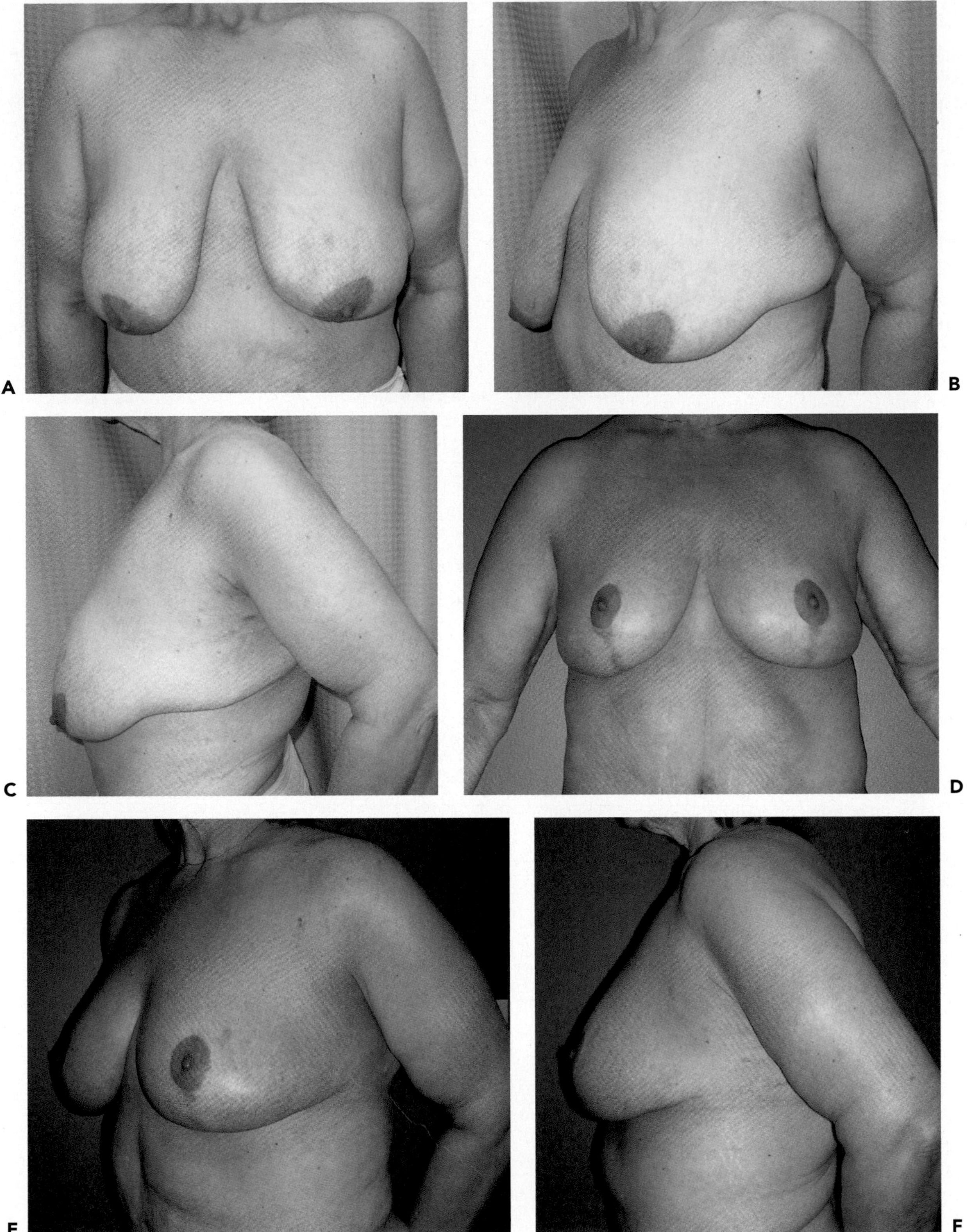

Figure 102.12. A 51-year-old woman with a 151-pound weight loss. **A–C:** Preoperative views. **D–F:** Postoperative views 18 months following mastopexy. The patient also underwent abdominoplasty and brachioplasty.

POSTOPERATIVE CARE

Gauze fluffs are placed over all incision lines, and the chest is wrapped with an elastic bandage. The dressing is taken down on postoperative day 4 or 5, and the patient is placed in a sports bra for 4 to 6 weeks. The bolster stitch is removed at 1 week, and the drains are removed once the daily output is less than 30 cc. The patients are instructed not to lift anything heavier than 10 pounds for the 3 weeks, after which they can slowly increase their activity. Underwire bras are to be avoided for at least 6 weeks. If mastopexy is performed as an isolated procedure, the patient can be discharged the same day.

COMPLICATIONS

This procedure has proven to be very durable and safe. Patient satisfaction with the procedure has been very high. Complications have included hematoma (1%), seroma (3%), and minor wound dehiscence at the triple point (5%). Wound issues can often be treated with local wound care. We have seen no cases of partial or total NAC necrosis, breast flap loss, or significant fat necrosis.

EDITORIAL COMMENTS

This chapter represents a solid introduction to the management of the breasts of a woman after massive weight loss. Whether presenting for an augmentation, mastopexy, augmentation/mastopexy, autoaugmentation, or reduction, these patients present both unique and challenging issues. With varying combinations of parenchymal loss, skin stretch, dislocation of normal landmarks, adjacent deformities, distortions, and often unrealistic expectations, these women require solutions not needed in the vast majority of other breast procedures.

Rubin and Michaels do a nice job of triaging these patients for us with special attention to the mastopexy, autoaugmentation, and reduction categories. The technique that they describe using all the tissues within the "Wise" pattern is unique to this group of patients and a wonderful way of harnessing all those displaced tissues that need to be removed or moved in order to recreate a more attractive breast.

Equally challenging is controlling the inframammary fold or skin stretch in patients receiving breast implants. For those patients, the use of alloplastic materials to support the implant and unweight the overlying skin and parenchyma may prove to be very important.

This chapter serves to shine a bright light on the management of the breast deformities in the massive weight loss patient. It is no doubt that improved understanding and additional techniques are soon to come.

REFERENCES

1. Song AY, Jean RD, Hurwitz DJ, et al. A classification of contour deformities after bariatric weight loss: the Pittsburgh Rating Scale. *Plast Reconstr Surg* 2005;116:1535–1544; discussion, 1545–1546.
2. Rubin JP. Mastopexy in the massive weight loss patient: dermal suspension and total parenchymal reshaping. *Aesthet Surg J* 2006;26:214–222.
3. Rubin JP, Khachi G. Mastopexy after massive weight loss: dermal suspension and selective auto-augmentation. *Clin Plast Surg* 2008;35:123–129.
4. Rubin JP, Gusenoff JA, Coon D. Dermal suspension and parenchymal reshaping mastopexy after massive weight loss: statistical analysis with concomitant procedures from a prospective registry. *Plast Reconstr Surg* 2009;123:782–789.
5. Hurwitz DJ, Agha-Mohammadi S. Postbariatric surgery breast reshaping: the spiral flap. *Ann Plast Surg* 2006;56:481–486.
6. Graf RM, Mansur AE, Tenius FP, et al. Mastopexy after massive weight loss: extended chest wall-based flap associated with a loop of pectoralis muscle. *Aesthet Plast Surg* 2008;32(2): 371–374.
7. Losken A, Holtz DJ. Versatility of the superomedial pedicle in managing the massive weight loss breast: the rotation-advancement technique. *Plast Reconstr Surg* 2007;120:1060–1068.
8. Hamdi M, Van Landuyt K, Blondeel P, et al. Autologous breast augmentation with the lateral intercostal artery perforator flap in massive weight loss patients. *J Plast Reconstr Aesthet Surg* 2009;62:65–70.
9. Kwei S, Borud LJ, Lee BT. Mastopexy with autologous augmentation after massive weight loss: the intercostal artery perforator (ICAP) flap. *Ann Plast Surg* 2006;57:361–365.
10. Rubin JP, Nguyen V, Schentker A. Perioperative management of the post-gastric bypass patient presenting for body contour surgery. *Clin Plast Surg* 2004;31:601–610.
11. American Cancer Society. Detailed guide: breast cancer. Available at: http://www.cancer.org/docroot/CRI/CRI_2_3x.asp?dt=5. Accessed July 12, 2009.

CHAPTER

103

Dennis J. Hurwitz

Strategies in Breast Reduction and Mastopexy After Massive Weight Loss

INTRODUCTION

After massive weight loss (MWL), breasts are often ptotic and project poorly. The tissues can become so deflated and lax that the breasts resemble pancakes (Fig. 103.1). Depending on residual breast volume, breast reshaping consists of reduction, mastopexy, or mastopexy with augmentation.

The poor quality of the tissues and severity of the deformity makes these breasts not only difficult to reshape, but also prone to recurrent deformity. Compounding the MWL breast deformity is the surrounding loose skin of the arms, axillas, and torso. Hence, the strategy for treatment of MWL breasts involves not only effective and long-term improvement of its varied deformities, but also correction of the surrounding soft tissues of the torso and upper extremity.

With the increased popularity of bariatric surgery and public acceptance of plastic surgery, this clinical challenge is becoming common. After nearly a decade of focused clinical activity, I present a comprehensive, effective, and safe approach to aesthetically contouring the breasts and upper torso. A brief discussion of obesity, weight loss surgery, the subsequent contour deformities, and their treatment introduces my approach to the MWL breast.

OBESITY AND WEIGHT LOSS

Obesity is approaching epidemic proportions and causes about 300,000 deaths per year in the United States (1). From 2003 to 2004, 66.3% of American adults were classified as either overweight or obese, 32.2% were obese, and 4.8% were morbidly obese (2). The values of body mass index (BMI) used to define overweight, obesity, and morbid obesity are 25.0 to 29.9, 30.0 to 39.9, and greater than 40.0 kg/m^2, respectively (3). Obesity is not only deforming, but it also is accompanied by a long list of adverse medical conditions that reduce the quality and length of life (4). While there are outstanding instances of massive weight loss by lifestyle change, weight loss surgery (WLS) is recognized as the effective long-term treatment for obesity and related comorbidities (5).

WLS results in a drastic reduction of food consumption by restrictive or malabsorptive means or by a combination of the two. The most common bariatric operations are laparoscopic adjustable banding (LAGB) and Roux-en-Y gastric bypass (RYGBP). LAGB is a restrictive procedure in which a small gastric pouch with a small outlet is created, resulting in early and prolonged satiety (6). Since the normal absorptive surface is left intact, specific nutrient deficiencies are uncommon, unless vomiting is induced or there are eccentric dietary restrictions. The RYGBP procedure involves both restrictive and malabsorptive components. The stomach pouch is decreased to less than 30 mL with a roughly 100-cm Roux limb. WLS produces weight loss within 1 year after surgery that is three to four times superior to what can be achieved with nonsurgical weight management programs (7). Depending on the procedure employed, patients typically lose about 25% to 40% of their initial weight at 12 to 18 months and maintain the majority of the lost weight for many years (7). These numbers clearly represent a much greater and lasting change compared to other weight loss options. Consequently, the number of bariatric operations has risen progressively, with more than 200,000 procedures performed in 2007 alone (8). Altered food intake and malabsorption lead to a variety of protein, vitamin, and mineral deficiencies that can have significant impact on outcomes of subsequent plastic surgery (9,10).

The recent success of bariatric surgery has led to increasing numbers of individuals with sagging skin and body contours. Just for the massive weight loss patients, there were more than 68,000 body-contouring procedures in 2006 (11).

WEIGHT LOSS DEFORMITY

MWL leaves a spectrum of body deformity (Figs. 103.1 to 103.11). The skin laxity relates to the rapidity of reduction, absolute change, and final BMI. The deflation is influenced by age, general health, and fitness, as well as by familial and gender-specific fat depositions, skin elasticity, skin to fascia adherences, muscular development, and skeletal form. The complexity of the etiology thwarts precise predictions.

The susceptible regions are the anterior neck, upper arms, breasts, lower back, abdomen, mons pubis, buttocks, and thighs. Characteristically there is a large, sometimes transversely septated abdominal pannus overlapping the pubic and groin regions, with smaller rolls about the back, and in the upper medial and lateral thighs. Skin rolls are partially emptied, localized deposits of fat defined by transverse adherence of dermis to deep fascia. Wrinkled skin is emptied of fat. A roll of an entire region or structure is considered ptosis. Ptosis occurs in the breasts, mons pubis, and buttocks. These contour changes androgenize women and feminize men.

The breast shape, texture, projection, and skin elasticity deteriorate. The breasts flatten, sag, and descend slightly down the chest. Superior pole fullness is diminished to absent. With reduced fat, the organ feels firm and gritty. Broad areas of dermal striae are common. The breasts are displaced and broadened by descended inframammary folds (IMF). The IMF descent progressively increases from medial to lateral. The nipple-areolar complexes (NACs) are ptotic and may be distorted.

Surrounding the breasts are cascading rolls of mid torso skin with shaping influenced by transverse subcutaneous fascial adherences to underlying muscular fascia. The flattened ante-

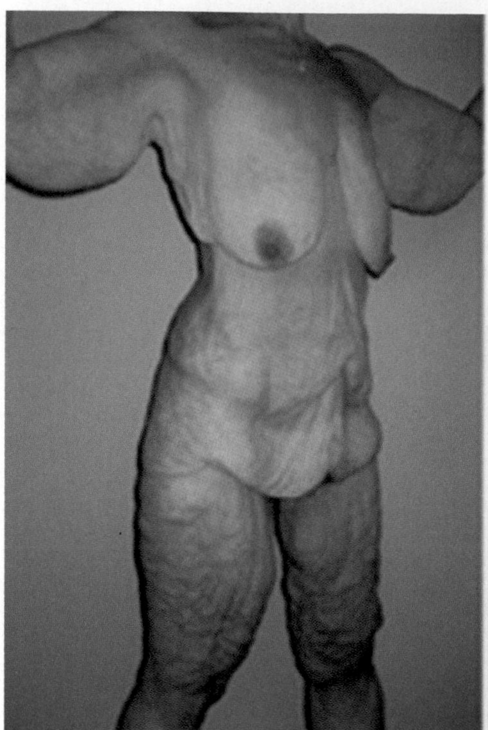

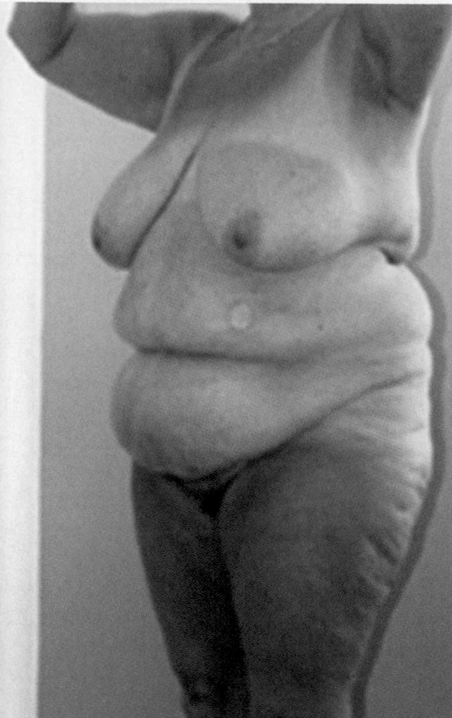

Figure 103.1. The wide range of massive weight loss deformity and body mass index (BMI) that is successfully treated with total body lift surgery and breast reshaping is depicted in these opposing oblique clinical views. **Left:** This 41-year-old, 5′6″ tall, 158-pound woman (BMI 26.6) lost 192 pounds from 350 pounds after gastric bypass performed 4 years earlier. She has sheets of skin hanging from her arms, thighs, and torso and pancake-shaped breasts. **Right:** This 54-year-old, 5′4″ tall, 195-pound woman (BMI 34.5) lost 150 pounds through lifestyle changes. She has multiple heavy skin rolls and severely ptotic and heavy breasts.

rior axillary line ends at a hyperaxilla (oversized and deep) and canopy-like sagging upper arm.

Overlapping skin traps moisture, with increased bacterial counts and mal odor. Skin irritation leads from intertrigo to abscesses. Flapping tissues inhibit athletic activity. Large pannus and ptotic regions may cause poor posture and back strain. Clothes fit poorly. The unclothed presence is often more objectionable to the patient after MWL.

PRINCIPLES OF BODY CONTOURING SURGERY

Body contouring surgery is the removal of excess tissue while improving gender-specific contours (Fig. 103.12). My appreciation of the surgical principles of body contouring surgery after MWL has evolved (12–14). The torso is shaped by the transverse removal of excess skin, leaving level, flat, and symmetric scars that are hidden from view in minimal clothing. The reliable positioning of incisions that result in such favorable scars requires a consistent marking plan that includes multiple body positions, vigorous manipulation of the tissues, artistic visualization, and willingness to redraw lines until they seem precisely correct. With consistency and experience, the surgeon will gain confidence in the accuracy of the planned excisions and make minimal intraoperative adjustments, facilitating efficiency and teamwork.

Closure across the widest diameters of the torso, the IMFs, and hips takes in some of the transverse excess. Vertical or oblique excisions of skin along the torso or thighs are reserved for severe gynecomastia, intervening scars, hernias, or massive transverse skin and fat excess. The fleur-de-lis abdominoplasty can be applied to the unscarred abdomen, if that is the only procedure used to shape the anterior-lateral torso.

With the preinfusion of epinephrine-containing solutions, large-blade scalpel incisions are made through the skin and subcutaneous fascia. Electrocautery is reserved for direct coagulation of vessels and undermining to avoid thermal injury to the superficial fascial system (SFS). Direct undermining is limited, relying on the Lockwood underminer, liposuction, and dissector dilators for more distant discontinuous skin release. The undermining is adequate when the dermis, not the deep fascial adherences, limits pulling the flap toward closure.

Secure closures depend on closely spaced broad inclusion of the multilayered SFS by large braided sutures. With poor skin elasticity, closure of the SFS must be tight. Even so, a tight abdomen on standing may have flaccid rolls of skin upon sitting. As permanent suture closure of the subcutaneous tissues was strongly advocated by the body lift pioneer Lockwood (15), at first I used them regularly. Subsequent to a single case of multiple delayed suture abscesses from permanent sutures, I abandoned their use in 2006. I found braided absorbable suture closure adequate. Concerned about strangulating fat necrosis within an overly constricting interrupted suture and for speed of closure, I moved toward running braided suture closure. Suture breakage with unraveling of the closure was a concern. Over the last few years, I have switched to double-needle two-direction barbed sutures called Quill SRS (Angiotech, Vancouver, Canada) for more rapid and secure two-layer closures. Lower-body lifts are generally closed with no. 2 Quill polydioxanone (PDO) 24-cm-long sutures. The dermis is aligned with rapid-absorbing 3-0 or 2-0 barbed Monoderm. The absence of knots reduces suture-related infections; however, spitting sutures do occur due to large-gauge suture placed near the dermis. The tension during closure should be minimized by flexing the region. Preliminary alignment and placement of cross-hatching aids in accurate closure of the wound with running sutures. When an undermined flap is to be advanced to a

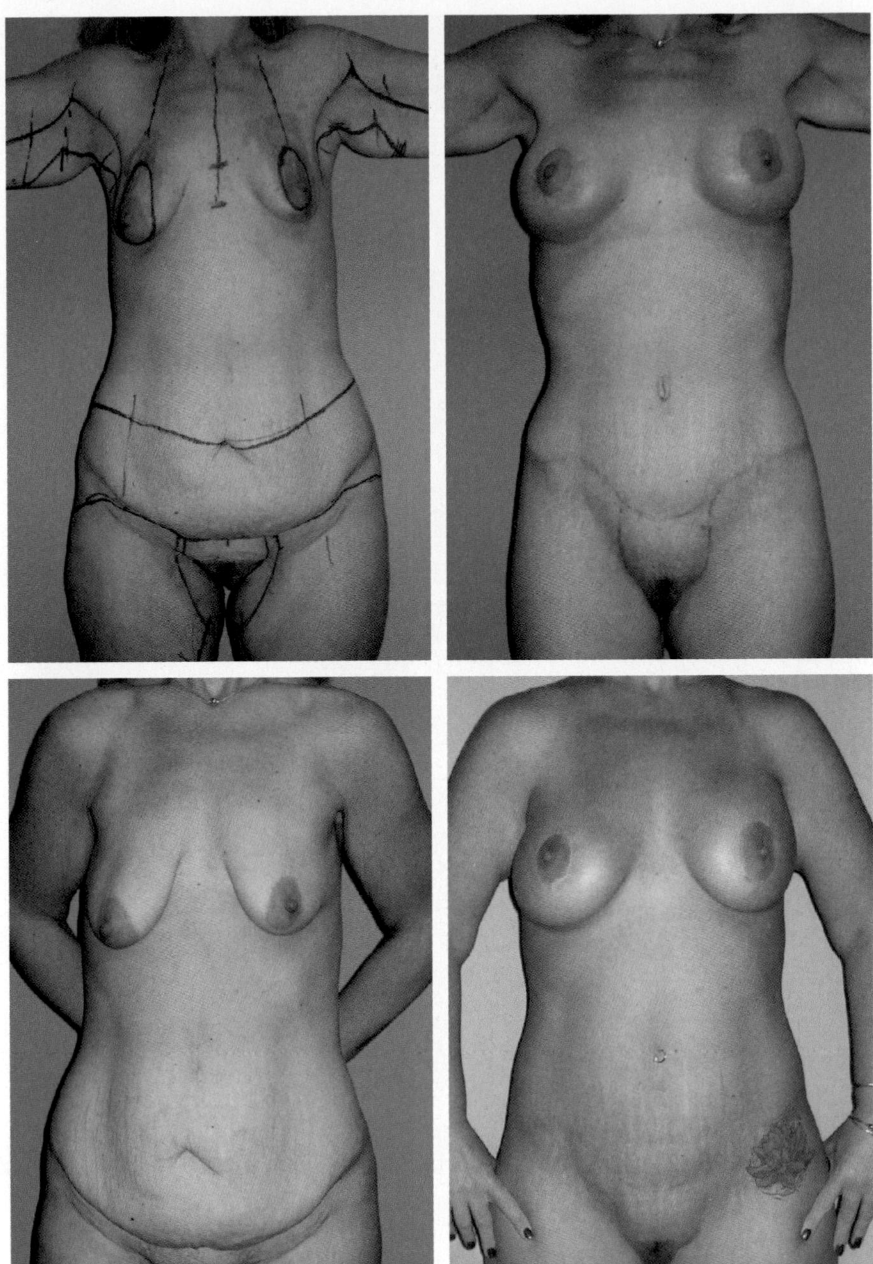

Figure 103.2. Preoperative and postoperative photographs of a 36-year-old woman. She is 5′6″ tall and weighs 165 pounds (body mass index 26.6) after losing 131 pounds through Roux-en-Y bypass. Her breasts were atrophied, but her inframammary folds were distinct and well positioned. Her skin redundancy was primarily in her lower trunk and thighs. After a total body lift consisting of L-shaped brachioplasties, concentric ring mastopexies, and partial subpectoral 350-cc, smooth-walled, gel-filled implant augmentation, internal suture fixation of the internal mammary folds, abdominoplasty, lower body lift, and bilateral vertical medial thighplasties were performed. Upper photos are frontal images with preoperative markings and 5 months after surgery. Lower photos are preoperative frontal images without markings and 2 years after surgery. While the soft tissue transitions from breast tissue to surrounding chest have improved, the breast implants and inframammary folds have descended slightly.

fixed point such as a reverse abdominoplasty flap to the sixth rib to create the new IMF or a medial thigh flap to the pubis, then all the interrupted sutures are placed first and later tied with the assistant pushing the tissues together.

Overresection of skin followed by excessively tight closure leads to wound dehiscence or later to broadly depressed tissues due to suture pullthrough, breakage, or premature dissolution. The etiology of the common suture abscess with exposure of the suture is multifactorial (16). Localized wound infection with suture abscesses may be due to incision ischemia, intraoperative hypothermia, vasoconstriction, bacterial contamination, foreign-body reaction, intraoperative or postoperative pressure sores, suture characteristics, excessive surgical trauma, and reduced immune status. Prompt drainage and removal of the offending material and debridement of necrotic tissue is essential, followed by appropriate wound care. Our initial series of total body lift patients, when closely examined for every delayed healing, experienced nearly a 75% wound-healing complication rate (16). There has been a steady downward trend of wound complications with better selection of patients, correction of preoperative nutritional deficiencies, and maintenance of adequate postoperative nutrition, as well as improved maintenance of body temperature and positioning (12,16).

Inadequate removal of skin and low closure tension lead to failure. Even when the skin tension at closure is high and an appropriate lift and contour correction appears for some months, significant recurrence can occur 6 months later. This disappointing and unpredictable event is treated by repeat surgery.

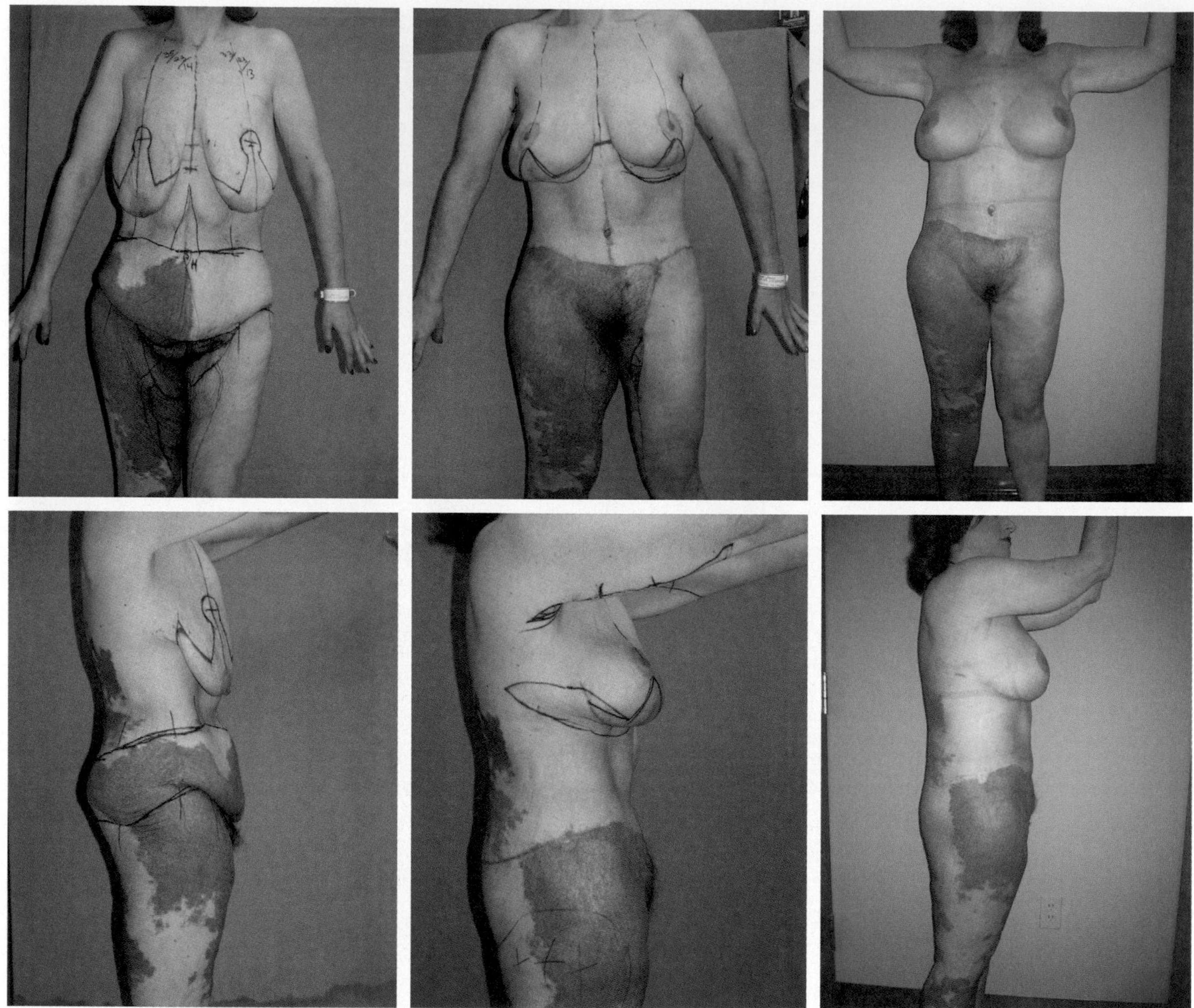

Figure 103.3. This case demonstrates the shortcomings of breast augmentation with mastopexy for the pancake breast and the potential help of a reverse abdominoplasty with elevation of the inframammary fold (IMF) in maintaining breast shape. This is a 5′5″ tall, 150-pound (body mass index 124.9) 34-year-old woman who lost 175 of her 325 pounds following gastric bypass. **Left:** These frontal and lateral images shows the markings for an abdominoplasty, lower body lift, vertical medial thighplasties, and Wise-pattern mastopexy with 325-cc, saline-filled silicone implant augmentation. **Middle:** Five months after her total body lift, these images show bottoming out of her breasts with loose epigastric skin. The superior poles are empty, and the nipple-areola complexes (NACs) are too high on the breast mounds. The immediate preoperative markings are for inverted-T excision revisions of the lower breast and reverse abdominoplasty that extends laterally to removal a small chest roll. As the vertical limb of her mastopexy was shortened to 5 cm, her IMF was raised 3 cm (to the transverse mark over the lower sternum). **Right:** These views are 2 years after her revision and 3 months into a pregnancy. Her improved breast shape with fullness of the superior pole and IMF positions have been maintained. Her NACs now lie at greatest projection of her breasts.

Gender-specific convexity and concavity are thoughtfully sculptured. The fullness of the female hips and gentle convexity of the mons pubis and lateral thighs need to be preserved or reconstructed if lost. Body contour flattens along the line of tight closure or between nearby transverse closures. Therefore, lower-body-lift incision closure is rarely along the lateral trochanters, which might obliterate their natural convexity. Yet, a high suture line along the waist is too exposed for most patients. The waist is maximally narrowed between the upper and lower body transverse closures of the total-body-lift operation. Convexity is created by preservation of subcutaneous fat and, if needed, by adipose flaps or lipoaugmentation. An appropriate amount of fat should be preserved in the midline distal abdominoplasty flap and over the lateral pelvis to create a gentle feminine suprapubic and hip fullness.

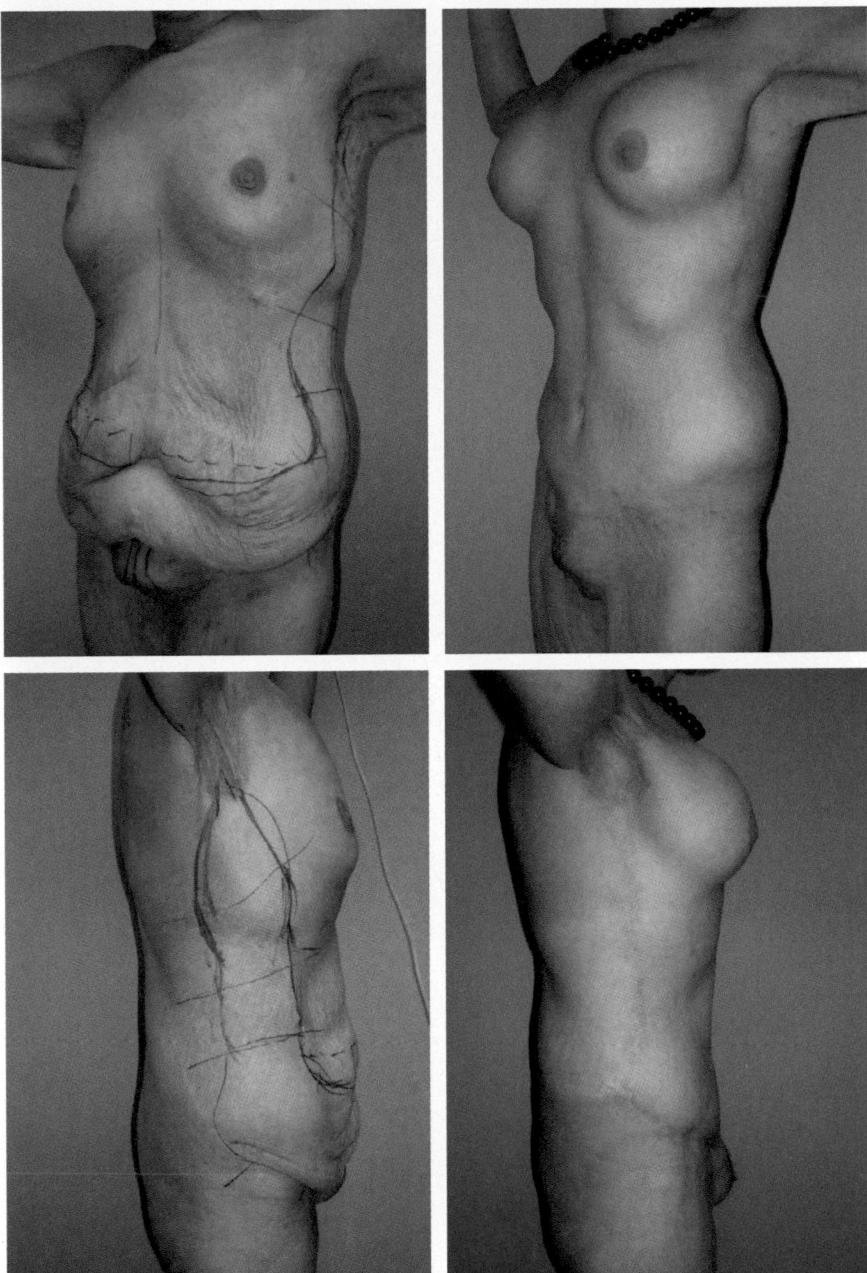

Figure 103.4. This 24-year-old, 5′3″ tall, 126-pound (body mass index 19.8) woman lost 120 pounds after Roux-en-Y gastric bypass surgery. These are the left oblique and right lateral images before and 15 months after a single-stage total body lift, consisting of a lateral torsoplasty with an abdominoplasty and placement of 425-cc, saline-filled implants in the partial subpectoral position and a midline pubic mons plasty. **Left:** Weight loss had flattened her breasts and hips and blunted her waist. There was little excess skin of her back, and she was unconcerned by her flat buttocks. The curvilinear lateral torso skin excision starts from her axilla and continues anteriorly to include the skin between the umbilicus and pubis as in a traditional abdominoplasty. The waist was narrowed to resecting maximum tissue at that level. Hip fullness was created by leaving as much subcutaneous tissue behind as possible. In order to not disturb the lateral border of the breasts, the advanced back flap was securely sutured to the serratus muscle. **Right:** The scars have faded and the loose torso skin removed as a sculptured feminine form was created. The inferior poles of the breasts are inadequately filled, and mild prominence of the mons persists.

REVIEW OF MASSIVE-WEIGHT-LOSS LITERATURE ON THE BREAST

After intestinal bypass surgery for obesity became popular in the 1970s, Zook opined that once all indicated surgical procedures were identified, a surgical plan was coordinated "so that as many [procedures] as possible can be done simultaneously" (17). With two or three teams working at the same time, the arms, breasts, and circumferential abdominoplasty were contoured (17,18). The aesthetic interrelationship between the breast deformity and the arms and trunk was not discussed. In fact, Zook later declared post–weight-loss body contouring nonaesthetic, primarily due to the extensive scars (18). He considered loosely hanging breasts as "an extremely difficult problem" (17). He cited others' and his experience, indicating that normally discarded flaps should be deepithelialized and placed behind the breasts. He favored the Pitanguy mastopexy with deepithelialization of the keyhole and the entire inferior breast, which was then turned upward to give the breast bulk and projection. For undesirable rolls and bulk, the inferior incision was carried around the trunk (17).

About the same time, Palmer et al. recommended procedures on only one area at a time because of the extent of each excision (19). Recognizing the skin folds below and lateral to the ptotic breasts, they built up the breast "using the loose tissue surrounding it" (19). They used the Wise pattern (20) and the popular McKissock (21) vertical deepithelialized bipedicle mammoplasty to gather the remaining glandular tissue under

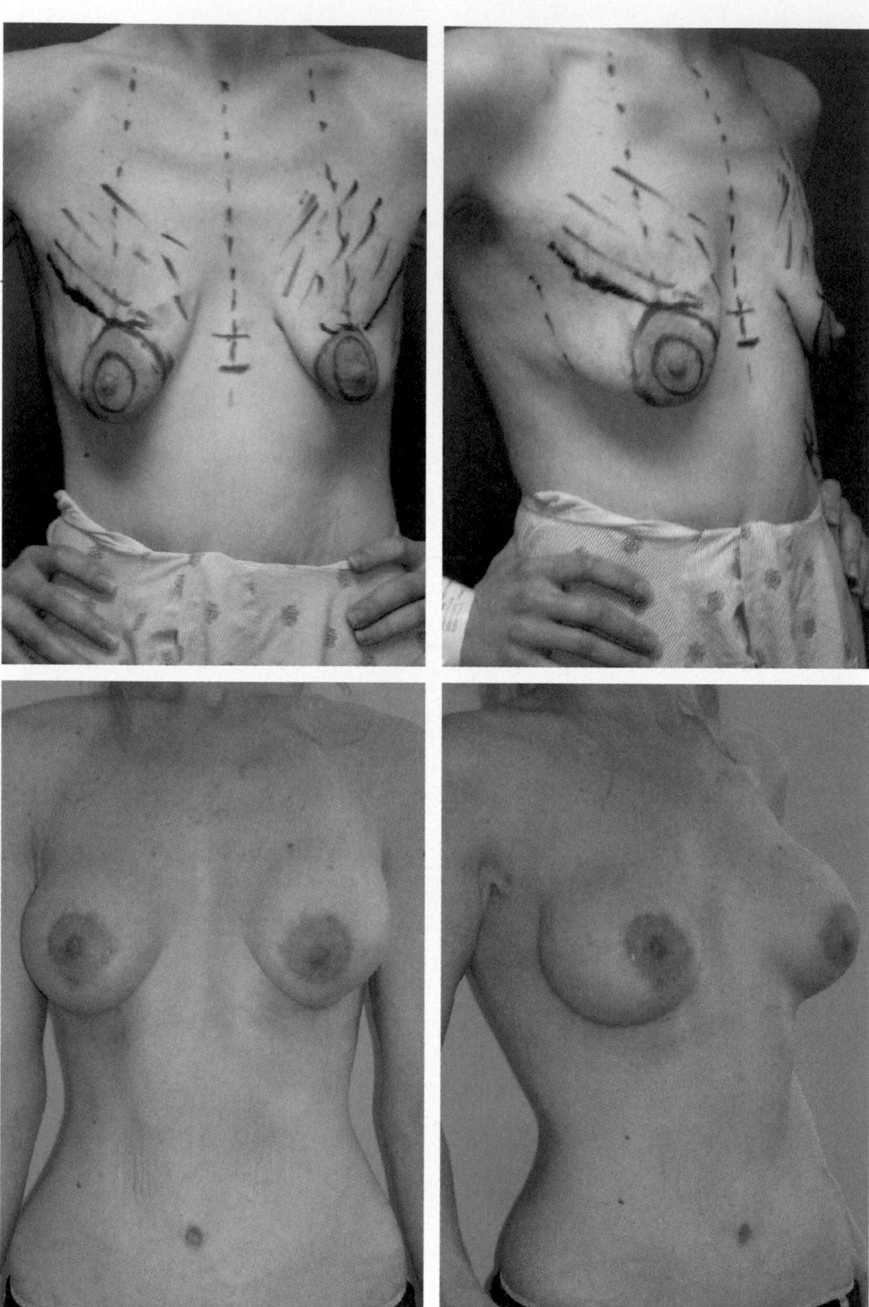

Figure 103.5. These are the frontal and right oblique preoperative and 8-month postoperative views of mastopexy augmentation with 325-cc silicone gel implants and acellular dermal sling for a 25-year-old, 5′9″ tall, 155-pound (body mass index 22.8) woman who lost about 150 of her 300 pounds by lifestyle changes. The operative markings show the concentric mastopexy skin incisions that remove excess pigmented areolar skin and elevate the nipples to the anticipated inframammary fold (IMF), which is at the lower transverse mark across her sternum. The Pectoralis muscle is indicated by the black harsh marks and a thicker line along the lateral border. The acellular dermis spans the lateral pectoral border and the IMF and lateral chest wall footprint, indicated by the dashed line over the serratus muscle. The breast shape has been maintained over these first 8 months with no evidence of lower pole excess.

the nipple. In all three reported patients, they combined this "with a wide excision of the submammary fold" (19). In 1979, Shons noted the variety of breast presentations after massive weight loss, preferring the McKissock technique with removal of excess skin through the Wise pattern (22).

During the 1980s, Lockwood elucidated the SFS and the need to approximate this multilayered fascia for high-tension closures of skin flaps (15). He stated that breast projection and scars were improved after reduction mammaplasty and mastopexy, when permanent suture closure of the SFS was performed (23). For tightening the loose IMF and improving breast projection, he advocated fixing the IMF at "the appropriate elevated position by nonabsorbable sutures from the SFS of the inferior skin wound edge to the underlying muscular fascia."

The more recent mastopexy references will be presented in the next sections.

EVOLUTION OF BREAST TECHNIQUE

Until 10 years ago, I treated the breast deformity in isolation, considering neither the poor aesthetics nor the reconstructive potential of nearby skin excess. It became clear that circumferential abdominoplasty with a lower body lift was inadequate to correct laxity about the upper torso. Moving the belt-like excision higher to the flanks improved the mid torso rolls but reduced the lift on the lateral thighs. Furthermore, patients preferred the hip-hugging to the mid-waist scars. Removal of

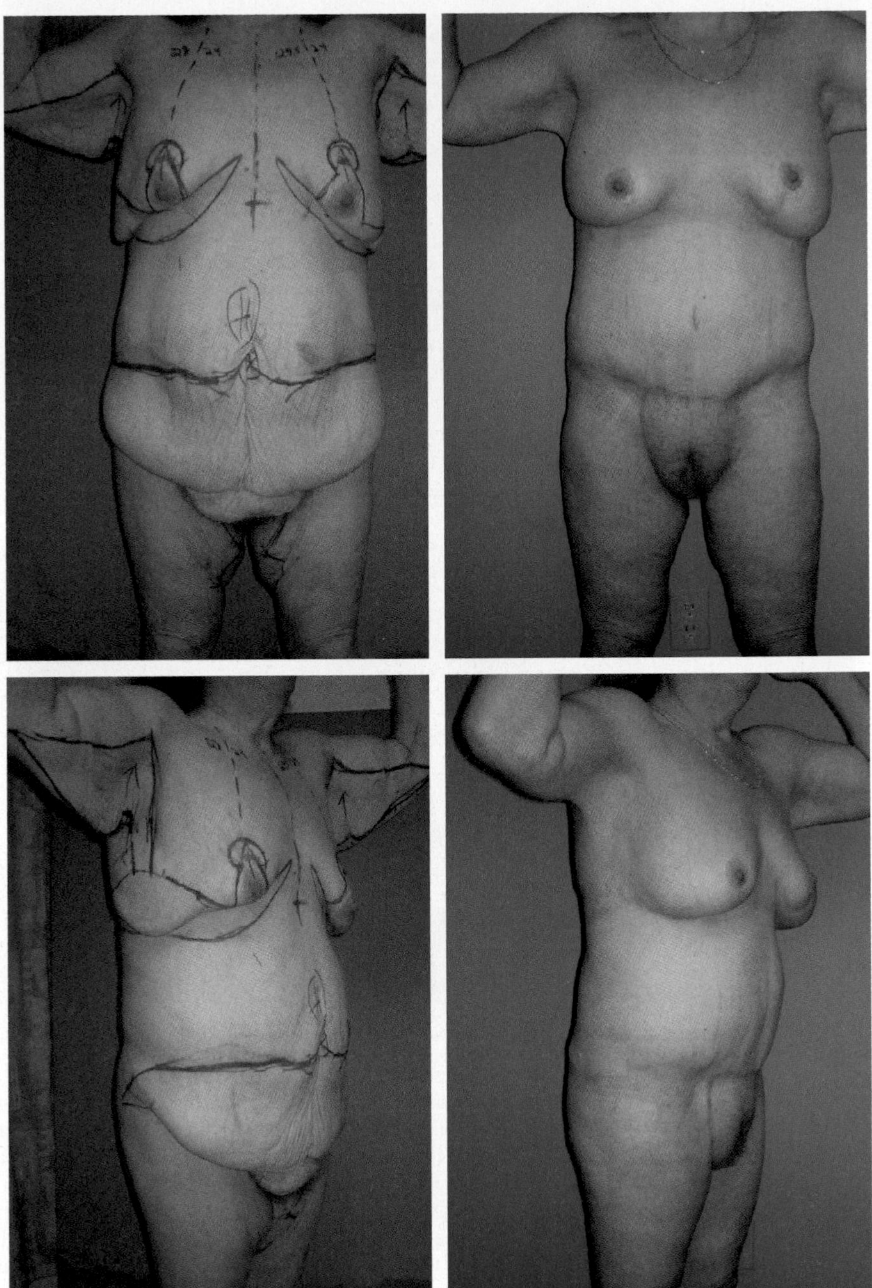

Figure 103.6. These are the preoperative and 3-year postoperative photos of a 48-year-old, 5′5″ tall, 176-pound (body mass index 28.20) woman who lost 150 from 326 pounds. In addition to hanging skin from the arms, torso, and thighs, her breasts were severely ptotic and constricted. She had a single-stage total body lift (TBL) consisting of an extended abdominoplasty, bilateral limited vertical thighplasties, upper body lift, brachioplasties, and breast reshaping using spiral flaps as seen in Figure 102.16. Her course was uncomplicated, and she returned to her job in the food-processing industry 6 weeks after her TBL. As seen 3 years later, her breasts have maintained their excellent shape and position.

the upper torso excess would be accomplished by a tight, nearly circumferential bra-line transverse excision of skin while preserving the flaccidity and projection of the breasts. The newly designed upper body lift would have to be in concert with the breast reshaping (24).

Coincident with seeking a solution to the breast and chest disorder, a better approach to the axilla and upper arms was needed. Leaving behind an oversized axilla, hanging arm skin, and a ptotic posterior axillary fold detracted from whatever breast improvement was achieved. An L-shaped brachioplasty was designed that addressed these issues and left a curvilinear inner arm scar that zigzags across the axilla to the lateral chest (25).

For breast atrophy, I relied on partial subpectoral placement of silicone breast implants, with usually a Wise-pattern mastopexy. Augmentation with mastopexy, complex and risk prone in the cosmetic patient, is described in the chapters of this text dealing with augmentation mammaplasty. The issues of recurrent ptosis, disassociation of implant, and gland and wound-healing complications are discussed by the experts. Currently, its relative simplicity, reliability, and surgeon familiarity make silicone implant augmentation with mastopexy a common method for increasing breast volume and improving shape. The problems with the MWL population are extreme atrophy and laxity, often with lowered breast position. An augmentation mastopexy for MWL patients usually leads to recurrent breast ptosis and bottoming out or displacement of the lower pole of the breast. Patients with good skin elastic recoil and smaller implants do better (Fig. 103.2).

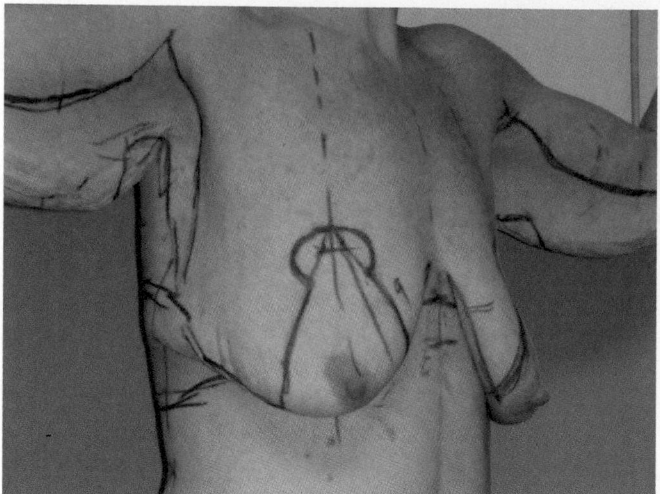

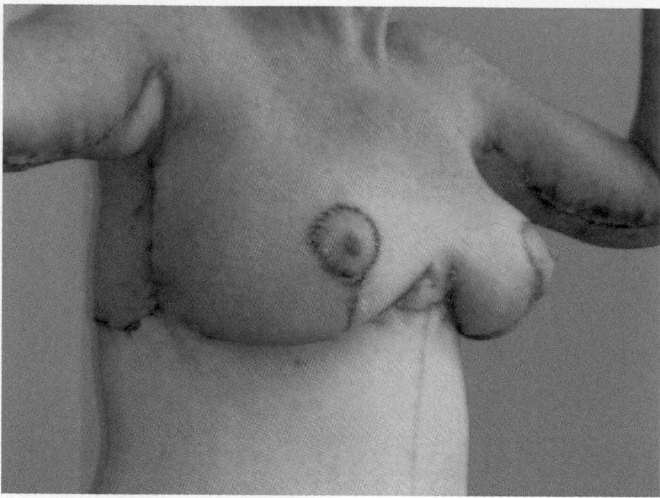

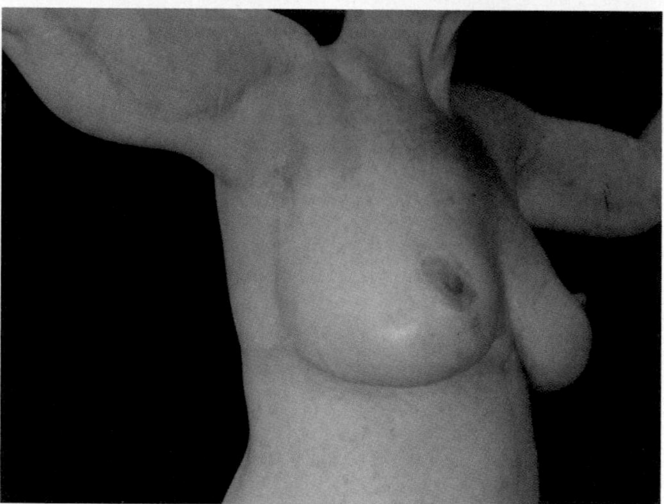

Figure 103.7. These are right anterior oblique views before and 3 days and 1 year after upper body lift, L-shaped brachioplasties, and spiral flap reshaping of the breasts in a 47-year-old 5′6″ tall, 207-pound (body mass index 33.80) woman. She had lost 220 of her 427 pounds through Roux-en-Y bypass surgery. Six months after her lower body lift, abdominoplasty, and vertical inner thighplasties, she had some minor revisions along with her upper body surgery. **Left:** The long vertical limb Wise pattern continues onto the epigastrium and lateral thorax as it passes the vertical descending lines of the L-shaped brachioplasties. The lower transverse line on the sternum registers the current level of the inframammary fold (IMF). The second transverse line is the projected new level of the IMF. **Right:** The reconstructed breasts and arms are tensely full. The nipple-areola complexes (NACs) are properly positioned at the prominence of the breasts with full superior poles. The fill of the lower poles required the entire 10 cm of vertical lines of the Wise pattern. **Bottom:** One year later the breasts and arms exhibit a more natural soft appearance with appropriate fill of the superior and inferior poles and no change in the position of the IMF or NACs.

Even the uncomplicated augmentation mastopexy can leave a compromised aesthetic result. With little parenchyma present, the new breast assumes the shape of the implant and its capsule. When the capsule is tight, the breasts are too round and firm. Even the best breast implant result fails to naturally taper the breasts into the axilla or along the sternum. These implanted breasts have a stuck-on appearance. Secondary lipoaugmentation along the perimeter of the reconstruction can mitigate this shortcoming. These unique tissue deficiencies in the MWL upper body led to exploration in the use of discarded flaps for autoaugmentation and support.

An epiphany case taught me that ignoring loose and descended IMF with loose skin epigastria can lead to inadequate upper body contouring and poor breast aesthetics (Fig. 103.3) The patient was a 5′5″ tall, 34-year-old woman who went from 325 to 150 pounds following gastric bypass surgery. She had a lower body lift, vertical medial thighplasty, and a Wise-pattern mastopexy with 325-cc, saline-filled silicone implants. Her implants bottomed out. A subsequent reverse abdominoplasty and secondary breast reshaping was maintained for more than 2 years and corrected epigastric skin excess (Fig. 103.13). This case was my beginning with the upper body lift, in concert with securing the IMF and longer-lasting shaping of the breast.

STRATEGY

My strategy for correcting the breast deformity in the MWL patient considers the degree of NAC ptosis, current and desired

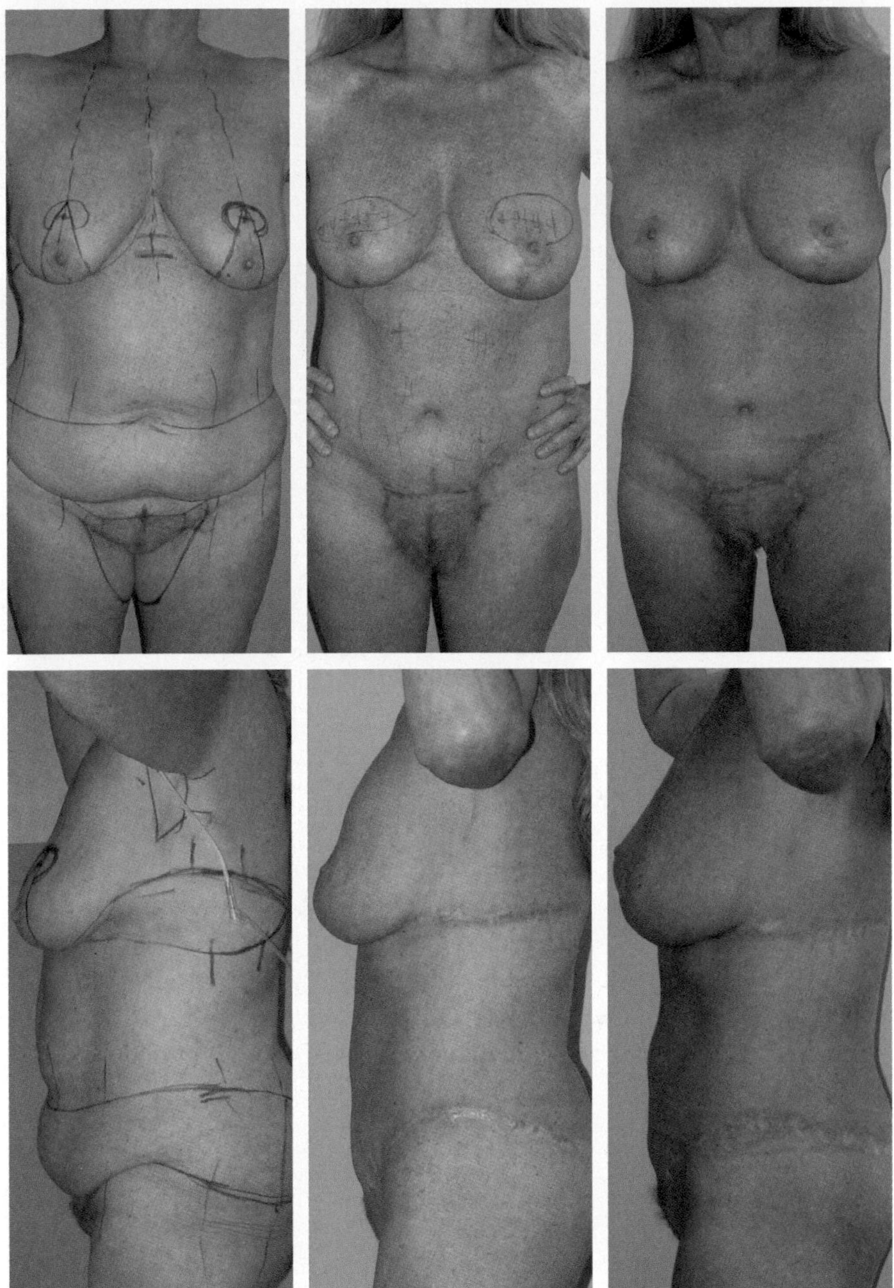

Figure 103.8. These are the preoperative, 6-month post total body lift (TBL), and 6-month post epigastric liposuction and lipoaugmentation of the breasts in a 47-year-old 5′6″ tall, 170-pound (body mass index 27.40) woman. She had lost 90 pounds after Roux-en-Y bypass surgery. **Left:** The markings for a TBL with spiral flaps and Wise-pattern mastopexy. **Middle:** She healed without complications, and 6 months later she returned and was marked for liposuction of her mid abdomen and lipoaugmentation of her breasts between the nipple-areola complexes and the superior pole of her breasts that were created by the lateral thoracic flaps. **Right:** The results 6 months later show improvements in both the abdomen and breasts.

breast volume and shape, skin quality and quantity, descent of the IMF, neighboring skin deformity and extent of available tissue excess for breast augmentation and suspension, and prior breast surgery. In many MWL patients, the breasts descend 1 to 4 cm on the chest. As the IMFs approach the costal margins, women admit that they have to uncomfortably pull up their brassieres to raise their breasts. The surface that the posterior aspect of the breast makes on the chest wall has been called a footprint, which is the "foundation for the overlying three-dimensional structure of the breast (26)." Blondeel et al. further subdivide the pertinent breast aesthetics into breast conus and skin envelope quality and quantity: "The breast conus refers to the three-dimensional shape, projection, and volume of the tissue (or implant) on top and anterior to the footprint of the breast" (26).

As the majority of MWL women have severe NAC ptosis and poor skin quality and excess, the determinate strategic issues are volume and shape (breast conus) and the breast footprint. The severity of the deformity, the need and acceptance of extensive incisions to correct the breast and neighboring tissues, and the availability of neighboring tissue for augmentation and suspension moved my conceptualization from cosmetic augmentation/mastopexy to breast reconstruction. The widespread MWL patient aversion to silicone implants and the poor results, along with willingness of patients to accept risks of flap reconstruction, are also important considerations.

Breast reshaping is offered to MWL women who desire body contouring. They are eligible as soon as 1 year after

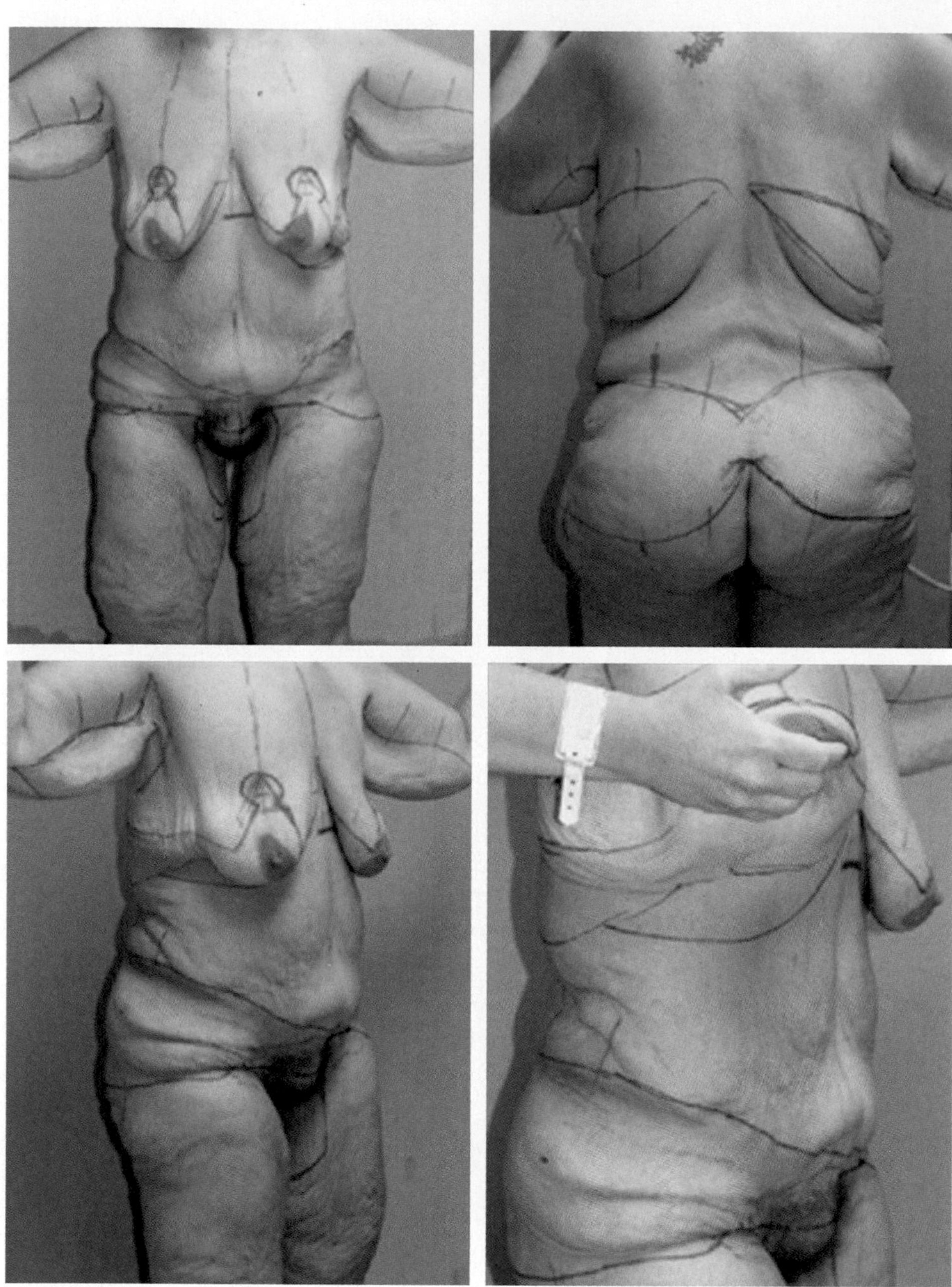

Figure 103.9. These are the markings for a total body lift that includes L-shaped brachioplasties, upper body lift with spiral flap reshaping of her breasts, lower body lift, and medial upper thighplasties in a 5′8″ tall, 195-pound (body mass index 29.6), 35-year-old manicurist who lost 180 pounds after gastric bypass. She had a prior abdominoplasty.

their bypass surgery if their weight loss has been stable for 4 months and if there is no expectation for further loss. A thorough review of their medical history, with emphasis on the evolution of obesity-related comorbidities, is important. The patient must be under optimal management of the remaining problems with no acute crisis. Overweight patients with BMI between 25 and 30 kg/m^2 are accepted. They will probably need liposuction as part of their treatment. Moderately obese patients with BMIs between 30 and 35 kg/m^2 are at greater risk for wound-healing complications, and efforts are made to reduce their weight. Patients with severe obesity must lose weight before they are candidates for sophisticated body contouring. While this group of patients tends to be appreciative and cooperative, there is a small subset that is unrealistic and hostile. One should consider body dysmorphic syndrome when the disabilities and distress are extreme.

The available procedures and the rationale follow.

VERTICAL BREAST REDUCTION

Macromastia with NAC ptosis is treated by breast reduction. For the still large but ptotic breast, reduction is usually conservative. The persistent large lower body is best counterbalanced with ample breasts. To improve projection and limit reliance on inelastic skin, I prefer a vertical pattern reduction. However, redundant inelastic skin often requires further elliptical skin excision along the IMF. Isolated breast reduction is indicated for patients who desire as few scars as possible and/or who fail to see the value of the upper body lift. Similarly, these patients

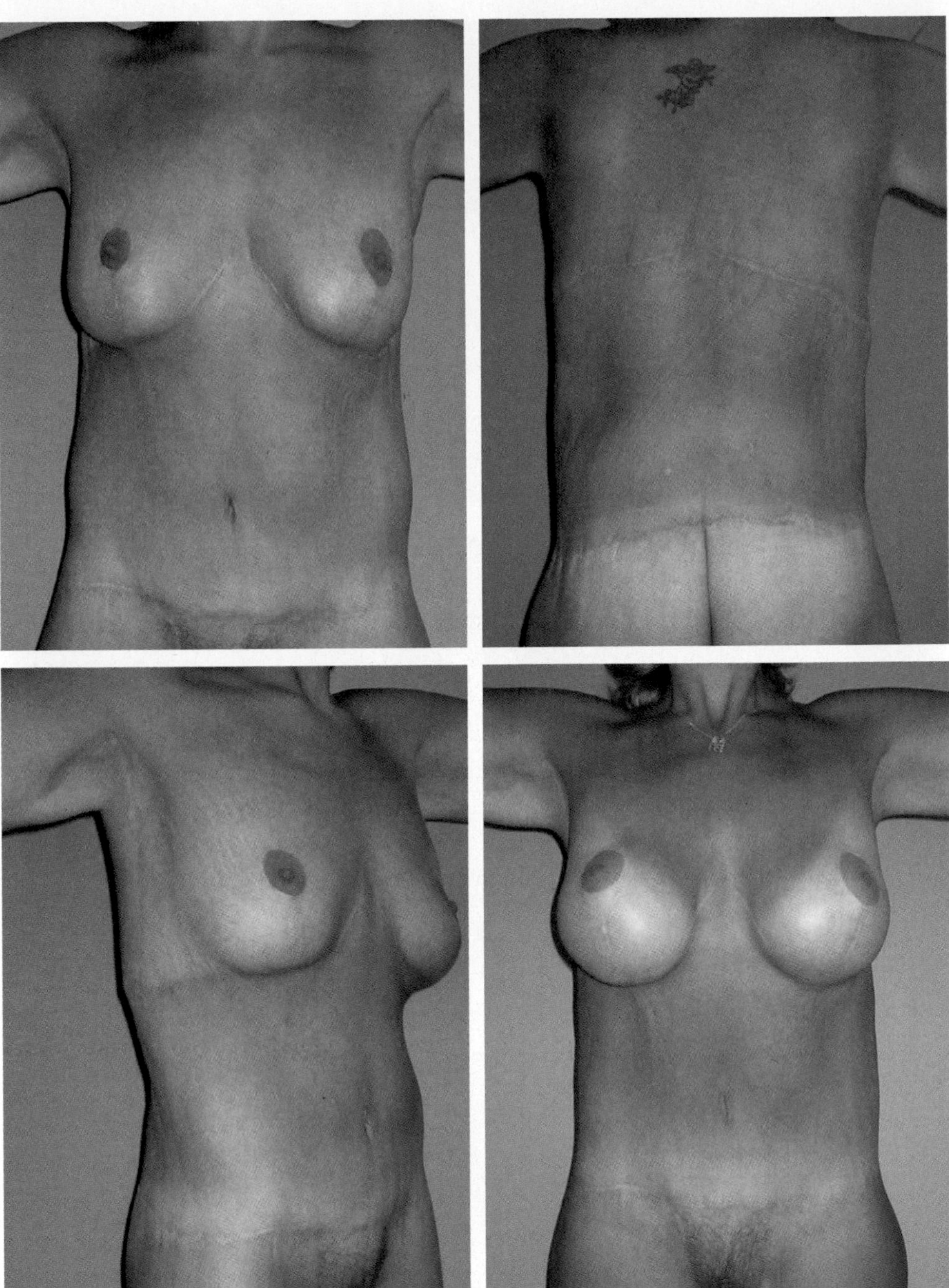

Figure 103.10. **Left:** The 1-year postoperative photographs of the patient shown in Figure 103.9. After 1 year, she desired 330-cc, saline-filled implant augmentation of her breasts and vertical medial thighplasty. **Right:** The results of both operative sessions. The contours are feminine, and the scars are inconspicuous.

prefer a standard abdominoplasty to the circumferential scars of a lower body lift. Even when warned of their compromises, these patients may regret their persistent mid torso and hip tissue excess.

DERMAL SUSPENSION MASTOPEXY

Ample-sized, properly positioned, and ptotic breasts are well treated with a dermal suspension mastopexy (27). An extensive dissection of the breast skin flaps is needed to suture suspend the deepithelialized superior extension to the NAC to the upper pectoral major muscle. My University of Pittsburgh colleague Peter Rubin, who includes breast reduction as an indication, presents his technique in Chapter 102. The medial and lateral extensions of the central pedicle are sutured to the suspended central flap with dermal imbricating suture shaping of the mound. With dependence on the inferior and central pedicle for blood supply, this procedure cannot be combined with a reverse abdominoplasty. Therefore excess upper abdominal skin, lowered IMF, and breast footprint are not treated. The Wise-pattern closure removes excess skin and helps shape the breast. I also find that meticulous and symmetric imbrications of the dermal flaps create a substantial mount. The early results are promising, but dermal suspensions have a way of stretching.

IMPLANT AUGMENATION WITH BODY LIFT

With no NAC ptosis, partial subpectoral silicone implant breast augmentation is an option during an upper body lift. An unusual approach for breast volume deficiency is silicone gel augmentation during bilateral lateral thoracoplasties with an

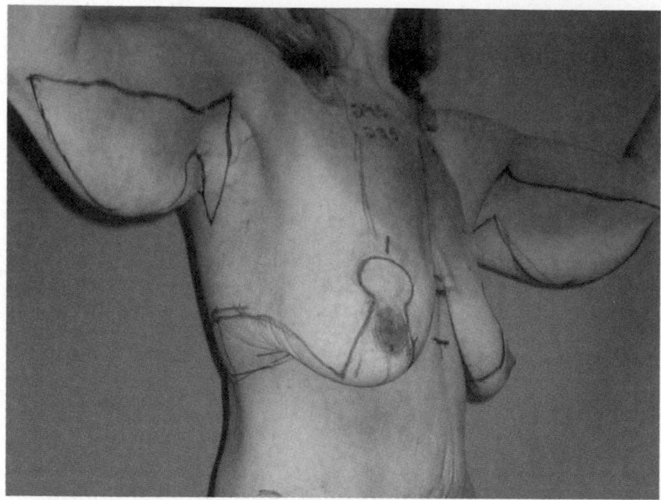

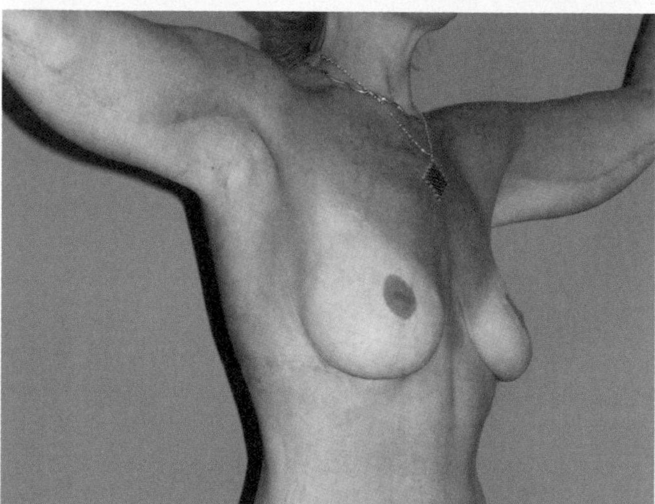

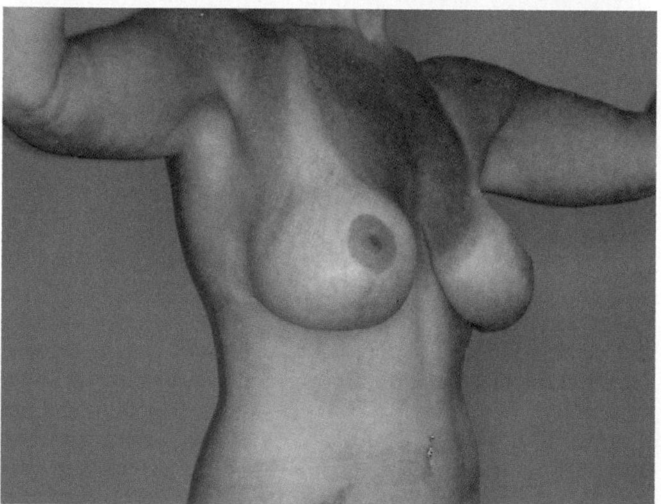

Figure 103.11. These are the right anterior oblique views pre and post total body lift of a 41-year old, 5′5″ tall, 157-pound woman (body mass index 27.5) who lost 160 pounds after gastric bypass. **Top:** Her markings for L-shaped brachioplasties, Wise-pattern mastopexies, and spiral flap reshaping of her breasts. **Middle:** The result 2 years later, when she presented for breast augmentation and further reduction of her arms. **Bottom:** The result 3 years after her 280-cc, saline-filled silicone submammary breast augmentation and brachioplasty revision and desiring no further surgery.

abdominoplasty (Fig. 103.4). Whether primary or secondary, lateral torso skin excisions are indicated to sculpture a broad and flaccid waist with narrow hips and minimal back excess.

IMPLANT AUGMENTATION MASTOPEXY

When the breast and nearby excess tissue volume is inadequate to fill the desired breast volume, then silicone gel implant augmentation is required. The optimal situation for implant augmentation with mastopexy is a distinct, appropriately positioned IMF and reasonable nearby skin contour and elasticity. A relatively small (250 to 400 cc) gel-filled implant with suture support of the IMF is performed (Fig. 103.2). Saline-filled implants are discouraged because the limited coverage leads to unnatural feel, rippling, and sagging.

IMPLANT AUGMENTATION MASTOPEXY WITH ACELLULAR DERMIS

Exceptionally thin, sagging breasts are unable to support large implants. When there is inadequate breast parenchyma, support of the implant and elevation of the IMF are integral to the augmentation mastopexy. A complete submuscular augmentation supports the implant but restricts breast projection and may dissociate the implant from the natural breast. The implant often rises high and the breast sags below the implant. Partial subpectoral augmentation allows more projection and is likely to have better implant-to-breast relationship. Unfortunately, the unsupported inferior portion of the implant will allow the implants to descend. Either the IMF falls or the breast bottoms out.

A preemptive internal support such as acellular dermis is a reasonable option. As in recent experience with implant reconstruction after mastectomy and implant exchange to the subpectoral position, broad slings of acellular dermis may be used to cradle implants between the lateral border of the pectoralis major muscle and IMF in augmentation mastopexy (28,29). I have started to apply approach this to the MWL patient, with early success in four patients (Figs. 103.5 and 103.14). I have found porcine grafts of either Strattice (LifeCell; Branchburg, NJ) or NeoForm (Mentor Corporation, Santa Barbara, CA) to equally support the implants. Small vacuum drains are placed between the dermal graft and breast for 1 week to prevent seromas. In my four cases, there has been no erythema or induration. The major problem with these materials is the high cost of $3,500 for the largest sheet, which is shared between the two breasts. I have found that lower-cost sheet alternatives such as Vicryl mesh allow unacceptable lower pole sag.

AUTOGENOUS TISSUE BREAST RESHAPING WITH UPPER BODY LIFT

Inadequate breast volume accompanied by sufficient nearby soft tissue calls for suspended autogenous tissue augmentation. Excess skin and fat of the epigastrium and lateral thorax are deepithelialized in continuity with the central breast mount and appropriately positioned, tailored, and buried under Wise-pattern flaps (14,24,30) (Fig. 103.15). The inevitable twisting and turning of this compound flap led to the name "spiral flap." The epigastric flap is an inferior extension of the central breast pedicle nourished through descending intercostal perforating vessels. The lateral chest flap is a tongue-like lateral

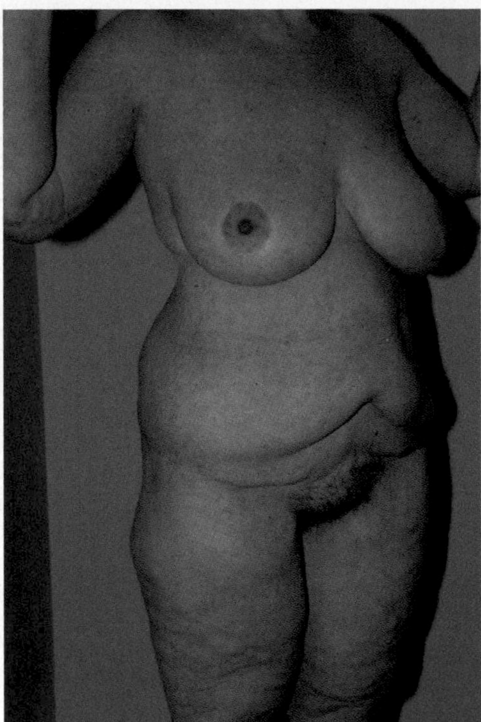
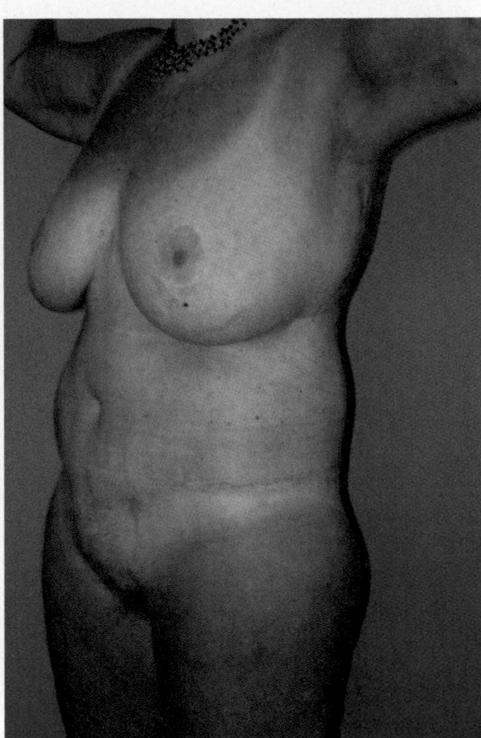

Figure 103.12. Left: This image is 4 years after a single-stage total body lift (TBL) of the woman in the left photo in Figure 103.1. She had L-shaped brachioplasties, upper body lift with spiral flap reshaping of the breasts, abdominoplasty, lower body lift and vertical medial thighplasties. Her gain of 50 pounds since the TBL further filled out her autogenous tissue breast augmentation and suspension. She developed a left-side abdominal hernia. **Right:** This image is 5 years after a two-stage TBL of the woman seen in the right photo in Figure 103.1. While her weight has fluctuated by as much as 30 pounds, at this time she is 10 pounds less than her preoperative weight. Her breasts are round and well shaped. For both patients, skin redundancy has been corrected, leaving feminine contours.

fasciocutaneous extension of the central pedicle, similar to the lateral thoracic flap described by Holstrom and Lossing in 1986 with confirmed utility and safety (31–34). It is a fasciocutaneous flap based on perforators through the serratus muscle. This donor site corrects the lateral chest and back roll, usual leaving a transverse closure along the bra line. Borud based his breast reshaping on this flap, which he referred to as the ICAP (intercostal arterial perforator) flap (35).

CONCEPTUALIZING THE SPIRAL FLAP AND UPPER BODY LIFT

The mastopexy with spiral flap augmentation integrates breast reshaping with the upper body lift (UBL). Fundamental to an UBL is correction of the mid torso skin rolls and contouring the waist through one of three patterns. If appropriate, the secondary component of the UBL is superior repositioning the breast footprint and IMF. The most common and effective UBL pattern is the bra-line excision, with the lift relying on a tight closure across the back, extending into the secured IMF. Narrowing of the waist is aided by flank liposuction. That technique will be presented in detail. The second pattern is for lesser degrees of back deformity or when the patient refuses a back scar. In this thoracoplasty, a wide, sickle-shaped vertical skin excision extending from the IMF to the axilla is performed. The lift is created by pushing skin upward and suture suspension into the serratus muscle and fascia lateral to the breast. The third and rarest pattern is the midlateral excision of skin from the axilla to the hip. There is no body lift, but as previously shown, the waist can be best narrowed by the lateral thoracoplasty (Fig. 103.4).

As seen in the next case drawings, the new IMF position, the reverse abdominoplasty, lateral thoracic flap harvest, and the Wise-pattern mastopexy are planned together (Figs. 103.6 to 103.10). With the patient standing, the ptotic breast is elevated, and the current IMFs are sighted and drawn under both breasts and registered over the sternum. Each breast and IMF is raised to the desired level, and the new IMF position, 1 to 4 cm superior, is now registered over the sternum. The excess skin of the upper abdomen is vigorously pushed superolateral. When all excess skin is gathered—the abdominal skin is tight and the umbilicus is pulled slightly cephalad—a mark is made where the gathered abdominal skin meets the new IMF position along the nipple line. With the tissues still suspended, the new parasternal and anterior axillary line attachments of the breasts are sighted and marked. The gathered tissues are dropped. The curvilinear incision line that serves both the reverse abdominoplasty and the new IMF is then drawn. This line starts at the marked parasternal breast attachment and descends to the upper abdominal marked nipple line point and then ascends to the marked point at the anterior axillary line. This line is similar to the IMF incision line of the Wise pattern, except that it includes all the redundant abdominal skin with the central breast pedicle. Obesity and/or excessive flare of the costal margins make this maneuver difficult to judge.

Obviously, the reverse abdominoplasty, which removes excess skin of the epigastrium not corrected by the standard complete abdominoplasty, can be performed without changing the location of the IMF. The IMFs are the upper line of excision of excess skin. The inferiorly based abdominal flaps are undermined to about the costal margins. The closure ends along the newly designated IMFs, and unless there is symmastia, it does not cross the sternum. Occasionally, too much upper midline skin excess remains, and then an inverted V of skin is excised secondarily over the sternum. The discontinuously undermined reverse abdominoplasty flap is advanced cephalically and secured along the sixth rib.

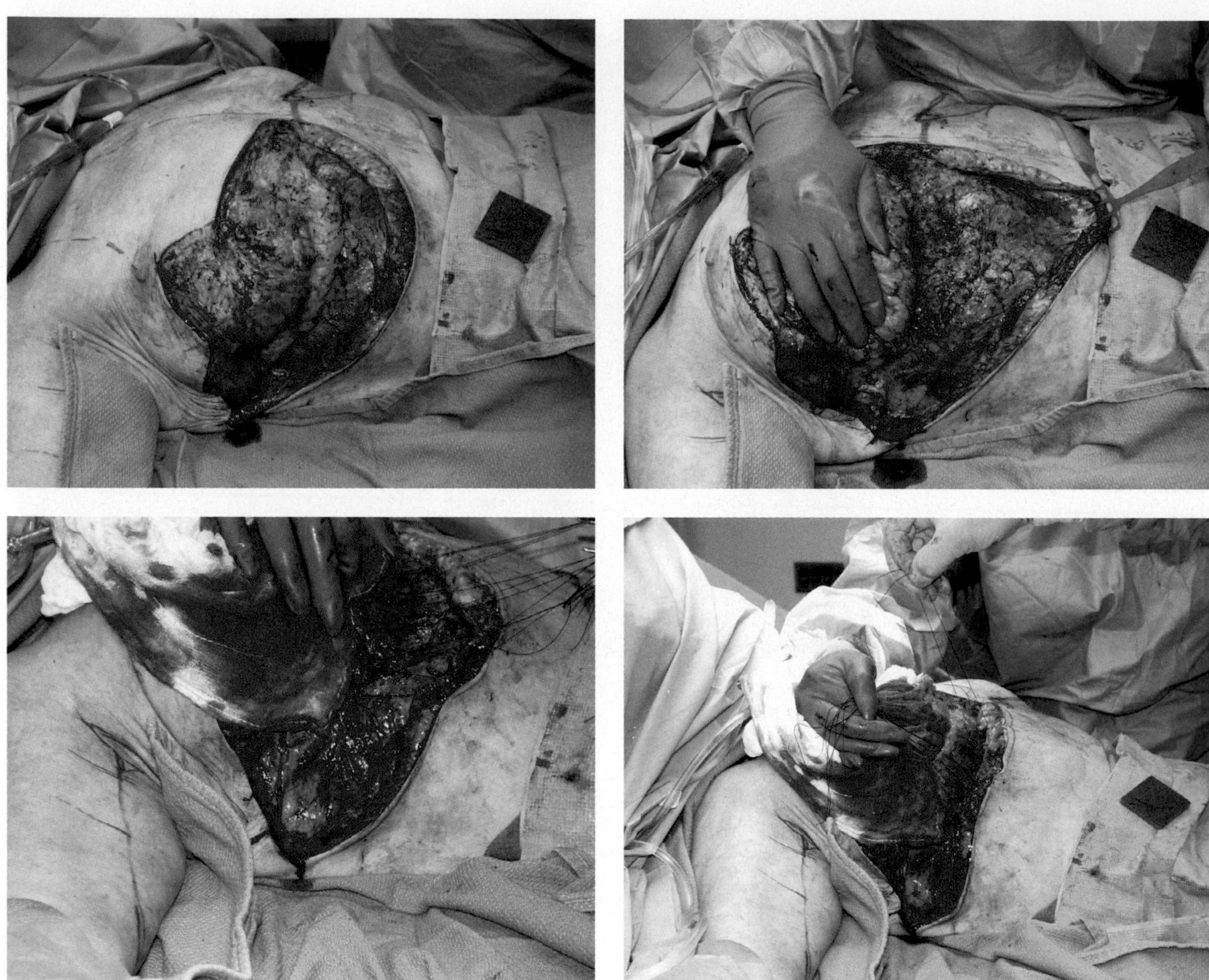

Figure 103.13. These are the major operative steps of the patient in Figure 103.3, who had inverted-T revision mastopexies and reverse abdominoplasty with elevation of her inframammary fold (IMF). **Top left:** Following the markings shown in the middle photos of Figure 103.3, the excess skin of the lower breast and upper abdomen was excised with the central inverted V of lower breast deepithelialized. The transverse mark over the lower sternum is the anticipated new location of the IMF. The yellow breast tissue can be seen 3 cm below that mark. **Top right:** The rake retracts the skin that has been undermined to the costal margin to expose muscular fascia. The right breast has been undermined to the sixth rib. A gloved right hand holds the breast in its new position. **Bottom left:** A row of 2-0 braided permanent sutures has been individually placed between the sixth rib and the superficial fascial system of the reverse abdominoplasty flap. **Bottom right:** The most medial suture is about to be tied as the remaining sutures are pulled up to approximate the reverse abdominoplasty flap to the new IMF.

Optimal recruitment of nearby soft tissue for breast reshaping requires precise preoperative determination of mid torso excess and aesthetic positioning of the breasts. With clinical experience, gather and pinch techniques faithfully present the excess available for deepithelialized flaps. Usually the Wise pattern is drawn with narrower and longer vertical limbs to accommodate the autogenous fill. In addition, the new NAC should not be placed too low, as it will descend slightly as the IMF is raised.

The position of the transverse incision considers the old and new IMF and epigastric excess being folded into the inferior breast mound. For the bra-line excision, the IMF and lateral Wise-pattern flap markings are continued parallel and posterior to just beyond the tip of the scapula. The width between the parallel incisions is that much tissue that can be pushed and pinched together to take up all the back slack. Only in the most severe cases does the excision cross the posterior midline, because there is no lax skin over the spinal column and scarring this area disrupts the contoured beauty and sensuality of the woman's mid back. One should position the incision lines and gauge the tension of closure to place the closure within the posterior bra line.

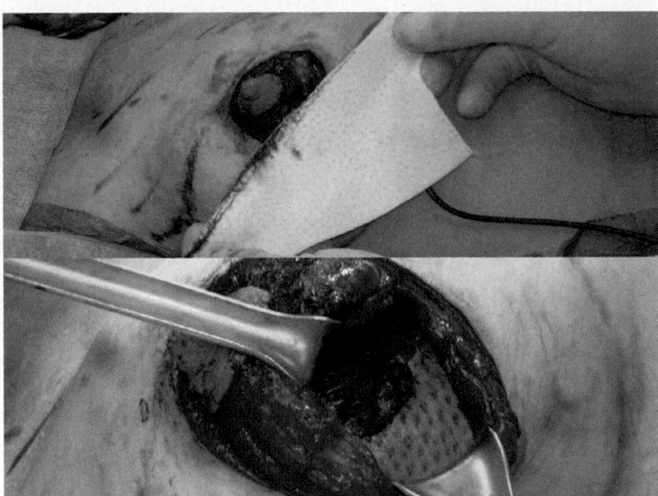

Figure 103.14. These are two intraoperative views of the patient in Figure 103.5. The concentric ring deepethialization of the right nipple-areola complex (NAC) has been done. Through a transverse infra-areolar incision a partial subpectoral space has been made for the gel implant. An 8 cm by 18 cm rectangular acellular dermis implant has been transected obliquely and oriented as shown to bridge the gap between the pectoralis muscle and the chest for the gel implant. With a sizer in place the dermal implant is first sutured to the chest wall and distal lateral pectoralis muscle. Through the retracted breast, the dermis implant is seen sutured to the pectoralis muscle over the gel implant. The breast parenchyma will be closed, followed by the purse-string closure of the NAC.

SPIRAL FLAP BREAST RESHAPING AND UPPER BODY LIFT OPERATION

The operation starts prone. After infusion with epinephrine-containing saline, the bra-line excision is deepithelialized using an electric dermatome set at 32,000th of an inch. After the perimeter incisions are made, the flap is raised from medial to lateral off the areolar tissue of the fascia overlying the latissimus dorsi (LD) muscle. Upon reaching the anterior border of the LD, the dissection plane includes serratus anterior muscle fascia. As the flap lies on the operating room table, the donor site is closed in two layers of absorbable barbed suture. Skin glue seals the closure.

The patient is turned supine (Fig. 103.6). The Wise-pattern deepithelialization, which extends inferiorly onto the abdomen, is again assisted by the electric dermatome. The lateral, superior, and medial Wise-pattern flaps are elevated superficially for 4 to 6 cm. The incision along the inferior margin of the extended Wise pattern is carried down to rectus muscular fascia from the parasternal margin to the inferior incision of the lateral back flap. The lateral flap incision of the Wise pattern is continued to the upper incision of the lateral back flap. Liberated by completion of the perimeter incisions, the lateral thoracic flap is sharply elevated from the serratus muscle until the intercostal perforators are visualized. The arterial pulsations between the anterior and mid axillary line can be confirmed by Doppler recordings. Effort is made to preserve these vessels from the third through the sixth intercostal vessels.

When the vascularity of the lateral thoracic flap is confirmed, the inferior breast with its superiorly based epigastric extension is elevated from its descended location near the eighth rib to the sixth. Despite severely descended NACs, this interruption of the inferior border of the breast has had no NAC vascular compromise. That is because our breast mobilization, Wise-pattern thin-skin flap elevation, and positioning of the spiral flaps have not interrupted the critical transverse blood supply to the breast along the fourth and fifth intercostal septa of the breast (36). We and others have anatomically and clinically confirmed Würinger's anatomic vision, making the distance of NAC elevation during mastopexy essentially irrelevant as long as the mid glandular septum is preserved (30,37).

Next, the lateral entry to a superior pole submammary position for the lateral thoracic flap is started with dissection laterally, superiorly, or medially. Laterally, the lateral margin of the pectoralis muscle is located over the fourth rib, and supramuscular dissection of the plane for the flap is made. With an effort made to avoid unnecessary trauma to lateral thoracic artery blood supple, grasping the skin and pectoralis muscle along the anterior axillary line assists in identifying this plane. Alternatively, an incision is made along the superior margin of the deepithelialized new NAC site and continued to the pectoralis fascia. Then the pocket for the flap over the third rib is developed from the lateral margin of the pectoralis to the parasternal region. Finally, the medial dissection under the medial Wise-pattern flap is extended superiorly to the superior pole of the breast, avoiding injury to the parasternal internal mammary perforators.

A pocket has been created over the pectoralis muscle for positioning of the deepithelialized lateral thoracic flap. Before the flap is placed, the descended breast is dissected from its location over the seventh and eight ribs with visual preservation of intercostal perforating vessels. The reverse abdominoplasty subcutaneous fascia is advanced to the sixth rib and serratus muscle with interrupted large braided permanent sutures. The secure IMF maintains the higher breast footprint.

Then, the medially based lateral thoracic flap, which remains attached to the central breast mound, is turned cephalad along the anterior axillary line. After cutting the distal tip to check for adequate blood supply, the flap is tunneled into the superior pole pocket. The distal end dermis and fat are sutured to the parasternal region about the third rib. The recent addition of the superior pole incision for exposure is very helpful here.

The mass of flap and breast tissue still flops laterally. To centralize the mound, the breast inferior dermal pedicle is advanced to the fifth intercostal cartilage and secured. Together with the secured lateral thoracic flap, a dermal flap sling is set to provide superomedial support. The lateral breast contour is improved by suturing the transposed flap to the lateral pectoralis major muscle. The flap is tailored and imbricated to optimally shape the breast. The tight closure of the lateral thoracic flap donor site from the axilla to the IMF appropriately flattens this lateral chest area and emphasizes the newly created lateral breast fullness and breast projection. The lateral chest donor-site closure is continuous with the advanced and stabilized new IMF.

The excess upper abdominal deepithelialized flap is usually flipped up and sutured to smoothly fill out the inferior breast. Dermal imbrication of the deepithelialized breasts and the spiral flap forms the desired contour. The Wise-pattern skin flaps are closed to each other and the new IMF. The NAC is fitted into the top of the keyhole pattern.

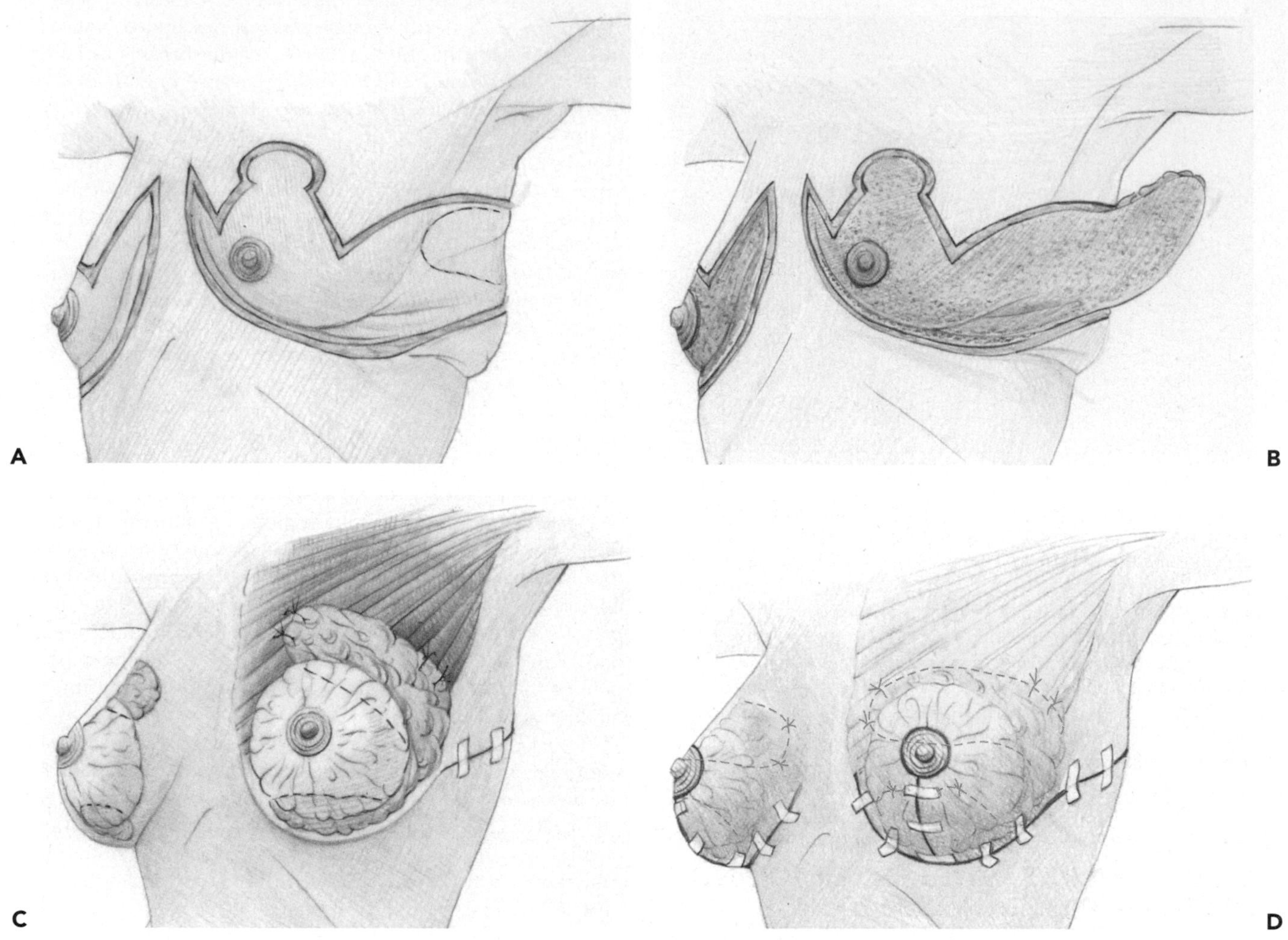

Figure 103.15. Diagrams for spiral flap reshaping of the breasts. **A:** An extended Wise pattern is drawn that includes excess epigastric skin and fat inferiorly, as well as a lateral thoracodorsal flap consisting of resected back roll. The lateral flap ends near the tip of the scapula. The vertical limbs vary from 7 to 10 cm in length in order to accommodate the spiral flap augmentation. **B:** All flap extensions are deepithelialized and elevated from the muscular fascia, leaving the nipple-areola complex island intact. **C:** The epigastric flap is folded on itself to augment the inferior breast. The lateral extension spirals around the pectoralis muscle to fit into a tunnel between the breast and muscle. Long-lasting suspension of the breast is achieved by tunneling of the superior flap and the suture suspension of this flap to the third rib cartilage and suture fixation of the inferior deepithelialized breasts flap to the sixth rib cartilage. The sutured sling centralizes the breast from its lateralized position. **D:** The suspended and reshaped breast with the Wise-pattern flaps sutured and skin strips in place.

Usually, an L-shaped brachioplasty is performed. The short descending limb excision of the L may extend to the bra-line closure. It awaits the breast closure because the lateral chest laxity is absorbed by the enlarged breast conus. The preoperative and postoperative upper body photographs of the procedure demonstrated in Figure 103.16 and including an L-shaped brachioplasty are shown in Figure 103.6. Four additional cases are presented (Figs. 103.7 to 103.11).

GENERAL MANAGEMENT AND INFORMED CONSENT

The chest and breast incisions are dressed in light gauze, a loosely applied surgical bra, and elastic sleeves on the arms without gauze. No constricting binder is place across the upper abdomen. After an upper body lift, the patient is admitted for at least 1 night's observation and care. Intake and output are closely monitored, with hemoglobin/hematocrit measured as needed. Blood transfusions are administered for symptomatic hypovolemia and/or hemoglobin under 6.5 g. Pain relief by patient-controlled analgesia through a pushbutton intravenous line is usually satisfactory. Intermittent calf pressure stockings are used until the patient resumes frequent ambulation. Because of the large wound area, thromboembolism chemoprophylaxis is reserved for moderate- to high-risk patients. A high-protein, low-salt diet with our customized amino acid, protein, mineral, and vitamin drink are encouraged on the first postoperative day (10).

With complete flap survival, the breasts are not only enlarged and well shaped, but they are also soft and shift naturally with change in body position. The constricted inferior breast is

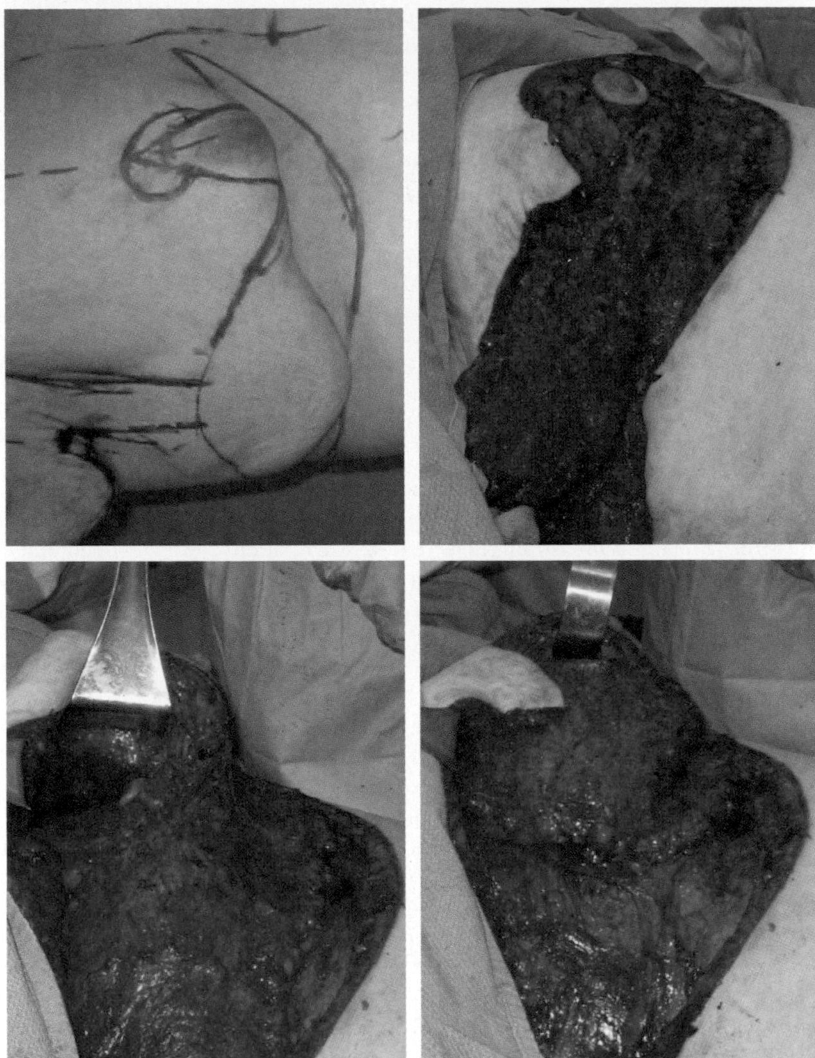

Figure 103.16. These are the essential operative steps in an upper body lift with spiral flap reshaping of the right breast. **Top left:** The markings for Wise pattern with epigastric and lateral thoracic flap extensions around sagging chest tissue. Both superior and inferior poles of the breast are severely deficient. **Top right:** The skin flaps have been deepithelialized. The Wise-pattern flaps have been incised and undermined. The lateral thoracic flap extension of the central breast mound has been incised and raised off the serratus fascia until the perforators along the anterior axillary line. **Bottom left:** The lateral border of the pectoralis major muscle has been identified and submammary space under the superior pole of the breast for the lateral flap, which lies in situ, has been created. The epigastric extension has been undermined to the new inframammary fold. **Bottom right:** The lateral thoracic flap has been advance and rotated into the submammary space as the epigastric flap is to be flipped up to augment the inferior pole of the breast.

corrected. The tapering of the breast into the axilla and superior pole fullness is limited only by the surgeon's artistry.

Informed consent is a process of physician and staff education and interaction with the patient. At the initial consultation, I introduce the upper body lift and breast reshaping, based on the strategy presented. Although the spiral flap reshaping has merit, due to the complexity of the procedure, unanticipated problems may occur. If recognized, they may be treated at the initial procedure, or revision surgery, including silicone implant insertion, may be appropriate later. Alternative and more conservative approaches with an implant augmentation and/or mastopexy are explained.

The UBL is often the second stage of total body lift surgery. For most patients, the upper body and breasts are secondary to the lower body issues. If not, at their request I will begin body contouring with the UBL. I prefer to complete the more invasive and arduous lower body lift first. When patients are satisfied, I have their trust and can proceed with the less conventional UBL and breast reshaping. We use the second operative opportunity to improve contours or scars from the first.

As soon as the UBL with breast reshaping was developed, measures were instituted to improve safety. There needs to be an effort to minimize blood loss, maintain normothermia, and reduce operative time. Efficiencies are gained by a consistent and logical plan with only one patient turn. Appropriate fluid management, autologous blood replacement, antiembolism prophylaxis, and patient warming are essential. Attentive hospital postoperative care discovers healing and medical problems early, before irreversible injury. The support, consistent teamwork, and reasonable pricing of Magee-Women's Hospital, a tertiary care facility of the University of Pittsburgh Medical Center, has been instrumental in improving outcomes.

The optimal treatment of the patient who had a prior breast reduction is complicated. These breasts are not only flat, but they also have extensive scars and unknown pedicles to the nipples. The nipple position is usually satisfactory, and if the scars are acceptable, then only the new IMF/reverse abdominoplasty incision is made. Improved breast projection is created by raising the IMF and autoaugmentation as just described. Secondary adjustments to the NAC may be necessary. In the five patients I have done, there was no NAC or skin necrosis.

SPIRAL FLAP COMPLICATIONS

While not a complication per se, the spiral flap takes up to an hour longer to perform for each breast than a comparable implant augmentation mastopexy with an upper body lift. The procedure is challenging and satisfying. The spiral flap has been harvested and used in each of the more than 50 cases treated. For the flap to suspend the breast, it is sutured under some tension to the costal cartilages. The breast skin flaps are closed under some tension over swollen tissues and the buried flaps. The initially tensely swollen breast softens by the end of the first postoperative week (Fig. 103.7). Since the spiral flap is buried, the incidence and extent of flap necrosis are unknown. In about 20% of cases there is palpable distal flap induration, suggestive of necrosis. Most areas of firmness resolve over time, leaving limited delayed debridement in 2 cases. One additional patient had operative debridement of the distal 50% of the flaps followed by insertion of saline-filled silicone implants. Two patients had revision of the back scar. Two patients disliked the shape and fill of their breast and have not returned for revision.

The most common aesthetic shortcomings of the spiral flap reshaping of the breasts are superior pole induration and depression and lateral breast bulges. A year or so of patience will allow for absorption of distal flap necrosis; however, debridement may be indicated for the more extensive pathology. Following those treatments and when there is a gap between the superior breast and the tunnels flap, limited lipoaugmentation through fat injections has been successful. The intentional retention of some localized fat deposits is a godsend for these aesthetic problems (Fig. 103.8). The lower portions of these reshaped breasts can be excessively broad due to the base of the lateral thoracic pedicle. After 6 months, direct excision of these lateral bulges and narrowing of the base of the breasts is effective and safe. Months to years later, desire for larger breasts has led to relatively small silicone implant submammary augmentation in 4 patients who wanted increased size (Figs. 103.9 to 103.11).

DISCUSSION

Until recently the consensus on treating breast deformity after weight loss was pessimistic. Although plastic surgeons have recommended using nearby deepithelialized flaps for more than 30 years, the technical details were scant and the results fair. I disagree with Zook that these procedures are unaesthetic because of the scars (18). The extensive scarring that follows these procedures can be hidden around the breasts and covered by underwear. Moreover, there is dramatic improvement in the breasts, torso, and arms. Although some scar hypertrophy occurs, most scars fade over several years. An active scar treatment program with a variety of modalities is essential. If the scars fail to regress after 8 weeks, we start a graded program with paper tape, silicone sheeting, microdermabrasion, Retin-A, and intense pulsed light. Adrucil (5-fluorouracil) injections are occasionally used (38). Adverse side effects limit steroid injections, except for keloids, which we have yet to encounter. Regardless of their appearance, the scars on the torso should to be level, symmetric, and hidden by underwear.

Whenever excess tissue is available, I favor the spiral flap for breast augmentation and suspension. For minimal breast deformity, the extra effort of flap deepithelialization and placement is questionable, whereas in the more difficult constricted and pancake breast, the spiral flaps and mastopexy are optimal therapy. The flaps are easy to raise, reliable, and flexible. The procedure fulfills a basic plastic surgery tenet to take from Peter to pay Paul only if Peter can afford it. The excess back tissue is removed and then aesthetically shaped with the deficient breast. Both the recipient and donor sites are naturally recontoured and improved. Patients are amazed and pleased that their previously offensive tissue excess can be recycled to create attractive and natural breasts. The surgeon should understand how to preserve the trans serratus muscle perforators to the lateral thoracic flap and the mid breast, transversely oriented septal blood supply to the parenchyma and NAC (31–37).

With better facility using silicone implants, I have broadened my approach to a comprehensive strategy presented in this chapter. With severe ptosis with atrophy, silicone implants with mastopexy and acellular sheet of dermis support should be considered. If not, there is likely to be a disconnect between the implant and breast or, worse yet, a bottoming out of the implant. It appears that breasts with good elastic recoil do not need that expensive acellular dermis, but that judgment can be difficult to make.

Regardless of the approach, positioning a proper and secure IMF is crucial. Many chapters in this book discuss the IMF. Chapters 41 to 43 are devoted to it. The IMF is a fascial condensation adhering dermis to the chest muscle fascia roughly along the sixth rib at the inferior extent of the breast footprint. The well-secured IMF establishes the end of the reverse abdominoplasty while maintaining the position of the breast. The new IMF raises the brassiere line and lowers the NAC. Proper IMF construction contributes to improved breast conus and footprint. It hides the reverse abdominoplasty scar under the breasts. It inhibits caudal migration of oversized silicone implants. It allows for maximum removal of redundant and lax mid torso skin flaps by a secure fixation to the chest wall.

Secure fixation is essential. The IMFs we have created approximate the SFS to muscular fascia and to rib cartilage and periosteum. Despite considerable tension caused by the reverse abdominoplasty, the IMF rarely drifts caudally. The anterior thoracic SFS is well defined with sparse fat. We minimize injury to the SFS by scalpel incision. The discontinuous suprafascial undermining goes to the coastal margin. We place interrupted permanent, large-braided sutures with generous vertical bites using tapered needles from just lateral to the sternum to the anterior axillary line. We tug on each suture to be sure of a secure placement. By forceful upward push on the reverse abdominoplasty flap, tension is relieved as the sutures are tied. They may temporarily dimple the skin.

A firmly secured IMF can have its problems. This closure is painful for weeks and sometimes many months. While no IMF scar under the breasts has hypertrophied, some of the medial and lateral chest extensions have. In several single-stage TBLs, the IMF has drifted down slightly. On a few occasions suture abscesses have required removal of the braided permanent sutures. In some patients the tight IMFs seemed to cause the implants to rise higher and form a higher pocket, as seen in Figure 103.4, which may need secondary pocket adjustment.

The L-shaped brachioplasty complements the upper body lift by reducing hyperaxilla, raising posterior axillary fold ptosis, and further reducing lateral chest rolls (25). The horizontal scar sweeps along the inferior medial aspect of the arm and then rises to the dome of the axilla and after bisecting the axilla drops vertically along the lateral chest. There is no restriction to the outstretched arms, which only accentuate the beauty of this region (Figs. 103.6, 103.7, 103.11, and 103.12). The aesthetics of the breasts are enhanced when the procedure is performed in concert with the L-shaped brachioplasty.

Zook correctly advised combining procedures with team surgery (17). Team surgery is possible by having several operators with assistants working on different parts of the body under the direction of the responsible surgeon. The surgeon must be confident in the preoperative markings and install a consistent plan of action so that his or her assistants, as well as the nurses, technicians, and anesthesiologists, are prepared and can anticipate. The surgeon must have stamina and prolonged concentration, moving fast during mundane tasks and more deliberately through the more creative facets. The breast reshaping tends to occurs toward the end of the lengthy surgery. As it is the most technically challenging, I tend to do that procedure myself. Its artistic demands help to keep me stimulated late into the case. What keeps me motivated through these exhausting procedures is the confidence that the result will be dramatic and well appreciated.

CONCLUSION

Despite the variety of clinical presentations, a strategy for managing the breast deformity after MWL has been developed that primarily relies on volume deficiencies and the usefulness of nearby tissue. The long-term aesthetics of silicone implants in the profoundly atrophied and sagging breast has been greatly improved with acellular dermis as a hammock. A variety of products are available, with no clear preference at this time. Clarification of the blood supply of the spiral flap and the septum of the breast has elucidated the vascular reliability of this technique even in the extreme deformity. The inset of the lateral thoracic flap portion of the spiral flap has been appreciably assisted by routinely using access to the pectoralis fascia through the superior opening for the advance NAC. Aesthetic shortcomings such as lateral bulge and uneven contours are readily corrected.

EDITORIAL COMMENTS

The field of breast and body contouring after massive weight loss represents a new frontier for the specialty of plastic surgery. This exciting and fertile area of surgery presents us with a patient population that has challenging body contouring problems that stimulate the imagination. One of the concepts presented in this chapter focuses on a unique aspect of the anatomy of these patients: management of the excess and redundant skin and fat. Although much attention has rightly focused on techniques for excision, innovative methods on harvesting these tissues safely and using them to strategically augment deficient areas of the body represent another level of refinement in the treatment of these patients. The breast is one of the major problem areas in these patients that might, more than any other area, benefit from "autoaugmentation" using these redundant tissues. In this chapter, Dr. Hurwitz describes a unique and effective method for accomplishing this goal. Use of the redundant local tissues under the arm and along the back not only recontours this very difficult and often ignored area, but also assists in filling out the redundant skin envelope of the breast, often without an implant. The reverse abdominoplasty strategy, although technically more difficult, also provides extra tissue for the breast. I agree completely with the attention directed at the IMF. This vital structure often requires resuspension and reinforces the fact that the "autoaugmentation" represents just one facet of the entire reshaping process these patients require. With time, even more options using this innovative strategy will be described, and multiple flap options for breast "autoaugmentation" will be described. It will be our task as plastic surgeons to find the most effective and safe options for these very challenging patients.

D.C.H.

REFERENCES

1. Wang Y, Beydoun MA. The obesity epidemic in the United States—gender, age, socioeconomic, racial/ethnic, and geographic characteristics: a systematic review and meta-regression analysis. *Epidemiol Rev* 2007;29:6–28.
2. Flegal KM, Carroll MD, Odgen CL, et al. Prevalence and trends in obesity among US adults, 1999–2000. *JAMA* 2002;288:1723.
3. Ogden CL, Carroll MD, Curtin LR, et al. Prevalence of overweight and obesity in the United States, 1999–2004. *JAMA* 2006;295:1549–1555.
4. National Institutes of Health. Clinical guidelines on the identification, evaluation, and treatment of overweight and obesity in adults: the evidence report. *Obesity Res* 1998;6(suppl 2):51.
5. Fisher BL, Schauer P. Medical and surgical options in the treatment of severe obesity. *Am J Surg* 2002;184(6B):9S.
6. Holloway JA, Forney GA, Gould DE. The Lap-Band is an effective tool for weight loss even in the United States. *Am J Surg* 2004;188(6):659–662.
7. Santry HP, Gillen DL, Lauderdale DS. Trends in bariatric surgical procedures. *JAMA* 2005;294(15):1909–1922.
8. American Society for Metabolic and Bariatric Surgery. Bariatric surgical society takes on new name, new mission and new surgery. Available at: http://www.asbs.org/Newsite07/resources/press_release_8202007.pdf. Accessed June 5, 2010.
9. Agha-Mohammadi S, Hurwitz DJ. Nutritional deficiency of post-bariatric body contouring patients: what every plastic surgeon should know. *Plast Reconstr Surg* 2008;122:604–613.
10. Agha-Mohammadi S, Hurwitz DJ. Potential impacts of nutritional deficiency of post-bariatric patients on body contouring. *Plast Reconstr Surg* 2008;122:19011–1914.
11. American Society of Plastic Surgeons. 2006 Cosmetic demographics. Body contouring after massive weight loss. Available at: http://www.plasticsurgery.org/Documents/Media/2006-Cosmetic-Demographics.pdf. Accessed July 5, 2010.
12. Hurwitz DJ, Zewert T. Body contouring surgery in the bariatric surgical patient. *Oper Tech Plast Surg* 2002;8:87–95.
13. Hurwitz DJ, Rubin JP, Risen M, et al. Correction of the saddlebag deformity in the massive weight loss patient. *Plast Reconstr Surg* 2004;114:1313–1325.
14. Hurwitz DJ. Single stage total body lift after massive weight loss. *Ann Plast Surg* 2004;52:435–441.
15. Lockwood TE. Superficial fascial system (SFS) of the trunk and extremities: a new concept. *Plast Reconstr Surg* 1991;87:1009–1015.
16. Hurwitz DJ, Agha-Mohammadi S, Ota K, et al. A clinical review of total body lift. *Aesthet Surg J* 2008;28(3):294–304.
17. Zook EG. The massive weight loss patient. *Clin Plast Surg* 1975;2:457–466.
18. Zook EG. Discussion of abdominoplasty following gastrointestinal bypass surgery by Savage RC. *Plast Reconstr Surg* 1983;74:508–509.
19. Palmer B, Hallberg D, Backman L. Skin reduction plasties following intestinal shunt operations for treatment of obesity. *Scand J Plast Reconstr Surg* 1975;9:47–52.
20. Wise RJ. A preliminary report on a method of planning the mammaplasty. *Plast Reconstr Surg* 1956;17:367–369.
21. McKissock PK. Reduction mammoplasty with a vertical dermal pedicle. *Plast Reconstr Surg* 1972;49:245–252.
22. Shons AR. Plastic reconstruction after bypass surgery and massive weight loss. *Surg Clin North Am* 1979;59:1139–1152.
23. Lockwood TE. Reduction mammaplasty and mastopexy with superficial fascial system suspension. *Plast Reconstr Surg* 1999;103:1411–1420.
24. Hurwitz DJ, Golla D. Breast Reshaping after massive weight loss. *Semin Plast Surg* 2004;18:179–187.
25. Hurwitz DJ, Holland SW. The L brachioplasty: an innovative approach to correct excess tissue of the upper arm, axilla and lateral chest. *Plast Reconstr Surg* 2006;117(2):403–411.
26. Blondeel PN, Hijjawi J, Depypere H, et al. Shaping the breast in aesthetic and reconstructive breast surgery: an easy three-step principle. *Plast Reconstr Surg* 2009;123:455–462.
27. Rubin JP, O'Toole J, Gusenoff JA, et al. Dermal suspension and parenchymal reshaping mastopexy after massive weight loss: statistical analysis with concomitant procedures from a prospective registry. *Plast Reconstr Surg* 2009;123:782–789.
28. Hochberg J, Margulies A, Yuen JC, et al. Alloderm (acellular human dermis) in breast reconstruction with tissue expansion. *Plast Reconstr Surg* 2005;116(suppl 3):126–128.

29. Mofid MM, Singh NK. Pocket conversion made easy: a simple technique using AlloDerm to convert subglandular breast implants to dual-plane position. *Aesthet Surg J* 2009;29(1): 12–18.
30. Hurwitz DJ, Agha-Mohammadi S. Post bariatric surgery breast reshaping: the spiral flap. *Ann Plast Surg* 2006;56:481–486.
31. Holstrom H, Lossing C. The lateral thoracodorsal flap in breast reconstruction. *Plast Reconstr Surg* 1986;77:933–941.
32. Woerdeman LAE, van Schijndel AW, Hage JJ, et al. Verifying surgical results and risk factors of the lateral thoracic flap. *Plast Reconstr Surg* 2004;113:196–203.
33. Levine JI, Soucid NE, Allen RJ. Algorithm for autologous breast reconstruction for partial mastectomy defects. *Plast Reconstr Surg* 2005;116:762–766.
34. Van Landuyt K, Hamdi M, Blondeel P, et al. Autologous augmentation of pedicled perforator flaps. *Ann Plast Surg* 2004;53(4):322–327.
35. Kwei S, Borud LJ, Lee BT. Mastopexy with autologous augmentation after massive weight loss: the intercostal artery perforator (ICAP) flap. *Ann Plast Surg* 2006;57:361–367.
36. Wuringer E, Mader N, Posch E, et al. Nerve and vessel supplying ligamentous suspension of the mammary gland. *Plast Reconstr Surg* 1998;101:1486–1491.
37. Hamdi M, Van Landuyt K, Tonnard P. Septum-based mammaplasty: a surgical technique based on Wuringer's septum for breast reduction. *Plast Reconstr Surg* 2009;123: 443–462.
38. Davison SP, Dayan JH, Clemens MW. Efficacy of intralesional 5-fluorouracil and triamcinolone in the treatment of keloids. *Aesthet Surg J* 2009;1:40–46.

CHAPTER

104

Frank Lista
Jamil Ahmad

Gynecomastia

INTRODUCTION

Gynecomastia is a benign proliferation of glandular breast tissue causing breast enlargement in males (1,2). There is a great deal of variation in the prevalence of gynecomastia reported in the literature. Prevalences ranging from 4% to 69% have been reported among adolescent males (3,4). Among adult males, prevalences between 32% and 65% have been reported (5,6). Comprehensive reviews of etiologic factors, including drugs that cause gynecomastia, have been published (1,2,7). Approximately 25% of patients experience idiopathic adult gynecomastia and 25% suffer from acute or persistent gynecomastia secondary to puberty (8). Other causes of gynecomastia include drugs (10% to 20%), cirrhosis or malnutrition (8%), primary hypogonadism (8%), testicular tumors (3%), secondary hypogonadism (2%), hyperthyroidism (1.5%), and renal disease (1%) (8). Gynecomastia results from an absolute or relative imbalance between estrogens, which stimulate development of breast tissue, and androgens, which antagonize this effect (9,10). During the initial period of gynecomastia development associated with puberty, ductal epithelium proliferates and stromal and connective tissue hyperplasia and edema occur (11–13). After this initial period of 1 to 2 years, less epithelial growth occurs, and there is deposition of dense, collagenous fibers causing periductal fibrosis and hyalinization (11–13). Once this occurs, surgical treatment is required to correct gynecomastia.

Surgical techniques using a variety of incisions, excisions, suction-assisted lipectomy, power-assisted liposuction, ultrasound-assisted liposuction, or some combination of these methods have been used to treat gynecomastia. Recently, several minimal-access excisional techniques have been described. In 1996, Morselli (14) first described the pull-through technique for treatment of gynecomastia. This technique involved the use of suction-assisted lipectomy to remove fatty breast tissue, followed by the use of a clamp to pull the remaining fibroglandular breast tissue through the two incisions used for liposuction. In 2003, Hammond et al. (15) reported consistently pleasing results obtained by combining ultrasound-assisted liposuction with the pull-through technique. In addition, Bracaglia et al. (16) reported their experience using suction-assisted lipectomy and the pull-through technique, and Ramon et al. (17) described the use of cross-chest power-assisted superficial liposuction with the pull-through technique under endoscopic visualization; both reported consistently good results. In 2008, we reported our initial experience combining power-assisted liposuction with the pull-through technique (18). We use several instruments that allow easier excision of fibroglandular breast tissue and make it possible to remove this tissue through a single incision located at the lateral aspect of the inframammary crease. Since first using this technique in January of 2003, we have successfully performed it in more than 200 patients. This technique has been used to treat patients with various degrees of gynecomastia and consistently produces a naturally contoured male breast while resulting in a single inconspicuous scar.

EVALUATION

Rohrich et al. (19) provide a comprehensive review of the management of gynecomastia and present a straightforward algorithm for its evaluation and treatment. Treatment of gynecomastia should begin, if possible, with identification of the underlying cause. Given that the majority of patients presenting for evaluation of gynecomastia have idiopathic adult gynecomastia or acute or persistent gynecomastia due to puberty, a detailed history and physical examination usually suffice to rule out other causes that may require further workup. Positive findings in the history or abnormal physical findings may necessitate further diagnostic investigations such as hormonal levels, imaging studies, and karyotyping, depending on the suspected etiology for gynecomastia (19).

During preoperative evaluation, an important differentiation should be made between gynecomastia and male breast cancer. Breast cancer in men accounts for approximately 1% of all cases of breast cancer (20). The mean age for male breast cancer is 65 years, but it may occur at any age (20). A family history of breast cancer increases the risk of male breast cancer, and this has been linked to both BRCA1 and BRCA2 genes (20). Although the association of gynecomastia and male breast cancer is of uncertain significance, high risk for male breast cancer has been established in certain states of relative estrogen excess to androgen deficiency such as Klinefelter syndrome, exogenous estrogen use, cryptorchidism, orchitis, or postorchiectomy (20). Exposure to ionizing radiation may also increase the risk of male breast cancer (20). Physical examination of the breasts may reveal signs that are suspicious for male breast cancer. Breast tissue in gynecomastia is usually soft or elastic and tends to be located bilaterally around the nipple-areola complex (1). In contrast, male breast cancer is usually hard or firm, may not be associated with the nipple-areola complex, and is typically unilateral (1). In addition, other clinical signs may include skin dimpling, nipple retraction, and bloody nipple discharge (1). If male breast cancer is suspected, the patient should undergo diagnostic mammography, which is 90% sensitive and specific for differentiating malignant from benign breast masses in males (1,21).

After ruling out other causes of gynecomastia, acute or persistent gynecomastia due to puberty is usually sufficiently treated with patience and reassurance, while patients with idiopathic adult gynecomastia persistent for more than 1 year are likely to benefit from surgical treatment.

Since 2003, we have combined power-assisted liposuction and the pull-through technique to treat all patients presenting for the treatment of gynecomastia (Figs. 104.1 and 104.2).

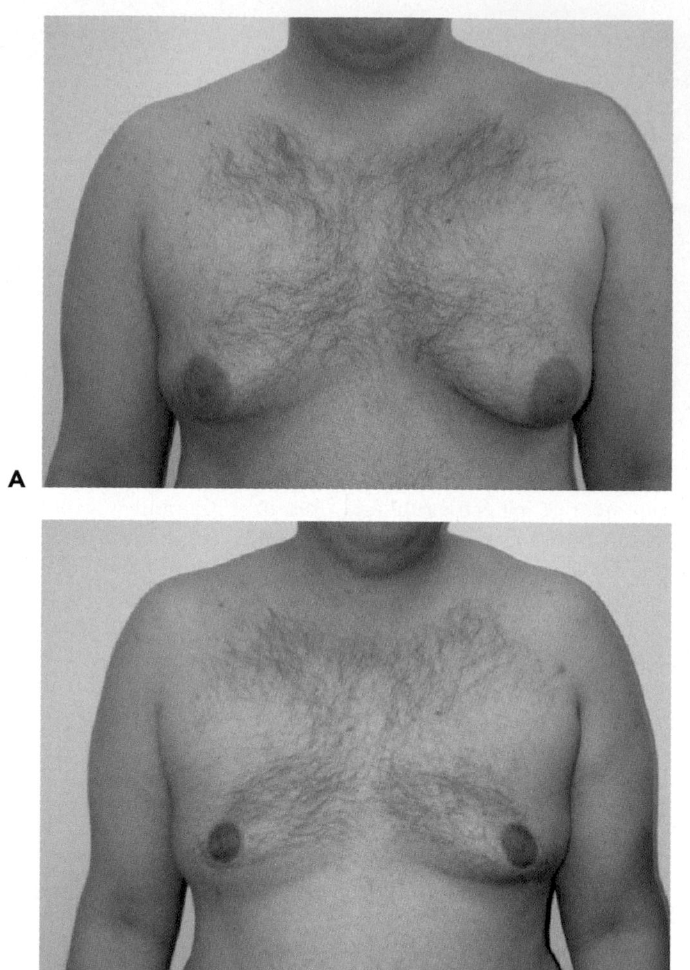
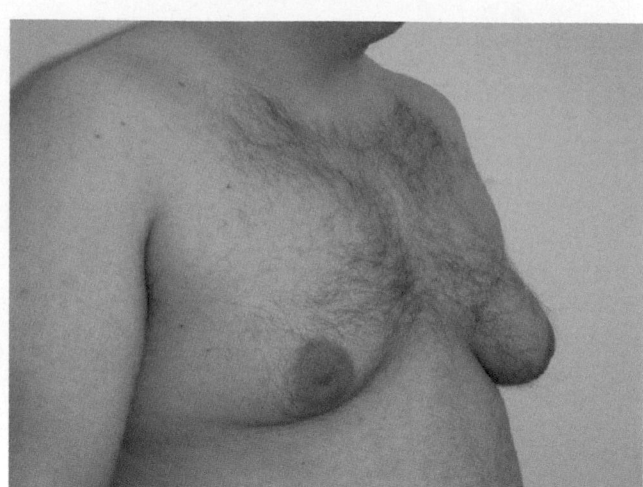

Figure 104.1. **A, B:** A 29-year-old man with bilateral gynecomastia. **C:** One month following power-assisted liposuction and the pull-through technique removing 800 mL from the right breast and 750 mL from the left breast.

In 2008, we reported the initial results using our technique in 99 consecutive patients (197 breasts) treated between January 2003 and November 2006 (18). In this clinical series, the average age of the patients was 29 years (range, 17 to 46 years) and the average body mass index was 28.0 kg/m^2 (range, 20.6 to 40.0 kg/m^2). Using power-assisted liposuction, the average volume aspirated per breast was 459 mL (range, 25 to 1400 mL), and between 5 and 70 g of tissue per breast was removed using the pull-through technique. The average operative time was 60 minutes (39 to 85 minutes). At 3-month follow-up, all patients expressed their satisfaction with the overall aesthetic result.

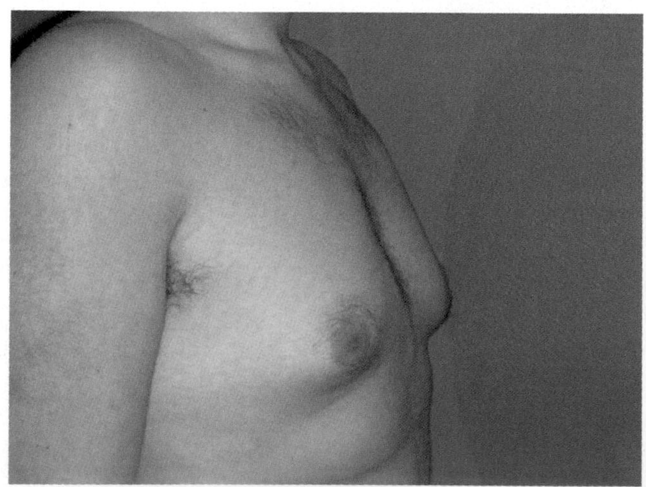
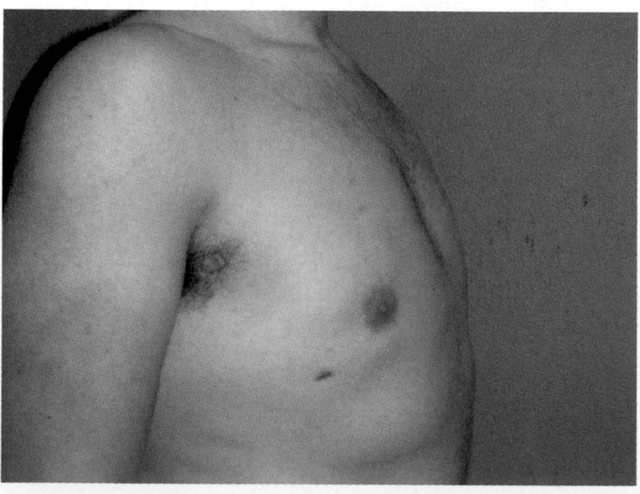

Figure 104.2. **A:** A 18-year-old man with bilateral gynecomastia. **B:** One month following power-assisted liposuction and the pull-through technique removing 200 mL from each breast.

TECHNIQUE

SKIN MARKINGS AND INFILTRATION

The patient is marked in the standing position. The areas where liposuction will be performed are topographically marked. In addition to treating breast tissue around the nipple-areola complex, we treat all areas of the chest that have excess fat and breast tissue. This extended contouring of the chest leads to an improved breast contour; blending the nipple-areola complex with the surrounding breast prevents the occurrence of a concave deformity of the nipple-areola complex.

We perform this procedure under general anesthesia. After the patient has been anesthetized and is placed in the supine position, a 4-mm stab incision is made at the inframammary crease where it intersects with the anterior axillary line. Infiltration is performed just deep to the skin and then within the breast parenchyma. Each breast is infiltrated with approximately 500 mL of a solution made with 1,000 mL of Ringer's lactate solution mixed with 40 mL of 2% lidocaine and 1 mL of 1:1,000 epinephrine.

POWER-ASSISTED LIPOSUCTION FOR REMOVAL OF FATTY BREAST TISSUE

Power-assisted liposuction is used to reduce breast volume arising mainly from fat by using the PAL-600E MicroAire power-assisted lipoplasty device (MicroAire Surgical Instruments, Charlottesville, VA). We prefer to use power-assisted liposuction because it aids in passing the liposuction cannula through the fibrous parenchymal framework of the breast, reducing operator fatigue. Before performing liposuction, a 4.5-mm Masaki skin protector (Dr. Masaki Clinic, Tokyo, Japan) is sutured to the stab incision to protect the surrounding skin from friction injury (Figs. 104.3). Liposuction of the entire breast is initially carried out in the middle layer of subcutaneous adipose tissue using the PAL-R407LL MicroAire helixed triport 4-mm cannula (MicroAire Surgical Instruments). Next, attention is focused on the breast tissue lying deep to the nipple-areola complex. Liposuction of this area is carried out in the subdermal plane, which we believe stimulates skin contraction in the postoperative period. Before we perform the pull-through technique, the Masaki skin guards are removed.

THE PULL-THROUGH TECHNIQUE FOR REMOVAL OF FIBROGLANDULAR BREAST TISSUE

The pull-through technique is performed using several instruments to sever the subdermal attachments of fibrous breast tissue and to divide the connections of the lactiferous ducts to the overlying nipple. Particular attention is focused on removing subdermal breast tissue deep to the nipple-areola complex. This tissue is then "pulled through" the incision used for liposuction. Fibroglandular breast tissue present in other areas of the breast is also removed using the pull-through technique. Using 19-cm straight Brand tendon tunnel forceps (Instrumentarium, Terrebonne, Quebec, Canada) through the incision used for liposuction, fibroglandular breast tissue is removed through this incision using a "grasp and pull" motion while the skin is pinched using the other hand (Fig. 104.4). When it is difficult to remove fibroglandular breast tissue in this manner, a Toledo V-dissector cannula (Tulip Products, San Diego, CA) and a special-order larger Toledo V-dissector cannula (Wells Johnson Company, Tucson, AZ) are used to sever the subdermal attachments of this tissue (Fig. 104.5). These attachments mainly consist of the lactiferous ducts and the suspensory ligaments of Cooper. The attachments of these structures to the deep fascia are weak, and it is unnecessary to perform any sharp dissection in this deep plane. Occasionally, curved, ebonized, micro ear scissors (Anthony Products, Indianapolis, IN) (Fig. 104.6) or a no. 12 blade scalpel are required to sever these attachments through the incision used for liposuction. Once these subdermal attachments have been adequately severed, the breast tissue is "pulled through" the incision used for liposuction using the Brand tendon tunnel forceps. After adequately removing fibroglandular breast tissue, the skin of the breast feels smooth and the underlying fibroglandular breast tissue is no longer palpable. It is possible to remove large amounts of fibroglandular breast tissue using these instruments (Fig. 104.7).

A

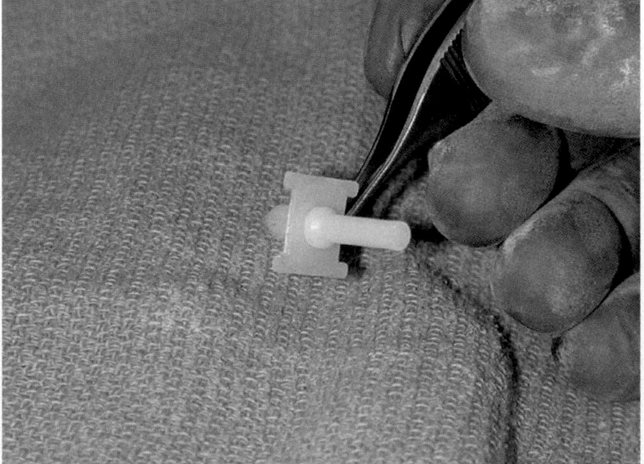

B

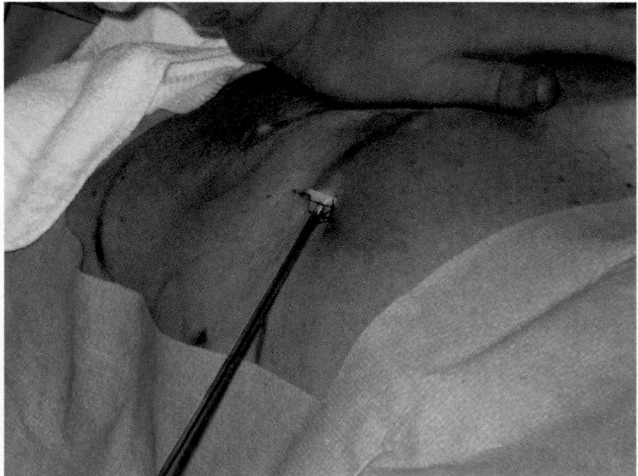

Figure 104.3. **A, B:** During power-assisted liposuction, a 4.5-mm Masaki skin protector with a 4.0-mm obturator is used to protect the skin edges from friction injury.

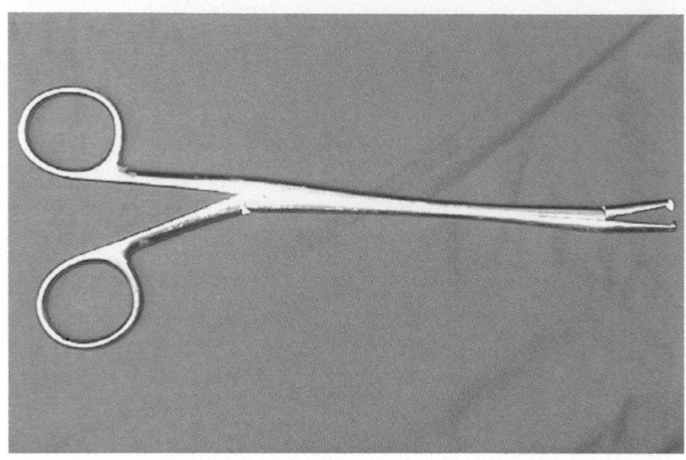

A

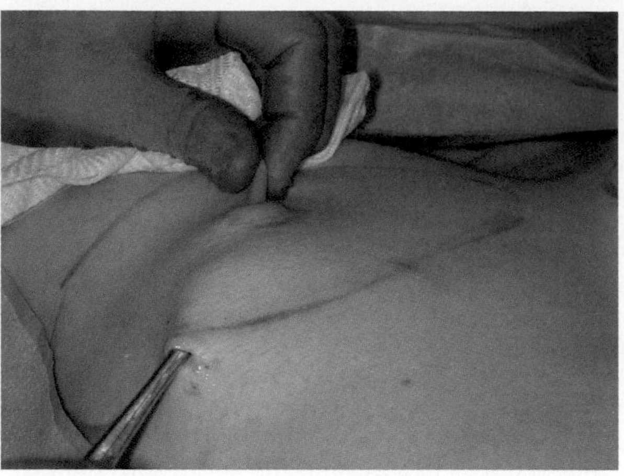

B

Figure 104.4. A, B: With the use of a 19-cm straight Brand tendon tunnel forceps through the incision used for liposuction, fibroglandular breast tissue is removed through this incision using a "grasp and pull" motion while the skin is pinched using the other hand.

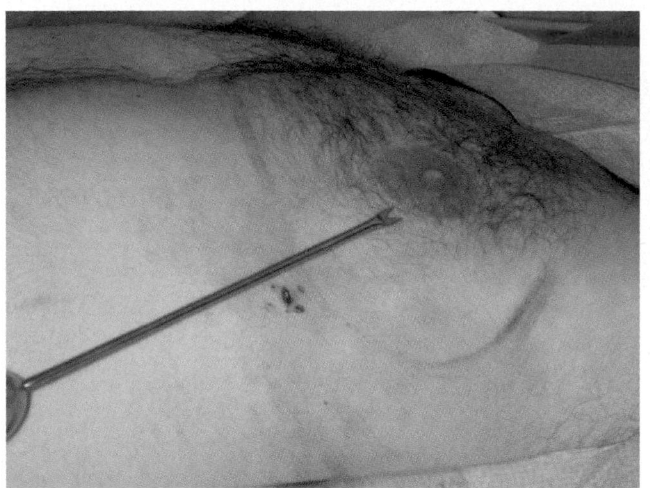

A

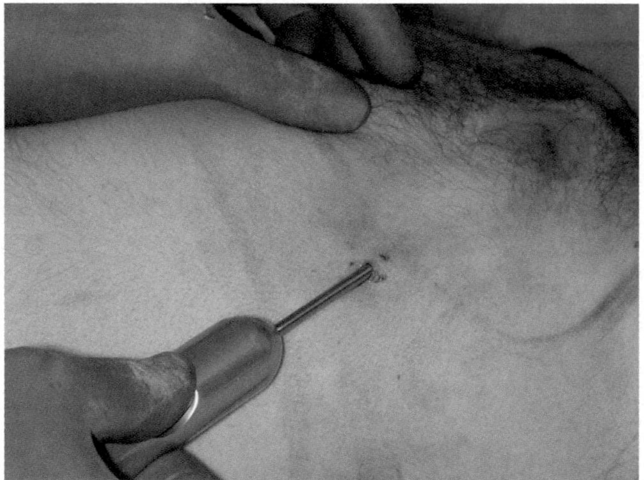

B

Figure 104.5. A, B: A special-order Toledo V-dissector cannula is used to sever the subdermal attachments of fibroglandular breast tissue.

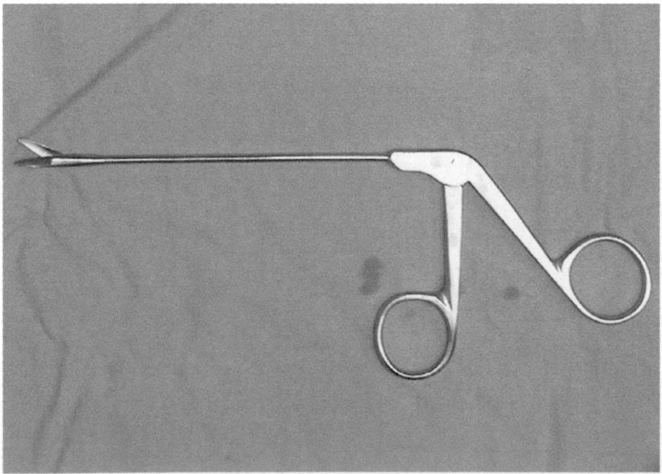

Figure 104.6. Curved, ebonized, micro ear scissors can be used to cut fibroglandular breast tissue.

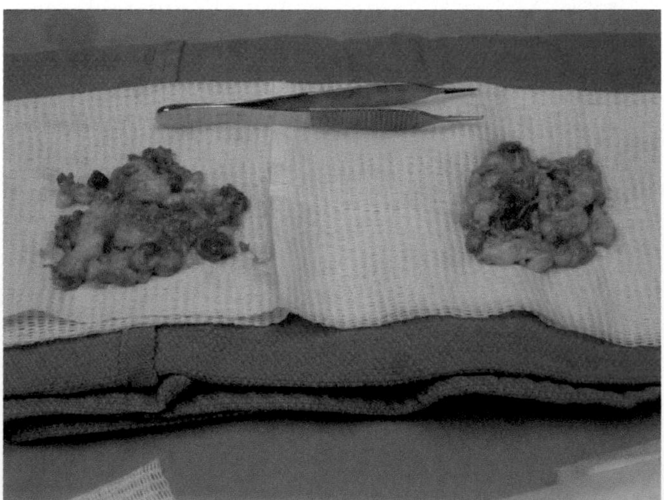

Figure 104.7. It is possible to remove large amounts of fibroglandular breast tissue using the pull-through technique.

POWER-ASSISTED LIPOSUCTION FOR CONTOURING BREAST TISSUE

After the pull-through technique is performed, power-assisted liposuction is used to feather the remaining breast tissue to soften the breast contour and blend the nipple-areola complex with the surrounding breast tissue. In addition, this final contouring is also necessary to remove fatty breast tissue that was dislodged after the dense parenchymal framework of the breast was removed using the pull-through technique. The incisions are closed using an inverted deep dermal 4-0 Monocryl suture (Ethicon, Somerville, NJ). The wounds are dressed with dry gauze, and a compression garment is applied.

POSTOPERATIVE CARE

Patients are typically seen on postoperative day 5 and then 2 weeks, 1 month, and 3 months postoperatively. The patient must wear a compression garment (Marena Group, Lawrenceville, GA) (Fig. 104.8) day and night for a total of 6 weeks to allow the skin of the breast to adhere to the underlying tissues. Patients should avoid strenuous activity for 3 weeks and then may return to their normal level of activity.

RISKS AND COMPLICATIONS

Since we began performing this technique in January 2003, we have not experienced complications such as hematoma, infection, contour irregularities, including a depressed nipple-areola complex, excessive scarring, or skin redundancy, which have been reported using other techniques to treat gynecomastia. Hematoma formation has likely been avoided by using a wetting solution containing epinephrine, limiting sharp dissection, and using a postoperative compression garment. Extended contouring of the chest using liposuction avoids contour irregularities and also prevents the occurrence of a concave deformity of the nipple-areola complex, which is a common result of some excisional techniques. We have found that our patients desire removal of as much breast tissue as possible, and as a consequence, sometimes the subcutaneous tissues of the chest can feel irregular in consistency following this procedure. This has not been an issue for our patients, but we feel that it is important to inform patients preoperatively that they may feel these irregularities. Patients may experience some temporary or permanent decrease in sensation to the nipple-areola complex or skin overlying the breast, but this too has not been a significant problem for our patients. A major disadvantage of excisional techniques is the resultant extensive scarring that has been the stigmata of male breast surgery in the past. The single, inconspicuous scar left after using the pull-through technique is a significant advantage of our technique.

On rare occasion, we have not been able to adequately excise fibroglandular tissue deep to the areola using power-assisted liposuction and the pull-through technique. In these cases, there was a single, large, solid mass of fibroglandular breast tissue responsible deep to the nipple-areola complex. Our procedure was modified using an inferior periareolar incision to adequately excise this fibroglandular breast tissue. The possibility of this type of excision should be discussed with the patient preoperatively.

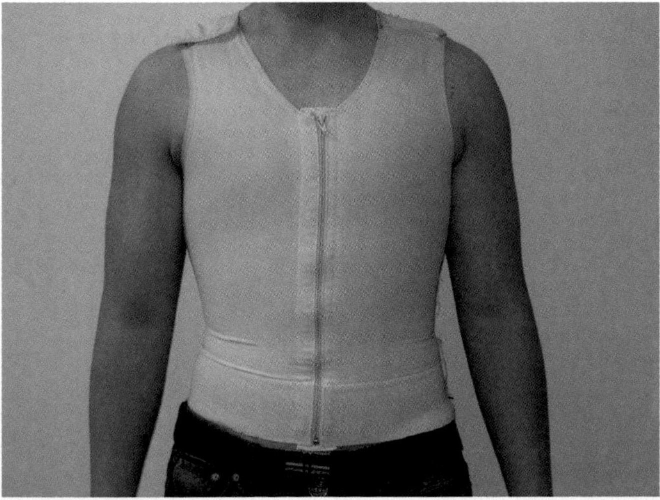

Figure 104.8. A compression garment is worn for 6 weeks postoperatively.

CONCLUSION

Since January 2003, we have used this technique to treat more than 200 patients presenting for treatment of gynecomastia. Combining power-assisted liposuction and the pull-through technique has proven to be a versatile approach for the treatment of gynecomastia. It consistently produces a naturally contoured male breast while resulting in a single inconspicuous scar, resulting in a high level of patient satisfaction.

EDITORIAL COMMENTS

Gynecomastia can present as a variable spectrum of breast enlargement. For patients who exhibit an isolated fibrous subareolar breast bud with minimal surrounding fibrofatty proliferation, the technique described in this chapter has limited applicability as it is too difficult to perforate through the dense mass of tissue. For these patients, who present most commonly with either adolescent gynecomastia without any level of associated obesity or drug (steroid) induced gynecomastia, direct excision through a periareolar approach is a better option. However a great many patients do present with a surrounding hypertrophy of the connective tissue stroma and adequate surgical correction must include recontouring of the peripheral portions of the breast and chest wall to be optimally effective. Most commonly these patients present with either adolescent gynecomastia in association with variable levels of obesity or are older men presenting later in life with a combination of subareolar fibrous proliferation along with generalized fatty hypertrophy. In these cases, the technique described in this chapter has great applicability. By accessing the breast through a small stab incision located either at the level of the inframammary fold as noted in the chapter, or along the inferior margin of the areola, or even laterally along the chest wall, recontouring of the fatty accumulation can be effectively performed without creating an unacceptable scar burden for the patient. In the process of performing the liposuction, the subareolar fibrous tissue is repeatedly perforated creating a honeycomb-like disruption of the integrity of this mass of tissue. Then, through the same incision used to perform the liposuction, the strands of excess fibrous tissue can be removed sequentially by pulling them through the incision until the desired level of subareolar recontouring is achieved. Using this combination approach affords precise control over the contour that is created on the chest and any tendency to over-resect in the subareolar area with the resultant creation of a saucer-like deformity is minimized. As noted in the chapter, complications are few and the results are typically quite good. Of particular advantage is the fact that the entire procedure can be accomplished through a small stab incision thereby avoiding the placement of any conspicuous telltale scars on the chest, a fact that is of great relief to adolescent boys and younger men where "breast" scars are viewed in an unfavorable light and can significantly detract from the overall success of the procedure. When removing the fat, any type of tumescent liposuction technique can be used, however the power assisted device described in the chapter or perhaps even more effective, the ultrasound assisted liposuction technique, will be more successful in breaking up the subareolar fibrous breast bud than traditional liposuction, thus easing the subsequent removal of the tissue using the pull through technique. Also, as noted in the chapter, it is advisable to treat all areas of fatty accumulation to achieve the best result, even those areas that extend superiorly as well as laterally around the thorax. Although these areas may not be in proximity to the major fibrofatty accumulation on the anterior chest wall, left untreated, persistent fullness in these areas can create results that have an out of proportion appearance possibly leading to patient dissatisfaction with the procedure.

In summary, the authors present a very useful technique for the treatment of gynecomastia that can optimize results and minimize complications for a wide variety of patient presentations.

D.C.H.

REFERENCES

1. Braunstein GD. Clinical practice. Gynecomastia. *N Engl J Med* 2007;328:1229–1237.
2. Neuman JF. Evaluation and treatment of gynecomastia. *Am Family Physician* 1997;55:1835–1844.
3. Harlan WR, Grillo GP, Cornoni-Huntley J, et al. Secondary sex characteristics of boys 12 to 17 years of age: the U.S. Health Examination Survey. *J Pediatr* 1979;95:293–297.
4. Lee PA. The relationship of concentrations of serum hormones to pubertal gynecomastia. *J Pediatr* 1975;86:212–215.
5. Carlson HE. Gynecomastia. *N Engl J Med* 1980;303:795–799.
6. Niewoehner CB, Nuttal FQ. Gynecomastia in a hospitalized male population. *Am J Med* 1984;77:633–638.
7. Glass AR. Gynecomastia. *Endocrinol Metab Clin North Am* 1994;23:825–837.
8. Biro FM, Lucky AW, Huster GA, et al. Hormonal studies and physical maturation in adolescent gynecomastia. *J Pediatr* 1990;116:450–455.
9. Edmondson HA, Glass SJ, Soll SN. Gynecomastia associated with cirrhosis of the liver. *Proc Soc Exp Biol Med* 1939;42:97–99.
10. Rochefort H, Garcia M. The estrogenic and antiestrogenic activities of androgens in female target tissues. *Pharmacol Ther* 1983;23:193–216.
11. Nicolis G, Modlinger R, Gabrilove J. A study of the histopathology of human gynecomastia. *J Clin Endocrinol Metab* 1971;32:173–178.
12. Bannayan G, Hajdu S. Gynecomastia: clinicopathologic study of 351 cases. *Am J Clin Pathol* 1972;57:431–437.
13. Hassan M, Olaizola M. Ultrastructural observations on gynecomastia. *Arch Pathol Lab* Med 1979;103:624–630.
14. Morselli PG. "Pull-through": a new technique for breast reduction in gynecomastia. *Plast Reconstr Surg* 1996;97:450–454.
15. Hammond DC, Arnold JF, Simon AM, et al. Combined use of ultrasonic liposuction with the pull-through technique for the treatment of gynecomastia. *Plast Reconstr Surg* 2003;112:891–895.
16. Bracaglia R, Fortunato R, Gentileschi S, et al. Our experience with the so-called pull-through technique combined with liposuction for management of gynecomastia. *Ann Plast Surg* 2004;53:22–26.
17. Ramon Y, Fodor L, Peled IJ, et al. Multimodality gynecomastia repair by cross-chest power-assisted superficial liposuction combined with endoscopic-assisted pull-through excision. *Ann Plast Surg* 2005;55:591–594.
18. Lista F, Ahmad J. Power-assisted liposuction and the pull-through technique for the treatment of gynecomastia. *Plast Reconstr Surg* 2008;121:740–747.
19. Rohrich RJ, Ha RY, Kenkel JM, et al. Classification and management of gynecomastia: defining the role of ultrasound-assisted liposuction. *Plast Reconstr Surg* 2003;111:909–923.
20. Niewoehner CB, Schorer AE. Gynaecomastia and breast cancer in men. *BMJ* 2008;336:709–713.
21. Evans GFF, Anthony T, Appelbaum AH, et al. The diagnostic accuracy of mammography in the evaluation of male breast disease. *Am J Surg* 2001;181:96–100.

CHAPTER

105

Scott L. Spear
Karen Kim Evans

Complications and Secondary Corrections After Breast Reduction and Mastopexy

INTRODUCTION

The relationship between reconstructive and cosmetic surgery is clearly at play in the case of breast reduction and mastopexy. The various methods of glandular excision, incision patterns, and type of neurovascular pedicle offer advantages and disadvantages for each patient. In the overwhelming majority of cases, the results of these techniques meet or even surpass patient expectation both in terms of symptomatic improvement and cosmetic outcome. Although proper patient selection for each method is a critical component for successful outcome, a thorough understanding of the complications of breast reduction and mastopexy and how to avoid them can also be very helpful. This is particularly true as surgeons attempt newer techniques, including shorter scars and different pedicle design.

NIPPLE LOSS

Although rare, nipple loss is one of the most devastating complications of breast reduction. The reported incidence varies from 0 to 10%, depending on whether the author includes partial nipple necrosis and complete nipple loss when determining the frequency of this mal-occurrence (1–14). As surgical skill, techniques, and understanding of the anatomy of the rich blood supply to the nipple from both cranial and caudal perforators have advanced, the incidence of nipple loss has decreased (15). Traditionally recognized "safer" and more familiar techniques, such as the inferior pedicle and free nipple grafting in very large reductions, have already become well accepted methods to minimize nipple loss. These techniques are the de facto benchmark standards that other techniques are measured against.

For moderate to large reductions, vertical scar patterns and/or superomedial pedicle techniques have been shown in some preliminary reviews to reliably protect the nipple (16,17). Nipple loss has been reported even in cases of mastopexy and especially in the setting of secondary procedures surrounding thin, poorly vascularized tissues. Of course, the combination of mastopexy with augmentation or mastopexy as a secondary procedure inherently increases complications such as nipple loss (18). It is generally recognized that secondary breast reduction should use the same pedicle as in the original procedure; however, more recent reports suggest that using a different pedicle may be "safe" (19–22). We would caution against this broad statement and suggest that it is imperative to maximize the blood supply to the nipple in the setting of secondary reduction mammaplasty by using the same pedicle if it is known and if the nipple is to be moved any significant amount. Moreover, we perform direct excision rather than undermining flaps and caution that previous scars, even within the breast parenchyma, are a permanent obstruction to blood flow (20). As a general principle, in secondary cases, it is wise to avoid creating risky pedicles or flaps and to maximize the blood supply to the nipple and flaps as much as possible.

Intrinsic patient risk factors, including smoking, diabetes, obesity, and hypertension, all of which are common in this patient population, further increase the risk of nipple loss. Avoiding nipple loss begins with patient selection and choosing the safest possible techniques in high-risk patients. Encouraging patients to lose weight and stop smoking could reduce the risk to some extent. Many times, insurance companies are reluctant to cover breast reduction for patients who are obese. In high-risk patients, including those with resections greater than 2 kg, severe ptosis, or with body mass index (BMI) greater than 35, reduction using free nipple graft should be considered, either as the primary or as a back-up procedure. Focusing on the quality of the recipient bed, careful handling of tissues and avoidance of hematoma or seroma under the graft should reduce the risk of nipple loss to 1 to 2%.

At the time of surgery, a doubtful or struggling nipple can be converted to a graft if the blood supply appears sluggish on the table. Even postoperatively, when in doubt, the nipple can still be converted to a nipple graft. Although it should be obvious that the sooner this is done, the better, there is no scientific evidence for a time limit to this opportunity for nipple salvage.

It is important to consider the etiology of an ischemic nipple, inspect the breast for hematoma, and release tight periareolar sutures. Some surgeons have even described using leech therapy or nitropaste on an early, struggling nipple. Rather than resort to early debridement, in the case of a struggling nipple, for the first few weeks, one should consider treating a compromised nipple conservatively. In addition to leeches and nitropaste, other conservative therapy includes hyperbaric oxygen, moist dressings, and systemic antibiotics to cover skin flora. Although lacking absolute scientific proof, we have been particularly gratified by the effects of hyperbaric oxygen if instituted within 24 hours of surgery and continued for 5 to 7 days. Debriding necrotic tissue should be done carefully and with deliberation because the nipple will often re-epithelialize from deeper dermal elements.

Once the wound has healed, the nipple-areola complex can be reconstructed using techniques similar to those used in breast reconstruction. These may include tattooing for the areola (Fig. 105.1), full-thickness skin grafting, contralateral nipple composite grafts, nipple reconstruction using local flaps (Figs. 105.2 and 105.3), dermal fat grafts, or filler injections into the nipple.

SCARS

Although nipple loss is a particularly devastating complication, unattractive or disfiguring scars are much more common and

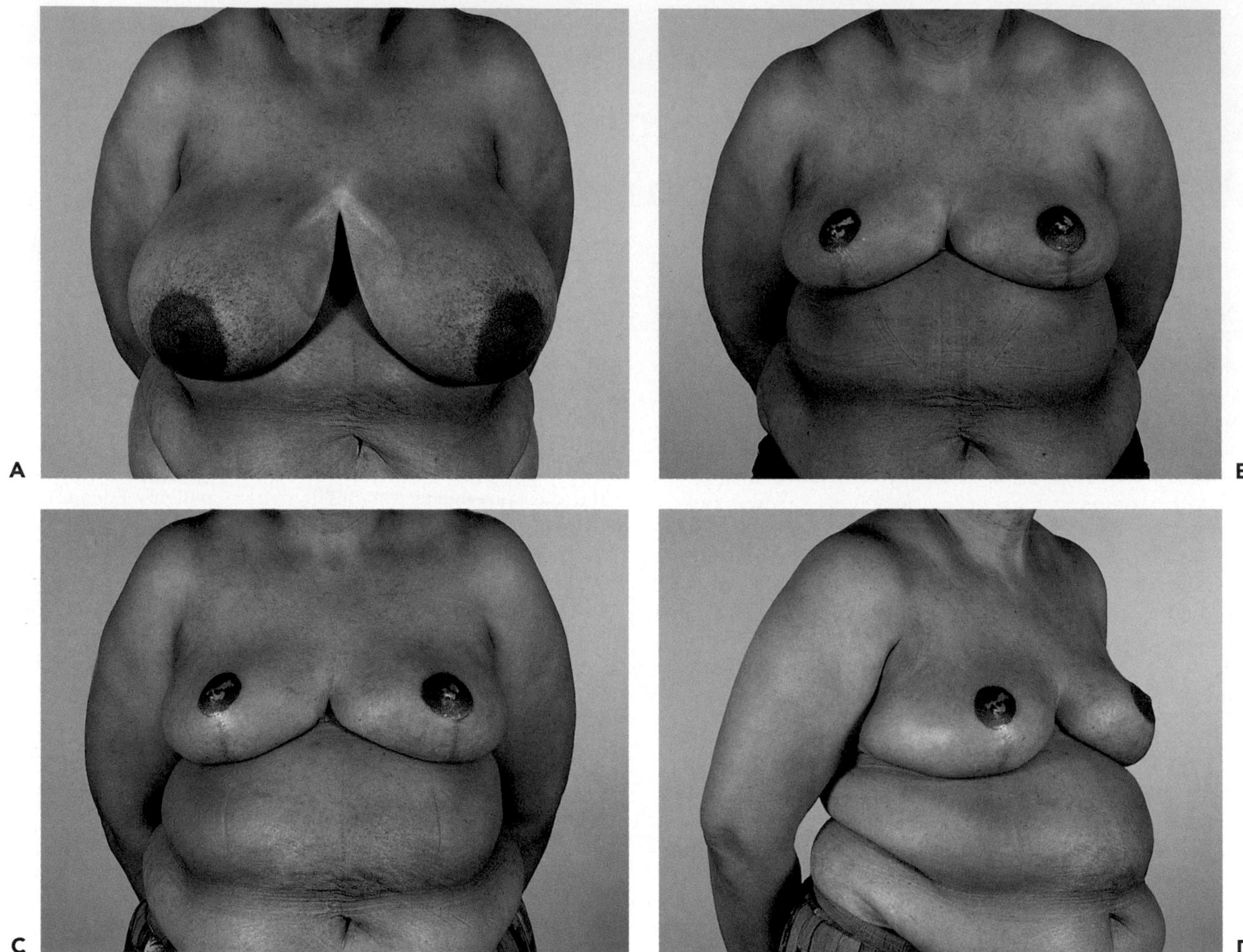

Figure 105.1. A 50-year-old with nipple depigmentation after free nipple graft reduction mammaplasty subsequently corrected by intradermal tattoo with brown and black pigment. **A:** Preoperative. **B:** After 1,500 g bilateral reductions and nipple transposition of 12 cm using the free graft technique. **C:** Mild postoperative vitiligo treated at 12 months with intradermal tattoo. **D:** Postoperative and posttattoo oblique view.

can also be a serious problem. Despite the universal desire of patients for scarless surgery, it is not possible. It is true that a number of abbreviated scar techniques are currently being used, and these all promote less or shorter scars, but they have not been proven to provide consistently better cosmetic results, or even better scars.

Although the choice of procedure and surgical skill are important, the underlying nature of the patient's tissues and skin are often the critical determinants of the quality of the scar. Young, dark-skinned or thick-skinned women, including Asian, African, and some Caucasian women, are often prone to poor scars. It is ironic that older patients with typically thinner skin, who usually care less about the scar, produce the best scars, whereas younger patients for whom scars are more critical often scar the worst. To help with the appearance of the scar, we have abandoned the use of braided Vicryl suture in the dermis due to its high inflammatory potential and use instead only monofilament dissolvable suture such as Monocryl.

The short-scar techniques, including vertical (Lassas or Lejour) reduction, Marchac, SPAIR, Spear modification of the SPAIR, L shaped (De Longis), Renault reduction, central pedicle, Hall Finlay's superomedial pedicle, and so on all attempt to shorten or avoid the inframammary component of the scar. Many reviews (3,7,11,12,14,16) suggest these techniques have evolved into safe, reliable methods of reduction with good aesthetic results and minimal major complications. The disadvantages to these types of minimal scar reduction include a steep learning curve, less reproducible outcomes, and the possibility of a high rate of "touch-up" procedures. Initially, there were reports of persistent vertical scar dog ears, teardrop nipple deformities, and persistent axillary fullness. It is safe to say that these techniques have their greatest appeal in the younger patient needing a moderate to small reduction, where obtaining significantly shorter or less scars is worth the added complexity.

We recommend standard postoperative scar management, including massage, silicone sheeting, topical vitamin E, and sunscreens. Poor scars, including keloids and hypertrophic scars, may be injected with dilute Kenalog or even managed with surgical revision (Fig. 105.4).

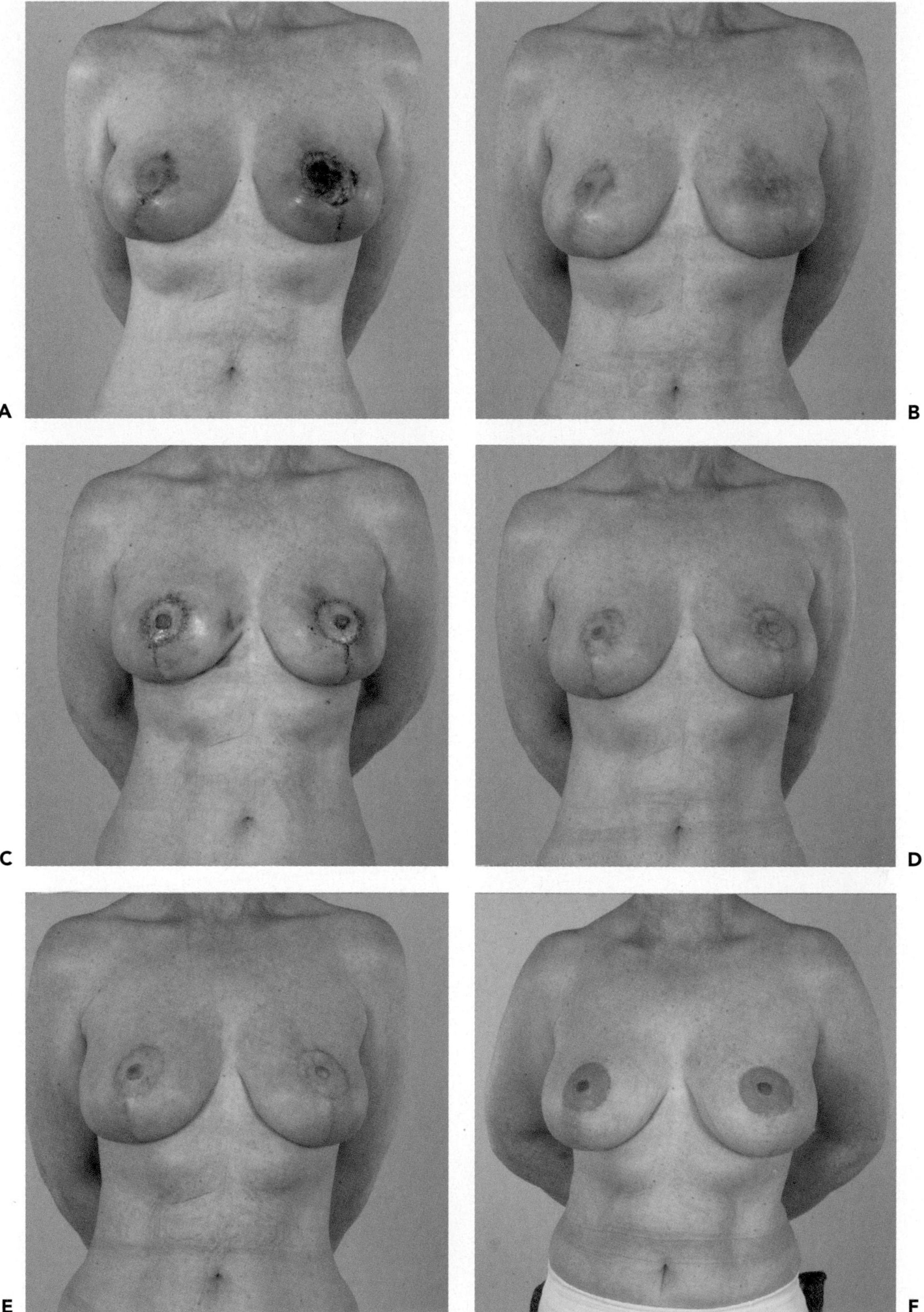

Figure 105.2. A 56-year-old who had a bilateral mastopexy at another institution with bilateral nipple necrosis. **A** and **B:** Preop photos showing nipple necrosis and following debridement and dressing changes. **C:** One week after bilateral nipple-areolar revision using the remaining nipple-areolar complex and full-thickness skin grafts and bilateral areolar tattoo. **D–F:** Three months, 6 months, and nearly 2 years postoperative.

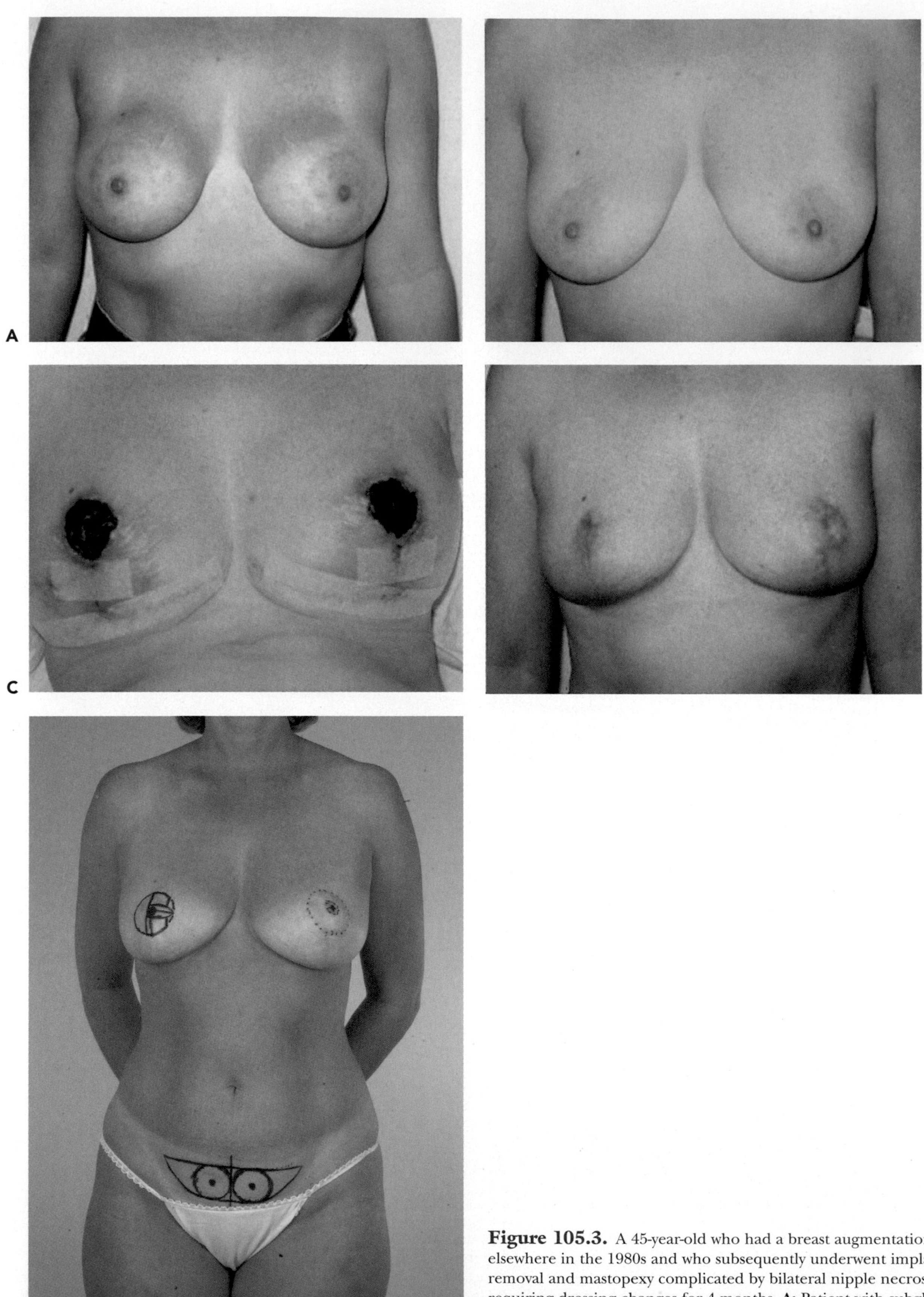

Figure 105.3. A 45-year-old who had a breast augmentation elsewhere in the 1980s and who subsequently underwent implant removal and mastopexy complicated by bilateral nipple necrosis requiring dressing changes for 4 months. **A:** Patient with subglandular implants placed in the late 1980s. **B:** After implant removal. **C:** After bilateral mastopexy with bilateral nipple loss. **D:** Following dressing changes. **E:** Preoperative plan for bilateral nipple reconstruction with full-thickness skin grafts. (*continued*)

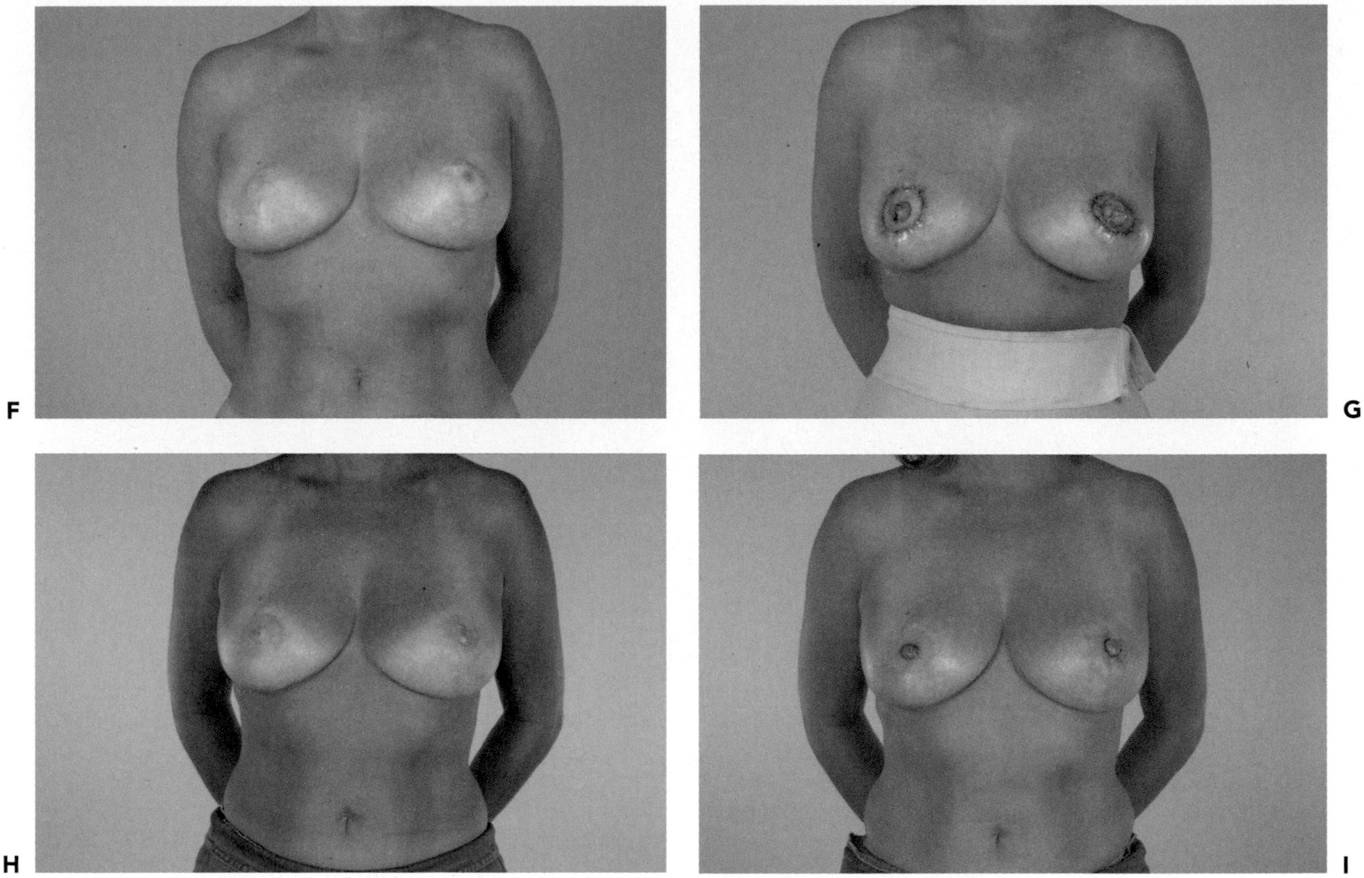

Figure 105.3. (*Continued*) **F:** Preoperative photo showing absence of the right nipple and severe scarring of the left nipple-areola complex. **G:** One week postoperative bilateral nipple reconstruction with full-thickness skin graft. **H:** Three months postoperative. **I:** Eight months postoperative.

FLAP NECROSIS

Some minor degree of flap necrosis or delayed wound healing is not uncommon. When performing breast reduction, raising the lateral flap, medial flap, and pedicle should be done carefully with attention to flap thickness. The medial flap rarely undergoes necrosis because it is usually left thick and is not undermined. The lateral flap however is the most likely site of distal flap loss. The most common area of flap necrosis occurs at the T junction, where the skin with the most distal blood supply occurs simultaneously at the point of highest tension. The use of a "W" incision or inferiorly based "triangular"

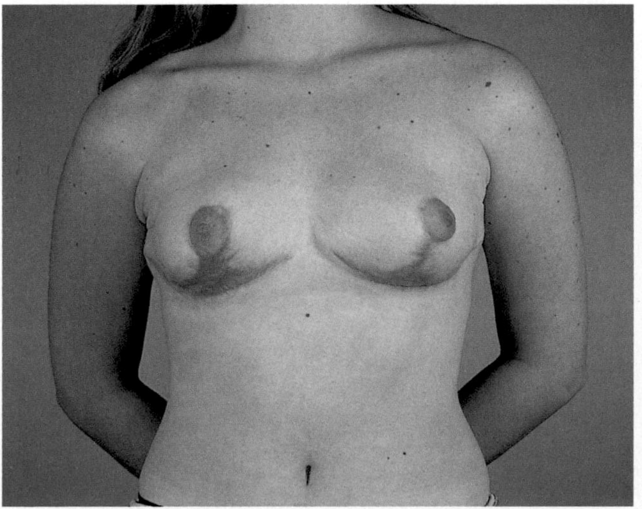

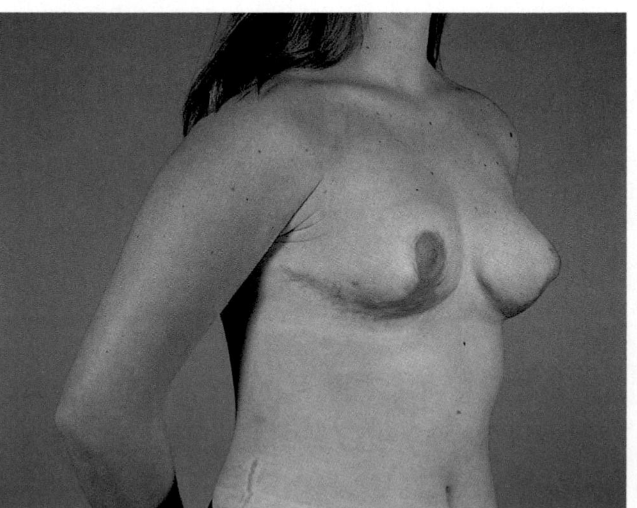

Figure 105.4. A 20-year-old after bilateral 500-g breast reduction performed elsewhere, resulting in asymmetry, nipple malposition, and poor scarring. **A** and **B:** Prerevision frontal and oblique views. (*continued*)

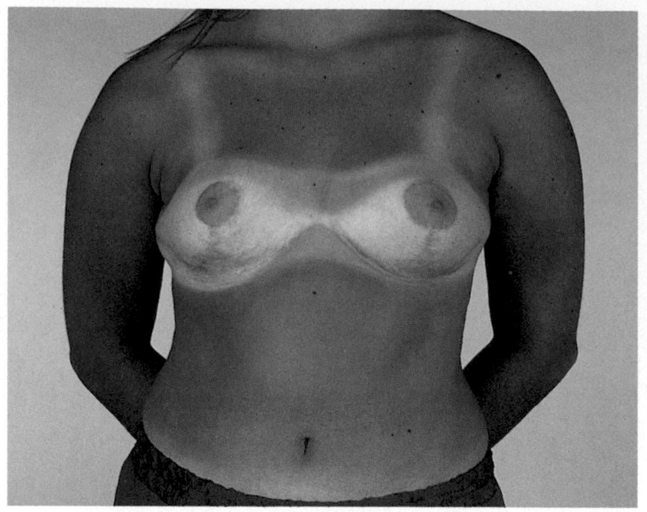

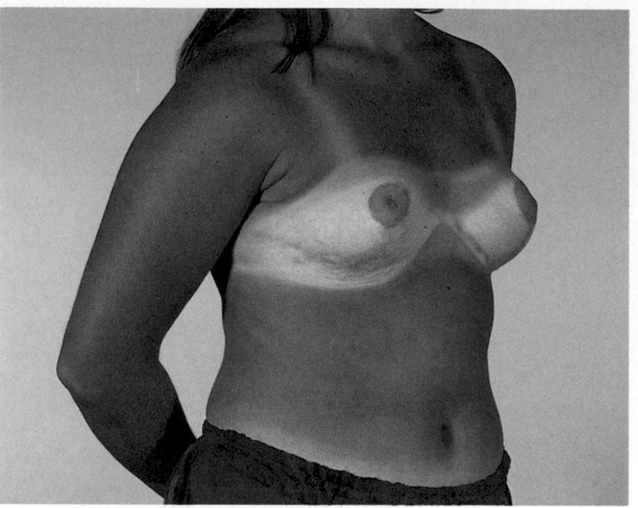

Figure 105.4. (*Continued*) **C** and **D:** Frontal and oblique views 18 months after scar revision, size adjustment, and nipple repositioning.

interposition flap has been recommended by some to help deal with this.

Flap loss is often a result of wound tension, ischemia, or both. Recognizing early flap ischemia is important and can be treated with greasy ointments, hyperbaric oxygen, and/or antibiotics. Any hematoma or seroma adding to the ischemia should be drained immediately. If the flap necrosis is of appropriate size and properly demarcated, it can often be excised and closed within the first 2 weeks of surgery to avoid delayed wound healing and secondary bacterial infection (Fig. 105.5).

NIPPLE MALPOSITION

Even when the nipple is healthy, the scars acceptable, and the flaps healthy, the overall result can still be disappointing. Poor cosmetic results can be the result of nipple malposition, asymmetry, poor aesthetic breast shape, overresection, or underresection. Classically, nipple position has been positioned at or near the inframammary fold during preoperative planning; however, all surgeons are aware that this must be altered from time to time and from patient to patient. Often, we adjust the level of the inframammary fold during the superior pedicle or superomedial technique, changing the nipple-to-fold distance. In addition, the absolute distance of the nipple-to-sternal notch should only be used as a guideline. The most important consideration is the nipple position on the breast itself, at or near the point of greatest projection. When planning, one should remember that it is much easier to raise a nipple that is too low than to lower a nipple that is too high.

It is advised to set the nipple at or just above the inframammary fold and then assess this height by visual inspection in addition to measurement and assessment of symmetry. The reduction pattern can then be centered on this chosen nipple height. On the table, fine-tuning of the nipple height can be achieved with the patient sitting up.

If nipple malposition does occur, revision should be delayed several months. An excessively low nipple can be elevated using upper skin excision and reconfiguration of the lower skin flaps. If the nipple is too high, correction is more complex (Fig. 105.6). If the breast mass has descended and bottomed out inferiorly, then the nipple can be left in place and the breast mass excised inferiorly through the old incisions (Figs. 105.7 and 105.8). However, if the breast mass itself is adequate and the nipple must be lowered, a V-Y advancement pattern inferiorly, flap transposition, or free nipple graft can be used (Fig. 105.9). The disadvantage is that these techniques will leave a scar above the nipple, and the patient must be counseled about that.

COSMETIC DISAPPOINTMENTS

Ultimately, the goal of breast reduction or mastopexy is to correct the size and shape of the breast and leave an attractive breast as a result. A misshapen breast or major asymmetry is a great disappointment and must be seen as a failure (Fig. 105.10). Although underresection is a disappointment, it is easily corrected with further resection. The incidence and degree of underresection can be reduced by careful preoperative consultation with the patient and appropriate execution of the planned procedure. Adequate reduction of a large breast generally requires removal of substantial amounts of lateral breast and narrowing of the pedicle enough to remove adequate amounts of tissue.

Overresection of the breast is a more difficult problem. Just as with underresection, this can usually be avoided by appropriate planning and attention to following that plan. If overresection has occurred, its correction may require balancing the remaining breast on one or both sides with an implant.

OTHER COMPLICATIONS

Other complications after breast reduction include fat necrosis, recurrent enlargement, infection, hematoma, seroma, loss of nipple sensibility, loss of the ability for lactation, nipple inversion, and galactorrhea. There are relatively few comprehensive reports on complications in the literature, but the

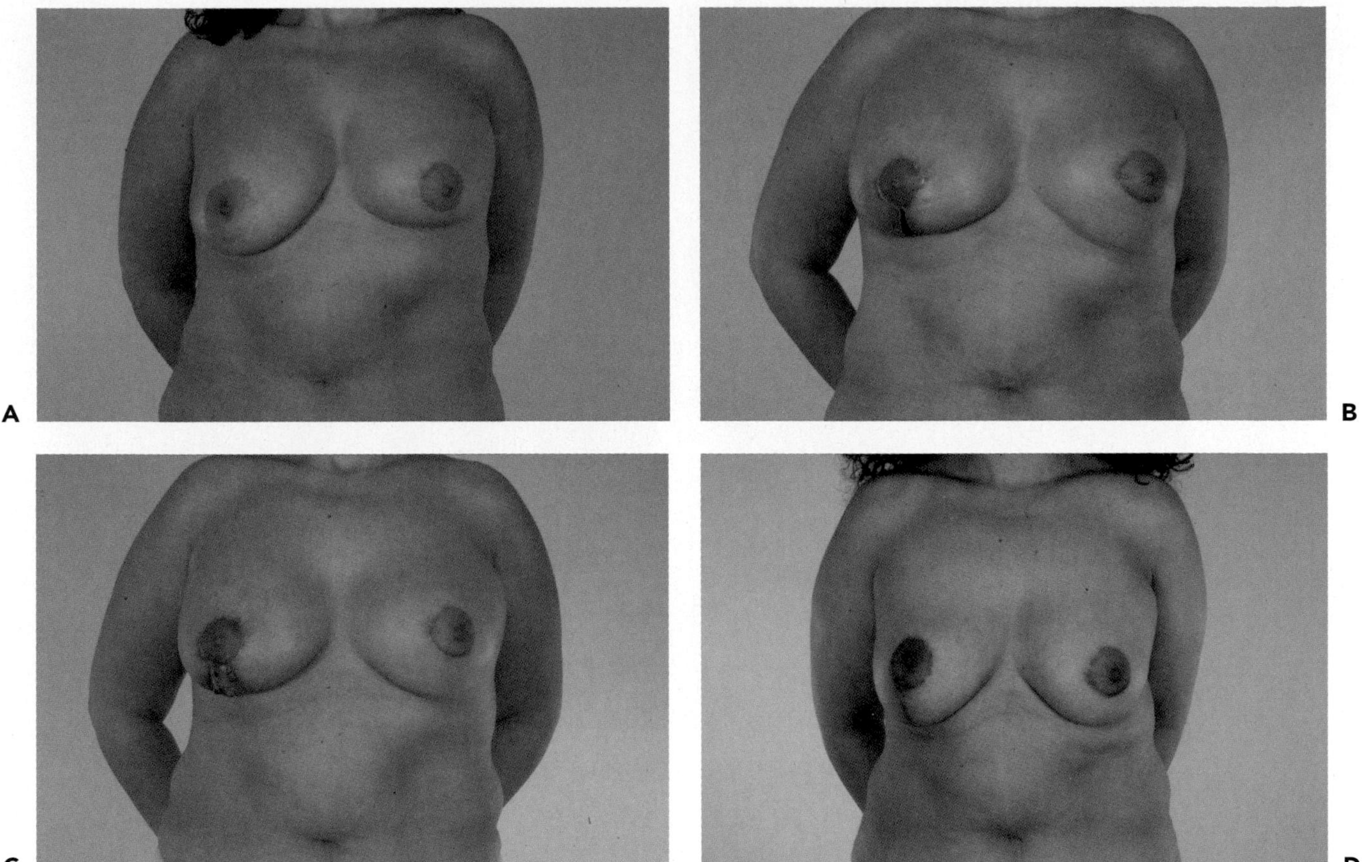

Figure 105.5. **A:** A 47-year-old with Poland's syndrome who had bilateral subpectoral breast augmentation elsewhere with double-lumen 225 gel, 25 saline (right) and 350 gel, 35 saline (left). **B** and **C:** Four and 6 months after bilateral reaugmentation with McGahn 110 360-cc, silicone gel implants with asymmetry, flap necrosis, and nipple malposition. **D:** Two months after left capsulorraphy, and right revision augmentation mastopexy exchanging to a smaller, 300-cc implant.

number is increasing, spurred by the controversy centered on the various vertical, short-scar versus inverted T reduction patterns. Dabbah reported a relatively high complication rate of 45% (retrospective study 185 patients) using the inverted T pattern, with the most common being infection/fat necrosis of 22% and wound dehiscence of 10% (2). An even higher overall complication rate of 53% was reported (406 patients) from a random group of breast reduction patients using a variety of techniques, most of them being minor complications (1).

Fat necrosis typically first becomes apparent 5 to 7 days after reduction and may appear similar to cellulitis with wound drainage, redness, and pain. Early debridement may be necessary to prevent abscess formation. Definitive resection of fat necrosis nodules may be necessary months later (Fig. 105.11). In rare cases, the breast may enlarge significantly postoperatively and has been described as true virginal hypertrophy. This hypertrophy has also been seen in the setting of pregnancy with "sudden severe gigantomastia" and may require mastectomy for treatment (Fig. 105.12) (23). Hematomas, seromas, and infection are fairly uncommon in our experience and can usually be treated without significant sequelae. There is ongoing controversy regarding the use of drains to prevent hematoma, without much evidence supporting their necessity (24).

Nipple sensation may be lost initially, but it usually recovers over time. Review of the literature produces conflicting conclusions regarding postoperative nipple sensibility (25–30). It is interesting that the breast reduction patient rarely complains of this postoperatively. Many patients with macromastia have preoperative decreased sensitivity that has been theoretically reported to be due to elongated, stretched nerves. Regardless of pedicle choice, leaving breast tissue intact along the chest wall is important to prevent loss of nipple sensitivity. Aside from nipple sensation, we believe lactation is usually spared after standard reduction (although not with free nipple graft). However, patients should be counseled on the possibility of lactation disturbance postoperatively.

BREAST REDUCTION IN THE DIFFICULT CIRCUMSTANCE

There has been an increased focus on the bariatric patient undergoing breast reduction/mastopexy. This is a unique group of patients with special circumstances both before and after significant weight loss. As the popularity of gastric bypass surgery increases, most patients with severe obesity (BMI

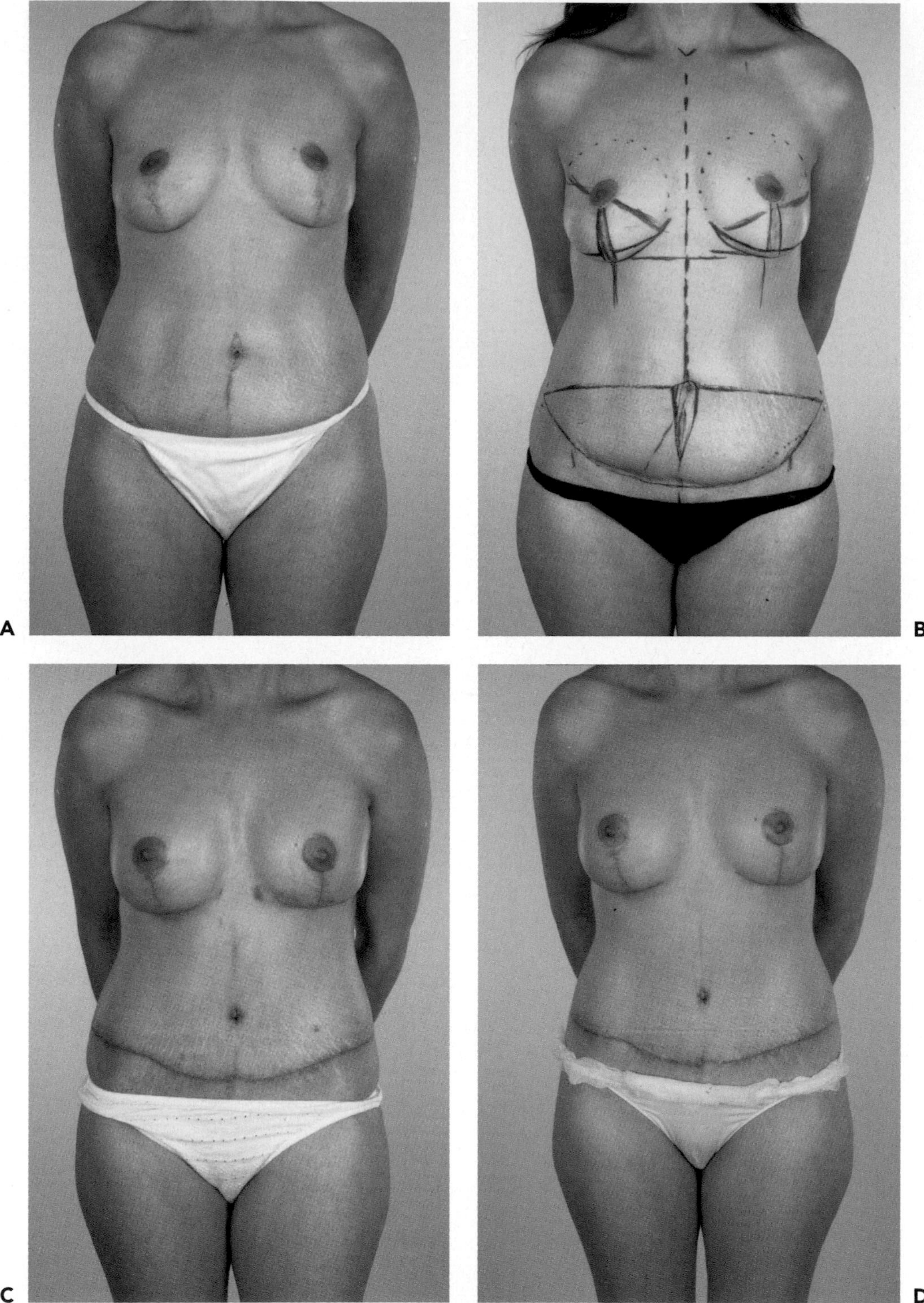

Figure 105.6. A 48-year-old who had a previous mastopexy and abdominoplasty performed elsewhere with nipples placed too high, left higher than right. **A:** Preoperative frontal view. **B:** Preoperative plan for revision mastopexy/augmentation placed in the dual plane. **C** and **D:** Four weeks and 2 months s/p revision mastopexy/augmentation using bilateral McGhan 68 LP, 200-cc implants and scar revision.

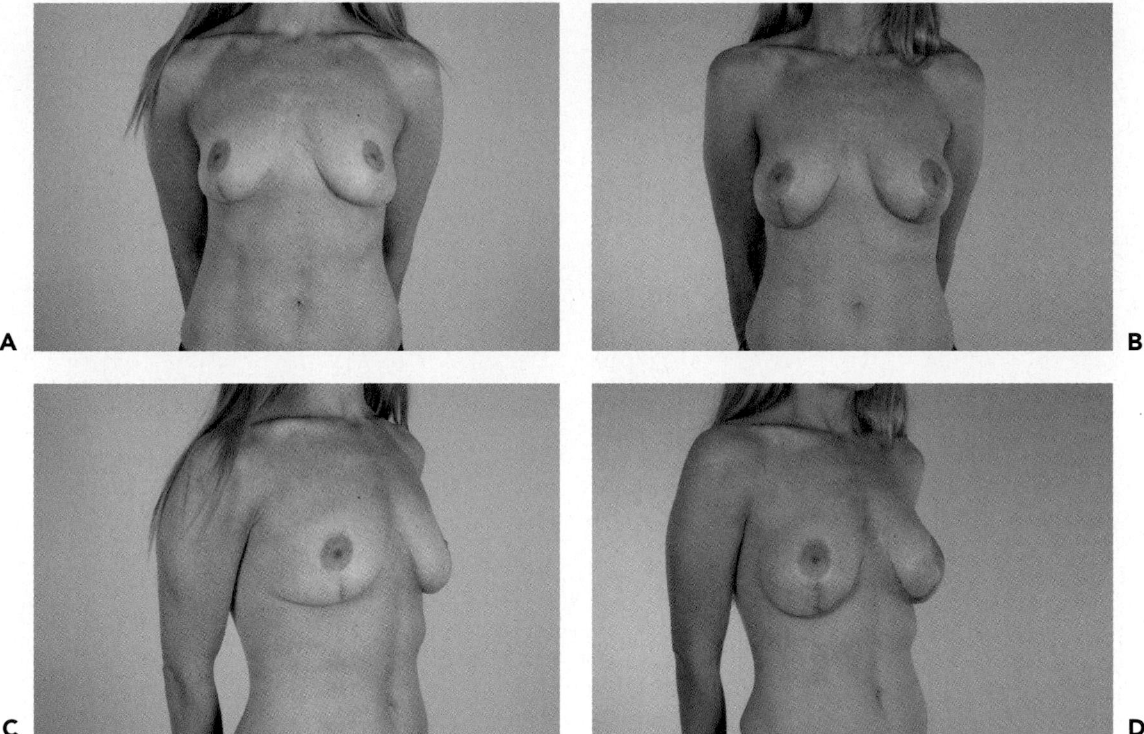

Figure 105.7. A 35-year-old who had a mastopexy performed elsewhere 6 years prior to presenting with complaints that her nipples appear too high. **A** and **B:** Preoperative photos showing a descent of breast tissue and the appearance of bilateral nipple elevation. **C** and **D:** Three months after bilateral revision augmentation mastopexy with subpectoral placement of McGhan 68 LP, 200-cc implants and excision of approximately 4 cm of the inferior "T" scar.

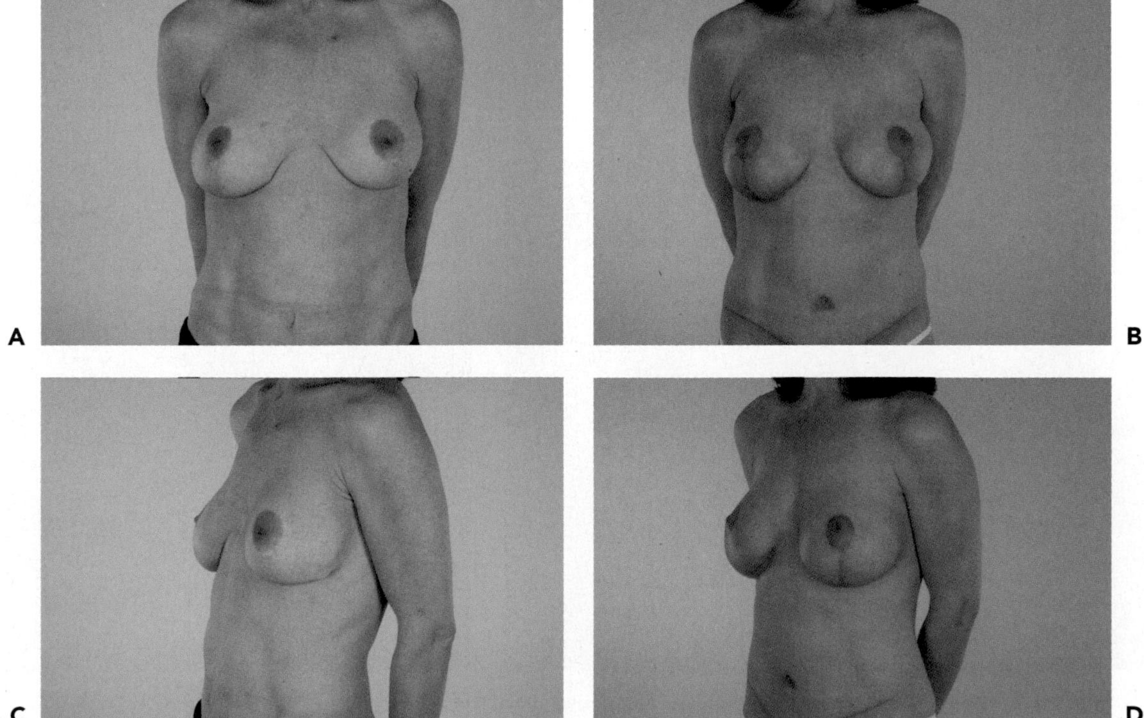

Figure 105.8. A 42-year-old who had a mastopexy/augmentation performed elsewhere with resulting asymmetry and nipple malposition. **A–C:** Preoperative frontal and oblique view. **B–D:** Two months after revision augmentation mastopexy using McGhan 40, 340-cc silicone gel implants placed in the dual-plane position.

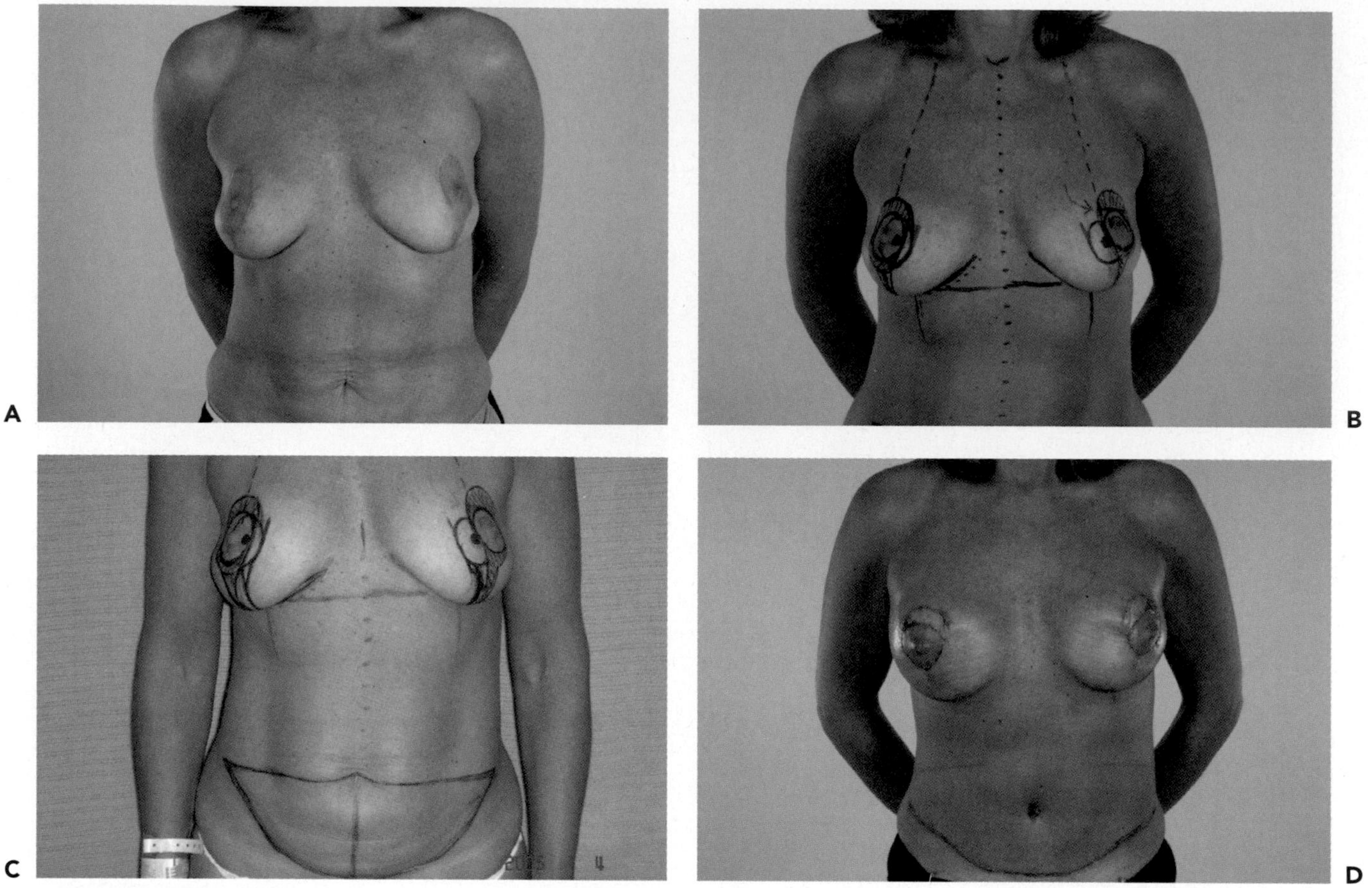

Figure 105.9. A 43-year-old with nipple malposition and large irregularly shaped areola after initial mastopexy performed elsewhere. **A:** Preoperative frontal view. **B** and **C:** Preoperative plan showing "Z" plasty transposition flaps to relocate and reshape the nipple areolar complexes and abdominoplasty. **D:** Two weeks postoperative.

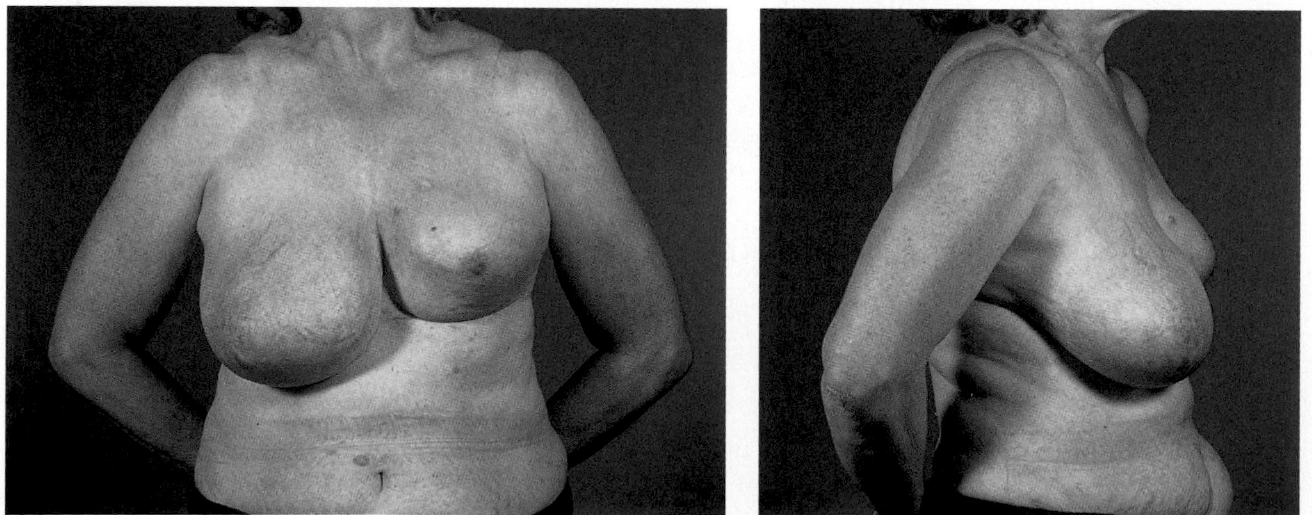

Figure 105.10. A 50-year-old with marked breast asymmetry. **A–C:** Preoperative photos. *(continued)*

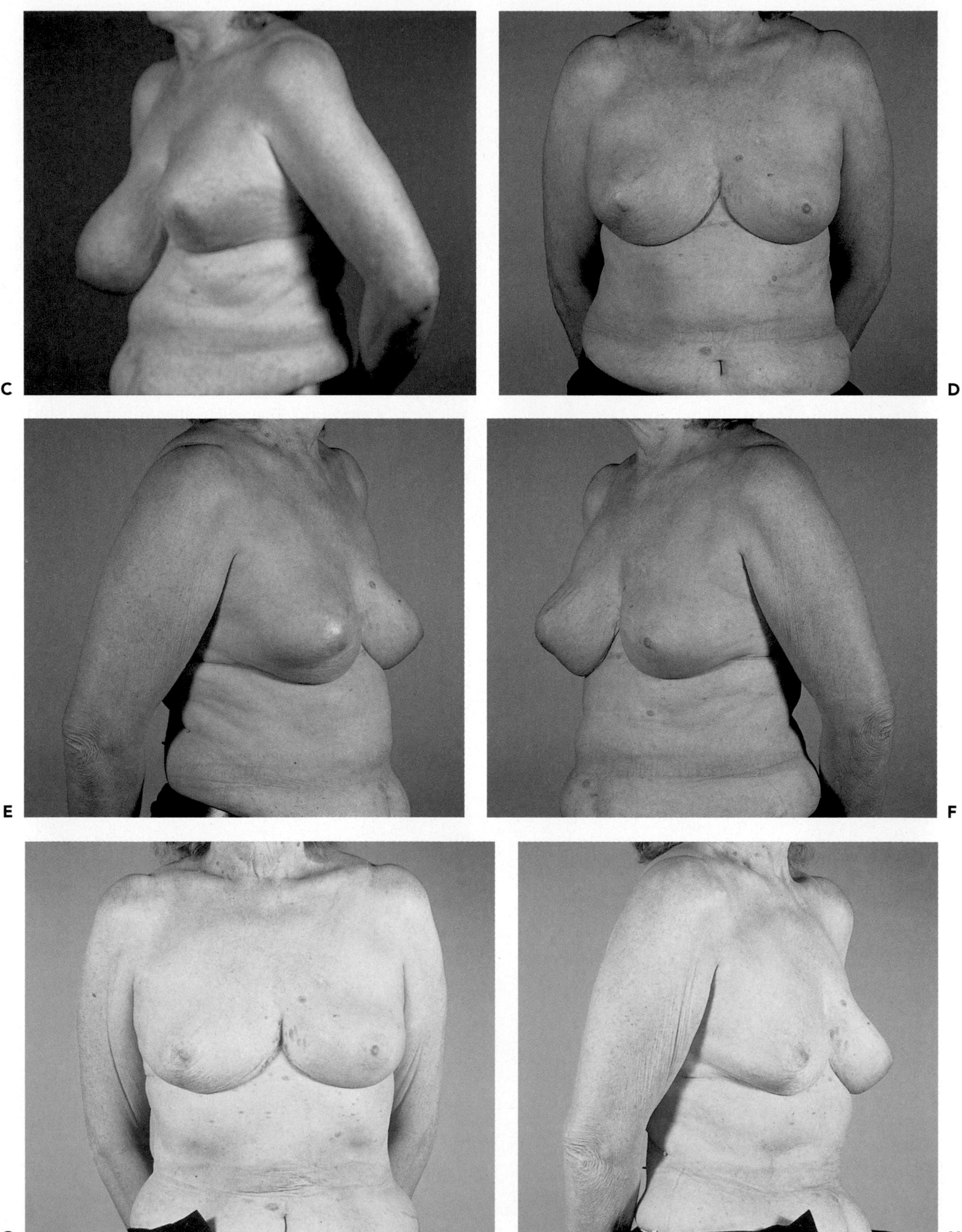

Figure 105.10. (*Continued*) **D–F:** After bilateral reduction of 500 g on the right using the McKissock technique and 200 g on the left using the central mound technique. The right breast developed swelling and redness and ultimately a large mass centrally. **G–I:** After excision of fat necrosis of the right breast, which corrected the asymmetry. (*continued*)

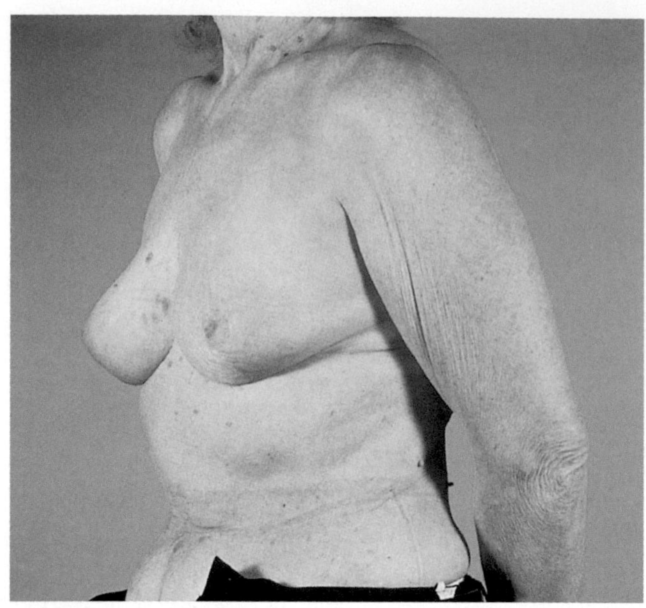

Figure 105.10. (*Continued*)

greater than 35) delay reduction or mastopexy until after bypass surgery and weight loss has stabilized. Prior to gastric bypass, these patients are at increased risk for complications related not only to the anesthetic risk of obesity, but also to the heightened complications associated with larger specimen weights. In a retrospective review of 395 patients, Zubowski et al. found an increased risk of complications in patients that are 5% above ideal body weight, but this higher risk did not increase with the degree of obesity. Interestingly, the specimen weight played a higher role in complications over the degree of obesity (9).

After massive weight loss, breast reduction/mastopexy is challenging indeed. In these patients, the large skin envelope with stretched glandular tissue is resistant to a lift without an implant. In addition, these patients are at higher risk for recurrent ptosis and bottoming out. It is important to note that breast tissue in these patients will likely fall to the inferior pole, thus appearing to raise the nipple over time. We recommend erring on slightly lower nipple placement centered on the breast tissue in these patients. Of course, most of these patients will require mastopexy augmentation rather than reduction mammaplasty. In addition, delaying breast reduction until weight loss is stabilized is important to avoid overresection.

A variety of other rare but important considerations in breast reduction surgery should be addressed. We have reported on the possibility of flap necrosis in patients with sickle

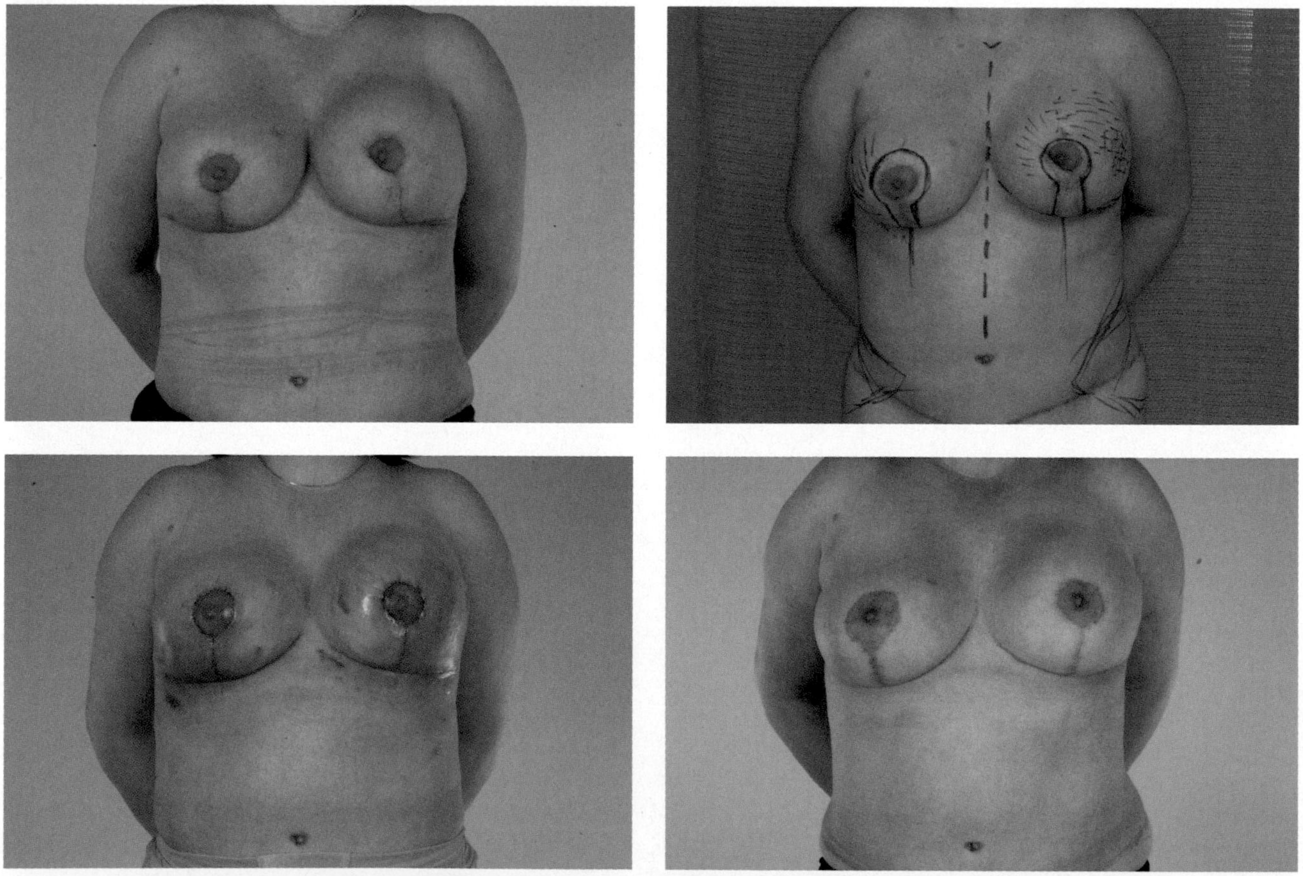

Figure 105.11. A 48-year-old who had a bilateral breast reduction performed elsewhere with left breast fat necrosis and scar contracture. **A:** Preoperative showing breast asymmetry, left breast fat necrosis, and nipple-areolar scar contracture deformity. **B:** Preoperative plan. **C:** One week postoperative. **D:** One year postoperative.

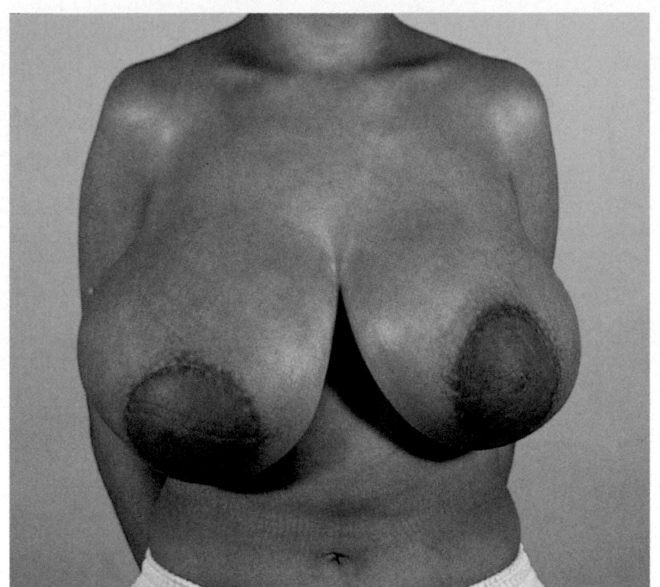
A

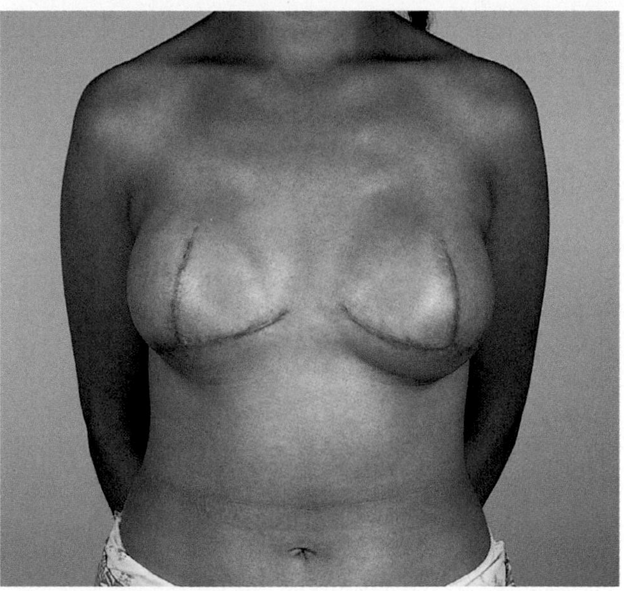
B

Figure 105.12. An 18-year-old who had undergone several previous reduction procedures with early, rapid, and tremendous regrowth of the breasts. Definitive treatment required bilateral mastectomies with implant reconstruction. **A:** After previous reduction procedures but before bilateral mastectomies. **B:** After bilateral mastectomies, with implant reconstruction.

cell trait in a case report of one patient who underwent routine bilateral reduction mammaplasty using a superior-medial pedicle and experienced flap necrosis requiring revision (31). Other rare complications include reports of severe postreduction pain syndromes that mimic reflex sympathetic dystrophy (32) and cases of necrotizing wound manifestations of pyoderma gangrenosum requiring corticosteroids (33).

BREAST CANCER AND BREAST REDUCTION SURGERY

Although not a complication of breast reduction or mastopexy, the unanticipated and rare occurrence of breast cancer within resected breast tissue is a concern. Six epidemiologic studies analyzing breast cancer risk after breast reduction surgery cite a relative risk between 0.2 and 0.7 (34–39). Also, there seems to be a relationship between specimen weight and the amount of breast cancer risk reduction. This concept parallels the reduction in breast cancer risk following prophylactic mastectomy in patients genetically susceptible to breast cancer. We routinely mammogram all patients older than ages 30 to 35 and consider mammography in younger, high-risk patients prior to undergoing reduction mammaplasty. Incidentally, postmastectomy breast reconstruction in patients who have previously had breast reduction or mastopexy are a special set of patients with increased complication risks. There is a report of successful tissue expansion and implant reconstruction in a small number of these patients (40); however, autologous tissue may be a better option to minimize flap necrosis.

CONCLUSION

Attention to preoperative markings and tailoring reduction/mastopexy patterns to each patient's needs should minimize complications. As more surgeons learn "newer" techniques of vertical pattern reduction and shorter scars, the special risks and complications of each method should be reviewed to help improve results.

EDITORIAL COMMENTS

I concur with Dr. Spear on the reduction mammaplasty as a predictable and safe procedure with a low rate of complications and a high degree of patient satisfaction. Complications do occur from time to time, despite the best operative planning and execution, and they must be remedied as he describes. Nipple malposition, almost always overelevation, is rarely a complication of surgery, but rather a result of poor or inappropriate planning. It continues to be seen far too often in postreduction mammaplasty results at a frequency that is particularly puzzling in the face of the invariable advice on the part of nearly every author on the subject to avoid it. I continue to position the nipple with respect to the inframammary fold and have found this method unfailingly reliable in avoiding unnatural position.

J.W.L.

REFERENCES

1. Davis GM, Ringler SL, Short K, et al. Reduction mammaplasty: long term efficacy, morbidity and patient satisfaction. *Plast Reconstr Surg* 1995;96(5):1106–1110.
2. Dabbah A, Lehman JA, Parker MG, et al. Reduction mammaplasty: an outcome analyst. *Ann Plast Surg* 1995;35:337–341.
3. Lejour M. Vertical mammaplasty: early complications after 250 personal consecutive cases. *Plast Reconstr Surg* 1999;104(3):764–770.
4. Schnur PL, Schnur DP, Petty P, et al. Reduction mammaplasty: an outcome study. Plast *Reconstr Surg* 1997;100(4):875–883.
5. Lassus C. A 30 year experience with vertical mammaplasty. *Plast Reconstr Surg* 1996;97(2):373–380.
6. Menke H, Eisenmann-Klein M, Olbrisch RR, et al. Continuous quality management of breast hypertrophy by the German Assoc of Plastic Surgeons: a preliminary report. *Ann Plast Surg* 2001;46(6):594–600.

7. Hammond DC. Short scar periareolar inferior pedicle reduction (SPAIR) mammaplasty. *Plast Reconstr Surg* 1999;103(3):890–901.
8. Berg A, Palmer B, Stark B. Early experience with the Lejour vertical scar reduction mammaplasty. *Br J Plast Surg* 1993;46:516–522.
9. Zubowski R, Zins JE, Foray-Kaplon A, et al. Relationship of obesity and specimen weight to complications in reduction mammaplasty. *Plast Reconstr Surg* 2000;106(5):998–1003.
10. Nahabedian M, Mofid MM. Viability and sensation of the nipple-areolar complex after reduction mammaplasty. *Ann Plast Surg* 2002;49:24–32.
11. Beer GM, Spicher I, Cierpka KA. Benefits and pitfalls of vertical scar breast reduction. *Br J Plast Surg* 2004;57:2–19.
12. Cruz-Korchin N, Korchin L. Vertical versus wise pattern breast reduction: patient satisfaction, revision rates, and complications. *Plast Reconstr Surg* 2003;112(6):1579–1581.
13. Ramon Y, Sharony Z, Moscana RA, et al. Evaluation and comparison of aesthetic results and patient satisfaction with bilateral breast reduction using the inferior pedicle and McKissock's vertical bipedicle dermal flap techniques. *Plast Reconstr Surg* 2000;106: 289–295.
14. Berthe JV, Massout J, Greuse M, et al. The vertical mammaplasty: a reappraisal of the technique and its complications. *Plast Reconstr Surg* 2003;111(7):2192–2199.
15. Wuringer E, Mader N, Posch E, et al. Nerve and vessel supplying ligamentous suspension of the mammary gland. *Plast Reconstr Surg* 1998;101(6):1486–1493.
16. Chen C, White C, Warren S, et al. Simplifying the vertical reduction mammaplasty. *Plast Reconstr Surg* 2004;113(1):162–172.
17. Hall-Findlay E. A simplified vertical reduction mammaplasty: shortening the learning curve. *Plast Reconstr Surg* 1999;104(3):748–759.
18. Spear SL. Augmentation/mastopexy: surgeon, beware. *Plast Reconstr Surg* 2003;112(3): 905–906.
19. Losee JL, Elethea H, Caldwell MD, et al. Secondary reduction mammaplasty: is using a different pedicle safe? *Plast Reconstr Surg* 2000;106(5):1009–1010.
20. Spear SL. Secondary reduction mammaplasty: is using a different pedicle safe? *Plast Reconstr Surg* 2000;106(5):1009–1010.
21. Würinger E. Secondary reduction mammaplasty. *Plast Reconstr Surg* 2002;109(2): 812–814.
22. Hudson DA, Skoll PJ. Repeat reduction mammaplasty. *Plast Reconstr Surg* 1999;104:401.
23. Vidaeff AC, Parks H. Gestational gigantomastia after reduction mammaplasty: complications or coincidence? *Plast Reconstr Surg* 2003;111(2):956–958.
24. Matarasso A, Wallach S, Rankin M. Re-evaluating the need for routine drainage in reduction mammaplasty. *Plast Reconstr Surg* 1998;102(6):1917–1921.
25. Ferreira MC, Costa MP, Cunha MS, et al. Sensibility of the breast after reduction mammaplasty. *Ann Plast Surg* 2003;51(1):1–5.
26. Mofid M, Dellon AL, Elias JJ, et al. Quantitation of breast sensibility following reduction mammaplasty: a comparison of inferior and medical pedicle techniques. *Plast Reconstr Surg* 2002;109:2283–2288.
27. Temple CL, Hurst LN. Reduction mammaplasty improves breast sensibility. *Plast Reconstr Surg* 1992;104:72–76.
28. Gonzalez F, Brown FE, Gold ME, et al. Preoperative and postoperative nipple-areola sensibility in patients undergoing reduction mammaplasty. *Plast Reconstr Surg* 1993;92:809–811.
29. Slezak S, Dellon AL. Quantitation on sensibility in gigantomastia and alteration following reduction mammaplasty. *Plast Reconstr Surg* 1993;91:1265–1267.
30. Terzis JK, Vincent MP, Wilkins LM, et al. Breast sensibility: a neurophysiological appraisal in the normal breast. *Ann Plast Surg* 1987;19:318–322.
31. Spear SL, Carter ME, Low M, et al. Sickle cell trait: a risk factor for flap necrosis. *Plast Reconstr Surg* 2003;112(2):697–698.
32. Hughes L. Post reduction pain syndrome. *Plast Reconstr Surg* 1999;103(5):1540–1541.
33. Gulyas K, Kimble FW. Atypical pyoderma gangrenosum after breast reduction. *Aesth Plast Surg* 2003;27(4):328–331.
34. Baasch M, Nielsen SF, Engholm G, et al. Breast cancer incidence subsequent to surgical reduction of the female breast. *Br J Cancer* 1996;73:961–965.
35. Brinton L, Malone KE, Coates RJ, et al. Breast enlargement and reduction: results from a breast cancer case control study. *Plast Reconstr Surg* 1996;97:269–273.
36. Boice JD, Friis S, McLaughlin JK, et al. Cancer following breast reduction surgery in Denmark. *Cancer Causes Control* 1997;8:253.
37. Brown MH, Weinber M, Chong N, et al. A cohort study of breast cancer risk in breast reduction patients. *Plast Reconstr Surg* 1999;103:1674–1677.
38. Boice JD, Perrsson L, Brinton L, et al. Breast cancer following breast reduction surgery in Sweden. *Plast Reconstr Surg* 2000;106:755.
39. Brinton LA, Persson L, Boice JD, et al. Breast cancer risk in relation to amount of tissue removed during breast reduction operations in Sweden. *Cancer* 2001;91:478–480.
40. Kilgo MS, Corderio PG, Disa JJ. Tissue expansion after inverted T mammaplasty: can it be performed successfully? *Ann Plast Surg* 2003;50(6):588–593.

SECTION

IV

Augmentation Mammaplasty

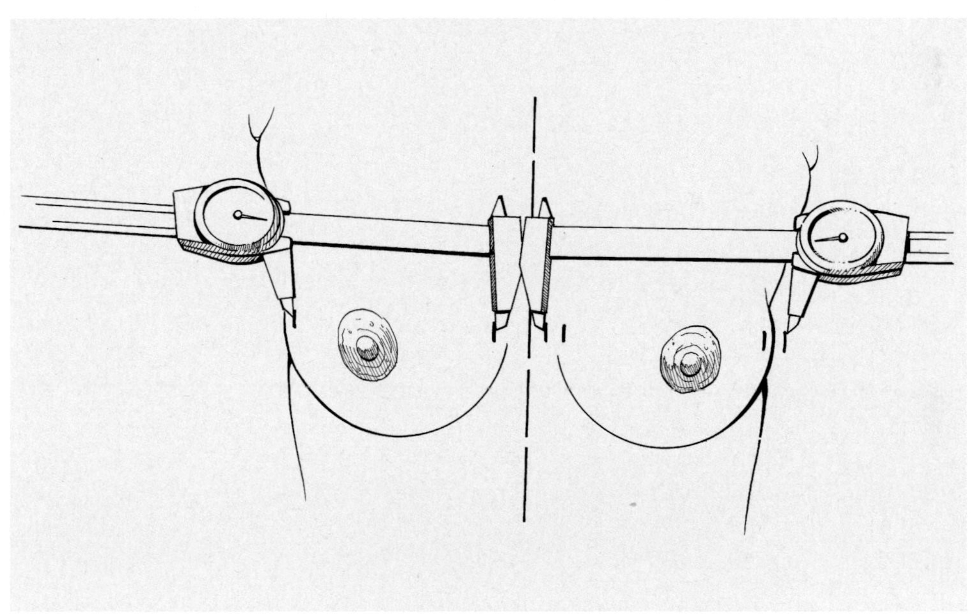

CHAPTER

106

G. Patrick Maxwell
Matthew B. Baker
Allen Gabriel

Augmentation Mammaplasty: General Considerations

INTRODUCTION

Glandular hypomastia may occur as a developmental or involutional process and affects a significant number of women in the United States. Developmental hypomastia is often seen as primary mammary hypoplasia or as a sequela of thoracic hypoplasia (Poland syndrome) or other chest wall deformity. Involutional hypomastia may develop in the postpartum setting and may be exacerbated by breast-feeding or significant weight loss. When compared to the norm, inadequate breast volume may lead to a negative body image, feelings of inadequacy, and low self-esteem (1). These disturbances may adversely affect a patient's interpersonal relationships, sexual fulfillment, and quality of life (2).

There has been a steady increase in breast augmentation surgery with the emerging importance of body image, changes in societal expectations, and the increasing acceptance of aesthetic surgery in the United States. Augmentation mammaplasty was performed 355,671 times in 2008 as the most frequently performed cosmetic surgical procedure in women in the United States (3). This is the first time that breast augmentations procedures have surpassed liposuction. In this chapter, we review the history of breast augmentation, operative planning and technique, and some perioperative and late complications of the procedure. The evolution of modern breast implants is described, and the controversy surrounding the use of silicone gel in breast augmentation is discussed.

HISTORY

The first report of successful breast augmentation appeared in 1895 in which Czerny described transplanting a lipoma from the trunk to the breast in a patient deformed by a partial mastectomy (4). In 1954, Longacre described a local dermal-fat flap for augmentation of the breast (5). Eventually, both adipose tissue and omentum were also used to augment the breast. However, the clinical results of using autogenous tissue for breast augmentation were often unpredictable and unacceptable (6).

During the 1950s and 1960s, breast augmentation with solid alloplastic materials was carried out using polyurethane, polytetrafluoroethylene (Teflon), and expanded polyvinyl alcohol formaldehyde (Ivalon sponge). Ultimately, the use of these materials was discontinued after patients developed local tissue reactions, firmness, distortion of the breast, and significant discomfort (7). Various other solid and semisolid materials have been injected directly into the breast parenchyma for augmentation, including epoxy resin, shellac, beeswax, paraffin, petroleum jelly, and liquid silicone. Liquid silicone (polydimethyl siloxane) was originally developed in the aeronautics industry during World War II. In 1961, Uchida reported the injection of liquid silicone into the breast for breast augmentation (8). Unfortunately, injection of liquid silicone resulted in frequent complications, including recurrent infections, chronic inflammation, drainage, granuloma formation, and even necrosis (9,10). Breast augmentation by injection of free liquid silicone was abandoned in the United States in light of these complications.

The modern breast implant is a two-component prosthetic device manufactured with a nearly impermeable silicone elastomer shell filled with a stable filling material, consisting of either saline solution or silicone gel. This shell plus filler implant was originally developed by Cronin and Gerow in 1963 using silicone gel as the filling material contained within a thin, smooth silicone elastomer shell (11). Since that time, both silicone gel– and saline-filled implants have undergone several technical alterations and improvements.

BREAST IMPLANT EVOLUTION

SALINE-FILLED IMPLANTS

The use of inflatable saline-filled breast implants was first reported in 1965 by Arion in France (12). The saline-filled implant was developed in order to allow the noninflated implant to be introduced through a relatively small incision, followed by inflation of the implant in situ (13). Although the incidence of periprosthetic capsular contracture was lower with the saline-filled implants compared to the earlier generation of silicone gel–filled implants, the deflation rate was initially quite high. The original saline-filled implants manufactured by Simiplast in France had a deflation rate of 75% at 3 years and was subsequently withdrawn from the market. In 1968, the Heyer-Schulte Company introduced its version of the inflatable saline-filled breast implant (Mentor 1800) in the United States.

The thin, platinum-cured shell and the leaflet-style retention valve were two features of the early saline-filled implants that contributed to their high deflation rate (14). The silicone elastomer shell of the saline-filled implant has been improved by making it thicker and by employing a new room-temperature vulcanization process. This process is used in the manufacture of all saline-filled implant shells currently available from Allergan (formerly Inamed Corporation and McGhan Medical) and from Ethicon [formerly Mentor Corporation (which acquired Heyer-Schulte)]. The original Heyer-Schulte saline-filled implant shell had a leaflet-style retention valve through which the implant was inflated (15). A more reliable diaphragm valve was developed and is currently incorporated into the shell of all modern saline-filled breast implants.

TABLE 106.1 Saline-filled Breast Implants

Model	Surface	Shape	Projection
Natrelle style 68LP	Smooth	Round	Low
Natrelle style 68MP	Smooth	Round	Moderate
Natrelle style 68HP	Smooth	Round	High
Natrelle style 168 Biocell	Textured	Round	Moderate
Natrelle style 468 Biocell BioCurve	Textured	Anatomic	Moderate
Natrelle style 363LF Biocell BioCurve	Textured	Anatomic	Full[a]
Mentor Smooth Round Moderate Profile	Smooth	Round	Moderate
Mentor Smooth Round High Profile	Smooth	Round	Full
Mentor Siltex Round Moderate Profile	Textured	Round	Moderate
Mentor Siltex Contour Moderate Profile	Textured	Anatomic	Moderate
Mentor Siltex Contour High Profile	Textured	Anatomic	Fill

[a]Style 363LF implants are designed with full projection and low height.

Saline-filled implants are manufactured with a range of recommended fill volumes. Mild breast asymmetry may be corrected by taking advantage of this range of recommended fill volumes during placement of the implants. Underfilling saline-filled implants may lead to increased deflation rates due to folding or friction subjected to the implant shell and is not recommended. Underfilling saline-filled implants may also lead to a wrinkled appearance or *rippling* with the breast in certain positions. Saline-filled implants have historically performed better when slightly overfilled and when placed under thicker soft tissue coverage. Although these implants may be slightly overfilled, aggressive overfilling may lead to a more spherical shape and *scalloping* along the implant edge with knuckle-like palpability and unnatural firmness. Another potential disadvantage of saline-filled implants is that the consistency of these implants on palpation is similar to that of water instead of the more viscous feel of natural breast tissue. Several saline-filled breast prostheses are available from both corporations with different surface textures, shapes, and degrees of projection (Table 106.1).

SILICONE GEL–FILLED IMPLANTS

Silicone Chemistry

Silicone is a mixture of semi-inorganic polymeric molecules composed of varying-length chains of polydimethyl siloxane [$(CH_3)_2$–SiO] monomers. The physical properties of silicones are quite variable, depending on the average polymer chain length and the degree of cross-linking between the polymer chains (16). *Liquid* silicones are polymers with a relatively short average length and very little cross-linking. They have the consistency of an oily fluid and are frequently used as lubricants in pharmaceuticals and medical devices. Silicone *gels* can be produced of varying viscosity by progressively increasing the length of the polymer chains or the degree of cross-linking. The consistency of silicone gels may vary widely from a soft, sticky gel with fluid properties to a firm, cohesive gel exhibiting shape retention or *form stability*, depending upon the polymer chain length and the degree of cross-linking. Extensive chemical cross-linking of the silicone gel polymer will produce a solid form of silicone referred to as an *elastomer* with a flexible, rubber-like quality. Silicone elastomers are used for the manufacture of facial implants, tissue expanders, and the outer shell of all breast prostheses. The versatility of these compounds has made them indispensable in aerospace engineering, medical devices, and the pharmaceutical industry.

Evolution of Silicone Gel–filled Implants

The first generation silicone gel–filled implant was introduced in 1962 by Cronin and Gerow and was manufactured by Dow Corning Corporation (11). The shell of the first-generation implant was constructed using a thick, smooth silicone elastomer as a two-piece envelope with a seam along the periphery (Table 106.2). The shell was filled with a moderately viscous

TABLE 106.2 Evolution of Silicone Gel–filled Breast Implants

First generation (1962–1970)	Thick, two-piece shell Smooth surface with Dacron fixation patches Anatomically shaped (teardrop) Viscous silicone gel
Second generation (1970–1982)	Thin, slightly permeable shell Smooth surface (no Dacron patches) Round shape Less viscous silicone gel
Third generation (1982–1992)	Thick, strong, low-bleed shell Smooth surface Round shape More viscous silicone gel
Fourth generation (1993–present)	Thick, strong, low-bleed shell[a] Smooth and textured surfaces Round and anatomically shaped More viscous (cohesive) silicone gel[a]
Fifth generation (1993–present)	Thick, strong, low-bleed shell[a] Smooth and textured surfaces Round and diverse anatomic shapes Enhanced cohesive and form-stable silicone gel

[a]In accordance with technical parameters established by the American Society for Testing Methodology.

TABLE 106.3 Silicone Gel-filled Breast Implants

Model	*Surface*	*Shape*	*Projection*
Natrelle style 10	Smooth	Round	Moderate
Natrelle style 15	Smooth	Round	Intermediate
Natrelle style 20	Smooth	Round	Full
Natrelle style 110 Biocell	Textured	Round	Moderate
Natrelle style 115 Biocell	Textured	Round	Intermediate
Natrelle style 120 Biocell	Textured	Round	Full
Natrelle style 410 BioDimensional	Textured	Anatomic	Matrix[a]
Mentor Smooth Round Moderate Profile	Smooth	Round	Moderate
Mentor Smooth Round Moderate Plus Profile	Smooth	Round	Intermediate
Mentor Smooth Round High Profile	Smooth	Round	Full
Mentor Siltex Round Moderate Profile	Textured	Round	Moderate
Mentor Siltex Round Moderate Plus Profile	Textured	Round	Intermediate
Mentor Siltex Round High Profile	Textured	Round	Full

[a]Style 410 and CPG implants are available in different combinations of low, moderate, and full height and low, moderate, full, and extra projection.

silicone gel. The implant was anatomically shaped (teardrop) and had several Dacron fixation patches on the posterior aspect to help maintain the proper position of the implant. Unfortunately, these early devices had a relatively high contracture rate that encouraged implant manufacturers to develop second-generation silicone gel–filled implants.

In the 1970s, the second-generation silicone implants were developed in an effort to reduce the incidence of capsular contracture with a thinner, seamless shell and without Dacron patches incorporated into the shell. These implants were round in shape (nonanatomic) and filled with a less viscous silicone gel to promote a *natural feel*. However, the second-generation breast implants were plagued by diffusion or *bleed* of small silicone molecules into the periprosthetic intracapsular space due to their thin, permeable shell and low-viscosity silicone gel filler. This diffused silicone may be encountered as an oily, sticky residue surrounding the implant within the periprosthetic capsule during explantation of older silicone-filled implants. Microscopic silicone particles have been shown to be present within the periprosthetic tissues and even within the draining lymphatics and axillary lymph nodes (17). The phenomenon of silicone bleed has *not* been shown to create significant local or systemic problems (18). However, long-term device failure issues have plagued these second-generation devices due to the thin, weak shell composition.

The development of the third-generation silicone gel-filled implants in the 1980s focused on improving the strength and integrity of the shell in order to reduce silicone gel *bleed* from intact implants and to reduce implant rupture and subsequent gel migration. The formerly Inamed Corporation (now allergen) developed a multilayer implant shell in which a patented barrier-coat material is sandwiched between two layers of silicone elastomer (Intrashiel). The formerly Mentor Corporation now ethicon also developed a shell for their silicone gel–filled breast implants, which consists of a multilayered silicone elastomer. These third-generation prostheses reduced gel bleed to an almost immeasurable level and significantly lowered device shell failure rate.

After the Food and Drug Administration (FDA) required the temporary removal of third-generation silicone gel implants from the U.S. market in 1992, the *fourth-generation* gel devices evolved for their market reintroduction. These silicone gel breast implants were designed under more stringent American Society for Testing Methodology and FDA-influenced criteria for shell thickness and gel cohesiveness. Furthermore, the fourth-generation devices were manufactured with improved quality control and with a wider variety of surface textures and implant shapes (Table 106.3).

The development of the anatomically shaped fourth generation of gel implants was based on recognition that breast augmentation must account for the individual patient's breast shape and chest wall dimensions in order to produce the most natural result. The shells of anatomically shaped breast implants are manufactured with a textured surface to encourage ingrowth and disorganization of the periprosthetic scar tissue and to reduce the incidence of implant rotation and resulting breast deformity (19). Figure 106.1 shows micrographs of the textured surface of several implants.

With the evolution of the *fifth-generation* silicone gel implants, the concept of anatomically shaped implants was carried to the next level. The BioDimensional Planning System in which a *matrix* of 12 possible combinations of implant height and projection was introduced for the specific needs of the individual patient. These anatomically shaped (style 410) implants are available with a range of volumes and any of the 12 combinations of low, moderate, and full *height* with low, moderate, full, and extra *projection* (Fig. 106.2). The Contour Profile Gel (CPG) implant has been designed by the Mentor Corporation with a more rounded and projecting lower pole and a flatter, more sloping upper pole to yield a more natural breast shape in breast augmentation and reconstruction.

It is believed that as the gel flows inferiorly with gravity, the upper portion of the implant collapses due to a relatively decreased volume in the upper pole. To combat this characteristic of silicone gel implants, efforts have been made to develop fifth-generation devices containing more *cohesive* silicone gel that exhibits less flow and more *form stability*. The development of these fifth-generation devices has resulted from advances in the technology of silicone gel.

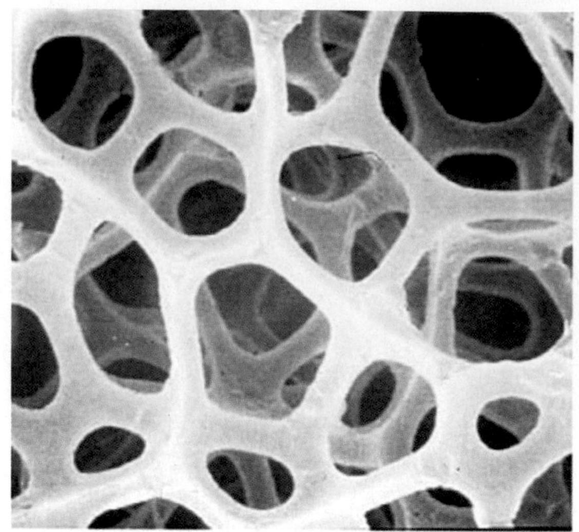

A

Polyurethane

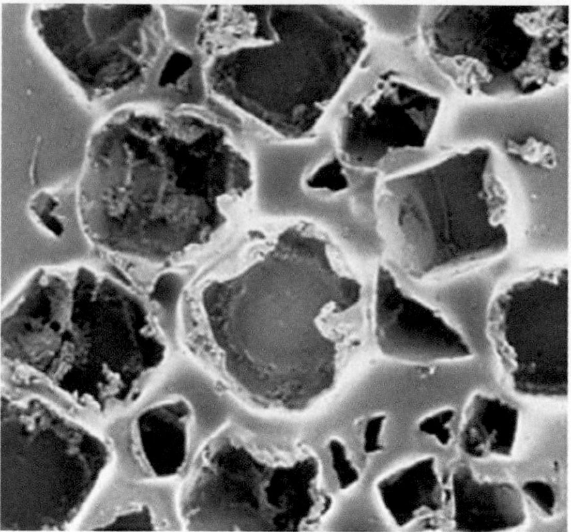

B

Biocell

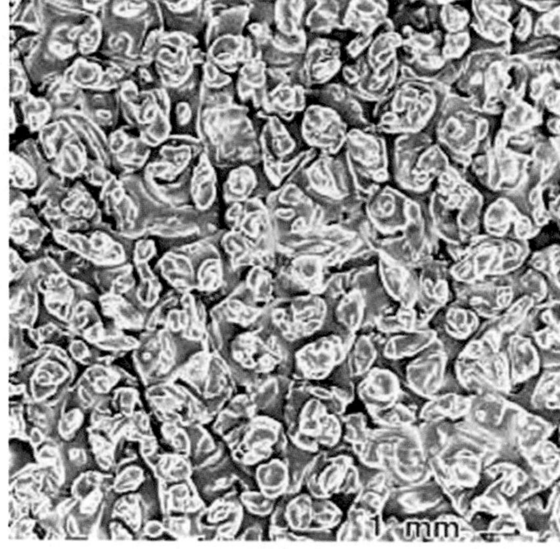

C

Siltex

Figure 106.1. **A:** Polyurethane foam gains tissue adherence and delaminates from the implant. No longer available in the United States, this texture fostered the development of textured silicone surfaces. **B:** Biocell is an aggressive silicone textured surface that adheres to surrounding tissue by an adhesive effect. **C:** Siltex is a less aggressive silicone textured surface that does not demonstrate any adhesive effect and does not gain tissue adherence. (From Maxwell GP, Hammond DC. Breast implants: smooth versus textured. *Adv Plast Reconstr Surg* 1993;9:209–220.)

The Approval of Silicone Gel Implants

In 1976, the U.S. Congress passed the Medical Device Amendment to the Food, Drug, and Cosmetic Act, which gave the FDA authority over implantable medical devices (14). Breast implants that were currently available at that time or those that were "substantially equivalent" were allowed to remain in use until the FDA could formally review their safety and efficacy. In 1988, the FDA called for the manufacturers of silicone gel–filled implants to submit Pre-Market Approval applications providing data that could substantiate the claim of safety and efficacy for these devices. In November 1991, the FDA convened an advisory panel of experts to evaluate the manufacturers' data and to hold public hearings. The advisory panel concluded that more research was needed to establish the safety and efficacy of silicone gel–filled breast implants but that these devices should remain available for use by the general population while the clinical trials were carried out.

Instead of ratifying the panel's recommendation, the FDA commissioner called for a *voluntary moratorium* on the use of all silicone gel–filled implants. Further evaluation by the advisory panel led the commissioner to rule in April 1992 that silicone gel breast implants were not necessarily unsafe, but that the law required more data than the manufacturers had supplied to establish the safety and efficacy of these devices (14). Although the news media and the general public regard this moratorium as a *ban* on the use of silicone gel–filled implants due to their supposed hazardous nature, their use has never been officially *banned*. From 1992 to 2006, the use of silicone gel–filled implants for aesthetic breast augmentation and breast reconstruction was restricted to patients with breast deformities who participated in clinical trials. Criteria and eligibility for enrollment in the silicone gel–filled breast implant Adjunct Study was developed both by Mentor (now Ethicon) and Inamed (now Allergan) (Table 106.4).

The manufacturers continued to improve their gel-filled products and presented the results of the silicone gel–filled breast implant Adjunct Study to the FDA. On November 17, 2006, the FDA approved the new and improved silicone gel–filled breast implants produced by the two manufacturers for breast reconstruction and for cosmetic breast augmentation. The approval was given with a number of conditions, including

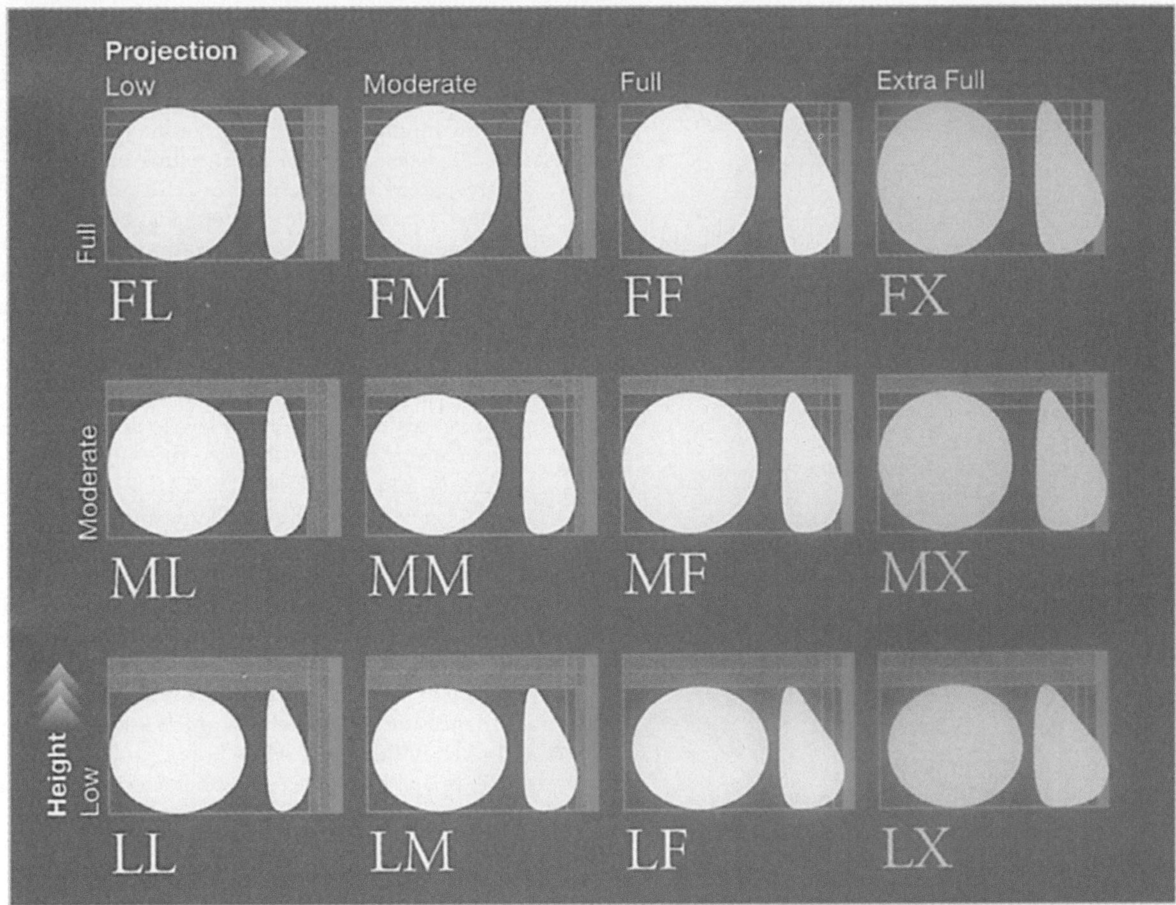

Figure 106.2. Style 410 matrix (Inamed) of enhanced cohesive silicone gel implants offers varying heights and projections of shaped devices for breast augmentation and reconstruction L, low; M, moderate; F, full; X, extra. (Courtesy of Inamed Corp., Santa Barbara, California.)

a requirement to complete 10-year studies on women who have already received the implants and a 10-year study on the safety of the devices in 40,000 women. The postapproval studies will be closely monitored and as of the writing of this chapter, both manufacturers have enrolled the minimum required number of patients.

Alternative Filling Materials

Manufacturers of breast implants have developed alternative filler materials in response to concerns about the safety of silicone gel (24). In 1991, the Bioplasty Corporation introduced the Misti Gold implant, which uses polyvinylpryrrolidone (PVP) as the filling material. The PVP filling material is described as a bio-oncotic gel and is believed to be more radiolucent than silicone. NovaMed acquired Bioplasty and still markets the PVP-filled implant under the name NovaGold outside the United States. The PIP Corporation in France developed breast implants filled with a hydrated polysaccharide gel (hydrogel). However, there have been reports of swelling of hydrogel and PVP-filled implants postoperatively due to the osmotic pressure gradient. In December 2000, the British Medical Devices Agency issued an alert citing a lack of studies that demonstrate the safety of these implants. In 1994, the LipoMatrix Corporation developed the Trilucent implant, which was filled with a triglyceride derived from soybean oil (24). However, problems developed with oil bleed, tissue irritation, and a foul, rancid odor. These implants were withdrawn from the market in 1999, and none of the alternative filling material implants are currently available in the United States.

The Absence of Evidence-based Medicine

Of interest, silicone-containing compounds are ubiquitous in everyday life. The general public has been exposed to them for more than 50 years in consumer products such as hairsprays, suntan lotions, and moisturizing creams. Silicones are extremely resistant to the action of enzymes when implanted into living tissue largely due to their hydrophobic nature (16). This makes silicone compounds extremely stable and inert. Silicones are often used in the consumer safety testing industry as the standard to which all other products are compared for biocompatibility (16). While elemental silicon and silicone particles are detected in periprosthetic tissues, the biologic significance of this finding remains undetermined and uncharacterized (25). In one study, no significant difference was found in levels of antisilicone antibodies between patients who had silicone elastomer tissue expanders and control subjects (26).

Several clinical studies have shown no difference in the incidence of autoimmune diseases in mastectomy patients receiving silicone gel implants compared to patients who had reconstruction with autogenous tissue (27–30). Even meta-analysis research combining data from more than 87,000 women has revealed no association between silicone breast implants and connective

TABLE 106.4 Inclusion Criteria for Participation in the Silicone Gel–filled Breast Implant Adjunct Clinical Study

I. Patient is female, 18 years of age or older, willing to sign informed consent, and willing to follow study requirements
II. Reconstructive breast surgery
  a. Postmastectomy or other oncologic surgery involving the breast
  b. Posttraumatic injury involving the breast
III. Congenital or developmental deformity of the breast
  a. Congenital breast absence
  b. Poland syndrome
  c. Thoracic hypoplasia
  d. Tuberous breast deformity
  e. Pectus excavatum/carinatum
  f. Scoliosis, isolated rib deformities
IV. Acquired deformity
  a. Severe ptosis requiring mastopexy
  b. Advanced periprosthetic capsular contracture (Baker grade III or IV)
V. Revision of ruptured breast implant
  a. Implant rupture after augmentation mammaplasty
  b. Implant rupture after reconstructive breast surgery
VI. Saline-filled implants deemed unsuitable for medical reasons
  a. Skin too thin
  b. Insufficient soft tissue coverage
  c. Severe wrinkling of skin

Based on Adjunct Study Enrollment Form 1 (McGhan Medical Corp.) and Preoperative Patient History Record CRF Page 2–1 (Mentor Corp.).

tissue diseases (31). In the modern era of evidence-based medicine, it seems that the only exception to the rule of science is in the use of silicone gel–filled breast implants, where lawsuits and hysteria supersede science. Notably, virtually all industrialized nations in the world except the United States use silicone gel implants almost exclusively for breast augmentation.

SURGICAL GOALS AND TREATMENT

PATIENT ASSESSMENT

The initial consultation for augmentation should begin with open-ended questions about the patient's goals and expectations for the procedure. Patients today have often spent some time researching the procedure either through friends or through the Internet. The surgeon should be able to form an impression of the patient as a well-informed, psychiatrically stable person with appropriately realistic expectations for the procedure. Any concerns about the patient's level of understanding, unrealistic expectations, or self-esteem issues should be fully explored prior to proceeding with surgery (1). Careful medical history and physical examination are essential for the assessment of risk factors and candidacy for breast augmentation. Preoperative mammography is recommended for patients older than 35 years of age or patients of any age with significant risk factors for breast cancer.

The *ideal* size and shape of the female breast is inherently subjective and relates to both personal preference and cultural norms. However, most surgeons will agree that there are certain shared characteristics that represent the aesthetic ideal of the female breast form. These characteristics include a profile with a sloping or full upper pole and a gently curved lower pole with the nipple-areola complex at the point of maximal projection (Fig. 106.3). The breast structure may be thought of as the breast parenchyma resting on the anterior chest wall surrounded by a soft tissue envelope made up of skin and subcutaneous adipose. Clearly, the resulting form of the breast after augmentation mammaplasty will be determined by the dynamic interaction of the breast implant, the parenchyma, and the soft tissue envelope (32).

A thorough physical examination begins with observation and careful documentation of any signs of chest wall deformity or spinal curvature. It is imperative to document and draw attention to any asymmetry of breast size, nipple position, or inframammary fold (IMF) position. Careful palpation of all quadrants of the breast and axilla is required to rule out any dominant masses or suspicious lymph nodes. While palpating the breast, the surgeon should carefully assess the quantity and compliance of the parenchyma and soft tissue envelope. The soft tissue pinch test is useful method of assessment in which the superior pole of the breast is gathered between the examiner's thumb and index finger and the thickness of the intervening tissue is measured. In general, a pinch test result of less than 2 cm will often indicate a need for subpectoral placement of the implant. It is also important to characterize the amount, quality, and distribution of the breast parenchyma as it may be necessary to reshape or redistribute the parenchyma to achieve the desired shape of the breast mound. The elasticity of the skin should also be characterized by observing its resistance to deflection and noting any signs of skin redundancy or stretch marks. Allergan has developed the BioDimensional preoperative planning system to facilitate patient assessment and implant selection (Table 106.5). Ethicon has also developed the bodyLogic breast implant sizing selection tool to enhance outcomes with ease of implant confirmation. In addition, a system for breast implant selection has been developed based on the patient's tissue characteristics (T), envelope (E), parenchyma (P), the implant (I), and the dynamics of soft tissue and implant interaction (D), referred to as the TEPID assessment system (33).

Precise measurements must be taken using the IMF, the nipple-areola complex, and the suprasternal notch as key landmarks (Fig. 106.4). The surgeon should measure the breast width (BW) at its widest point, the breast height (BH), and the distance from the nipple-areola complex to the inframammary

TABLE 106.5 Preoperative Planning and Dimensional Analysis in Augmentation Mammaplasty

1. Carefully analyze and measure the dimensions and shape of the existing breasts.
2. Analyze the character and evaluate the adequacy of the soft tissue envelope.
3. Develop an anatomically well-defined goal for the breast shape after augmentation (e.g., more or less upper pole fullness).
4. Select implant size, shape, height, width, and projection to accomplish the individual patient's goals.
5. Select surgical approach (incision) and implant pocket location (i.e. subpectoral, subglandular, subfascial).

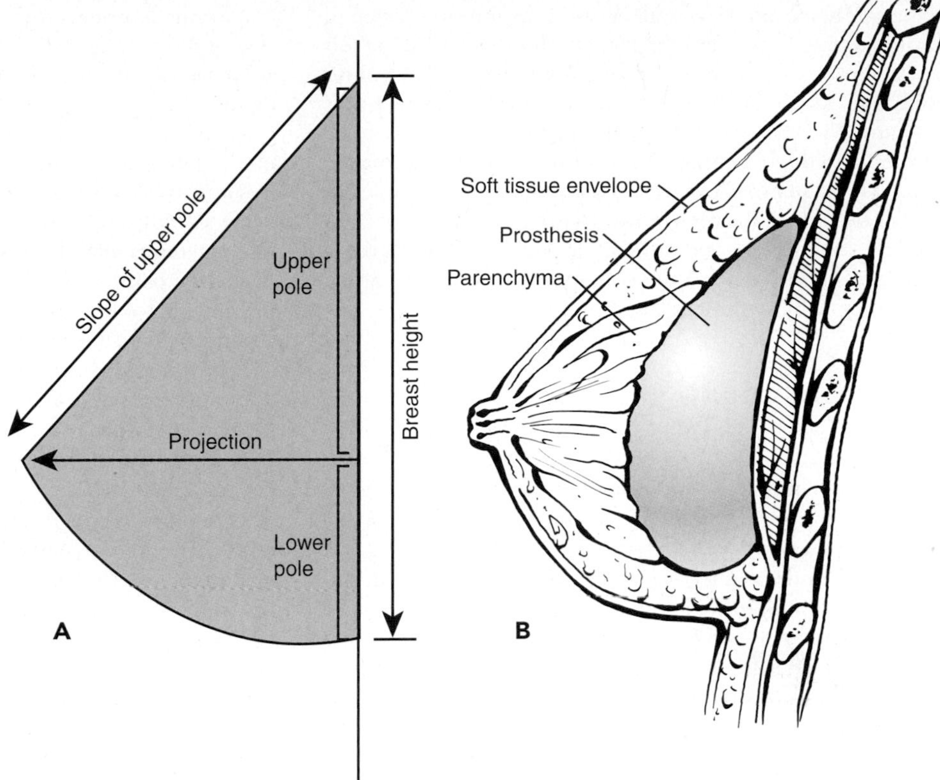

Figure 106.3. **A:** Measurable parameters that comprise the aesthetic breast form. **B:** Following breast augmentation, the resultant breast form is composed of the interaction among the character and compliance of the soft tissue envelope, the volume and quality of the breast parenchyma, and the dimensions, volume, and characteristics of the breast implant. (Redrawn from Maxwell GP, Hartley W. Breast augmentation. In: Mathes SJ, Hentz VR, eds. *Plastic Surgery*. 2nd ed. Philadelphia: Elsevier; 2006.)

fold (N:IMF). The distance from the suprasternal notch to the nipple-areola complex (SSN:N) and the intermammary distance (IMD) should also be documented. It is often helpful to make markings on the patient in the seated position with a permanent marker just prior to surgery. It is imperative to mark the original IMF, and it is a good idea to mark the true midline of the anterior chest.

In addition to manual measurements, three- and four-dimensional systems are available to facilitate the measurement process in addition to enhancing the patients overall experience by increasing physician–patient interaction in selecting the appropriate implant. The visual display of the implant selected increases the confidence of the patient in the results that will be achieved. The four-dimensional imaging system (Precision

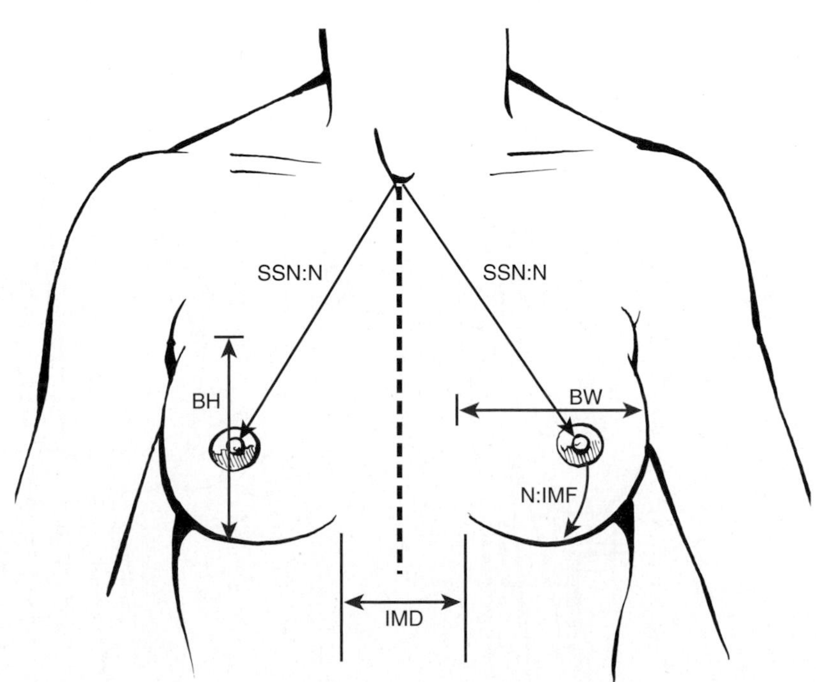

Figure 106.4. Preoperative assessment includes the measurements from supersternal notch to nipple (SSN:N), nipple to inframammary fold (N:IMF), breast width (BW), breast height (BH), and intermammary distance (IMD). The soft tissue thickness and quality is also assessed with a soft tissue pinch test and further tissue characterization. (Redrawn from Maxwell GP, Hartley W. Breast augmentation. In: Mathes SJ, Hentz VR, eds. *Plastic Surgery*. 2nd ed. Philadelphia: Elsevier; 2006.)

Light, Los Gatos, CA) automatically measures and characterizes both the soft tissue and chest wall, as this is an important step in surgical planning. There are times that minor chest wall or soft tissue asymmetries are missed by manual measurement and visualization. This new system captures all of the asymmetries preoperatively so that appropriate preoperative planning can be performed and the patient is advised with an accurate informed consent. This system is based on biodimensional principles as previously described. As we continue to pursue this approach to increasing patient safety and satisfaction while decreasing reoperation rates, this system will serve as another tool in our armamentarium to achieve these goals.

OPERATIVE PLANNING

Implant Position

The breast implant may be positioned in the *subglandular* position between the breast parenchyma and the pectoralis major muscle or in the *subpectoral* position between the pectoralis major muscle and the chest wall (Fig. 106.5). In general, the position of the implant will be determined by the adequacy of the nascent breast tissue. Subglandular implant placement should be considered for patients with mild glandular hypomastia and an adequate soft tissue envelope. Patients who undergo subglandular augmentation have less perioperative discomfort and a shorter period of convalescence than those undergoing subpectoral placement. Subglandular augmentation is believed to yield a more natural-looking breast form because the overlying breast tissue is less distorted than with subpectoral positioning. An additional advantage of subglandular augmentation is that activation of the pectoralis major muscle does not cause unnatural movement or deformation of the implant as is often seen with subpectoral implants in active women (34). However, thin patients with severe hypomastia will be at risk for palpability and even visibility of the implant if it is placed in the subglandular position. This accounts for the predominance of subpectoral implant placement in thin patients.

During subpectoral placement of the implant, it is often necessary to either partially or totally release the inferior portion of the pectoralis major muscle origin in order to achieve the needed expansion in the lower pole of the breast. Frequently, implants placed in the subpectoral position are in reality only covered with pectoralis major muscle in the superior and medial two thirds of the implant. This common situation may be more accurately characterized as the *partial subpectoral* position (35). Infrequently, it may be necessary to place the implant under both the pectoralis major muscle and the serratus anterior muscle, which is called the *total submuscular* position.

In some cases, the interaction between the breast parenchyma and the pectoralis major muscle may adversely affect the appearance of the resulting augmented breast. For example, the breast mound may appear to hang anteriorly and inferiorly off the pectoralis muscle, resulting in the *Snoopy-nose* breast deformity (6). It is then necessary to perform a partial release of the breast parenchyma from the pectoralis muscle, creating a plane of dissection in both the subpectoral *and* subglandular planes (32). This *dual-plane* dissection allows the pectoralis muscle to retract superiorly or *window-shade* upward while the breast parenchyma is redraped over the inferior portion of the implant, avoiding deformity of the resulting augmented breast (Fig. 106.6).

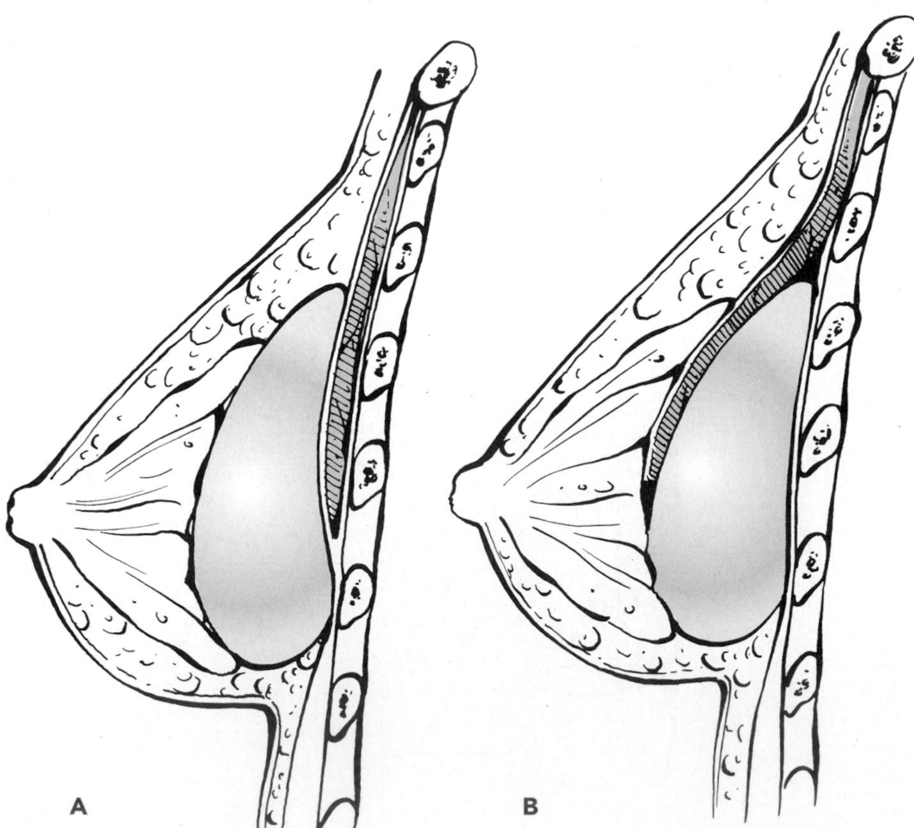

Figure 106.5. **A:** When ample soft tissue is present, the implant may be placed over the pectoral muscle in the subglandular or subfascial position. **B:** When inadequate soft tissue is present, the implant is placed beneath the pectoral muscle in the subpectoral or dual-plane position. (Redrawn from Maxwell GP, Hartley W. Breast augmentation. In: Mathes SJ, Hentz VR, eds. *Plastic Surgery*. 2nd ed. Philadelphia: Elsevier; 2006.)

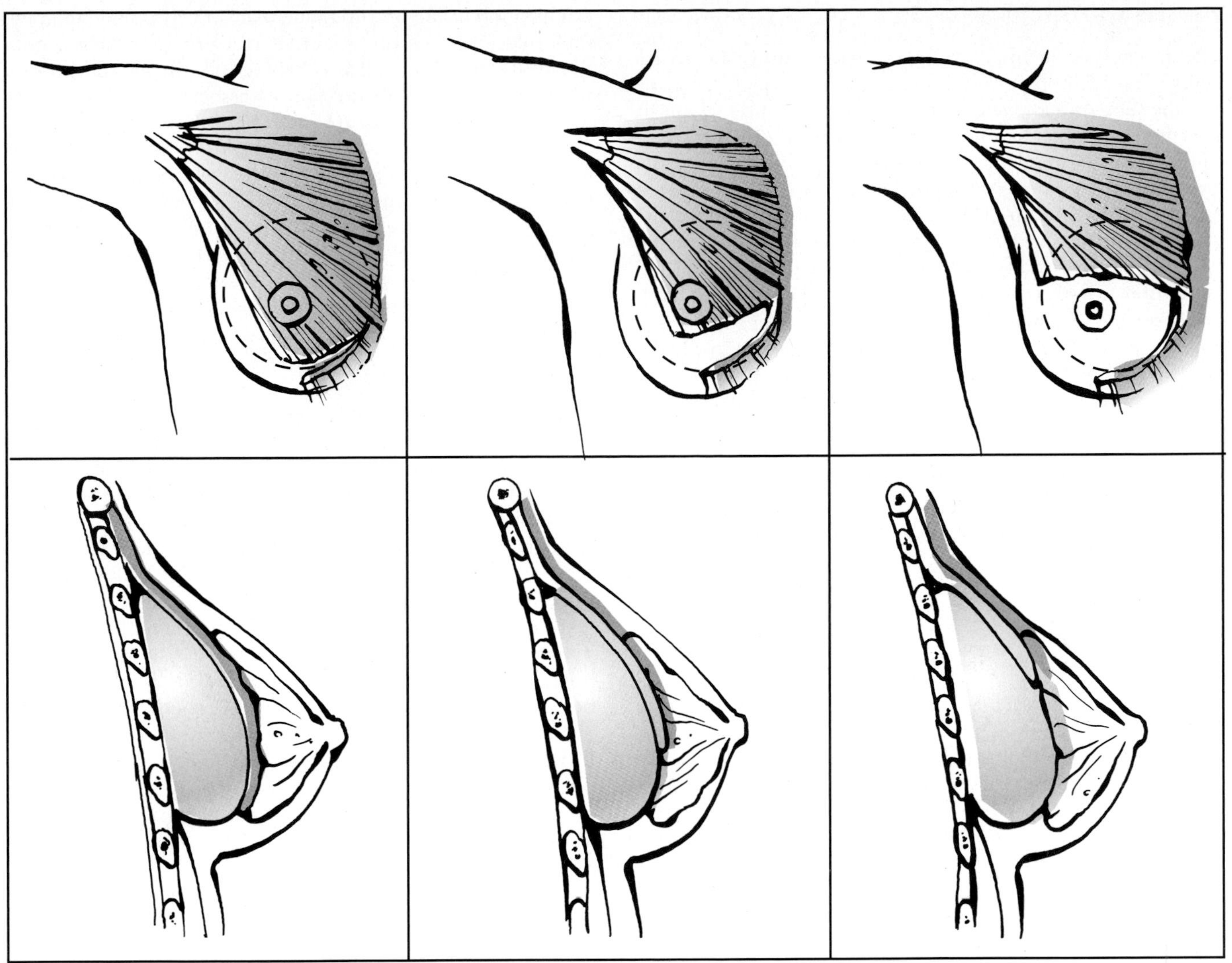

Figure 106.6. Subpectoral implant placement generally involves the release of the pectoralis major muscle. This results in varying degrees of muscle coverage of the upper portion of the implant and mammary glandular coverage of the lower portion. The degree and location at which the pectoral muscle is divided will determine the amount of relative muscle and glandular implant coverage. The term "dual plane" has been used to describe this implant positioning. (Redrawn from Maxwell GP, Hartley W. Breast augmentation. In: Mathes SJ, Hentz VR, eds. *Plastic Surgery*. 2nd ed. Philadelphia: Elsevier; 2006.)

Recently, a *subfascial* implant position has been advocated for augmentation mammaplasty in certain patients (36,37). Theoretically, placement of the implant in the subfascial position between the anterior fascia of the pectoralis major and the muscle itself may provide additional support to the overlying soft tissue envelope, causing less distortion of the breast form and decreasing mobility of the implant within the pocket. The long-term outcome studies of breast augmentation employing this position are not yet available, but the procedure is gaining popularity worldwide.

Implant Selection: Filling Material

Since the reintrocution of silicone implants to the US market, the number of the their placements as compared to saline implants has gradually been increasing. In our experience, breast augmentation with silicone gel–filled implants consistently produces a softer, more natural feel on palpation and an appearance that is superior to augmentation with saline-filled implants. The superiority of silicone gel–filled implants seems to be widely accepted internationally and silicone gel implants are used almost exclusively for primary breast augmentation.

Even though the safety of silicone implants have been shown in several studies and the link to immunological disorders have been disproven (23), many patients still have the impression that saline-filled implants are somehow *safer* than silicone-filled implants despite the lack of any scientific data to support this notion. Saline-filled implants are a good alternative for those patients who are convinced that silicone gel–filled implants are potentially dangerous.

Implant Selection: Implant Size

The selection of the implant size is initiated during the preoperative consultation period based on both the patient's goals and the surgeon's assessment. In general, the critical factors in selecting a specific implant size are the dimensions of the nascent breast, the compliance and characteristics of the soft tissue envelope, and the desired volume for the resulting augmented breast. The base width of the breast is related to the width of the patient's chest and is proportional to the overall body habitus. It is imperative that this dimension is respected during augmentation in order to maintain the normal anatomic landmarks such as the lateral breast fold in the anterior axillary line and the IMD. The same is true for breast height but to a lesser degree than for breast width. Violation of these landmarks may yield an unnatural and deformed appearance. Generally, the surgeon should select an implant that is slightly less wide than the existing breast (Fig. 106.7). Fortunately, implant manufacturers are now producing implants with varying degrees of projection for a given base width. In this way, the surgeon should be able to attain the desired amount of projection by choosing a low-profile, moderate-profile, or high-profile implant while preserving the normal aesthetic proportions of the breast.

Implant Selection: Implant Surface Texture

In 1970, Ashley reported a dramatically reduced incidence of capsular contracture when using a silicone gel implant coated with a thin layer of polyurethane foam for breast reconstruction (38). The textured surface was originally designed to promote ingrowth of the surrounding tissue and help to maintain the position of the implant on the chest wall. Microscopic examination of the polyurethane foam (PUF) reveals an open, trabecular structure (Fig. 106.1A). This structure elicits aggressive tissue ingrowth, which is believed to disrupt and prevent the circumferential linear fibrosis associated with periprosthetic capsular contracture (39). Examination of the PUF-coated prostheses after implantation frequently revealed delamination of the coating and limited mobility of the silicone gel–filled implant within the capsule. Despite this fact, the periprosthetic capsules that formed were soft and did not produce clinically relevant contractures. During the next two decades the PUF-coated implants (Natural-Y, Même, Replicon) enjoyed increasing popularity with plastic surgeons due to the aesthetically pleasing results and remarkably low rates of capsular contracture (40–42). Concerns about the safety of PUF-coated implants arose in response to the findings of a National Cancer Institute study published in 1979 finding that mice fed extremely high doses 2,4-toluenediamine showed an increased incidence of breast cancer (43). Ultimately, the manufacturer of the PUF-coated implants (Surgitek/Bristol-Meyers-Squibb) failed to attain FDA premarket approval in April 1991, and these implants were withdrawn from the U.S. market.

In light of safety concerns associated with PUP-coated devices, implant manufacturers developed processes to create a textured surface on the silicone elastomer shell of breast prostheses and tissue expanders. In 1986, McGhan Medical (now Allergan) introduced the Biocell textured surface, available on both silicone gel–filled and saline-filled breast implants (Fig. 106.1B). The Biocell textured surface is created using a lost salt technique and produces a coarse, open-pore surface with a variable pore size of 300–600 μm and average density of 3.1 pores/ mm^2 (39). This surface has been shown to induce an aggressive tissue response, which causes adherence of the

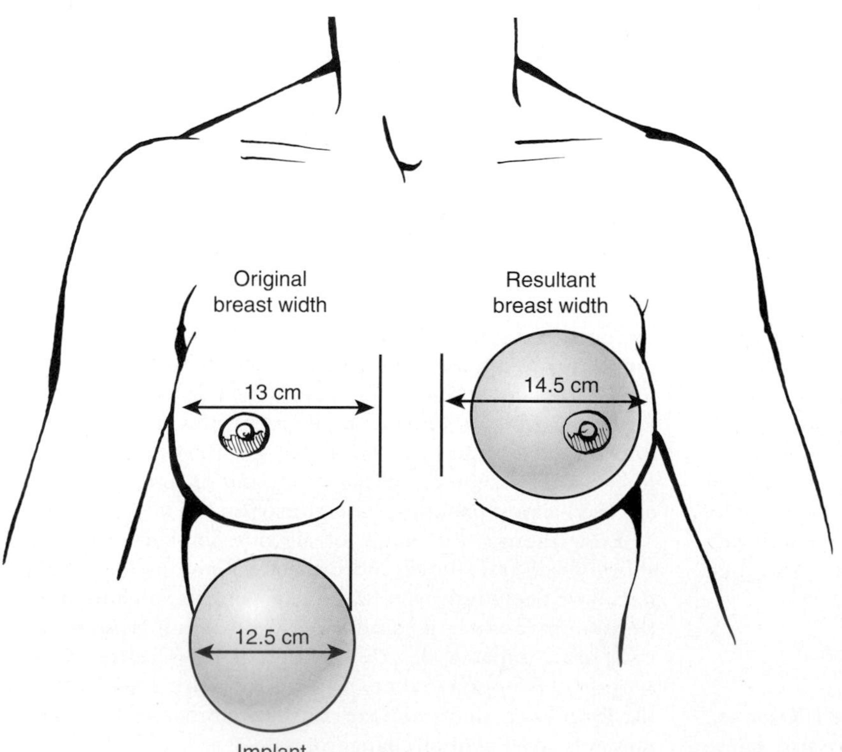

Figure 106.7. The width of the selected implant generally should not exceed the width of the patient's breast tissue. In this illustration, the breast width is 13 cm. An implant is selected 12.5 cm in width and placed beneath the patient's tissue. This gives a resultant postoperative breast form of approximately 14.5 cm in width with similar resultant dimensional changes in breast height and projection. (Redrawn from Maxwell GP, Hartley W. Breast augmentation. In: Mathes SJ, Hentz VR, eds. *Plastic Surgery*. 2nd ed. Philadelphia: Elsevier; 2006.)

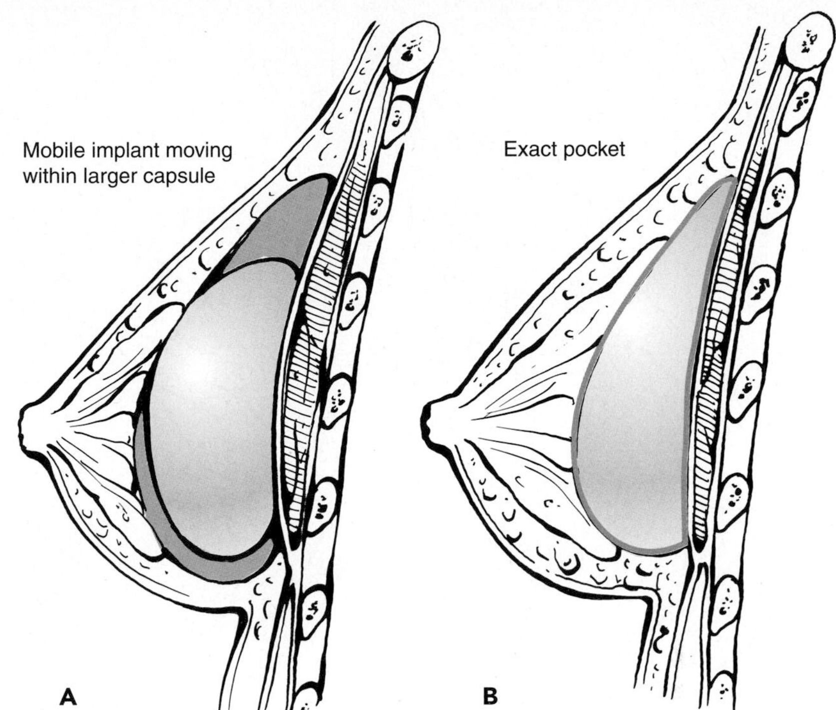

Figure 106.8. Pocket dissection is implant specific. **A:** When round, smooth implants are used, a large pocket is dissected to allow implant mobility within the resultant bursa. **B:** When anatomic implants are used, the pocket should be dissected very precisely around the base dimensions of the implant, promoting tissue adherence and implant immobility. (Redrawn from Maxwell GP, Hartley W. Breast augmentation. In: Mathes SJ, Hentz VR, eds. *Plastic Surgery*. 2nd ed. Philadelphia: Elsevier; 2006.)

implant to the periprosthetic capsule (44). This *adhesive effect* seen with the Biocell textured implants is similar to that seen with the PUP-coated implants but differs in that the textured surface does not delaminate from the implant. Ultimately, the Biocell textured prosthesis remains relatively immobile within the implant pocket but generally produces a soft, noncontracted periprosthetic capsule. This was the genesis of the concept of *immobility with softness.* The principle of immobility with softness yields a relatively fixed location of the implant within the precisely fitted pocket and contrasts dramatically with the great mobility of a smooth implant within a significantly larger capsule pocket (Fig. 106.8). Several clinical studies have shown a significantly lower incidence of capsular contracture with Biocell textured surface implants than with smooth surface implants (39,44–46).

In 1989, the Mentor corporation (now Ethicon) introduced the Siltex textured surface on an inflatable saline breast prosthesis and on tissue expanders, as shown in Figure 106.1C (47). The Siltex textured surface is created as a negative imprint by contact with a texturing foam that produces a dense pattern of raised irregular nodules ranging in height from 65 to 150 μm and in width from 60 to 275 μm. The Siltex textured surface is less coarse than the Biocell textured surface, as it does not exhibit the same degree of adherence to the periprosthetic capsule seen with the Biocell implant. Therefore, the Siltex textured surface implants exhibit more mobility within the pocket but theoretically also reduce the risk of rippling visible on the breast surface. Of importance, clinical studies have shown a significantly lower incidence of capsular contracture with Siltex textured surface implants than with smooth surface implants (47).

Implant Selection: Implant Shape

It is important to reiterate the principle that the shape of the natural female breast is not a semicircle or a hemisphere. Dimensional analysis of the aesthetically pleasing breast form reveals a gently sloping upper pole and a curved lower pole with the nipple-areola complex at the point of maximum projection (Fig. 106.3). The typical round breast implant has its greatest projection centrally with the remainder of the volume distributed evenly along the base of the implant (Fig. 106.9A). In contrast, anatomically shaped breast implants have a flatter upper pole with the majority of the volume and projection in the lower pole (Fig. 106.9B). Thus, the anatomically shaped implant of a given base width and volume will produce less upper pole convexity than a round implant of the same base width and volume. This characteristic of anatomically shaped implants can be extremely useful when the patient desires a significant volume augmentation but has a relatively narrow breast width (48–50).

Both manufacturers have developed anatomically shaped breast implants to address the need for more naturally shaped breast prostheses in breast reconstruction and augmentation mammaplasty. Allergan has developed the BioDimensional style 410 anatomically shaped, silicone gel–filled breast prosthesis (Table 106.3). The Mentor Corporation has developed the Contour Profiles series of saline-filled breast implants with either a moderate or a high level of projection (Table 106.1). Obviously, it is imperative that anatomically shaped implants be relatively immobile within the implant pockets since rotation or inversion would produce a significant breast deformity (51). Therefore, all anatomically shaped implants are produced with a textured surface to promote either sufficient friction or tissue ingrowth between the implant and the periprosthetic capsule to ensure immobility of the implant.

OPERATIVE TECHNIQUE

SURGICAL APPROACH

Preoperative markings are made with the patient in the upright position and are useful as a reference point during the actual procedure (Fig. 106.4). The surgeon should mark

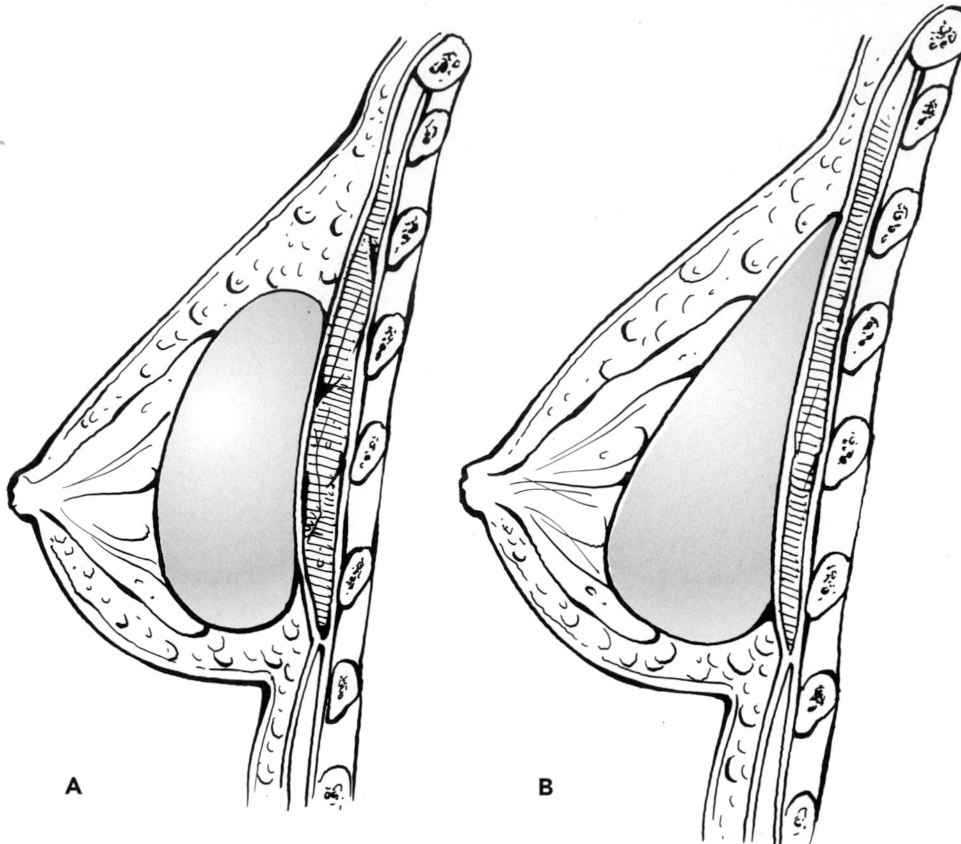

Figure 106.9. **A:** When there is acceptable preoperative breast form, a round implant may suffice for volumetric enhancement. **B:** When there is inadequate breast form as well as volume deficit, an anatomic implant is preferable. (Redrawn from Maxwell GP, Hartley W. Breast augmentation. In: Mathes SJ, Hentz VR, eds. *Plastic Surgery.* 2nd ed. Philadelphia: Elsevier; 2006.)

the chest midline in the frontal view from the suprasternal notch to the xiphoid process, the existing inframammary folds, and the likely position of the new inframammary folds as the proposed limits of the dissection. The patient is then placed in the supine position, centered on the operating table with the pelvis directly over the flexion point of the bed. The arms must be well secured to the arm boards, which are placed at 90-deg angles to the torso. These preparations are required so that the patient may be placed in the upright seated position as often as needed during the procedure. The sterile preparation and draping of the anterior chest must provide visualization of the patient's shoulders as an important anatomic reference point.

The three types of incision that are commonly employed in augmentation mammaplasty are inframammary, periareolar, and transaxillary incisions (52). While the patient's preference should be taken into consideration, the ultimate choice of incision must allow the surgeon optimal visualization, control of the dissection, and precise control of the implant. The potential advantages and limitations of each approach should be discussed with the patient (Table 106.6). The surgeon should become facile with each technique so that the surgical approach can be tailored to the individual patient's anatomy.

The inframammary approach permits complete visualization of the implant pocket with either subglandular or subpectoral placement, and was popularized by Cronin and Gerow (11). The incision should be placed in the predicted location of the new inframammary fold, which is typically 1 to 2 cm below the existing fold. Smaller incisions (1 cm than 3 cm) may be used for inflatable saline-filled implants, but prefilled implants (silicone gel or saline) often require incisions up to 5.5 cm in length. The incision should be designed with the majority of the incision lateral to the breast midline, as this will place the resulting scar in the deepest portion of the new IMF.

The periareolar approach for augmentation mammaplasty was described by Jenny in 1972 and currently enjoys widespread use by plastic surgeons (53). The periareolar incision is placed along the inferior portion of the areolar-cutaneous juncture. The principal advantage of this incision is that the resulting scar is usually well camouflaged and quite inconspicuous. The periareolar approach allows easy adjustment of the IMF and direct access to the parenchyma for scoring and release when the lower pole of the breast is constricted. However, visualization and control of the dissection are typically inadequate with the periareolar incision in patients with areolas less than 3 cm in diameter. Other disadvantages of this approach include the potential risk of contamination if the lactiferous ducts are transected, the increased risk of changes in nipple sensitivity, and the risk of a hypopigmented scar in patients with darkly pigmented areolas.

The transaxillary approach was described by Hoehler in 1977 and popularized by Bostwick and others (54). This procedure can be performed either bluntly using the Montgomery dissector or using an endoscope for precise visualization, together with dissection of the implant pocket. The transaxillary approach avoids incisional scarring directly on the breast and places the incision in the inferior and anterior area of the axilla. The transaxillary incision usually provides adequate access when placing an inflatable round breast implant, and while not

TABLE 106.6 Incision Options in Breast Augmentation

Factor	Axillary	Periareolar	Inframammary
Implant plane			
Submuscular	+	+	+
Subglandular	−	+	+
Implant type			
Saline round	+	+	+
Saline shaped	−	+	+
Silicone round/shaped	−	+	+
Preoperative breast volume			
High (>200 g)	+	+	+
Low (<200 g)	+	+	−
Preoperative breast base position			
High	+	+	+
Low	−	+	+
Breast shape			
Tubular	−	+	−
Glandular ptosis	+	+	+
Ptosis (grade I–II)	−	+	−
Areolar characteristics			
Small diameter	+	−	+
Light/indistinct	+	−	+
Inframammary crease			
None	+	+	−
High	+	+	−
Low	+	+	+
Secondary procedure	−	+	+

+, applicable; –, not generally recommended.
Adapted from Hidalgo DA. Breast augmentation: choosing the optimal incision, implant and pocket plane. *Plast Reconstr Surg* 2000;105(6):2202–2216.

it does not preclude it, it is more difficult for placement of a large, prefilled implant or an anatomically shaped device.

CREATING THE IMPLANT POCKET

The incision is made in the location determined during the preoperative consultation period. The superficial fascial system (Scarpa's), which is contiguous with the inferior and lateral edge of the breast parenchyma, is divided and the dissection is beveled cephalic to avoid fold tissue disruption down to the anterior fascia of the pectoralis major muscle. Meticulous hemostasis is maintained using the Bovie electrocautery device. A variety of fiberoptically lighted retractors are available to aid visualization during the procedure. The surgeon may wish to use a fiberoptically lighted headlight to illuminate the operative dissection instead of a lighted retractor. Once the anterior fascia of the pectoralis major muscle is identified, the dissection will proceed either above or below the muscle, depending upon the planned position of the breast implant. Alternatively, the dissection plane may be developed between the anterior fascia of the pectoralis major and the muscle itself in order to place the implant in the subfascial position.

When placing the implant in the subpectoral position, it is necessary to identify the lateral border of the pectoralis major muscle as a key anatomic landmark. The lateral edge of the muscle is carefully elevated to gain access to the subpectoral pocket. This plane is developed superiorly, medially, and inferiorly by dividing the loose areolar connective tissue between the muscle and the chest wall. Perforating branches of the internal mammary artery are frequently encountered medially within the pocket and need to be carefully coagulated using the extended tip on the electrocautery or the insulated DeBakey forceps. The inferior origin of the pectoralis major muscle may need to be partially or totally divided in order for the pocket to accommodate the subpectoral implant (Fig. 106.6). The extent to which the inferior origin of the pectoralis muscle is divided (or attenuated) is determined by the location of the origin in the individual patient, the dimension of the patient's breast, and the height of the implant. Conversely, the lateral portion of the implant pocket should be developed using a blunt dissection technique. In this way, the third, fourth, and fifth intercostal cutaneous nerves, which provide sensory function to the nipple-areola complex, may be preserved.

The subpectoral implant pocket is then copiously irrigated with a triple antibiotic-containing saline solution or a povidone-iodine solution. The pocket is carefully inspected again to ensure meticulous hemostasis. When placing prefilled implants, it is generally helpful to first insert an adjustable implant sizer, inflate it to planned volume, and place the patient in a seated position. Careful observation at this point will allow confirmation of the appropriate implant volume and identification of minor asymmetries intraoperatively. The prefilled implant or the deflated implant is then placed in the implant pocket, making sure that the point of maximal projection is centered beneath the nipple. Once the implant is in the proper position and inflated to the appropriate volume, a multilayer closure is accomplished using absorbable suture material and sterile paper tape is applied longitudinally over the incision. Typical results of augmentation mammaplasty with round, smooth, saline-filled implants placed in the subpectoral position are shown in

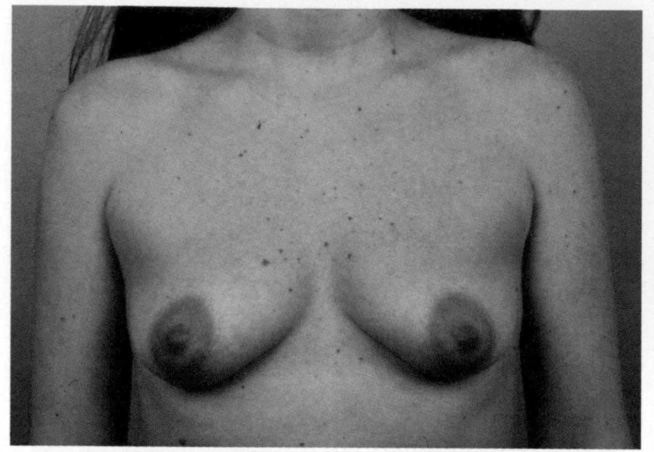

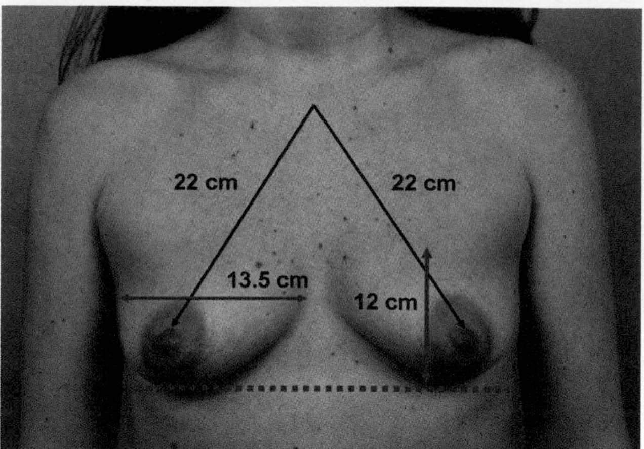

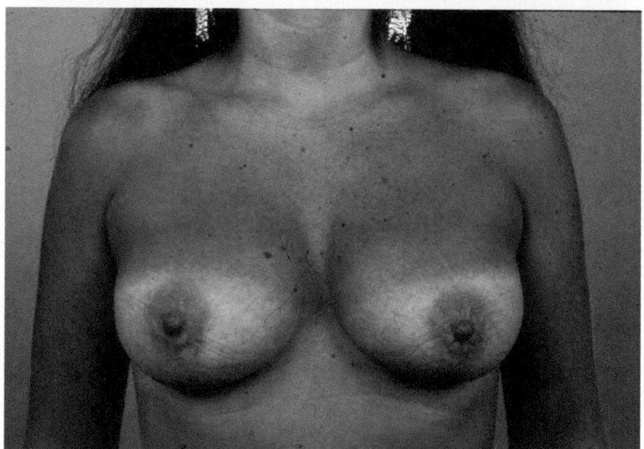

Figure 106.10. **A:** The patient is shown preoperatively **B:** Supersternal notch-to-nipple measurements are 22 cm, breast widths are 13.5 cm, and breast heights are 12.5 cm. Based on these dimensions and the patient's desire for saline implants, implants of 12.7 cm are selected from the data chart. These are 360-cc implants filled to 375-cc per side. The implants are placed subpectorally with pectoral release. The implants are placed subpectorally due to a soft tissue pinch test of less than 2 cm. **C:** The result is shown with the round, smooth saline implant in the dual plane.

Figure 106.10. Results following breast augmentation with round, smooth, silicone gel–filled implants placed in the subpectoral position are shown in Figure 106.11.

In patients with adequate soft tissue coverage, the subglandular position may yield the optimal aesthetic result (Fig. 106.12). Placement of the implant in the subglandular position involves development of the plane between the posterior aspect to the breast parenchyma and the anterior fascia of the pectoralis major muscle. It is imperative to maintain meticulous hemostasis and avoid injury to the lateral intercostal cutaneous nerves during the dissection. A larger pocket is created for smooth, round implants to allow mobility of the implant within the pocket (Fig. 106.8A). For textured anatomically shaped implants, the pocket is precisely dissected to snugly accommodate the implant. Selection of the final implant volume, adjustments of the implant pocket, irrigation, and closure are carried out in the fashion described previously.

POSTOPERATIVE CARE

In the overwhelming majority of cases, augmentation mammaplasty is performed as an outpatient procedure. Patients are given prescriptions for oral analgesics and a 3-day course of prophylactic oral antibiotics. Patients are allowed to remove operative dressings and shower as desired starting on postoperative day 2. The first follow-up visit is scheduled for 3 to 5 days after the procedure. If smooth (nontextured) implants were used, initiation of implant mobility exercises is recommended at this time. If the patient is at risk for superior implant displacement, a circumferential elastic strap may be used to apply continuous downward pressure during the early postoperative period. Patients are usually able to return to work a few days after surgery but are not permitted to resume rigorous exercise for 2 to 3 weeks. Additional follow-up visits are scheduled at 4 to 6 weeks, 3 months, and 1 year. The importance of postoperative photographic documentation and critical analysis of the operative outcomes cannot be overemphasized.

MANAGEMENT OF THE AUGMENTED PATIENT

PERIOPERATIVE COMPLICATIONS

Alterations of nipple sensitivity after augmentation mammaplasty may be manifested as either anesthesia or hyperesthesia and are believed to result from traction injury, bruising, or transection of the lateral intercostal cutaneous nerves. The incidence and severity of nipple sensation changes vary considerably with the surgical approach employed. The periareolar approach is generally associated with the highest rate of changes in nipple sensation, while the transaxillary approach is associated with a significantly lower incidence. The frequency of changes reported in the literature varies widely, but patients should be advised that the risk of *permanent* alterations in nipple sensitivity is about 3% to 5% for all approaches (55).

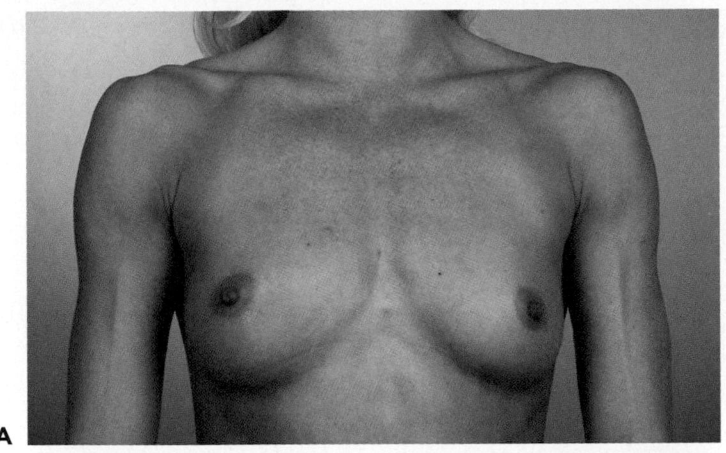

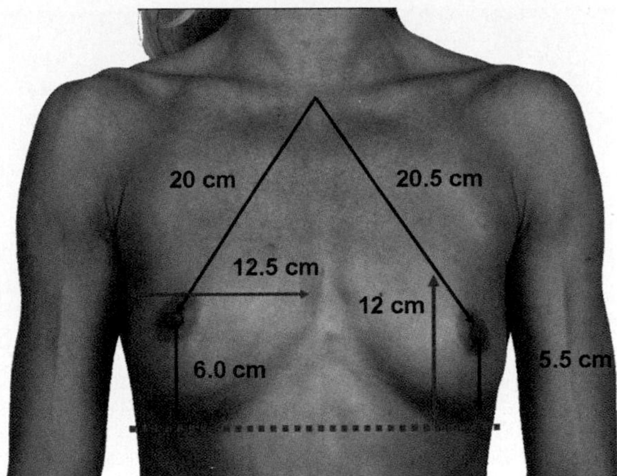

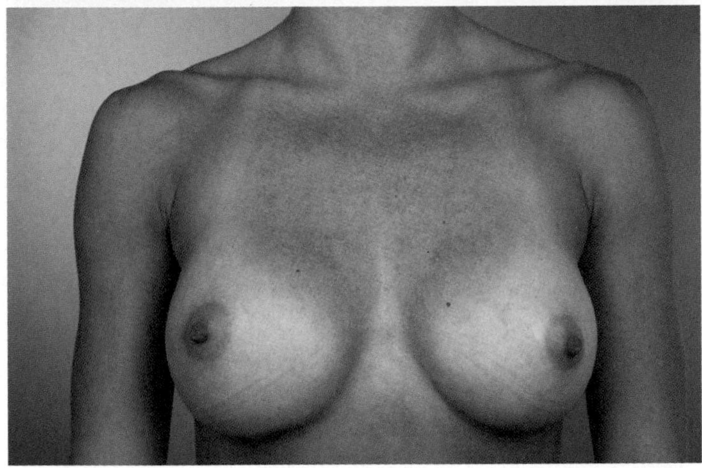

Figure 106.11. **A:** This athletic patient desiring proportionate breast enhancement is shown preoperatively. **B:** Supersternal notch-to-nipple dimensions are 20 and 20.5 cm, nipple intermammary fold asymmetries are 6.0 and 5.5 cm, breast widths are 12.5 cm, and breast heights are 12 cm. **C:** The resultant breast form meets the patient's aesthetic and functional goals.

Periprosthetic seroma fluid is usually resorbed by the soft tissues within the first week of surgery (56). Persistent seromas, although very rare in primary augmentation, may require ultrasound-guided aspiration or drainage catheter placement. Diluting the antibiotic irrigation solution and minimizing use of the electrocautery may help to prevent seroma formation. The development of a hematoma after breast augmentation has several deleterious effects in both the early and late postoperative periods, including pain, blood loss, disfigurement, and capsular contracture (57). Preoperatively, patients should receive a list of prescription and over-the-counter medications that may contribute to excessive postoperative bleeding. It is imperative that the patient discontinue any medications that impair clotting or platelet function at least 1 week prior to surgery. Obviously, maintenance of meticulous hemostasis during the procedure is critically important, and blunt dissection is to be used sparingly if at all to avoid hematoma formation. If a hematoma does develop in the perioperative period, immediate evacuation of the hematoma and exploration of the pocket is recommended. Unfortunately, the source of the hematoma is only rarely identified at the time of the exploration. Patients may occasionally present with a delayed hematoma 1 to 2 weeks or even months to years after augmentation, and frequently a history of breast trauma is elicited. Expanding hematomas require exploration and drainage regardless of the length of time from the augmentation. Nonoperative management of small, nonexpanding hematomas is one option but places the patient at a higher risk of subsequent periprosthetic capsular contracture (57).

Postoperative wound infection may present with a spectrum of severity ranging from a mild cellulitis of the breast skin to a purulent periprosthetic space infection. The organism *Staphylococcus epidermidis* is part of the normal skin flora and is the most frequently identified pathogen in postoperative wound infections. Patients are given prophylactic antibiotics intraoperatively and postoperatively to reduce the risk of infection. Sterile technique is maintained during the procedure, and the implant pocket is irrigated with triple antibiotic solution containing 50,000 units of bacitracin, 1 g of cefazolin, and 80 mg of gentamicin per 500 mL of saline. Further reduction of risk for bacterial contamination may be achieved by employing the *no-touch* technique in which only the surgeon handles the implant with fresh, powder-free gloves. The implant is then inserted carefully with surgeons choice of insertion technique. Our patients are also asked to shower with antimicrobial soap (Hibiclense) three days prior to the operation followed by 5–10 days during the postoperative period. A significant number of postoperative wound infections will respond to oral or intravenous antibiotics if therapy is initiated very early in the course of the infection (56). If the infection persists or progresses, then the implant should be removed and the wound should be allowed to heal by secondary intention. Once the infection has totally cleared, a secondary augmentation and scar revision should be planned.

Mondor disease is a superficial thrombophlebitis of the breast that may occur in up to 1% to 2% of augmentation patients (56). This process usually affects the veins along the inferior aspect of the breast and occurs most frequently with the

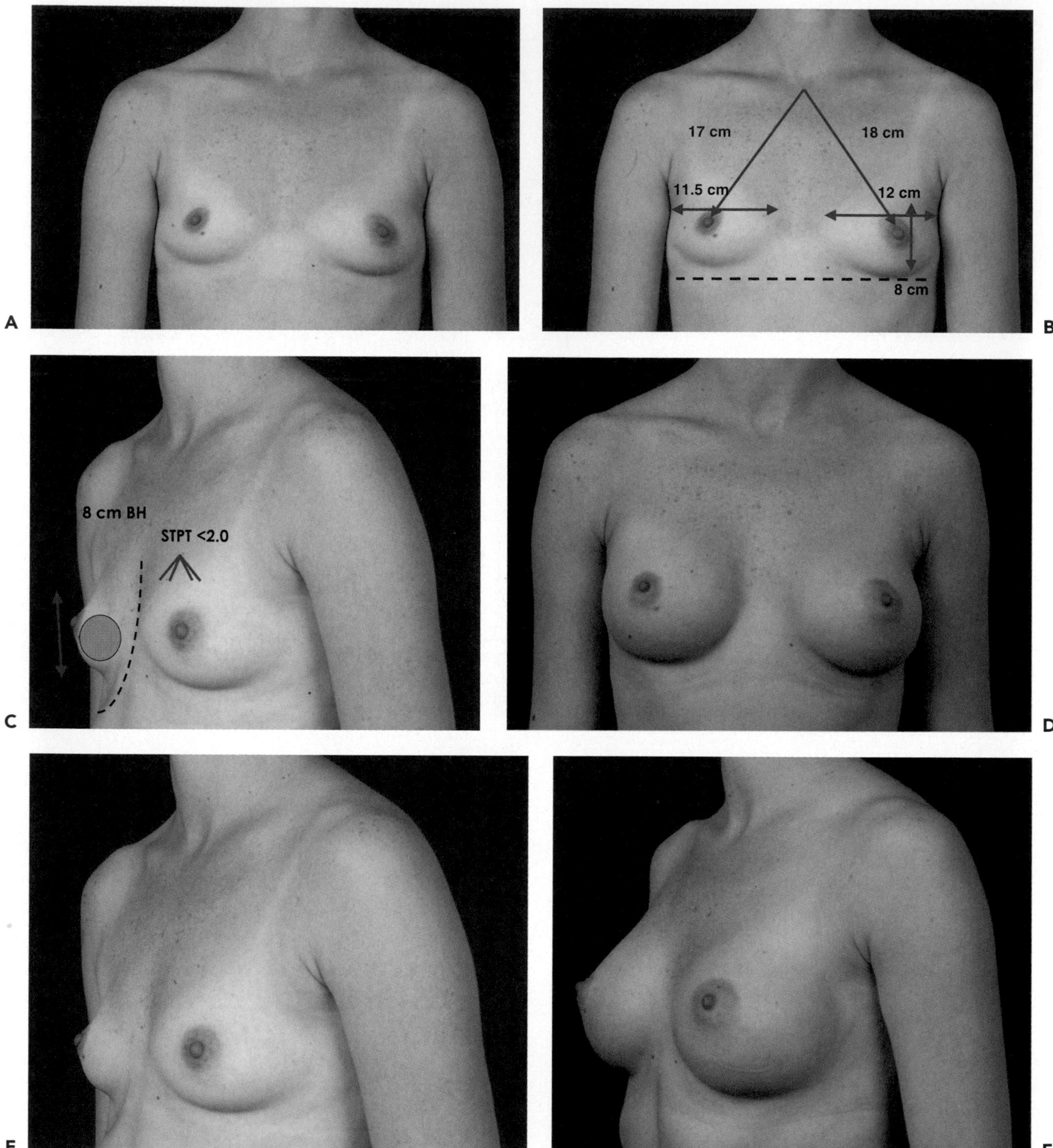

Figure 106.12. **A:** This young patient presented with significant bony, musculoskeletal, and breast asymmetry. She desired a natural aesthetic breast form with improvement in symmetry. **B:** Assessment shows nipple-to-supersternal notch distances of 17 and 18 cm, breast widths of 11.5 and 12 cm, and the obvious discrepancy in inframammary fold locations. **C:** The patient's breast height of 8 cm is noted with the significant depression in the chest wall. The right breast has a constricted lower pole. The soft tissue pinch test is less than 2 cm. **D:** The asymmetric augmentation result was accomplished with a 255-g style 410 MF implant and a 245-g 410 MM implant in the left, placed through inframammary incisions in the subpectoral or dual-plane location. **E:** Preoperative oblique appearance. **F:** Postoperative result with enhanced aesthetic breast form and better breast symmetry.

inframammary approach. Fortunately, this is a self-limiting process that usually resolves with warm compresses over a period of several weeks.

DELAYED COMPLICATIONS OF AUGMENTATION MAMMAPLASTY

Periprosthetic Capsular Contracture

One of the most common delayed complications of augmentation mammaplasty is the development of a palpable and deforming periprosthetic capsular contracture. All surgical implants undergo some degree of encapsulation due to the natural foreign-body reaction by the surrounding tissues. Clinically significant periprosthetic capsular contracture is characterized by excessive scar formation that leads to firmness, distortion, and displacement of the breast implant. Histologic examination of these contractures reveals circumferential linear fibrosis, which is especially severe when formed in response to smooth shell implants (39). In 1975, Baker proposed a clinical classification system of capsular contracture after augmentation that is still commonly used to describe periprosthetic contractures (58). This classification system is summarized in Table 106.7. Capsular contracture remains one of the most common and most problematic complications of augmentation mammaplasty, with an incidence reported between 0.5% and 30%.

While several factors have been identified that contribute to capsular contracture, the precise etiology remains unknown. The hypertrophic, circumferential linear scar probably involves stimulation of myofibroblasts that are known to be present within the periprosthetic capsule. Irritation caused by periprosthetic hematoma, seroma, or silicone gel bleed may incite the capsular contracture (59). Other foreign-body particles such as glove powder, lint, or dust may also contribute to the process.

Several studies have suggested an infectious etiology for periprosthetic capsular contracture (60,61). This theory describes a chronic subclinical infection located immediately adjacent to the implant shell within a microscopic biofilm that is relatively inaccessible to cellular and humoral immune function (62,63). The appropriate treatment for the infectious etiology would be total capsulectomy and placement of a new sterile breast implant. The use of perioperative prophylactic antibiotics theoretically reduces the risk of bacterial contamination and has become standard in augmentation.

Many strategies have been employed to prevent periprosthetic capsular contracture. One strategy has been the creation of a large implant pocket and maintenance of this oversized pocket with implant displacement exercises. The use of implants with textured surfaces has been described earlier in this chapter and has been shown to reduce the rate of capsular contracture in breast augmentation. Other efforts have focused on minimizing operative trauma in order to reduce the risk of seroma or hematoma formation. Seromas, hematomas, and even blood staining of the periprosthetic tissues may incite capsular contracture. Any bleeding that does occur during the dissection needs to be controlled, and the staining of the tissues with blood should be diluted with copious irrigation fluid.

Some evidence has accumulated that leukotriene receptor antagonists, which are used to treat asthma, may prevent and reverse the formation of a periprosthetic capsular contracture (64). Specifically, zafirlukast (Accolate) and montelukast (Singulair) have been shown to reverse clinical signs of capsular contracture in patients taking the medication for asthma.

Treatment of established capsular contractures usually requires operative intervention. Open capsulotomy involves scoring the capsule circumferentially and anteriorly to adequately release and expand the soft tissue envelope. With very thick fibrous capsules or with calcified capsules containing silicone granulomas, it is often necessary to perform either a partial or complete capsulectomy to correct the deformity (70,71). This is often extremely effective in treating advanced grade IV capsular contractures, especially when the implant is replaced with a saline-filled or a no-bleed silicone gel–filled implant. Implant site change surgery has become popular for treating established or recurrent capsular contracture. Recent evidence also shows that the use of Acellular Dermal Matrix (ADM) may be helpful in both treating and possibly preventing capsular contractures. Although long term follow up is still needed, use of ADM is showing promise in treating the most common reason that the patients present for revisionary breast surgery. The workhorse of revisionary breast surgery for the authors are the use acellular dermal matrix (ADM) with or without the creation of the neopectoral pocket (76,77). For those patients whose original implants were subglandular, a pocket change to a subpectoral plane and lower pole coverage with acellular dermal matrix should be preformed. For those patients whose original implants were in a subpectoral, a neopectoral pocket with the addition of acellular dermal matrix should be performed. Patients who did have adequate breast tissue a subfascial pocket with ADM sling should be performed. This allows the newly placed implant to be positioned in contact with normal, well-vascularized tissue instead of residual scarred tissues.

TABLE 106.7 Baker Classification of Capsular Firmness in Augmented Breasts

Grade	Description
Grade I (no palpable capsule)	The augmented breast feels as soft as an unoperated one
Grade II (minimal firmness)	The breast is less soft, and the implant can be palpated but is not visible
Grade III (moderate firmness)	The breast is harder, the implant can be palpated easily, and it (or distortion from it) can be seen
Grade IV (severe contracture)	The breast is hard, tender, and cold; distortion is often marked

Implant Rupture and Deflation

Any defect in the silicone elastomer shell of a saline-filled breast implant will ultimately result in *deflation* of the implant. The saline filling material leaks out of the implant and is harmlessly absorbed by the surrounding tissues. Clinical recognition of deflation is usually made by the patient and virtually always requires surgical explantation and replacement of the implant. A history of recent trauma is frequently elicited with deflation, and true *spontaneous* failure of the implant shell is relatively rare. Both manufacterers submitted their 7-year deflation rates for saline-filled breast implants as part of the FDA postmarket approval process (66). The 7-year deflation rate reported for the Mentor saline-filled implants was 16.4% in 1,264 patients with a 50% follow-up rate. The Inamed data were somewhat different, with a reported 7-year deflation rate of 9.8% in 876 patients with a 85% follow-up rate. It is important to note that the statistical significance of these data was not provided in the press release. However, the surgeon should advise any patient considering augmentation mammaplasty with saline-filled implants to expect a deflation rate of approximately 10% to 15% over a 7-year period.

The spontaneous rupture rates for silicone gel–filled prostheses have been significantly more difficult to monitor (67,68). It is often difficult to distinguish between silicone gel *bleed* and minor silicone gel *leak* when both produce nearly identical clinical findings. Actual failure of the shell may result in only a small amount of gel leak into the periprosthetic intracapsular space. Leakage of silicone gel into the extracapsular tissues may occur only as small herniations in isolated areas. Certainly, patients who have undergone closed capsulotomies are at greater risk for gel leakage into the surrounding tissues. Of interest, the constrictive force of the periprosthetic capsular contracture itself may contribute to extrusion of the gel into the extracapsular space. In the majority of gel implant ruptures, significant deformity of the breast is not clinically obvious, with only a small amount of intracapsular or extracapsular gel leakage (68). Instead, there may be only very subtle changes in the implant shape or firmness even when frank rupture of the gel implant shell is present.

Magnetic resonance imaging (MRI) of the breast is considered the state-of-the-art technique for evaluating breast implant integrity. However, false positives and false negatives occur when using breast MRI to assess silicone gel–filled implants (69). The finding of silicone residue between the implant shell and the periprosthetic capsule on MRI may often be misinterpreted as evidence of implant *rupture*. Upon explantation, however, the implant shell is often actually found to be *intact* and the residue represents only gel bleed.

Hölmich et al. showed that the majority of the second-generation implants examined by MRI showed evidence of rupture despite the fact that the patients were asymptomatic with this finding (69). Patients with evidence of ruptured silicone gel implants on MRI did not have increased symptoms, autoimmune disease, or autoantibodies compared to patients without MRI evidence of rupture. The authors concluded that silicone gel–filled implant rupture is a relatively harmless condition, which only rarely progresses and gives rise to notable symptoms (69).

Modern silicone gel is substantially more cohesive than the second-generation gel and less likely to leak into the surrounding tissues, even when the implant shell is ruptured. This cohesive silicone gel is described as being form stable or as having shape retention with little or no gel flow and immeasurable gel bleed. This raises the question of whether an actual rupture of a modern silicone gel implant shell is relevant, since both gel leak and gel diffusion are unlikely to occur even in the face of shell failure.

Recently, both manufacturers reported their long-term follow-up data. The results were very strong and supportive. Mentor's Core MemoryGel 10-year study included 1,008 women at 6 years' follow-up with 9.8% capsular contracture (72), whereas Allergan's 10-year core study included 940 women at 6 years' follow-up with 14.8% capsular contracture for augmentation mammaplasty (73).

Both manufacturers had less capsular contractures with the highly cohesive gel implants. The Mentor Contour Profile Gel study at 2-years' follow-up showed a 0.8% capsular contracture in augmentation mammaplasty (74). On the other hand, Allergan's style 410 highly cohesive breast implant core study at 3 years showed a 1.9% capsular contracture rate (75).

The data provided by both manufacturers demonstrate safety and efficacy of these medical devices. The journey is yet not over, and we have to strive to provide continuous data and science followed by extensive education and improvement of surgical techniques for improved clinical outcomes in the future.

CONCLUSION

We have reviewed the history and development of breast augmentation in the United States. In addition, our aim has been to provide a method for patient assessment, operative planning, and technique. Currently, there are several alternatives when selecting the surgical approach and the specific type of breast implant for a given patient. Ultimately, decisions about the size, shape, surface texture, and filling material must be made in conjunction with the recommendations of the surgeon and the desires of the patient. However, there is not one strategy for achieving all of the goals of breast augmentation for every patient. Recognizing that augmentation mammaplasty is both a science *and* an art, it is imperative that the surgical approach, the creation of the implant pocket, the implant selection, and the implant position must always be tailored to the individual patient.

EDITORIAL COMMENTS

Drs. Maxwell, Baker, and Gabriel have provided an in-depth review of the history of breast implants and provide numerous clinical pearls that will be useful to the plastic surgeon performing augmentation mammaplasty. With regard to the history of breast implants, I have one additional comment. It was very interesting to perform a PubMed Internet search of "silicone gel breast implants." Prior to 1990, there were 8 indexed references, and from 1990 to 2009, there were 874 indexed references. The safety and efficacy of these devices have been clearly demonstrated based on the myriad of scientific publications.

Currently, the FDA permits the used of smooth, round silicone gel implants for breast augmentation. Final approval for the use of anatomic silicone gel implants for breast augmentation is pending. Many women have decided to pursue breast augmentation using silicone gel devices. The use of saline devices continues; however, interest in these devices is slowly declining.

The remainder of this chapter was concerned with patient and implant selection, operative technique, and postoperative care. It provided a thorough discussion of the relevant issues regarding breast augmentation from one of the leading authorities in the world. It is wonderfully prepared, with outstanding illustrations and relevant references.

M.Y.N.

REFERENCES

1. Shipley RH, O'Donnell JM, Bader KF. Personality characteristics of women seeking breast augmentation, comparison to small-busted and average-busted controls. *Plast Reconstr Surg* 1997;60(3):369–376.
2. Baker JL Jr, Kolin IS, Bartlett ES. Psychosexual dynamics of patients undergoing mammary augmentation. *Plast Reconstr Surg* 1974;53(6):652–659.
3. American Society of Plastic Surgeons. Press release: More than 8.7 million cosmetic plastic surgery procedures in 2003—up 32% over 2002. Available at: http://www.plasticsurgery.org/Media/Press_Releases/More_Than_87_Million_Cosmetic_Plastic_Surgery_Procedures_in_2003.html. Accessed July 9, 2010.
4. Czerny V. Plastic replacement of the breast with a lipoma [in German]. *Chir Kong Verhandl* 1895;2:216.

5. Longacre JJ. Correction of the hypoplastic breast with special reference to reconstruction of the "nipple type breast" with local dermofat pedicle flaps. *Plast Reconstr Surg* 1954;14:431.
6. Picha GJ, Batra MK. Breast augmentation. In: Achauer BM, Eriksson E, Guyuron B, et al, eds. *Plastic Surgery: Indications, Operations, and Outcomes.* 1st ed. St. Louis, MO: Mosby; 2000:2743–2756.
7. Institute of Medicine. *Safety of Silicone Breast Implants.* Washington, DC: National Academy Press; 1999.
8. Uchida J. Clinical application of crosslinked dimethylpolysiloxane, restoration of the breast, cheeks, atrophy of infantile paralysis, funnel-shaped chest, etc. *Jpn J Plast Reconstr Surg* 1961;4:303.
9. Boo-Chai K. The complications of augmentation mammaplasty by silicone injection. *Br J Plast Surg* 1969;22:281.
10. Ortiz-Monasterio F, Trigos I. Management of patients with complications from injections of foreign materials into the breasts. *Plast Reconstr Surg* 1972;50(1):42–47.
11. Cronin TD, Gerow FJ. Augmentation mammaplasty: a new "natural feel" prosthesis. In: *Transactions of the Third International Congress of Plastic Surgery.* Amsterdam: Excerpta Medica; 1963;41–49.
12. Arion HG. Presentation d'une prothese retromammaire. *J Soc Fr Gynecol* 1965;35:421.
13. Regnault P, Baker TJ, Gleason MC. Clinical trial and evaluation of a proposed new inflatable mammary prosthesis. *Plast Reconstr Surg* 1972;50:220.
14. Young VL, Watson ME. Breast implant research. *Clin Plast Surg* 2001;28(3):451–83.
15. Lavine DM. Saline inflatable prostheses: 14 years' experience. *Aesthet Plast Surg* 1993;17:325–330.
16. Brody OS. Silicone technology for the plastic surgeon. *Clin Plast Surg* 1988;15(4):517–520.
17. Barnard JJ, Todd EL, Wilson WG, et al. Distribution of organosilicone polymers in augmentation mammaplasties at autopsy. *Plast Reconstr Surg* 1997;100(1):197–203.
18. Thomsen JL, Christensen L, Nielsen M, et al. Histologic changes and silicone concentrations in human breast tissue surrounding silicone breast prostheses. *Plast Reconstr Surg* 1990;85(1):38–41.
19. Baeke JL. Breast deformity caused by anatomical or teardrop implant rotation. *Plast Reconstr Surg* 2002;109(7):2555–2567.
20. Miyoshi K, Miyamura T, Kobayashi Y. Hypergammaglobulinemia by prolonged adjuvanticity in men: disorders developed after augmentation mammaplasty. *Jpn Med J* 1964;9:2122.
21. Endo LP, Edwards NL, Longley S. Silicone and rheumatic diseases. *Semin Arthritis Rheum* 1987;17:112.
22. Spiera H. Scieroderma after silicone augmentation mammaplasty. *JAMA* 1988;260:236.
23. Van Nunen SA, Gatenby PA, Basten A. Post-mammoplasty connective tissue disease. *Arthritis Rheum* 1982;25:694.
24. Spear SL, Mardini S. Alternative filler materials and new implant designs: what's available and what's on the horizon? *Clin Plast Surg* 2001;28(3):435–443.
25. Schnur PL, Weinzweig J, Harris JB, et al. Silicon analysis of breast periprosthetic capsular tissue from patients with saline or silicone gel breast implants. *Plast Reconstr Surg* 1996;98(5):798–803.
26. Robrich RJ, Hollier LH, Robinson JB. Determining the safety of the silicone envelope: in search of a silicone antibody. *Plast Reconstr Surg* 1996;98(3):455–458.
27. Edworthy SM, Martin L, Barr SG, et al. A clinical study of the relationship between silicone breast implants and connective tissue disease. *J Rheum* 1998;25(2):254–260.
28. Gabriel SE, O'Fallon WM, Kurland LT, et al. Risk of connective-tissue diseases and other disorders after breast implantation. *N Engl J Med* 1994;330(24):1697–702.
29. Park AJ, Black RJ, Sarhadi NS, et al. Silicone gel-filled breast implants and connective tissue diseases. *Plast Reconstr Surg* 1998;101(2):261–268.
30. Schusterman MA, Kroll SS, Reece GP, et al. Incidence of autoimmune disease in patients after breast reconstruction with silicone gel implants versus autogenous tissue: a preliminary report. *Ann Plast Surg* 1993;31(1):1–6.
31. Sanchez-Guerrero J, Colditz GA, Karison EW, et al. Silicone breast implants and the risk of connective-tissue diseases and symptoms. *N Engl J Med* 1995;332(25):1666–1670.
32. Tebbetts JB. Dual plane breast augmentation: optimizing implant-soft-tissue relationships in a wide range of breast types. *Plast Reconstr Surg* 2001;107(5):1255–1272.
33. Tebbetts JB. A system for breast implant selection based on patient tissue characteristics and implant-soft tissue dynamics. *Plast Reconstr Surg* 2002;109(4):1396–1409.
34. Biggs TM, Yarish RS. Augmentation mammaplasty: retropectoral versus retromammary implantation. *Clin Plast Surg* 1988;15(4):549–555.
35. Regnault P. Partially submuscular breast augmentation. *Plast Reconstr Surg* 1977;59(1):72–76.
36. Graf RM, Bernardes A, Auersvald A, et al. Subfascial endoscopic transaxillary augmentation mammaplasty. *Aesthet Plast Surg* 2000;24:216–220.
37. Graf RM, Bernardes A, Rippel R, et al. Subfascial breast implant: a new procedure. *Plast Reconstr Surg* 2003;111(2):904–908.
38. Ashley FL. A new type of breast prosthesis: preliminary report. *Plast Reconstr Surg* 1970;45(5):421–424.
39. Barone FE, Perry L, Keller T, et al. The biomechanical and histopathologic effects of surface texturing with silicone and polyurethane in tissue implantation and expansion. *Plast Reconstr Surg* 1992;90(1):77–86.
40. Capozzi A, Pennisi YR. Clinical experience with polyurethane-covered gel-filled mammary prosthesis. *Plast Reconstr Surg* 1981;68(4):512–518.
41. Gasperoni C, Salgarello M, Gargani G. Polyurethane-covered mammary implants: a 12-year experience. *Ann Plast Surg* 1992;29(4):303–308.
42. Herman S. The Même implant. *Plast Reconstr Surg* 1984;73(3):411–414.
43. Hester TR, Tebbetts JB, Maxwell GP. The polyurethane-covered mammary prosthesis: facts and fiction (II). *Clin Plast Surg* 2001;28(3):579–586.
44. Burkhardt BR, Eades E. The effect of Biocell texturing and povidone-iodine irrigation on capsular contracture around saline-inflatable breast implants. *Plast Reconstr Surg* 1995;96(6):1317–1325.
45. Hakelius L, Ohisén L. Tendency to capsular contracture around smooth and textured gel-filled silicone mammary implants: a 5-year follow-up. *Plast Reconstr Surg* 1997;100(6):1566–1569.
46. Tarpila E, Ghassemifar R, Fagrell D, et al. Capsular contracture with textured versus smooth saline-filled implants for breast augmentation: a prospective clinical study. *Plast Reconstr Surg* 1997;99(7):1934–1939.
47. Burkhardt BR, Demas CP. The effect of Siltex texturing and povidone-iodine irrigation on capsular contracture around saline inflatable breast implants. *Plast Reconstr Surg* 1994;93(1):123–128.
48. Bronz G. A comparison of naturally shaped and round implants. *Aesthet Surg J* 2002;22(3):238–246.
49. Hobar PC, Gutowski K. Experience with anatomic breast implants. *Clin Plast Surg* 2001;28(3):553–559.
50. Niechajef I. Mammary augmentation by cohesive silicone gel implants with anatomic shape: technical considerations. *Aesthet Plast Surg* 2001;25:397–403.
51. Panettiere P, Marchetti L, Accorsi D. Rotation of anatomic prostheses: a possible cause of breast deformity. *Aesthet Plast Surg* 2004;28:348–353.
52. Hidalgo DA. Breast augmentation: choosing the optimal incision, implant and pocket plane. *Plast Reconstr Surg* 2000;105(6):2202–2216.
53. Jenny J. The areolar approach to augmentation mammaplasty. *Int J Aesthet Plast Surg* 1972(fall).
54. Hoehler H. Breast augmentation: the axillary approach. *Br J Plast Surg* 1977;26:373.
55. de Cholnoky T. Augmentation mammaplasty: survey of complications in 10,941 patients by 265 surgeons. *Plast Reconstr Surg* 1970;45:573.
56. Handel N. Managing local implant-related problems. In: Spear SL, ed. *Surgery of the Breast: Principles and Art.* 1st ed. Philadelphia: Lippincott-Raven;1998:953–968.
57. Williams C, Aston S, Rees TD. The effect of hematoma on the thickness of pseudosheath around silicone implants. *Plast Reconstr Surg* 1975;56:194.
58. Baker JL Jr. Classification of spherical contractures. Presented at the Aesthetic Breast Symposium, Scottsdale, Arizona, 1975.
59. Barker DE, Retsky MI, Schultz S. "Bleeding" of silicone from bag-gel breast implants, and its clinical relation to fibrous capsule reaction. *Plast Reconstr Surg* 1978;61(6):836–841.
60. Burkhardt BR. Fibrous capsular contracture around breast implants: the role of subclinical infection. *Infect Surg* 1985;4:469.
61. Courtiss EH, Goldwyn RM, Anastazi GW. The fate of breast implants with infections around them. *Plast Reconstr Surg* 1979;63:812–816.
62. Dobke MK, Svabn JK, Vastine VL, et al. Characterization of microbial presence at the surface of silicone mammary implants. *Ann Plast Surg* 1995;34(6):563–569.
63. Virden CP, Dobke MK, Stein P, et al. Subclinical infection of the silicone breast implant surface as a possible cause of capsular contracture. *Aesthet Plast Surg* 1992;16:173–179.
64. Schlesinger SL, Ellenbogen R, Desvigne MN, et al. Zafirlukast (Accolate): a new treatment for capsular contracture. *Aesthet Surg J* 2002;22(4):329–336.
65. Spear SL, Carter ME, Ganz JC. The correction of capsular contracture by conversion to "dual-plane" positioning: technique and outcomes. *Plast Reconstr Surg* 2003;112(2):456–466.
66. Inamed. News release. Inamed files 7-year deflation rate data for its saline-filled breast implants post approval survey study with FDA; August 12, 2004.
67. Cohen BE, Biggs TM, Cronin ED, et al. Assessment and longevity of the silicone gel breast implant. *Plast Reconstr Surg* 1997;99(6):1597–1601.
68. Cook RR, Bowlin SJ, Curtis JM, et al. Silicone gel breast implant rupture rates: research issues. *Ann Plast Surg* 2002;48(1):92–101.
69. Hölmich LR, Vejborg TM, Conrad C, et al. Untreated silicone breast implant rupture. *Plast Reconstr Surg* 2004;114(1):204–214.
70. Maxwell GP, Hammond DC. Breast implants: smooth versus textured. *Adv Plast Reconstr Surg* 1993;9:209.
71. Maxwell GP, Hartley W. Breast augmentation. In: Mathes SJ, Hentz VR, eds. *Plastic Surgery.* 2nd ed. Philadelphia: Elsevier; 2006:1–34.
72. Cunningham B, McCue J. Safety and effectiveness of Mentor's MemoryGel implants at 6 years. *Aesthetic Plast Surg.* 2009;33(3):440–4.
73. Spear SL, Murphy DK, Slicton A, et al. Inamed silicone breast implant core study results at 6 years. *Plast Reconstr Surg* 2007;120:8S.
74. Cunningham B. The Mentor study on contour profile gel silicone MemoryGel breast implants. *Plast Reconstr Surg* 2007;120:33S.
75. Bengtson BP, Van Natta BW, Murphy DK, et al. Style 410 highly cohesive silicone breast implant core study results at 3 years. *Plast Reconstr Surg* 2007;120:40S.
76. Maxwell GP, Gabriel A. Use of the acellular dermal matrix in revisionary aesthetic breast surgery. *Aesthet Surg J* 2009;29(6):485–93.
77. Maxwell GP, Birchenough SA, Gabriel A. Efficacy of neopectoral pocket in revisionary breast surgery. *Aesthet Surg J* 2009;29(5):379–85.

CHAPTER

107

William P. Adams Jr.

The High Five Process: Tissue-based Planning for Breast Augmentation

INTRODUCTION

Breast augmentation has recently been reported to be the first or second most common surgical procedure in plastic surgery (1). Within the last 5 years, the discipline of breast augmentation has been recognized as being not just a surgical procedure but as a process that involves four subprocesses (2):

1. Patient education
2. Tissue-based preoperative planning
3. Refined surgical technique
4. Defined postoperative care

Tissue-based preoperative planning is the second of the four components of the process of breast augmentation that is essential to obtaining reproducible results in breast augmentation while at the same time minimizing the reoperation rate (2). Although preoperative planning has historically been performed subjectively by surgeons, in the last 15 years the reoperation rate at 3 years in multiple premarket approval Food and Drug Administration (FDA) studies has been 15% to 20%, reflecting the unscientific and often arbitrary approach to implant selection. Recent advances in tissue-based planning have demonstrated not only a simplified method of planning, but also one that matches implants to patient tissues and breast dimensions; it has produced superior patient outcomes. There are different "systems" for implant selection; most are not true tissue-based systems that take a set of breast measurements and then use those data directly to derive options for implant selection that "fits" that breast. Actually, very few systems can claim to be tissue-based systems based on that definition. The most recently described tissue-based planning system is the "high five" process (3). The high five process was developed over 15 years, and this third-generation system codifies the five most important decisions surgeons make during the preoperative planning phase that affect patient outcomes.

Accurate planning is not unique to breast augmentation but is relevant in all professions and results in success in areas from business ventures to sporting endeavors. Surgeons often ask, "How do I pick the implant?" "What implant gives the best results?" "What implant do patients like best?" The truth is that it is not about the implant, but rather the process, or more specifically the process of breast augmentation (2). In fact, in a recent FDA implant premarket approval application (PMA) hearing, although the devices were discussed, the next most visible concerns were about complications in patient reoperation rates.

The bottom line in selecting breast implants is that it is about "wishes versus tissues." In other words, patients wish they looked like a actress or a model on the cover of a magazine, or want to have breast implants the same size as their friend, who may have a totally different breast/body type. However, what really matters is their tissues and to assess these objectively and to match the implant to the tissues specifically.

The concepts of tissue-based planning are well established in the plastic surgery literature. In published and peer-reviewed series as well as national presentations in the last few years, there have been more than 2,500 primary breast augmentations (4–6) performed with similar concepts to tissue-based preoperative planning with reoperation rates of less than 3% with 6- to 7-year follow-up, compared to the reoperation rate of 15% to 20% within 3 years in all the PMA studies in the last 15 years.

The immediate predecessor to the high five process was a tissue-based planning system developed by Tebbetts (7). This was the first tissue-based system of its kind. It prioritized the tissues of the patient as the most important factor, contrary to previous generations such as the McGhan BioDimensional system, which prioritized the desired result (i.e., desired intermammary distance, or desired breast projection) of the patient or surgeon over the tissue. The TEPID system (tissue characteristics of the envelope, parenchyma, and implant and dimensions and filler dynamics of the implant) was primarily a tool to determine tissue-based implant volume, and some aspects of the acronym were difficult for many surgeons. In the current third-generation high five process the five critical preoperative decisions that determine outcomes have been codified and put into a simple, easy-to-follow algorithm for patient assessment that can be performed in less than 5 minutes.

THE HIGH FIVE PROCESS: HOW IT WORKS IN CLINICAL PRACTICE

The five critical decisions in the high five process include the following:

1. Implant coverage/pocket planning
2. Implant size/volume
3. Implant type
4. Inframammary fold position
5. Incision

The high five process has been found to be safe and simple. It leaves the control totally up to the surgeon and gets the surgeon "on base." The process is applicable to all implant types, including regular gel, highly cohesive form-stable gel, and saline implants. It is effective and proven, and, most important, it is transferable, meaning that surgeons, residents, patient coordinators, and even patients have successfully used this system to objectively select implants appropriately for a given patient's breast.

There are four primary measurements:

1. Pinch thickness in the superior (SPP) and inferior pole (IPP) of the breast. These measurements assess tissue coverage.

Consideration of a subglandular or subfascial pocket should only be entertained for a SPP of 3 cm or greater. The original high five paper used 2 cm as a cutoff; however, it is clear that even 2 cm may not be adequate 3 to 5 years postoperative. The inferior pole pinch assesses the tissue thickness along the inframammary fold (IMF). If IPP is less than 5 mm, consideration may be given to not dividing the inferior pectoralis origins (dual plane 1) but instead a traditional retropectoral pocket plane to maximize inferior coverage. (See Fig. 107.1A, B.)

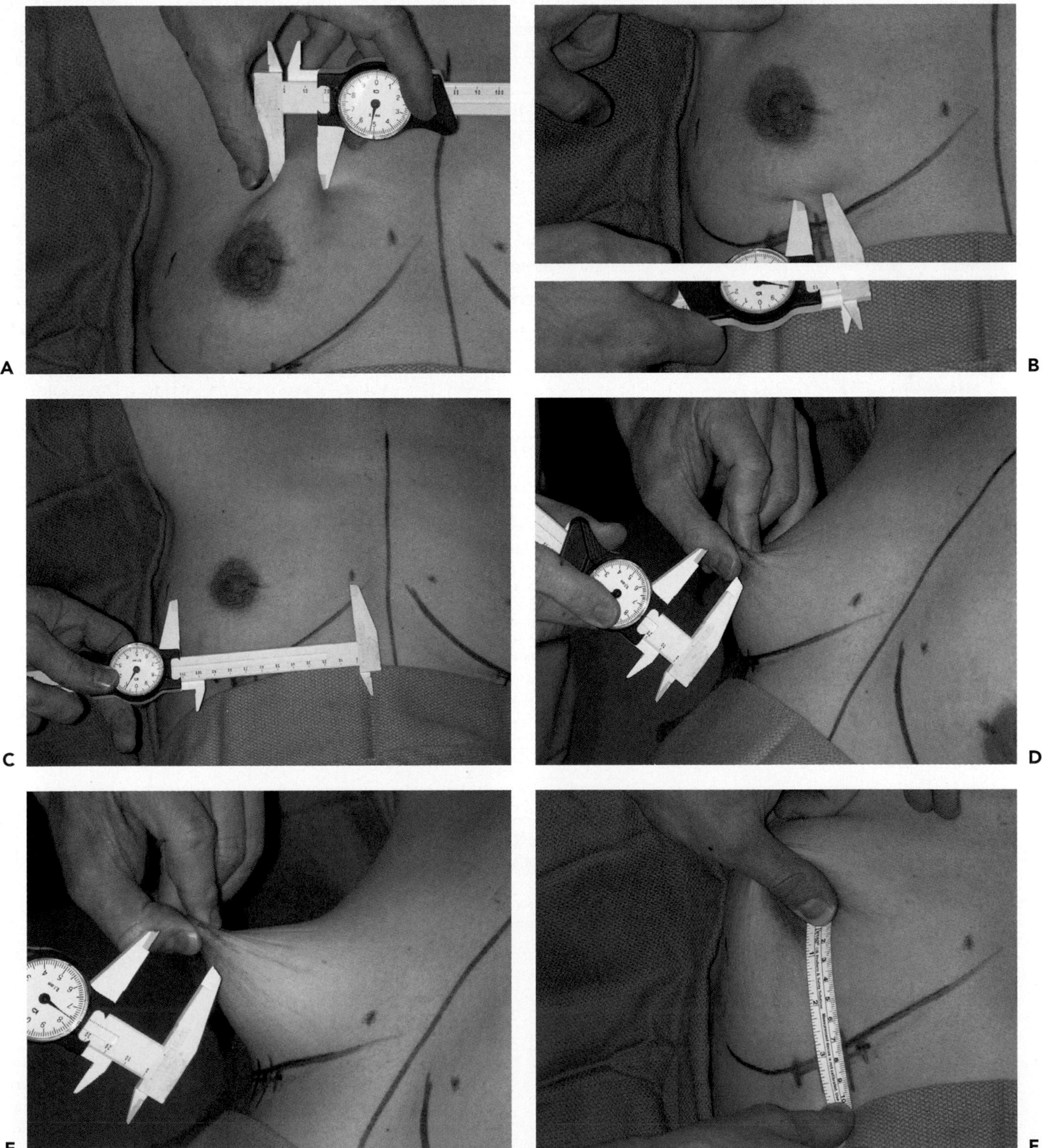

Figure 107.1. **A, B:** Pinch thickness in the superior pole (SPP) and inferior pole (IPP) of the breast to assess tissue coverage. **C:** Breast base width (BW), the cornerstone measurement and the first of two key measurements to determine implant volume. **D, E:** The second of the two measurements for implant selection. This is an objective measurement of the skin envelope. **F:** Nipple-to-inframammary fold on stretch.

High Five^{TM} Tissue Analysis and Operative Planning

Patient Name:		**Date:**	
1. COVERAGE - Selecting Pocket Location to Optimize Soft Tissue Coverage Short- and Long-Term			
SPP		If <2.0 cm., consider dual plane (DP) or partial retropectoral (PRP, pectoralis origins intact across IMF)	DP 1 2 3 PRP RM/SG
IPP		If STPTIMF <0.5 cm, consider subpectoral pocket and leave pectoralis origins intact along IMF	
POCKET LOCATION SELECTED BASED ON THICKNESS OF TISSUE COVERAGE			

2. IMPLANT VOLUME/ WEIGHT - Selecting an Estimated Implant Volume for Optimal Envelope Fill													
		Estimating Desired Breast Implant Volume Based on Breast Measurements and Tissue Characteristics											
Base Width		B.W. Parenchyma (cm)	10.5	11.0	11.5	12.0	12.5	13.0	13.5	14.0	14.5	15.0	
		Initial Volume (cc)	200	250	275	300	300	325	350	375	375	400	cc
$APSS_{MaxStr}$		[2]If APSS < 2.0, - 30cc; If APSS > 3.0, + 30cc; If APSS > 4.0, +60cc Place appropriate number in blank at right											cc
$N:IMF_{MaxSt}$		If N:IMF > 9.5, + 30cc Place appropriate number in blank at right											cc
PCSEF %		If PCSEF < 20%, + 30cc; If PCSEF > 80%, - 30cc Place appropriate number in blank at right											cc
Pt. request													cc
[7]**NET ESTIMATED VOLUME** TO FILL ENVELOPE BASED ON PATIENT TISSUE CHARACTERISTICS													cc

3. IMPLANT DIMENSIONS, TYPE, MANUFACTURER- Selecting specific implant characteristics					
Implant Manufacturer	Implant Style/Shape/Shell/Filler Material	Implant Vol/wt (cc/ g)	*Implant Base Width	Breast Base Width[1]	Implant Projection
		Cc/Gm	cm.	cm.	cm.
*For optimal long-term coverage, implant base width should not exceed base width of patient's existing parenchyma, even if wider IMD results.					

4. IMF LOCATION- Estimating desired postoperative inframammary fold position										
(Circle Volume closest *to net estimated implant volume* calculated above, and *circle suggested N:IMF* in the cell beneath that volume)										
		Volume closest to calculated "total estimated implant volume" above	200	250	275	300	325	350	375	400
		Recommended new N:IMF distance (cm.) under maximal stretch ▶	7.0	7.0	7.5	8	8.25	8.5	9.0	9.5
*Planning Level of New Inframammary Fold**		Transfer the patient's $N:IMF_{MaxSt}$ measurement from above to corresponding cell at right. Then transfer the Hi-5 recommended new N:IMF to the corresponding cell at right. If the patient's preop N:IMF is shorter than the Hi-5 recommended new N:IMF, consider lowering the fold. If the patient's preop N:IMF is equal to or greater than the Hi-5 recommended new N:IMF, no change in IMF position is indicated.			Patient's Preop $N:IMF_{MaxSt}$		Hi-5 Recomded $N:IMF_{MaxSt}$		Change In Fold Position	Lower Fold
					cm.		cm.		Yes /No	cm.
*Other factors may affect optimal IMF level and require surgeons to modifiy the recommendations for N:IMF										

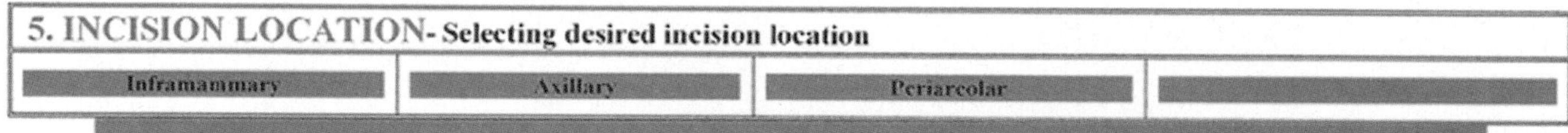

5. INCISION LOCATION- Selecting desired incision location			
Inframammary	Axillary	Periareolar	

Figure 107.2. The high five tissue analysis and operative planning sheet, which can be used to summarize the findings of the measurements and to make decisions.

2. Breast base width (BW). This is the cornerstone measurement and the first of two key measurements to determine implant volume. This should be measured as if it represents the actual width of the pocket in which the implant will rest. The BW is measured from the parasternal border at the pectoralis major origins transversely using a caliper to a point just medial to the most lateral part of the breast at the widest transverse aspect of the breast (usually across the nipple). The BW is actually always smaller than the actual true width of the breast. The caliper yields a linear measurement. Using a tape measure over the dome of the breast will yield a falsely increased BW and should be avoided. (See Fig. 107.1C.)
3. Skin stretch (SS). This is the second of the two measurements for implant selection. This is an objective measurement of the skin envelope. Many surgeons tend to characterize the skin envelope as tight or loose; however, these are too subjective and do not allow consistent evaluation. This measurement is easily taken by grasping the medial areolar border and then pulling anteriorly on maximum stretch (within patient comfort level) and measuring the anteroposterior excursion with a caliper. A measurement of 2 to

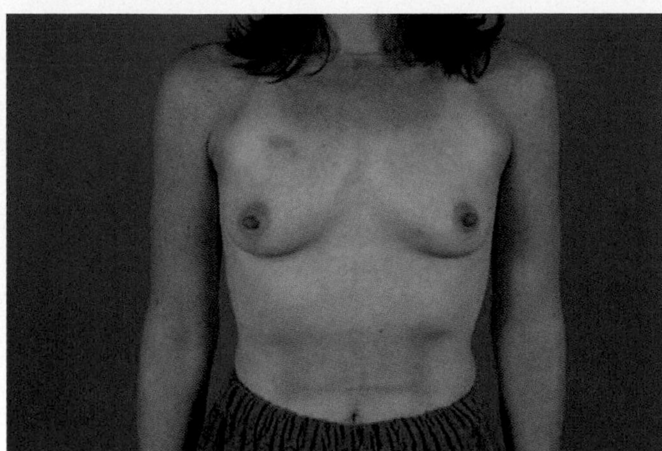

Figure 107.3. Anteroposterior view of a 31-year-old woman who desires breast augmentation. Superior pole thickness is 2.5 cm, base breast width is 12.5 cm, skin stretch is 1.5 cm, nipple-to-inframammary fold distance is 6.5 cm, and parenchyma to stretched envelope file is 50%.

3 cm is normal, less than 2 cm is tight, and 3 to 4 cm is loose. A measurement of greater than 4 cm may indicate a degree of laxity that is incompatible with getting an adequate result with an augmentation alone without a skin-tightening procedure. (See Fig. 107.1D, E.)

4. Nipple to IMF on stretch. This measurement is taken with a flexible tape measure under maximum stretch from the midnipple to the IMF at the center of the breast. The measurement assesses skin laxity, as well as provides information for incision planning. (See Fig. 107.1F.)

The high five tissue analysis and operative planning sheet can be used to summarize the findings of the measurements and to make decisions (Fig. 107.2). Figure 107.3 shows the critical measurements of a 31-year-old woman desiring breast augmentation.

DECISIONS TO BE MADE

1. Coverage. This is the most important decision because the consequences of inadequate implant coverage are very difficult to correct. This decision is primarily based on the pinch thickness in the upper pole. If pinch thickness is less than 2 cm, a subpectoral or dual plane-type pocket plan is advisable to try to maintain adequate coverage over the implant, particularly long term. If the pinch thickness in the upper pole is greater than 2 cm, preferably greater than 3.0 cm, a subglandular pocket plane may be considered. However, it is my practice to generally place most implants in the dual-plane position, given the trade-offs of the subglandular versus the subpectoral position. (See Fig. 107.4.)
2. Implant volume. Implant volume is determined by the high five nomogram that is provided in the system. The base width is measured as demonstrated in the planning sheet. There is an initial implant volume associated with a given base width. Next, adjustments of the implant volume are made based on the skin stretch and the amount of parenchyma present. Adjustments may also be made based on patient requests, whether a patient is asking to be larger or smaller. These values are totaled, and a net estimated volume to optimally fill the given breast envelope is obtained. (See Fig. 107.5.)
3. Implant type. The implant type is selected. This is based on patient request and surgeon recommendation. The implant volume from step 2 is used as a reference. The implant spec sheets may be reviewed, and the patient's base width is compared in an implant that is similar to or slightly less in width than the patient's base width of similar volume, as calculated in step 2, and the implant type is selected. (See Fig. 107.6.)
4. Selection of the optimal IMF position. This is based on some consistent relationships between the width of the breast and the nipple-to-fold length. It is important to know where the IMF position will be postoperatively. When using the IMF incision this information allows the surgeon to place the incision directly in the postoperative IMF. The high five system provides these relationships, and this can simply be followed based on the measurements. The details can be found in the original report (3). Some surgeons have a difficult time following this concept; however, after 10 cases following these simple steps, the ease, predictability, and reproducibility of the procedure should be evident. (See Fig. 107.7.)
5. Incision. The final decision is the incision. Although this is frequently talked about, the incision is the least important of all five and is again based on patient request, surgeon recommendation, and surgeon skill set. (See Fig. 107.8.)

CONSEQUENCES

Using this system, all important preoperative decisions may be made in approximately 5 minutes, allowing the surgeon to very reproducibly match the implant to the given patient's breast tissues and dimensions. This allows for several important

High Five™ Tissue Analysis and Operative Planning

Patient Name: JP		Date: 4-20-2006	
1. COVERAGE - Selecting Pocket Location to Optimize Soft Tissue Coverage Short- and Long-Term			
SPP	2.5	~~If <2.0 cm, consider dual plane (DP) or partial retropectoral (PRP, pectoralis origins intact across IMF)~~	DP 1 2 3
IPP	1	If STPTIMF <0.5 cm, consider subpectoral pocket and leave pectoralis origins intact along IMF	PRP
POCKET LOCATION SELECTED BASED ON THICKNESS OF TISSUE COVERAGE			RM/SG

Figure 107.4. The superior pole pinch is 2.5 cm. A dual-plane, one-pocket plane is selected.

2. IMPLANT VOLUME/ WEIGHT - Selecting an Estimated Implant Volume for Optimal Envelope Fill													
		Estimating Desired Breast Implant Volume Based on Breast Measurements and Tissue Characteristics											
Base Width	12.5	B.W. Parenchyma (cm)	10.5	11.0	11.5	12.0	12.5	13.0	13.5	14.0	14.5	15.0	
		Initial Volume (cc)	200	250	275	300	300	[illegible]	[illegible]	[illegible]	[illegible]	[illegible]	300 cc
$APSS_{MaxStr}$	1.5	[2]If APSS < 2.0, - 30cc; If APSS > 3.0, + 30cc; If APSS > 4.0, +60cc Place appropriate number in blank at right											-30 cc
$N:IMF_{MaxSt}$	6.5	If N:IMF > 9.5, + 30cc Place appropriate number in blank at right											- cc
PCSEF %	50%	If PCSEF < 20%, + 30cc; If PCSEF > 80%, - 30cc Place appropriate number in blank at right											- cc
Pt. request	-												cc
[7]NET ESTIMATED VOLUME TO FILL ENVELOPE BASED ON PATIENT TISSUE CHARACTERISTICS													270 cc

Figure 107.5. Base breast width is 12.5 cm for an initial implant volume of 300 cc. A reduction of 30 cc is subtracted for a tight envelope, indicated by a skin stretch less than 2 cm (1.5 cm in this case). The total represents the optimal fill volume for that individual breast tissue type.

3. IMPLANT DIMENSIONS, TYPE, MANUFACTURER- Selecting specific implant characteristics					
Implant Manufacturer	Implant Style/Shape/Shell/Filler Material	Implant Vol/wt (cc/ g)	*Implant Base Width	Breast Base Width[1]	Implant Projection
Inamed	Style 10	270 Gm	12.2 cm.	12.5 cm.	3.3 cm.
*For optimal long-term coverage, implant base width should not exceed base width of patient's existing parenchyma, even if wider IMD results.					

Style 10		
Implant Volume (cc)	Diameter (CM)	Projection (CM)
120	9.4	2.5
150	10.1	2.7
180	10.7	2.9
210	11.2	3.0
240	11.7	3.2
270	12.2	3.3
300	12.6	3.5
330	13.0	3.6
360	13.4	3.7
390	13.6	3.8
420	14.0	3.8
450	14.4	3.9
480	14.8	3.9

Style 15		
Implant Volume (cc)	Diameter (CM)	Projection (CM)
213	10.6	3.5
234	10.9	3.6
265	11.4	3.7
286	11.7	3.8
301	11.9	4.0
339	12.4	4.0
371	12.9	4.1
397	13.1	4.2
421	13.3	4.3
457	13.7	4.5
492	14.0	4.6
533	14.4	4.7
575	14.8	4.8

Style 20		
Implant Volume (cc)	Diameter (CM) A	Projection (CM) B
325	11.2	4.6
350	11.4	4.9
375	11.7	4.9
400	11.9	5.0
425	12.0	5.2
450	12.4	5.2
475	12.6	5.5
500	13.0	5.2
550	13.5	5.6
600	13.8	5.7
650	14.2	5.9

Figure 107.6. The desired volume (step 2) is 270 cc. The implant specification sheets are reviewed. The patient desired a round silicone gel implant. The data sheets for the Inamed/Allergan styles 10, 15, and 20 implants are depicted. The best match of an implant about 270 cc with a base diameter of 12.5 cm or less is chosen: style 10, 270 cc, implant base width 12.2 cm.

4. IMF LOCATION- Estimating desired postoperative inframammary fold position										
(Circle Volume closest *to net estimated implant volume* calculated above, and *circle suggested N:IMF* in the cell beneath that volume)										
		Volume closest to calculated "total estimated implant volume" above	200	250	275	300	325	350	375	400
		Recommended new N:IMF distance (cm.) under maximal stretch▶	7.0	7.0	7.5	8	8.25	8.5	9.0	9.5
*Planning Level of New Inframammary Fold**	Transfer the patient's $N:IMF_{MaxSt}$ measurement from above to corresponding cell at right. Then transfer the Hi-5 recommended new N:IMF to the corresponding cell at right. If the patient's preop N:IMF is shorter than the Hi-5 recommended new N:IMF, consider lowering the fold. If the patient's preop N:IMF is equal to or greater than the Hi-5 recommended new N:IMF, no change in IMF position is indicated.		Patient's Preop $N:IMF_{MaxSt}$		Hi-5 Recomded $N:IMF_{MaxSt}$		Change In Fold Position		Lower Fold	
			6.5 cm.		7.5 cm.		Yes /No		1 cm.	
*Other factors may affect optimal IMF level and require surgeons to modifiy the recommendations for N:IMF										

Figure 107.7. Determining the inframammary fold position with objective data.

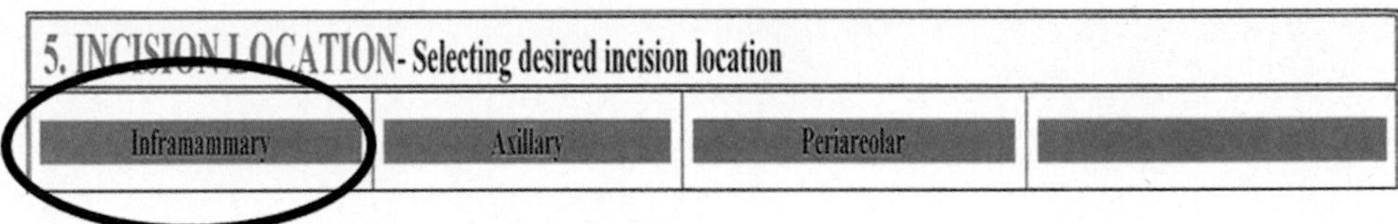

- Patient desires/ input
- Surgeon's key points
  - Control of the procedure for surgeon
  - Minimizing tissue trauma
  - Avoiding injury to neural and vascular structures
  - Effect on implant

Figure 107.8. Incision and key factors.

consequences, which include allowing the patient's surgeon to go to the operating room with all of the important decisions made. This allows the third step (the operative technique) of the process of breast augmentation to proceed in a very logical fashion. See Figure 107.9 for the final result.

DISCUSSION

The high five process allows the surgeon to make all important decisions that determine outcomes preoperatively. Included in this system is a tissue-based system for selecting breast implant size to match the implant to the patient's breast tissues and dimensions. Although different methodologies have been proposed for implant selection, it is important to make a distinction regarding what systems are actually tissue based.

A tissue-based planning system directly uses the data from the breast analysis to lead the surgeon to appropriate choices of implants. Unfortunately, if one looks critically at many of the popular methodologies, one sees that they do not lead to implant choices based on objective data. The concept that a surgeon could choose a low-, moderate-, or high-profile implant all of the same 12-cm BW for a given breast with a BW = 12 cm is a common fallacy and one derived from the typical implant manufacturer implant families or recommendation from non–tissue-based systems. The volumes for this family are typically 250 to 450 cc. The long-term effects and consequences of this range of implant size would be vastly different in a given breast, and this is the precise reason the high five analysis uses primarily the BW and the SS to fine tune the implant volume. In a tight breast envelope a lower volume (approximately 30 cc) should be considered to optimally fill the breast. This recommended volume may be adjusted on the basis of patient request and surgeon judgment. Of interest, the high five process allows the surgeon to adjust the volume on the basis of patient request, and I have found a significant increase of complications when

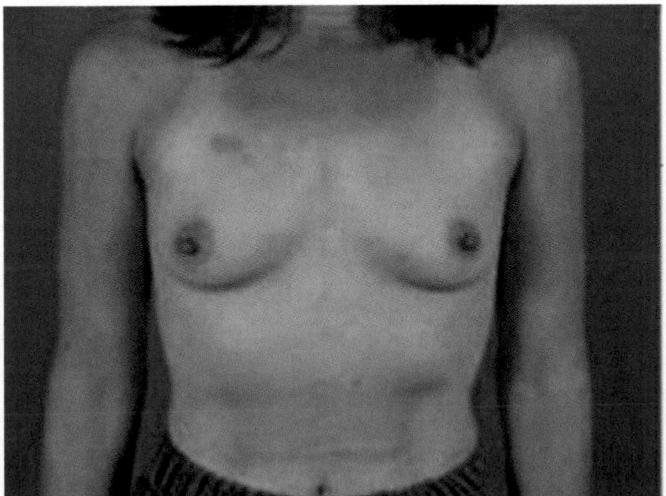

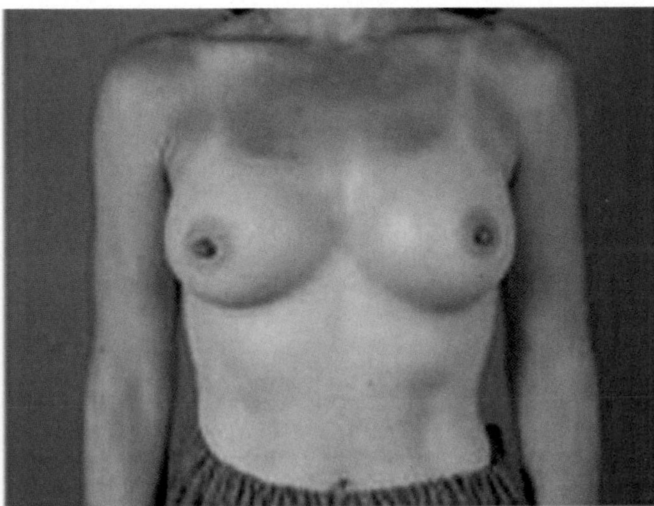

Figure 107.9. Final postoperative result at 1 year. *(continued)*

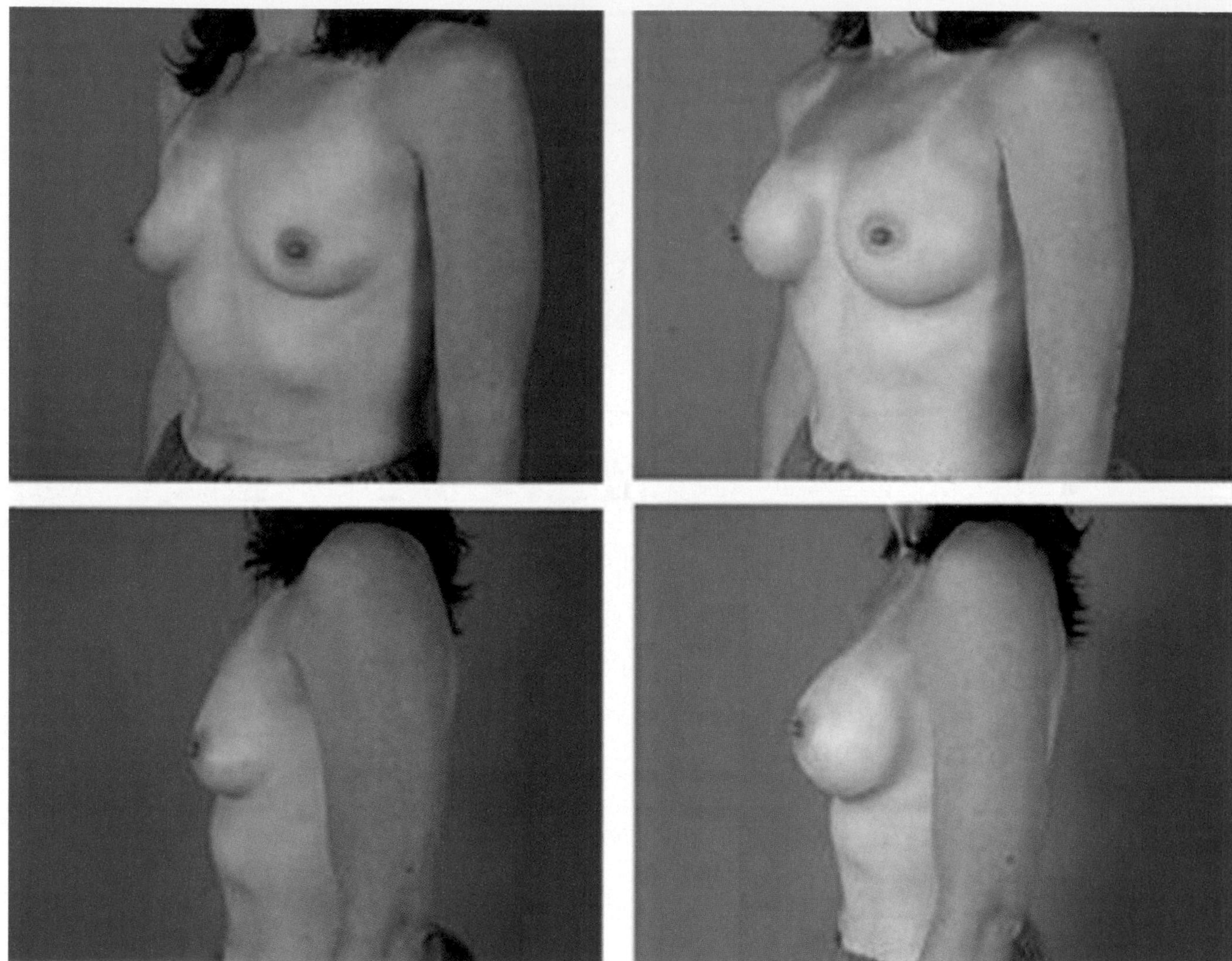

Figure 107.9. (*Continued*)

volume is added above the high five recommended volume, particularly in high-risk patients, that is, those with a narrow BW (less than 11.5 cm) and a tight envelope (SS less than 2 cm) (8).

Tissue-based planning allows the surgeon to easily determine the optimal fill volume of the breast that will give the best shape and cosmetic result, but also the most minimal risk for complication and reoperation based on peer-reviewed and published data. On the basis of this type of planning, patient outcomes, including reoperation rates and recovery, have been optimized. Over time, surgeons will find the use of this system very advantageous for delivering optimal results to their patients.

EDITORIAL COMMENTS

Dr. Adams has provided an excellent overview on the Tebbetts/Adams High 5 Process for planning breast augmentation surgery. The relevance of this system is that it is based on more than 15 years of surgeon experience and placement of thousands of breast implants. The real benefit of this system is that it provides the plastic surgeon with a framework by which to proceed when planning a breast augmentation. It is safe because it is relatively conservative, and it is effective because it is reproducible and patient satisfaction is high. That said, I am sure that there are some surgeons who feel that these concepts do not necessarily apply to their practice. This is because patient expectations following breast augmentation are not uniform; in fact, they are highly variable. On the basis of this system, a surgeon may calculate that a 300-cc device would be optimal, given the properties of a given breast; however, the patient may have been expecting something larger.

The high five protocol was originally described in 2005; however, in this updated version, there have been some changes that should be useful. The basics of the protocol are as follows: (a) coverage is based on tissue thickness; (b) implant volume is based on breast width, which can be adjusted with regard to pinch test, amount of parenchyma, and patient expectations; (c) implant type (round vs. contoured) is based on patient and surgeon factors; (d) there is proper positioning of the IMF; and (e) incision choice is based on patient and surgeon factors. The primary measurements include upper and lower pole pinch thicknesses, base width, skin stretch, and nipple-to-IMF stretch distance. Important recommendations are reviewed. When considering subglandular implant placement, the previous recommendation was for a 2-cm upper pole pinch test. It has now been changed to 3 cm. Skin stretch in excess of 4 cm will usually require an augmentation-mastopexy.

Overall, this is a useful chapter that will usually lead to satisfied patients and surgeons. The concepts are helpful, beneficial, and effective.

M.Y.N.

REFERENCES

1. American Society of Plastic Surgery. 2009 Plastic Surgery Procedural Statistics. Available at: http://www.plasticsurgery.org/Media/Statistics.html. Accessed July 11, 2010.
2. Adams WP Jr. The process of breast augmentation: four sequential steps for optimizing outcomes for patients. *Plast Reconstr Surg* 2008;122:1892.
3. Tebbetts JB, Adams WP Jr. Five critical decisions in breast augmentation. Using five measurements in 5 minutes: the high five decision support process. *Plast Reconstr Surg* 2005;116:2005.
4. Bengtson B. Experience with 410 implant. Presented at the American Association of Aesthetic Plastic Surgery Meeting, New Orleans, Louisiana, April 2005.
5. Jewell M. S8 Breast Education Course. Presented at the American Association of Aesthetic Plastic Surgery Meeting, New Orleans, Louisiana, April 2005.
6. Tebbetts JB. Achieving a zero percent reoperation rate at 3 years in a 50-consecutive-case augmentation mammaplasty premarket approval study. *Plast Reconstr Surg* 2006;118:1453.
7. Tebbetts JB. Breast implant selection based on patient tissue characteristics and dynamics: the TEPID approach. *Plast Reconstr Surg* 2002;190(4):1396–1409.
8. Adams WP Jr. Consequences of implant-soft tissue mismatch in breast augmentation. Manuscript in preparation.

CHAPTER

108

Rebecca Cogwell Anderson
Jason C. Levine

The Augmentation Mammoplasty Patient: Psychological Issues

The breast is a universal symbol representing nourishment, nurturing, love, femininity, and sexuality. The symbolic function of the breast dates to artifacts found in cave drawings (1). By 3,000 BC, external breast prostheses similar to brassieres and corsets were being used by women as a means of altering breast appearance in a culturally desirable manner (2). Throughout history, every civilization has established its standards regarding physical appearance. In American culture (with the exception of the flat, boyish chest popular during the 1920s), full, firm breasts have almost always been considered ideal as a physical attribute for women (3). The vital statistics of the first Miss America in 1921 were 30-25-32. In 1970, they were 34-21-34, and more contemporary winners have reported measurements of 36-21-36 (4). A view of Western culture clearly indicates that prizing women for their appearance is many centuries old. The size and shape of the breasts have classically been included in these appearance standards. The petite early Victorian figure, with its hourglass shape, grew taller and sturdier through the 19th century. In the 20th century, the perfect beauty became tall and statuesque, and breasts were emphasized in the well-developed bosom (5). Allen and Oberle observed that as early as 1946, in an issue of *Cosmopolitan*, an advertisement referred to the lines of a woman's figure as her "Lifeline . . . target of all eyes." The advertisement further implied that a wrong line above the waist could spoil a first impression, impairing the way a woman feels and works. The Life bra was touted as a product that "lifts, holds, corrects, and molds" (6). In 1962, also in a *Cosmopolitan* advertisement, the Bleumette bra was hailed as "the ultimate in bosom loveliness" for it lifted and built "youthful, high lines" (6).

With such a cultural and media focus on the breast, it is not difficult to understand why women have opted to undergo breast enhancement procedures such as augmentation mammoplasty. This chapter deals with the psychological profile of the woman seeking breast augmentation, as well as possible reasons for seeking the procedure. It assesses patient satisfaction with the procedures, both short and long term, and discusses the evolution of the breast implants.

PSYCHOLOGICAL PROFILE OF WOMEN SEEKING AUGMENTATION MAMMOPLASTY

Numerous studies have assessed personality factors associated with patients seeking augmentation mammoplasty. Beale et al. (7) attempted to evaluate the effect of augmentation mammoplasty on women seeking the procedure. They looked for predictors of women who would benefit most from the procedure, and their findings indicated that women who received augmentation mammoplasty were a homogeneous group who experienced very similar breast difficulties. The augmentation mammoplasty patients were noted to be different from the control group in terms of personality and childhood experience. Beale et al. concluded that with the use of personality tests it would be possible to predict which women would benefit most from augmentation mammoplasty. They further concluded that those who scored low on a scale of neurotic tendencies were most likely to be satisfied with the results. Meyer and Ringberg (8) reported that augmentation mammoplasty patients were not psychologically abnormal, apart from their negative evaluation of their physical attractiveness. The augmentation mammoplasty patients in their study generally came from insecure homes with conflicts between parents and unsatisfactory emotional relationships with parents.

Descriptions of women seeking augmentation mammoplasty are very consistent, with a common thread being their doubts about their femininity, which motivate them to request the surgery. It is further postulated that preoccupation with breast size in women seeking augmentation mammoplasty does not arise suddenly, but usually either dates to adolescence or develops after childbirth (1,4,9). Among women seeking augmentation mammoplasty, there is a higher incidence of divorce, unhappy marriages, emotional discomfort, diminished feelings of femininity, and elevated levels of depression than in the general population (1,4,9). Most women seeking augmentation mammoplasty do so while in their 30s and are likely to report concerns about their appearance and preoccupation with inadequate breast size. The typical augmentation mammoplasty patient usually presents as articulate, stylishly dressed, and charming; she is usually wearing a padded brassiere. She projects self-confidence that is believed by some to conceal her insecurities (10,11).

In 1981, Goin and Goin (12), in their comprehensive text regarding the psychological effects of plastic surgery, indicated that it is difficult to truly understand the nature of the augmentation mammoplasty patient. They described the typical patient as likely to be in her early 30s and to have one or more children. She is frequently middle to upper middle-class socioeconomically and has experienced at least one previous aesthetic surgical procedure. They further reported that many augmentation mammoplasty patients have experienced depressive episodes, and they identified three concerns regarding these patients:

1. They believed that an unrecognized depression was often masked by the patient's fixation regarding her breasts.
2. They believed that these patients tended to think obsessively about their physical appearance and to view their self-worth in terms of the physical body.

3. They described these individuals as charming, attractive, outgoing, and socially secure, but noted that this demeanor may act as a protective shell to guard them from their underlying lack of self-esteem.

Sarwer et al. evaluated body image concerns of augmentation patients. They hypothesized that breast augmentation candidates would report greater dissatisfaction with their breasts, greater avoidance of social situations, more frequent appearance-related teasing, and lower self-esteem (13). Results indicated that breast augmentation patients reported a greater investment in their physical appearance. They also reported greater frequency of appearance-related teasing than controls and suggested that this may represent a variable that describes women who seek cosmetic surgery. The majority of breast augmentation patients (77%) reported a significant life change in the year prior to seeking the operation, and 87% reported experiencing increased stress, anxiety, or depressive symptoms during that time, suggesting that the vast majority of breast augmentation candidates may be experiencing psychological distress, which should be assessed and evaluated preoperatively. Cash et al. demonstrated that, despite the fact that women seeking cosmetic breast augmentation often experience body image issues and psychological concerns prior to surgery, they experience improvements in body image following breast augmentation (14).

Most research examining the presence of psychopathology of the breast augmentation candidate has relied heavily on clinical interviews and self-report questionnaires. The findings are limited due to methodological problems and challenges to validity (15) and therefore should be interpreted with caution. Research using actuarial data from the Minnesota Multiphasic Personality Inventory and spanning 34 years has found little or no significant differences in personality and/or clinical psychopathology between breast augmentation candidates and controls (16). Nonetheless, breast augmentation candidates were found to have higher rates of previous psychiatric hospitalizations (17) and higher rates of outpatient psychotherapy and/or psychopharmacologic treatments than other women in the general population (16).

Kjoller et al. cited characteristics of women with cosmetic breast implants compared with women with other types of cosmetic surgery and population-based controls in Denmark (18). They discovered that women with breast implants had a significantly lower body mass index and reported a twofold greater incidence of chronic smoking than the general population and women who had other cosmetic surgery. Women with implants were not statistically more likely to report a history of diseases, including connective tissue diseases, cancer, or depression, before their implant surgery.

In summary, there seems to be a common thread of preexisting depression identified in the research regarding augmentation mammoplasty patients (8,12,13). In addition, low self-esteem and difficulty with social relationships were also identified (1,19,20). Edgerton et al. (1) and Edgerton and McClary (20) suggested that difficult childhoods, particularly those involving conflict with the parents, and lack of security in childhood were common in women seeking augmentation mammoplasty. With these factors in mind, an examination of the motivations reported by women for seeking breast augmentation is warranted. However, at this time, the literature finding a common thread of unfavorable mental health characteristics conflicts with the limited number of studies using actuarial data.

MOTIVATIONS OR REASONS FOR SEEKING AUGMENTATION MAMMOPLASTY

Each individual reports a variety of factors that impact self-esteem and body image. When conflicts arise between the idealized body image and the perceived body image, psychological distress, lower self-esteem, and elevated depression frequently occur (20). Cash (21) indicated that the psychology of physical appearance can be divided into two perspectives: (a) the external or social body image of the individual and (b) the individual's subjective appearance or personal body image. Sexual differences may also affect body image and body attitudes. In 1969, Kurtz (22) hypothesized that women should have a more clearly differentiated notion of their bodies because women are able to draw a finer evaluative distinction about various aspects of their bodies and are less inclined to respond to their bodily appearance in a global manner. Thompson and Thompson (23) documented that a significant global distortion of body image was negatively correlated with self-esteem in women, noting that the higher the distortion, the lower is the individual's self-esteem. Women, therefore, appear to be more sensitive to body image changes and react to them with heightened monitoring of the affected area.

The average augmentation mammoplasty patient has had concerns about the appearance of her breasts since adolescence (10). When asked about her motivation for surgery, she frequently responds, "to look better in clothing" or "to look more normal." Most women are not seeking to outdo other women in breast size; rather, they want to catch up. A number of researchers have evaluated the reasons that women seek augmentation mammoplasty, which cluster around the basic theme of doubts regarding femininity. Most women seeking breast augmentation have had small breasts since their teens, with a second, smaller group becoming concerned about the appearance of their breasts after giving birth and/or breast-feeding.

Goin and Goin (12) described three distinct groups of women seeking augmentation mammoplasty:

1. Those uncertain about their femininity, feeling incompletely realized as women. These women may have felt inadequate because of their small breast size.
2. Those who considered their breasts to have been adequate before pregnancy but found them to have diminished as a result of postpartum involution. These women seek to restore their breasts to an earlier state.
3. Those patients who seek augmentation for purposes of exhibitionism.

Kaslow and Becker (24) reported that common psychological reasons for seeking breast implants included the following: (a) to increase the size of breasts that are small, (b) to acquire better shape when firmness is lost due to childbearing and/or weight gain or loss, (c) to increase self-confidence, (d) to look better in clothing, (e) to improve physical appearance, (f) to feel more feminine, (g) to obtain better proportions, and (h) to increase sex appeal and look better in the nude. Of interest, many women seeking augmentation mammoplasty admit to feeling uncomfortable in the nude, either with their spouse or significant other or with other women, such as in gym class or when trying on clothing (25). Anderson (26) reported that women seeking augmentation mammoplasty do so for a variety of reasons, including increasing sexual self-confidence, satisfying

TABLE 108.1	Questions to Consider When Evaluating the Potential Augmentation Mammoplasty Patient

- Does the patient have difficulty describing the desired change?
- Does the patient have only minimal deformity?
- Is the patient's support system (friends and family) opposed to the procedure?
- Does the patient display bizarre behavior suggestive of possible schizophrenia or psychosis? (Such behavior might include lack of appropriate affect, hallucination, or failure to orient in time and space.)
- Does the patient have unreasonable expectations, make frequent demands of surgeon and/or staff, and display a sense of urgency?
- Does the patient appear extremely depressed or anxious, as evidenced by psychomotor retardation or agitation?
- Is the patient in the midst of a major life change or crisis?
- Has the patient had a history of dissatisfaction with cosmetic surgery or frequent cosmetic procedures?
- Does the patient have concerns regarding gender/sexual identity issues?
- If the answer to one or more of these questions is yes, a follow-up appointment for clarification before scheduling surgery is recommended.

Adapted from Anderson RC. Aesthetic surgery and psychosexual issues. *Aesthet Surg Q* 1996;16(4):227–229, with permission.

their partners, expanding clothing options, enhancing their sense of femininity and sexual identity, providing a more proportionate figure, and improving self-confidence. She stressed that evaluation of the potential augmentation mammoplasty patient should include assessment of her motivation for surgery, discussion regarding her expectations of surgical outcomes, consideration of her satisfaction with her life in general, recognition of signs of depression or anxiety, and evaluation of potential difficulties associated with body image. Anderson proposed a list of questions for the aesthetic surgeon to consider when evaluating the potentially concerning patient. These are given in Table 108.1.

In addition, Matarasso (27) identified two categories for rejecting a patient seeking aesthetic surgery: anatomic unsuitability and emotional inadequacy. Matarasso suggested that potential problem patients included the patient with unrealistic expectations, the obsessive-compulsive patient, the patient acting on a sudden whim, the indecisive patient, the rude patient, the overflattering patient, the patient with minimal or imagined deformity, the poor historian, the self-important patient, the uncooperative or noncompliant patient, the depressed patient, the "plastic surgaholic" patient, and the patient involved in litigation.

In short, many women seek augmentation mammoplasty, and most report satisfaction with the results. This procedure seems to offer women an answer to some significant concerns regarding body image.

PATIENT SATISFACTION WITH AUGMENTATION MAMMOPLASTY

The overwhelming majority of women who undergo augmentation mammoplasty report satisfaction with the results (7,12–14,18,19). Schlebusch and Mahrt (19) designed a study to determine the long-term psychological sequelae in the augmentation mammoplasty patient. Their results indicated that most patients benefited psychologically from augmentation mammoplasty and experienced improvement in psychological functioning as well as body image. The results also indicated less anxiety and depression postoperatively. Although not all patient expectations were met and basic personalities remained unchanged, most women had no regrets and indicated they would recommend the procedure to other women in similar situations. However, Schlebusch and Mahrt (19) found that most women had not seriously contemplated the possibility of an unsatisfactory postoperative result. Kilmann et al. (28) reported that women perceived the surgery to have had a significant positive effect on their attractiveness and on their body and self-image. The women viewed their partners as significantly more interested in sexual activity than they had been before the surgery. In the women's perception, their partners considered them significantly more attractive after the augmentation and believed the sexual relationship to be enhanced. Kilmann et al. inferred from this that the women had received a great deal of positive feedback from their partners associated with the augmentation. At a 1-year follow-up examination, patients indicated that the operation exceeded their expectations for positive benefits. After surgery, patients did report less distress and shyness (29). Hetter (30) found that a relatively small number of patients reported dissatisfaction, and this was due to physical discomfort. Ninety-six percent of the 165 patients in Hetter's study felt that the operation met their expectations, 88% were satisfied with the results, and almost 97% indicated they would undergo the procedure again.

Clearly, the majority of women opting to undergo augmentation mammoplasty are pleased with the results and believe that it has a positive effect on their body image. Most reports of satisfaction have been by patient self-report (7,12–14,18,19,29). The Breast Evaluation Questionnaire has been validated to assess patient satisfaction with breast attributes (31). According to Anderson et al. (31), this assessment (which has been translated into several languages) may be used to assess clinical satisfaction and for research purposes.

MORTALITY ISSUES

Studies have sought to ascertain mortality data among augmentation mammoplasty patients. The first, published in 2001 in the journal *Epidemiology*, looked at mortality among augmentation mammoplasty patients (32). In this study, epidemiologic data were reviewed in a retrospective cohort study of 13,488 women receiving breast implants and 3,936 with other types of plastic surgery. Mortality was compared with U.S. general population rates for both implant and comparison subjects. Results indicated that patients seeking plastic surgery are generally healthier than their peers. Implant patients, however, experienced a higher risk of death than the general population for brain cancer and suicide. It was further indicated that suicide attempts were correlated with a number of characteristics, including marital difficulties, depression, and emotional disorders, all of which have been noted among patients with breast implants. The authors further speculated that low self-esteem, which is commonly reported among breast implant patients, may have contributed to the higher suicide rates (1,4,8,9,12,13). They summarized their findings by noting that women with breast implants have slightly higher mortality risks than patients with other types of plastic surgery but that both groups have substantially lower mortality rates than the general population.

In a Swedish study published in 2003 in the *British Medical Journal,* the potential mortality risk among Swedish women with cosmetic breast implants was assessed (33). This study was based on the premise that a desire for cosmetic surgery suggested underlying psychopathology in some patients; therefore, it was hypothesized that death due to suicide may be overrepresented in the augmentation population (34). Fifteen women committed suicide, compared with the expected 5.2 deaths from suicide. Additional excess deaths were due to malignant disease, primarily lung cancer, and the number of deaths from all the causes was close to that expected. In their comments, the authors suggest that women who undergo cosmetic surgery for augmentation purposes are more likely to commit suicide than women from the general population. In this study, the deaths due to lung cancer were linked to smoking, and this was previously demonstrated in a cohort study (35).

A third mortality study published in 2003 examined the potential mortality risk among Finnish women with cosmetic breast implants (36). The results of this study indicated that 32.1 deaths (from all causes) were expected and 31 were observed. No excess of cancer mortality was observed. Ten women committed suicide, compared with an expected 3.1 deaths. The authors suggested that underlying psychopathology represents a possible explanation for these observed excesses of suicide among women who had breast augmentation.

An internationally recognized expert in the field of suicide, however, actually calculated somewhat higher expected suicide rates than those observed in these three mortality studies based on demographic and other preoperative characteristics of breast augmentation patients. These characteristics, which have been documented to be associated with elevated rates of suicide, were summarized by Joiner (37):

1. The prototypical breast augmentation patient is white and between the ages of 25 and 44 years.
2. Although most breast augmentation patients are behaviorally and interpersonally stable before surgery, differences exist between these women and others with regard to divorce, heavy alcohol and tobacco use, and the symptoms of mood, eating, and appearance-related disorders.
3. More impulsive personality features may be present among these patients.
4. Other differences likely exist between breast augmentation patients and others.

Further evidence that preexisting factors contribute to the observed elevation in suicide rates is provided by a 1987 study that included an evaluation of preoperative psychiatric and psychosocial characteristics in a group of Swedish women prior to augmentation mammoplasty (8). In this study, attempted suicide (predating surgery) was reported in 18% of patients preparing to undergo augmentation mammoplasty as compared with 3% of control group patients preparing to undergo surgery for benign skin tumors of the face and neck.

As previously mentioned, many of the factors associated with suicide are present prior to surgery in the augmentation mammoplasty patient, despite the fact that most augmentation mammoplasty patients report significant satisfaction with the outcome (14). Joiner suggested that observed suicide rates among these patients might be higher if they had not undergone breast augmentation. He further maintained that there are consistent findings that, before surgery, breast augmentation patients are "body dissatisfied" (at least with regard to their breasts) and that body dissatisfaction is a risk factor for mood and eating disorders. Both affective and eating disorders represent strong risk factors for suicide. Because breast augmentation appears to ameliorate body dissatisfaction for many patients, Joiner postulated that the procedure may suppress suicidality because of the protective effects of increased body image satisfaction (37).

There may be a subset of patients for which the surgery is too little, too late. In fact in a letter of response to the study regarding mortality in Swedish women with cosmetic breast implants, Klesner described a subset of cosmetic surgery patients who might be at higher risk for suicide (38). He pointed out that in body dysmorphic disorder, which is a form of somatoform disorder that involves a preoccupation with a defect in appearance that is either imagined or present but slight, the patient's concern is excessive. This disorder is estimated to occur in between 6% and 15% of patients having cosmetic surgery or dermatologic procedures. Klesner recommended that cosmetic surgeons seek mental health consultations when concerns are present preoperatively in order to rule out body dysmorphic disorder. Klesner suggested that if body dysmorphic disorder is identified and treated, the suicide rate associated with breast implants might be diminished.

Early studies investigating the risk of unfavorable health outcomes following breast augmentation using silicon gel–filled implants influenced the Food and Drug Administration (FDA) to issue a moratorium on the use of silicon gel–filled breast implants in 1992. The FDA reversed the decision in 2006 after new evidence suggested no increased physical or psychological risk (39). The largest cohort study to date, consisting of 25,588 Canadians (40), found a higher-than-expected mortality rate for suicide in breast augmentation patients. Taken from these studies, the rate of suicide is believed to be twofold to threefold greater than in the general population (41). Secondary findings suggest that the age of the patient and life of implant may be associated with risk of suicide (32,40,42). A longer life of an implant and being 40 years or older at the time of receiving cosmetic breast augmentation may be associated with the risk of suicide.

Epidemiologic evidence has shown an increase in mortality rate for suicide following breast augmentation. However, a causal relationship between breast augmentation surgery and suicide is premature and should not be made due to the nature of correlational research. Sarwer et al. (16) recommended that well-controlled prospective trials are necessary before conclusions about causal relationships can be drawn. Nonetheless, explanations for this phenomenon in epidemiologic research have investigated the type of relationship between suicide and breast augmentation (e.g., direct, indirect) and have focused on underlying risk factors associated with demographic and descriptive risk factors (e.g., sexual promiscuity, alcohol and tobacco use), the role of preoperative personality characteristics and psychopathology (e.g., body image dissatisfaction), preoperative motivations and expectations (e.g. internal vs. external motivations), and psychological functioning and postoperative complications (e.g., body image, quality of life) (16).

THE SILICONE BREAST IMPLANT CONTROVERSY AND ITS IMPACT ON BREAST AUGMENTATION PATIENTS

Since 1992, when the popular media first reported the FDA's recommendation for a moratorium on silicone implants, safety has been an issue for women with implants. Most of the information obtained by women came from the popular media (43,44). A bias or lack of accuracy of information has been reported by several researchers (43,44). Researchers have consistently reported common concerns expressed by women in the studies. These concerns included capsular contracture, leakage, and autoimmune disease. Other concerns were related to difficulty with the reading of mammograms and increased risk of cancer (43–46).

Palcheff-Weimer et al. (45) conducted research to evaluate how women with breast implants felt about the media coverage. They found that satisfaction with the decision to have implants decreased from 98% of the sample before the moratorium to 71% for augmentation patients and 79% for reconstruction patients after the moratorium. In May 1992 at the meeting of the American Society of Plastic Surgeons in Vancouver, British Columbia, Concannon et al. presented research regarding perceptions of the accuracy of the media in reporting on the silicone implant topic (43). Sixty-three percent of patients with breast reconstruction believed that the information was somewhat or very inaccurate, whereas 54% of the patients with breast augmentation believed that the information was somewhat or very inaccurate. Most women surveyed indicated that their attitudes about implants had not changed after exposure to media coverage.

In 1994, Larson et al. (44) conducted research to assess the public's attitude regarding silicone breast implants in the wake of the media publicity regarding their safety. The results of their research indicated that television was the primary source of information for all groups, followed by newspapers and magazines. Only 10% of their respondents indicated medical journals as a source of information. Eighty-eight percent of those surveyed believed the balance of media coverage was strongly or somewhat against the use of silicone implants, whereas only 6% believed the media coverage was objective. Almost all women polled indicated that they believed that women should have the right to choose silicone breast implants after being allowed the opportunity to give informed consent. Larson et al. asked if women with implants believed their willingness to undergo routine or recommended mammography had changed as a result of the publicity. Only 3% indicated they would not have mammography, whereas 40% responded that their feelings about mammography were unchanged, and 53% indicated they would definitely have the recommended mammography. Of interest, the Larson study surveyed the general population and discovered much hesitancy in the use of implants. Seventy-eight percent of the general population reported significant hesitancy in the use of the implants or indicated that they would not have implants at all as a result of information obtained from media coverage. When compared with the general population, those women who had silicone implants reported much less anxiety, and the majority indicated that they would submit to the procedure again.

Merkatz et al. (47) reported that during the highly publicized FDA deliberation period, the FDA received thousands of letters from women with breast implants. The majority of the letters were from satisfied women; however, a small group of women reported dissatisfaction. A qualitative analysis of letters was completed by the FDA, and of the 112 negative responses examined for psychosocial content, the following four patterns were identified:

1. Women believed that they did not receive adequate information before surgery.
2. Women believed that they were not taken seriously by their physicians when they complained of pain or other symptoms.
3. Women reported having difficulty maintaining their normal activities.
4. Women expressed concerns about the future and difficulty gaining information.

The FDA also completed a descriptive analysis of 271 letters from women who reported health problems that they believed to be associated with their implants. The most commonly cited problems were breast pain (40%), rupture of implants (31%), capsular contracture (29%), joint pain (39%), and fatigue (35%) (48).

Anderson and Larson (49) conducted a study among women with implants to evaluate anxiety responses evoked by the media coverage. They concluded that the media exposure was clearly a concern to women who had undergone breast reconstruction or augmentation mammoplasty. All the patients surveyed were aware of controversy over silicone breast implants, with varying levels of anxiety reported among breast reconstruction and augmentation mammoplasty patients. Anxiety over the media coverage, despite its being judged as not objective, did seem to be associated with hesitancy to use the implants by some of the respondents.

In summary, most researchers in this area agree that concerns related to silicone implants are an issue of importance to women and, in fact, the media has exerted an effect on these women. Based on a review of the literature, the majority of women with implants are satisfied with them and would undergo the procedure again (43–45,49).

STATUS OF LEGISLATION REGARDING BREAST IMPLANTS

The FDA recognizes three types of breast implants, all of which are intended for breast augmentation, reconstruction, and revision. The types of implants considered by the FDA are saline-filled breast implants, silicone gel–filled breast implants, and alternative breast implants. In 1993, manufacturers of saline-filled breast implants were notified by the FDA that the agency would require data on their product safety and effectiveness. The implants remained on the market while manufacturers conducted required studies. In August 1999, the FDA asked manufacturers to submit evidence in a premarket approval (PMA) that saline-filled breast implants were safe and effective, and in March 2000, the FDA's General and Plastic Surgery Devices Panel met to review PMAs for saline breast implants. Two of the three implant manufacturers were approved by the panel, and in May 2000, the FDA granted approval to these two manufacturers. The FDA reported that, despite complications, the majority of women studied by these two manufacturers indicated that after 3 years they were satisfied with their implants. To date, all other saline-filled breast implants are considered investigational (50).

In April 1991, the FDA asked manufacturers to submit evidence in a PMA application that silicone gel–filled implants were safe and effective. The FDA determined that manufacturers did not have enough data regarding safety and effectiveness; therefore, silicone gel breast implants were removed from the market. In January 1992, a voluntary moratorium on the use of silicone gel–filled implants pending safety information to be reviewed by the panel was issued. Three months later, the voluntary moratorium on breast implants was lifted by the FDA, and they announced their decision to allow silicone gel–filled implants on the market but only under controlled clinical studies for reconstruction after mastectomy, correction of congenital deformities, or replacement of ruptured silicone gel implants due to medical or surgical reasons. In 1998, one of the manufacturers received approval from the FDA for silicone gel–filled implants for augmentation, reconstruction, and revision for a limited number of patients at a limited number of sites. Approval followed in 2000 for another manufacturer to study silicone gel–filled implants under the same conditions (51). An FDA advisory panel recommended market approval for one of the manufacturers of silicone gel–filled breast implants in October 2003. However, rather than accept the panel's advice, in January 2004 the FDA deferred a decision on the implants pending submission of additional information. Although some interpreted the FDA's response as a denial of silicone gel–filled implants for use in the United States, the FDA clearly specified that approval be withheld pending submission of additional information regarding safety of the device (52). Documents filed with the FDA by that manufacturer indicate that patient satisfaction remains high despite complications (53). In April 2005, the FDA convened an advisory panel to review the PMAs of two manufacturers. In July and September 2005, each manufacturer received an approval letter from the FDA; in November 2006, the PMAs for silicone gel implants of both manufacturers were approved by the FDA (54). PMAs for contoured implants are currently under review by the FDA.

CONCLUSION

Clearly, the breasts, which represent nurturing, femininity, and sexuality, have been a focus of the female anatomy dating back thousands of years. Small breasts or breast deformities have been associated with feelings of low self-esteem and diminished femininity. In an effort to address this problem, women have sought changes through external prostheses such as brassieres and corsets. With the advent of augmentation mammoplasty, many women have sought to surgically change the size and contour of their breasts. Most women do so in an effort to enhance their body image, their sense of self-esteem, and their ability to feel more proportionate and wear a greater variety of clothing styles. The quality and safety of implants continue to advance, and surgical techniques have improved medical and aesthetic outcomes. Most women seeking and undergoing augmentation mammoplasty report satisfaction with the procedure. With continued focus on the female breast, comprehensive medical and psychological assistance to those women seeking augmentation mammoplasty must continue to be provided.

EDITORIAL COMMENTS

Dr. Anderson's chapter on the psychology of breast augmentation provides an appropriate insight into both the augmentation patient and the psychological effects of the silicone gel implant controversy. She reminds us that the average augmentation patient is a woman in her thirties who has had concern about the appearance of her breasts since adolescence. This patient typically and simply seeks to look better in clothing or to look more normal. A subgroup among these women are those who have become concerned about their breasts more recently subsequent to childbirth or breast-feeding. Dr. Anderson also mentions a third group of women who are seeking augmentation not for appearing normal but rather for purposes of exhibitionism. These are women who may be in the arts or who are simply exhibitionistic.

We are also reminded that there are certain patients that need to be approached carefully: those who are anatomically unsuitable and others with emotional problems. Included in the group with emotional difficulties are those with unrealistic expectations, the obsessive-compulsive patient, those acting impulsively, the indecisive patient, the rude patient, the overflattering patient, the patient with minimal or imagined deformity, the poor historian, the VIP, the uncooperative or noncompliant patient, the depressed patient, the "surgaholic" patient, and the patient involved in litigation.

The evidence seems compelling that most patients who have undergone breast augmentation have been satisfied with the outcome both physically and psychologically. Whereas the typical patient who seeks augmentation has suffered primarily from a negative body image associated with her breasts, the vast majority of patients obtain correction of that negative body image and therefore achieve their initial emotional goals.

Dr. Anderson's review of the silicone breast implant controversy also proves to be enlightening. We learn from this section of the chapter that the public in general had its perception of silicone breast implants worsened as a result of the media coverage of the silicone controversy of the early 1990s. Furthermore, whereas the general public had a significantly more negative impression about silicone than previously, those patients with silicone implants actually felt less negative about silicone implants than the public at large. Dr. Anderson's review of the FDA patient letters is very interesting. She reports that the majority of women who wrote to the FDA were satisfied with their implants. Among the smaller group of women who were dissatisfied, the dissatisfaction was related either to inadequate preoperative information, the perception that the surgeon did not take the patient's complaints seriously, some difficulty with routine physical activity, and concerns about attaining future accurate information.

Dr. Anderson's review of the psychology of the augmentation patient is reassuring. We get the sense that the desire for breast augmentation or improvement of the feminine figure has been around for thousands of years; that the motivation by these patients to achieve a larger, more shapely bosom appears to be a normal one; and that most patients are helped by this surgery.

S.L.S.

REFERENCES

1. Edgerton MT, Meyer E, Jacobson WE. Augmentation mammoplasty. II. Further surgical and psychiatric evaluation. *Plast Reconstr Surg* 1962;21:279–302.
2. Peters WJ. Plastic surgery of the breast. *Mod Med* 1981;6:37–41.
3. Schalk DN. The history of augmentation mammaplasty. *Plast Surg Nurs* 1988;8:88–90.
4. Schlebusch L. Negative body experience and prevalence of depression in patients who request augmentation mammoplasty. *S Afr Med J* 1989;75:323–326.

5. Steele V. *Fashion and Eroticism: Ideals of Feminine Beauty from the Victorian Era to the Jazz Age.* New York: Oxford University Press; 1985.
6. Allen M, Oberle K. Augmentation mammoplasty: a complex choice. *Health Care Women Int* 1996;17:81–90.
7. Beale S, Hambert G, Lisper HO, et al. Augmentation mammoplasty: the surgical and psychological effects of the operation and prediction of the results. *Ann Plast Surg* 1984;13:279–297.
8. Meyer L, Ringberg A. Augmentation mammaplasty: psychiatric and psychosocial characteristics and outcome in a group of Swedish women. *Scand J Plast Reconstr Surg Hand Surg* 1987;21(2):199–208.
9. Goin MK. Psychological reactions to surgery of the breast. *Clin Plast Surg* 1982;9:347–354.
10. Walsh KC. Breast augmentation: your patient's adjustment to a new body image. *Today's OR Nurse* 1986;8:20–25.
11. Shipley RH, O'Donnell JM, Bader KF. Personality characteristics of women seeking breast augmentation. *Plast Reconstr Surg* 1977;60:369.
12. Goin JM, Goin MK. *Changing the Body: Psychological Effects of Plastic Surgery.* Baltimore: Williams & Wilkins; 1981.
13. Sarwer D, LaRossa D, Bartlett S, et al. Body image concerns of augmentation patients. *Am Soc Plast Surg* 2003;112(1):83–90.
14. Cash T, Duel L, Perkins L. Women's psychosocial outcomes of breast augmentation with silicone gel filled implants: a two-year prospective study. *Plast Reconstr Surg* 2002;109: 2112.
15. McGrath MH. The psychological safety of breast implants for augmentation mammaplasty. *Plast Reconstr Surg* 2007;12:120.
16. Sarwer DB, Brown GK, Evans DL. Cosmetic breast augmentation and suicide. *Am J Psychiatry* 2007;164:1006–1013.
17. Jacobsen PH, Hölmich LR, McLaughlin JK. Mortality and suicide among Danish women with cosmetic implants. *Arch Intern Med* 2004;164(22):2450–2455.
18. Kjoller K, Holmich L, Fryzek J, et al. Characteristics of women with cosmetic breast implants compared with women with other types of cosmetic surgery and population based controls in Denmark. *Ann Plast Surg* 2003;50(1):6–12.
19. Schlebusch L, Mahrt I. Long-term psychological sequelae of augmentation mammoplasty. *S Afr Med J* 1993;83:267–271.
20. Edgerton MT, McClary AR. Augmentation mammoplasty: psychiatric implications and surgical indications. *Plast Reconstr Surg* 1958;21:279–305.
21. Cash TF. Physical appearance and mental health. In: Graham JA, Kligman A, eds. *Psychology of Cosmetic Treatments.* New York: Praeger Scientific; 1985:196–216.
22. Kurtz RM. Sex differences in variations in body attitudes. *Consult Clin Psychol* 1969;35:625–629.
23. Thompson JK, Thompson CM. Body size distortion and self-esteem in asymptomatic, normal weight males and females. *Int J Eat Disord* 1986;5:1061–1068.
24. Kaslow F, Becker H. Breast augmentation: psychological and plastic surgery considerations. *Psychotherapy* 1992, 29:467–473.
25. Birtchnell S, Whitfield P, Lacey JH. Motivational factors in women requesting augmentation and reduction mammaplasty. *J Psychosom Res* 1990;34:509–514.
26. Anderson RC. Aesthetic surgery and psychosexual issues. *Aesthet Surg Q* 1996;16:227–229.
27. Matarasso SL. Introduction to cosmetic surgery. *Semin Dermatol* 1994;13:60–63.
28. Kilmann PR, Sattler JI, Taylor J. The impact of augmentation mammaplasty: a follow-up study. *Plast Reconstr Surg* 1987;80(3):374–378.
29. Sihm F, Jagd M, Perse M. Psychological assessment before and after augmentation mammaplasty. *Scand J Reconstr Surg* 1978;12:295–298.
30. Hetter GP. Satisfactions and dissatisfactions of patients with augmentation mammaplasty. *Plast Reconstr Surg* 1979;64:151–155.
31. Anderson RC, Cunningham B, Tafesse E, et al. Validation of the breast evaluation questionnaire. *Plast Reconstr Surg* 2006;118(3):597–602.
32. Brinton L, Lubin J, Cay Burich M, et al. Mortality among augmentation mammaplasty patients. *Epidemiology* 2001;12(3):321–326.
33. Koot V, Petters P, Granath F, et al. Total and cause specific mortality among Swedish women with cosmetic breast implants: perspective study. *BMJ* 2003;326(7388):527–528.
34. Hasan JS. Psychological issues in cosmetic surgery: a functional overview. *Ann Plast Surg* 2000;44:89–96.
35. Fryzek J, Weiderpass E, Signorello L, et al. Characteristics of women with cosmetic breast augmentation surgery compared with breast reduction surgery patients and women in the general population of Sweden. *Ann Plast Surg* 2000;45(4):349–355.
36. Pukkala E, Kulmala I, Hovi SL, et al. Causes of death among Finnish women with cosmetic breast implants, 1971–2001. *Ann Plast Surg* 2003;51(4):339–342.
37. Joiner TE Jr. Does breast augmentation confer risk of or protection from suicide? *Aesthet Surg J* 2003;23(5):370–375.
38. Klesner J. Mortality in Swedish women with cosmetic breast implants, body dysmorphic disorder should be considered [Letter]. *BMJ* 2003;326:1266–1267.
39. McLaughlin JK, Lipworth L, Murphy DK, et al. The safety of silicone gel–filled breast implants: a review of the epidemiologic evidence. *Ann Plast Surg* 2007;59:569–580.
40. Villeneuve PJ, Holowaty EJ, Brisson J, et al. Mortality among Canadian women with cosmetic breast implants. *Am J Epidemiol* 2006;164:334–341.
41. Crerand CE, Infield AL, Sarwer DB. Psychological considerations in cosmetic breast augmentation. *Plast Surg Nurs* 2007;27(3):146–154.
42. Brinton LA, Lubin JH, Murray MC, et al. Mortality rates among augmentation mammoplasty patients: an update. *Epidemiology* 2006;17:162–169.
43. Concannon MJ, Weimer MS, Puckett CL. Media impact on breast implant patients. Paper presented at the American Association of Plastic Surgeons, Vancouver, British Columbia, Canada, May 1992.
44. Larson DL, Anderson RC, Maksud D, et al. What influences the public perception of silicone breast implants? *Plast Reconstr Surg* 1994;94:318–325.
45. Palcheff-Wiemer ME, Concannon MJ, Conn VS, et al. The impact of the media on women with breast implants. *Plast Reconstr Surg* 1993;92:779–785.
46. Anderson RC, Larson DL. Patient concerns related to media coverage of silicone implants. *Plast Surg Nurs* 1995;15:89–91.
47. Merkatz RB, Bagley GP, McCarthy EJ. A qualitative analysis of self-reported experience among women encountering difficulties with silicone breast implants. *J Women's Health* 1993;2:105–109.
48. McCarthy EJ, Merkatz RB, Bagley GP. A descriptive analysis of physical complaints from women with silicone breast implants. *J Women's Health* 1993;2:111–115.
49. Anderson RC, Larson DL. Reconstruction and augmentation patients' reaction to the media coverage of silicone gel-filled implants: anxiety evaluated. *Psychol Rep* 1995;76:1323–1330.
50. U.S. Food and Drug Administration. FDA breast implant consumer handbook—2004. Available at: http://www.fda.gov/cdrh/breastimplants/indexbip.html. Accessed July 8, 2005.
51. U.S. Food and Drug Administration. Breast implants: an information update 2000. Available at: http://www.fda.gov/cdrh/ breastimplants/bichron.html. Accessed March 5, 2004.
52. CBS News. FDA rejects silicone implants. January 8, 2004. Available at: http://www.cbsnews.com/stories/2003/11/05/health/ main581986.shtml. Accessed July 8, 2005.
53. INAMED Corporation. Making an informed decision: saline-filled breast implant surgery: 2004 Update. Available at: http://www.fda.gov/cdrh/breastimplants/labeling/inamed_patient_labeling_5900.html. Accessed July 8, 2005.
54. U.S. Food and Drug Administration. (2009). Silicone gel–filled breast implant timeline. Available at: http://www.fda.gov/MedicalDevices/ProductsandMedicalProcedures/ImplantsandProsthetics/BreastImplants/ucm064461.htm. Accessed April 8, 2009.

CHAPTER

109

Caroline A. Glicksman

Patient Education in Breast Augmentation

INTRODUCTION

The start of the new millennium proved to be a difficult time for breast augmentation surgeons. For those who were witness to the U.S. Food and Drug Administration (FDA) silicone gel advisory panels, it was evident that, for better or worse, the decision to undergo breast augmentation surgery has had a significant impact on the lives of hundreds of thousands of U.S. women. As devices have evolved over the last 45 years, their improved longevity and reliability have been well documented (1). However, despite these technological advances, the most recent premarket approval application (PMA) data suggest that surgical outcomes, as reflected by revision rates, still lag far behind (2,3).

Considerable effort has been placed on redefining breast augmentation as more than just a surgical procedure. Peer-reviewed publications confirm that markedly improved long-term outcomes can be achieved when there is effective communication between the physician and the patient. The first step in accomplishing improved outcomes in breast augmentation is *comprehensive* patient education (4). Decisions made by both the surgeon and the patient during the consultation phase of the breast augmentation process may have more of an impact on the quality of the outcome and its longevity than the device selected or the augmentation procedure itself. It is during this educational process that surgeons have the best opportunity to introduce informed-consent documents that will hold patients accountable for their decisions. An effective educational process must link understanding with accountability, and what really matters is whether the patients understand, accept, and take responsibility for their decisions (5).

This chapter focuses on analyzing the current informed-consent issues and how they relate to patient education in breast augmentation. It reviews essential content suggested in the initial consultation, presented in a format that patients will understand while simultaneously integrating informed-consent documents into the patient's educational experience. Useful educational tools that can be used both in and out of the office are recommended, as well as suggested steps to be taken preoperatively to clearly document the patient's accountability for decisions made. Finally, this chapter reviews methods that will help manage patient expectations with regard to the financial responsibilities of potential complications or staged procedures, as well as suggested long-term follow-up as both the patient and the devices age.

PATIENT EDUCATION AND INFORMED CONSENT

In the medical setting, the term "informed consent" arose in the United States in 1957. This terminology shifted the physician–patient relationship away from the medical paternalism that had encompassed medicine and surgery for centuries toward that of a duty to respect patient autonomy. The U.S. court case of *Cobb vs. Grant* (1972) noted that the doctrine of informed consent is "anchored" in four postulates. First, patients are generally ignorant of medicine. Second, patients have a right to control their body and decide about their medical treatment. Third, consent to treatment must be informed to be effective. Fourth, patients depend on their physicians for truthful information and must trust them (6). Informed consent in breast augmentation, therefore, should have two main aims. The foremost goal should be to respect and promote the patients' autonomy; the second should be to be truthful and protect them from harm. If we assume the provision that accurate, detailed information has been provided in an understandable format, patients should be assured of both of these aims. Only if the patient obtains a comprehensive understanding of the possible benefits, harms, and alternatives to the procedure can she give adequate informed consent. In addition, with respect to breast augmentation, we must also convey the fact that there remain unknown risks associated with the procedure.

Successful communication plays the central role in physician–patient relationships, and it has been shown to influence positively patient satisfaction, compliance, medical outcomes, and the overall quality of the patient experience (7). It is especially important for informed consent, where patients are allowed, and expected, to participate in the decision-making process by weighing the benefits against the risks of recommended options (8). To be able to become true and knowledgeable decision makers, patients need to understand the basis and significance behind those recommendations and discuss them with their physicians properly. The current practice of obtaining informed consent is often centered on the legal duty of having the patient sign a form. Signing does not always represent patient understanding. Furthermore, the U.S. Department of Health and Human Services now requires that all consent forms be "in language understandable to the subject or their representative." Many states require culturally sensitive informed-consent documents, as this process has also been shown to be compromised when language or cultural barriers are present. It is also recommended that documents and brochures be provided in writing that is understandable to the reading level of eighth grade or lower (9).

One of the roles of the physician is to become an effective communicator. Physicians and their staff must be able to deliver information in language that is familiar to their patients and easy to understand, using common words from everyday language. Studies have shown that medical language and everyday language are seen as two separate languages (10). Most physicians and caregivers can translate the necessary medical information into a language that the patients can understand. An interactive communication loop between the patient and physician or nurse educator should be used to frequently check comprehension and recall while clarifying and tailoring the information in repeated cycles to improve comprehension (11). Some studies suggest that patient understanding might be improved if the consent forms were short and easy to read. They suggest modifications to consent forms with regard to content, writing style, format, and length (12). Others conclude that these modifications are no more successful than other approaches to improving patient comprehension (13). In addition, the term "fully" informed consent would require that every piece of information available would be provided to every patient. No *rational* patient desires all the information about a procedure or a device, nor is there sufficient time. It is also particularly difficult to obtain true informed consent in breast augmentation because there remain unknowns that have yet to be identified (14). Patients should be provided with "reasonable" and "adequate" information, which will always be less than *all* of the available information (15). In breast augmentation, we must also further define risks as either surgical- or implant-related risk (16).

Although the patient's signature on a single surgical consent document might represent agreement, it does not always imply understanding. An attempt to assess understanding should be made at varying steps throughout the educational process and documentation recorded at each step. Several options have been suggested that create an integrated approach to patient education and the informed-consent process (5). In addition to providing multiple, short, readable documents in a staged approach, physicians and their staff should frequently check the patient's level of understanding. The method of "teach back" can confirm understanding. The physician or staff can ask the patient to say in her own words what has been described, and ask again if the patient's words show incomplete or inaccurate understanding. Probably the most important factor in ensuring a high level of patient understanding is the quality of the time spent with the patient. When the surgeon and the staff are dedicated to providing their patients with a breast augmentation process that is specifically designed to ensure safe, predictable, long-lasting results with the lowest chance of unnecessary revisions, patients should be given the necessary time to make well-informed decisions. Many patients make their surgical decisions too quickly and select surgical options without taking the time to process the information they have received. Patients should, if possible, always be given the opportunity to return for a second consultation. Between the two visits they should be encouraged to read any educational materials provided, search the Internet, and even seek another surgical opinion if they desire. For women who want to be involved in the surgical decisions entailed in breast augmentation, it is crucial that they are reassured that they have time to evaluate their surgical options.

Much of the research focusing on the quality of patient decisions in surgery has been associated with clinical trials of patient decision aids and other decision support tools. The preoperative decisions in breast augmentation are known as "preference-sensitive" decisions to reflect the fact that although medical evidence is necessary to make decisions, it may not be sufficient. The patient's preferences are also necessary to make the appropriate decision. It follows, however that "preference-sensitive" clinical decisions can be defined as the extent to which the implemented choices reflect the considered preferences of the *well-informed* patient. Therefore patients should be given ample opportunity to become well informed (17). There has been a great deal of discussion in the plastic surgery literature and at scientific meetings surrounding the balance between patient autonomy, that is, the physician's obligation to create the conditions necessary for autonomous choice and an individual's right to self-determination, and beneficence, which is the physician's responsibility to do what is best for the patient. Beneficence is also the belief that physicians are expected to refrain from causing harm in addition to having an obligation to help their patients. While there has been a long tradition in Western medical ethics toward focusing on autonomy, that prioritization has now been critiqued (18,19). The ethical debate in breast augmentation arises when the patient's autonomous decisions conflict with the physician's beneficent duty to look out for the patient's best interest, for example, if the physician wishes to prevent avoidable breast augmentation complications that may eventually result in potentially uncorrectable deformities. Both surgeons and patients may sense this as a return to an era of paternalism and reject the concept of "doctor-knows-best" with regard to patient education in breast augmentation. However, if we accept that there are quantifiable guidelines that can minimize revision surgeries and optimize long-term results, then there is a need to incorporate beneficent actions in the preoperative education process. Patients may still proceed with autonomy during the informed-consent process involved in breast augmentation, provided they are accurately informed and fully understand the long-term consequences of their decisions. They must then also be willing to be held accountable for those decisions.

THE INITIAL PATIENT CONSULTATION

The education process in breast augmentation can actually begin before the first consult, at the time of the initial contact between the patient and the physician's office. The opportunity to set in motion a comprehensive process of patient education starts before the patient even steps foot into the physician's office. Verbal information presented by the office staff will establish a pattern to be followed throughout the breast augmentation experience. Printed material can be mailed to the patient and website information should be suggested for review prior to the first office visit. Both physicians and patients routinely use the Internet as a source of health-related information; however websites are not monitored, and therefore the quality of information is variable. Prospective breast augmentation patients need to be taught to distinguish between sponsored websites, in which advertisers pay for placement, and unsponsored ones, which do not provide payment to the search engine. A physician's website, if current, can be an excellent source of information and should include links to additional sites that are both sponsored and unsponsored. The information on the Internet, however, is not intended to replace information provided by the physician. In addition, the sites visited by the patient before the initial consult should be reviewed by the physician or nurse educator at the first visit to correct any inaccuracies encountered (20).

If patient education is to be a staged repetitive learning process, it will require participation from several members of the surgeon's staff. Many large practices have a patient educator who plays an active role in the educational process. For smaller practices, it may be the responsibility of the surgeon and a well-trained staff member to develop a detailed precise approach to patient education and informed consent. Extremely well thought out programs that integrate patient education and informed consent have been published (6). Comprehensive informed-consent documents have been developed that are incorporated directly into the preoperative educational process. These documents are specifically designed to verify the patients understanding of content and their acceptance of responsibility for their decisions. These documents are available for downloading from the *Plastic and Reconstructive Surgery* website (21) and can be modified to meet the needs of individual practice styles (Fig. 109.1). There is a substantial quantity of information that will be transferred to the patient.

An approach to education that documents decisions made between the surgeon and patient after each topic has been discussed may produce a more valid informed consent than a single consent document signed at the time of payment for the procedure. It is also extremely important to document whether a spouse, significant other, or relative will be involved in the decision-making process. That individual should be present for at least one of the office educational visits if he or she is to be allowed to participate in any postoperative discussions on the surgical outcome (5,6). Although it may not be the preference or style of all breast augmentation practices to interject the signing of multiple documents throughout the patient's preoperative experience, there should be a verbal discussion with clear written documentation preoperatively that the patient understands the alternatives offered and accepts trade-offs, risks, and possible short- and long-term complications associated with her decisions. In addition, there should be written documentation of the financial responsibilities that the patient may encounter postoperatively either for possible untoward complications or for future radiologic imaging and eventual replacement of her implant.

PATIENT EDUCATION IN BREAST AUGMENTATION: TOOLS, TECHNOLOGY, AND THE SENSES

Most surgeons develop their communication skills over the years are turning with increasing frequency to tools and technology as aids in the patient education process. From use of a simple illustration to the use of interactive digital education, there is a perceived need to reach out to patients with better educational tools so they can make better-informed decisions (22). Most women seeking breast augmentation are highly motivated to learn about the breast augmentation process. Many practices offer patients printed materials or a Web-based introduction to the practice that includes their philosophy on breast augmentation and can be read before the first consultation. These materials are then reviewed by the patient educator or the physician during the initial consultation.

Many patients present with little or no knowledge concerning the history of breast implants and may have biases based on the media, personal experiences, or the experiences of friends or relatives. By incorporating the patient's senses into the learning experience, physicians can utilize both visual and tactile tools to reinforce the messages presented. Visuals have proven to be an important asset in improving patient–physician communications, enhancing education, and advancing the informed consent process. Visuals can increase patient satisfaction and comprehension while reducing the amount of time a physician needs to spend explaining specifics, such as implant designs or fill. Visual tools have also been shown to overcome virtually any literacy or cultural barriers that a patient may display (23). The use of older-generation silicone implants as educational tools can be invaluable when discussing the important changes that have occurred in implant technology over the last 45 years (24,1). The 1992 FDA moratorium on silicone breast implants generated a cohort of women who still maintain a preconceived notion on the safety of breast implants to this day (25). A great deal of misunderstanding can be eliminated when patients are given the opportunity to see and feel the older devices and compare them to the latest generation of saline, round, and form-stable gel devices. Women seeking breast augmentation are increasingly aware of the many implant choices available to them. Providing the patient the opportunity to hold an optimally filled saline device, a round gel, and a shaped form-stable, highly cohesive gel implant may be far more informative than merely describing the differences in shape, shell, and fill. Patients hold on to much more information when it is presented repeatedly, and combining educational modalities has been shown to enhance both written and verbal communication. Most important, patients can be educated to the benefits and trade-offs of each device that they may be considering. In a study designed to evaluate a patient's acceptance of softer or firmer implants, patients were given the opportunity to observe round or shaped saline implants filled to optimal volume. This hands-on demonstration was combined with scripted information regarding implant fill issues and their possible effect on the tissues over time. Patients were then allowed to select a device based not only on their sense of feel, but also on the knowledge of potential outcomes of that decision. Given the choice of implant, along with information describing the possible long-term consequences of each device, the majority of patients in the study chose the optimally filled implants, despite their firmer feel (26). Patients must eventually decide on the fill and shape of their implant and should be informed of their options as well as the trade-offs of each choice. Utilizing actual implants as an educational tool creates a more engaged and informed patient.

A more common approach to patient education in breast augmentation has been the use of "before" and "after" photos as both educational and marketing tools. As of June 2009, a Google search revealed close to two million sites on the Internet with breast augmentation photographs. Images can increase patient comprehension, as well as the retention of information. What most patients fail to understand is that pictures cannot document the tissue characteristics or the quantitative measurements that make each patient unique. Viewing images with a patient can, however, provide invaluable insight into her desires and is an opportunity to educate women with respect to the need to reconcile those desires with their individual tissues and dimensions. Moreover, most patients have only a vague understanding of the possible short- and long-term risks that may be a direct result of the choices made preoperatively, for example, when the patient desires an implant far wider than her tissues will accommodate, or when a mastopexy may also be recommended. Quality images can be used to help patients understand terms like capsular contracture, skin stretch, implant malposition, symmastia, and visible wrinkling (Fig. 109.2A, B). The use of images may also aid the discussion of the incision locations and potential wound-healing problems. These visual counseling tools are also useful

Patient Educator Consultation Checklist

Patient Concerns

Additional Questions for [Surgeons name]

Have you had any type of Plastic Surgery before?
- ❑ **Are you happy with your results?**
- ❑ **My role in your care**
- ❑ **Our commitment to patient education**
- ❑ **What we'll talk about today**
- ❑ **Have you read the information we provided you?**
- ❑ **Clinical evaluation sheet medical history and patient preferences**
- ❑ **Brief history of augmentation**
- ❑ **Alternatives versus a single approach**
- ❑ **Do implants cause disease? The research and sources**
- ❑ **Breast implants and breast cancer**
- ❑ **Breast implants and mammography**
  - All implants interfere with mammograms
  - Implants may require imaging as they age to detect rupture and patients may be responsible for all costs
  - ❑ Prophylactic antibiotics may be suggested for all future dental work
- ❑ **Breast implant technology**
  - ❑ Constantly changing alternatives- current alternatives
  - ❑ Limitations of implants- no implant is without tradeoffs
- ❑ **Summarizing the alternatives**
  - ❑ Incision alternatives- inframammary, axillary, periareolar, axillary
  - ❑ Implant pocket locations- retromammary, retropectoral, dual plane, totally submuscular
  - ❑ Current implant choices Saline- Smooth round, textured round, textured shaped - types and manufacturers
  - ❑ Fitting the procedure and implant to your tissues to minimize long-term risks and compromises

- ❑ **Determining the best size**
  - ❑ If you could just pick a size, what would it be?
  - ❑ Which is more important, size or problems long-term?
  - ❑ Common misconceptions
  - ❑ How implant size affects your tissues- now and later
  - ❑ Bra cup sizing-we can't guarantee cup size
  - ❑ Balancing your breast with your figure
  - ❑ Measuring your breast, understanding your tissues
  - ❑ Concentrating on shape, fill, dimensions
  - ❑ Photos and planning the operation

- ❑ **The operation- what's it like**
  - ❑ Day surgery routine
  - ❑ The facility and facility personnel
  - ❑ Anesthesia
    - Safety of anesthesia, misconceptions, risks
    - Local versus general anesthesia
    - Our anesthesia personnel
- ❑ **During surgery**
  - ❑ What will occur, expected time frame

- ❑ **After surgery**
  - ❑ Waking in recovery, then to stepdown with caregiver
  - ❑ **Detailed instructions will be given to you**
    - Tells you and your caregiver what to expect and do
    - What we do simplifies your instructions

- ❑ **Recovery and activity**
  - ❑ Importance of resuming normal activity
  - ❑ What we do and what we need you to do
  - ❑ No bandages, bras, straps, drains or special devices
  - ❑ Nothing aerobic for 2 weeks

- ❑ **Risks of augmentation**
  - ❑ This is a totally elective operation with risks and uncontrollable factors
  - ❑ Bleeding
  - ❑ Infection
  - ❑ Sensation compromise
  - ❑ Capsular contracture
  - ❑ Unsatisfactory aesthetic results or scarring
  - ❑ Interference with cancer detection
  - ❑ Complications may require additional surgery, longer recovery, additional costs
  - ❑ Reviewed risks on consent forms & documents
- ❑ **Capsular contracture and breast firmness**
  - ❑ What is it?
  - ❑ How a capsule forms
  - ❑ Controlling the capsule
  - ❑ How often does it occur?
  - ❑ Correcting the hard breast
- ❑ **Factors that the surgeon cannot predict or control**
  - ❑ Capsular contracture
    - ❑ Different degrees, if severe, requires reoperation
    - ❑ Surgeon alone makes finaldecisions re: reoperation
    - ❑ All costs are patient's responsibility, no insurance
    - ❑ Tissue stretch problems- increase with implant size
    - ❑ Stretch allowing implant shift downward or outward
    - ❑ Stretch allowing implant rotation
    - ❑ Traction rippling
    - ❑ Your request for a different size implant after surgery

❑ **All costs for any surgery relating to factors the surgeon cannot predict or control are the patient's responsibility (surgeon fees, facility fees, anesthesia, lab, time off work)- includes capsular contracture, infection, stretch deformities, implant size changes.**

- ❑ **Importance of communicating with us**
  - We want to do what you want
  - You must be honest with us at all times
  - The surgeon cannot read your mind

- ❑ **What you can expect from [Surgeon name]**
  Type of care, Written materials, Photos, The operation, Your care.

- ❑ **[Surgeon's]Qualifications**
  Surgical training, board certification, professional affiliations, scientific publications, other.

- ❑ **Patient has read all information material provided (Yes/No) _____ Pt. initial.**
- ❑ **Discussed any significant other's involvement, gave patient copy of Will There Be Anyone Else Involved.**
- ❑ **Written information provided patient was discussed in detail with patient, answered patient's questions to patient's satisfaction.**

- ❑ **All informed consent documents discussed in detail with patient, answered patient's questions.**

_______**Pt. (Initial)** _______**Dr./educator**

Figure 109.1. Patient educator checklist for patients. (Adapted from Tebbetts JB, Tebbetts TB. An approach that integrates patient education and informed consent in breast augmentation. J *Plast Reconstr Surg* 2002;110(3):971–978, with permission.)

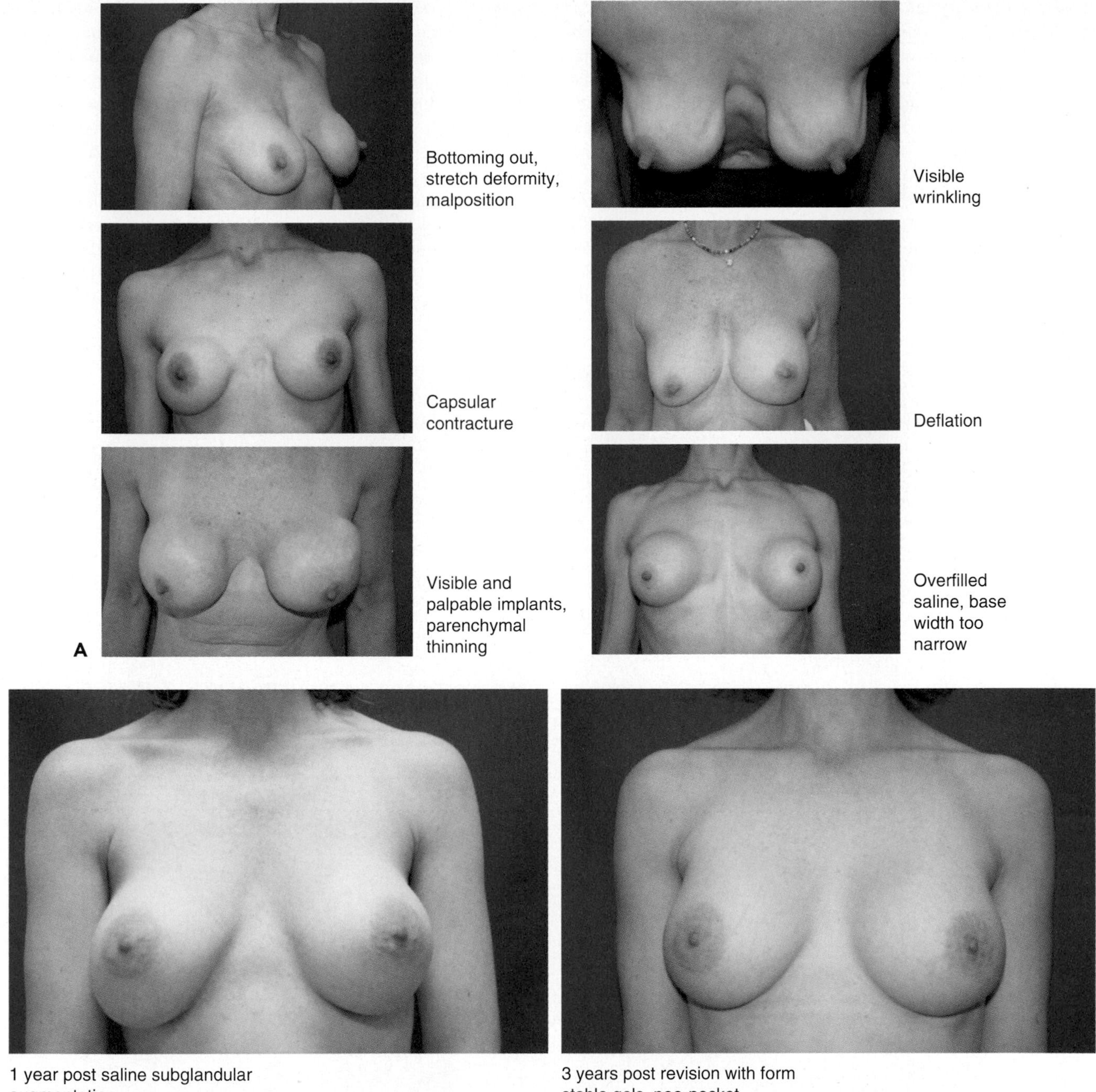

Figure 109.2. **A:** Images can be used as an educational tool to help patients visualize common breast augmentation complications and increase their understanding of the possible short- and long-term risks that may be a direct result of the choices made preoperatively. **B:** Patient educational tools can include a visual demonstration of the possible consequence of selecting an oversized implant placed in the subglandular position. Terms such as stretch deformities, malposition, and parenchymal thinning, as well as the concept of correctable and uncorrectable deformities, can be explained through images. Physicians can then demonstrate revision surgery of a complication using implants and techniques that prioritize implant–soft tissue relationships.

in demonstrating unclear concepts such as parenchymal thinning, skin stretch, and implant malposition. What is more, images can be shown depicting revision procedures necessary to correct some of the discussed potential complications, as well as those problems that may be uncorrectable. The goal of using images in patient education is not to discourage the patient from undergoing a breast augmentation, but to enhance the patient's knowledge base, thereby making her better able to make informed choices.

In an effort to further broaden the educational experience of women seeking information on breast augmentation, the leading implant manufacturers have developed websites that are designed to help inform patients about specific shells, shapes, fills, and sizes. Patients are becoming more savvy with respect to the language of implants, using terms such as "memory gel (Mentor Corporation) and "gummy bears" (Natrelle style 410), clearly a result of well-designed, direct-to-consumer marketing campaigns. Tools designed to streamline the selection of devices have been available for physicians for decades (27,28). Patient education in breast augmentation may be enhanced with the assimilation of these tools into the implant selection process during the consultation with the patient. In addition to printed device catalogs, manufacturers have developed highly specific implant selector tools that can be used in a verbal format, offered as a numeric list, or presented in a more visual format for patients (Fig. 109.3). Interactive implant selector tools have also been designed. The physician can incorporate the patient's desires (larger, smaller, optimal) with this modality, which, when used during a patient consultation, may help produce a more knowledgeable patient. Eager to enhance the patient learning experience even further, other manufacturers have developed interactive surgical simulation software integrated with image capture technology. This three-dimensional technology is designed to help physicians and their patients predict possible surgical outcomes (29).

Patients must eventually decide upon an implant type and size, pocket location, and location of the incision. Every surgeon can decide which of these educational modalities works best for his or her practice in an efficient manner, ensuring an effective transfer of information to breast augmentation

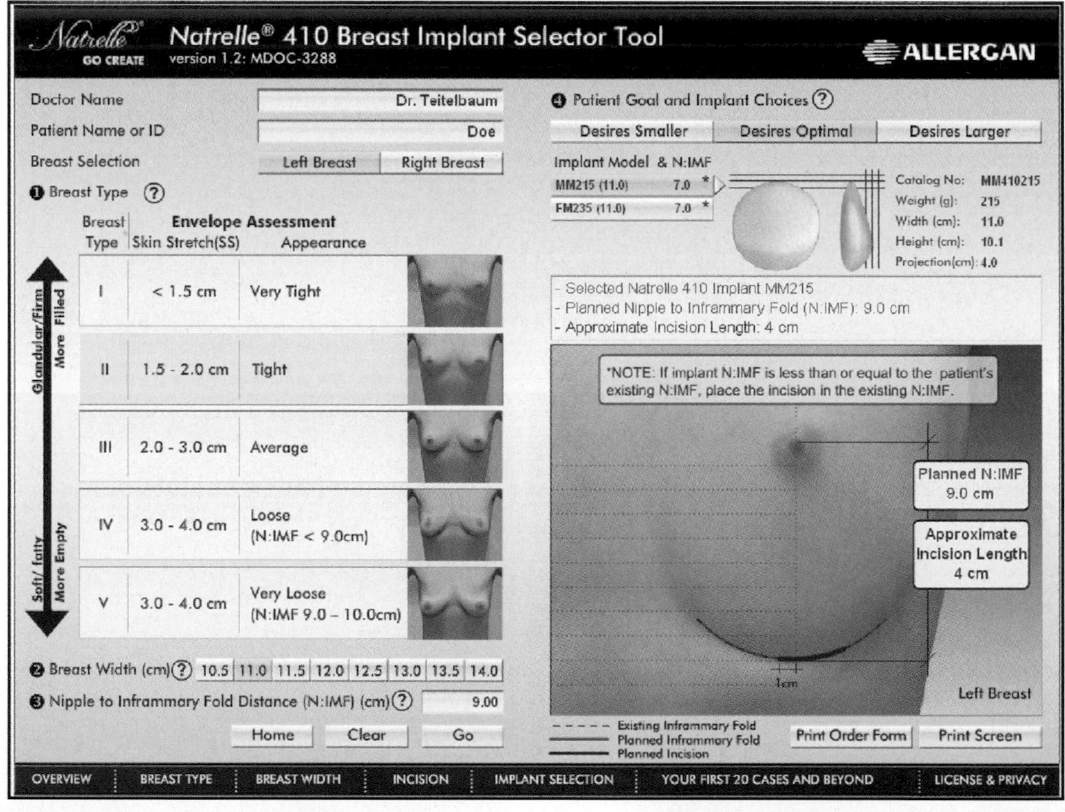

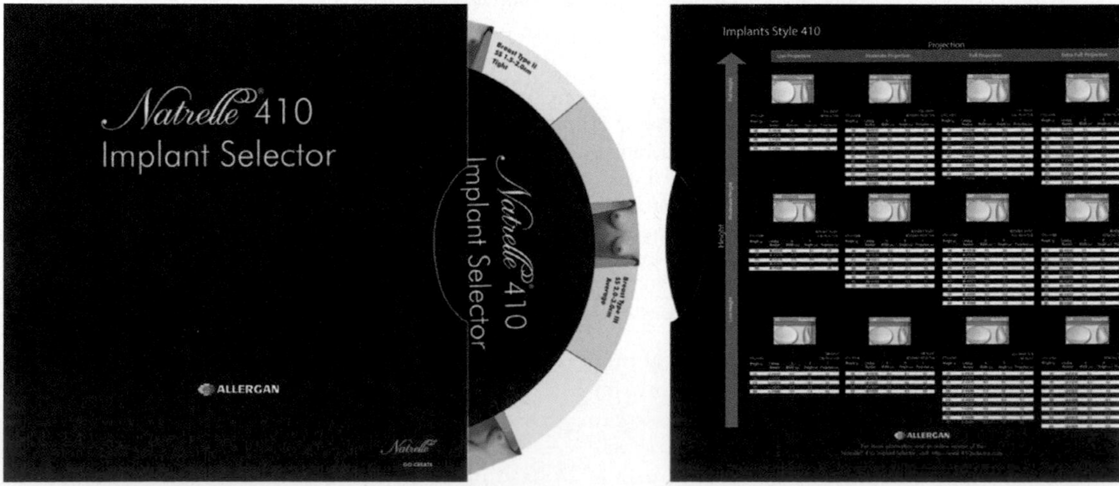

Figure 109.3. Natrelle 410 implant selector: print and interactive formats. Manufacturer's implant selector tools may be useful as both numeric and visual aids in patient education. (Courtesy of William P. Adams Jr., Dallas, Texas.)

patients. In addition, all of the tools can be of great value in the management of patient expectations and help distinguish the realistic from the unrealistic patient. The educational tools described can be used repetitively to address vital issues and make certain that there is effective communication of risk. The expectation is that a well-educated patient is going to make better lifelong decisions and be willing to be held accountable for those decisions.

CONVEYING LIFELONG RISK IN BREAST AUGMENTATION

A key factor in any communication of risk is whether the patient pays attention to the details. In general it is believed that the greater the elaboration of risk messages, the greater is the likelihood that the resulting perception of risk will influence behavior (30). The decision to undergo a breast augmentation is entirely elective, and patients should be presented with useful information to be able to make well-informed decisions. Information should be provided in a clear, positive, and personally relevant format. It is recommended that all information provided, as well as the decisions made between the surgeon and the patient, should be completely and thoroughly documented (5,6).

THE LONGEVITY OF BREAST IMPLANTS

It should be conveyed that despite the advances in technology, no device, saline or silicone, will last forever. Patients must be provided with the manufacturer's package insert, informed-consent documents, and implant warranty information, if the manufacturers offer them. The FDA website also includes current information from the Centers for Devices and Radiological Health, including patient labeling information from both Allergan and Mentor (31). The direct link to the manufacturer's website is also available for the most recent data on rupture and capsular contracture rates, and patients should be provided with these links so they can view them again at home (32). Breast augmentation surgeons who routinely follow their patient's outcomes should be able to provide long-term data on their own revision rates, including surgeries for capsular contracture and other complications. Patients should then be given the opportunity to compare data, focus on realistic risks, and make better choices. Data on rupture and capsular contracture rates can be overwhelming for many patients, but providing the information through visuals, numerically, and verbally will improve the process of risk communication.

BREAST IMAGING FOR CANCER SCREENING AND EVALUATION OF SILICONE GEL IMPLANTS

Several studies have addressed the question of whether breast implants interfere with mammography and therefore delay cancer detection in women with breast augmentation (33,34). Patients need to be informed that the presence of breast implants may interfere with standard mammography. Silicone gel–filled breast implants are radiopaque, and the physical presence of the implant may obscure part of the breast tissue and deform breast structure. The amount of interference varies depending on a variety of factors, including the position of the implant. Although there is evidence that subpectoral placement of the implant may improve the amount of tissue visible on mammography as compared with subglandular placement, the effect that the placement of the implant has on the sensitivity and specificity of screening needs further study (34). Breast implants are not, however, associated with an increased risk of breast cancer incidence or death. Patients should be advised that studies have shown that women with breast augmentation had tumors with better prognostic characteristics, including smaller size, lower grade, and more favorable estrogen receptor status (35,36). This may be due to the fact that augmented women have less natural breast tissue or because the implant provides a firm surface to palpate against (36). The best information that we can provide to breast augmentation patients suggests that although the sensitivity of screening mammography is lower in asymptomatic women with breast augmentation, there is no evidence that this results in more-advanced disease at diagnosis compared with women without augmentation (35,38). To increase sensitivity, patients need to be informed that they may require displacement-type views and possible additional images (39). Under ideal conditions, up to 90% of the breast may be visualized using these modified mammography techniques, but women with breast implants may also require longer mammographic examinations with additional views and a subsequent increase in exposure to radiation. Patients also need to recognize that capsular contracture may make imaging not only more difficult, but also more painful (40).

All patients who opt for silicone gel implants need to be informed of the FDA guidelines on breast imaging with magnetic resonance imaging (MRI) for the detection of rupture. Although some implant ruptures can be diagnosed on physical exam, the sensitivity of plastic surgeons who routinely perform breast augmentation to diagnose rupture by clinical exam has been reported at 30% (41), compared to 89% for MRI (42). For that reason, patients need to be informed that clinical examination is an insufficient screening method, and they will need to have regular MRIs over their lifetime to screen for silent rupture even if they have no problems. The FDA suggests that the first MRI should be performed at 3 years postoperatively, then every 2 years thereafter. Diagnostic procedures will add to the cost of having breast implants, and patients should be told that these costs may exceed the cost of their initial surgery over their lifetime, as they may not be covered by insurance carriers (43). Patients can be advised that newer diagnostic tools including four-dimensional ultrasound imagery may be on the horizon and may be a less expensive option for the long-term evaluation of gel implants.

Women considering breast augmentation need to be encouraged to participate in long-term follow-up studies to help evaluate the long-term safety and benefits of breast implants. Ten-year postapproval studies have been implemented to collect data on women receiving saline and silicone breast implants. These studies provide financial incentives to both the patient and the surgeon who monitors the implants (44,45).

EDUCATION AND ITS ROLE IN THE MANAGEMENT OF PATIENT EXPECTATIONS

If the preoperative educational experience is to be complete, a significant portion of the consultation should be devoted to the management of the patient's postoperative expectations. Time spent prior to surgery should include a discussion of what factors the surgeon can and cannot predict or control. Patient expectations related to breast size are perhaps the most common early postoperative area of potential conflict between patient and surgeon. The FDA PMA data from 2004 revealed that reoperation for size change accounted for almost one third of all reoperations. Allergan's core study data from the FDA PMA studies, updated in 2007, disclosed that patient request for size change, reported at 23.4%, was the second-most-common reason for revision surgery at 4 years (30,45). Reoperation for incorrect size can mean either that a patient desires a larger size after surgery than was agreed on before surgery or the patient is unhappy with implants that have been oversized for her tissues. Furthermore, physicians need to inform their patients that no method of breast augmentation exists that can accurately determine an exact postoperative breast cup size. The current accepted system of determining bra size is so inaccurate and varies so often it is of no true value. If one includes the many different styles of bras, fabrics, and elastics and the lack of standardization among brands, it is understandable why women struggle to find a comfortable, well-fitting bra. Determining the correct bra size is more a matter of educated guesswork and trial and error than of precise measurements (47). Bra sizing varies worldwide and differs considerably among manufacturers. In addition, many bra manufacturers, designers, and bra shop fitters have their own techniques for sizing and fitting. Patients often are given misleading information concerning both their back measurements and cup size. Confusion exists when patients either underestimate or overestimate their back size, and very few understand the concept of sister sizes; for example, a 34C is equivalent to a 36B bra. In the United States, the US Standard Clothing Size sets some guidelines, but there is no formal standard inch-based brassiere sizing system in the United States (48). Studies have demonstrated, however, that reoperations for size change can be virtually eliminated when the surgeon places a high value on patient education and decision-making processes that emphasize potential long-term complications over postoperative cup size (5,6).

Patients, who share in the selection of their breast implants based on their individual tissue measurements make decisions that are knowledge based and patient centered. Communication is crucial during the informed-consent process, as is the absolute need to document the patient's implant selection in writing. The education process can also continue postoperatively if patients question their size or shape after surgery. Quality preoperative photos are invaluable as teaching tools postoperatively. Patients often forget "how small" or "how asymmetric" they were before surgery. Side-by-side photography offers patients the opportunity to validate the decisions that were made together with the surgeon. Patients who understand and participate in the implant selection process by and large accept their improvements in breast size and shape postoperatively.

Before surgery, patients should also be provided with a clear and forthright dialogue that addresses the very issues that can drain the gratification out of the physician–patient relationship after surgery. One of these issues concerns who will be responsible financially for the possible known and unknown events that might occur after surgery (49). Financial responsibilities after surgery may include surgical or implant-related complications (Table 109.1), costs associated with radiologic evaluation of the implants as they age, and eventual replacement or removal of breast implants. Defining the potential financial risks that may occur over the patient's lifetime and whether the surgeon or patient will be financially responsible is imperative before breast augmentation. These important issues should be delineated in writing during the informed-consent process. Finally, patients should be aware of the physician's policy on "out-points," defining when implant removal without replacement would be recommended to decrease further surgical and financial risks (50).

TABLE 109.1 Implant and Surgery-Related Risks

Implant-Related Risks	*Surgery-Related Risks*
Implant failure: rupture or deflation, including silent rupture	Bleeding
Capsular contracture	Seroma
Malposition deformities	Infection
Tissue stretch	Scarring
Calcification	Allergic reactions
Extrusion	Anesthesia
Chest wall irregularity	Nipple or skin sensation loss
Asymmetry	Thrombosed veins
Gel bleed	Pain
Surface contamination: late infection or capsular contracture	Malposition deformities
Interference with mammography	Suture problems
Unusual occupations	Delayed wound healing
Personal financial expenses	Skin discoloration
Unknown risks	Cardiac complications
	Pulmonary complications
	Shock

Adapted from Jewell M. S8 Breast Education Course. Presented at the American Society for Aesthetic Plastic Surgery Meeting, New Orleans, Louisiana, April 29, 2005.

CONCLUSION

For decades preoperative decisions in breast augmentation, including implant selection, pocket location, and incisions, were based on either a surgeon's subjective preferences or the desires of the patient. Although physicians were responsible for obtaining informed consent prior to the procedure, there failed to be a means to assess whether the decisions made by the patient were fully informed and reflected the patients preferences based on an adequate communication of risk by the physician and staff. Data suggest that breast augmentation surgeons should try to better understand the patient's knowledge base and decision quality so as to address any gaps in comprehension before surgery. Patient decisions in breast augmentation are considered "preference-sensitive" clinical decisions and should reflect decisions made by a *well-informed* patient. Furthermore, debate continues with regard to a plastic surgeon's beneficent duty to recommend that the patient reconcile her desires within the limitations of her tissues if data suggest that doing otherwise may increase risks of revision surgeries and potential uncorrectable deformities. In addition, the simultaneous introduction of informed-consent documents into the educational process will help hold patients accountable for autonomous decisions while preserving their right to self-determination. Patient consultations are now turning toward more interactive learning experiences, with the inclusion of verbal, visual, and tactile tools in order to create a more engaged and informed patient. Considerable media attention has been focused on the safety of breast implants, and many women seeking breast augmentation may have unsubstantiated biases that may require a multimodality educational approach to surmount. The management of patient expectations should also include what factors a surgeon can and cannot control and who will be financially responsible for possible untoward results.

Finally, the physician must convey to patients the lifelong risks of breast augmentation, which may be complicated by the natural aging process. Events such as weight gains and losses, childbearing and breast-feeding, breast cancer risks, and eventually menopause are all natural events in a woman's life. Furthermore, patient education in breast augmentation does not end with the surgical procedure and should continue over the years as both the patient and the implants age. Plastic surgeons should be aware that the most frequent complaint of women who reported dissatisfaction with breast augmentation surgery to the FDA was that they felt they had not received adequate information before surgery (51). It is unlikely that the government or the media will ever turn their attention away from this issue. Physicians can, however, make a difference by assuring that their patients are *well informed* with regard to the known and unknown risks of breast augmentation surgery.

EDITORIAL COMMENTS

Dr. Glicksman has provided an excellent account of the informed-consent process as it relates to breast augmentation. She has described the importance of effective communication on the part of the surgical team and comprehension on the part of the patient and emphasized the concept of realistic expectations and its role in short- and long-term outcome. Education is critical. Fortunately my practice is very much in sync with what Dr. Glicksman espouses. Photography as an educational tool is invaluable. Patients should be shown good, average, and poor outcomes. I especially enjoyed reading the section on bras because prospective patients overly emphasize desired bra size. The problem is that bra size is not directly correlated to breast volume. It is more reflective of body habitus, breast shape, and proportion. A woman with a 44B cup will usually have a larger volume of breast tissue than a woman with a 34D cup. Thus informed consent is not just about signing a piece of paper that states one understands the nature of the operation; it is about proper education and counseling to minimize the chance of a poor outcome.

Although I agree with all of the concepts reviewed by Dr. Glicksman, there are a few caveats to all of this. The first is that most plastic surgeons are excellent communicators but fewer are good educators. The second is that not all patients are rocket scientists, and thus some may lack the capacity to assimilate a relatively large amount of new information. This, coupled with the fact that some plastic surgeons are biased when it comes to breast augmentation because they want to perform the operation to a far greater degree than they want to deny it, can lead to unrealistic expectations and poor surgical outcomes. The unfortunate reality is that in a few practices, it is the job of the surgeon and staff to "sell" the operation. The feeling is that if they do not, another plastic surgeon will, and rarely does that plastic surgeon want to lose the business. Complicating this further is that some patients often arrive at the consultation with preconceived notions of what they want based on what they have learned from their friends, the Internet, societal tends, magazines, and television. This sets the stage for choices that may be less than optimal. It has been my experience that a few patients know exactly what they want and are not open to the idea of choosing a device or approach that may be better suited for them based on body and tissue characteristics and what is recommended. In these cases, the surgeon should put aside his or her bias and deny the operation. In the ideal world, which is the world we would like to live in, it is the responsibility of the surgeon and staff to redirect patients' expectations from unrealistic to realistic.

M.Y.N.

REFERENCES

1. Adams WP, Potter JK. Breast implants: materials and manufacturing past, present, and future. In: Spear SL, ed. *Surgery of the Breast: Principles and Art.* 2nd ed. Baltimore: Lippincott Williams & Wilkins, 2006:424–437.
2. Mentor Corporation. Silicone gel and saline implant PMA clinical trials. Available at: http://www.fda.gov/cdrh/breastimplants/index.html. Accessed February 12, 2009.
3. Inamed Corporation. Silicone gel and saline implant PMA clinical trials. Available at: http://www.fda.gov/cdrh/breastimplants/index.html. Accessed February 12, 2009.
4. Adams WP. The process of breast augmentation: four sequential steps for optimizing outcomes for patients. *J Plast Reconstr Surg* 2008;122(6):1892–1900.
5. Tebbetts JB, Tebbetts TB. An approach that integrates patient education and informed consent in breast augmentation. *J Plast Reconstr Surg* 2002;110(3):971–978.
6. Cobb v Grant [1972]. 8 Cal3rd 229, 104 Cal Rptr 505, 502 P21.
7. Stewart M. Effective physician–patient communication and health outcomes: a review. *Can Med Assoc J* 1995;152:1423–1433.
8. Whitney SN, McGuire AL, McCullough LB. A typology of shared decision making, informed consent, and simple consent. *Ann Intern Med* 2004;140:54–59.
9. Davis TC, Crouch MA, Willis G, et al. The gap between patient reading comprehension and the readability of patient education materials. *J Family Pract* 1990;31:533–538.
10. Ong LML, de Haes JCJM, Hoos AM, et al. Doctor–patient communication: a review of the literature. *Soc Sci Med* 1995;40:903–918.
11. Kusec S, Oreskovic S, Skegro M, et al. Improving comprehension of informed consent. *Patient Educ Couns* 2006;60:294–300.
12. Beardsley E, Jefford M, Mileshkin L. Longer consent forms for clinical trials compromise patient understanding: so why are they lengthening? *J Clin Oncol* 2007;25:e13–e14.
13. Flory J, Emanuel E. Interventions to improve research participants understanding in informed consent for research: a systematic review. *JAMA* 2004;292:1593–1601.
14. Wood S, Spear S. What do women need to know and when do they need to know it? *Plast Reconstr Surg* 2007;120(7):135S–139S.
15. Veatch R. Implied, presumed and waived consent: the relative moral wrongs of under and over-informing. *Am J Bioeth* 2007;7(12):39–54.
16. Jewell M. Managing patient expectations in breast augmentation. S8 Breast Education Course (with permission). Presented at the American Society for Aesthetic Surgery meeting, New Orleans, La., April 29, 2005)
17. Sepucha K, Ozanne E, Silvia K, et al. An approach to measuring the quality of breast cancer decisions. *Patient Educ Couns* 2007;65:261–269.
18. Schneider CE. *The Practice of Autonomy: Patients, Doctors, and Medical Decision.* New York: Oxford University Press; 1998:307.
19. Tauber AI. *Patient Autonomy and the Ethics of Responsibility.* Cambridge, MA: MIT Press; 2005:328.
20. Yermilov I, Chow W, Devgan L, et al. How to measure the quality of surgery-related Web sites. *Am Surg* 2008;74:997–1000.
21. American Society of Plastic Surgeons. *Plastic and Reconstructive Surgery.* Available at: http://www.plasreconsurg.org. Accessed July 12, 2010.
22. Heller L, Parker P, Youseff A, et al. Interactive digital education aid in breast reconstruction. *Plast Reconstr Surg* 2008;122(3):717–727.
23. Noland K, Juhn G. *The Visual Health Experience: Tools, Technology, and Information for Providers and Their Patients.* Atlanta, GA: ADAM; 2001.
24. Young VL, Watson ME. Breast implant research: where we have been, where we are, where we need to go. *Clin Plast Surg* 2001;28(3):451–483.
25. Palcheff-Weimer ME, Concannon MJ, Conn VS, et al. The impact of the media on women with breast implants. *Plast Reconstr Surg* 1993;92:779–785.
26. Tebbetts, J. Patient acceptance of adequately filled breast implants using the tilt test. *Plast Reconstr Surg* 2000;106(1):139–147.

27. Allergan. Natrelle. Breast augmentation and breast enhancement. Available at: http://www.natrelle.com/1.2_find_fit.aspx. Accessed July 12, 2010.
28. Mentor. BodyLogic system. Available at: http://www.mentorcorp.com/global/physician-information/bodylogic.htm. Accessed July 12, 2010.
29. Axisthree. Available at: http://www.axisthree.com/welcome. Accessed July 12, 2010.
30. Lipkus IM. Numeric, verbal, and visual formats of conveying health risks: suggested best practices and future recommendations. *Med Decis Making* 2007;27:696–713.
31. U.S. Food and Drug Administration. Labeling for approved breast implants. Available at: http://www.fda.gov/MedicalDevices/ProductsandMedicalProcedures/ImplantsandProsthetics/BreastImplants/ucm063743.htm. Accessed July 12, 2010.
32. Mentor. Important information for augmentation patients about Mentor MemoryGel™ silicone gel–filled breast implants. Available at: http://www.mentorcorp.com/pdf/approved/Augmentation.pdf. Accessed February 23, 2009.
33. Allergan. Breast implant answers: understanding silicone gel–filled breast implants. Available at: http://www.breastimplantanswers.com/. Accessed July 12, 2010.
34. Miglioretti DL, Rutter CM, Geller BM, et al. Effects of breast augmentation on the accuracy of mammography and cancer characteristics. *JAMA* 2004;291:442.
35. Handel N, Silverstein MJ, Gamagami P, et al. Factors affecting mammographic visualization of the breast after augmentation mammaplasty. *JAMA* 1992;268:1913–1917.
36. Deapen D. Breast implants and breast cancer: a review of incidence, detection, mortality, and survival. *Plast Reconstr Surg* 2007;120(suppl 1):70S.
37. Handel N, Silverstein MJ. Breast cancer diagnosis and prognosis in augmented women. *Plast Reconstr Surg* 2006;118(3):587–593.
38. Clark CP III, Peters GN, O'Brien KM. Cancer in the augmented breast. Diagnosis and prognosis. *Cancer* 1993;72(7):2170–2174.
39. Eklund GW, Busby RC, Miller SH, et al. Improved imaging of the augmented breast. *Am J Roentgenol* 1988;151:469–473.
40. Brown SL, Todd JF, Luu HD. Breast implant adverse events during mammography: reports to the food and drug administration. *J Women's Health* 2004;13:371.
41. Hölmich LR, Fryzek JP, Kjøller K, et al. The diagnosis of silicone breast implant rupture. Clinical findings compared to findings at magnetic resonance imaging. *Ann Plast Surg* 2005;54(6):583–589.
42. Hölmich LR, Vejborg I, Conrad C, et al. The diagnosis of breast implant rupture: MRI findings compared to findings at explantation. *Eur J Radiol* 2005;53:213–225.
43. Allergan. INAMED silicone gel-filled breast implants. Smooth & BIOCELL texture. Directions for Use. DFU Inamed Rev. Santa Barbara, CA: Allergan; November 3, 2006. Available at: http://www.fda.gov/cdrh/pdf2/P020056c.pdf. Accessed January 12, 2009.
44. Allergan. BIFS. Breast Implant Follow-up Study. Available at: http://www.bifs.us/. Accessed January 12, 2009.
45. Mentor. MemoryGel™ breast implants. Post-approval study. Available at: http://www.memorygel.com/PAS.aspx. Accessed January 12, 2009.
46. Spear S, Hedén P. Allergan's silicone gel breast implants. *Expert Rev Med Devices* 2007;4(5):699–708.
47. Pechter EA. A new method for determining bra size and predicting post-augmentation breast size. *Plast Reconstr Surg* 1998;102(4):1259–1265.
48. Apparel Search Company. US standard clothing sizes. Definition for the clothing industry. Available at: http://www.apparelsearch.com/Definitions/Miscellaneous/US_standard_clothing_sizes.htm. Accessed July 12, 2010.
49. Spear S. What women need to know and when do they need to know it? *Plast Reconstr Surg* 2007;120:135S–139S.
50. Tebbetts JB. "Out points" criteria for breast implant removal without replacement and criteria to minimize reoperations following breast augmentation. *Plast Reconstr Surg* 2004;114:1258–1264.
51. Merkatz RB, Bagley GP, McCarthy EJ. A quantitative analysis of self-reported experience among women encountering difficulties with silicone breast implants. *J Women's Health* 1993;2:105–109.

CHAPTER

110

Dennis C. Hammond

The Inframammary Approach to Augmentation Mammaplasty

INTRODUCTION

When planning a breast augmentation, there are generally three preoperative decisions that must be made. These include choosing the size and style of the breast implant, choosing the pocket plane into which the implant will be placed, and selecting an incision location to gain access to the breast. With respect to the choice of incision, any incisional strategy for breast augmentation must balance the sometimes competing goals of providing comfortable access to the breast, while placing the incision in the most inconspicuous location possible. To this end, several different approaches have been described, including incisions located around the areola, through the nipple, in the axilla, and in the umbilicus. However, for many surgeons, it is the inframammary fold approach that provides the best balance between these two aspects of incision location. Perhaps the most important advantage of the inframammary fold approach is that direct access to the breast is provided, which facilitates accurate creation of the dimensions of the pocket and precise control of bleeding. The resultant scar then falls strategically within the inframammary fold crease where it remains unseen unless the breast is lifted or the patient lies supine. The other incisions tend to variably compromise operative exposure for dissection of the breast pocket either due to incision length, as can be the case with periareolar or transnipple incisions, or due to their remote location, as with the transaxillary and periumbilical techniques. In addition, with these other incisions, pocket dissection is often performed in a blunt fashion, which can compromise precise pocket development and hemostasis. Also, if any patient develops complications such as hematoma, capsular contracture, or shape distortion, the inframammary approach may then be necessitated anyway to provide adequate exposure to correct the problem. Therefore, despite the relatively inconspicuous appearance of the other resulting scars, many surgeons find the inframammary fold approach to be the most attractive option when comparing operative exposure with scar quality and location.

INCISION PLANNING

Placing the incision so it will eventually fall directly in the resultant inframammary crease requires that many factors be taken into account. Perhaps the easiest situation to deal with is the patient who preoperatively has enough breast volume to form a defined crease and enough skin to accommodate the breast implant without recruiting upper abdominal skin to assist in forming the lower pole of the breast. This also assumes the inframammary fold location will not change. In these cases, the incision is diagrammed directly in the fold, and it is made long enough to allow adequate exposure for accurate pocket dissection and placement of the breast implant. Incision length for saline implants ranges from 3 to 4 cm in most cases, and for silicone gel implants, 4 to 5 cm. When the more cohesive anatomically shaped silicone gel implants are used, incisions of up to 7 cm in length may be required for larger implants. In these types of patients, the scar will consistently and reliably fall directly in the fold postoperatively, and in most cases, will be almost imperceptible (Fig. 110.1). When the existing skin envelope of the breast is not adequate to easily accommodate the proposed breast implant, skin from the periphery of the breast will be recruited, and a new inframammary fold location will generally be created. This must be taken into account when planning incision location. Direct measurement of the base diameter of the proposed breast implant can assist in placing the new fold. By using the radius measurement of the implant, a measurement from the nipple to the proposed fold can be made to approximate the location of the new fold. The elasticity of the skin must also be taken into account. Assuming the lower pole breast skin will stretch to accommodate the breast implant, this measurement is optimally made with the lower pole skin under stretch to attempt to predict this proposed effect. Alternatively, a maneuver I have found to be helpful in these types of patients is to gently lift the breast skin envelope away from the chest wall, with mild tension directed from above and with the patient supine, and observe where the new fold tends to form. Placing the incision at the lower margin of this fold ensures the resulting scar will fall in the new fold formed after the breast implant is inserted (Fig. 110.2). In cases of severe restriction of the skin envelope of the breast preoperatively, placement of the inframammary fold incision can be difficult to gauge accurately. The location of the fold is almost always lowered in these patients, and the lower pole breast skin tends to be relatively inelastic so the stretch effect will be limited. As a result, direct measurement of the distance from the nipple to the proposed fold is the best method to predict the ultimate location of the new inframammary fold. This measurement is again guided by the radius measurement of the width of the proposed breast implant. There is still a tendency for the incision to ride up on the lower pole of the breast in these types of patients, and an additional 0.5 to 1 cm lowering of the planned incision is generally used to increase the likelihood that the scar will fall directly in the subsequent fold (Fig. 110.3).

After the location of the desired fold is determined, the actual incision can be located anywhere along this line. A common strategy to position the incision is to drop perpendicular from the medial aspect of the areola or the nipple to the proposed fold and then measure the desired distance laterally along this line. I have found that an even more lateral location can be desirable in some patients. By measuring from the lateral margin of the areola and then extending laterally, the scar

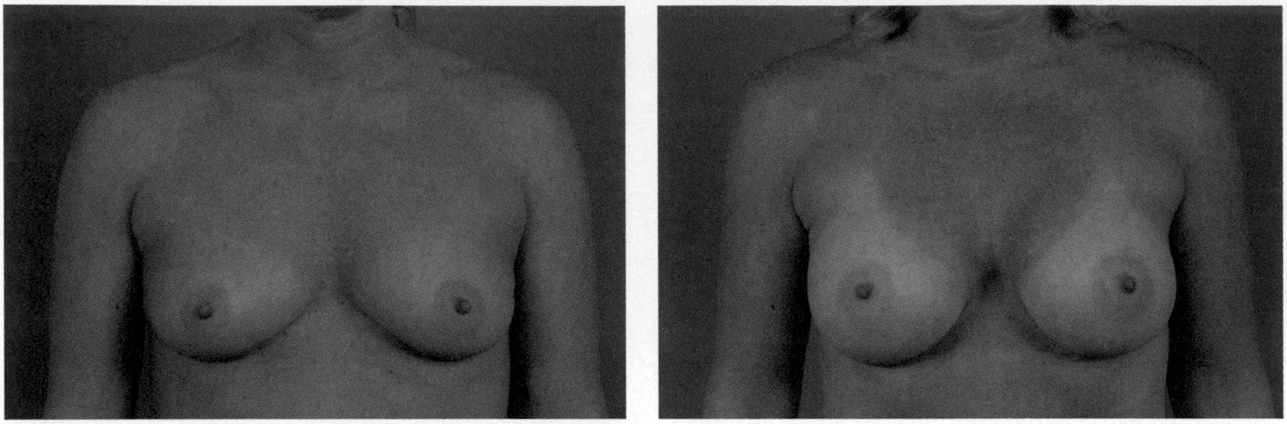

Figure 110.1. **A:** Preoperative appearance of a woman with moderate breast volume prior to breast augmentation through an inframammary fold incision. **B:** At 1 year, the augmented breast falls over the fold, concealing the scar. **C:** Only with the breast lifted and by looking from below can the well-healed scar be seen.

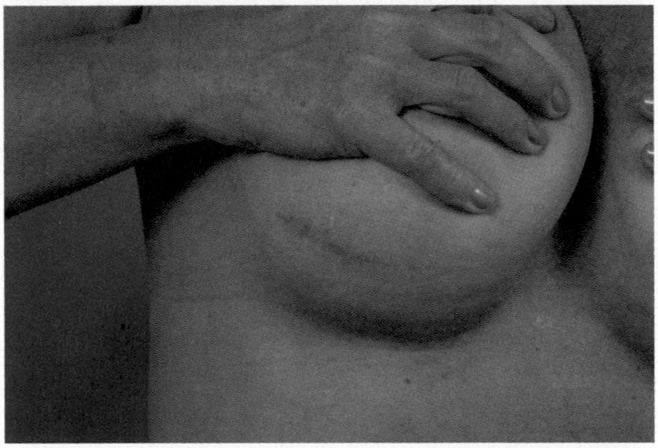

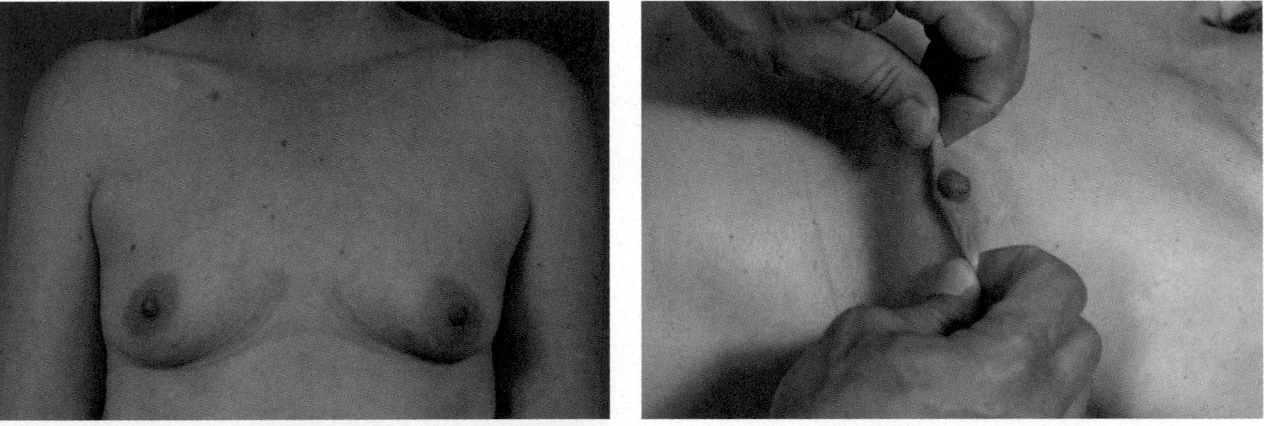

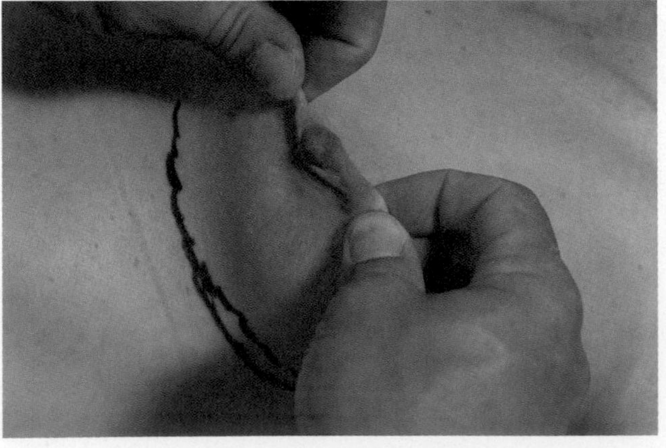

Figure 110.2. **A:** Preoperative appearance of a woman with minimal breast volume and a short inframammary fold-to-nipple distance prior to breast augmentation. **B:** By lifting the breast away from the chest wall, the redundancy in the skin can be taken up to simulate what effect the breast implant will have on the soft-tissue envelope. **C:** By applying slight pressure from above, the exact location of the new inframammary fold can be seen, which allows for accurate placement of the incision so the resulting scar will fall precisely in the fold.

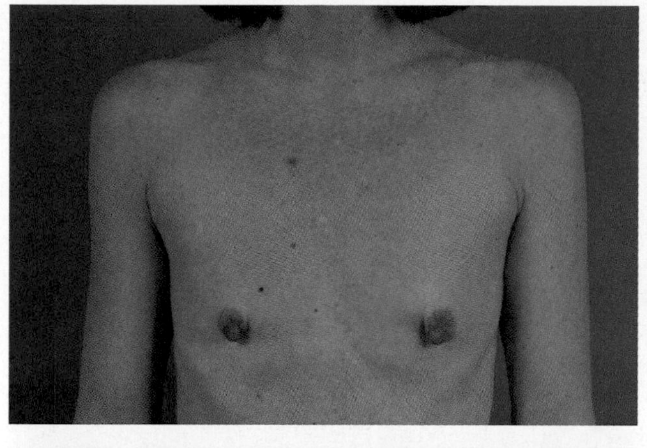

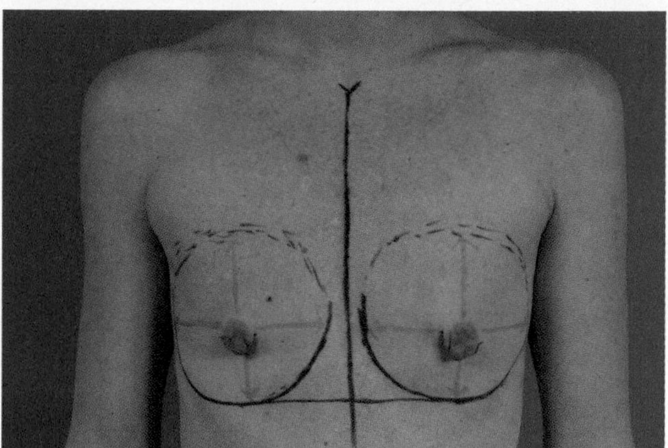

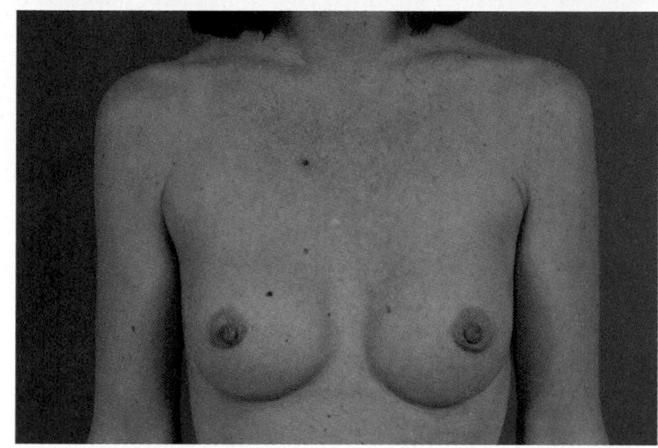

Figure 110.3. A: Preoperative appearance of a woman with essentially no breast volume and no defined inframammary fold. **B:** Measurements based on the radius of the proposed breast implant are made in each direction centered on the nipple. In this fashion, the location for the new fold can be estimated. **C:** Postoperative result showing accurate placement of the fold with good symmetry.

is even more difficult to see as the breast falls over the fold (Fig. 110.4). This approach also has the added benefit of allowing more of the inframammary fold to be addressed surgically from above and to the side rather than when the incision is located directly in the midportion of the fold. Accurately dissecting the fold to a desired level is easier to do from this more remote location than when the incision is directly in the center of the fold (Fig. 110.5).

In cases where the native inframammary folds are asymmetric, it is generally easier to maintain the position of the lowermost fold and then drop the position of the higher fold as needed (Fig. 110.6). The effect of lowering the fold on the position of the nipple and areola must also be taken into account. In cases of significant fold asymmetry, the high fold cannot be lowered to such a degree that the nipple areola complex (NAC) becomes malpositioned superiorly on the breast mound, relative to the other contours of the breast. Here, it is best to raise the opposite fold, manipulate the NAC position with periareolar surgery, or simply accept a persistent mild, but improved, fold asymmetry.

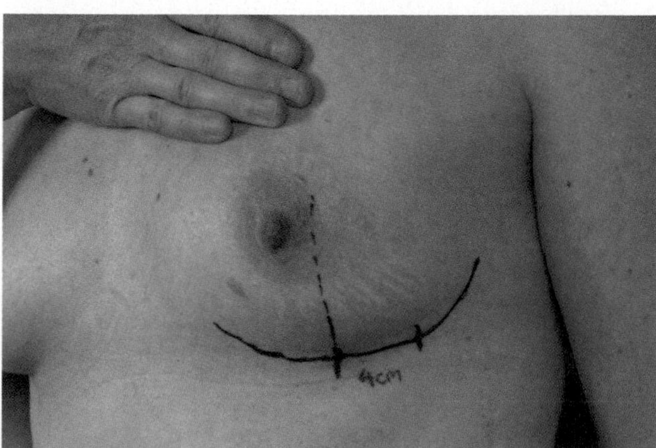

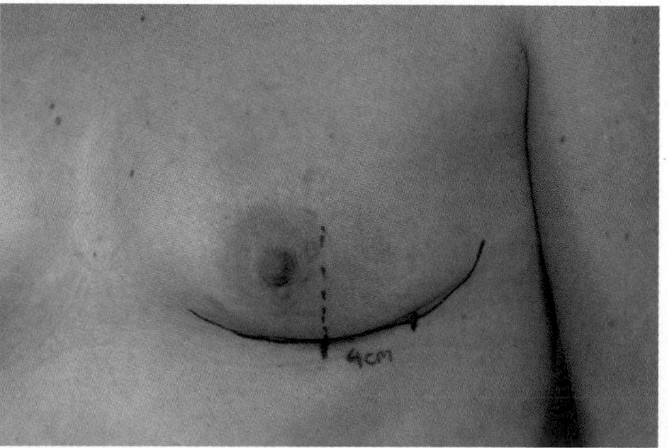

Figure 110.4. A and **B:** A line is drawn extending from the lateral aspect of the areola to the proposed inframammary fold. An incision of the desired length is then measured along the fold laterally. This places the resulting scar low and lateral, which is a location that heals well and is difficult to see postoperatively.

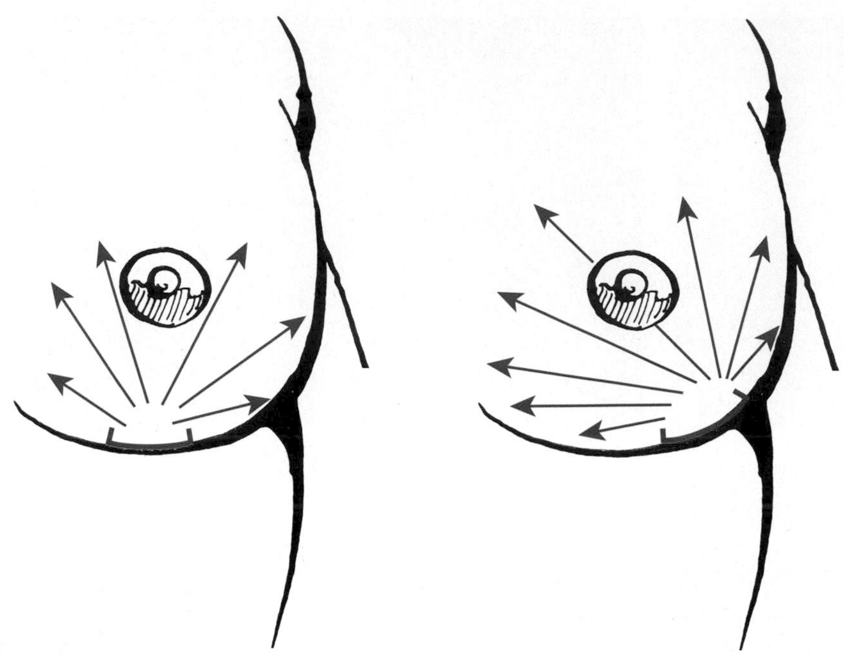

Figure 110.5. **A:** Working through an incision in the middle of the inframammary fold can sometimes be cumbersome when it comes to controlling the dissection space and positioning the location of the fold. Due to the proximity of the fold to the incision, it is easy to lower the fold position too much and end up with an implant that has a "bottomed out" appearance. **B:** By moving the inframammary fold incision to a more lateral location, the same access to the breast is provided, but it is easier to directly dissect the implant pocket as it relates to the fold, which can provide for greater control of fold location.

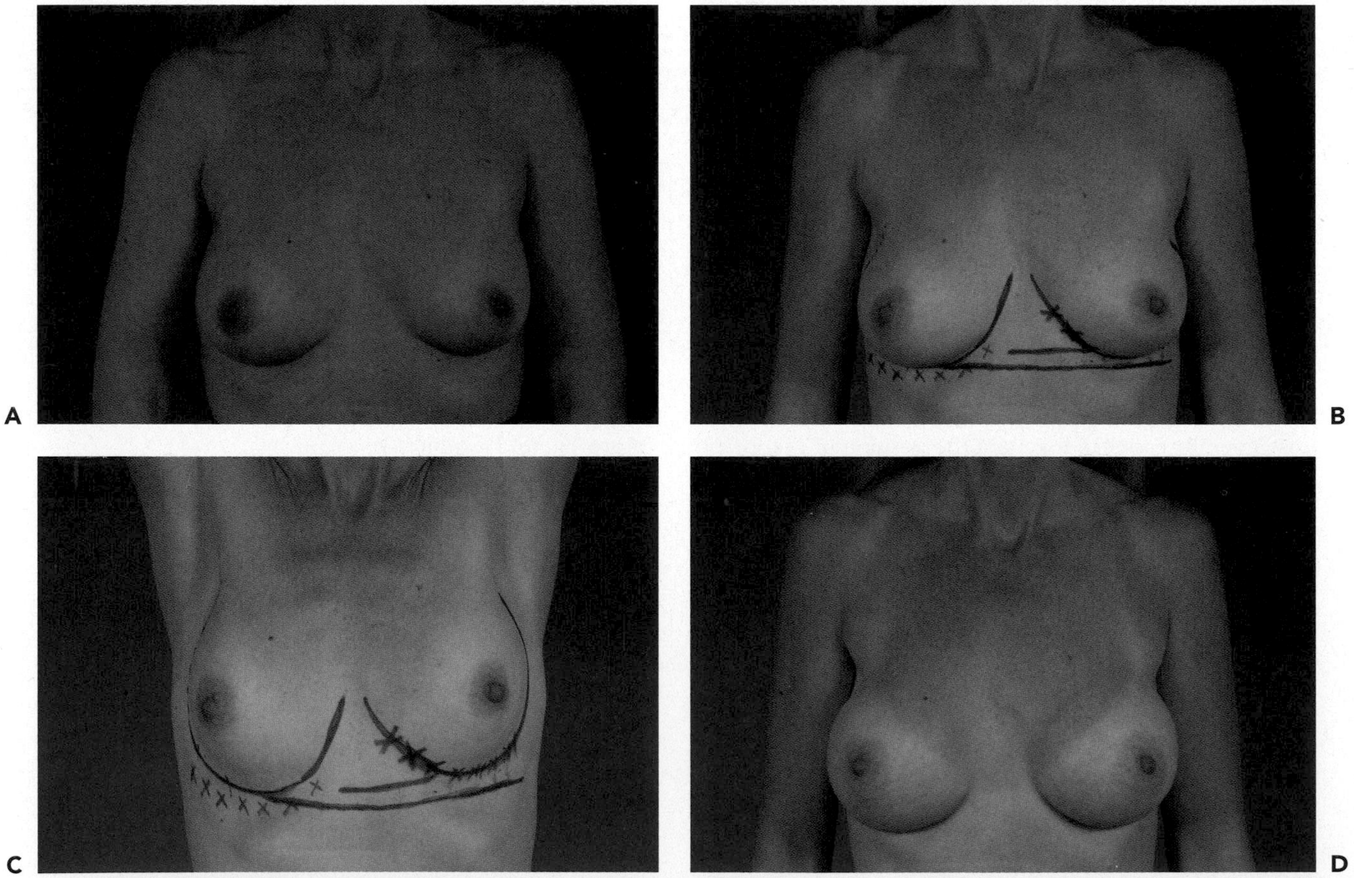

Figure 110.6. **A:** Preoperative appearance of a woman with an inframammary fold asymmetry. **B** and **C:** At surgery, the left inframammary fold will be lowered to match the fold on the right. **D** and **E:** Postoperatively, after placement of smooth round saline implants, the fold levels are symmetric with the breasts in repose and with the arms elevated. (*continued*)

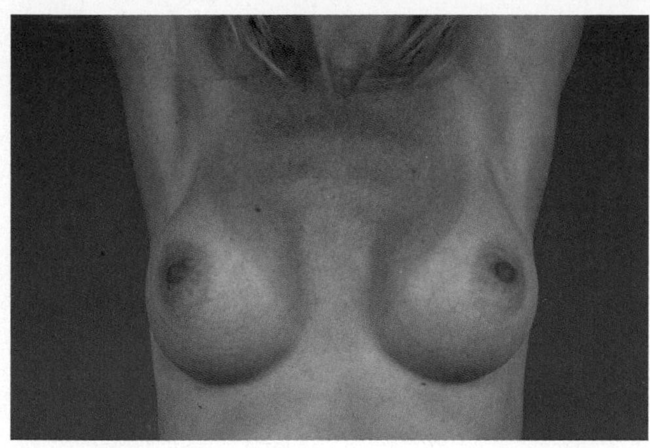
E

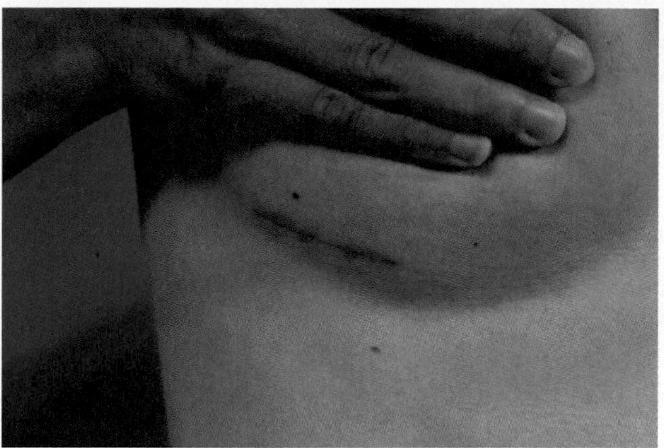
F

Figure 110.6. (*Continued*) **F:** The low and laterally placed scar has been correctly positioned directly in the fold.

OPERATIVE TECHNIQUE

Utilization of an incision in the inframammary fold affords direct visualization of the dissection plane required for breast augmentation. All types of pocket dissection techniques are facilitated using this approach, including subglandular, subfascial (1,2), partial subpectoral, dual-plane (3–6), and completely submuscular dissection spaces. After infiltrating the skin with a dilute solution of local anesthetic with epinephrine, incision is made through the skin. By angling upward to the underside of the breast, inadvertent lowering of the inframammary fold can be avoided. A lighted retractor is inserted and the desired pocket dissection is begun by expanding the superior dissection in all directions for several centimeters. For partial subpectoral or submuscular pockets, direct superolateral dissection will expose the lateral margin of the pectoralis major muscle. The underside of the muscle is elevated and then, by working from medial to superior to lateral, the pocket is opened. Laterally, care must be taken to avoid inadvertent overdissection because this space tends to open up easily. Through this incision, the pectoralis major muscle can be easily and under direct vision released along the inferomedial border of the pocket as desired. In addition, if dual-plane release of the overlying soft tissues is desired, the lower edge of the muscle can be released from the overlying breast as needed. Subcutaneous and subfascial pocket dissection also proceeds directly and easily through an inframammary incision. The limits of pocket dissection are readily identified and precise control of potential bleeding points is accomplished without difficulty. In addition, structures that are optimally preserved can be readily identified through the inframammary incision. In particular, the large second intercostal perforator off the internal mammary artery in the superomedial portion of the pocket, as well as the lateral intercostal nerves, can be visualized and protected. The pocket dissection is continued until the dimensions of the pocket approximate the dimensions of the desired implant. This is particularly important with respect to the medial and lateral extent of the pocket dissection. If the pocket is too wide, the implant will tend to fall off laterally under the arm when the patient is supine and create a medial concavity in the breast. This finding can be a great source of dissatisfaction in selected patients. After the pocket is developed, insertion of the implant also proceeds without difficulty because the incision and the pocket are in such close proximity. This is particularly advantageous with silicone gel implants, which have a fixed volume and must be coaxed into the pocket with gentle manipulation. In addition, with the anatomically shaped cohesive silicone gel implants, ensuring proper orientation and positioning of the shaped devices is facilitated because the orientation dots on the device can be easily visualized and palpated through the incision. Textured devices can sometimes be difficult to insert and position through remote incisions due to friction between the rough implant surface and the soft tissues of the breast. Again, the proximity of the breast pocket to the incision can help ease implant insertion in these cases. After the pocket has been developed and the implants properly positioned, the surgical wound is closed in layers, first closing the deep fascia and dermis with interrupted 3-0 or 4-0 absorbable monofilament sutures, and finally closing the skin incision with a running subcutaneous suture.

CONCLUSION

When performing breast augmentation, precision and control of pocket dissection and proper implant positioning are key factors in obtaining aesthetic results with few complications. To this end, the inframammary fold incision provides excellent operative exposure to accomplish both of these goals. The scar heals well and is unobtrusive because it is hidden in the inframammary crease. Thus, the inframammary approach is recommended as a consistent and widely applicable method for performing augmentation mammaplasty.

EDITORIAL COMMENTS

The inframammary approach to augmentation mammaplasty is perhaps the technique most used to access the subpectoral or subglandular plane. Having personally used the inframammary, periareolar, and axillary approach, I have come to the conclusion that the inframammary approach has distinct advantages over the other approaches. These include visualizing and accurately creating the implant pocket, hiding and modifying the length of the incision in the inframammary fold, and allowing the surgeon to easily place the implant in the subglandular or subpectoral position. Although the other techniques are effective, the inframammary technique has been predictable and satisfying in my hands. In addition, it is a very forgiving approach in the event of complications.

Dr. Hammond elegantly points out the subtleties of augmentation mammaplasty using the inframammary approach. His expertise on this subject is evident in his description of the operation. He reviews the importance of the inframammary fold based on placement and incision properties. That is, it is important to gauge where the final location of the inframammary fold should lie based on the size of the breast, proposed implant volume, and length of the torso. Lowering the inframammary fold will allow for increased compliance of the breast envelope and better positioning of the device. I agree with Dr. Hammond that the dimensions of the pocket should reflect those of the implant. I have had the occasion to reoperate on women with implants that migrate within a smooth, nonadherent pocket, and this is always a high source of patient dissatisfaction.

M.Y.N.

REFERENCES

1. Graf RM, Bernardes A, Rippel R, et al. Subfascial breast implant: a new procedure. *Plast Reconstr Surg* 2003;111:904–908.
2. Góes JC, Landecker A. Optimizing outcomes in breast augmentation: seven years of experience with the subfascial plane. *Aesthetic Plast Surg* 2003;27:178–184.
3. Tebbetts JB. Dual plane breast augmentation: optimizing implant—soft-tissue relationships in a wide range of breast types. *Plast Reconstr Surg* 2001;107:1255–1272.
4. Tofield JJ. Dual plane breast augmentation. *Plast Reconstr Surg* 2001;108:2162–2164.
5. Ramirez OM, Heller MDL, Tebbetts JB. Dual plane breast augmentation: avoiding pectoralis major displacement. *Plast Reconstr Surg* 2002;110:1198.
6. Spear SL, Carter ME, Ganz JC. The correction of capsular contracture by conversion to "dual-plane" positioning: technique and outcomes. *Plast Reconstr Surg* 2003;112:456–466.

CHAPTER

111

Scott L. Spear
Jeffrey M. Jacobson
Elan Reisin

The Periareolar Approach to Augmentation Mammaplasty

INTRODUCTION

The periareolar incision for augmentation mammaplasty allows for excellent, direct access with an inconspicuous scar, making this a particularly versatile approach. First described in the 1970s (1–4), this method provides central access to the implant pocket and is compatible with all planes of dissection and most types of implants (5). It is equivalent to or better than an inframammary approach at preserving nipple sensation (6,7). The nipple-areola junction appears to be a privileged area for scars; the resultant scar is often inconspicuous. In fact, in our experience, very few patients have expressed dissatisfaction with their scars. This is in contrast to our earlier experience with inframammary incisions, where dissatisfaction with scars was more common (8). The location of the periareolar incision is independent of the inframammary fold. Furthermore, it is an excellent choice when lowering of the inframammary fold is desired either at the first operation or subsequent operations (5). This incision does not interfere with breast biopsies or mastectomy incisions performed through or around the areola and is compatible with future mastopexy incisions by simply extending the periareolar incision around the entire areola (3–5,8–14). Finally, should the patient require revisionary surgery, the periareolar approach can be used again for most procedures (15).

This approach does violate some breast parenchyma and may create scarring within the breast, but in practice this is rarely a problem clinically or radiographically (9,10,12,14). A periareolar scar may be more visible than an inframammary scar in the upright patient but tends to be less visible when the patient is supine. The scar is only visible when the entire breast is exposed; otherwise the scar is hidden by even the most minimal amount of clothing. The periareolar approach can be used in virtually all women, in breasts with or without ptosis, and with most small or large areolas. As the amount of breast parenchyma increases, the periareolar incision becomes less desirable because of the increasing amount of breast tissue that must be traversed to reach the retromammary space. One concern of going through the breast near the nipple is the increased likelihood of contamination of the implant with breast bacterial flora. Such contamination has been speculated to be a risk factor for infection or capsular contracture (16).

In breast augmentation, the choice of incision must be considered along with several other decisions, including subpectoral versus subglandular pocket placement, smooth versus textured and round versus anatomic implant choice, and accompanying mastopexy or not. A periareolar incision facilitates a future mastopexy, whereas a previous inframammary incision does not help and may in fact interfere. If the patient's areola is large or the inframammary fold is high, the periareolar approach is similarly appealing. Even if the areola is small or the fold is diminutive or absent, it may be desirable to use the existing areola edge rather than estimate the location of the incision at the site of the new fold to be created by the breast implant. In patients with minimal or no ptosis and an existing inframammary fold 4 to 6 cm below the caudal edge of the areola, the periareolar approach has no major cosmetic advantages over the inframammary incision. Although remote incision placement, such as transaxillary and transumbilical, may carry certain cosmetic advantages, in many situations it is more difficult and potentially less accurate than the periareolar approach, even with the help of an endoscope. The periareolar approach is direct, easy, and user friendly and does not require special equipment (18).

TECHNIQUE

The preoperative markings are performed with the patient facing forward, sitting or standing upright, with her arms at her sides. The breast meridian, inframammary fold, and the location of the planned inframammary fold are marked. In the operating room, before the infiltration of an epinephrine-containing local anesthetic, the periareolar incision is marked precisely at the junction of the areola and surrounding unpigmented breast skin. It is important that this be performed prior to infiltration of any local anesthetic and/or epinephrine-containing solution because these can distort or obscure this border and make it more difficult to place the skin incision correctly. The incision is placed directly inferior for most dissections (4). In general, we try to avoid making the incision above the equator of the areola, and we center the skin incision at the 6 o'clock position (13). Perioperative antibiotics are recommended as in most procedures involving prostheses, but their use is optional.

The patient is positioned in the akimbo position or with the arms abducted no more than 90 deg on padded arm boards. It is essential that the patient's shoulders be level to best judge the intraoperative result when the patient is sat upright during the operation. Adequate lighting is crucial for this procedure; use of an endoscope, headlight, lighted retractor, or lighted electrocautery is recommended.

The region to be incised is infiltrated with a local anesthetic solution containing epinephrine. After allowing adequate time for the epinephrine to take effect, the skin incision is made through the dermis with a scalpel, and electrocautery is then used to incise into the breast tissue (Fig. 111.1). Skin hooks are placed on either side of the wound to provide the necessary retraction. The dissection through the breast tissue proceeds either directly posteriorly or by beveling inferiorly toward the chest wall (13) (Fig. 111.2). This maneuver leaves adequate breast tissue caudally to facilitate wound closure and preserves the skin and the breast contour. Rake retractors followed by Army/Navy retractors are used as the dissection proceeds

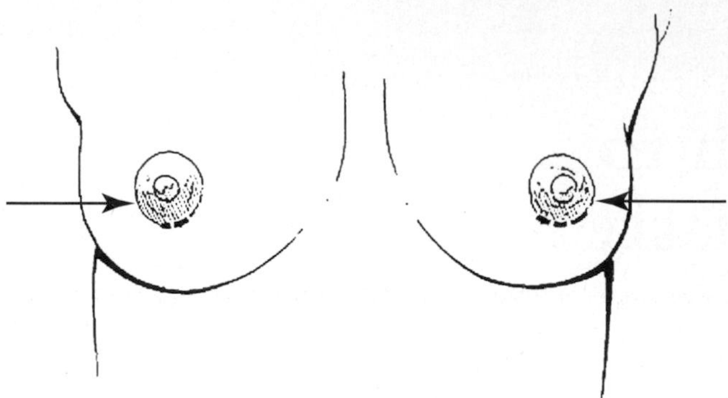

Figure 111.1. It is crucial to make the periareolar incision precisely along the edge of the areola. If done accurately, this produces a nearly invisible scar over time. The incision should be centered over the 6 o'clock position.

deeper into the breast, toward the chest wall. When the pectoralis fascia is reached, the breast tissue is mobilized off this layer, exposing the underlying fascia and muscle in an area corresponding to the lower pole of the breast from the inframammary fold inferiorly, to a point superiorly, which may vary depending on the existing skin envelope and degree of ptosis (Fig. 111.3). Inferiorly and inferolaterally, the dissection is

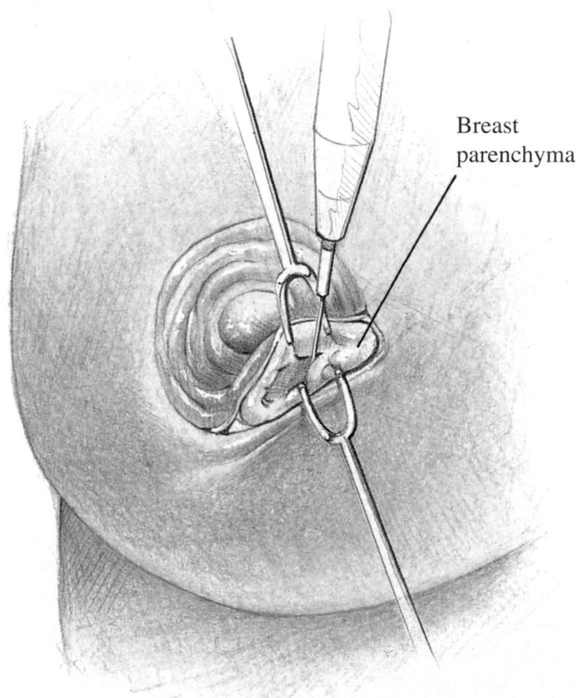

Figure 111.2. After the skin incision has been made, dissection begins with an electrocautery cutting either directly posteriorly or obliquely through the breast, aiming inferiorly while deepening the incision. For subpectoral augmentation, the dissection proceeds more medially. We recommend against an initial superficial dissection just beneath the skin, which is more likely to produce visible subcutaneous scar distortion. As the dissection deepens, it is prudent to use a scalpel or heavy, sharp scissors to completely divide the deeper aspect of the breast down to the pectoral fascia in order to create a tunnel to perform the operation.

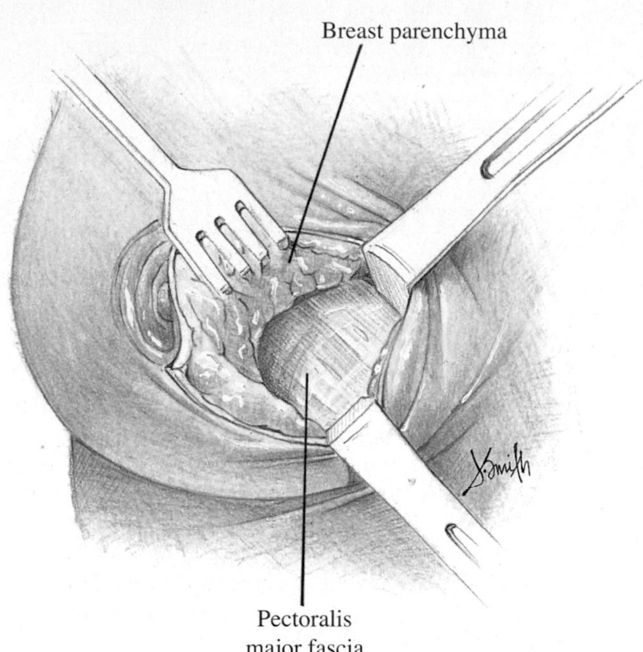

Figure 111.3. After the fascia has been identified, the breast is reflected off the underlying pectoralis major using cautery or sharp dissection. For subglandular breast augmentation, the dissection continues until the entire planned pocket has been created. A tissue expander or an inflatable implant can be used and inflated with saline or air to help with the dissection and to identify areas that need further release. For subpectoral augmentation, the breast inferior to the pectoralis muscle should be dissected first, lifting that portion of the breast off the muscle just as in a subglandular augmentation. The free inferior edge of the pectoralis muscle should be exposed to allow access beneath it.

subcutaneous down to the level of the desired inframammary fold (Fig. 111.4). If a subglandular approach is to be used, the remainder of the pocket is then precisely dissected under direct vision with electrocautery, fiber-optic lighting, or endoscopy, and Deaver retractors.

When performing a subpectoral augmentation, the inferior edge of the exposed pectoralis muscle is then grasped with an

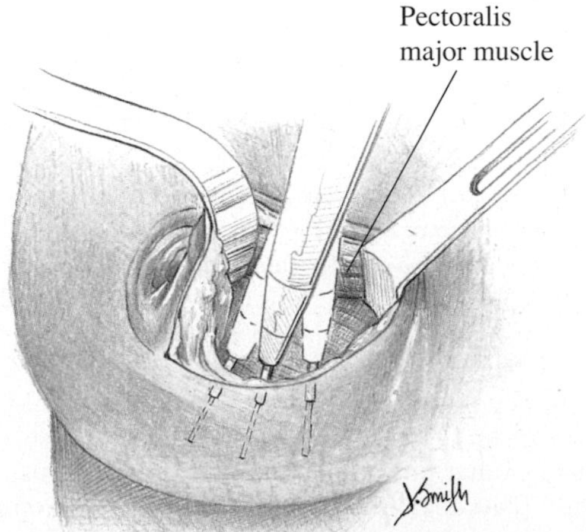

Figure 111.4. The inferior portion of the pocket should be created using primarily sharp cautery dissection under direct visualization. Subtle adjustments can then be made with blunt finger stretching and pulling or pushing movements. Anterior traction on the overlying tissues helps with these maneuvers. Subglandular dissection should proceed inferiorly down to the fold.

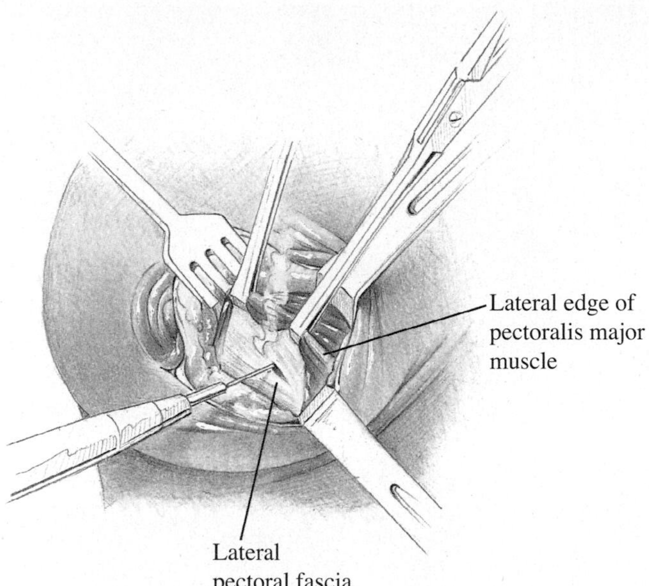

Figure 111.5. For subpectoral augmentation, the free edge of the pectoralis major muscle is grasped using one or two Allis clamps and lifted up out of the wound through the tunnel that has already been created.

Allis clamp. The lower edge of the muscle is lifted up and separated from the underlying chest wall by first creating a tunnel in the central portion of the subpectoral space. This step provides access to the subpectoral plane (Fig. 111.5). The subpectoral pocket is precisely enlarged using a combination of electrocautery and minimal blunt dissection (Fig. 111.6). Care is taken to cauterize perforating blood vessels before they are cut. Throughout this dissection, it is essential that the utmost care be taken to avoid lifting either the serratus anterior or the pectoralis minor muscles. The completed pocket is created by releasing the entire length of the lower edge of the pectoralis major muscle so it is confluent with the previously created lower pole subglandular pocket. After the muscle has been completely divided along its lower border, the subglandular dissection is finalized. Hemostasis is confirmed with fiberoptic lighting and precision use of electrocautery, followed by irrigation of the wound with a triple antibiotic and/or dilute Betadine solution. The skin around the incision should then be reprepped and the single surgeon who will be handling the implant should don new, powder-free gloves.

In the case of inflatable implants, air is aspirated from the prostheses, and they are then rolled like a cigar from each side toward the valve and inserted into the pocket. The implants are filled with the proper amount of saline or other fluid, and with the fill tubes left in, the incision is tacked together with skin staples and the patient is placed in the sitting position. The breasts are assessed for symmetry in terms of size, position, contour, inframammary fold, and nipple height.

After the surgeon is satisfied, the fill tubes are removed, and valve closure is verified under direct vision. The breast gland is then repaired with several interrupted 2-0 or 3-0 PDS sutures on a taper needle. A 3-0 or 4-0 absorbable monofilament suture is then used for buried, interrupted dermal sutures. Finally, a 3-0 or 4-0 absorbable monofilament suture is used for a running intradermal closure. External tissue glue is then applied to the wound as a surface dressing (14).

DISCUSSION

The periareolar approach works well with all types of implants: silicone or inflatable, round or anatomic, textured or smooth. Because of its excellent versatility and exposure, it often can adequately accommodate anatomic implants. The use of inflatable implants allows the effective use of a periareolar incision, even with the smallest of areola. Even in a small areola of 25 mm diameter, a semicircular incision around the areola measures approximately 4 cm in length (10) (Figs. 111.7 to 111.9). It is the logical choice when eventual mastopexy is suspected but is

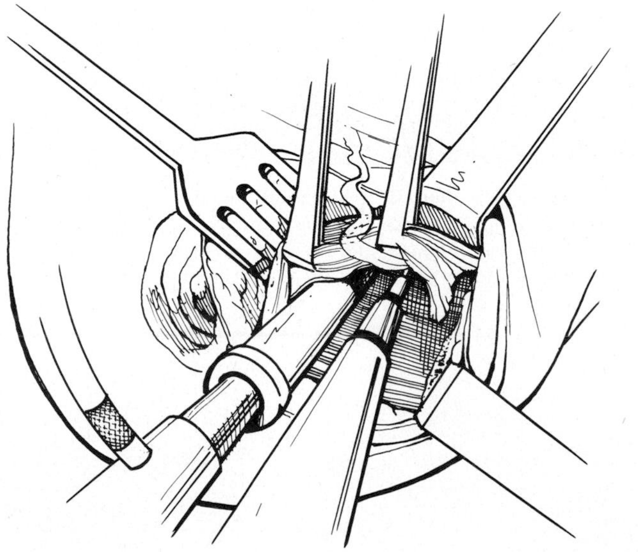

Figure 111.6. Using fiberoptic lighting or an endoscope, the muscle is sharply and carefully released using the electrocautery medially and inferiorly to create a pocket with the desired shape.

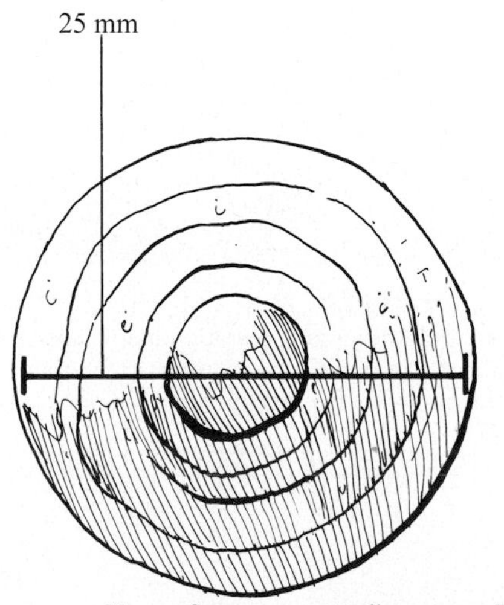

Figure 111.7. Although there are legitimate drawbacks to all incisions, including the periareolar one, this approach does not limit the size of incision, even in patients with a small areola. Even with an areola measuring 25 mm (about the size of a quarter), this allows the easy creation of a 4-cm incision along one half of the areola circumference.

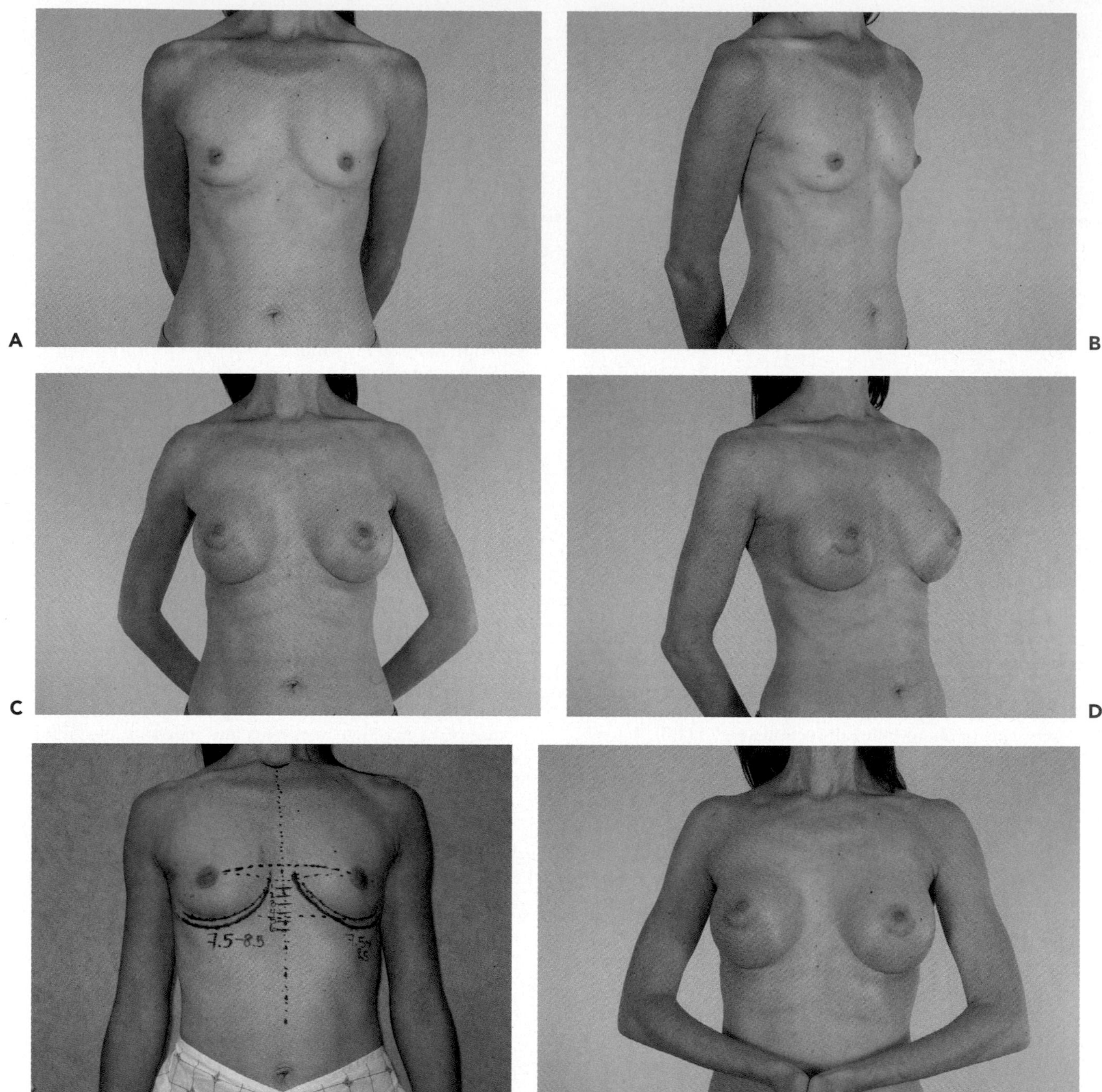

Figure 111.8. **A, B:** A 51-year-old, 5′7″ tall woman before breast augmentation. **C, D:** The same patient 3 months after augmentation mammaplasty with a 375-mL silicone gel implant placed in a dual-plane pocket through a periareolar incision. **E:** Preoperative markings. Note that the inframammary fold is lowered from 7.5 cm to 8.5 cm. **F:** Patient at 3 months postop flexing her pectoral muscles to show her level of animation deformity.

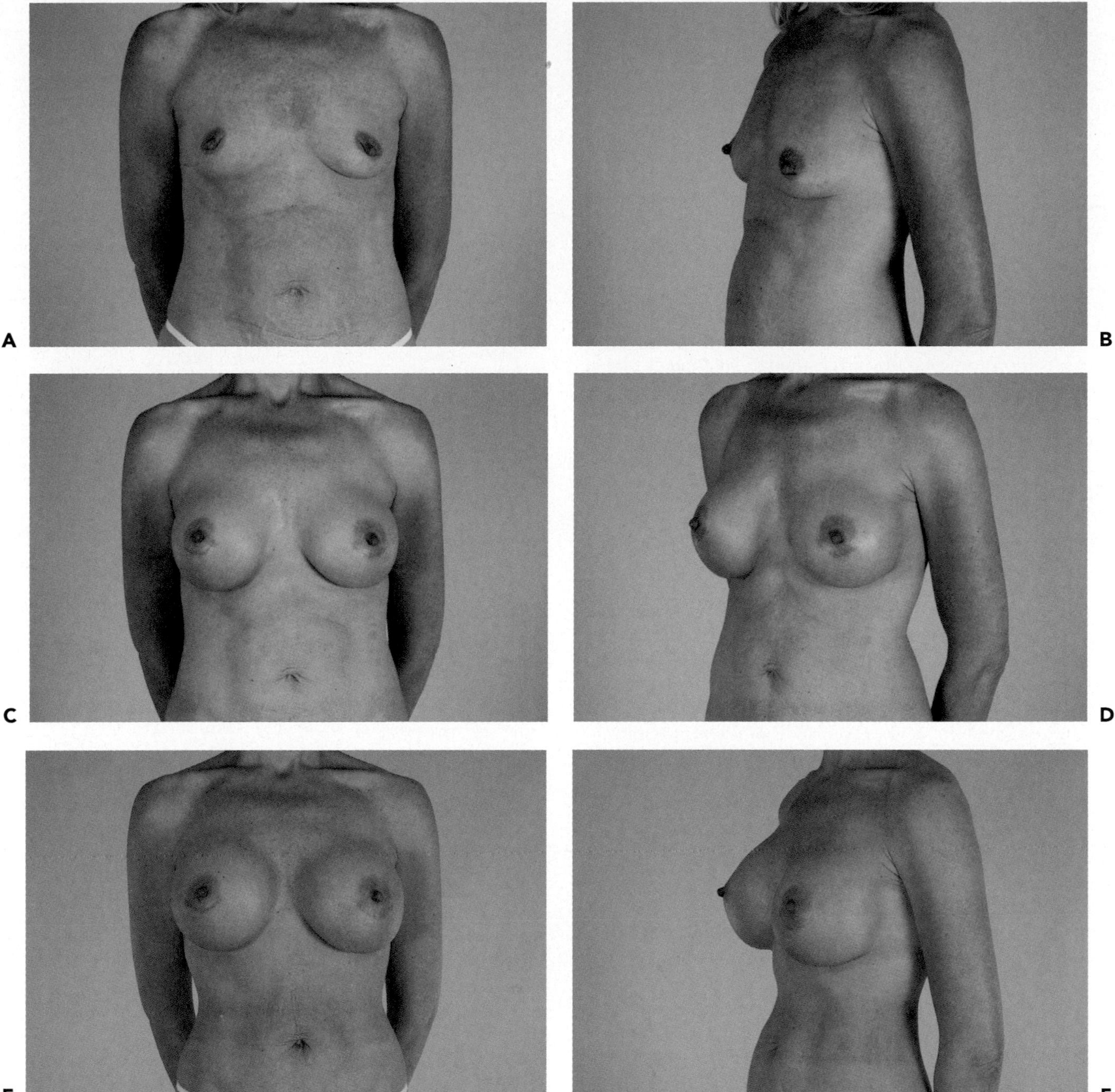

Figure 111.9. **A, B:** A 41-year-old, 5′10″ tall woman before breast augmentation. **C, D:** The same patient 6 months after augmentation mammaplasty with a 425-mL high-profile, saline-filled implant placed in a dual-plane pocket through a periareolar approach. **E, F:** The same patient 3 months after bilateral implant exchange to a 700-mL high-profile, saline-filled implant placed in a dual-plane pocket through a periareolar approach.

not certain preoperatively (5). This approach is also the best in cases of tubular breast hypomastia because it affords the possibility of periareolar skin or breast parenchymal excision, if necessary (5). Secondary procedures requiring capsulectomy, implant exchange, unilateral augmentation for symmetry, pocket size adjustments, and correction of implant malposition can all be performed through the periareolar incision.

EDITORIAL COMMENTS

The periareolar incision frequently provides good access to the subglandular or subpectoral plane. In my practice this approach is limited to women with a large areolar diameter. It is also recommended for women with a tuberous breast contour or when the inframammary fold needs to be lowered. One limitation of this approach is that it may be difficult to insert prefilled silicone gel devices through these sometimes-limited-length incisions. It is my preference to use an inframammary approach when inserting prefilled devices that are greater than 400 cc. As mentioned in the chapter, the dissection can proceed directly through the parenchyma or through the subcutaneous plane along the lower pole of the breast. Bacterial translocation can be a concern following the parenchymal approach, and this may predispose toward capsular contracture. When this approach is used, women are routinely placed on oral antibiotics for 1 week. Studies comparing periareolar versus inframammary approach have demonstrated a higher incidence of capsular contracture (16). However, this is minimized when the devices are placed in the subpectoral position (19). Studies comparing sensitivity of the nipple-areolar complex have demonstrated no significant difference between the periareolar and inframammary approaches (7).

REFERENCES

1. Williams JE. Experiences with a large series of silastic breast implants. *Plast Reconstr Surg* 1972;49:253.
2. Jenny H. Areolar approach to augmentation mammaplasty. *Plast Reconstr Surg* 1974;53:344.
3. Jones FR, Tauras AP. A periareolar incision for augmentation mammoplasty. *Plast Reconstr Surg* 1973;51:641.
4. Gruber R, Friedman GD. Periareolar subpectoral augmentation mammoplasty. *Plast Reconstr Surg* 1981;67:453.
5. Hidalgo DA. Breast augmentation: choosing the optimal incision, implant, and pocket plane. *Plast Reconstr Surg* 2000;105(6):2202–2216.
6. Okwueze MI, Spear ME, Zwyghuizen AM, et al. Effect of augmentation mammaplasty on breast sensation. *Plast Reconstr Surg* 2006;117:73–83.
7. Mofid MM, Klatsky SA, Singh NK, et al. Nipple-areola complex sensitivity after primary breast augmentation: a comparison of periareolar and inframammary incision approaches. *Plast Reconstr Surg* 2006;117:1694–1698.
8. Becker H. The intra-areolar incision for breast augmentation. *Ann Plast Surg* 1999;42(1): 103–106.
9. Biggs TM, Humphreys DH. Augmentation mammaplasty. In: Smith JW, Aston SJ, eds. *Grabb and Smith's Plastic Surgery*. 4th ed. Boston: Little, Brown; 1991:1145–1156.
10. Spear SL, Matsuba H, Little JW. The medial periareolar approach to submuscular augmentation mammaplasty under local anesthesia. *Plast Reconstr Surg* 1989;84:399.
11. Riefkohl R. Augmentation mammaplasty. In: McCarthy JG, ed. *Plastic Surgery*. Vol. 6. Philadelphia: Harcourt Brace; 1990:3879–3844.
12. Biggs TM, Cukier J, Worthing JF. Augmentation mammaplasty: a review of 18 years. *Plast Reconstr Surg* 1982;69:445.
13. Spear SL, Bulan EJ. The medial periareolar approach to submuscular augmentation mammaplasty under local anesthesia: a 10 year follow up. *Plast Reconstr Surg* 2001;108(3):771–775.
14. Courtiss EH, Goldwyn RM. Breast sensation before and after plastic surgery. *Plast Reconstr Surg* 1979;58:1.
15. Hammond D. The periareolar approach to breast augmentation. *Clin Plast Surg* 2009;36 (1):45–48.
16. Wiener TC. Relationship of incision choice to capsular contracture. *Aesthet Plast Surg* 2008;32:303–306.
17. Mladick RA. Breast augmentation: ease of dissection with the periareolar technique. *Aesthet Surg J* 1999;19(2):162–164.
18. Yavuzer R, Basterzi Y, Tuncer S. Using tissue adhesives for closure of periareolar incisions in breast reduction surgery. *Plast Reconstr Surg* 2003;112:337.
19. Hendricks H. Complete submuscular breast augmentation: 650 cases managed using an alternative surgical technique. *Aesthet Plast Surg*. 2007;31:147–153.

CHAPTER

112

Ruth Maria Graf
Maria Cecília Closs Ono
André Ricardo Dall'Oglio Tolazzi

Subfascial Breast Augmentation

INTRODUCTION

The number of breast augmentation procedures has increased over the years (1,2). Along with this increase have come controversies regarding surgical approach, implant selection, and especially the issue of implant plane or pocket plane. There are basically two pocket planes into which to put a silicone implant: above (subglandular) and behind (submuscular) the pectoralis major muscle. Both have advantages and disadvantages.

The subglandular approach gives better projection to the breast and usually fulfills the expectations of patients who want to augment their breasts. In very thin patients, however, this approach ends up with an artificial look of the breasts, with the entire implant contour being visible under the skin. In this type of patient, the submuscular breast augmentation offers more natural results with round implants. It also reduces the incidence of clinically visible capsular contractures, once the pectoralis action helps to prevent the capsular restriction around the implant, and also serves as an anatomic barrier for mild distortions. The submuscular approach has some drawbacks as well. It has more limitations on the volume to be used, because the pocket is a little bit smaller than the subglandular one. In the middle and long term postoperatively, pectoralis muscle action can move the implant when the patient is exercising, which looks unpleasant and can also cause displacements of the implants. Due to muscle action, the implant usually does not follow the breast parenchyma descent, which drops over the implant, resulting in a "double-bubble" appearance.

In order to better compensate for the pros and cons of subglandular and submuscular breast augmentation, we have been using the subfascial approach since 1998. This chapter describes in detail three different accesses for performing a subfascial breast augmentation and discusses some advantages compared with the subglandular and submuscular approaches.

OPERATIVE TECHNIQUES

PREOPERATIVE MARKINGS AND ANESTHESIA

Preoperative markings are done with the patient in the upright position. The limits of the breast pocket are marked, passing at least 1 to 2 cm lateral to the mid-sternum line, not extending laterally to the anterior axillary line, and connecting superiorly at the level of second intercostal space. The natural inframammary fold and the future inframammary crease are marked, considering the nipple-areola complex (NAC) position, the implant base diameter (radius), the subcutaneous thickness, and the skin stretchiness (Fig. 112.1).

The operation can be performed under general anesthesia, epidural, intercostal, or local anesthesia, and sedation. We prefer epidural blockage associated with sedation. Patients are positioned with the arms abducted 90 deg and the dorsum slightly elevated. The incision and pocket limits are infiltrated with a normal saline-epinephrine solution (1:300,000), but the whole pocket area is not infiltrated, to avoid difficulty in dissecting the fascia.

AXILLARY ACCESS

An S-shaped, 4-cm-long incision is made in the main axillary fold, about 1 cm behind the lateral border of the major pectoralis muscle. It is important never to cross beyond the lateral edge of the pectoralis muscle, keeping the scar hidden in the axilla. Transaxillary breast augmentation can damage lymphatic vessels during subcutaneous tunnel dissection and insertion of the implant into the breast pocket. To minimize lymphatic injuries, a subcutaneous tunnel should be dissected up to the superior lateral border of the muscle, preserving an inferior lateral triangle of soft tissue containing most of lymphatic structures (Fig. 112.2) (3,4).

The pectoralis fascia is incised, and the subfascial breast pocket is dissected with electrocautery. This can be done using an endoscopic retractor or through direct view using long, lighted retractors (Figs. 112.3 and 112.4).

AREOLAR ACCESS

Periareolar breast augmentation can be performed with or without mastopexy. Skin is usually incised in the lower half of the areolar margin, preserving the upper half as a superior pedicle for the NAC. If a mastopexy is planned, a donut-shaped area of skin is deepithelialized, also preserving the upper half of the dermis. The outer limits of the deepithelialization area are as follows: new superior areola position (point A), 9 to 10 cm from midline (medially), about 12 cm from anterior axillary line (laterally), and 5 to 8 cm from the future inframammary fold (inferiorly). The inferior pole of the breast is dissected in an oblique direction, between the breast parenchyma and the subcutaneous tissue. Once the pectoral fascia is reached, it is incised about the nipple level, and the subfascial pocket is created in all directions up to the marking limits (Figs. 112.5 to 112.7).

Another option of incision is the transareolar approach, which can be indicated for patients with an areolar diameter of at least 3.5 cm. A geometric broken line incision is done horizontally in the areola, merging and not transecting the nipple, without disturbing the lactiferous ducts or mammary gland (5). Dissection of the breast is performed as in the periareolar approach.

INFRAMAMMARY ACCESS

A 4-cm incision is made in the future inframammary crease. The new inframammary fold and the incision should be carefully planned in order to have a good-quality and well-placed scar. The site of the new inframammary fold and future scar should consider the implant diameter, the subcutaneous

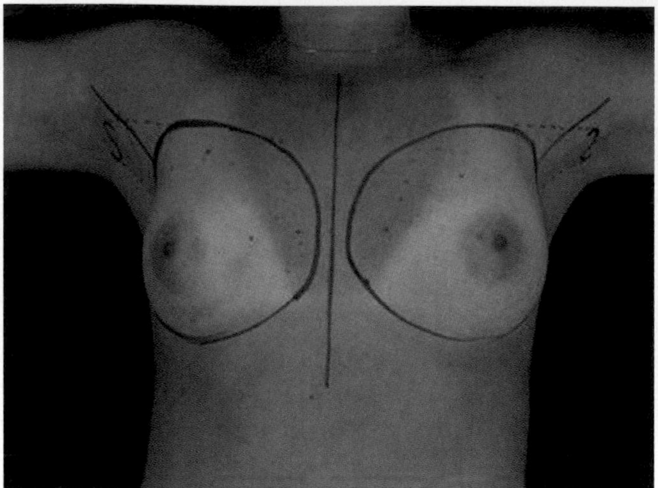

Figure 112.1. Preoperative markings.

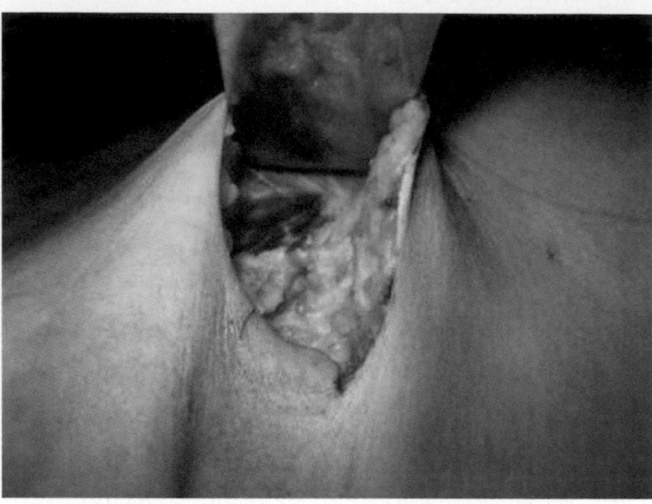

Figure 112.3. Incision of the pectoralis fascia.

thickness, and the skin elasticity. Gently stretching up the NAC, the new inframammary fold distance from the nipple is marked, adding the implant radius size and the subcutaneous thickness. This distance (nipple–new inframammary fold) usually ranges from 5 to 8 cm. After the skin and subcutaneous tissue are incised, the pectoral fascia is identified, and the subfascial pocket is dissected superiorly (Figs. 112.8 and 112.9).

SUBFASCIAL BREAST POCKET DISSECTION

There are some important details regarding the creation of a subfascial pocket (6,7). After the incision, the undermining of the subfascial plane should be done very carefully to avoid fascia injury, and, if there is doubt about the plane of dissection, some muscle fibers may be lifted up with the fascia. We dissect the breast pocked using the electrocautery device with a thin tip, set in the pure coagulation or blend cut mode. We prefer not to use the pure cut mode nor blunt nor scissor dissection because of the

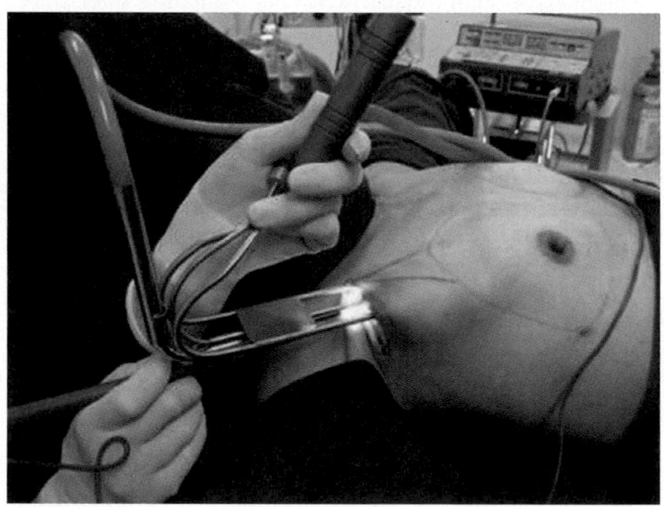

Figure 112.4. Dissection using an illuminated retractor.

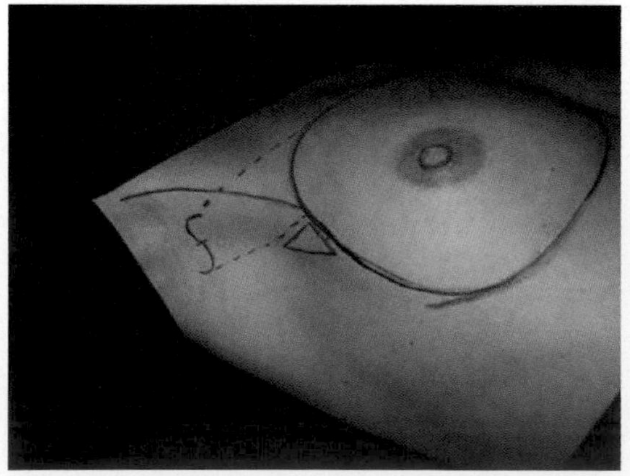

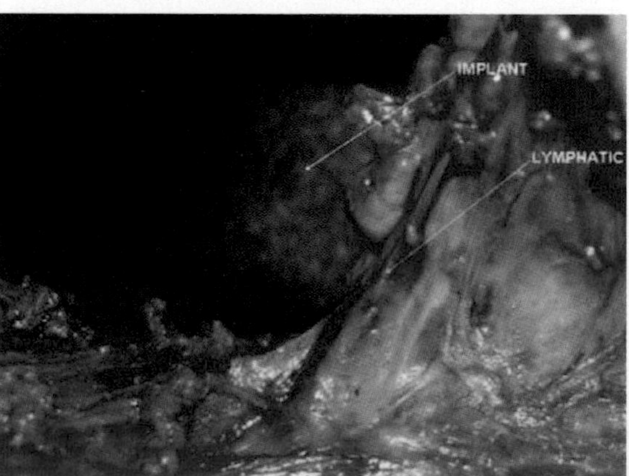

Figure 112.2. Preservation of the lymphatic structures.

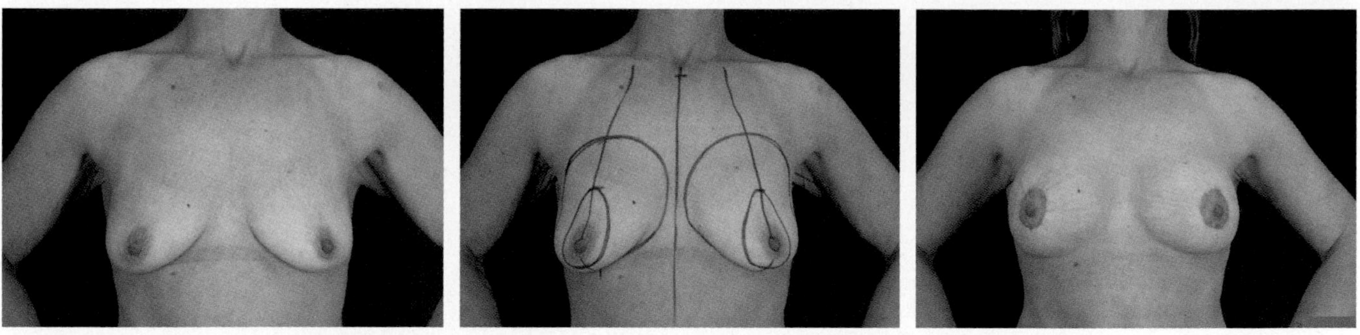

Figure 112.5. Preoperative view, preoperative markings, and 1-year postoperative view.

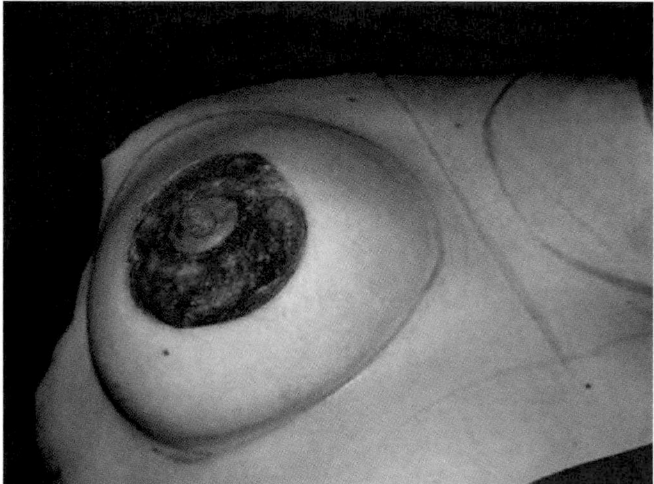

Figure 112.6. Deepithelialization of an periareolar approach.

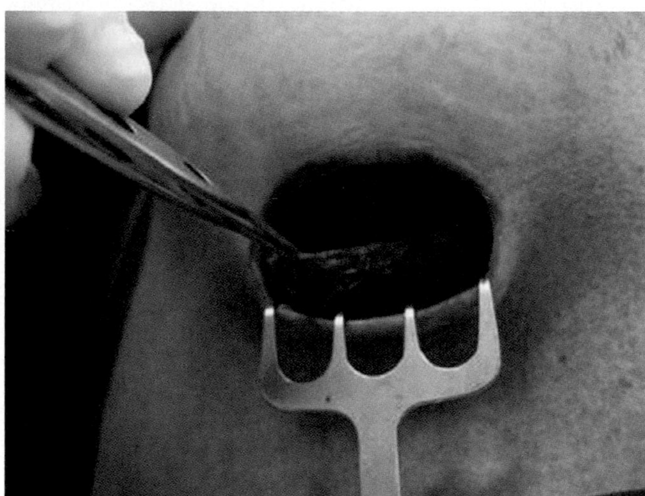

Figure 112.8. Access to the pectoralis fascia.

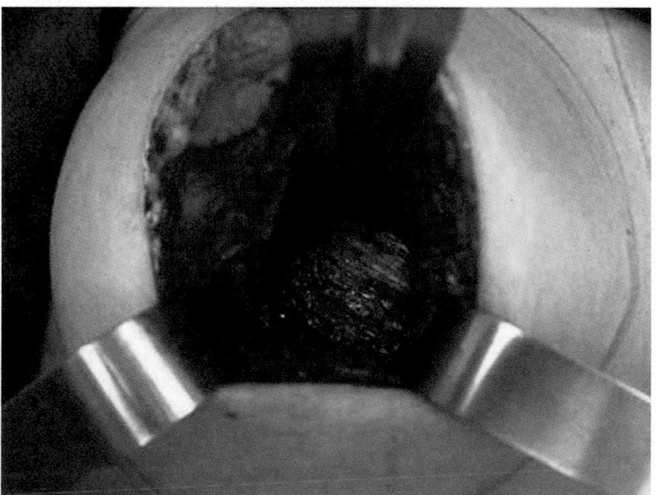

Figure 112.7. Reaching the pectoralis fascia.

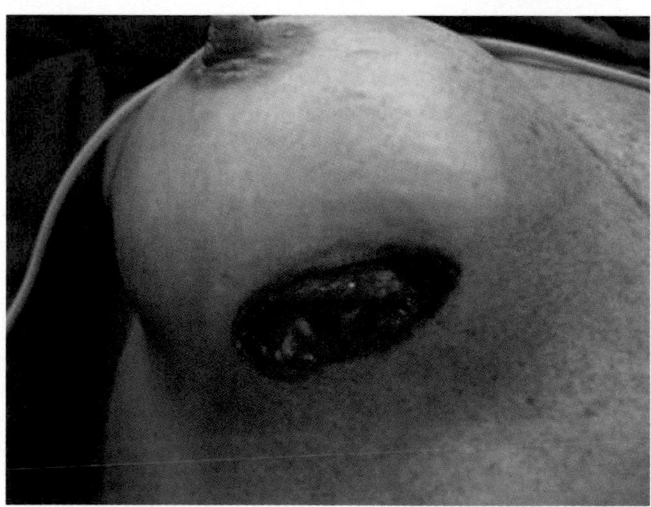

Figure 112.9. Closure of the fascia, protecting the implants.

risk of bleeding. Once a bleeding vessel retracts into the muscle, hemostasis and clear dissection become difficult. With adequate surgical technique, it is possible to use the cautery cut mode very selectively, preventing additional unnecessary tissue damage.

The use of traction upward is necessary and facilitates the procedure, in both video-assisted and direct vision approaches. Limits for dissection are the second intercostal space (superiorly), 1 to 2 cm from the midsternum line (medially), 5 to 8 cm below the NAC (new inframammary fold), and the anterior axillary line (laterally). The distance between implants should not be less than 2 to 3 cm to prevent the occurrence of synmastia (8).

Once dissection is completed, a meticulous evaluation for bleeding is carried out, and the implant is inserted into the pocket. Careful hemostasis is mandatory to avoid bleeding complications and late capsular contractures. To avoid leaving debris and foreign body in the pocket, it is not recommended to use gauze or cotton pads to clean up the space, but it should be washed using normal saline solution. Implant sizers may be used to precisely choose the most appropriate implant. We routinely change and wash the new gloves just before handling the implants and again clean the skin around the incision with the antiseptic solution just before inserting the implants. We prefer not to use drains due to the risk of infection (9).

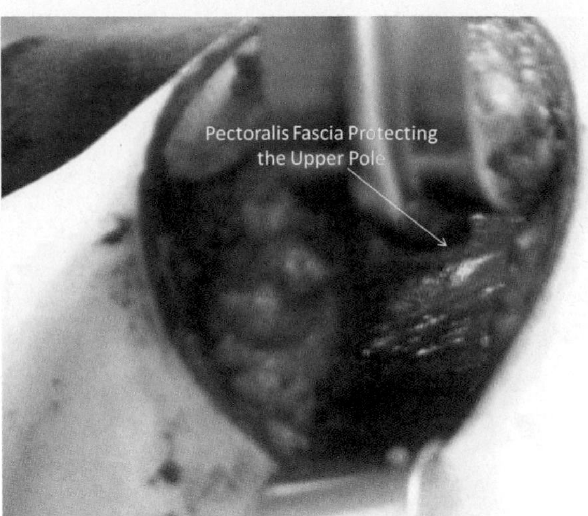

Figure 112.10. Pectoralis fascia, protecting the upper pole.

DISCUSSION

The breast is essentially a skin appendage contained within layers of the superficial fascia. The superficial layer of this fascia is near the dermis and is not distinct from it. The deep layer of the superficial fascia is more distinct and is identifiable when the breast is elevated in a subglandular augmentation mammaplasty (10). There is a loose areolar tissue between the deep layer of the superficial fascia and the fascia that covers the pectoralis major and continues to cover the adjacent rectus abdominis (11).

In our practice, we have seen several advantages of subfascial breast augmentation. Once the pectoral fascia is a firm and relatively inelastic tissue, it causes some pressure over the round edges of the implants, helping to give a smoother transition in the upper pole of the breast. As it is firmly attached to the pectoralis muscle, it raises upward some peripheral muscle fibers when the implant is placed, also contributing to a gradual transition of the implant edges in slim patients. (Fig. 112.10) (6,7,12). Exceptions include very thin patients who desire relatively large implants. In these situations it is better to use round implants in the submuscular pocket or anatomic/naturally shaped implants subfascially (Fig. 112.11). Some other clinically noted possible advantages with subfascial breast augmentation still need to be investigated. We have the impression that this approach also reduces postoperative breast ptosis and rippling due to better implant support by the fascia. Being in direct contact with pectoralis muscle could also reduce the incidence of capsular contracture. Moreover, placing the implant over the muscle avoids future displacements when exercising.

Transaxillary subfascial breast augmentation can be indicated for every patient who does not need mastopexy. Augmenting the breasts without leaving a scar on them is the major advantage in this technique and has been frequently required by young patients (Fig. 112.12) The possibility of creating a scar in a low-tension area far from the breasts makes this approach the preferred technique in patients with history or risk factors for hypertrophic scars and keloid. Preoperative conversation regarding axillary lymphatic drainage of the breasts and sentinel node implications is advisable. Recent studies published by our group showed that the sentinel node in axilla can be preserved after transaxillary breast augmentation if some technical details during dissection are respected (3,4). This technique requires special instruments (long, lighted retractors or video-endoscopic apparatus) and has a longer learning curve. Any kind of implant can be used through this access; however, special attention should be given to avoiding misplacement of anatomic/naturally shaped implants.

The periareolar approach can be indicated for patients with medium-size or large areolas once the lower half perimeter of the areola has to permit an incision of at least 4 cm. A well-defined transition between areola and breast skin is also important to have a less visible scar. Breasts with mild ptosis that will probably not be corrected by the breast implant chosen are good candidates for periareolar mastopexy (Fig. 112.13). Patients with tuberous breasts usually present with lower pole hypoplasia and some degree of NAC weakness and prolapse. In these cases we have also indicated the periareolar approach with nylon round-block suture to improve NAC herniation. The subfascial pocket is created, but the fascia is radially incised in the lower breast in order to allow more skin distention. Round implants can be used for mildly tuberous breasts; however, in more severe cases anatomic shaped implants are better indicated to obtain greater lower pole projection.

The inframammary breast augmentation is the simplest and most direct access for inserting silicone gel implants. It is not limited by the size of the implant, and the incision can be extended if necessary. It is also the most conservative approach regarding breast parenchyma and lymphatic drainage preservation. The scars are usually of good quality and hidden under the brassiere. A correct planning of the incision is important to have a final scar positioned correctly in the new inframammary fold. This approach can be indicated for every patient not a candidate for periareolar mastopexy and without a history of hypertrophic scar or keloid. Disadvantages include a visible scar when the patient is lying down and greater risk of implant exposure compared to other approaches.

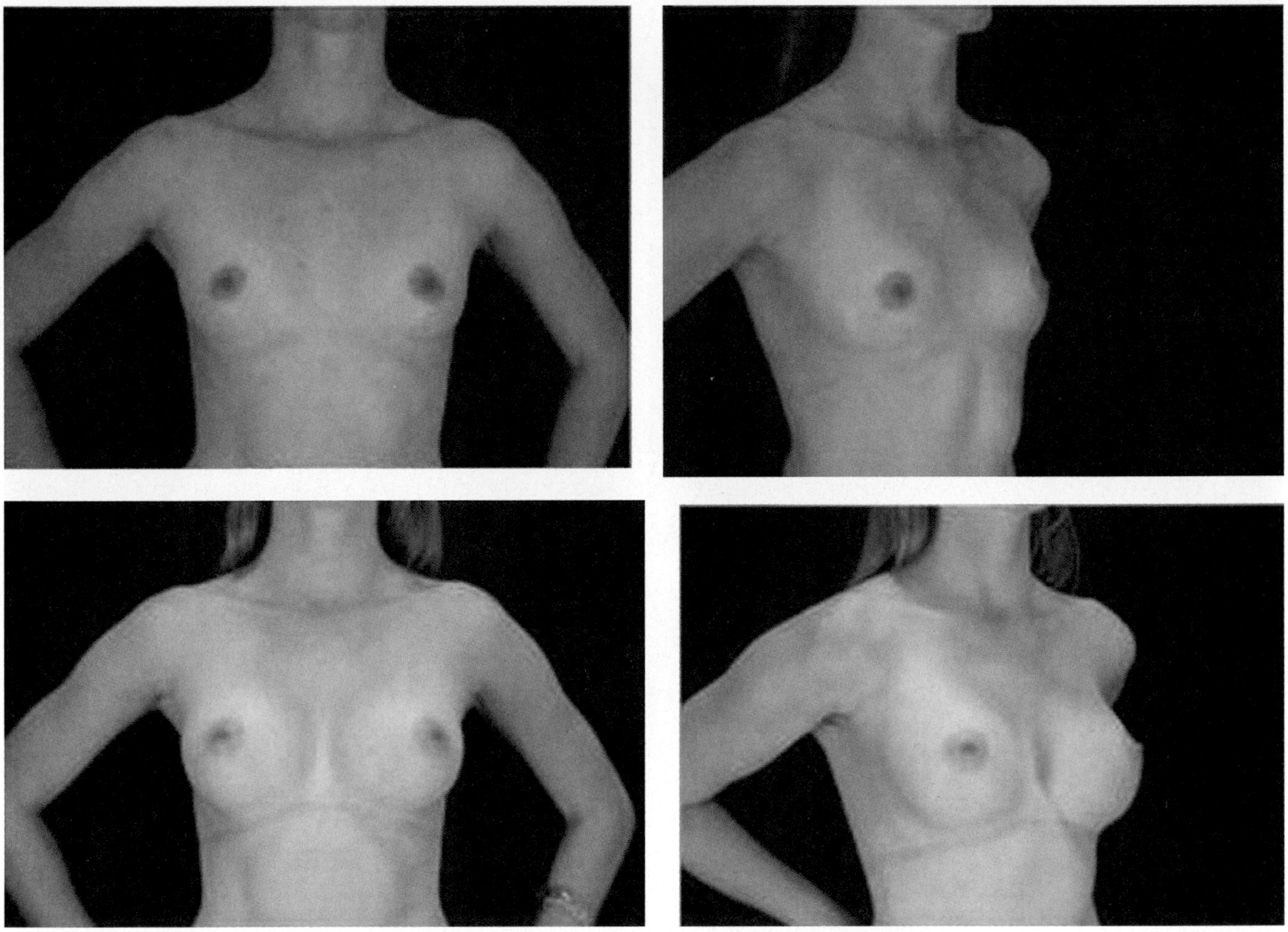

Figure 112.11. A very thin patient treated with subfascial anatomic implants, preoperative and 1-year postoperative views.

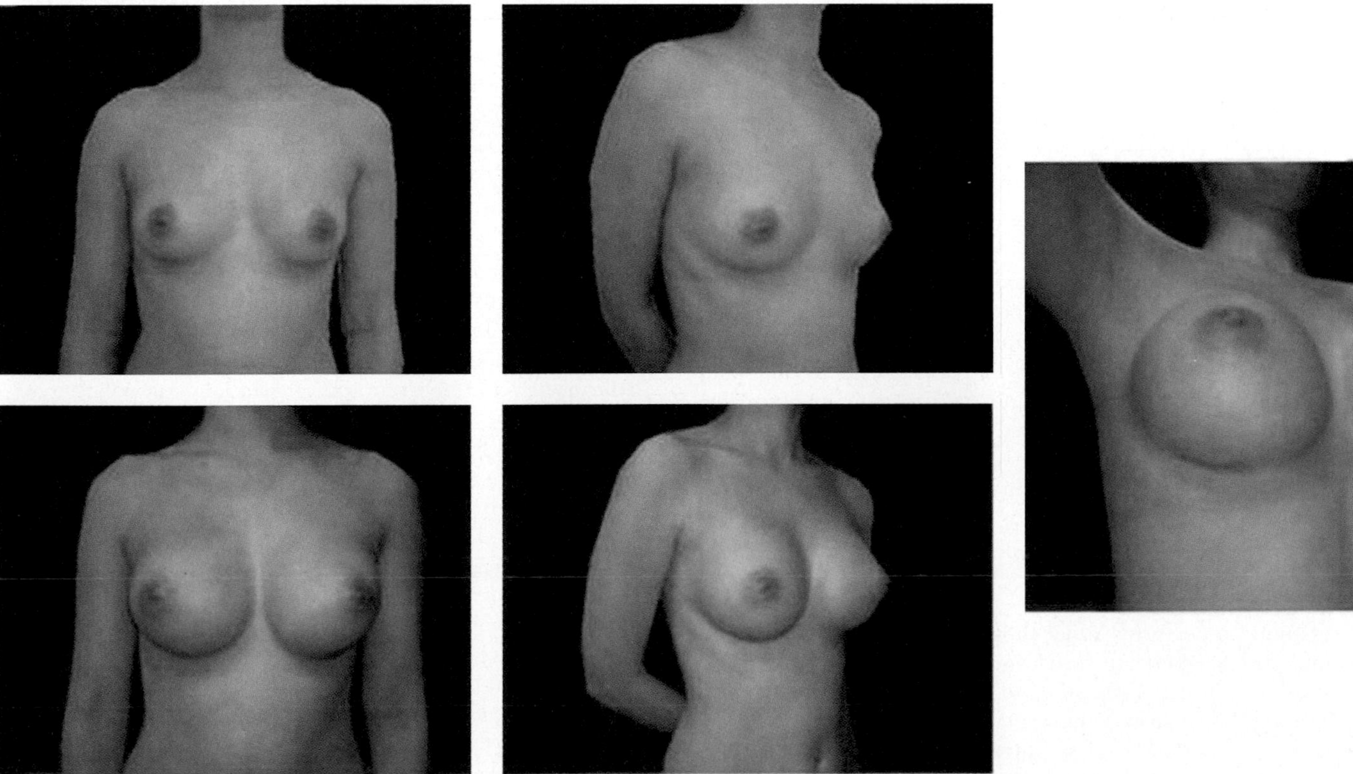

Figure 112.12. A young patient, round implants, preoperative and 1-year postoperative views.

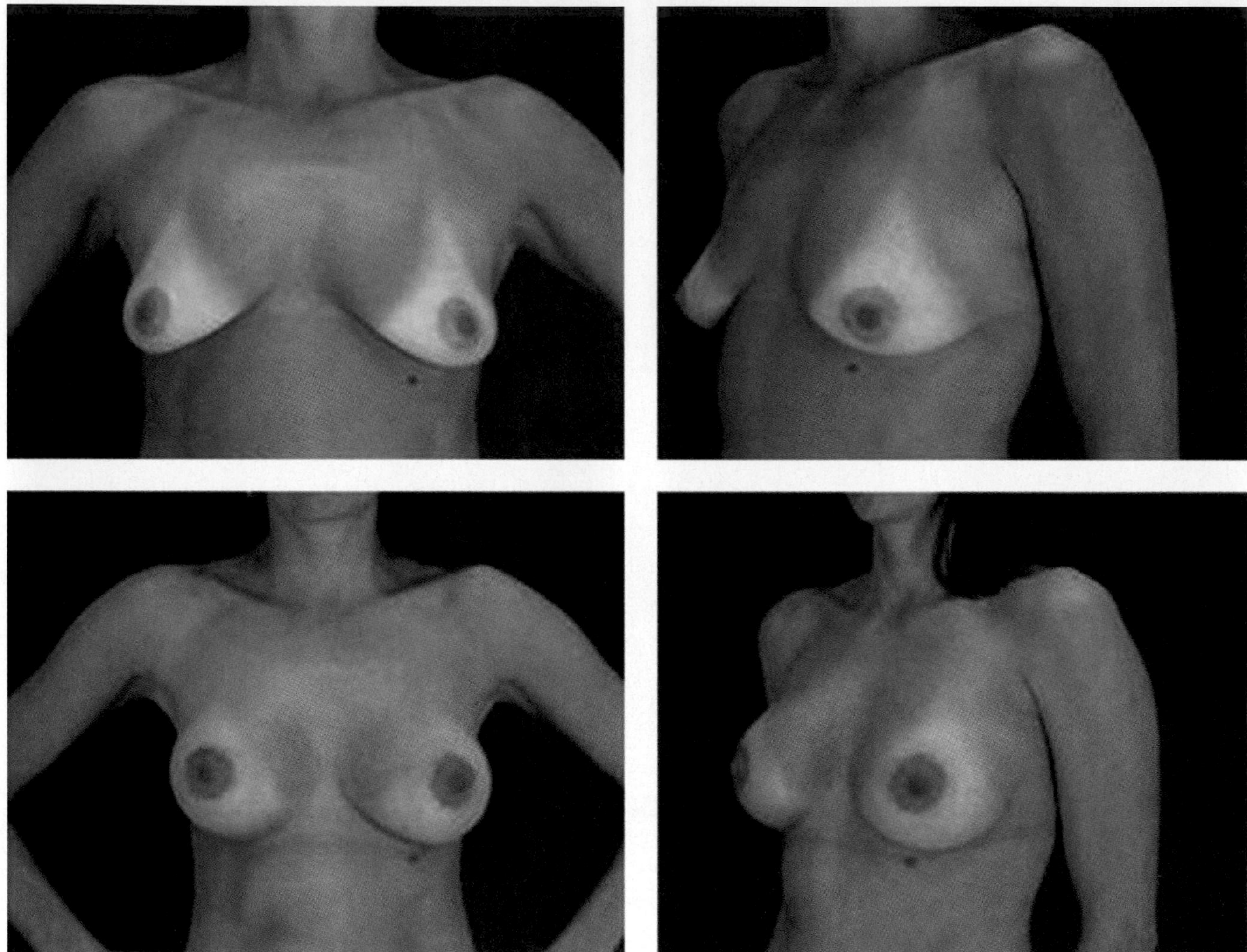

Figure 112.13. A case of mild ptosis, treated with round implants, preoperative and 2-year postoperative views.

CONCLUSION

Subfascial breast augmentation is a relatively new approach that combines several advantages of the subglandular and submuscular techniques. It uses the pectoralis fascia to cover and support the implant and can be performed through most of the incision accesses. The clinical impression of surgeons who have been using this approach suggests that better aesthetic outcomes with less visible implant edges and reduced rates of complications (rippling, capsular contractures, implant ptosis, and displacements) have been achieved with this technique. Controlled studies should be done to confirm these subjective findings.

EDITORIAL COMMENTS

As one who performs either subglandular or subpectoral implant placement for breast augmentation, I found this chapter of interest. Dr. Graf and colleagues have been performing the subfascial augmentation since 1998 and have been very pleased with outcomes. They have nicely described the technique and have shown excellent clinical outcomes. Approaches to the subfascial plane include periareolar, inframammary, and transaxillary. They have noticed that certain sequelae such as visible implant edges, rippling, implant ptosis, displacement, and capsular contracture appear to be reduced, resulting in better aesthetic outcomes. The lower capsular contracture rate has been confirmed in an independent study in which Baker III capsular contracture rates following a periareolar approach were less with subfascial placement (1.5%, smooth surface device) than with the submuscular (4.5%, textured and 1.9%, smooth) and subglandular (14.4%, textured) approaches (13).

Although I have not performed a subfascial placement of a breast implant, I am compelled to try this. My concern has typically been that the pectoralis fascia is too thin and would be traumatized by this approach; however, this does not appear to be the case, as it is acceptable to sometimes raise slips of the muscle with the fascia. The reported results are excellent and certainly warrant giving this operation a try.

M.Y.N.

REFERENCES

1. Spear SL, Bulan EJ, Venturi ML. Breast augmentation. *Plast Reconstr Surg* 2006;118(7 suppl):188S–196S.
2. Hidalgo DA. Breast augmentation: choosing the optimal incision, implant, and pocket plane. *Plast Reconstr Surg* 2000;105(6):2202–2216.
3. Graf RM, Canan LW Jr, Romano GG, et al. Re: implications of transaxillary breast augmentation: lifetime probability for the development of breast cancer and sentinel node mapping interference. *Aesthet Plast Surg* 2007;31(4):322–324.
4. Sado HN, Graf RM, Canan LW, et al. Sentinel lymph node detection and evidence of axillary lymphatic integrity after transaxillary breast augmentation: a prospective study using lymphoscintography. *Aesthet Plast Surg* 2008;32(6):879–888.
5. Tenius FP, da Silva Freitas R, Closs Ono MC. Transareolar incision with geometric broken line for breast augmentation: a novel approach. *Aesthet Plast Surg* 2008;32(3): 546–548.
6. Graf RM, Bernardes A, Auersvald A, et al. Subfascial endoscopic transaxillary augmentation mammaplasty. *Aesthet Plast Surg* 2000;24(3):216–220.
7. Graf RM, Bernardes A, Rippel R, et al. Subfascial breast implant: a new procedure. *Plast Reconstr Surg* 2003;111:904.
8. Spear SL, Bogue DP, Thomassen JM. Synmastia after breast augmentation. *Plast Reconstr Surg* 2006;118(7 suppl):168S–171S.
9. Araco A, Gravante G, Araco F, et al. Infections of breast implants in aesthetic breast augmentations: a single-center review of 3,002 patients. *Aesthet Plast Surg* 2007;31(4):325–329.
10. Hwang K, Kim DJ. Anatomy of pectoral fascia in relation to subfascial mammary augmentation. *Ann Plast Surg* 2005;55(6):576–579.
11. Würinger E, Mader N, Posch E, et al. Nerve and vessel supplying ligamentous suspension of the mammary gland. *Plast Reconstr Surg* 1998;101(6):1486–1493.
12. Góes JC, Landecker A. Optimizing outcomes in breast augmentation: seven years of experience with the subfascial plane. *Aesthet Plast Surg* 2003;27(3):178–184.
13. Stoff-Khalili MA, Scholze, R, Morgan WR, et al. Subfascial periareolar augmentation mammaplasty. *Plast Reconstr Surg* 2004;114:1280–1288.

CHAPTER

113

Louis L. Strock

Transaxillary Breast Augmentation

The transaxillary approach for breast augmentation has the appeal of allowing for a breast implant to be placed with no incisions on the breast. The approach was first reported in 1973 by Hoehler, who described the placement of an implant in a partial subpectoral pocket using mainly blunt dissection (1). While other early reports provided encouragement for this approach based on short-term results, technical limitations became readily apparent that limited its popularity (2). This led Tebbetts to describe a series of technical refinements based on anatomic studies and long-term follow-up, seeking to limit complications using this approach (3). Despite these efforts, this early approach, which depended completely on blunt technique with limited or no tissue visualization, had limited appeal because of problems with implant asymmetry and a general lack of technical control compared with the more conventional inframammary and periareolar approaches.

The addition of endoscopic assistance to the transaxillary approach, as first described by Price et al., allowed for direct visualization of the tissue layers to be released, helping to overcome the greatest limitation of the previous transaxillary approaches that were based on blunt technique with no tissue visualization (4,5). The improved visualization allowed for improved hemostasis, improved control of inframammary fold level and shape, and the ability to precisely divide specific tissue layers according to the needs of each patient. The added technical control afforded by endoscopic assistance to the transaxillary approach for breast augmentation has been reflected in multiple patient series reports (4–12). This combined experience with improved technical control suggests that the endoscopic approach for transaxillary breast augmentation has become the standard for implant placement using a transaxillary incision.

I am a strong advocate for the use of endoscopic assistance when the transaxillary approach is used for breast augmentation due to the added technical control afforded by visualization of the specific tissue layers to be divided. This chapter presents this approach in detail, followed by a discussion of the nonendoscopic approach, where the technique differs in the tissue release phase of the procedure.

MARKINGS

Markings are routinely placed in the preoperative holding area with the patient in the sitting position and include breast and chest wall width, tissue thickness, inframammary fold position, inframammary fold position planned, and exact incision location (Fig. 113.1) The anatomic chest midline and midbreast meridian at the inframammary fold are marked with the patient in the sitting position and reconfirmed when the patient is supine under anesthesia on the operating table.

POSITIONING

The patient is placed in a supine position with the arms secured onto arm boards at 90 deg. The procedure is performed under general anesthesia with the aid of short-acting muscle relaxation. Draping is performed as with routine breast augmentation, except that the surgeon must be able to work above and below the shoulder on each side. The anesthesia machine is located at the head of the bed, also with enough space to allow for the surgeon to perform a majority of the procedure from a position above the shoulder, facing the endoscopic equipment at the foot of the bed. In addition to the endoscopic tower, all cautery and suction lines are directed toward the foot of the bed (Fig. 113.2).

EQUIPMENT

The equipment used is that described by Price et al., consisting of an endoscopic tower with monitor, endoscopic light source, recorder, and camera. The camera is mounted to a 10-mm downward-angled endoscope that slides into an Emory Breast Retractor (Cardinal Health, Dublin, OH) sheath with a grooved handle that holds the fiberoptic light cord (4,5). I prefer use of Agris-Dingman dissectors for blunt dissection (5,8,12) (Fig. 113.3A, B).

INCISIONS

The incisions for the procedure differ depending upon whether saline or silicone gel implants are to be used. For saline augmentation, an incision 2.5 to 3 cm in length is marked in the axillary apex, within an existing skin crease (Fig. 113.4A). Alternatively, for silicone gel augmentation, an incision 5 cm in length is used. The markings for this incision begin with a dot marked in the axillary apex. A line is then drawn anteriorly, in an existing skin crease, just short of the posterior boundary of the pectoralis major muscle. The posterior portion of the incision, beginning at the dot in the axillary apex, is marked in a posterior and slightly superior direction. There marks are carefully made to be confined within the axilla (Fig. 113.4B). These marks are usually made in the preoperative holding area with the patient in a sitting position to ensure proper incision placement behind the anterior axillary fold. While some prefer the exposure for the initial dissection provided by the longer incision, regardless of implant type to be used, I strongly prefer use of the longer incision only for silicone gel implants. In my experience, the short incision as used routinely for saline augmentation is visible for up to 6 months, as compared with 9 months for the longer incision routinely used for silicone gel augmentation (Fig. 113.5).

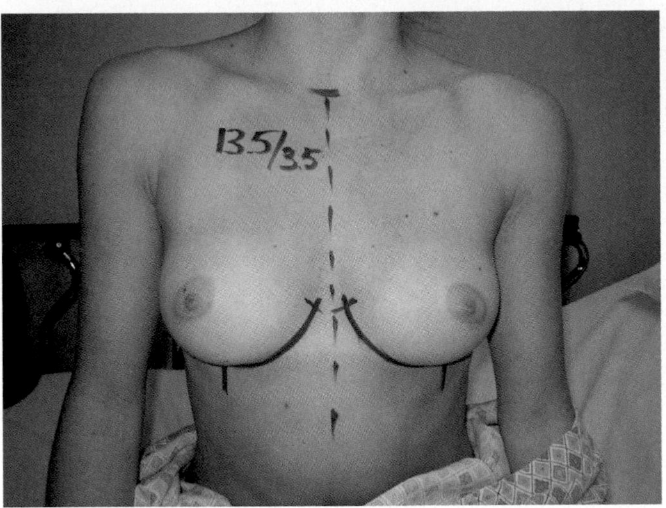

Figure 113.1. Preoperative markings.

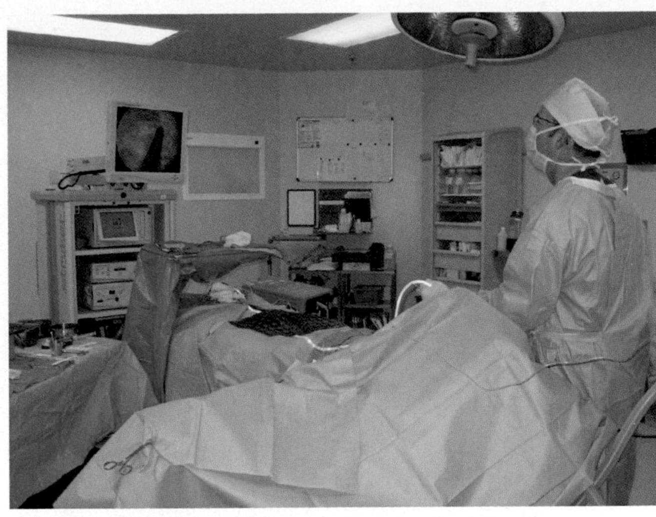

Figure 113.2. Patient is positioned with arms out, allowing room for the surgeon to perform the procedure from above the shoulder. Note the endoscopic tower at the foot of the operating room bed.

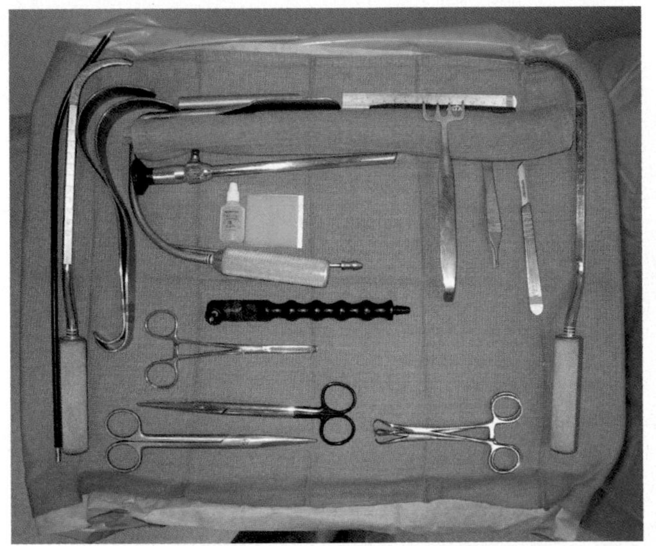

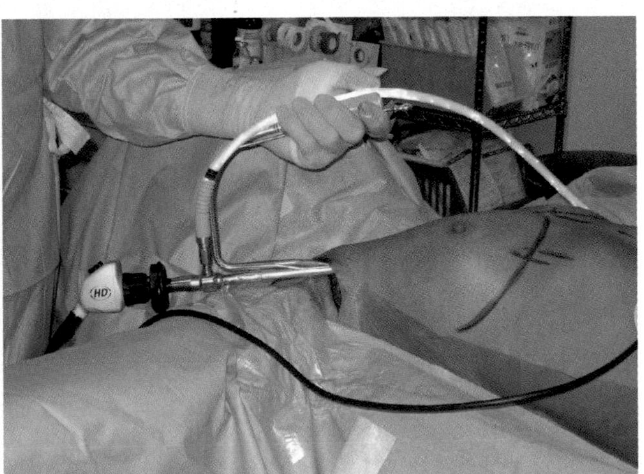

Figure 113.3. **A:** Endoscopic instruments. **B:** Endoscopic setup with the camera mounted to the endoscope, the light source above into endoscope, and the cord held in the groove in the Emory Endoscopic Retractor (Cardinal Health, Dublin, OH).

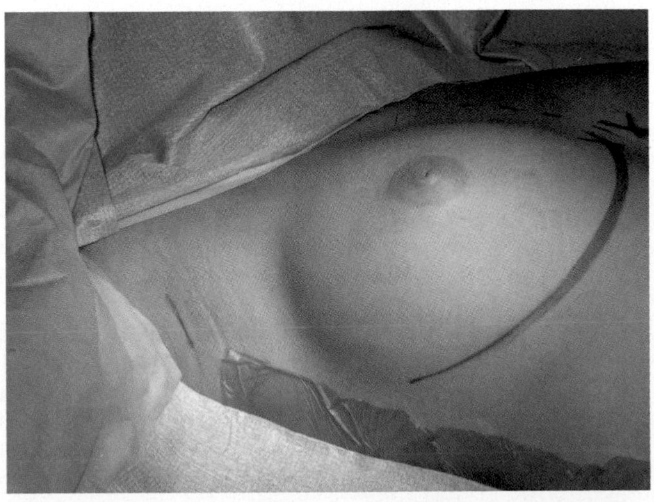

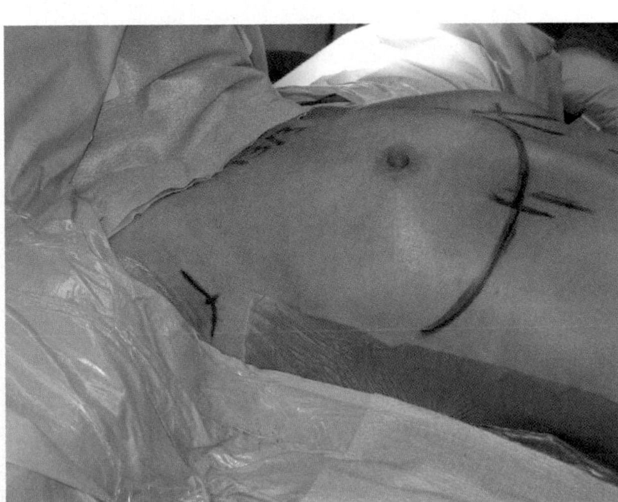

Figure 113.4. **A:** Saline augmentation incision 2.5 to 3 cm, located in existing axillary crease. **B:** Silicone gel augmentation incision 5 cm, extending from mark in the axillary apex. This longer incision can be used for saline for improved visualization.

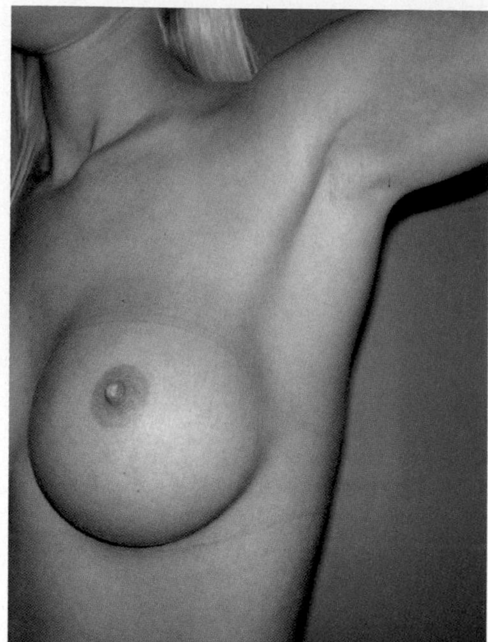

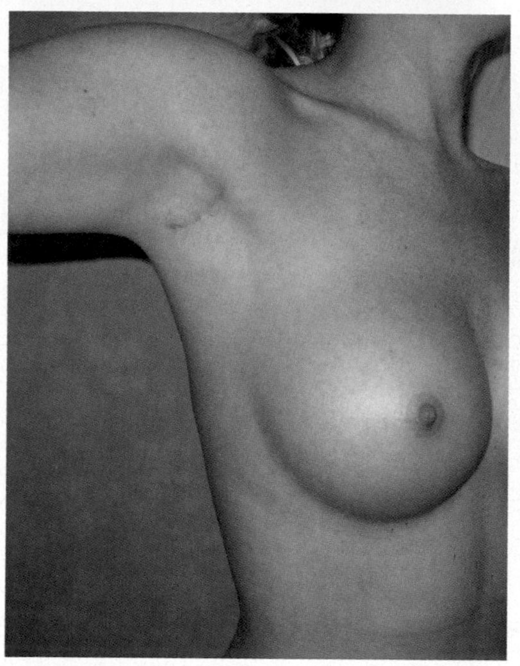

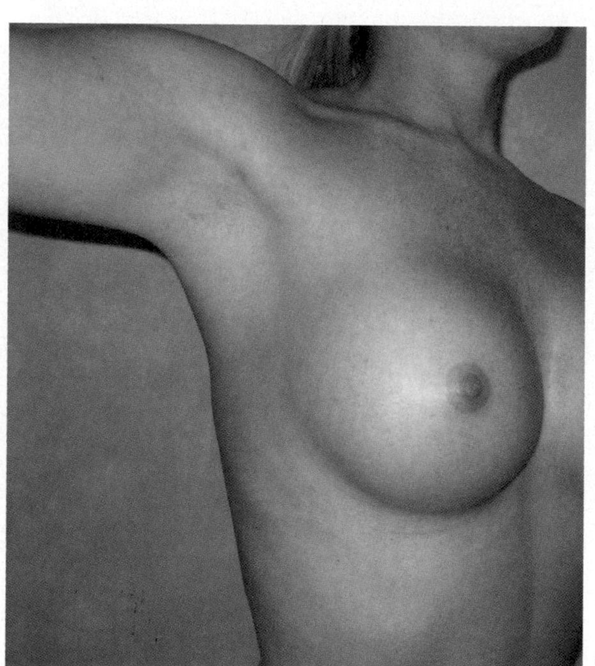

Figure 113.5. **A:** Saline augmentation incision at 6 months. **B:** Silicone gel augmentation incision at 4 months. **C:** Silicone gel augmentation incision in the same patient as in panel B at 1 year.

INITIAL DISSECTION

After incision placement, the initial dissection is performed in an immediate subcutaneous plane, in an anterior direction, first using the electrocautery and then scissor dissection, until the lateral border of the pectoralis major muscle is reached. Dissection in this superficial plane is important to prevent damage to the intercostobrachial nerve (Fig. 113.6). The subpectoral space is then entered using facelift scissors, developing the plane between the pectoralis major and the pectoralis minor muscles. Alternatively, using the longer incision, a fiberoptic retractor is used to enter the subpectoral space under direct vision. Gentle blunt finger movement is used to provide additional limited dissection of the subpectoral space.

SUBPECTORAL DISSECTION

The subpectoral dissection is an important phase of the procedure that largely determines the ease of the endoscopic release of the pectoralis major muscle. Emphasis is placed on creation of a clear optical field with little or no blood staining. While the initial description of the endoscopic approach states preference for blunt dissection to the pectoralis major muscle at the inframammary fold, I prefer to avoid the occasional blood staining of tissue that can be seen with that approach (4). I prefer creation of the optical cavity by sharp endoscopic dissection, releasing the areolar plane just deep to the pectoralis major muscle using electrocautery with blended current (12) (Fig. 113.7). This is accomplished by initial placement of the Emory retractor into the subpectoral space, followed by placement of the endoscope through

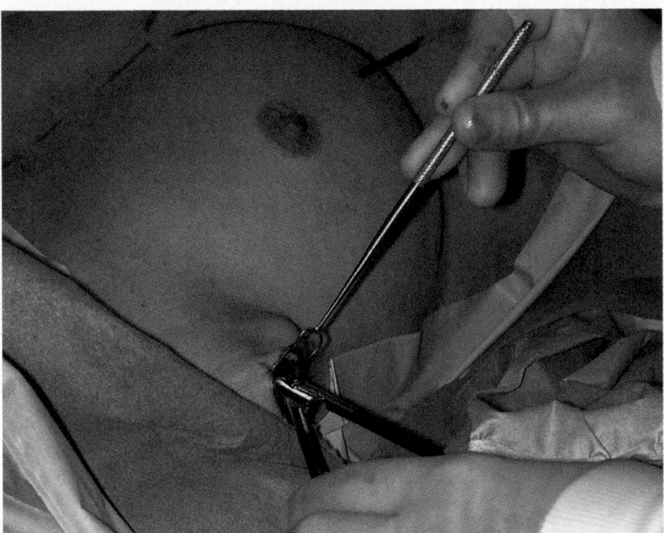

Figure 113.6. Superficial dissection plane from the incision to the lateral border of the pectoralis major muscle.

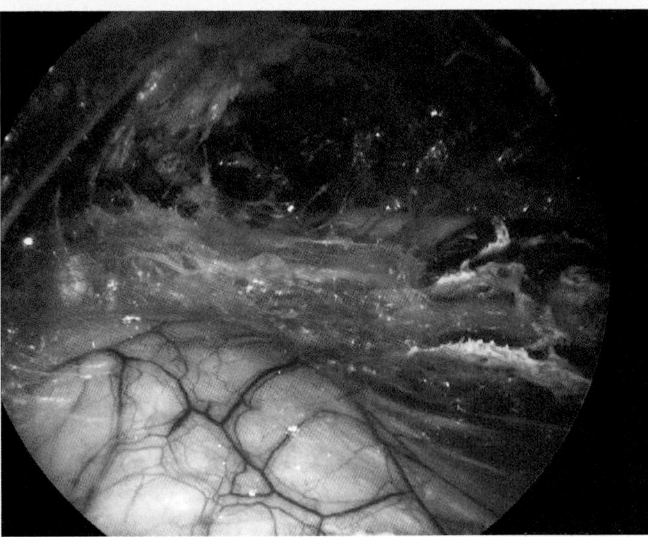

Figure 113.8. The optical field is created to allow for visualization of the main body of the pectoralis major muscle for release.

the retractor sheath after contact with defogging solution. The spatulated cautery rod, with a J shape oriented outward in a lateral direction, is used for the dissection. Suction is attached to the posterior end of the cautery handle for smoke evacuation. This sequence is used for all endoscopic portions of the procedure. Orientation is maintained by identification of a rib, following which the tissue is released until the main body of the pectoralis major muscle is identified clearly in all areas to be addressed with the main muscle release (Fig. 113.8).

PECTORALIS MAJOR MUSCLE RELEASE

The release of the pectoralis major muscle is started medially, carefully correlating internal anatomy seen endoscopically with external reference markings (Fig. 113.9A, B). This ensures that the release will be performed at the intended level relative to the inframammary fold, a critical issue whether the fold level is to be maintained or lowered. The pectoralis release then proceeds from medial to lateral, carefully rechecking the level of the muscle release relative to the inframammary fold. Hemostasis is meticulously maintained during the tissue release. The retractor is elevated in a toe-up position to expose the tissue release. The excellent visibility afforded by the combination of endoscopic magnification and proper retractor elevation allows for specific release of muscle and fascia layers as needed in a given patient (Fig. 113.9C, D). The release is continued laterally to just past the base toward the lateral breast or the lateral edge of the pectoralis major muscle. While the sharp dissection is performed laterally in some patients, this is carefully monitored to always avoid overrelease. Sharp dissection is always carefully limited laterally so as to avoid damage to the sensory nerves in this area. Light blunt technique in this area is preferred. Agris-Dingman dissectors are then used to confirm the medial and lateral extent of the tissue release, which can then be refined with additional endoscopic inspection and release. Hemostasis is carefully rechecked with the aid of the endoscope at this time. The extent of the medial release is rechecked with the endoscope, addressing any persistent accessory muscle slips that may require division (Fig. 113.10). The medial release is rarely extended above the level of the nipple. It is critically important that the main body of the pectoralis major muscle not be overreleased medially, as significant deformity can result that can be difficult to repair. The release site is irrigated with antibiotic solution and local anesthetic agents per routine.

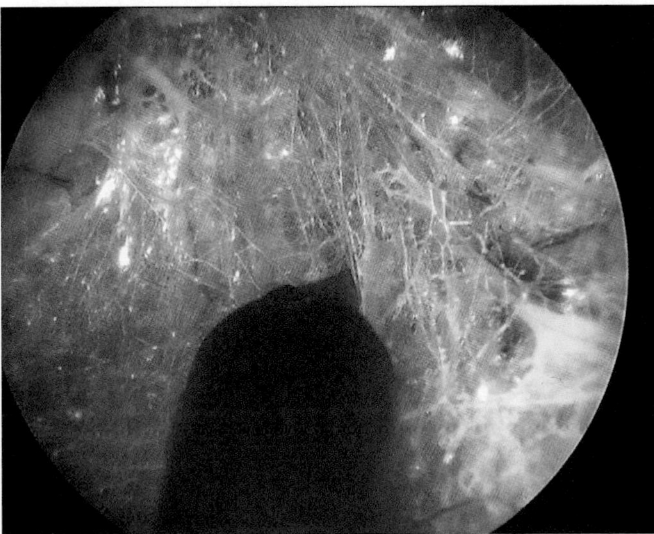

Figure 113.7. Initial dissection in the subpectoral space as seen immediately following placement of the endoscope. For orientation, the view is of the right breast pocket, medial is left, lateral is right, and ribcage is at the lower end of the field.

The release of the pectoralis major muscle using endoscopic assistance is straightforward if attention is paid to maintaining a clear optical field at all stages of the procedure. This demands that attention be paid to the method for entry into the subpectoral space, the method used for subpectoral dissection to reach the main body of the pectoralis major muscle, and the method of muscle release. Smoke evacuation must be working at all times to maintain visibility, and hemostasis must be meticulously

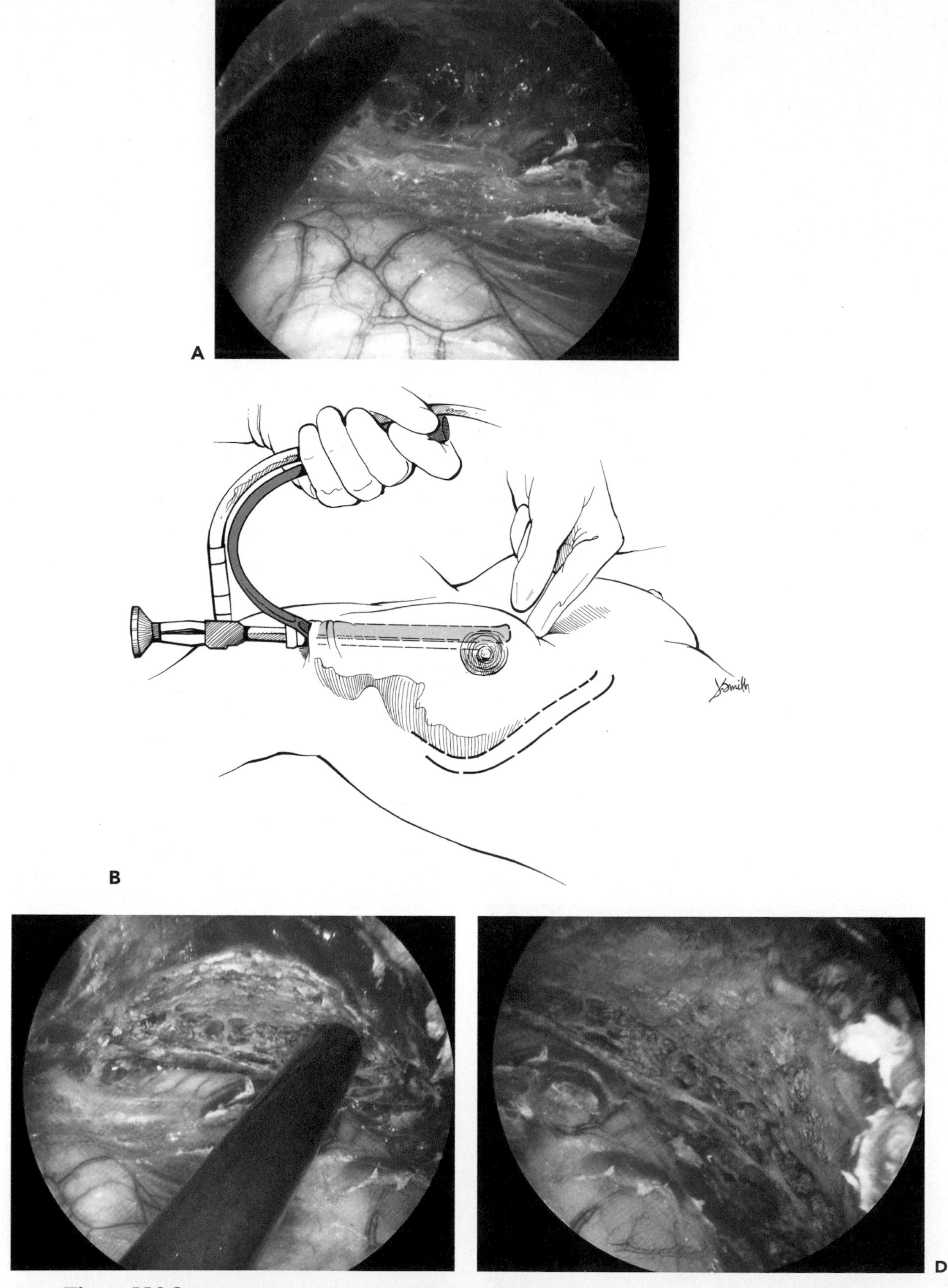

Figure 113.9. **A:** Internal endoscopic view, correlating internal anatomy with external landmark of the start of release medially. The level of the inframammary fold is checked and rechecked during release to confirm the correct level of release. For orientation, right breast pocket, medial left, lateral right. **B:** External marking correlated with start and level of internal muscle release. (From Jones GE, Nahai F. Transaxillary breast augmentation. In: Spear SL, ed. *Surgery of the Breast: Principles and Art.* 2nd ed. Philadelphia: Lippincott Williams & Wilkins; 2006; 1311–1318.) **C:** Release is performed from medial to lateral, with visualization to allow for specific tissue layer division. **D:** Release completed.

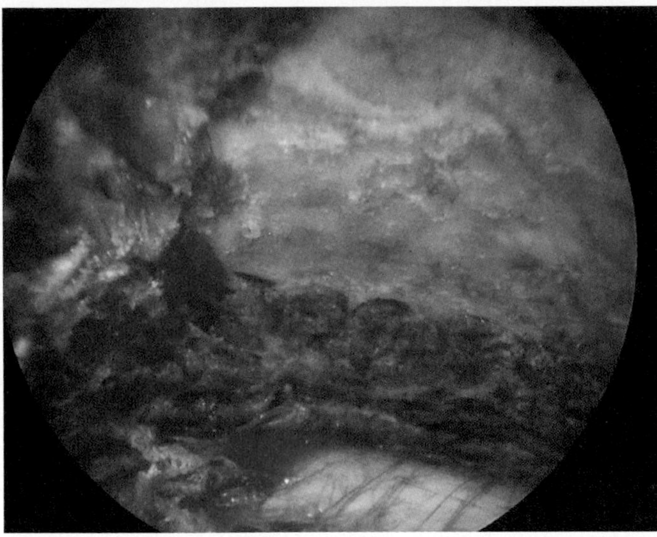

Figure 113.10. Medial muscle release is rechecked, preserving the main pectoralis major muscle superior to external reference marking. Correlation of internal anatomy and external marking is reconfirmed.

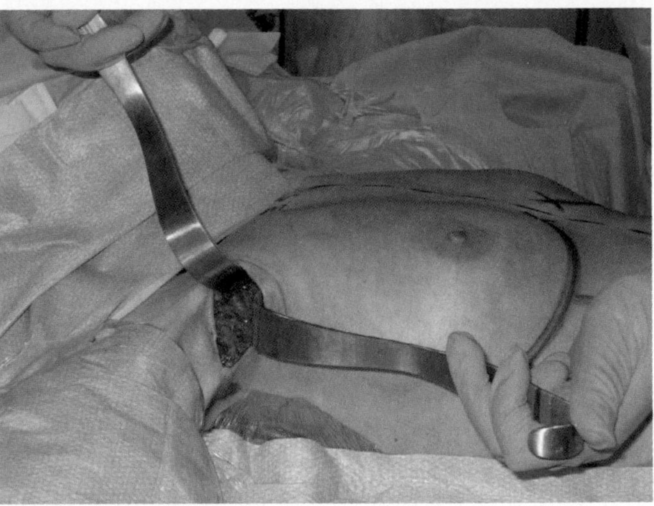

Figure 113.12. Silicone gel implant placement technique with two 1-inch Deaver retractors placed at right angles to open space for gel implant insertion.

maintained during the tissue release and rechecked following blunt refinements medially and laterally. An adequate muscle cuff must be maintained in the direction of the chest wall to allow for control of bleeding during release of the pectoralis major muscle.

IMPLANT PLACEMENT

The technique for saline implant placement begins with evacuation of air from the device, followed by placement into antibiotic solution. A narrow Deaver retractor is placed thorough the incision and into the subpectoral space, pointed inferiorly and medially, toward the medial aspect of the base of the breast. The implant is rolled with the fill tube in the center facing up and then placed beneath the retractor and into the soft tissue pocket (Fig. 113.11). The device is then carefully unrolled and filled to the desired volume. The patient is placed in the 45- and 80-deg sitting position, allowing for the level and shape of the inframammary fold to be checked. Minor adjustments can be made using smooth edge dissectors. Alternatively, the device can be deflated and removed, the pocket adjusted with endoscopic visualization, and the implant replaced. As the surgeon gains more experience with the technique, this is rarely if ever needed. The identical procedure is performed on the contralateral side, with any adjustments performed as needed for optimal symmetry.

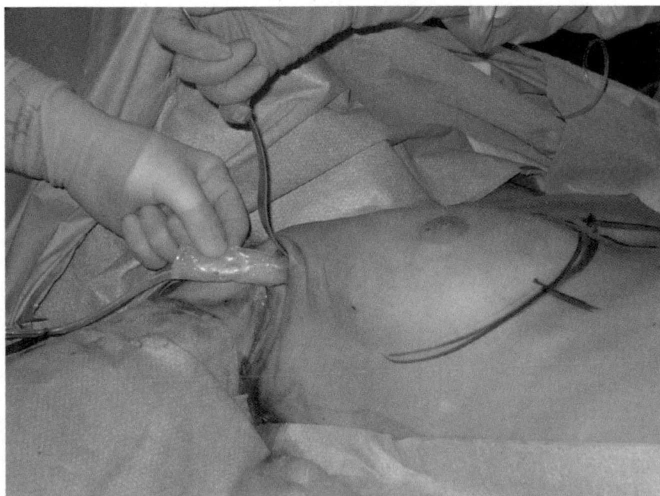

Figure 113.11. Saline implant placement with implant rolled beneath a single Deaver retractor.

The technique for silicone gel implant placement differs because the device is placed with full volume. I prefer to use two 1-inch Deaver retractors placed perpendicular to one another, one parallel to the clavicle, the other parallel to the lateral chest wall, pulled simultaneously apart to permit introduction of the implant in a rolling motion (Fig. 113.12). Correct placement and position is confirmed manually. Inspection is then performed as described, with the patient's back raised to 45- and 80-deg sitting position to adequately inspect pocket dimensions and inframammary fold level and shape and to fully evaluate for the symmetry of the augmented breasts. Layered closure of incisions is then performed, followed by placement of a pressure dressing.

POSTOPERATIVE CARE

An important aspect of the transaxillary approach is that the space in the upper area of the subpectoral space used for implant placement is not otherwise needed and must be addressed in the early postoperative period by the use of external pressure. This serves to close that space that would otherwise tend to collect fluid or allow the implant to migrate superiorly into an undesirable position. To obliterate this space, a pressure dressing is placed in the operating room and maintained for 24 to 48 hours, followed by use of an elastic wrap, which is then used to maintain downward pressure for 5 to 7 days (Figs. 113.13 and 113.14). Other complications are

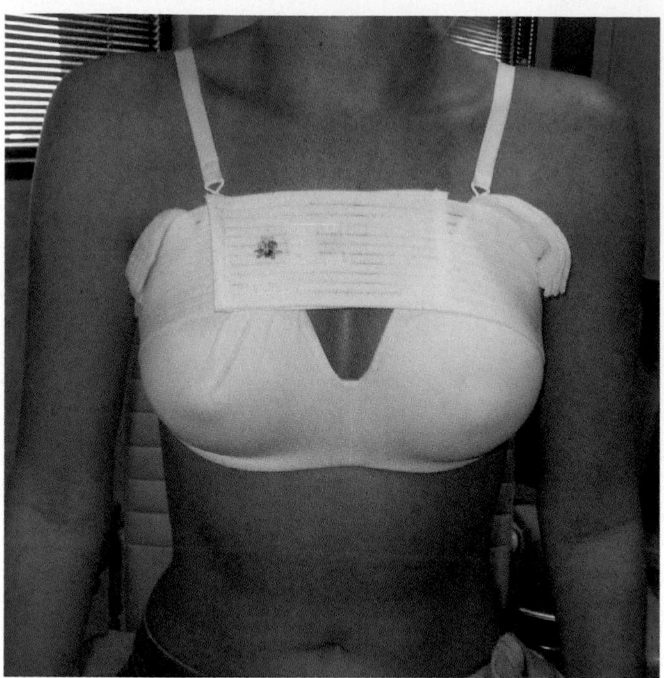

Figure 113.13. Postoperative implant space stabilization using bra and elastic wrap.

essentially all those seen with any of the other traditional inframammary or periareolar approaches to breast augmentation.

NONENDOSCOPIC APPROACH

The nonendoscopic technique can performed in an identical fashion to the technique just described, except that the tissue release is performed using entirely blunt dissection. Once the subpectoral space is entered, Agris-Dingman dissectors are used to complete development of the subpectoral space to the main body of the pectoral muscle. After the initial pocket is created, the pectoralis major muscle is bluntly separated using the Agris-Dingman dissectors to the 6 o'clock position. Further blunt refinement of the lateral pocket is then performed in a similar fashion. The inframammary fold level and shape are checked with the patient in the sitting position. Hemostasis is then checked with a long fiberoptic retractor. Once satisfactory soft tissue pocket dimensions and hemostasis have been accomplished, the implants are then placed (5).

DISCUSSION

The transaxillary endoscopic approach to breast augmentation provides the precision and technical control need to obtain consistent and reliable results when a transaxillary approach is selected for breast augmentation. Endoscopic tissue visualization provides the consistent ability to perform specific tissue release and control inframammary fold level and shape in a way that is very difficult to accomplish without direct tissue visualization. Experience with the transaxillary endoscopic technique permits this approach to be used in patients with a variety of tissue types, patients with varying needs for inframammary fold position maintenance or modification, and patients seeking augmentation with saline or silicone gel breast implants (Figs. 113.15 to 113.18). The transaxillary endoscopic approach to breast augmentation can provide results as consistent as those seen with the more traditional inframammary and periareolar approaches, with the distinct advantage of leaving no incisions on the breast.

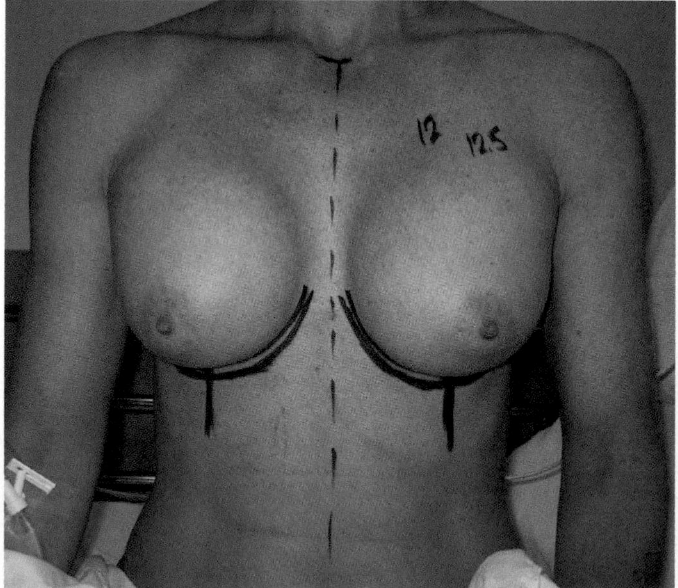

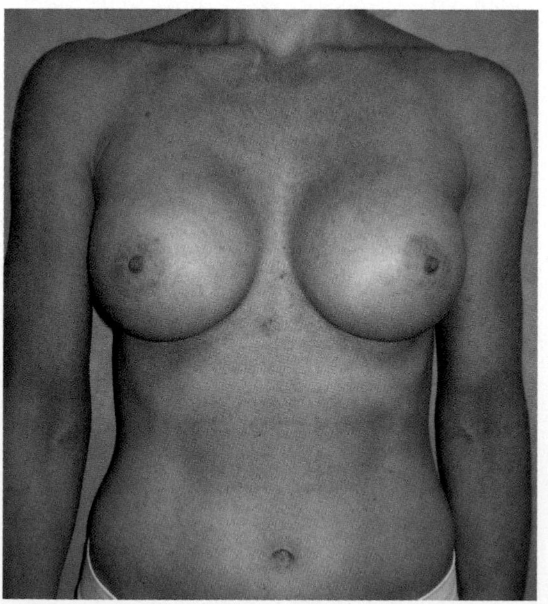

Figure 113.14. **A:** Preoperative markings of a 44-year-old woman who presented seeking revision of her saline implants with superior malposition placed using transaxillary approach. **B:** Postoperative view 1 year following transaxillary endoscopic open capsulotomy, saline implant exchange using 420-cc, high-profile implants with lowering of inframammary fold. The postoperative routine shown in Figure 113.13 is intended to prevent this problem.

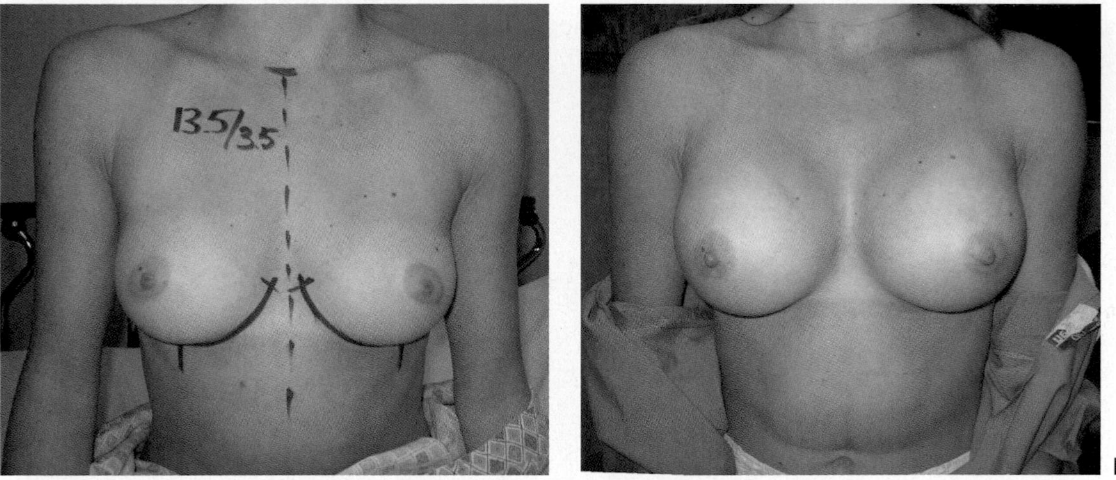

Figure 113.15. **A:** A 21-year-old woman shown in technique photos, with moderate soft tissue envelope. Preoperative markings show the plan to maintain the level of the inframammary fold during the transaxillary endoscopic procedure for saline implant placement. **B:** Early postoperative view shows symmetry of implants with maintenance of inframammary fold position, following placement of 380-cc, high-profile saline implants in a partial subpectoral pocket using a transaxillary endoscopic approach.

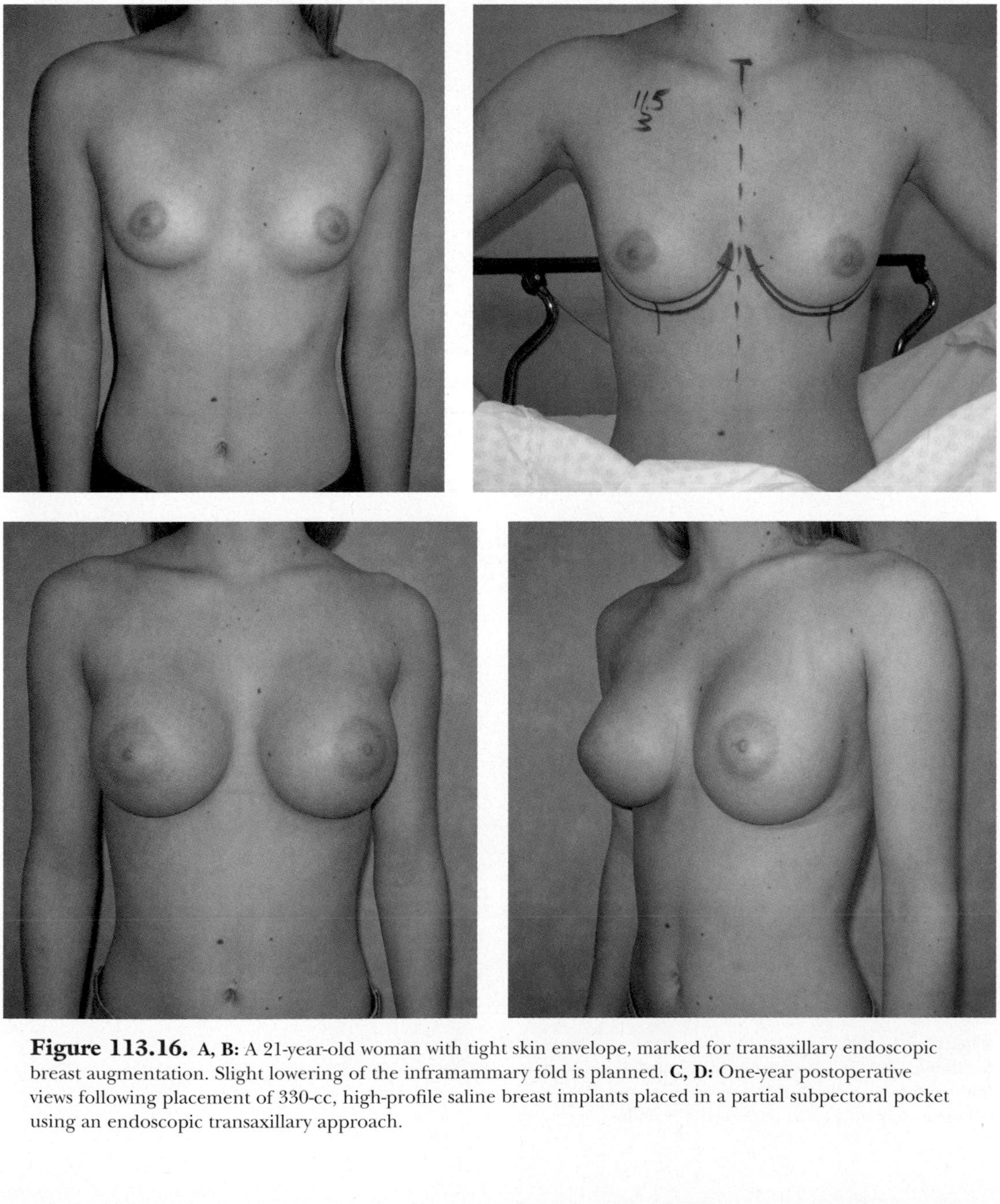

A B C D

Figure 113.16. **A, B:** A 21-year-old woman with tight skin envelope, marked for transaxillary endoscopic breast augmentation. Slight lowering of the inframammary fold is planned. **C, D:** One-year postoperative views following placement of 330-cc, high-profile saline breast implants placed in a partial subpectoral pocket using an endoscopic transaxillary approach.

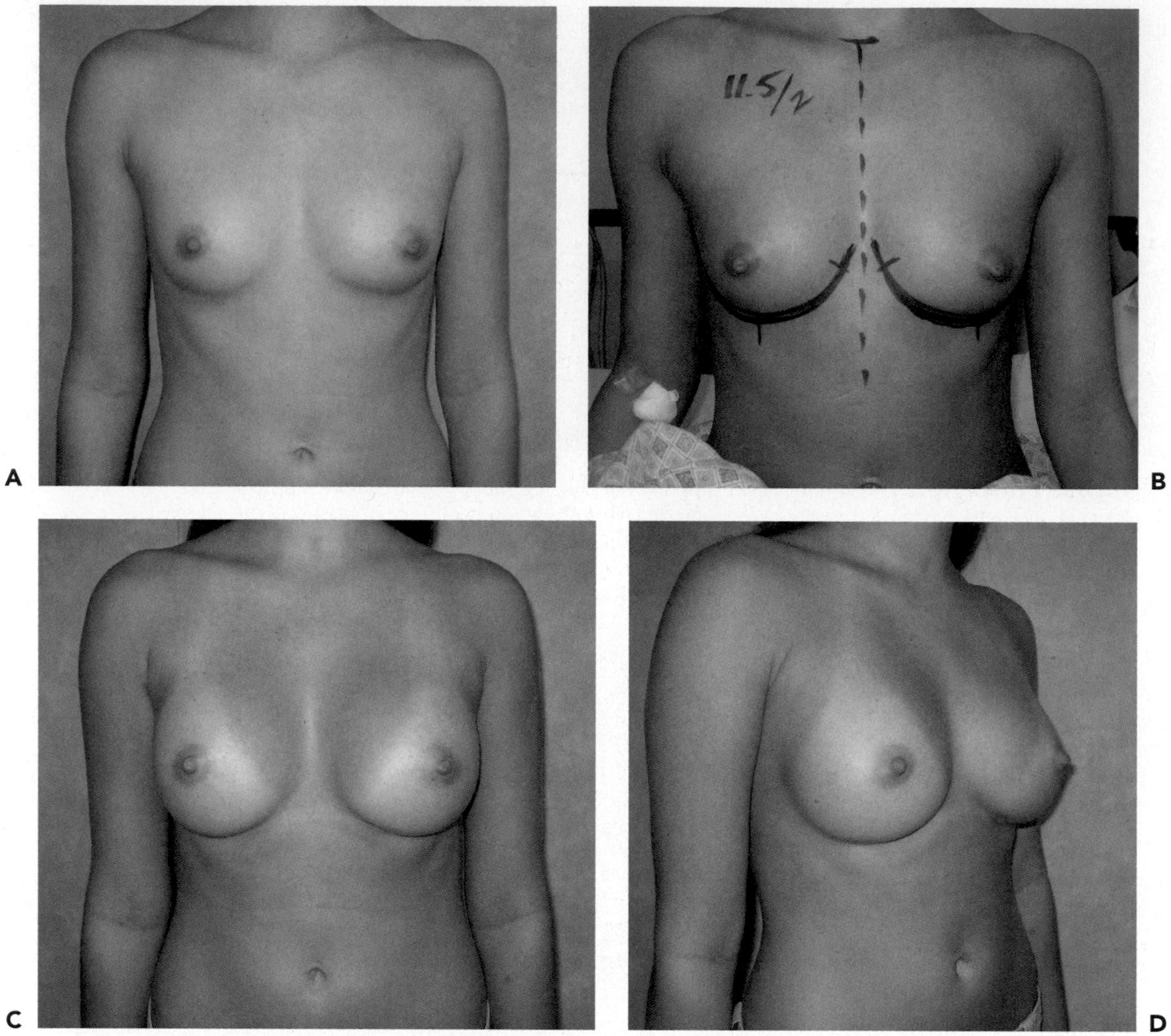

Figure 113.17. **A, B:** A 29-year-old woman with tight skin envelope, marked for transaxillary endoscopic silicone gel breast implant placement. Slight lowering of inframammary fold is planned. **C, D:** Five-month postoperative views following placement of 250-cc moderate plus–profile silicone gel implants in a partial subpectoral pocket using a transaxillary endoscopic approach.

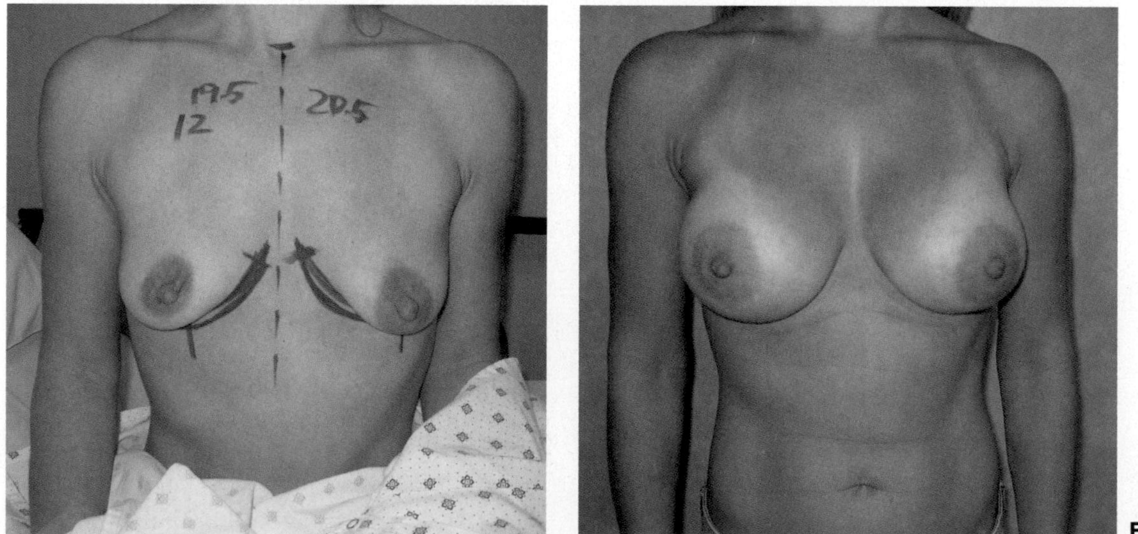

Figure 113.18. **A:** A 41-year-old woman with loose skin envelope and high inframammary folds, marked for transaxillary endoscopic breast augmentation. Note the plan for significant lowering of the inframammary fold levels bilaterally. **B:** Eight-month postoperative view following placement of 350-cc, high-profile silicone gel breast implants using a transaxillary endoscopic approach.

EDITORIAL COMMENTS

Dr. Strock has presented an excellent description of the technique of transaxillary breast augmentation. In this chapter he reviews the endoscopic and nonendoscopic approach. It is clear that the endoscopic approach confers significant advantage in terms of visibility, hemostasis, and pocket dissection. Common to both techniques are the markings, patient positioning, and incision location. Differences between the two techniques include the equipment and the dissection. The nonendoscopic approach is performed using a blunt technique, whereas the endoscopic approach is performed using electrocautery. Incision length depends on the type of implant. When a saline device is used, a 2.5- to 3-cm incision is created, whereas when a silicone gel device is used, a 5-cm incision is created. Dr. Strock has several illustrated results with outstanding results.

M.Y.N.

REFERENCES

1. Hoehler H. Breast augmentation: the axillary approach. *Br J Plast Surg* 1973;26:373.
2. Wright JH, Bevin AG. Augmentation mammaplasty by the transaxillary approach. *Plast Reconstr Surg* 1976;58(4):429–433.
3. Tebbetts JB. Transaxillary subpectoral augmentation mammaplasty: long-term follow-up and Refinements. *Plast Reconstr Surg* 1984;74(5):636–647.
4. Price CI, Eaves FF, Nahai F, et al. Endoscopic transaxillary subpectoral breast augmentation. *Plast Reconstr Surg* 1994;94(5):612–619.
5. Jones GE, Nahai F. Transaxillary breast augmentation. In: Spear SL, ed. *Surgery of the Breast: Principles and Art.* 2nd ed. Philadelphia: Lippincott Williams & Wilkins; 2006:1311–1318.
6. Eaves FF. Breast augmentation: enhanced visualization with the endoscopic transaxillary technique. *Aesthetic Surg J* 1999;19:162.
7. Graf RM, Bernardes A, Auersvald A, et al. Subfascial endoscopic transaxillary augmentation mammaplasty. *Aesthet Plast Surg* 2000;24:220–220.
8. Strock LL. Technical refinements and complication avoidance in transaxillary endoscopic breast augmentation. Presented at the American Society for Aesthetic Plastic Surgery Meeting, Boston, Massachusetts, 2003.
9. Serra-Renom JM, Garrido MF, Yoon T. Augmentation mammaplasty with anatomic soft, cohesive silicone implant using the transaxillary approach at a subfascial level with endoscopic assistance. *Plast Reconstr Surg* 2005;116(2):640–645.
10. Giordano PA, Roif M, Laurent B, et al. Endoscopic transaxillary breast augmentation: clinical evaluation of a series of 306 patients over a 9-year period. *Aesthet Surg J* 2007;27(1):47–54.
11. Tebbetts JB. Axillary endoscopic breast augmentation: processes derived from a 28-year experience to optimize outcomes. *Plast Reconstr Surg* 2006;118(7S):53S–80S.
12. Strock LL. Technical refinements and complication avoidance in transaxillary endoscopic breast augmentation: an updated experience. Presented at the American Society for Aesthetic Plastic Surgery Meeting, San Diego, California, 2008.

CHAPTER

114

Richard V. Dowden
Marianne A. Fuller

Transumbilical Breast Augmentation

HISTORY AND BACKGROUND

Attempts to find a procedure to satisfy a woman's desire for larger breasts without a breast incision have a long history. Inserting breast implants during operation upon the abdominal wall was reported in 1976 by Planas (1) and again in 1980 by Barrett (2). The idea of inserting breast implants through the navel was conceived and developed by Johnson in 1991 and published soon thereafter, revealing a very low complication rate (3). Subsequent to the initial publication the procedure has undergone several significant modifications (4–6), has been proven safe and effective both for patients (7) and for implants (8), is now widely used (9–14), and has become an integral part of the standard of care. Transumbilical breast augmentation makes use of established techniques with which most plastic surgeons are familiar, such as suction-assisted lipectomy, operative endoscopy, and tissue expansion, but which are combined in a way that was novel 16 years ago.

A few words are in order concerning terminology. The accepted correct term is transumbilical breast augmentation (TUBA). Other terms have been suggested but have been rejected for inaccuracy, such as "periumbilical" or "transabdominal." These are misleading and should be discarded. Just as transaxillary means through the axilla, transumbilical means through the navel—peri means around, and neither periumbilical nor periaxillary would be correct. Transabdominal is worse, because it implies a procedure done through the abdominal cavity, still an occasionally encountered misconception. Even when the incision is made through an abdominal scar or when the procedure is done during an abdominoplasty, the term TUBA should be used because what most distinguishes this method from all others is the unique set of technical principles involved rather than the precise location of the incision.

Except for the scar, the transumbilical approach produces final results not unlike the successful results of any other method of inserting saline-filled implants, but the TUBA has a few distinct advantages over those other methods (15). Those who perform the procedure have consistently noted a low rate of complications, minimal pain, a fast recovery, and very high patient satisfaction. Our experience has reflected those observations as well. Most important, we find that especially for asymmetric breasts, TUBA gives the best control over the final position, shape, and symmetry of the breasts. The recovery is remarkably rapid after the TUBA procedure, especially if prepectoral. As the choice of prepectoral or subpectoral is left to the patient, it is not surprising that patients are equally satisfied with the results of the plane they chose. The consistently minimal bleeding with the TUBA procedure is probably due to the fact that there is no cutting in, or behind, the breast (3). The remarkably low level of pain after the transumbilical augmentation has not been fully explained, but one hypothesis is that the implant is exerting no tension upon the healing incision; that characteristic is of course shared with transaxillary augmentation, but the TUBA has the added advantage over the transaxillary approach that the incision is located in an immobile area not moved or stretched by arm raising. Another advantage of TUBA is the surgeon's freedom to use quite large implants without fear of a wound dehiscence or symmastia, despite the considerable tension that may be exerted on the breast skin.

The TUBA is a blunt expansion technique, requiring no cutting and no cauterization within the pocket. It does not require insertion of gauze or sponges inside the pocket, avoiding the chance of retention thereof. Some authors (16) have speculated that such blunt expansion might result in more pain than cutting or cautery techniques, yet that hypothesis has been disproven in practice. Of course, assessment of patient pain levels is highly subjective, and attempting to compare pain levels between different incisions is nearly impossible; moreover, it is highly unlikely that any true controlled study can or will ever be done.

Another advantage of the TUBA method pertains to drains. Many surgeons believe that serosanguineous fluid collections around the implants may be a major factor leading to capsular contracture. For this reason, some advocate use of drain tubes, while others avoid doing so because they are uncomfortable with the concept of a drain connecting the skin to the surface of the implant. One advantage of the TUBA procedure is that the tunnels provide a dependent reservoir for any seroma that might otherwise collect around the implant, or at least provide a location for drain tubes that need not be in contact with the implants.

The TUBA method has some advantages in terms of implant protection. Manufacturer representatives are well aware of four types of potential intraoperative damage to implants, which can occur with any augmentation technique: damage from use of an implant as a tissue expander, contact with sharp-edged instruments, rupture during forced insertion of filled implants, and needle puncture during closure. These modes of injury cannot occur with the TUBA technique, in which the implants are not used as expanders, the implants do not contact any instruments, the implants must be empty when inserted, and the closure sutures are far distant from the implant.

If the TUBA has so many advantages, one might ask, why have not more surgeons learned how to perform it? Several possible reasons include that surgeons may be afraid to learn something new or may be wary of something unfamiliar, or they may see no justification for expanding their current practice methods in light of the cost of the equipment and the time needed to learn the TUBA technique. It is conceivable that some surgeons may be resentful that someone else has devised an excellent method that they cannot offer the patient and wish to hold on to their established methods. Perhaps it is an example of the maxim due to Thomas Szasz stating that "Every act of conscious learning requires the willingness to suffer an injury to one's self-esteem" (17). It is historically noteworthy that negativity and reluctance also attended the introduction of endoscopic methods for performing other traditionally open procedures, such as cholecystectomy, splenectomy, hernia repair, and carpal tunnel, to name but a few of the hundreds of procedures now done primarily endoscopically.

Another possible reason for reluctance to learn the TUBA method may be a lack of the requisite endoscopic ability or at least a lack of understanding of the way the endoscope is used for transumbilical breast augmentation. In any breast enlargement technique there must be adequate visualization to ensure that the critical portions of the procedure are done correctly and safely (18). In some techniques, this is accomplished by direct vision using lighted retractors, and in other techniques this visibility is enhanced by use of endoscopes. If the navel is chosen, implant plane and orientation, absence of bleeding, adequacy of pocket formation, and valve integrity can be verified *only* through the use of an endoscope. Therefore, proper performance of the TUBA procedure requires that the surgeon possess strong endoscopic skills. The surgeon must be comfortable relating what the hands are doing to what is seen on the monitor and relating the monitor view to the reality of the anatomy (19). It is important to note that, in contrast to every other endoscopic breast procedure, in the transumbilical augmentation *the endoscope is not used during pocket formation*, for which internal hydraulic expansion is used instead, with external monitoring by observing the position and shape of the breasts. The endoscope is only used at key points to verify the status of the pocket. Nevertheless, there are some surgeons who perform the TUBA without an endoscope in order to shorten the operating time; this is inadvisable. In addition, it would be a mistake to change the procedure to one involving sharp dissection under endoscopic visualization, as has been suggested from time to time by various surgeons not thoroughly conversant with the TUBA technique.

Many surgeons are under the misconception that using endoscopic techniques might void the implant warranty. This is a false assumption based on the implant brochures, which state that the manufacturers do not recommend the transumbilical or any other endoscopic method (which therefore precludes transaxillary as well). A little history is in order concerning that unfortunate implant brochure wording. At the U.S. Food and Drug Administration (FDA) implant approval hearings, the TUBA procedure was mentioned briefly in passing. Although there were two plastic surgeons present, unfortunately neither was knowledgeable about TUBA. Due to the absence of information, the FDA committee members heard a false statement that implants are "wadded up and shoved in through an endoscope" (20), and as a result of that misunderstanding it was suggested by one of the plastic surgeons that the FDA not approve endoscopic methods, which in turn led to the inappropriate wording in the brochures. Federal law prohibits the *manufacturer* from recommending that any product be used "off label," that is, in any manner not approved by the FDA. Because the manufacturers cannot recommend the transumbilical approach, one might think that the plastic surgeon might be barred from using the TUBA or axillary approaches. In fact, however, there is no legal obstacle to a physician using any product in an off-label application (21). Therefore, there are no legal limitations on plastic surgeons regarding the TUBA procedure. *When performed as specified in this chapter*, there would be no basis for voiding the warranty, and in fact the manufacturers have continued to honor their warranties. More to the point, both of the U.S. manufacturers whose implants are FDA approved have provided written assurance that their implant warranties are fully in effect after using the transumbilical approach (22), and both manufacturers provide extra-long fill tubes specifically designed for the TUBA method.

The TUBA method has been the subject of a variety of other criticisms. Careful examination of each of those criticisms reveals that most are at best misconceptions, or at worst intentional falsehoods (19), but in any case all are unquestionably false. Some of the worst misunderstandings need to be clarified. The entire TUBA procedure takes place external to the anterior rectus fascia, in the subcutaneous plane, and does not involve abdominal muscles, the abdominal cavity, or internal organs. No actual cutting takes place behind or within the breast. The surgeon is able to see externally the exact shape of the breasts, as well as the position of the implants, during the expansion phase, so there is no guesswork involved in pocket formation or implant positioning. Implant pocket creation is actually easier than with any other method. We find that the TUBA method facilitates correction of breast asymmetry, and modest degrees of tubular breasts as well, because of the ability to pressure expand the skin without fear of dehiscence.

Surgeons who intend to offer the TUBA method must be prepared to counter with true information all such false criticisms that the patients may have heard or read. These criticisms generally originate from surgical colleagues, and are usually just an indication of ignorance about the procedure, although in some instances they could represent a desire to discredit the TUBA method. For example, some surgeons disparage this blunt expansion technique by describing it using emotionally charged negative terms intended to alarm patients. They use terms such as "ripping" or "tearing" or "avulsing," despite the time-honored role of blunt techniques in other commonly performed procedures such as face lift, abdominoplasty, rhinoplasty, and liposuction, in connection with which those same surgeons do not use such pejorative terms. Surgeons may also attempt to cast aspersions on the TUBA by saying that it is a "blind" technique, ignoring the fact that we commonly perform other blind techniques such as rhinoplasty and liposuction, in which progress is assessed externally rather than from the inside. Patients need clear information to counteract such misguided influences.

Having said all that, the legitimate disadvantages of the TUBA procedure also warrant discussion. The TUBA cannot be used for prefilled implants, silicone or saline, because the atraumatic insertion of implants through a narrow passageway and their confinement within the appropriately dimensioned pocket require the ability to shape them into a small cross section for insertion. A method for inserting silicone gel implants transumbilically may be developed in the future, as research is ongoing toward that end. Another drawback is that the TUBA method may be less than ideal for placement of nonround implants because creating the appropriate nonround pocket might be difficult, possibly increasing the chance of later rotation, but here too research is being done.

One disadvantage of the TUBA procedure is the need for a significant investment in equipment not otherwise required for breast augmentation, including the endoscope, video camera, monitor, light source, Johnson instrument set (Fig. 114.1), and two full sets of intraoperative expanders. The endoscope is a standard 10 mm × 34 cm–long, rigid, 0-deg nonoperating

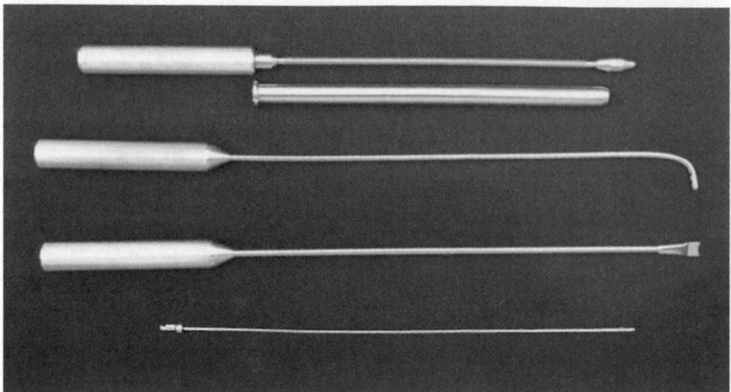

Figure 114.1. Transumbilical breast augmentation instruments. From above downward, the Johnson obturator, Johnson tube, Johnson blunt hockey stick, Johnson pusher (rarely used), and the infusion/aspirator wand. Note that the Johnson obturator has a blunt tip for safety. See text for details.

gynecology type. Note again the key principle that there is no dissection taking place under endoscopic view, only verification at key points during the procedure, hence the nonoperating scope.

Johnson instrument sets can be obtained directly from the Wells Johnson Company (Tucson, AZ). They offer two different calibers of tube and obturator, a 19-mm and a 24-mm outside diameter. We use the 19-mm size for almost all implants, but the 24-mm size may be needed for the larger Allergan implants, which are somewhat bulky when rolled. The Johnson tube and matching obturator are essential for establishing the correct plane of placement and for endoscopic verification at critical points during the procedure. To maximize safety, we strongly contend that the obturator tip should be slightly blunt rather than sharply pointed (Fig. 114.2), which may require that some modification be performed. The Johnson hockey stick, a long, blunt rod bent at the end, with blunt notches near the tip, is also used on every case. We use the straight, notched pusher

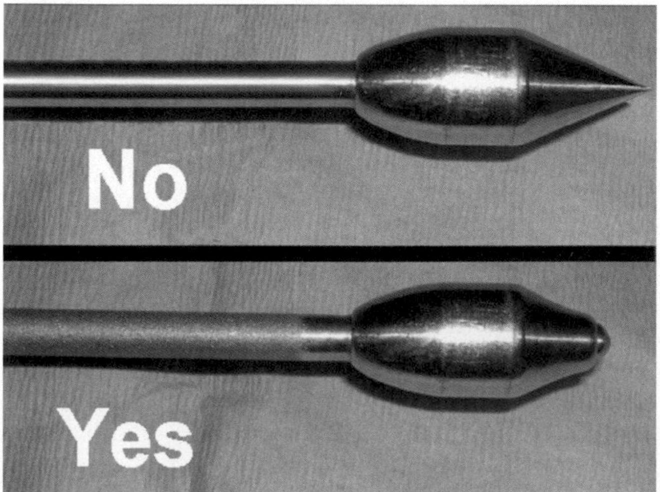

Figure 114.2. Close-up views of obturator tips, both the incorrect (sharp) shape and the correct (blunt) shape. If the only shape available is the sharp type, any machine shop should be able to modify the shape appropriately. Note that the shaft should be roughened for a better grip.

about once every 50 cases to push a fibrous band out of the way. A long, thin (3/32 inch) suction tube, blunt at the tip with a locking connector, is part of our set as well; although not part of the standard set, it can be supplied by Wells-Johnson. It is important to note here that the Johnson tube is *not* used to push the implant into position as was portrayed in the original publication (3). Of course, it never was recommended to pass the implant *through* any instrument, the erroneous FDA testimony to the contrary. It is sufficient, and safer, for the implant to be advanced solely by external manipulation by the surgeon.

In the original description of the technique (3), the implant itself was used as the device that initially overexpanded the pocket, which was then left in place. To avoid expansion trauma to the implants, the procedure was changed in 1992, requiring a preliminary step to create the pocket using strong, saline-filled expanders. These expanders permit precise and symmetric development of the pockets and are then removed. The expanders used should have the same volume and dimensions as the implant. Usually, except in highly asymmetric patients, the expanders are not used as "sizers" to decide which implants are to be used, a decision that is best made in advance. The expander is generally inflated to 150% to 170% of final volume for prepectoral and from 150% to 200% for subpectoral placement; the greater levels of temporary overinflation are used if the skin envelope is very tight. The expanders should be transparent, not opaque, in order to permit inspection of the interior of the pocket *through* the expander itself. If no transparent expanders are available, a set can be easily fabricated by taking standard smooth implants and securely bonding their fill tubes using a commercial grade of room temperature–curing silicone adhesive and then heating in an autoclave.

Far more important than the instrumentation, the main prerequisite for the TUBA technique is proper training of the surgeon. The TUBA is not a procedure to be attempted on the basis of reading articles or books, attending lectures, and watching a few cases. Once mastered, the TUBA procedure is very safe and straightforward, but the learning curve can be steep, and there are many ways that an inadequately trained individual can get into problem situations. Proper training includes lectures, visual aids, endoscopic practice, and cadaver lab sessions, as well as an extensive review of videotapes about the recognition and management of potential problems. It is worth reemphasizing that endoscopic skill is an absolute requirement for performing this ingenious and effective procedure safely and well (4).

Out of 2,796 breasts that we originally augmented via the navel, we reoperated on 117 breasts (4.1%), most via the navel, chiefly for size change, and other indications as listed in Table 114.1. On a patient basis, 4.4% of patients were reoperated, over half being elective patient choice.

PATIENT SELECTION

In our practice, once it has been determined which incision locations would be feasible for her, the patient decides on the incision site. Nearly all patients are suitable candidates for the transumbilical approach, even those with significant deformity of the chest wall and those with a flared rib cage, as well as those who have pectus excavatum or carinatum. It is suitable for augmenting breasts with moderate degrees of tubular breast deformity, and contrary to popular folklore, the TUBA is

TABLE 114.1	Reoperated Breasts (117)
Via navel incision: 87	
With implant replacement: 83	
Change to larger size (with capsulotomy): 18	
Change to smaller size: 22	
Deflations: 19	
Obsolete implant styles: 10	
Nonobsolete implant styles: 9	
Elective replacement: 24	
Without implant replacement: 4	
Capsulotomy: 2	
Explantation: 2	
Via other incisions: 30	
With implant replacement: 24	
Much larger size or silicone: 16	
Deflations: 6	
Obsolete implant style: 4	
Nonobsolete implant style: 2	
Capsulectomy: 2	
Without implant replacement: 6	
Capsulotomy: 1	
Mastopexy: 1	
Increase the fill volume: 2	
Explant alone: 2	

excellent for correcting breast asymmetry. As opposed to an opinion in the literature (11), we have had no problem lowering the inframammary fold, even as much as 3 cm. Use of the TUBA simultaneously with a mastopexy has not yet been reported, but it would be possible. Some might argue that since a mastopexy would require incisions on the breast anyway, doing a TUBA procedure would have little merit. However, doing the TUBA first would permit accurate assessment of the degree of remaining ptosis without the distortion produced by a fresh breast incision. The "tailor-tack" approach could then be done without concern that any subsequent flap necrosis would necessarily expose the implant. It is noteworthy that prior breast surgery has not interfered with the TUBA technique; we have used the TUBA method for patients who had prior biopsies, mastopexies, explantations, radiation, and breast reduction surgery. Less ideal candidates for TUBA include those with severe tubular breast deformity or those whose nipples require relocation, because for them a great deal of modification of the surface of the breast would be required.

We have encountered no difficulty from abdominal scars due to C-sections, liposuction, abdominoplasties, laparoscopies, or laparotomies, including scars that actually cross the paths of the tunnels, such as from cholecystectomy, gastrectomy, or splenectomy. For many of our patients with abdominal scars it has even been straightforward to use those scars rather than make a navel incision. Patients with scleroderma have posed no obstacle even when a patch of atrophic sclerodermatous skin lies directly over the path of the tunnels. One contraindication to the TUBA procedure is an upper abdominal hernia positioned in the path of the tunnels and likely to interfere with passing the obturator. Obesity per se is not a contraindication to the TUBA procedure, but if a patient's abdominal fat layer were too thick to permit detection of such an upper abdominal hernia, she would not be a candidate without further studies to exclude such a hernia. An umbilical hernia is not a contraindication; in fact, an ideal opportunity to repair an umbilical hernia is at the completion of the TUBA. We have done that on numerous occasions; however, it does increase the postoperative pain.

Navel rings are no impediment to the TUBA procedure, as the incision is simply detoured behind the jewelry hole. Some surgeons prefer to leave such navel jewelry in place during the procedure, even using it as a retractor, whereas our preference is to have it removed a few days in advance rather than work around it. The device can be sterilized and reinserted after the completion of the procedure if the patient so desires (7); as an alternative, a polypropylene suture loop can be placed to use as a retractor and to later keep the jewelry track from closing. The TUBA procedure also combines quite well with other simultaneous procedures, such as abdominoplasty, liposuction, or tubal ligation. Two of our patients had a unilateral TUBA procedure done at the time of postmastectomy reconstruction of the opposite side, both patients having felt strongly that they did not want any scar on their remaining breast. As mentioned earlier, another disqualification for TUBA is the choice of prefilled saline or silicone implants, and it is questionable whether the shaped implants are suitable for the TUBA method due to an increased possibility of rotation. We did use textured, round implants in two patients early in our TUBA experience, but because textured, round implants have not been proven to have any long-term advantage over smooth ones, we no longer use them for any breast augmentations.

PLANNING

Because the transumbilical breast augmentation does not lend itself to trying various sizes of implants intraoperatively, size determination is done in advance, using any of the customary methods. Our preference for doing so is the use of adjustable volumetric sizers within the patient's chosen bra size, in conjunction with a dimensional approach with particular attention to the transverse diameter of the breast and the thickness by pinch test at the top of the breast and at the inframammary fold (23). It should be kept in mind that because the TUBA procedure permits insertion of larger sizes of implant without fear of dehiscence, the surgeon must accurately assess the patient's tissue characteristics in order to fully discuss with her the consequences and trade-offs that her desired size may involve; this is often a very lengthy discussion (24). Our philosophy is to permit the patient to make her own choices, which of course places upon us the responsibility of educating her about the trade-offs involved in all those choices (25).

Accordingly, the decision of whether to place the implants in front of or behind the pectoralis muscle must also be made in advance, and since May 19, 1999, when the senior author started doing the subpectoral TUBA technique, he has given patients who request the incision in the navel their choice of placement plane. Since the date when both procedures were offered, about 60% have chosen prepectoral placement and 40% have chosen subpectoral placement. A full discussion of the pros and cons of prepectoral versus subpectoral placement is beyond the scope of this chapter, other than to point out two very important aspects: first, that the incidence of capsular contracture in our practice has been the same for prepectoral and subpectoral implants, provided that prepectoral patients do daily compression (not displacement) massage; second, that just as studies have shown that implanted women are not more likely to get breast cancer than those without implants (26), there has never been any reported difference in the accuracy of mammographic breast cancer detection, nor any difference in prognosis, between prepectoral and subpectoral augmentation (27), theoretical mammographic considerations notwithstanding. Having said that, it should be pointed out that some radiologists find it faster to read mammographic films of subpectoral implants than prepectoral ones, and other the contrary.

On rare occasion, for patients with great asymmetry, we have recommended that on one side the implant be placed prepectoral and on the other side subpectoral. As no convincing evidence has ever been presented showing any advantage to subfascial or subserratus/rectus augmentation, we have not attempted either via the navel but speculate that either might be somewhat challenging to perform via the navel.

In our practice, several separate informed-consent documents are used. These include the general augmentation consent; an "off-label consent" for any endoscopic procedure (transumbilical or transaxillary); a consent for the drawbacks of implants of greater than 400-cc volume; and an "optimal fill consent" for bringing the implant volume to its optimal value even if that volume exceeds the manufacturer's specified maximum for that implant (28), resulting in "overfill." We prefer to have these documents understood and signed well in advance of the operation; therefore they are completed in the office, giving the patient an opportunity to address any areas of concern with the surgeon or the office nurse.

PATIENT PREPARATION

We advise patients to exercise preoperatively to strengthen the abdominal muscles. All medications that inhibit coagulation, including vitamin E and herbal remedies, are discontinued 2 weeks prior to the procedure. As is our practice for any operation done under general anesthesia, to help prevent postoperative constipation, it is a kindness to patients to have them empty the gastrointestinal tract preoperatively with stool softeners and laxatives. Patients are instructed to do meticulous cleansing of the navel with antimicrobial soap the day before the operation. Any navel jewelry must be removed 2 days before operation.

On the operative day, an intravenous antibiotic is administered. Prior to any sedation being given, the patient is visited in the holding area and prepares her skin with alcohol, including cotton-tipped applicators inside the navel. With the patient standing, the markings are then done: first the midline is drawn from sternal notch to xiphoid, and then the existing inframammary creases. A second semicircular line is then drawn below the breasts, using as the radius from the anticipated breast center the sum of the radius of the implant plus the thickness of the lower breast tissues as determined by the pinch test. The vertical pocket limits are also indicated on each upper breast. To indicate the paths of the tunnels, on each side a line is drawn from the umbilicus toward the medial edge of the areola for prepectoral procedure or toward the head of the pectoral muscle for subpectoral procedure. As has been discussed in the literature (29), often the navel is not in the midline; this can have medicolegal consequences, so it is worthwhile pointing that out to the patient preoperatively, along with any other asymmetries.

To best ensure that the incision scar is well hidden within the navel, that too should be drawn with the patient standing. A variety of configurations can be used (Fig. 114.3), whichever is best hidden entirely within the specific contours of the patient's navel, as long as the incision has sufficient length to comfortably allow insertion of the Johnson tube with no resistance. As a rough guide, the incision length, when stretched, should equal one half of the circumference of the Johnson tube. For the 19-mm diameter tube this is usually on the order of about 2 cm total length before stretching of the incision. We have not yet encountered a navel too small to allow an adequate incision to be completely hidden within it.

IMPLANT PREPARATION

The implants and the expanders are inspected and prepared on a separate back table *before* the patient is under anesthesia, thereby providing the opportunity to cancel the procedure in the unlikely event of finding faulty devices. It is important to check the imprinted markings on the implants, as it has happened that a correctly marked box actually contained the wrong implant. Rather than filling with saline and watching for fluid leaking, testing the implants by watching for air bubbles when they are immersed in saline is a far superior method, with the caveat that no additional (potentially unsterile) room air is ever added. We use fresh, powder-free gloves whenever handling the implants. It is a noteworthy reflection upon the manufacturer's acceptance of the transumbilical technique that Allergan supplies extra-long fill tubes in the implant boxes, and Mentor now makes long fill tubes available. (The long fill tubes can be ordered separately: Mentor #600975-002 and Allergan #2955-02). Shorter fill tubes would require a sterile extension tube; if desired, a silk tie can be used to secure the tubing junction, but a tight twist fit suffices. Using a completely closed system, about 50 mL of saline is instilled into each implant to permit removal of all the air. A closed system greatly reduces the possibility of introducing pathogens into the implant and will likely become the standard of care, if not an FDA requirement. The implant is rolled as the remaining saline is removed, allowing the implant to hold its rolled-up shape as it traverses the slippery subcutaneous tunnel, and in fact the implant usually maintains its orientation without difficulty. Both the implants and the expanders are rolled in the same manner, like a scroll from side to side inward to protect the fill tube (Fig. 114.4) rather than in a cigar shape as described in the original article, to assist in maintaining orientation while transversing the tunnel. The expanders are prepared in a similar manner, again verifying the size marks on the devices, immersion testing for leaks, instilling a small amount of saline, and rolling them up during saline withdrawal. Because expanders are supplied with long tubing, they do not require extensions, but they *do* require a silk tie to secure their connector to the fill tube, as the hydraulic pressures involved in pocket creation can cause the locking connector to pop off of the fill tube. After preparation, the implants are returned to their sterile containers.

OPERATIVE TECHNIQUE

The operating room setup is fairly standard (30); a right-hand-dominant surgeon will likely prefer to stand on the patient's

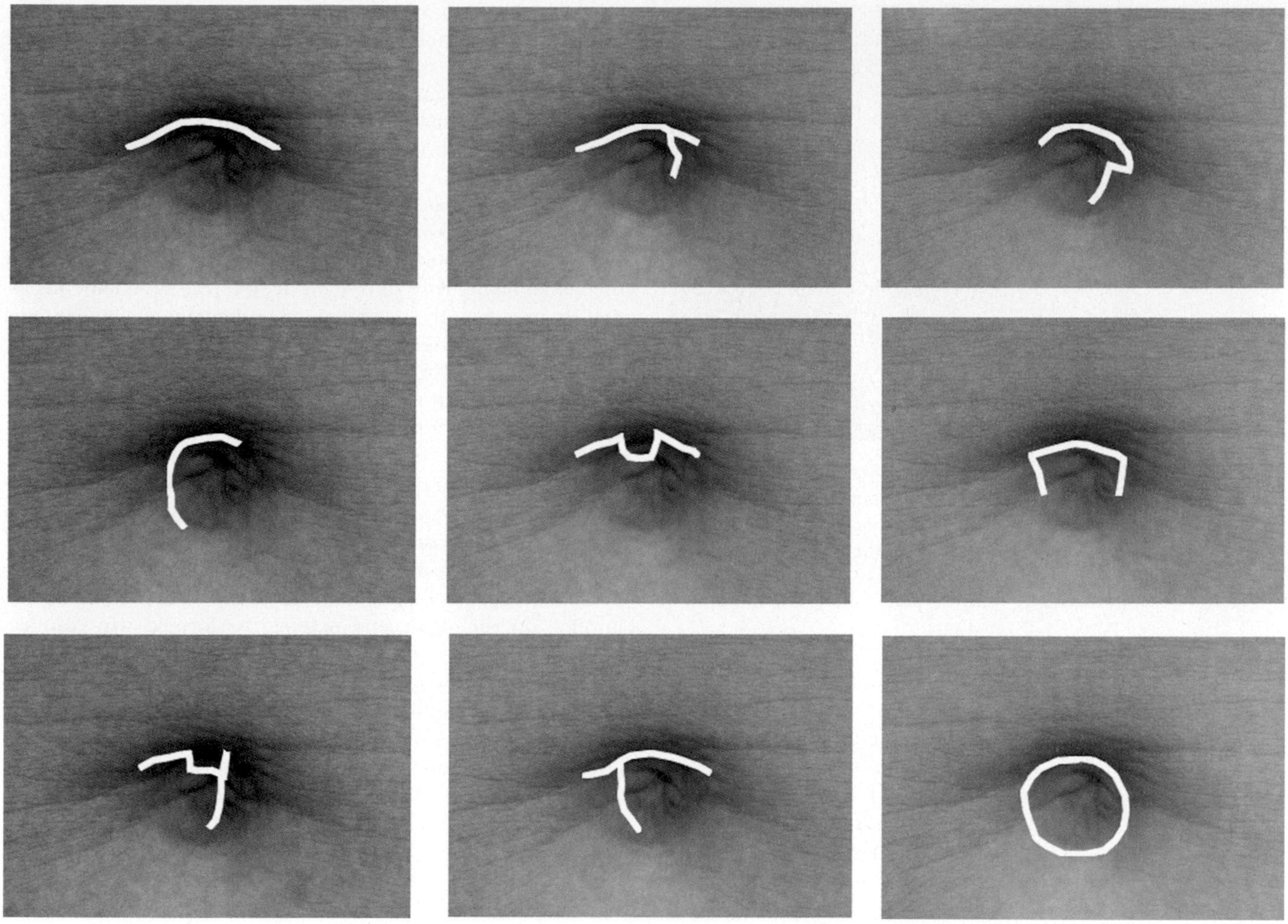

Figure 114.3. The navel incision can have a wide range of configurations, even detouring around a jewelry hole. The circumference must accommodate the Johnson tube. The markings should be done with the patient upright to ensure that they are contained within the navel and well hidden.

right side with the monitor near the patient's left shoulder. The operating table is preheated with warm air. As soon as the patient arrives in the operating room, a cotton ball soaked in iodophor is placed in the navel and left there until the prep. The patient is positioned supine with arms at 90 deg for prepectoral or 70 deg for subpectoral procedure. The knees are kept flat, no pillow or other object behind them, to avoid obstructing the instruments. We favor use of a warming blanket and pneumatic stockings. Sedation and local can be used for the TUBA, but with the excellent agents now available, we prefer general anesthesia for all breast augmentations. The laryngeal mask (LMA) is ideal for both prepectoral and subpectoral TUBA. We prefer that nitrous oxide not be used for operations such as TUBA, abdominal liposuction, or abdominoplasty because it can cause abdominal distension. Monitoring includes pulse oximetry, blood pressure, electrocardiogram, and often a bispectral index neurologic monitor. Muscle relaxation *should not* be present during initial tunnel formation in order to keep the rectus muscles taut and flat. Later, for subpectoral augmentation only, a short-acting relaxant can be given *after* the obturator has reached the inframammary crease.

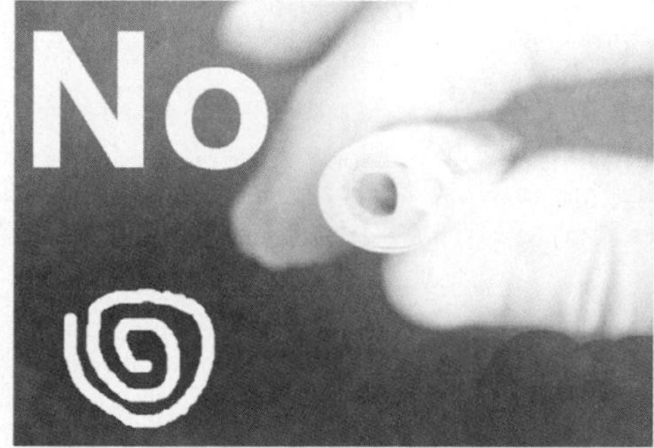

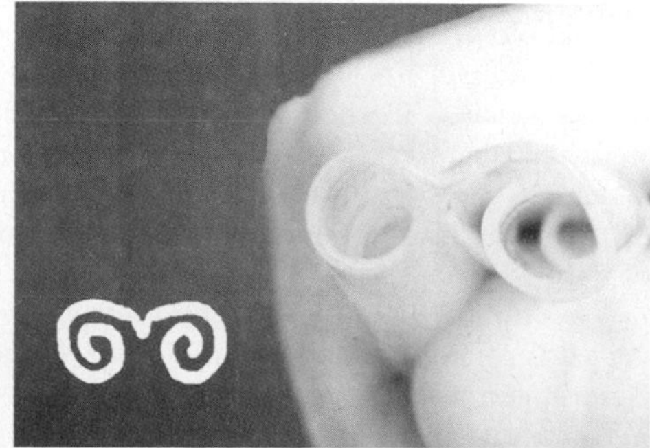

Figure 114.4. To assist in maintaining implant orientation during passage up the tunnels, the implant should be rolled not as a cigar shape, but rather as a scroll form the two sides. The fill tube is protected between the two rolled sides.

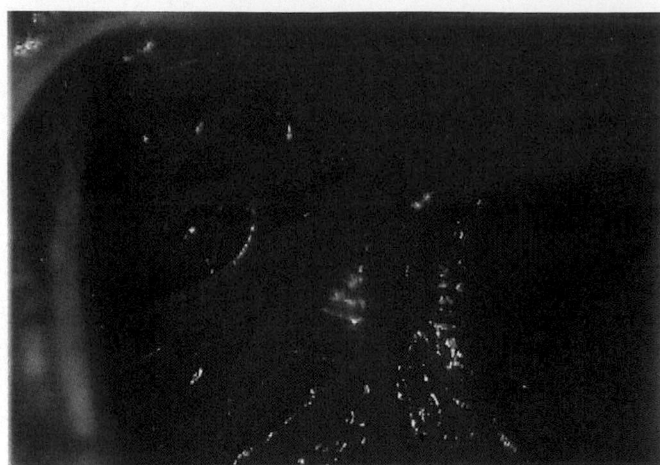

Figure 114.5. Endoscopic view after abdominal liposuction showing the multiple tunnels that could make implant passage difficult. When abdominal liposuction is performed along with augmentation, the liposuction should be deferred until after the implants are in place.

Skin prep extends from neck to pubis and to the posterior axillary line on each side. If there is a hole for navel jewelry, that is prepped by passing through it a braided silk suture soaked with prep solution. The drapes are positioned to leave exposed the entire anterior chest and abdomen and must be flat over the pelvis in order to not interfere with the long instruments. A slight head-down tilt of the table will help prevent air accumulation within the pockets, to avoid postoperative implant sounds (31). We apply a transparent plastic film to each nipple to keep any discharge off the field. If abdominal liposuction is also to be done, that should be deferred until *after* the TUBA; otherwise the multiple tunnels (Fig. 114.5) impede implant insertion. When we combine TUBA with abdominoplasty, we do the TUBA prior to, or at the midpoint of, the abdominoplasty.

Long-acting local anesthetic is infiltrated superficially for the incision. Some surgeons infiltrate or tumesce the entire path of the tunnels with local anesthetic and epinephrine, but with general anesthesia we do not consider that helpful. The navel incision is the only time any sharp instrument is used during the procedure. Skin hooks may assist in stabilizing the skin for this incision. Round-tipped scissors are then used to spread bluntly downward onto the surface of the rectus fascia. To avoid entry into an unsuspected umbilical hernia, this spreading should initially be directed laterally on each side, then progressing more medially on the fascial surface. Using an Army-Navy retractor, along with caudal tension on the skin, a large blunt scissors is used to begin each tunnel on the fascial surface, about 5 cm up, spreading minimally to avoid creating blind pockets. Direct vision confirms that the tunnel is directly on the fascia, care being taken to not penetrate the rectus sheath in the rare case where its fibers are thin and only loosely attached. The right index finger is used to verify that the first few centimeters of the tunnels are of adequate caliber and free of fibrous obstructions.

The tip of the Johnson obturator (without the tube) is passed through the incision and up the tunnel. The obturator is advanced in the plane between rectus fascia and subcutaneous tissue, while the skin and subcutaneous tissue are gathered up and supported with the opposite hand staying just ahead of the obturator tip. It is important that this advancement be done in increments only, about 4 cm per step, and not in one continuous steady forward push as per the original article. The obturator must not be gripped by the handle at its end, but rather along its shaft, about 4 cm from the incision; this prevents an improperly directed stroke from traveling any great distance. It is important not to back up and restart the obturator, which can create small dead-end tunnels that could cause difficulty when passing the tissue expander and implant (Fig. 114.6). The Johnson obturator is advanced on the surface of the fascia, taking care to remain deep to the subcutaneous tissue to prevent any postoperative subcutaneous irregularity (a complication often mentioned but which the senior author has not seen in 1,402 cases over a 16-year span).

If the placement will be subpectoral, before crossing the inframammary crease we instill a chilled, dilute 1:1,000,000 epinephrine mixture behind the pectoralis for hemostasis. To do this, the short-acting muscle relaxant is given, and then the tip of the suction/irrigation wand is passed up through the tunnels to the inframammary crease. While lifting up on the breast to elevate the pectoral muscle origin, the wand is then advanced across the inframammary crease, about 60 mL of the epinephrine mixture instilled on each side, and massage performed. (In contrast, some surgeons use a tiny skin incision below the inframammary crease on each side to instill the epinephrine solution, but this will leave a small scar that some patients dislike.) One must be certain when doing this that the irrigation is not being instilled anterior to the muscle, or the result will be firm edematous swelling that will make assessment of symmetry difficult.

The obturator is then advanced farther. For prepectoral placement, when crossing the inframammary crease one must not lift up on the breast, as this in turn elevates the pectoral muscle and increases the likelihood of passage into the subpectoral plane (Fig. 114.7). That is why for subpectoral placement, the breast is deliberately lifted during obturator passage. Passage across the denser tissue at the inframammary crease is signaled by a decrease in resistance. The prepectoral and subpectoral advancement give the surgeon distinctly different tactile feedback, and this is one of the reasons cadaver experience

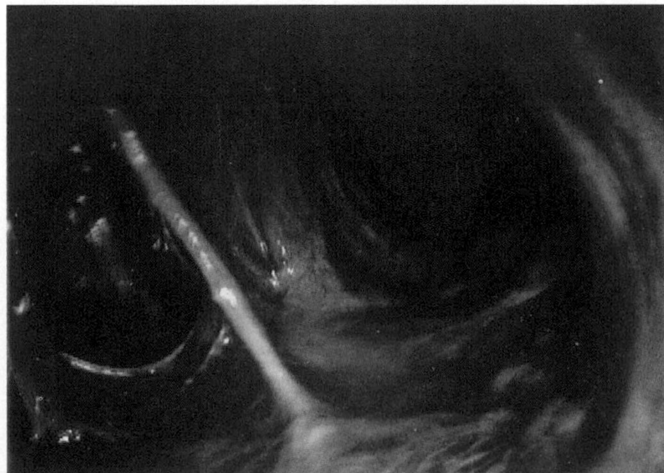

Figure 114.6. Endoscopic view showing a blind or false passage on the left resulting from backing up the obturator and then resuming forward motion. Also visible is a blood vessel traversing obliquely down from the upper left. Such vessels do not need to be divided. The false pocket will be avoided by transcutaneously manipulating the implant by hand.

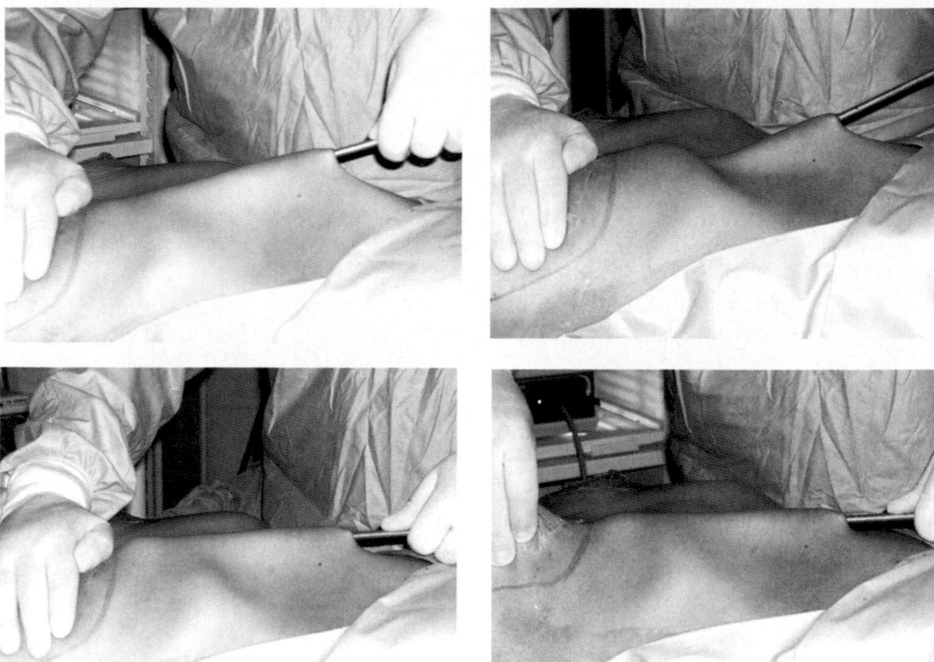

Figure 114.7. The manner of holding the obturator is crucial for safety and for obtaining the desired result. The error in the top left view is that the obturator is not parallel to the chest wall. The top right view shows an egregious error in which the shaft is directed toward the retrocostal plane; in addition, the handle is being held rather than the shaft as required. The left lower view shows the correct technique for prepectoral passage, and the right lower view shows the correct technique for subpectoral passage. Note the position of the other hand in holding the breast.

is so important (7). Prepectoral passage gives a somewhat granular or gritty sensation and continued resistance, whereas with subpectoral advancement there is a smooth, slippery feeling and very little resistance. The obturator is then advanced to the premarked position above the nipple. As with any subpectoral augmentation or reconstruction, contact with the ribs should be avoided to minimize postoperative periosteal pain.

Next the combined Johnson tube and obturator are advanced through the passageway. Some lubrication is helpful for each insertion of the tube, for which we use Shur-Clens (E.R. Squibb & Sons, Princeton, NJ). The obturator is then withdrawn from the tube, and the endoscope is used to verify the proper plane relative to the muscle, as well as to confirm that there is no significant bleeding (Fig. 114.8). For prepectoral placement, the undersurface of the breast will appear a glistening yellow-white color in the upper visual field, with the pectoralis major muscle having a reddish-brown color and a distinct linear pattern in the lower visual field (Fig. 114.9). For subpectoral placement, the reddish-brown striated pectoralis (often with a layer of fat encompassing the vessels) (Fig. 114.10) will be apparent in the upper visual field, with the whitish transverse ridges of the ribs seen in the lower visual field. With subpectoral placement, the fibers of the pectoralis attached to the ribs caudally are seen as sloping pillars at the sides of the visual field (Fig. 114.11).

The endoscope and tube together are then slowly withdrawn while inspecting the entire passageway. It is remarkable how little bleeding there is. Any blind passages, tissue bands

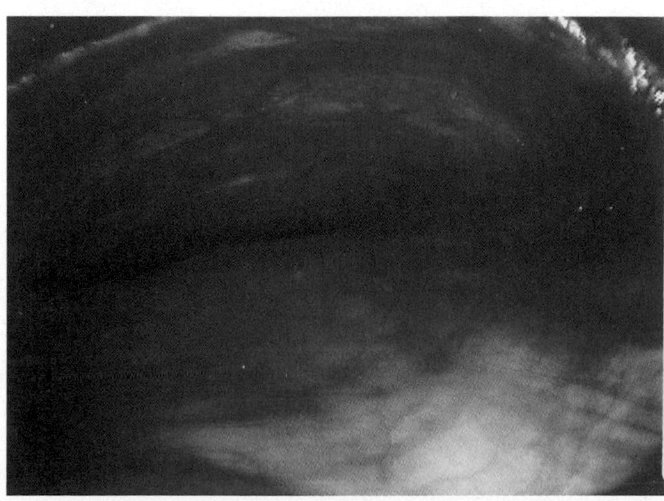

Figure 114.8. Endoscopic view of a typical tunnel, directly on the surface of the rectus fascia, with the subcutaneous tissues above. Note the absence of bleeding or blood staining.

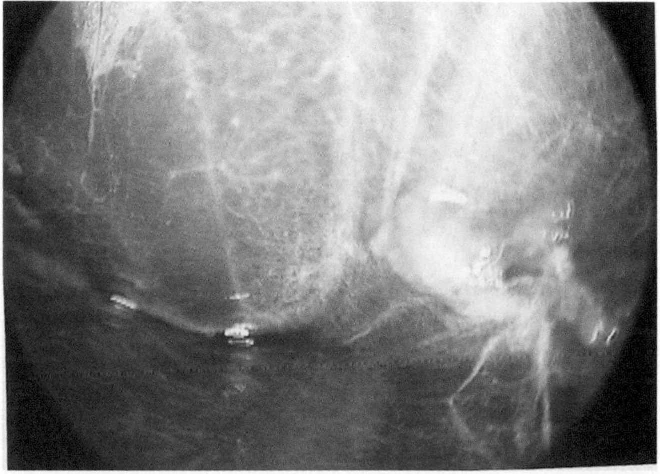

Figure 114.9. Endoscopic view of prepectoral passage, with pectoralis major muscle fibers in the lower visual field and the posterior aspect of the breast tissue in the upper field. Note the separation of the breast tissue from the muscle and the absence of bleeding or blood staining of tissues.

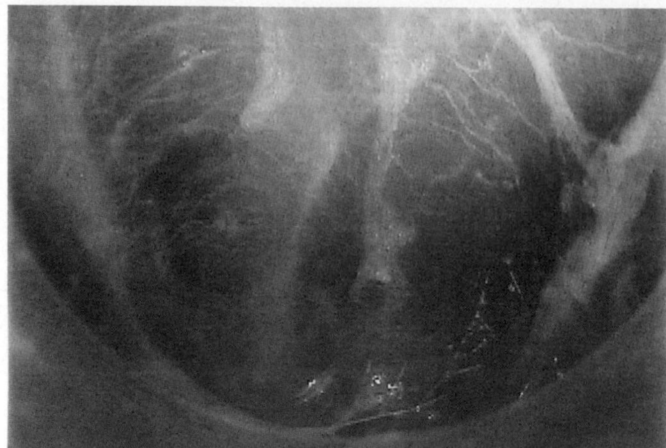

Figure 114.10. Endoscopic view of subpectoral passage, with pectoralis major muscle fibers in the upper visual field, sometimes with linear streaks of fat and vessels. Note the absence of bleeding.

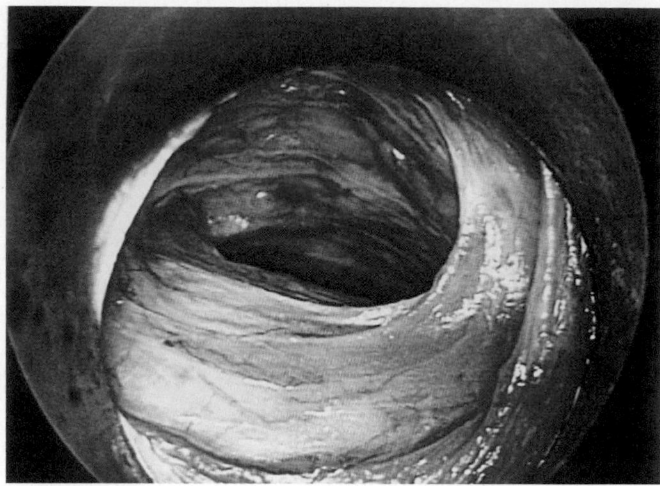

Figure 114.12. Endoscopic view of the tunnel, showing a tissue band encroaching slightly from the right side. This band may well contain and be protecting a vessel and need not be divided, as the implant can easily be steered around it. The band should be indicated on the skin.

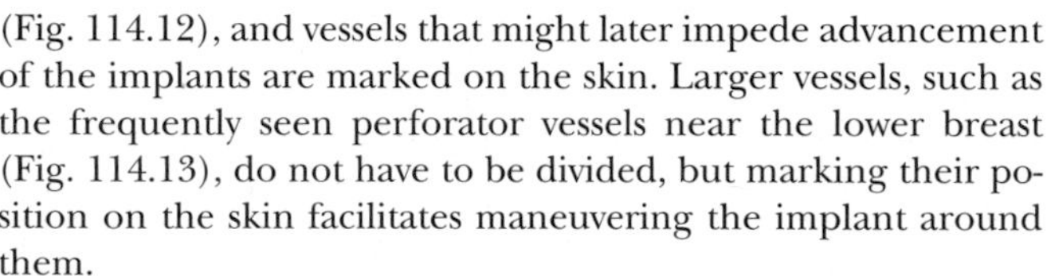

(Fig. 114.12), and vessels that might later impede advancement of the implants are marked on the skin. Larger vessels, such as the frequently seen perforator vessels near the lower breast (Fig. 114.13), do not have to be divided, but marking their position on the skin facilitates maneuvering the implant around them.

Next the Johnson blunt right-angled instrument is used to begin separating the tissues for a limited distance medially and laterally in the desired plane. For subpectoral placement, this separation should include detaching the caudal fibers of the pectoralis. As with any subpectoral procedure, actual contact between the instruments and the rib periosteum should be avoided to reduce postoperative pain. To help avoid symmastia, care must be taken not to detach the parasternal muscle fibers, and we stop the medial detachment at the 4 and 8 o'clock positions. An additional irrigation of 60 mL of epinephrine solution (chilled for vasoconstriction if desired) is then instilled, and the breasts are massaged. The reason that bleeding is minimal and brief in the transumbilical procedure is presumably because there is no sharp cutting of tissues. From time to time, critics unfamiliar or uncomfortable with the TUBA procedure have suggested changing the technique to one involving sharp tissue dissection and cautery; however, that would negate many of the advantages of the TUBA and create some disadvantages where none now exist. This operation is not "broken" and it does not need "fixing."

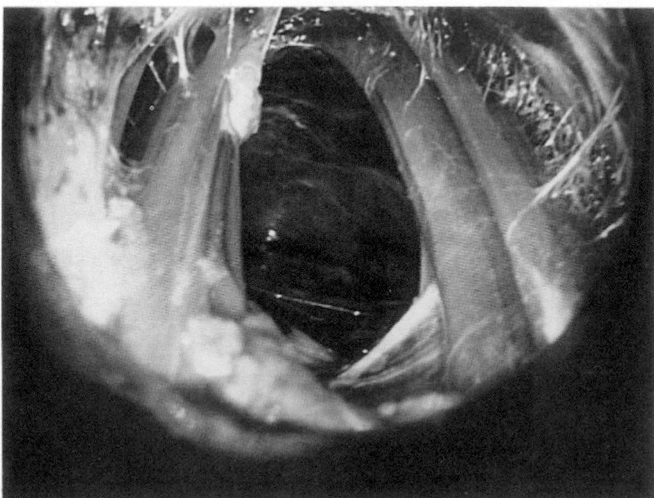

Figure 114.11. Endoscopic view near the lower pole of the breast early during a subpectoral approach, as the tube and endoscope are withdrawn from the subpectoral pocket, showing the pectoralis fibers like pillars on either side, originating from the ribs, with the subpectoral pocket seen beyond. These fibers will shortly be detached from the ribs.

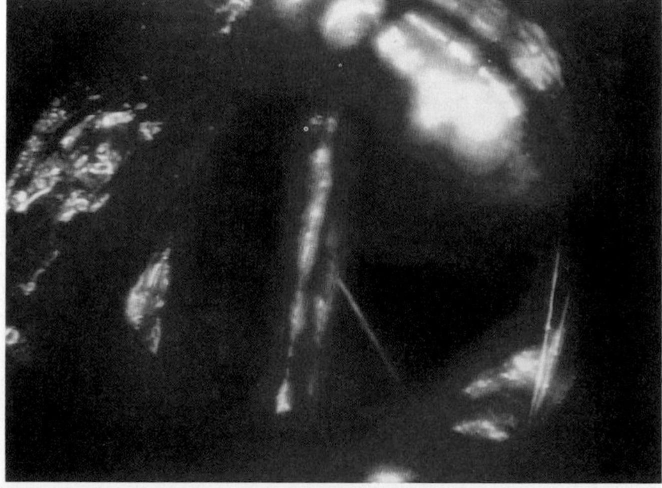

Figure 114.13. Endoscopic view of a large vessel complex, which need not be divided, but marking its location on the skin will permit the expander and the implant to be externally manipulated past it.

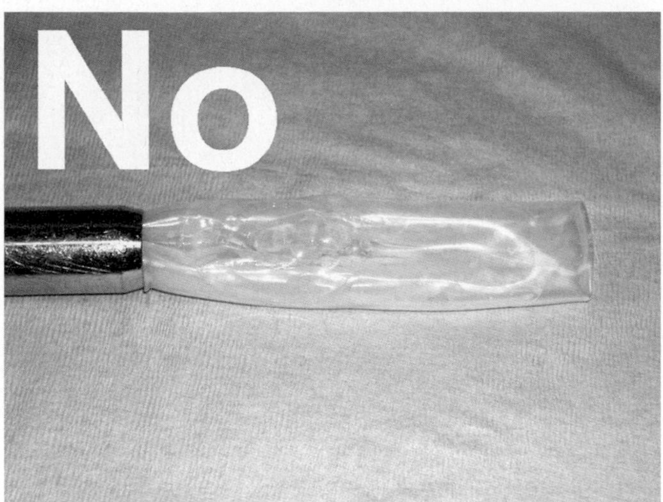

Figure 114.14. The original article described using the Johnson tube to push the implant through the tunnel. This maneuver is not necessary, and to protect implants, it should not be done.

Everything should now be ready for insertion of the expanders. As mentioned, the expander tubing needs to be secured with a silk tie to its plastic connector, and the strength of this connection needs to be verified. Illustrations in Johnson's original publication showed the end of the rolled implant lodged a few centimeters into the open end of the Johnson tube for advancement, but that is not necessary for either expanders or implants, and it is not recommended (Fig. 114.14). The expander is simply introduced through the umbilical incision, and advanced up the tissue tunnel, solely through external digital manipulation (Fig. 114.15). Note that neither the expander nor later the implant is passed through or has any contact with the tube, the endoscope, retractors, or any other solid object. Once the expander is in the pocket a closed fill system is used to inject sterile saline. Some surgeons use a pressurized pump for this; we prefer the syringe method. Saline, not air, is preferred for this expansion because the compressibility of air compromises the ability to achieve full, smooth, symmetric expansion, and use of air may cause the expander to not expand precisely where expanding is most needed. It is no coincidence that the surgeons who prefer to use air for expansion in TUBA also report a high rate of reoperation for asymmetry. Moreover, using saline rather than air facilitates a clear endoscopic view right *through* the expander, as will be outlined in the next section. The saline should be warm to help maintain the patient's core temperature.

The quality of the final result rests on the next step. One great advantage of augmentation procedures using remote incisions is that the final shape of the breasts is actually observed intraoperatively. As the expanders are being filled, manual external pressure is used to control the development of the pockets, defining both shape and position. This step is critical and requires the full attention of the surgeon to the evolving shape so that the pocket does not become too large in an undesired area, yet does expand adequately where needed. Considerable compressive force may be required to control the developing pocket, as well as to counter the natural tendency for tissues to expand where resistance is least, where expansion may be unnecessary. It is because of the forces needed for this step that the junction of the expander tubing and its plastic connector needs to be tied securely. It is during this expansion that any scoring of the posterior breast capsule and/or caudal pectoralis muscle fibers can be performed, as will be outlined later.

After checking that its tip is cool, the endoscope is inserted (without the Johnson tube) and advanced to touch the surface of the expander, which permits viewing the inside of the pocket right through the saline-filled expander to verify a proper prepectoral plane (Fig. 114.16), without any muscle fibers having been raised up, or subpectoral plane with muscle above and ribs below (Fig. 114.17), to locate any bands that require release (Fig. 114.18), and to confirm proper release of any persistent muscle fibers, especially near the lower pole. Some muscle bands may be clearly demonstrated only during this expander phase (Fig. 114.19). All the muscle fibers originating above the inframammary fold (Fig. 114.20) must be released

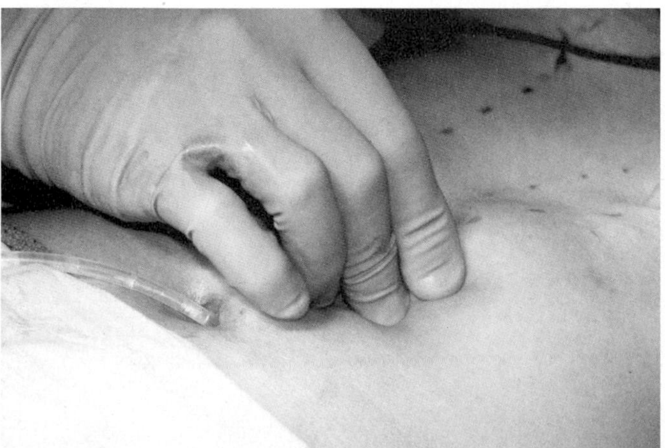

Figure 114.15. Rather than push the implant using any instrument, external digital manipulation is perfectly adequate for causing the implant to traverse the tunnel. The assistant ensures that the fill tube does not snag or catch during this advancement.

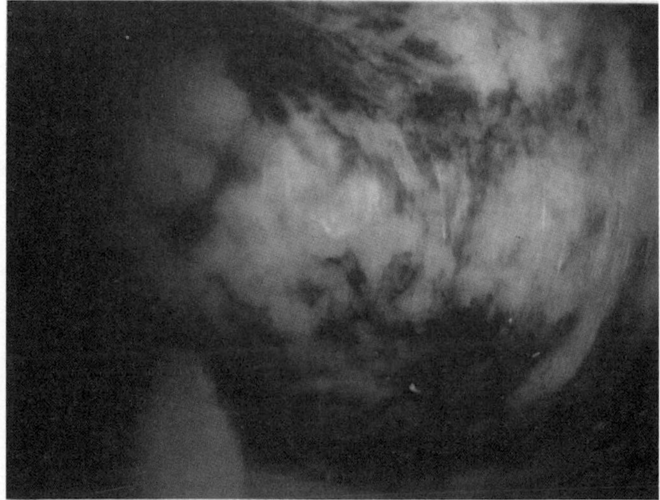

Figure 114.16. Endoscopic view through the prepectoral expander showing the posterior aspect of the breast tissue with minimal bleeding or blood staining of tissues.

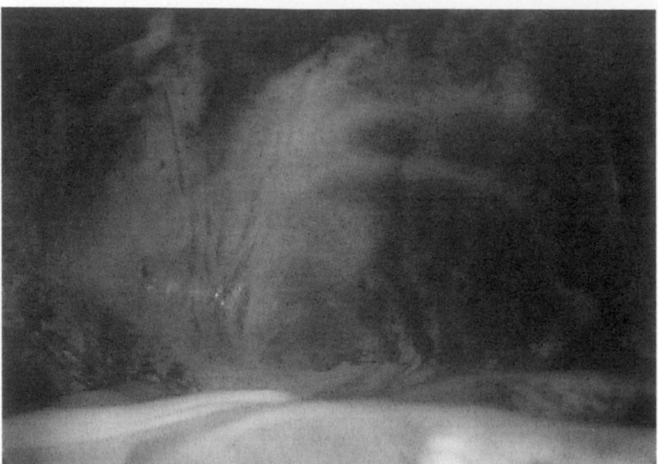

Figure 114.17. Endoscopic view through the subpectoral expander showing the posterior aspect of the pectoralis muscle with its vascular pedicle surrounded by fat. The whitish transverse ridges in the lower field are the ribs. The expander can touch the ribs, but metal instruments should not.

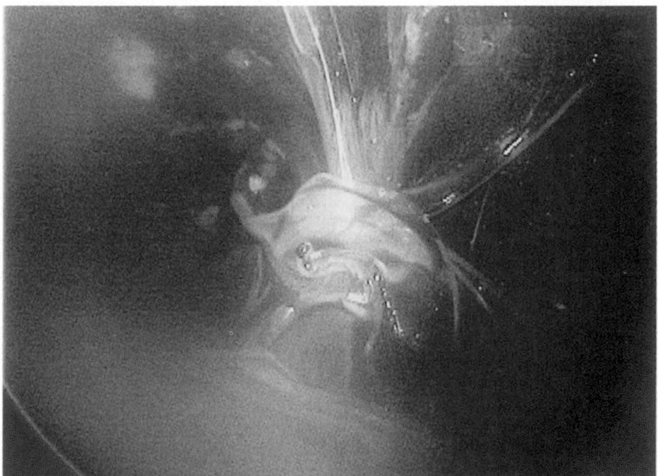

Figure 114.18. Endoscopic view through the expander of a muscle band requiring release. This is easily accomplished using the Johnson blunt hockey stick.

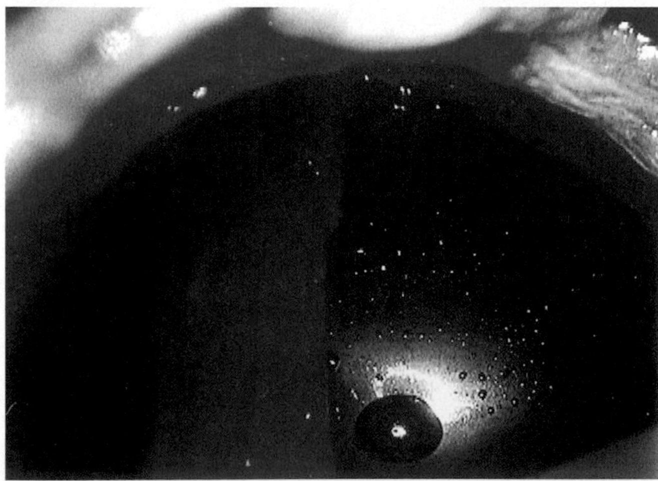

Figure 114.19. Endoscopic view looking at the lower pole of a subpectoral expander, showing a muscle band that must be divided to prevent later upward migration of the implant.

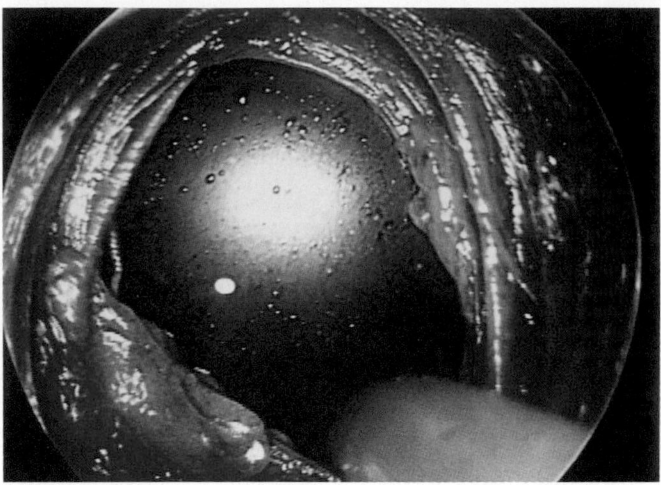

Figure 114.20. Endoscopic view of the lower pole of a subpectoral expander, showing persistent muscle fibers of origin both left and right of the tunnel. The hockey stick is used to divide these bands in order to prevent upward migration of the implant.

for subpectoral placement to avoid the upward shift of the implant that is often seen after failure to divide those fibers. Occasionally one sees so-called "accessory pectoralis" fibers originating well down on the anterior rectus sheath caudal to the inframammary fold, and these do not require dividing. Even moderately large vessels at the inframammary fold do not usually need division (Fig. 114.21), but division of any such vessels should be done bluntly rather than sharply, in order for any bleeding to cease quickly. It is often necessary during this pocket development to use the blunt right-angle instrument to release small bands or restrictions. Care must be taken to avoid damaging the expander with these instruments; it is important to effect complete band release at this expander stage in order to avoid the need to use any instrumentation within the pocket later adjacent to the implant. We inflate the expander with saline (not air) to 150% to 170% of the final desired volume of

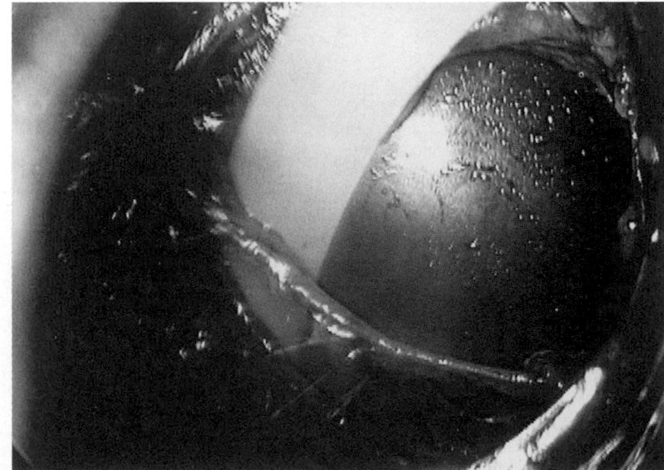

Figure 114.21. Endoscopic view of a prepectoral expander, showing a moderately large vessel near the inframammary crease. This vessel does not require division, but marking its position on the skin will assist in maneuvering the implant around it.

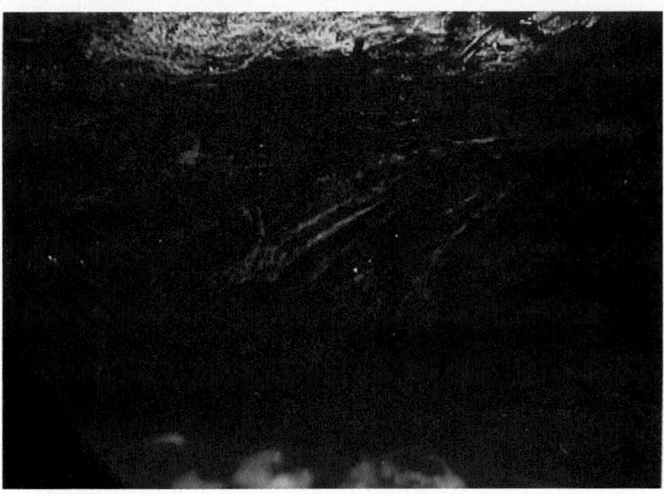

Figure 114.22. Endoscopic view of the subpectoral pocket after withdrawal of the expander, showing the typical absence of any significant bleeding.

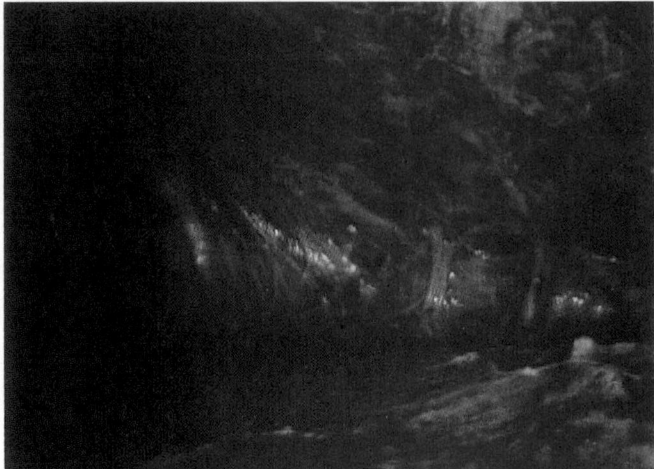

Figure 114.23. Endoscopic view of the prepectoral pocket after withdrawal of the expander, showing the typical absence of any significant bleeding. The linear light-colored structure to the right of center is the preserved fourth intercostal nerve, supplying the nipple.

the implant for prepectoral and 150% to 200% for subpectoral procedure. With larger implants, particular care may be required to avoid medial overdissection that could lead to dislocation or to symmastia. The overexpanded devices are left in place for several minutes for both intraoperative expansion and hemostasis. The view through the expander should be crystal clear. If it is cloudy or particulate, that may mean that the expander has a leak, most commonly at its fill-tube junction, and it needs to be replaced to ensure an accurate pocket dimension.

The volume in the expanders is then reduced to the final desired implant volume, and the head of the table is elevated to bring the patient nearly upright. Symmetry is verified, adjusting the volume as necessary, and the patient is returned to the supine position. The expanders must not be removed until the size, shape, position, and symmetry are optimal. Then the saline is evacuated, and the expanders are removed by traction on their fill tubes when they are almost but not completely empty. (If all the saline were to be removed before the expander is started down into the tunnel, the stiffened expanders would resist the deformation needed for easy passage, making removal more difficult.) Once the expanders are partially down the passageways, they can then be fully deflated for removal.

The Johnson tube and obturator combination is then reinserted, the obturator withdrawn, the endoscope introduced, and the pockets inspected, again verifying absence of any significant bleeding (Fig. 114.22). Often when inspecting the pockets for bleeding, the nerve to the nipple can be clearly seen (Fig. 114.23). If there is more bleeding than usual, it is at this point that we make the commitment to use drains, and we proceed with drains later even if the bleeding has abated. It has not been necessary to cauterize within the implant pockets. In 2 early cases of the 1,402, after dividing large vessels that we would not now divide, a bleeding point was identified, but by the time the equipment was prepared for cauterization, the bleeding had almost stopped; cauterization was done anyway even though superfluous. At this point we irrigate with 0.25% bupivacaine, 10 mL per side, for postoperative comfort. Of course the pockets can now be irrigated with any type of antibiotic or antiseptic solution desired.

After changing to fresh powder-free gloves and isolating the skin incision edges as desired, the surgeon inserts the implant through the incision, pushing it up the passageway with the index finger. Care must be taken to avoid dislodging the fill tube as the finger is withdrawn. The surgeon then uses only external manipulation to advance the implant, milking the implant up through the passageway (Fig. 114.15). To facilitate this, the assistant applies slight negative pressure with the syringe to stiffen the implant. It is a hallmark of the current TUBA technique that the implants need touch nothing whatsoever other than the patient's soft tissues and the surgeon's gloves, specifically not the endoscope and not the tube (Fig. 114.14). The implant is advanced, but before it is pushed all the way free of the tunnel into the pocket, its orientation is verified as correct using the endoscope *without the Johnson tube* (Fig. 114.24). If it needs to be reoriented, it is manipulated (not pulled by its tubing) back down the tunnel and adjusted.

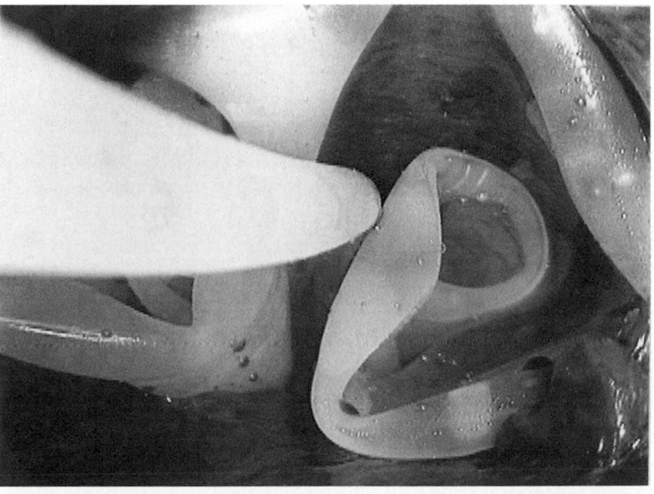

Figure 114.24. Endoscopic view showing the properly rolled posterior valve implant poised at the upper end of its tunnel, not yet fully inside the pocket. Implant filling can now begin.

Following complete advancement of the implant into the pocket, it is inflated to the specified volume via a closed system using sterile intravenous saline (no dextrose!) warmed to approximately 40°C to help maintain the patient's core temperature, without any external compression being performed. Some surgeons use an open basin and a pump to fill the implants, but our preference is to minimize the risk of contamination by using a closed system; in fact this may soon be mandated by the FDA. The patient is again brought to nearly upright position, and minor volume adjustments are made as desired for symmetry. If the surgeon wants to view the implant while its fill tube is in place, the endoscope can safely be introduced, provided that the Johnson tube is not used (Fig. 114.25), which could cause premature fill tube separation on withdrawal; even with the endoscope alone, care must be taken not to dislodge the fill tube until the volume is finalized. Each fill tube is removed by traction while holding back the implant with the other hand.

If an umbilical hernia is present, this is the moment to repair it, using standard techniques. The sac is delineated, the ring cleared, and a two-layer closure performed. If the surgeon is concerned about bleeding from the pockets, it is a simple matter to leave a thin suction drain, about 10-French size, in each passageway, exiting through tiny incisions within the umbilicus. One advantage of the TUBA procedure is that the tunnels provide a dependent reservoir for any seroma that might otherwise collect around the implant and provide a place for drain tubes that do not contact the implants. If abdominal liposuction is to be done, this is the point at which we tumesce the tissues for that procedure.

After final inspection of the pockets, implants, valves, and passageways, any remaining air is manipulated toward the passageways from around the implants and suctioned out from within the passageways to help prevent crepitus or other postoperative sounds (31), and then the navel incision is closed with subcuticular absorbable suture. Sterile adhesive strips are applied, any navel jewelry reinserted if the patient desires, and a small gauze applied, secured by a transparent film dressing. If abdominal liposuction is to be done, that procedure is performed now; the periumbilical area can be better contoured with liposuction if the navel incision has been fully closed first. As is our practice for most breast augmentations, a 3-inch-wide elastic band is positioned across the upper half of the breasts as shown (Fig. 114.26). This helps to hold the implants immobile, helps eradicate any of the old inframammary crease in certain cases, helps keep the pocket stretched, and begins the implant compression that will eventually help avoid contracture. An elastic abdominal band provides comforting support.

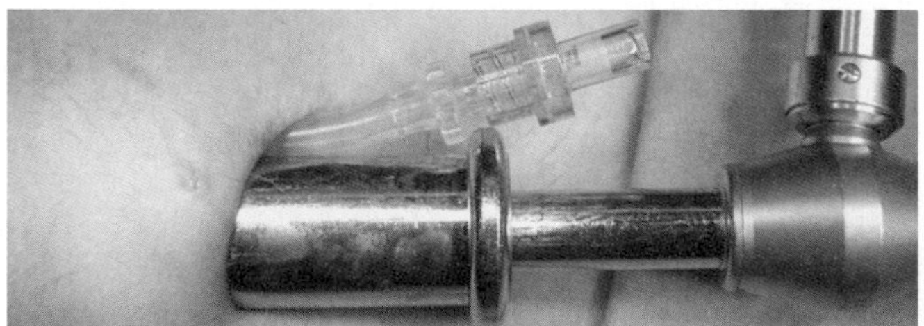

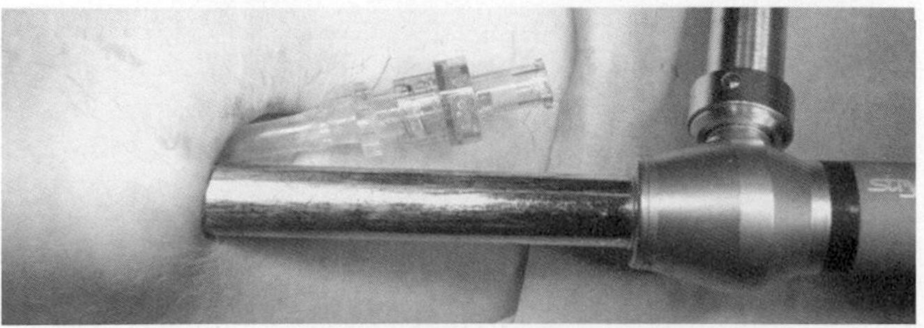

Figure 114.25. Once the implant is in place, every effort must be made to avoid premature fill tube separation. The upper photo shows what not to do, because the Johnson tube will likely pull out the fill tube. Instead, the endoscope is inserted without the Johnson tube as in the lower photo.

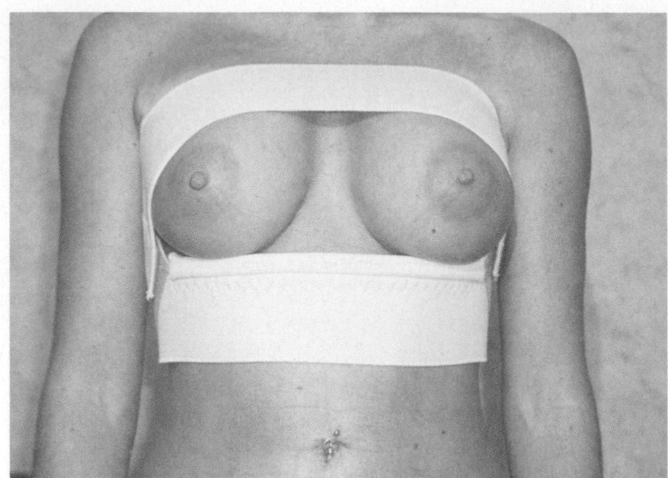

Figure 114.26. Patients often seem to be more comfortable in the early postoperative period if a mildly compressive elastic strap is placed across the upper breasts.

VARIANCES

In about 5% of cases, the surgeon must deal with minor difficulties. As will become apparent, detection of these problems clearly requires use of an endoscope. Those who perform the TUBA without an endoscope are leaving some of these problems undiagnosed and untreated, as evidenced during our revisions of transumbilical augmentations done by surgeons who did not use an endoscope, and unfortunately during medicolegal reviews of such cases. Passage into the undesired plane is one of these problems. We have seen patients whose implants were put into a different plane than intended, which remained undetected intraoperatively because no endoscope was used.

Diagnosing formation of the tunnel in the wrong plane is easy, as the endoscope discloses muscle fibers in the incorrect part of the visual field (Fig. 114.27). It is essential that this problem be corrected before the pocket is developed further, or the correction would become very difficult. Although an instrument has been designed (32) to change the plane of insertion, we have not found any special instrument necessary. Correcting an undesired incorrect tunnel plane begins with first determining at what point entry into the wrong plane occurred. Then the obturator is readvanced into the correct plane, all the way to the top of the pocket. The endoscope will then disclose that there are two tunnels separated by the pectoral muscle and fascia, which appears as a transverse band (Fig. 114.28). Then the long, blunt Johnson hockey stick instrument is passed, tip directed medially, into the correct plane tunnel and repeatedly

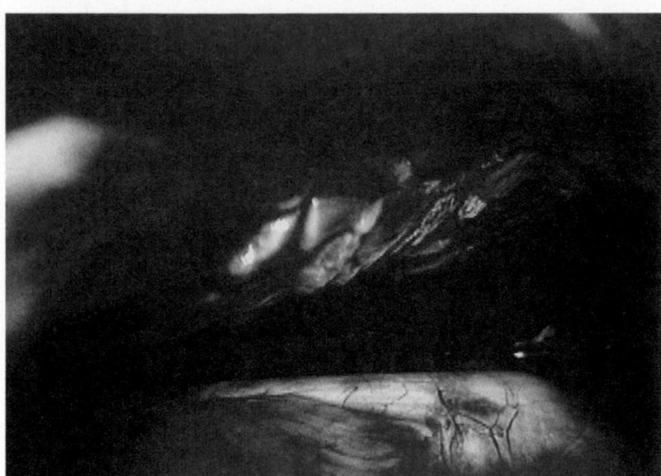

Figure 114.27. Endoscopic view of a subpectoral passage. The small blood-stained spot on the rib was caused by instrument contact, which should be avoided to decrease postoperative pain.

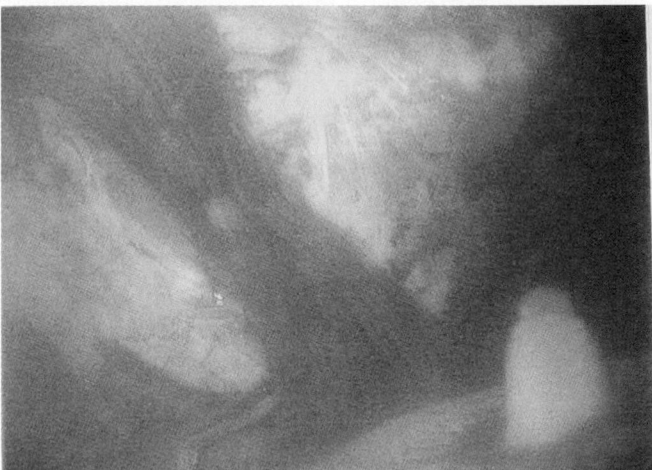

Figure 114.29. Endoscopic view through the prepectoral expander showing that a narrow band of muscle has been elevated. This occurred following a conversion of a subpectoral tunnel to a prepectoral tunnel and indicates that these fibers were incompletely released. The Johnson hockey stick can resolve this if it is considered significant.

drawn caudally, loosening the tissues a little at a time, especially caudally near the opening to the tunnel. Next the tip is rotated up and over so it points laterally, and the instrument is pulled caudally several times to define the new plane laterally. This is repeated as needed to bluntly make a wider pocket, necessary in this situation to preventing the expansion from separating the muscle fibers. There will be somewhat more bleeding temporarily if this step has been needed.

Transexpander endoscopic visualization may reveal errant muscle fibers (Fig 114.29) or bands in the upper breast (Fig. 114.30) or in the inframammary regions (Fig. 114.31), that may need separation by use of the Johnson hockey stick unless very minor. Persistent inferior muscle bands may not become apparent until after the expander has been filled (Fig. 114.19). Failure to recognize such persistent muscle inferiorly will increase the likelihood of subsequent upward migration of the implant. This too, is something we have found when reoperating on patients whose surgeons did not use an endoscope. Such bands are divided bluntly using the blunt right-angle instrument. There is no need to divide all vessels present at the inframammary fold (Fig. 114.32); noting their position on the skin allows the implant to be diverted around them.

One frequent objection to the TUBA procedure, voiced by those who do not understand it, is that it is "too difficult to control the bleeding from so far away." Contrary to what one might expect, bleeding vessels requiring cautery in the tunnel or pocket have turned out to be quite rare. We have occasionally cauterized just under the navel skin incision, but have never encountered bleeding in the tunnels themselves, which are remarkably dry (Fig. 114.33). As mentioned earlier, in only 2 early cases was it thought that the cautery should be used inside the pocket, a tiny bleeding vessel having been noted, but

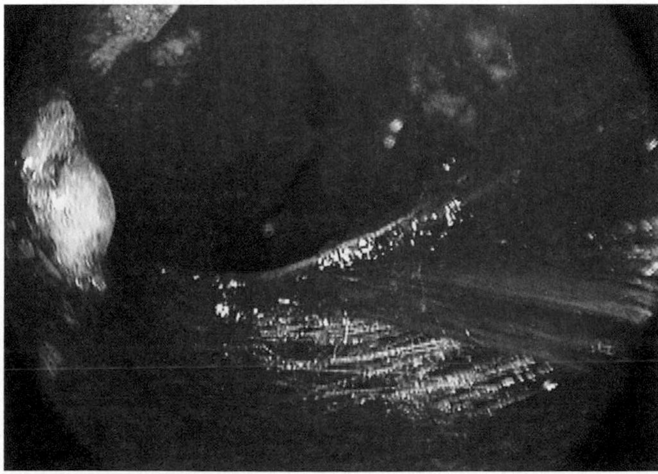

Figure 114.28. Endoscopic view of a prepectoral passage, but showing in addition that elevation of some pectoralis muscle fibers has occurred. The Johnson hockey stick will be used to resolve this problem as described in the text.

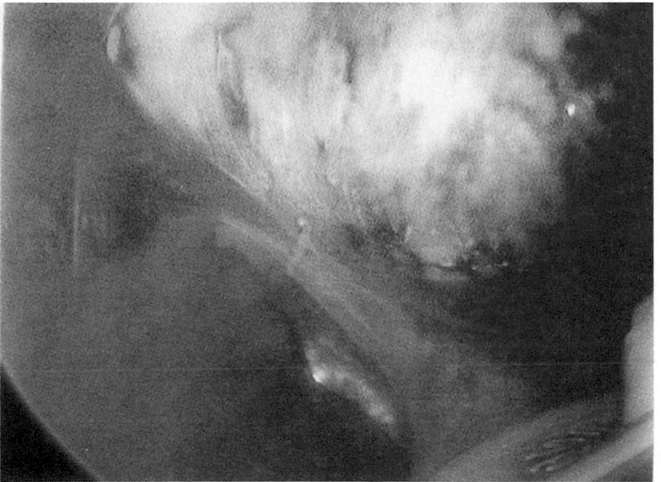

Figure 114.30. Endoscopic view through the prepectoral expander showing a portion of the expander trying to expand deep to a muscle band in the upper outer quadrant. The etiology and the treatment are as outlined in Figure 114.30.

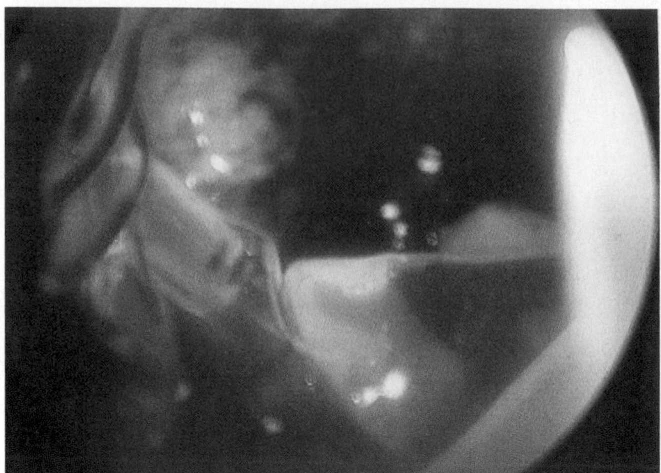

Figure 114.31. Endoscopic view through the prepectoral expander showing persistent fibers near the lower pole that need to be divided. In this instance this band is partly made up of pectoralis muscle fibers remaining from incomplete resolution of a subpectoral entry. Correction by the hockey stick in this area is mandatory.

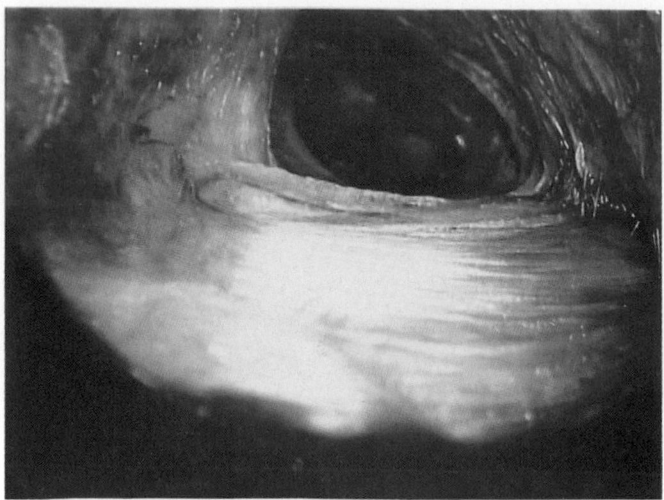

Figure 114.33. Endoscopic view of the tunnel, showing the subcutaneous tissues cleanly separated off the rectus sheath. The absence of significant bleeding is a hallmark of the transumbilical breast augmentation procedure.

in fact by the time the equipment to deal with it was prepared, the bleeding had virtually stopped and cauterization was no longer really needed. The equipment needed for such cauterization is a right-angled operating endoscope and a long, insulated suction cautery tip. Such bleeding has not been encountered again, but were it to occur, we would now likely treat it by pressure and waiting, followed by drain insertion. Again, of course, detection of such a bleeding site mandates the use of an endoscope.

Regardless of the incision used for access, with any subpectoral plane augmentation (and sometimes even with prepectoral for tubular breasts), the preexisting inframammary crease may persist as a transverse indentation across the lower breast. This indentation does improve with the passage of time, but resolution is hastened by a specific intraoperative maneuver that the TUBA procedure facilitates, similar to the scoring of the posterior aspect of the breast employed with open augmentation techniques. For that, the right-angled instrument is introduced (during the expansion phase, not later when the implant is in place), superficial to the expander, tip pointing anteriorly, and drawn downward in line with the muscle fibers in several locations. This separates the fibers and can even score the breast fascia as well, to facilitate expansion of the old crease over some 4 to 6 months. In a subpectoral augmentation, this instrument can even effect separation of the muscle from the breast parenchyma caudally, a useful maneuver for breasts exhibiting a degree of glandular ptosis and/or loose stretched lower pole breast tissue (33), a maneuver sometimes described as a “dual-plane” release.

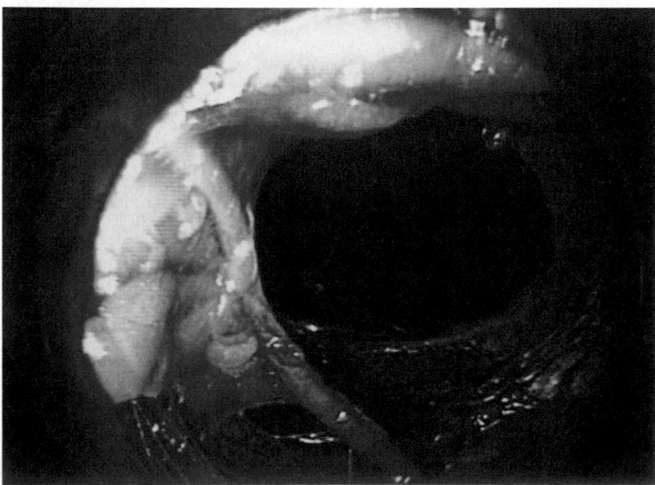

Figure 114.32. Endoscopic view of a large vessel near the lower pole of the breast. The position of this vessel should be marked on the skin so that it can be preserved and avoided.

Several other minor difficulties are occasionally encountered and are also easily prevented or treated. One such problem, premature detachment of the implant fill tubes, is easily prevented by avoiding traction on the tubes, and in particular by not inserting the Johnson tube while the implant fill tube is present in the tunnel. There is no extra space between the Johnson tube and the tunnel walls, so the Johnson tube could pull the fill tube out with it (8). If the fill tube does get pulled out prematurely, the implant might have to be punctured and replaced. However, it is possible to reconnect an anterior diaphragm fill tube via a tiny periareolar incision through which the fill tube is inserted into the valve under endoscopic control.

Theoretically, the initial abdominal tunnel could be made too superficially, within the subcutaneous tissue rather than in the proper plane below it, but we have not had this occur. This problem would also be more likely to occur if the obturator had a pointed tip. Such a pointed obturator might also pass into or through the rectus sheath. Sometimes, one can see with the endoscope that a few fibers of the anterior sheath have separated and lifted slightly even with the use of the blunt obturator (Fig. 114.34). This is yet another justification for requisite use of an endoscope.

Inversion of the implant is prevented by checking its orientation endoscopically (Fig. 114.35) *before* it is pushed clear of the tunnel and into the pocket, prior to inflation, while there is

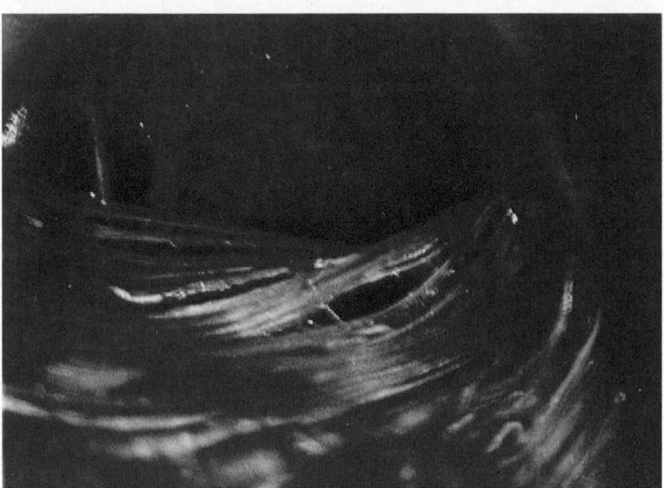

Figure 114.34. A rarely seen endoscopic view showing that some fibers of the rectus sheath have lifted slightly. It is clear that a sharp obturator tip might penetrate the rectus sheath. Note the vessels farther over to the left. These do not need dividing, but they should be marked on the skin.

still an opportunity to milk the implant back down the tunnels and reorient it. Using the endoscope also permits direct observation of the valve for leakage; if encountered, the implant will have to be drained, removed, and replaced.

POSTOPERATIVE CARE

The postoperative patient will experience varying degrees of chest and upper abdominal discomfort. For prepectoral implants this is usually mild, less than that after use of the other incisions, but subpectoral implantation patients may experience muscle cramps and spasms, for which we prescribe diazepam for several days. Occasionally, mild abdominal distention, lasting about a week, may occur. This may be due to pain medication, reflex relaxation of the rectus muscles, the use of nitrous oxide, which we discourage. Most patients describe the abdominal soreness as comparable to having done too many sit-ups. The sensibility of the nipples may be altered initially but for most patients will return to normal over time. Bleeding has been minimal, so usually there is little ecchymosis (6). All patients are prescribed pain medication and an oral broad-spectrum antibiotic for a few days. Without a breast incision under tension, there is little fear of incision edge necrosis that could lead to exposure of the implant; nevertheless we advise patients not to use nicotine for 1 week postoperatively.

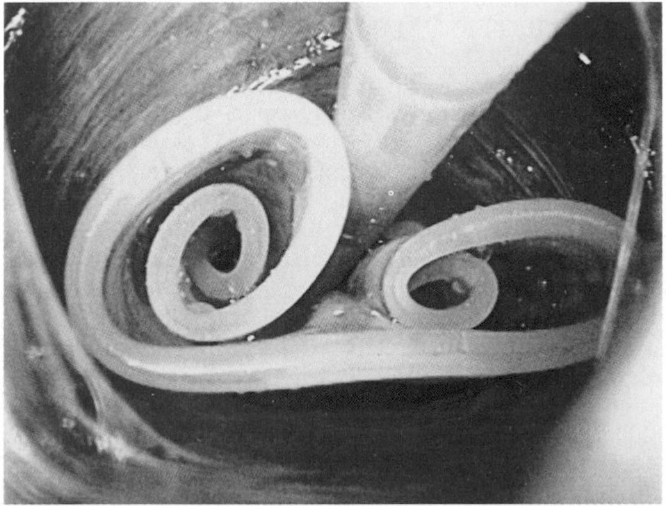

Figure 114.35. Endoscopic view of a properly oriented anterior-valve implant, which has been advanced up the passageway and almost fully into the pocket. Verification of orientation permits an upside-down implant to be pushed back down the passageway where it can easily be realigned.

The TUBA method is one of the techniques encompassed by the term "rapid recovery methods." Starting the first night, we encourage full range of arm motion without force after both prepectoral and subpectoral augmentation. The subpectoral patient will be more comfortable if the patient does not use her arms to push or pull herself up in positioning or exerting force in getting into or out of bed. The patient should not engage in any strenuous activities but can do a reasonable range of normal activities as tolerated. Patients must also wait until they are no longer taking their diazepam or prescription pain medications before driving or using machinery.

The main postoperative complaint has not been pain, but rather a feeling of pressure. We prefer that the elastic band stay in place until the patient is seen the next morning, when the bandages are removed, her choice of bra is applied, and she can begin removing the band for frequent short intervals throughout the day. Underwire bras are perfectly acceptable because there are no inframammary incisions. If there is more upper pole fullness than the patient desires, or if the old inframammary fold persists as a transverse crease, the upper elastic band and/or upper compression massage are used. There is no contraindication to allowing the patient to shower or bathe immediately, and full arm motion is encouraged. Running, aerobics, and heavy lifting are delayed, depending on the individual's rate of recovery and the plane of the implants; unrestricted activity is permitted as soon as the patient is comfortable doing so. Breast massage of the compression type can be encouraged early, depending upon patient comfort and surgeon preference. Vitamin E (200 IU per day) and MSM (2,000 mg per day) can be used if desired (34). Drains are not often used, but if so, they are removed after a few days. None of our TUBA patients developed Mondor's cords.

The duration of band use and manual upper pole compression is based on whether the patient has achieved her contour goals. The breasts may at first appear quite rounded superiorly, especially with prepectoral implants. With superior pole compression, the lower pole tissues stretch, and the implants settle into final shape within weeks to months. If the patient wants the breasts to appear flatter superiorly or if the old inframammary crease persists, then compression of the upper hemisphere of each breast is continued as needed. Once the patient is satisfied with the contour of her breasts, she can dispense with upper breast compression. As with any breast augmentation, mild soft tissue edema is common for a few weeks, and patients need to be reminded not to become accustomed to their temporarily larger size. There can be some temporary crepitation from subcutaneous air. With any subpectoral smooth implant procedure, patients may experience bourdonnement or "squeaking," which will eventually resolve (31). Patients with subpectoral implants generally note visible indenting and displacement of the implants during strong pectoralis contraction that persists long term. We normally schedule postoperative visits at 1 week, 2 months, 6 months, 12 months, and earlier as needed, and we strongly advocate continued annual evaluations for breast augmentation patients.

TRANSUMBILICAL IMPLANT REPLACEMENT

Plastic surgeons who offer transumbilical augmentation will also want to understand, and be adept at, replacing the implants via the navel. Patients for whom the umbilical location of the scar was important in the first place usually want their eventual implant replacement to be done via the navel as well. Replacement of a failed saline implant through the navel is a straightforward procedure, provided it is done promptly after the deflation (35) or performed electively. At the outset, it should be stressed that what is being discussed here is replacement in a timely manner with the same-size or smaller implant, not replacement with a much larger implant nor major correction of a capsular contracture or replacement a long time after the deflation.

The equipment for replacement includes all the standard transumbilical augmentation instruments, plus these additional items: gynecologic right-angle operating endoscope (e.g., #26034A, Karl Storz Gmbh, Tuttlingen, Germany), a long endograsper forceps (e.g., #5DSG, Ethicon, Cornelia, GA) (note that the grasper does not pass through the endoscope), and any long, insulated cautery tip. A means of evacuating the saline from the implants is also needed; although one could use an 18-gauge needle percutaneously, we prefer doing it endoscopically with a sharpened endoscopic cautery tip. As an alternative, a standard aspirator (such as the Karl Storz #26175P) can be used, although with that instrument the aspiration is done blindly because it is not long enough to be used through the endoscope. The operating room setup is the same as that used for the transumbilical breast augmentation.

Except for a few steps described in what follows, the secondary technique is nearly the same as for a primary augmentation. As is true of the primary transumbilical breast implant, the replacement implant size is best decided upon in advance. The markings, made while the patient is standing in the preop holding area, are the same as those used for primary TUBA, with the exception that the two tunnels are aligned to run from the navel directly to the nearest point on the inframammary crease. The initial operative steps are also identical to those previously described for primary TUBA. The prior navel scar is opened, and then blunt spreading is used to reach the fascia and continued a short distance toward each breast on the anterior surface of the rectus sheath. Next the Johnson obturator is advanced incrementally in the usual manner. Just as with the transumbilical breast augmentation procedure, one must be careful not to create any false passageways that would make insertion of the new implants difficult. We have encountered no problems resulting from scarring due to either the previous operation or a prior abdominoplasty.

To this point there has been no great divergence from the original transumbilical breast augmentation technique, but now the differences begin. Normally, the obturator would be advanced deep to the breast directly on the muscle or on the chest wall, of course keeping the instrument parallel to the chest wall. For replacement, however, doing that would make the tunnel pass behind the capsule, leading to a capsular opening that is too far posterior to be useful. Therefore once the tip of the obturator has arrived near the inframammary crease, the tip must be forcefully elevated away from the chest wall as the obturator is being advanced in order to contact the capsule directly at its lower pole. (If the implant has deflated completely, upward traction on the breast will be required in order to present the lower pole of the capsule at a right angle to the chest wall and obturator.) After the obturator abuts against the lower pole of the capsule, it is removed. Following this, the Johnson tube-and-obturator combination is advanced to the same position, the obturator withdrawn, and the endoscope used to confirm that the tube is indeed right up against the capsule (Fig. 114.36). The operating scope is inserted. There are no differences between prepectoral replacement and subpectoral replacement because in the subpectoral transumbilical augmentation the fibers of origin of the pectoralis major should have already been elevated off the ribs inferiorly.

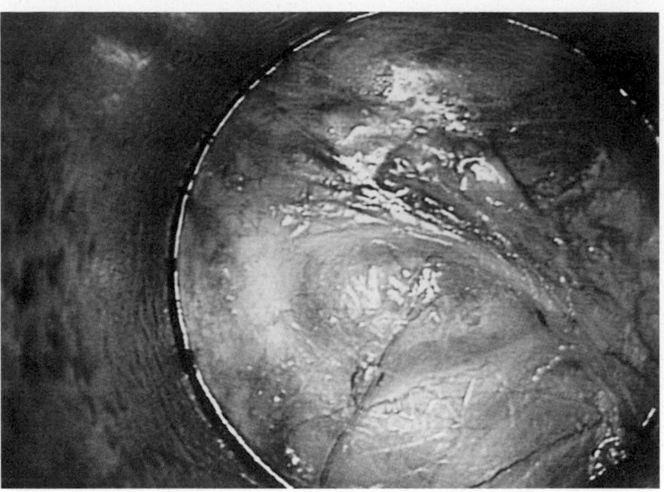

Figure 114.36. Endoscopic view during transumbilical revision, showing the lower pole of the breast capsule, ready for electrocautery incision and withdrawal of the implant for replacement.

The next step is another departure from the primary TUBA procedure. One of the strengths of the TUBA technique is that there is absolutely no cutting, sharp or cautery, within the pocket, and hence no need to try to endoscopically observe the process of pocket formation. For replacement however, an endoscopically controlled cutting cautery is used to open the lower pole of the capsule, and this requires endoscopic monitoring. Short strokes and brief current times are used in order to prevent excessive tip heating that might further damage the implant and interfere with the manufacturer's device analysis. We prefer to make an X-shaped capsular incision with each of the two limbs about the same length as the diameter of the Johnson tube in order to avoid impeding passage of the new implants. During this capsulotomy, care must be taken to verify that there is no intruding skin fold at risk from the cautery.

The implant is then almost fully evacuated (which may require puncture), leaving inside a small amount of saline to ease deformation of the implant to a small cross section allowing for easy withdrawal through the tunnel. During evacuation it is important to gently squeeze on the breast to mold the deflating implant into a narrow, elongated shape. The obturator and tube are advanced together through the capsule right into the pocket. The obturator is withdrawn, the endoscope reintroduced, and the cautery used to divide any remaining capsular bands or folds that constrict the opening. Using external manipulation, the deflated implant is maneuvered into position right at the end of the Johnson tube. At this point we formerly used an endograsper to remove the implant, but that often damaged the implant, so now we use suction to remove it as follows. The endoscope is withdrawn, and then clear plastic tubing (as used for liposuction) is inserted through the tube, slid down to contact the implant, and then the strong suction machine turned on. Even though this is done blindly, it is not difficult. The suction tubing is pulled back until the implant abuts against the distal end of the Johnson tube, and then tubes and implant are withdrawn together. Just as in the original transumbilical breast augmentation procedure, no attempt is made to pass any implant *through* the Johnson tube, not even for removal.

After implant removal, the interior of the pocket is examined endoscopically, and if necessary, the insulated cautery instrument can be used to perform a limited capsulotomy under endoscopic visualization, anywhere from about the 8 o'clock position on the breast, over the top and down, to about the 4 o'clock position on the breast. Unlike the transumbilical breast augmentation procedure, in which the endoscope is used only intermittently to verify progress during the procedure but not while creating the pocket, such a capsulotomy procedure requires continuous monitoring with the endoscope and, just as in any open capsulotomy, care to avoid penetration of the skin. We have developed a technique for lower pole capsulotomy between 8 and 4 o'clock, but that is outside the scope of this chapter.

Normally we put the replacement implant into the original pocket. However, on one occasion, when doing a replacement for a patient who had had some capsular contracture, a principle described by Hedén et al. (36) was used in which the new implant pockets were created superficial to the old capsules. Therefore, before opening of the capsule, the obturator tip was elevated and passed superficial to the old capsule, creating the tunnel that would become the start of the new pocket. There was no difficulty passing the implant into the newly created pocket.

If the implant being inserted is a little larger than the previous one or if the deflation had been long-standing, the pocket will need to be expanded, whether or not a definitive capsulotomy has been required. Just as with the original transumbilical augmentation, the implant is never used for pocket expansion. We put in an expander with the same dimensions as the new implant and hydraulically expand the pocket, which in the case of a deflation or a modest size increase will accomplish an internal capsulotomy. The shape of the enlarging pocket is monitored by external observation of the breast, using compression where appropriate.

After expander removal, the pocket is inspected and hemostasis obtained if needed. As discussed earlier, with primary transumbilical augmentation, hemostasis within the pocket is rarely, if ever, needed because of the hydraulic manner of pocket creation. By contrast, with replacement for deflation or a size increase, the necessary capsular incision increases the likelihood of needing cauterization. After the pocket is judged suitable, local anesthetic is instilled, and the new implants are inserted, during which once again the implant is not pushed by, passed through, or touched by any instrument whatsoever, only the surgeon's gloves and the patient's sterile subcutaneous tissues. If internal capsulotomy has been done, we usually use drains (e.g., round 10 French) extending up to just below the inframammary crease, exiting via tiny navel incisions. No sutures are necessary if an adhesive plastic film is applied.

Recovery from transumbilical implant replacement is rapid, with the patient returning to her usual activities within a day or two. Incisional pain is minimal, as there is no tension on the incision site, but soreness along the tunnel pathways is expected, as well as pain at the site of any capsulotomy. Because the approach to the pocket is made at its lower pole where there are no muscle fibers, neither muscle pain nor spasms has been a problem postoperatively, even with subpectoral implants. Postoperative bruising has occurred more often after revision than after primary TUBA.

Replacement via the navel should pose no difficulty for the surgeon already familiar with transumbilical augmentation. The skills mastered for the primary technique will serve well for replacement of the implants via the navel following the guidelines given here, and an additional training course should not be necessary.

RESULTS

The risks of the TUBA procedure performed by a well-trained plastic surgeon are no greater than those seen after any breast augmentation. A truly controlled study, in which the TUBA method is done on one side while another incision is done on the other, is quite unlikely to ever be done. The most valid report of outcomes was the study by Johnson et al. (37), in which independent reviewers found that the incidence of infection was 0.4%, postoperative hematoma 0.8%, decreased nipple sensibility 0.8%, and tunnel seroma 0.6%. The senior author's experience certainly corroborates that study's conclusion that the TUBA procedure is extremely safe and effective. From January 1, 1993, until the date of writing this chapter (March 10, 2009), I performed 1,001 prepectoral TUBA procedures and 401 subpectoral TUBA procedures (all since May 19, 1999), for a total of 1,402 cases. There have been zero hematomas, zero infections, no implants damaged during the procedures, and no instances of conversion to an open procedure. There have been no cases of Mondor's cords. No persistent track deformities, indentations, irregularities, or scars on the abdomen have been encountered, nor have I ever seen photographs of these, although there have been anecdotal reports of them occurring with untrained surgeons. Nine prepectoral TUBA patients and 11 subpectoral TUBA patients have had small (10 to 30 cc) accumulations of serous fluid within the tunnels, and although such a small amount would no doubt have been absorbed spontaneously with compression, it was chosen to aspirate them in the office (Fig. 114.37). This small volume could not have been recognized, nor could aspiration have been performed safely, had there not been tunnels available as dependent reservoirs. This leads to speculation about whether such small seromas are also occurring unrecognized with other types of augmentation, possibly contributing to capsular contracture. This presents an area that deserves more study.

The representative cases depicted (Figs. 114.38 to 114.43) show preoperative and postoperative views of patients with prepectoral and subpectoral TUBA. As can be seen in these

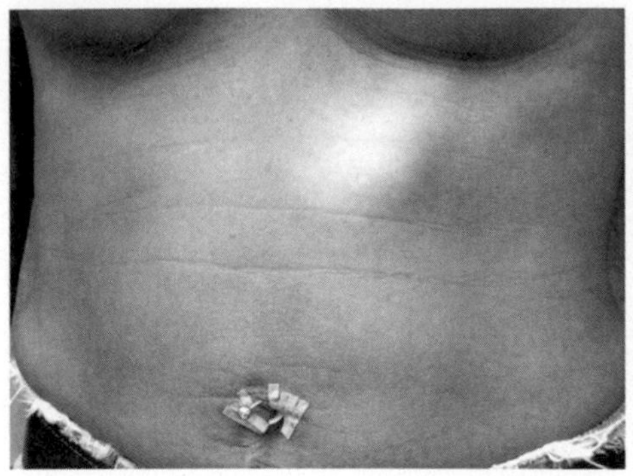

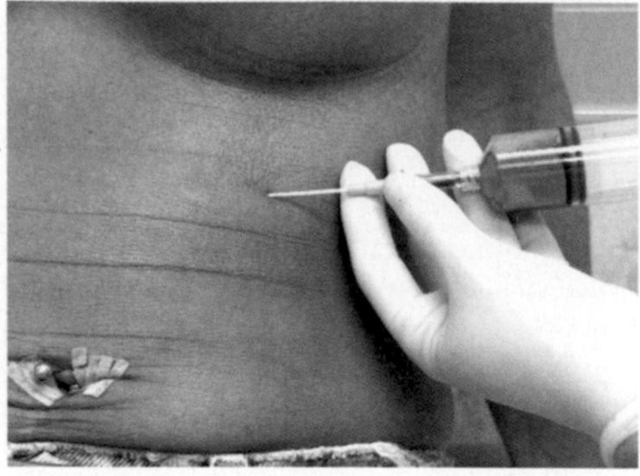

Figure 114.37. In contrast to our other techniques of breast augmentation, a minute volume of serous accumulation has an outlet whereby it can manifest and be safely aspirated. This small volume would no doubt absorb spontaneously, but for patient comfort, it is usually aspirated.

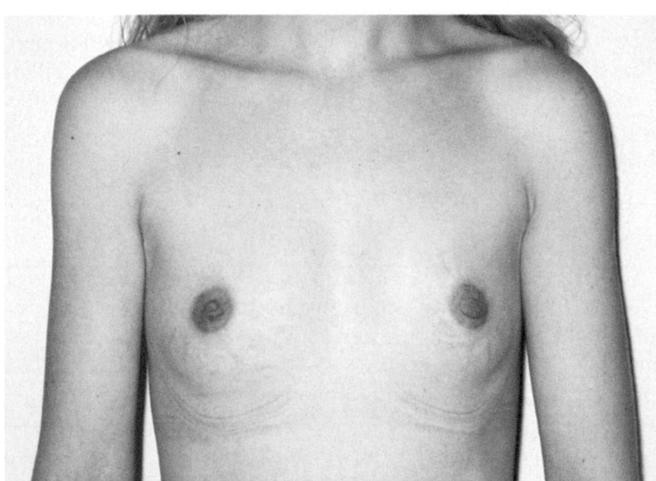

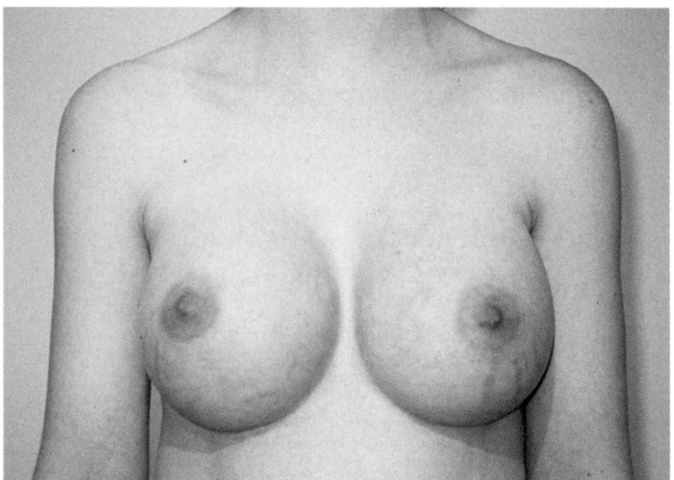

Figure 114.38. This patient had prepectoral transumbilical breast augmentation using smooth, round (475–570) implants filled to within the optimal volume range (570 mL) on each side. As with any augmentation, minor discrepancies in nipple position are magnified. The patient's stretch marks did not increase.

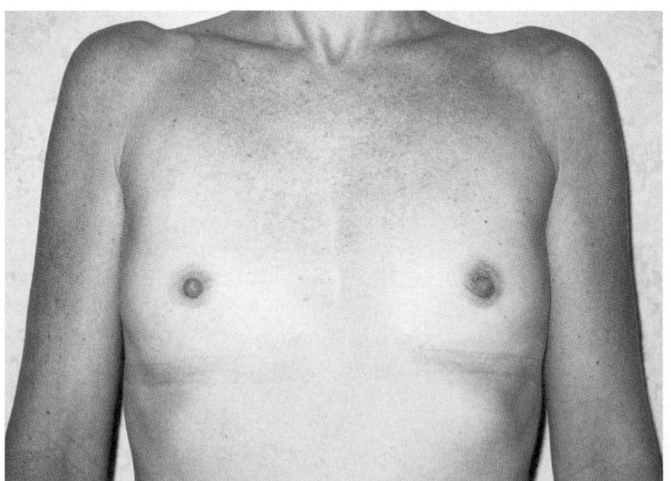

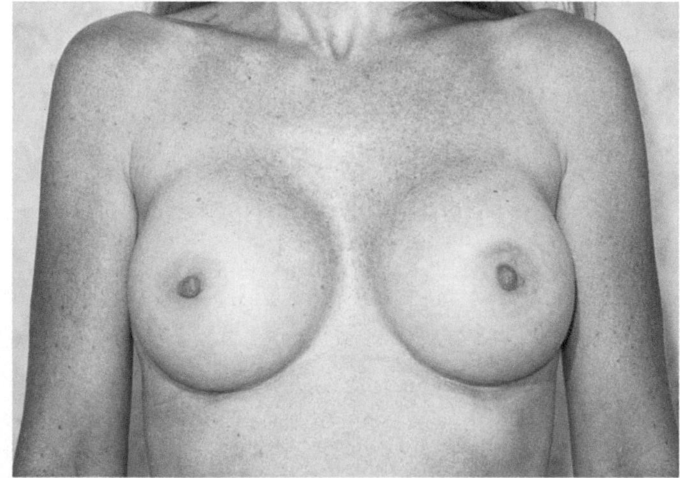

Figure 114.39. This patient with minor asymmetry had subpectoral transumbilical breast augmentation using smooth, round (375–390) implants filled to within the optimal volume range (390 mL right, 375 mL left).

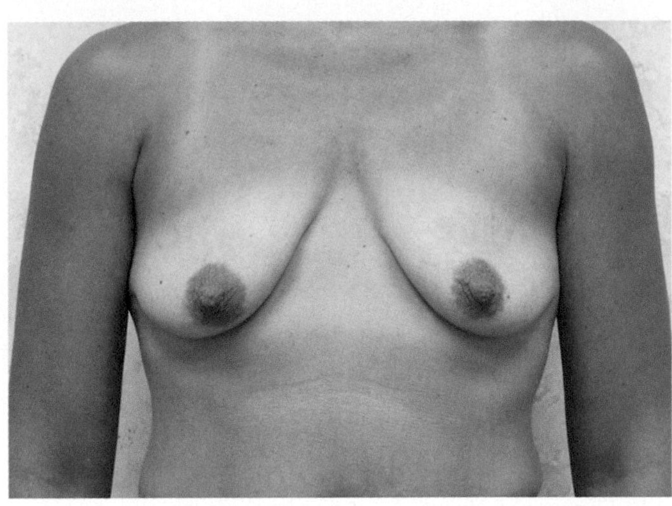

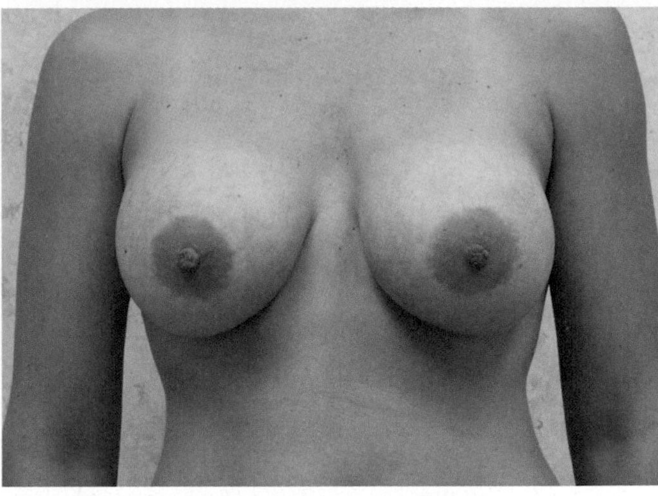

Figure 114.40. This patient had moderate ptosis and underwent prepectoral transumbilical breast augmentation using smooth, round, high-profile (560–675) implants filled to within the optimal volume range (650 mL). Had the implants been subpectoral, this patient might well have had the "double-bubble" look.

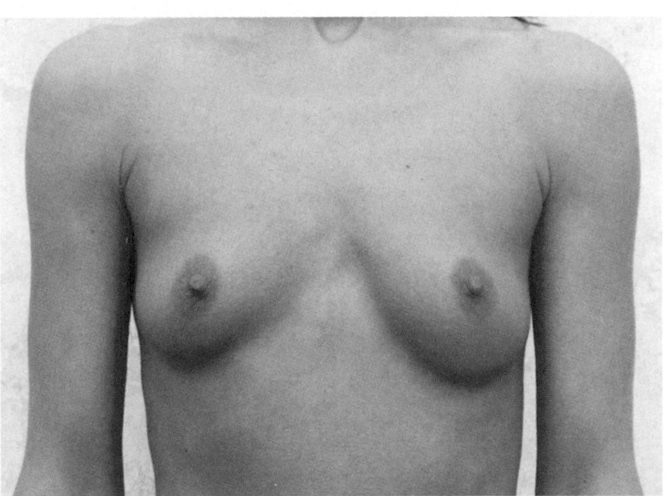

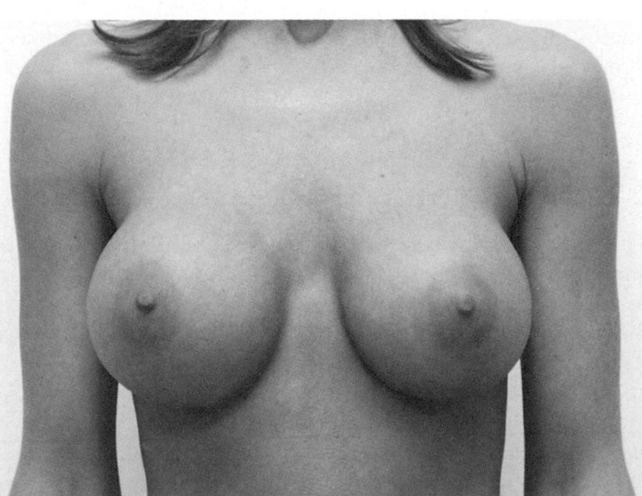

Figure 114.41. This patient had prepectoral transumbilical breast augmentation using a smooth, round (375–450) implant filled to within the optimal volume range (450 mL right) and a 325–390 implant filled to within the optimal volume range (390 mL left). The very great degree of control that the transumbilical breast augmentation procedure gives the operator permits correction of fairly dramatic asymmetries of breast volume and position. No known technique permits adequate repositioning of the nipples without incisions.

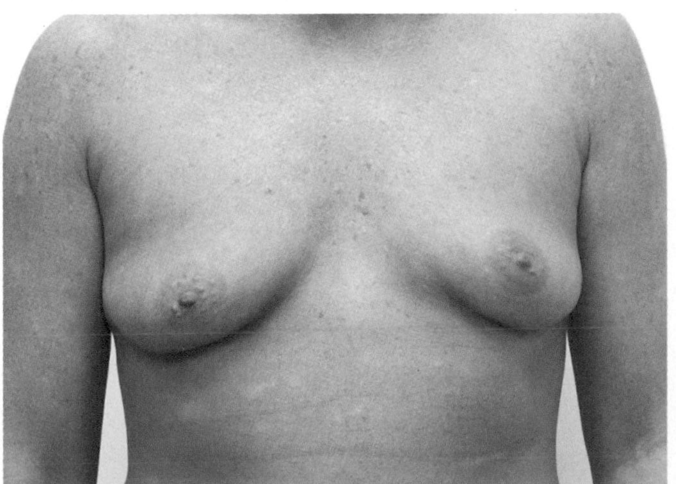

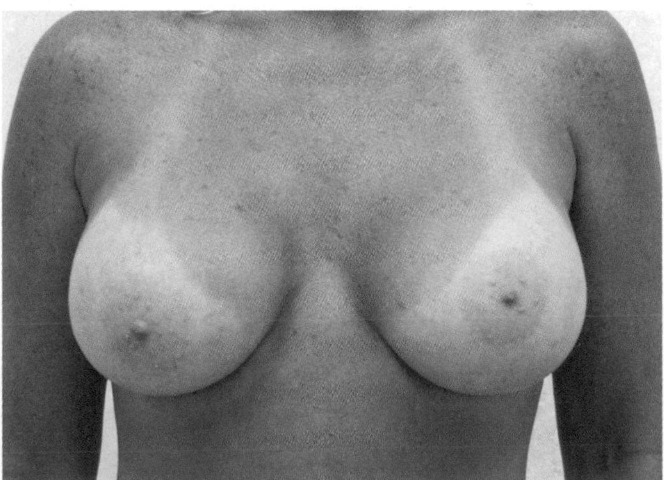

Figure 114.42. This patient had prepectoral transumbilical breast augmentation (TUBA) using smooth, round (475–570) implants filled to within the optimal volume range (570 mL) on each side. Although no augmentation technique can correct discrepancies of nipple position without external incisions, the TUBA procedure permitted correction of this patient's differences in contours and inframammary crease levels.

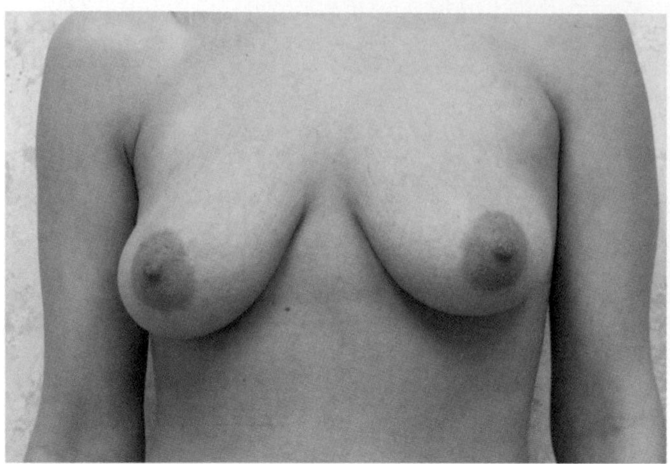
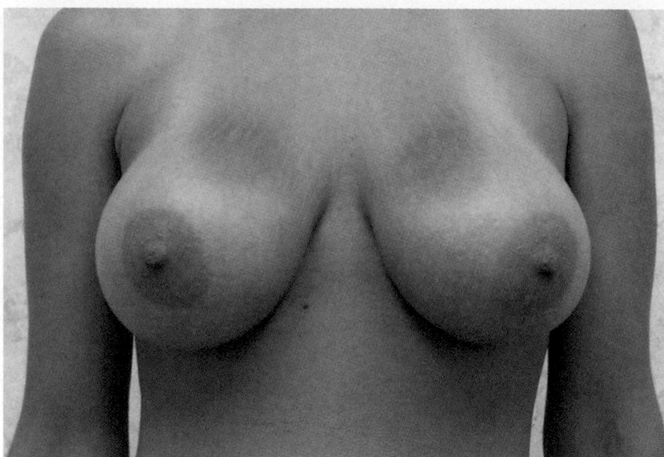

Figure 114.43. This patient had prepectoral transumbilical breast augmentation using smooth, round implants (475–570) filled to within the optimal volume range (550 mL right, 570 mL left).

photos, the TUBA procedure permits the surgeon to correct significant asymmetries of breast volume and position, as well as differences in contours and inframammary crease levels.

CONCLUSION

The TUBA is a safe procedure and an excellent alternative for the patient who is a candidate for it. The technique requires of the surgeon both skill and patience, and it is not a procedure for the hurried or the easily frustrated. The transumbilical breast augmentation is a reliable, safe procedure, and, once learned, it is quite straightforward (38). However, as is true of any technically complex procedure, there are many details that must be mastered to achieve reliability and safety, and a greater incidence of complications might be expected early in a surgeon's experience (39). The senior author has served on the faculty of formal 3-day teaching courses, training about 30 surgeons in the TUBA method, which courses included endoscopic practice sessions, cadaver laboratory procedures, and numerous videotapes showing how to avoid or correct problems. Based on that experience, he is convinced that anything short of such a formal course is inadequate for patient safety and implant protection. Although the transumbilical breast augmentation method appears conceptually simple, technical pitfalls await the inadequately trained and the careless. Transumbilical breast augmentation, like much of plastic surgery, is not learned through books, articles, or lectures. As Rohrich put it, "if we provide plastic surgeons with a template for formalized advanced training in new areas of interest, we automatically improve the quality of care for our patients" (40). It is the learning surgeon's responsibility to seek training, preferably through a formal course, but at least from a properly qualified teacher who has performed the technique a number of times, can teach the procedure effectively, has the appropriate cadaver laboratory facilities for teaching the requisite skills, has a videotape library of the diagnostic points during the procedure, and is prepared to give the equivalent of a formal course to that surgeon. The TUBA is a very safe augmentation procedure, provided all precautions are taken as outlined here, starting with the proper skills, qualifications, training, and certification of the surgeon and extending to the proper equipment, judicious patient evaluation, and consistent attention to the details of the technique.

EDITORIAL COMMENTS

The editors are extremely grateful for this comprehensive review of the TUBA technique. For those who are interested in this operation, this chapter should be an excellent start and preliminary guide to developing a good understanding of the principles and technique associated with this surgery. Within this text on the surgery of the breast, we have some diverging points of view and strategies associated with many areas of breast surgery and, in particular, breast augmentation. This is probably no better illustrated than in the juxtaposition of this chapter on TUBA and Dr. Tebbetts's chapter on quantitative tissue assessment and planning in breast augmentation.

The approach espoused by Dr. Dowden is for all practical purposes a blunt procedure done from a distance using hydraulic expansion techniques combined with blunt dissection and endoscopic visualization primarily for confirmation. The chapter by Dr. Tebbetts is part of a scheme of fairly precise measurements combined with meticulous sharp dissection using electrosurgical techniques and precise pocket creation around an implant.

Judging by Dr. Dowden's and others' reported data, we must believe that using this blunt and somewhat blind technique, in expert hands, one is able to achieve a high rate of success with low complications. I want to emphasize that this is particularly in the short run. As I read through this chapter, I was struck by the sophistication of the procedure described. TUBA may appear to be simple, but in fact there are many steps along the way in this procedure as described here that require careful attention to detail and avoidance of missteps. In fact, evidence for the possibility of missteps is in the frequent mention of patients that Dr. Dowden has seen done by others attempting TUBA but failing to achieve good results. It is worth noting that the results shown in the figures in this chapter are generally quite good. Five of the six, however, are prepectoral breast augmentations, and all of these cases are remarkable for fairly large implants that truly change the dimensions and boundaries of the breasts. As we travel down the road of the effects of breast augmentation, it should be noted that using implants of these dimensions and volumes in patients such as those described here does pose the question about the long-term effects of the implants on the patient's soft tissues. In the chapter by Tebbetts, we are offered an alternative approach, where the surgery is done preferentially within the boundaries of the existing breast so as to avoid long-term negative effects on the soft tissues. I want to finish this commentary by congratulating the authors for providing such a thorough and accurate description of this technique and showing its potential for achieving an attractive result that is comparable to what most surgeons would achieve with a round, large-volume implant placed through whatever incision. I have offered TUBA to my patients and have done it on a handful of patients over the last few years. I think what the authors show is that for those who are truly interested in this technique, it is possible to produce high-quality outcomes. The difference in philosophy, technique, and outcomes both short term and long term, however, between this technique and that espoused by Tebbetts is indeed extraordinary and certainly challenges surgeons to pick and choose which way they want to proceed.

S.L.S.

REFERENCES

1. Planas J. Introduction of breast implants through abdominal route. *Plast Reconstr Surg* 1976;57:434.
2. Barrett BM Jr. Combined abdominoplasty and augmentation mammoplasty through a transverse suprapubic incision. *Ann Plast Surg* 1980;4:286.
3. Johnson GW, Christ JE. The endoscopic breast augmentation: the transumbilical insertion of saline-filled breast implants. *Plast Reconstr Surg* 1993;92(5):801–808.
4. Dowden RV. Technical update on transumbilical breast augmentation. *Aesthet Surg J* 2000;22:240–242.
5. Johnson GW, Dowden RV. Breast augmentation: umbilical approach. In: Ramirez OM, Daniel RK, eds. *Endoscopic Plastic Surgery*. New York: Springer, 1995:156–175.
6. Johnson GW, Dowden RV. Breast augmentation: transumbilical retroglandular approach. In: Fodor PB, Isse NG, eds. *Endoscopically Assisted Aesthetic Plastic Surgery*. St. Louis, MO: Mosby; 1995:145–166.
7. Dowden RV. Keeping the transumbilical breast augmentation procedure safe. *Plast Reconstr Surg* 201;108(5):1389–1400; discussion, 1401–1408.
8. Dowden RV. Why the transumbilical breast augmentation is safe for implants. *Plast Reconstr Surg* 2002;109(7):2576–2579.
9. Songcharoen S. Endoscopic transumbilical subglandular augmentation mammaplasty. *Clin Plast Surg* 2002;29(1):1–13.
10. Pound EC III, Pound EC Jr. Transumbilical breast augmentation (TUBA): patient selection, technique, and clinical experience. *Clin Plast Surg* 2001;28(3):597–605.
11. Sudarsky L. Experience with transumbilical breast augmentation. *Ann Plast Surg* 2001;46(5):467–472; discussion, 472–473.
12. Caleel RT. Transumbilical endoscopic breast augmentation: submammary and subpectoral. *Plast Reconstr Surg* 2000;106(5):1177–1182; discussion, 1183–1184.
13. Pandeya NK. Transumbilical insertion of saline-filled breast implants. *Plast Reconstr Surg* 1997;99(4):1198.
14. VilaRovira R. Breast augmentation by an umbilical approach. *Aesthet Plast Surg* 1999;23:323–330.
15. Dowden RV. Endoscopic breast surgery. In: Achauer BM, Eriksson E, Guyuron B, et al., eds. *Plastic Surgery: Indications, Operations, Outcomes*. Philadelphia: Mosby; 2000:2757–2767.
16. Tebbetts JB. Achieving a predictable 24-hour return to normal activities after breast augmentation part II. *Plast Reconstr Surg* 2002;109:293–305.
17. Szasz TS. *The Second Sin*. New York: Doubleday; 1973.
18. Fisher J, Maxwell GP. Selection of technique for augmentation mammaplasty. In: Noone RB, ed. *Plastic and Reconstructive Surgery of the Breast*. Philadelphia; Mosby-Year Book; 1991.
19. Dowden RV. Dispelling the myths and misconceptions about transumbilical breast augmentation. *Plast Reconstr Surg* 2000;106(1):190–194.
20. U.S. Food and Drug Administration, Medical Devices Advisory Committee. General and Plastic Surgery Devices Panel, Meeting, March 1, 2000. Panel discussion: Clinical; 2000:492–503. Available at: http://www.fda.gov/ohrms/dockets/ac/00/transcripts/3596t1.rtf. Accessed July 13, 2010.
21. Dowden RV, Reisman NR, Gorney M. Going off-label with breast implants. *Plast Reconstr Surg* 2002;110(1):323–329; discussion, 330.
22. Letter confirming implant warranty for transumbilical augment. Available at: http://breastimplant.net/faqs/McGhanLg.html. Accessed July 13, 2010; Letter confirming implant warranty for transumbilical augment. Available at: http://breastimplant.net/faqs/MentorLg.html. Accessed July 13, 2010.
23. Tebbetts JB. *Dimensional augmentation mammaplasty*. Santa Barbara, CA: Allergan Medical Corporation; 1994.
24. Tebbetts JB. A system for breast implant selection based on patient tissue characteristics and implant-soft tissue dynamics. *Plast Reconstr Surg* 202;109:1396–1409.
25. Dowden RV. Who decides the breast augmentation parameters? [Editorial]. *Plast Reconstr Surg* 2003;112:1937–1940.
26. Miglioretti DL, Rutter CM, Geller BM, et al. Effect of breast augmentation on the accuracy of mammography and cancer characteristics. *JAMA* 2004;291:442–450.
27. Skinner KA, Silberman H, Dougherty W, et al. Breast cancer after augmentation mammoplasty. *Ann Surg Oncol* 2001;8(2):138–144.
28. Dowden RV, Reisman NR. Breast implant overfill, optimal fill, and the standard of care. *Plast Reconstr Surg* 1999;104(4):1185–1186.
29. Rohrich RJ, Sorokin ES, Brown SA, et al. Is the umbilicus truly midline? Clinical and medicolegal implications. *Plast Reconstr Surg* 2003;112:259–263.
30. Dixon P, Dowden RV, Connor P, et al. Transumbilical breast augmentation. *AORN J* 2000;72(4):615–625.
31. Dowden RV. Bourdonnement and other benign temporary breast implant sounds. *Ann Plast Surg* 1999;43(6):589–591.
32. Rey RM Jr. Transumbilical breast augmentation: a new instrument. *Plast Reconstr Surg* 2001;15(107):1310–1311.
33. Tebbetts JB. Dual plane breast augmentation: optimizing implant-soft-tissue relationships in a wide range of breast types. *Plast Reconstr Surg* 2001;107:1255–1272.
34. Baker JL. The effectiveness of alpha-tocopherol (vitamin E) in reducing the incidence of spherical contracture around breast implants. *Plast Reconstr Surg* 1981;68:696.
35. Dowden RV. Transumbilical breast implant replacement. *Aesthet Surg J* 2003;23(5):364–369.
36. Hedén P, Jernbeck J, Hober M. Breast augmentation with anatomical cohesive gel implants: the world's largest current experience. *Clin Plast Surg* 2001;28:531–552.
37. Johnson G, Black J, Spira M. Endoscopic augmentation mammoplasty. Presentation at the 1994 Senior Residents Conference, Boston, Massachusetts, May 27, 1994.
38. Dowden RV. Transumbilical breast augmentation is safe and effective. In: Hollier LH, Hallock GG, eds. *Seminars in Plastic Surgery*. New York: Thieme; 2008:51–59.
39. Brennan WA, Haiavy J. Transumbilical breast augmentation; a practical review of a growing technique. *Ann Plast Surg* 2007;59:243–249.
40. Rohrich RJ. Lessons learned from a botulinum toxin type A survey. *Plast Reconstr Surg* 2004;113:1435–1437.

CHAPTER

115

Per Hedén

Breast Augmentation With Anatomic, High-cohesiveness Silicone Gel Implants (European Experience)

The desire of women to have more youthful and shapely breasts can be traced a long way back in human history. The female breast is strongly connected to human sexuality and under appropriate conditions sends a signal of fertility and youth to the opposite sex. It is therefore not surprising that breast augmentation surgery for cosmetic reasons was performed already in the late nineteenth century (1). Since the introduction of silicone gel breast implants in 1964 (2), a steadily increasing demand for these procedures has followed.

Traditionally and throughout the first three decades of silicon implant breast augmentation, the approach to the procedure was volumetric. However, a clear trend toward more dimensional thinking in breast augmentation has evolved since the 1990s. Breast augmentation in the twenty-first century is at a turning point. In the traditional techniques, implant selection was based more on the surgeon's experience and the patient's desires than on measurements and tissue analysis. The preoperative planning of the implant's positioning was also fairly arbitrary, based on the surgeon's experience. Implant alternatives were limited to round, smooth ones with one or few shapes. In the new era of breast augmentation surgery, implant selection is much more precise, based on a careful analysis of the chest and glandular tissue. Instead of implant selection based on volume, three-dimensional thinking is applied. Implant positioning during surgery is no longer arbitrary and is much more precise, based on careful analysis and measurement. Many different implants are also available. Besides the traditional round ones, anatomic and asymmetric implants are available. Implants can have a smooth or textured surface and are available in several different shapes with varying heights, widths, and projections.

Current filling material in breast implants, however, has changed little since the 1960s. In the United States saline is still the dominant filler due to the silicone moratorium imposed by the Food and Drug Administration (FDA) in 1992. Silicone-filled implants have recently been reintroduced in the United States, and a rapid growth in their use has been noted. Silicone gel dominates as implant filling material in the rest of the world. During the 1990s the characteristics of silicon fillings changed, however, resulting in implants with higher cohesiveness. This has resulted in greater shape-retaining properties. Thus the fundamental difference between traditional silicone gel–filled implants and these new high-cohesiveness silicone implants is their form stability. Recently round, high-cohesiveness silicone gel implants have also been introduced.

This chapter discusses how to select form-stable implants and make preoperative markings, as well as how much the implant shape and filling material matter. It is important to realize that form-stable implants behave considerably differently than non–form-stable implants. Surgeons who use them in similar ways are bound to have more complications and increase the risk for reoperations. Indeed, not only are the implant selection and surgical technique different, the patient communication, the preoperative markings, and the postoperative recommendations also differ. Form-stable implants provide much better chances to control the shape of the new breast, and we in the twenty-first century have entered into a new breast-shaping era as opposed to the old breast-stuffing era.

ANATOMIC, HIGH-COHESIVENESS SILICONE GEL BREAST IMPLANTS: MANUFACTURERS

In 1994 the McGhan Corporation (later Inamed and now a part of Allergan) was the first manufacturer to introduce anatomic, high-cohesiveness silicon breast implants (AHCSI). The brand name was Style 410. This was followed by the introduction of a family of different shapes of these implants (the Matrix system). The first eight patients in the world were operated with this Matrix system at Akademikliniken in Stockholm in 1997, and since then our group has gained leading international experience with these implants. In 2008 more than 10,000 of these had been implanted, and several international postgraduate courses, workshops, and demonstration operations had been held. The Allergan Matrix Style 410 implants are filled with a highly cohesive silicone gel, which results in the stability of their form. The implant shapes are tear dropped, anatomic, and available in 12 different sets of heights and projections (a given combination of height and projection is called a cell). Height varies from low to moderate to full, and projection from low to moderate to full to extra projecting. Thus, a moderate-height implant with a low projection is called an ML implant, and a full-height implant with extra projection is called an FX model (Fig. 115.1). These implants are soft but slightly firmer than regular low-cohesiveness (responsive) silicone gel implants. When these AHCSI implants are cut in half, the material is slightly sticky on direct contact but shape retaining. In contrast to a standard silicone gel breast implant, the material will not leave the shell during manual compression of a cut implant. Much of the discussion in this chapter is based on experience in the use of Allergan Style 410 implants but is also applicable to other types of implants. Since McGhan/Allergan introduced AHCSIs, other manufacturers (e.g., Mentor, Eurosilicone, Polytech/Silimed, Perthese, and Arion) have also introduced AHCSIs. The Matrix system with 12 different

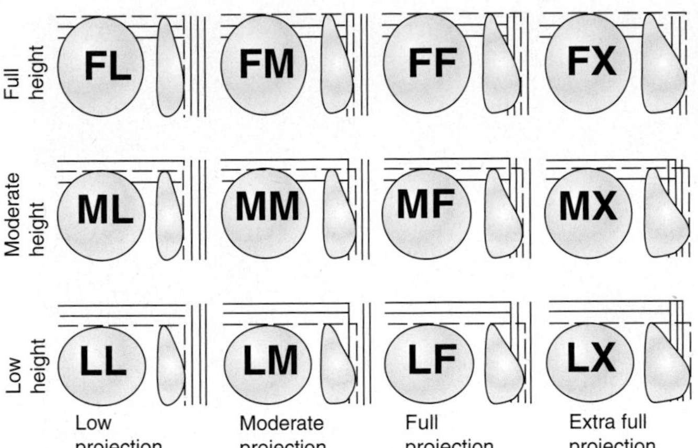

Figure 115.1. Schematic illustration of the Matrix breast implant system.

implant cells is exclusive to Allergan, but other manufacturers have systems of form-stable anatomic implants with varying heights and projection. Mentor, which recently became a part of Johnson & Johnson, has an anatomic, high-cohesiveness silicone gel implant style called CPG (Contour Profile) available in five different shapes with varying heights and projection. Allergan has also introduced a new type of form-stable anatomic implant called Style 510. This implant contains two different cohesive silicone gels. The ventral part is considerably firmer than the posterior part, with the aim to maintain extra projection in the nipple-areola complex. AHCSIs of different manufacturers have different properties of the silicone gel, and the cohesiveness characteristics may vary from one type of implant to another. No standardized nomenclature describing the degree of cohesiveness has been developed by the industry, and thus it is difficult to make comparisons among manufacturers. A degree of confusion exists regarding "cohesive" silicone gel implants because all silicone implants by definition are cohesive. The liquid state only exists where molecules are relatively free from each other as in water or saline solution. Thus even a silicone gel implant that has "flowing" properties is cohesive. However, it is low in cohesiveness. A simple way to get an idea of the degree of cohesiveness of a silicone breast implant is to do a so-called tilt test: The implant is placed flat in the horizontal hand of the examiner and then turned vertical by tilting the tip of the implant with the fingers; the degree of shape-retaining properties is then noted. The lower the cohesiveness, the more one will note collapses of the upper pole of the implant.

To minimize the risk for rotation of anatomic implants, the surface of the implant shell is textured. The purpose of this texturing is to allow tissue in-growth, immobilization, and a reduced frequency of capsular contraction. Indeed, surface texturing may permit tissue in-growth and adherence to the surrounding tissue, thereby facilitating implant immobility (3–5). Texturing also prevents circumferential linear fibrosis associated with capsular contraction (6). This effect is only clear in studies of implants in the subglandular position. Different manufacturers of AHCSIs have different techniques to produce the texturing of their implants. To aid tissue in-growth and adherence, a pore diameter of greater than 300 μm is regarded as a prerequisite (7). The BioCell surface of Style 410 implants has a pore size between 250 and 750 μm and a mean pore diameter of 500 μm. The Mentor implant has a pore size of less than 300 μm in its textured Siltex surface, which does not permit tissue in-growth. However, there is no indication that the pore size has any effect on the degree of capsular contracture.

INDICATIONS FOR HIGH-COHESIVENESS SILICONE GEL BREAST IMPLANTS

The main indications for AHCSIs are primary breast augmentations in women who desire a proportionate breast augmentation. This augmentation may be of greater, lesser, or moderate extent but still proportionate to the dimensions of the chest and glandular tissue. AHCSIs are not suitable for women who desire a very large and nonproportionate breast augmentation with an artificial appearance. AHCSIs are also useful in secondary breast augmentation but may be more technically demanding than standard low-cohesiveness breast implants or liquid-filled implants. In a secondary breast augmentation it is recommended that a new implant pocket be created to minimize the risk for rotation of the implant. If severe capsular contraction is present, it is possible that the atrophy of the glandular tissue is pronounced. If this is the case, it may be difficult to fill the dead space after the old implant with a high-cohesiveness filler. The use of implants without shape-retaining properties may be advantageous in these cases. An alternative may be to use a combined mastopexy augmentation and an AHCSI. A third clear indication for AHCSI is breast reconstructive surgery. The wide variety of implant shapes provides a greater degree of individualization and variation than other implants on the market. This is of extra value when correcting breast asymmetries. Congenital deformations such as Poland syndrome (Fig. 115.2) and postmastectomy defects are examples of very pronounced asymmetries that can benefit from the great range of choices of different implant shapes. The stable mound of a high-cohesiveness silicon implant also permits better skin redraping and contracture after a subcutaneous mastectomy than a low-cohesiveness implant or liquid filler, which would tend to flow out into the lower part of the dissected pocket (Figs. 115.3 and 115.4).

ADVANTAGES AND DISADVANTAGES OF HIGH-COHESIVENESS SILICONE GEL BREAST IMPLANTS

The large number of form-stable implant shapes available makes a more customized breast augmentation possible compared to the traditional breast augmentation technique. This is obviously better, as a great variation exists in patient desires, thoracic shapes, and amount of glandular tissue. An obvious advantage of this variation in shapes exists in the treatment of breast asymmetries. By careful analysis of the thoracic and glandular differences between right and left sides, the prerequisites for different implant shapes can be established. A computed tomography scan can be useful in evaluating thoracic asymmetries for detailed analysis of the chest wall shape (Fig. 115.5). A newer tool in the analysis of breast shapes is three-dimensional imaging.

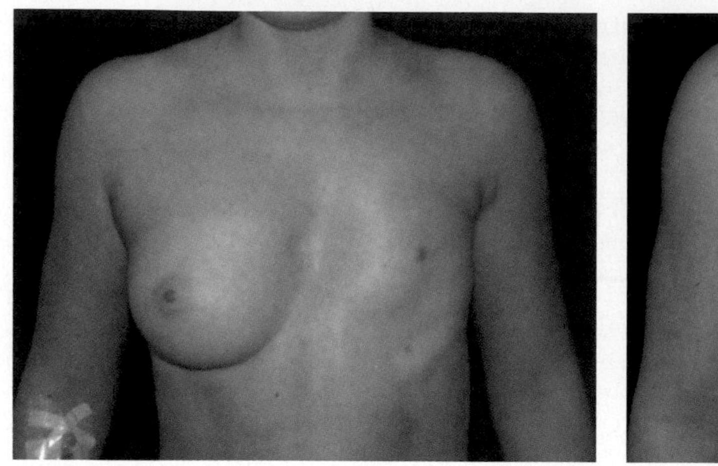

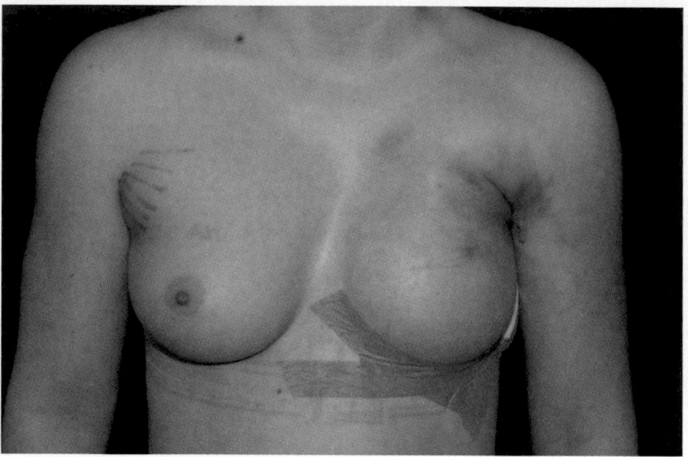

Figure 115.2. Pronounced Poland syndrome with extremely tight tissue. Before and early after Style 410 MF model, 335-g and latissimus dorsi muscle transfer with reinsertion of its tendon in the ventral humerus.

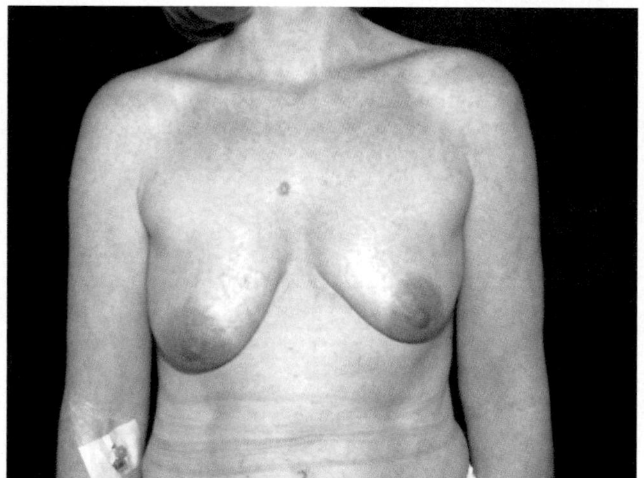

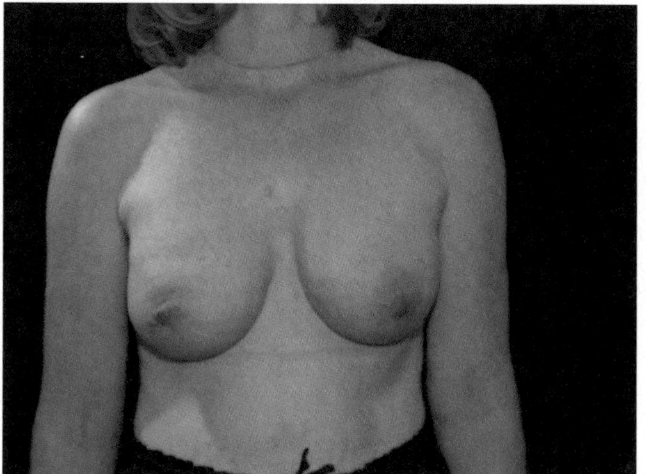

Figure 115.3. Before and 6 months after subcutaneous mastectomy and reconstruction with Style 410 FF model, 475 g. The form-stable, highly cohesive filler permits contraction of the skin on this stable mold. Note right nipple elevation without mastopexy. A low-cohesiveness filler would likely fill the empty skin pocket in the lower pole and produce a considerably different result.

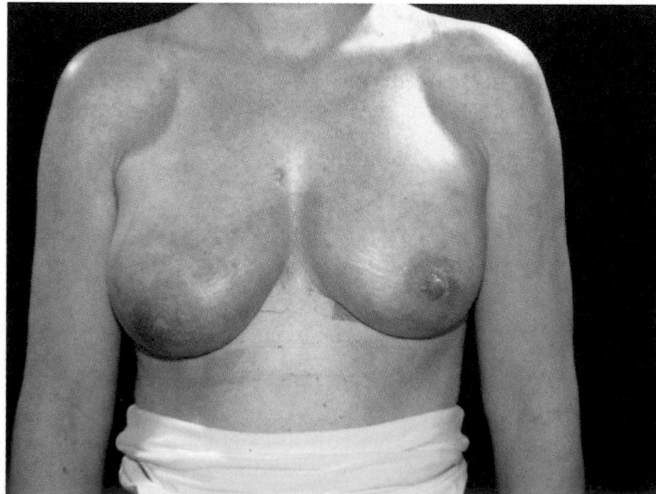

Figure 115.4. Same case as in Figure 115.3 at 1 week after surgery. Note the nipple position and compare it to the situation 6 months later (Fig. 115.3B).

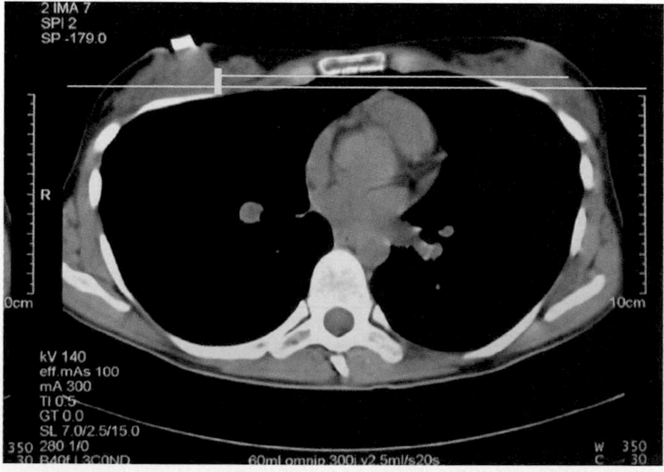

Figure 115.5. In evaluating thoracic asymmetries a computed tomography scan of the chest wall may be useful. Minute analysis of asymmetries at different heights on the chest wall is possible. These differences can then be transferred into different shapes of high-cohesiveness implants.

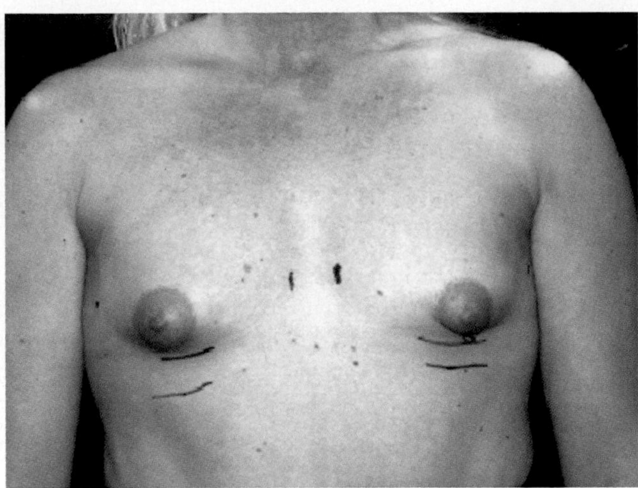

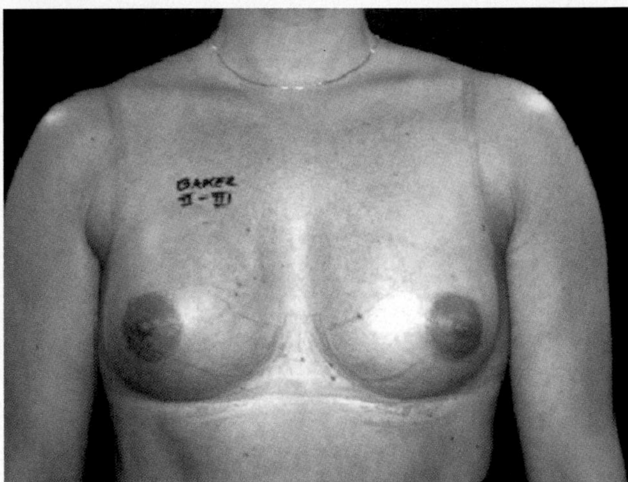

Figure 115.6. Before and after augmentation with high-cohesiveness silicon breast implants. Capsular contracture on the right side (Baker III firmness but less deformity; note a small narrowing of the base). The left side is soft.

Today this permits analysis of existing breast shape, and systems for prediction of the outcome of a breast augmentation using differently shaped implants are under development. This could be an extremely valuable tool for the planning of a breast augmentation, as well as for patient communication in advance of surgery (Fig. 115.6).

The FDA moratorium on silicone gel implants in 1992 raised three main concerns:

1. Risk for breast cancer
2. Risk for autoimmune disease
3. Implant rupture

Since 1992 it has clearly been documented that breast augmentation does not increase the risk for breast cancer (8–11). It has also been well documented in large epidemiologic studies that no increased risk for autoimmune disease exists after implantation of silicone gel implants (12–15). However, the true frequency of implant rupture is unknown and varies greatly with the generation of implants. One advantage with AHCSIs is that there is less movement of the implant shell due to the nature of the filling material. Implants with less movement of the shell are likely to wear less and may have a longer life expectancy. We have demonstrated a very low rupture frequency of high-cohesiveness silicone gel implants with implantation time of up to 9 years. Comparison of the results from this magnetic resonance imaging study with the rupture frequency of low-cohesiveness silicone-filled implants with similar implantation time shows that low-cohesiveness fillers may have between 5 and 30 times higher rupture risk (16). If a shell rupture occurs in an implant with a high-cohesiveness filler, it is even possible that this may not produce negative effects because the form-stable filling material is less likely to leak out through small holes in the shell. Another advantage with AHCSIs is that more force is needed to deform the implants compared to a low-cohesiveness or liquid filler. If capsular contraction occurs, this is likely to result in less deformation, and this has also been our clinical experience (Fig. 115.7). Implants with low-cohesiveness fillers are easily deformed into a spherical shape when compressed (Fig. 115.8).

High-cohesiveness implants also have less tendency to wrinkle even if surface irregularities can been seen. The upper pole of an AHCSI is the area that is most prone to irregularities because this is the thinnest part of the device. Due to their shape, full-height implants with low projection have the weakest upper pole, and these are the models with the highest risk for upper pole irregularities. The risk increases if the upper pole of the implant pocket is underdissected and implants are placed in the subglandular position in thin patients. A more pronounced irregularity with buckling of the upper pole has been reported (17) and may be attributed to the aforementioned factors.

If similar-shaped breasts with similar amounts of glandular tissue are treated with implants of different shapes and the implants are placed in the same implant position in relation to the pectoralis muscle and are found to be without capsular contraction on late follow-up, it has been noted that anatomic implants produce a more natural upper pole than round ones (Fig. 115.9). It has been claimed that round implants change into anatomic shape in the standing position (18). This is only true if the device is underfilled and filled with a low-cohesiveness or liquid filler and if no capsular contraction is present. However, this also results in collapse of the upper pole with irregularities of the shell. This situation is also likely to result in more envelope wear and probably long-term increased rupture risk. If a capsular contraction develops, these implants will deform into a spherical and unnatural shape. If the devices are overfilled to reduce these problems, they become more rounded and unnatural in shape. They will also be firmer. Thus the implant shape and filling material clearly make a difference in the final outcome of a breast augmentation procedure.

What are the indications for round breast implants? The primary indication is the patient's preference, especially in women who desire a more rounded and artificial appearance. It may also be an economic consideration for the patient because most AHCSI implants are considerably more expensive than round ones. For patients who desire the softest implant available, a low-cohesiveness, round silicone implant may also be offered. The patient should be informed, however, that a common small degree of capsular contraction activity is much

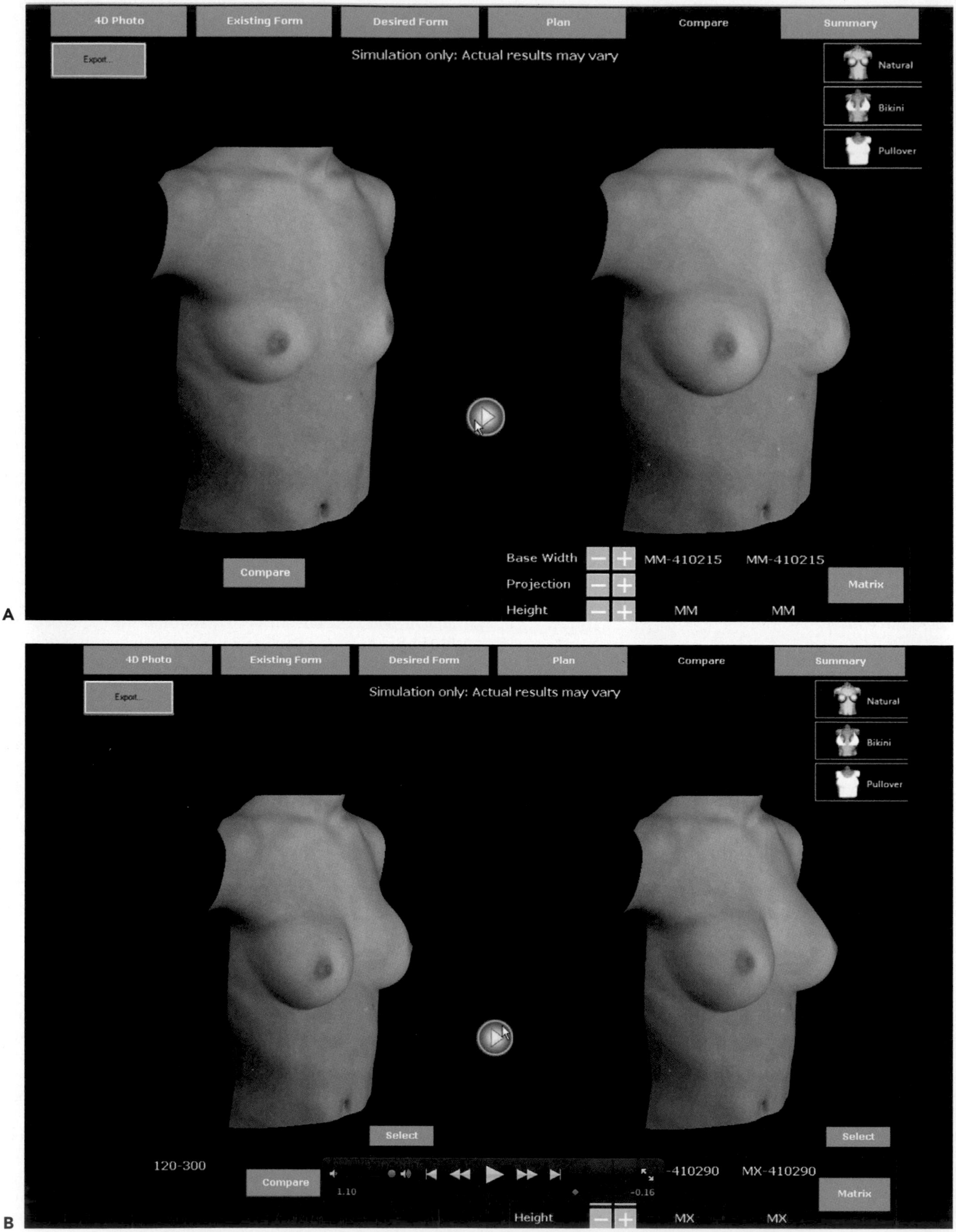

A

B

Figure 115.7. A new three-dimensional simulation tool (Precision Light) illustrating **(A)** the calculated outcome of a Style 410 MM, 215-cc implant (right) compared with the preoperative situation (left), and **(B)** the difference between a round Style 120, 300-g implant (left) and an anatomic Style 410 MX, 290-g implant (right).

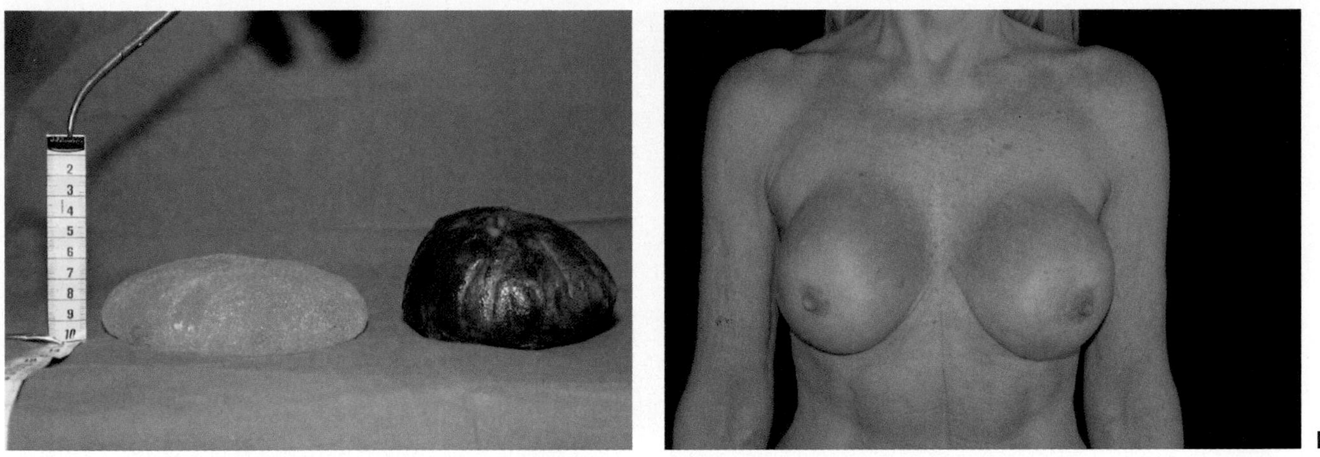

Figure 115.8. **A:** Implants with low-cohesiveness fillers are easily deformed into a spherical shape when compressed. Baker III contraction. On the right the implant is seen with its intact capsule. The capsule on the left implant has been removed. The implants (Inamed Style 110) are of equal shape size and type. **B:** Low-cohesiveness silicone gel implants (Style 110) and a similar degree of firmness as the right breast in Figure 115.7 but considerably more deformed.

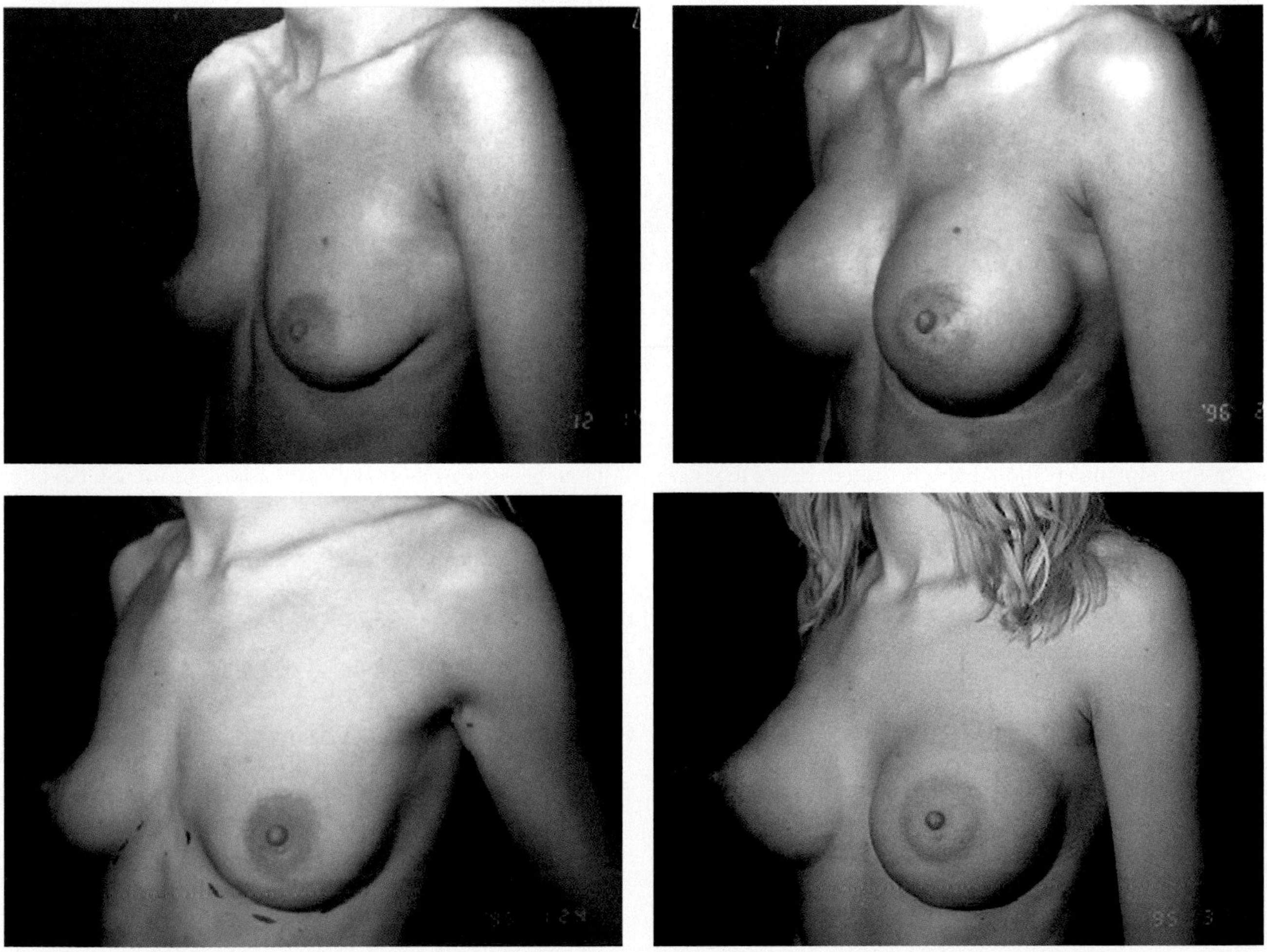

Figure 115.9. If similar types of breasts are treated with the same type of surgical technique and the same amount of capsular activity is noted at the late follow-up, the anatomic implants produce a more natural upper pole compared to round ones. **A, B:** Before and after augmentation with subglandular high-cohesiveness silicon breast implants. **C, D:** Before and after augmentation with subglandular round Style 110 implants. Both patients have soft breasts. The benefits of anatomic implants is most apparent in patients with poor upper pole cover. (*continued*)

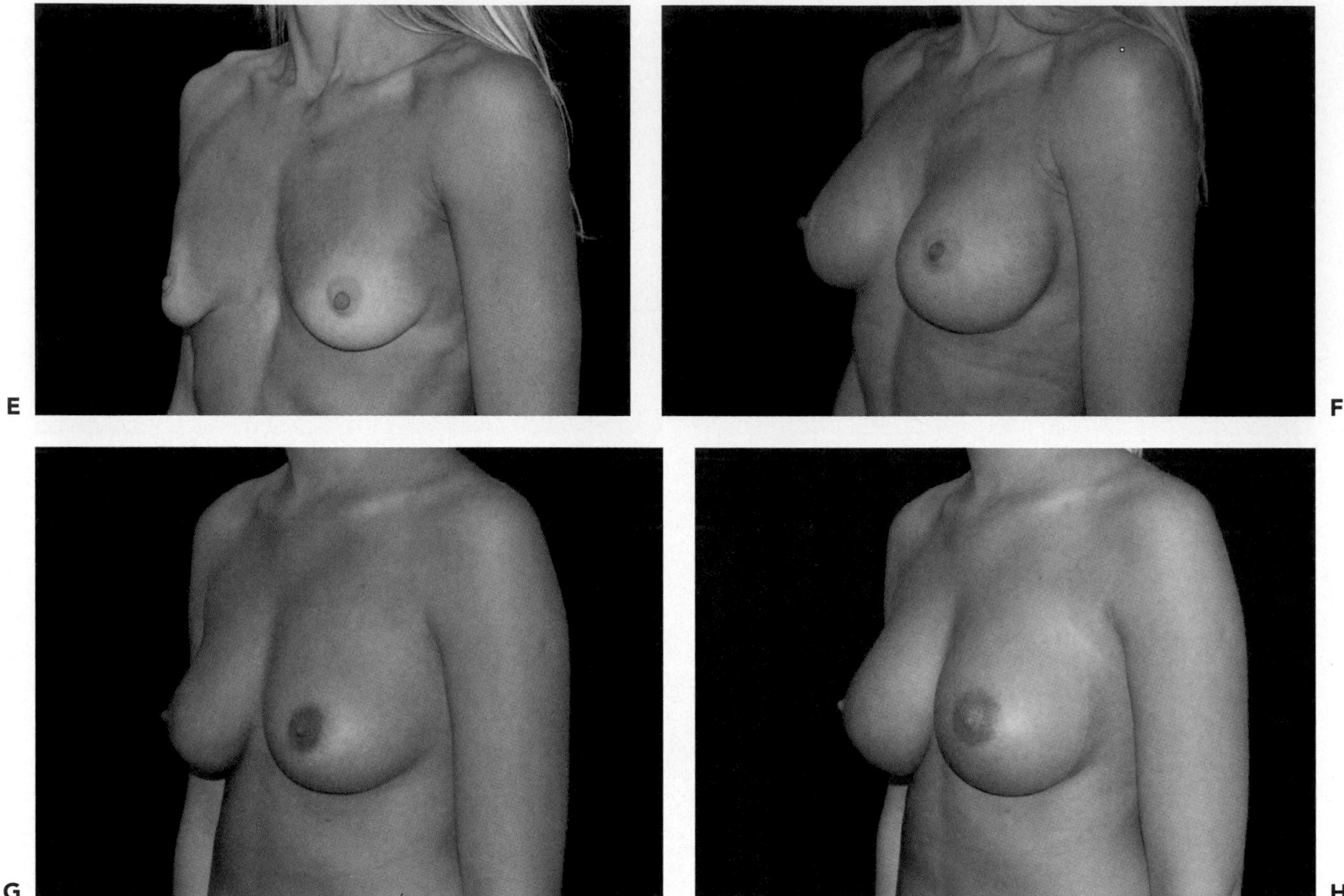

Figure 115.9. (*Continued*) **E, F:** Before and after Allergan Style 410 MM 280-g implants in dual-plane II-III submuscular position. In patients with good upper pole cover, the upper pole appearance may look natural and anatomic even with round implants. **G, H:** Before and after implantation of round, high-cohesiveness silicone gel implants (Inspira TSM 240 g) in subfascial position.

more important for the firmness of the breast than the consistency of the implants. It should also be noted that AHCSIs are available with different degrees of firmness (e.g., the Allergan Style 410 Soft Touch implant). Another indication for round implants is recurrent rotation of anatomic implants. Round implants may also be recommended in selected secondary cases, especially, as mentioned earlier, in severe unilateral capsular contraction cases. In these cases low-cohesiveness filler or a combination of cohesiveness filler with mastopexy may be recommended. Recently, round, form-stable implants (e.g., Allergan Inspira TRM, TRF, and TRX) have been introduced. These behave similar to anatomic form-stable, high-cohesiveness implants, but due to their shape obviously do not have the risk for rotational problems. They may also be favored in situations in which patients want a fuller upper pole.

Other disadvantages of AHCSIs include higher costs and more technically demanding procedures with a steeper learning curve. Incisions also need to be a slightly longer (4 to 6.5 cm, averaging 5.5 cm, depending on implant dimensions and size) because of the characteristics of the filling material. High-cohesiveness implants should not be forced through a too-small hole. AHCSIs are also firmer in Baker I cases and not suitable for exaggerated and nonproportionate augmentations. Finally, a risk for rotation exists with these implants. However, the frequency has been reported to be as low as 0.42% (19). It also has to be recognized that nonadhesion of tissue on the implant surface does not always result in rotation. A textured implant surface with a pore size larger than 300 μm is a prerequisite for in-growth of tissue and fixation of the implant. Some anatomic form-stable implant surfaces (e.g., the Siltex of Mentor/Johnson & Johnson implants) have a pore size smaller than 300 μm and thus do not permit tissue fixation (7). However, despite this, it is rotation is also relatively uncommon with these anatomic high-cohesiveness, form-stable implants.

Most rotations were seen in secondary cases, and to avoid these problems anatomic implants should not be implanted into old implant pockets in secondary augmentation surgery. This is especially true if the implant pocket has been formed around a smooth-walled implant. It is believed that the smooth-walled pocket does not permit tissue in-growth into the texturing of the implant and thus rotation is facilitated. Rotation may also be seen in primary augmentation surgery. In these cases the implants are not immobilized, and this may have several possible explanations. The reasons for poor tissue immobilization of the implants are not clearly known, but several possible explanations can be offered. The problem may be related to poor surgical technique with dissection of a too-large implant pocket. To minimize this risk for an overdissected implant

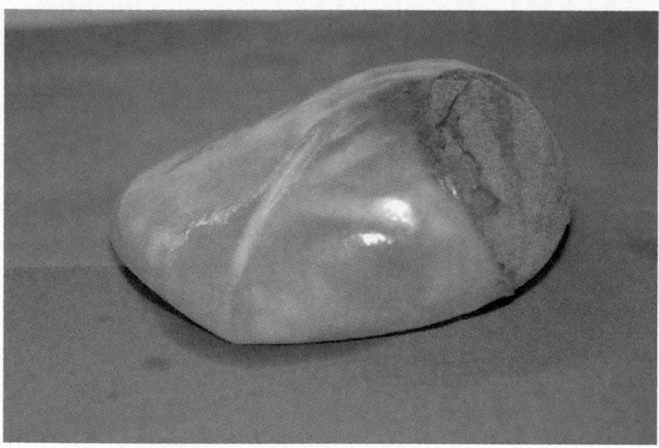

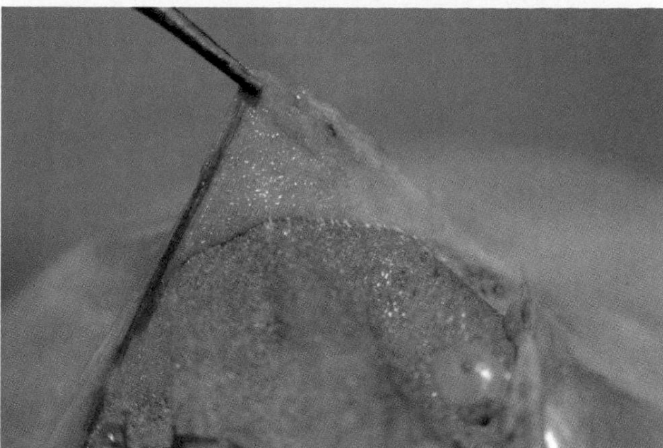

Figure 115.10. High-cohesiveness silicon breast implant with double-capsule formation. The inner capsule is sticking on the implant surface, but this has separated from the outer layer of the capsule, and the implant is thus movable in the breast.

pocket, it could be checked with a ruler during the procedure. The goal is a snug-fitting implant pocket. The width of the pocket only marginally should exceed the implant width. Less than 1 cm of dissection on each side is recommended. However, the height of the implant pocket should exceed the implant height by at least 2 cm or slightly more to allow good redraping of the tissues in the upper pole of the implant. Other possible explanations for late rotations of anatomic implants may be the formation of a so-called pseudocapsule or double capsule (Fig. 115.10). This is clinically noted as a complete separation of the capsule into two layers. The inner one is complete or partial and sticks on the walls of the textured implant. A small amount of serous material may be noted between the two layers of the capsule. No explanation of these phenomena is available in the literature, but several possible hypotheses may be offered. One is that a subclinical infection with the formation of a biological film on the implants is present. In support of this theory is the observation that only one side may be affected and that the situation can be effectively treated with the creation of a new implant pocket and exchange of the implant. Another possible explanation is that seroma is formed around the implant early after implantation, and contributing to this could be a poor surgical technique with creation of too large an implant pocket or traumatic blunt dissection. The dissection should be sharp, bloodless, and without overdissection. The use of tungsten carbide needle cautery (Colorado tip) is recommended. In the setting of submuscular implantation, the loose connective tissue between ribs and muscle should be left on the ribs to minimize seroma formation. Another possible explanation for rotation of anatomic implants is trauma or excessive motion. Support for this theory comes from noting that this has been mostly observed in patients with loose parenchyma and an envelope where the implant has more opportunity for movement. It has also been noted in secondary cases that the smooth patch on the back side of Style 410 implants often is surrounded by a slightly larger area of nonadhesion. It could be argued that this is a weak point of the implants and could be the starting point for seroma formation and dissection of the implant capsule into two separate layers.

Common arguments against the use of anatomic implants include that these are too expensive and that patients are happy with traditional round, less cohesive gel-filled implants. It has also been stated that high-cohesiveness fillers are too firm and do not move naturally on the chest wall. AHCSIs are indeed more expensive. However, as these implants appear to have a longer life span, they may actually be cheaper per time unit. Dividing the extra cost of AHCSIs by the number of years that such implants are likely to be in place results in a fairly small annual cost. This argument is easily accepted by patients, and most prefer an extra cost for something they "wear" every day. It is also true that most patients are happy with traditional round silicone gel implants, but it should been remembered that many patients are happy with inferior results and that this is no reason plastic surgeons should refrain from improvements. In fact it is their obligation as surgeons to try to do their best. Patients should be happier with an even better result.

Careful analysis of the consistency of an augmented breast reveals that a low grade of capsular activity is more common than usually noted by the surgeon or patient. If a breast judged to be without capsular contraction is compressed and this is compared to the implant material external to the body, it is commonly noted that the breast is slightly firmer. This much more commonly results in firmness of the breast than the actual firmness of the implant. It has also been noted that the grade of capsular activity is a much more important factor for the movement of the breast on the chest wall than the firmness of the implant itself (Fig. 115.11). The AHCSI without clear capsular contracture moves as freely on the chest wall as any other implant type. I conclude this section on the advantages and disadvantages of the AHCSI by stating that in my 30 years of experience in breast augmentation surgery, this type of implant has given higher patient satisfaction and a lower frequency of complications than all other implant types and techniques I have used.

IMPLANT SELECTION: PREOPERATIVE ANALYSIS AND MEASUREMENTS

In spite of the fact that dimensional thinking was introduced in breast implant surgery during the early 1990s (19,20), it is still very difficult to get patients, nurses, and plastic surgeons to

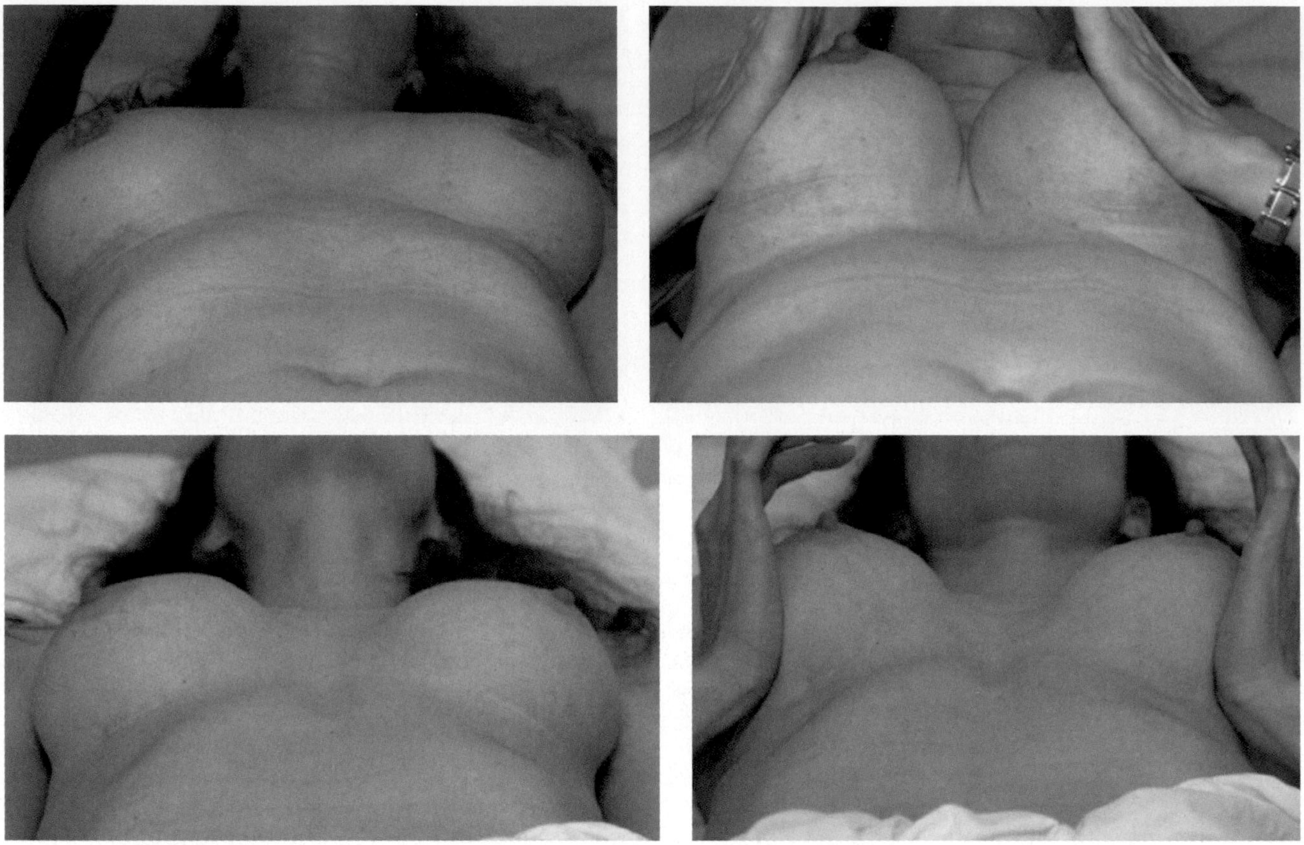

Figure 115.11. **A, B:** High-cohesiveness silicon breast implants without capsular contraction. Manual manipulation moves these breasts more than the low-cohesiveness silicone gel implants **(C, D)**. These latter implants have a Baker II firmness.

stop thinking of implant volume as the most important factor in implant selection. Many surgeons still arbitrarily select and suggest an implant volume based on feelings and experience rather than on measuring and analyzing the breast prior to implant selection. Today, however, breast augmentations are much more about proportions and dimensions than implant volume. This can be illustrated by comparing patients with a large-looking breast but a small implant volume and patients with a moderately sized breast but a larger implant volume (Fig. 115.12). Patients should be led to understand that the final appearance of the augmented breast is highly related to the initial amount of breast tissue, its dimensions, and the size of the chest wall and that they should not select an implant based on a preconceived idea about a suitable volume. Many

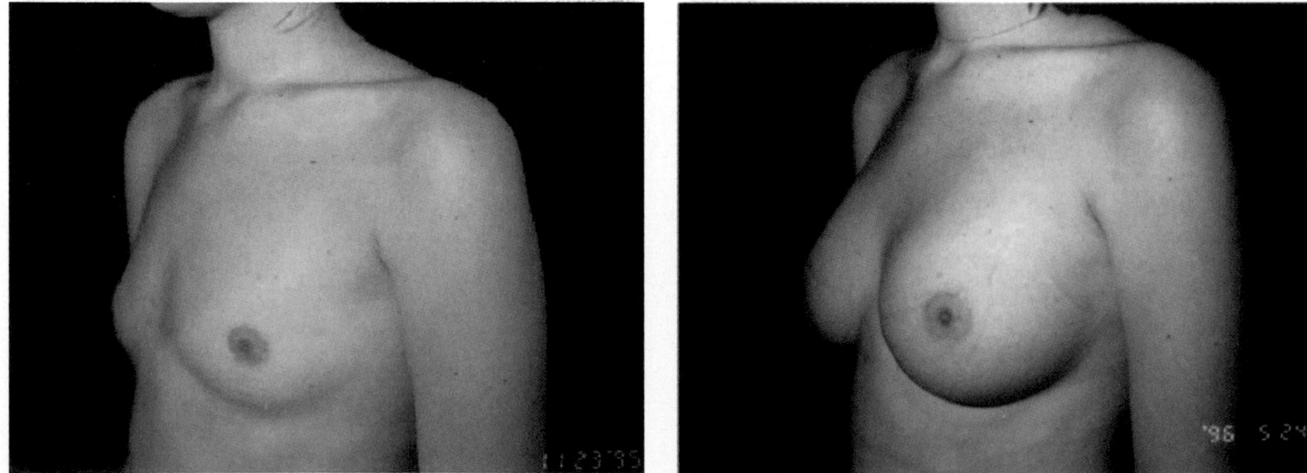

Figure 115.12. The patient in Figure 115.9B after augmentation with Style 410 implant, 340 g, has considerably larger looking breasts than the patient here **(B)** after implantation of Style 410 FM, 395 g. **A:** Before the operation. The reason for this is that the patient here is shorter, has a smaller thorax, and has more glandular tissue to begin with.

patients have reviewed the Internet before a consultation, and therefore it is not uncommon that they have a faulty idea about the desired implant volume. It is fundamentally important that patients understand that implants have to suit the biological conditions and that implant selection has to be tissue based.

Advantages with preoperative measurements include increased accuracy and awareness. Measurement also permits patient participation and documentation. This leads to better evaluation and more predictable results. Patients also have more realistic expectations, which finally should lead to improved patient satisfaction. When dimensional analysis of the breast prior to augmentation surgery was proposed by John Tebbetts, a large number of different measurements were suggested. To many surgeons this was confusing, and it has been found that these measurements can be greatly simplified. However, some measurements are still of great importance. These include the width of the existing breast and the desired width of the new breast. The position of the submammary fold and the position of the fold after augmentation should also be calculated and considered when selecting a suitable implant shape. These measurements are employed in a consultation that varies greatly from the traditional type of breast augmentation consultation. In the conventional consultation, an implant volume was estimated and suggested to the patient. Some surgeons confirmed the accuracy of the selected implant with measurements. In the biodimensional consultation, a reversed way of getting the ideal implant volume is adopted. By calculating suitable implant width and height and taking the patient's desires into consideration, the surgeon can suggest a suitable implant type. The width of the selected implant is noted in the manufacturer's chart, and this finally provides information about the volume of the implant.

Selecting the ideal AHCSI can be divided into several fundamentally different steps. The first is to examine the breast and the thorax. Most patients with small asymmetries are unaware of these but may note them after surgery. As most patient have asymmetries of different kinds, it is important to point these out for the patient. It should also be stated that these still will be present after the procedure and that it is neither possible nor desirable to correct minor asymmetries. More prominent asymmetries can be minimized by measurement and careful analysis of the situation. By selection of different implants dimensions and/or shapes it may be possible to correct the asymmetry.

Other important observations that have to be made during the examination of the existing breast and thorax are the characteristics of the envelope and gland. The laxity of the envelope is of importance when selecting implant projection. Examination of laxity can be done with an anterior pull-stretch of the envelope, measuring the extensibility, or by measuring the lower pole dimension during maximum stretch of the tissues. The shape and consistency of the gland are also of great importance. A contracted tight glandular tissue increases the risk for a double-bubble deformity of the lower pole, and especially if the nipple–inframammary fold distance is short, it is extremely important to consider the implant height that should be selected. In patients with short nipple–inframammary fold distance preoperatively, a low-height implant may be favored to minimize the risk for a double-bubble deformity.

The shape of the upper breast is also of importance. If the distance to the clavicle is short and/or if the upper thorax if bulging, full-height implants may be unfavorable, whereas if the upper thorax is depressed, full-height implants may provide better upper pole shape. Another important consideration during the examination of the preoperative conditions is the shape of the bony cage, as prominence in the bony structures may be exaggerated when using form-stable implants. However, asymmetries here can also be compensated with differently shaped anatomic implants.

Having examined the biological conditions properly, the second step in selecting implants is to determine a suitable implant width. Usually a proportionate breast should have an intermammary distance between 2 and 3 cm. Laterally the new breast should respect the anterior axillary fold. By displacing the breast medially and laterally in front of the mirror, it is possible to communicate the desired and suitable width of the new breast with the patient. This can then be measured with a caliper. By subtracting the tissue cover, the appropriate implant width can be calculated. The tissue cover is measured with a pinch medially and laterally at the border of where the implant is expected to be positioned. This pinch should be done at nipple height, and as this is a double fold of tissue, the sum of the lateral and medial pinches should be divided by 2 to provide information on how much the gland adds to the width of the new breast. Having calculated ideal implant width, it is important to correlate this to the existing breast width. If the desired implant width is wider than the existing breast width, this may increase the risk for palpability and visibility of the implant. However, in patients with narrow breasts the width of the implant may have to exceed the existing breast width to provide a natural appearance of the breast. In most cases, however, the selected implant respects the width of the existing breast.

The next step in implant selection is to decide on a suitable implant height. Obviously, if a round implant is selected, this is equal to the selected width. With anatomic implants, however, the height of the implant can be varied. The height of the implant should be selected in relation to the position of the existing inframammary fold and the shape of the upper pole of the breast. The position of the nipple-areola complex after the augmentation can be predicted by arm elevation of 45 deg (see preoperative markings discussed later). This maneuver preoperatively helps to calculate where the upper and lower poles of different implant heights will be positioned. Usually half of an anatomic implant is positioned above the nipple-areola complex after the areola complex and half below. Thus the height of different implants could be divided in two and this distance measured proximal to the nipple-areola complex with arms elevated above the horizontal plane 45 deg and half measured distally. The height is then selected depending on where the existing inframammary fold is positioned. In some cases it is safe to lower this inframammary fold, but in others there is a high risk for a double-bubble deformity, and therefore it may be recommended to select a lower-height implant to come in closer connection with the existing inframammary fold than what a full-height implant might provide. After a suitable implant height and width have been selected, this is then recommended to the patient. Obviously, this "footprint" of the implant is without any volume. The volume will be provided by the selection of the suitable projection of the implant.

The next step in the selection of a suitable implant is the projection. When selecting implant projection (low, moderate, full, or extra in the Allergan Matrix system), the patient's desires and the amount of glandular tissue should be taken into consideration. An important part of the implant selection process is to communicate different implant projections by showing the patient the estimated outer border of the new breast in front of a large mirror. With the patient standing obliquely in front of the mirror, with the breast parallel to and furthest away from it, the projection of the different available implants can be demonstrated with a caliper and a cupped hand. Remember that the breast tissue will be compressed and flattened by the implant, and thus the caliper has to be pushed into the glandular tissue when projection is demonstrated. It should also be remembered when selecting a suitable implant that this has to fit the envelope. Thus if the patient has laxity, she may need more implant projection than she actually desires to fill the envelope, and in these circumstances an alternative is to combine a low-projecting implant and a mastopexy. For patients with tight envelopes who desire extra-projecting implants, these may provide tight conditions initially; however, tissues will expand over time, and it is not a contraindication to use an extra-projecting implant in a relatively flat patient. Patients should be well informed about these conditions preoperatively.

When selecting implants it is important to evaluate the patient's desires. It may be difficult to evaluate patient goals, but this is a key to success in aesthetic surgery. A well-informed patient with realistic expectations is the basis for a successful outcome. Improved patient communication can be obtained with the aid of patient educators. These specially trained nurses have more time to spend with patient, and many patients describe that situation as more relaxed compared to the usual doctor's consultation. Reviewing pictures in books and magazines can also give a better idea of the patient's preferences. A patient education book has also been written to improve communication (21). This contains a large number of before and after pictures and describes the procedures in detail, including postoperative events, risks, and complications. In our experience, it has been extremely helpful in preparing the patient for surgery. A final step in the consultation to create confidence and trust in the patient when it comes to having selected the suitable implant is to test the selected implant volume in a tight-fitting sports bra. Positioning of the actual implant into the sports bra is accurate only if the patient is completely flat. If the patient has a larger amount of glandular tissue, placement of the implant in a sports bra will provide a false picture, especially when it comes to the width of the new breast. In these cases it is better to use special sizers provided by the manufacturer (Allergan). As mentioned earlier, an important part of the definition of the patient's desires is to stand in front of a mirror together with the patient and demonstrate the estimated dimensions and borders of the new breast (Fig. 115.13).

In the early days of dimensional breast augmentation a decision tree to facilitate implant selection was developed (19). With the present approach as described here of implant selection this has become redundant. It is likely that new three-dimensional analysis and prediction systems will provide additional improvements in the implant selection process and patient communication.

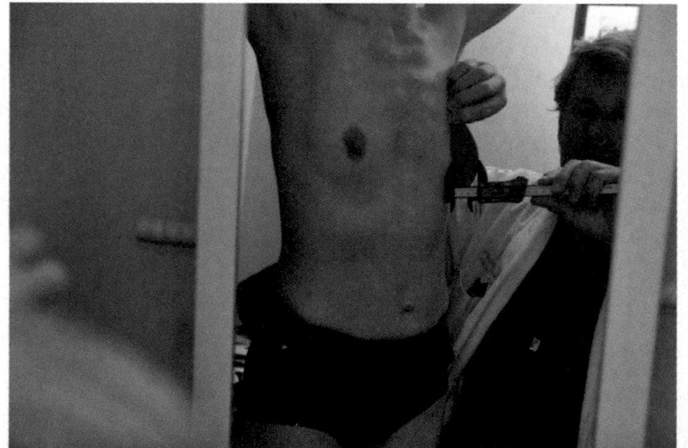

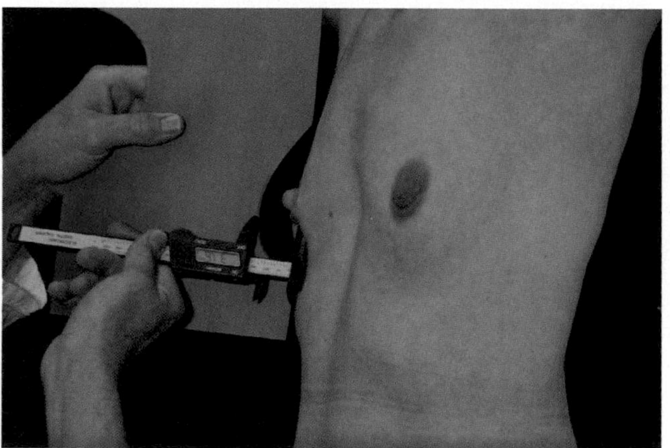

Figure 115.13. Having defined the ideal width and height of the implant, the final step in the implant selection process is to select the projection that will result in an implant volume. The projection of different implants is demonstrated for the patient in front of the mirror. **A:** When measuring tissue thickness or illustrating the projection of different implants with a caliper, mimic the effect of the implant on the breast tissue. Thus, one must compress the gland. Usually the patient can easily determine whether she desires a low-projecting **(B)** or **(C)** an extra-projecting implant.

PREOPERATIVE MARKINGS: THE AKADEMIKLINIKEN METHOD

Traditionally, breast augmentation surgery has been a relatively arbitrary procedure based on each surgeon's experience and artistry. Dimensional analysis and preoperative measurements according to the so-called Akademikliniken (AK) method have the goal of making this surgery much more precise.

Preoperative markings should answer two important questions:

1. Where on the thoracic wall should the implant be positioned? The vertical position of the implant in relation to the nipple-areola complex is of great importance for the postoperative appearance of the breast. If the implants are placed too low, the breasts will be too full in the lower pole and the nipples will point upward. For most patients, an even worse and more unnatural appearance is achieved if the implants are too high on the chest wall, resulting in downward-pointing nipple-areola complex and too-full upper poles.
2. How much skin should the lower pole of the breast have? Prediction of suitable and ideal nipple-inframammary crease distance (N-IMF) provides information on where to position the new inframammary crease, and if a submammary fold incision is to be used, the position of this is also provided. In the early days of breast augmentations surgery it was frequently stated that it is better that a submammary fold scar be located on the lower pole of the breast than on the thoracic wall. This may be true, but the best position of a submammary scar is exactly in the crease, where it is most inconspicuous. The reason that old submammary scars often ended up on the lower pole of the breast was that no good methods were available to exactly calculate the ideal amount of skin in the lower pole of the breast.

VERTICAL POSITIONING OF THE IMPLANT ON THE CHEST WALL: NIPPLE–STERNUM LINE TO IMPLANT LOWER POLE MARKINGS

When the biodimensional system for breast augmentations was introduced, a chart providing suitable areola–inframammary fold distance in relation to implant base width was provided by the manufacturer (McGhan/Allergan). These figures were based on the experiences of John Tebbetts. These areola inframammary fold (A-IMF) measurements were, however, also fairly arbitrary and based on clinical experience. Thus there was a clear need for more exact biodimensional planning. This inspired me to develop the method presented here. In the mid 1990s, two fundamental and important observations for this method were made:

1. A breast augmentation elevates the nipple-areola complex, and this elevation can be simulated by arm elevation preoperatively.
2. If a line is drawn from this predicted and new position of the nipple-areola complex to the sternum (NS), this line can be used to calculate how to position the lower pole of the implant (ILP).

See Figs. 115.14 and 115.15.

The NS line is also a valuable guide during surgery. By pressing down the breast when the patient is lying flat on her back so the NS line becomes horizontal, the appearance of the breast is visualized in spite of the fact that the patient is lying on her back. It also provides information on the level to which the muscle should be divided during a dual-plane dissection (the muscle should never be divided higher than 2 cm distal to this line). The ILP line is a valuable guide on how to position the lower pole of the implant during surgery. Measurements along the fixed sternal tissue along the midline are more exact, as they are not influenced by glandular tissue and envelope characteristics of the breast.

In a careful evaluation of several hundred breast augmentation patients it was noted that the amount of nipple elevation achieve by a breast augmentation can be accurately simulated preoperatively by the elevation of the arms 45 deg above the horizontal plane and that this only varied slightly if low to moderate full or extra-projecting implants were used (2 mm to maximum 5 mm). A simplified way to predict the new nipple position is to let the patient close her hands on top of her head (Fig. 115.16). With this position maintained, a horizontal line is then drawn between the nipple and the sternum. After most breast augmentations with implants, the nipple should ideally project centrally on the implant for the most natural postoperative appearance of the breast. Thus, knowledge of the dimensions and base plate of the

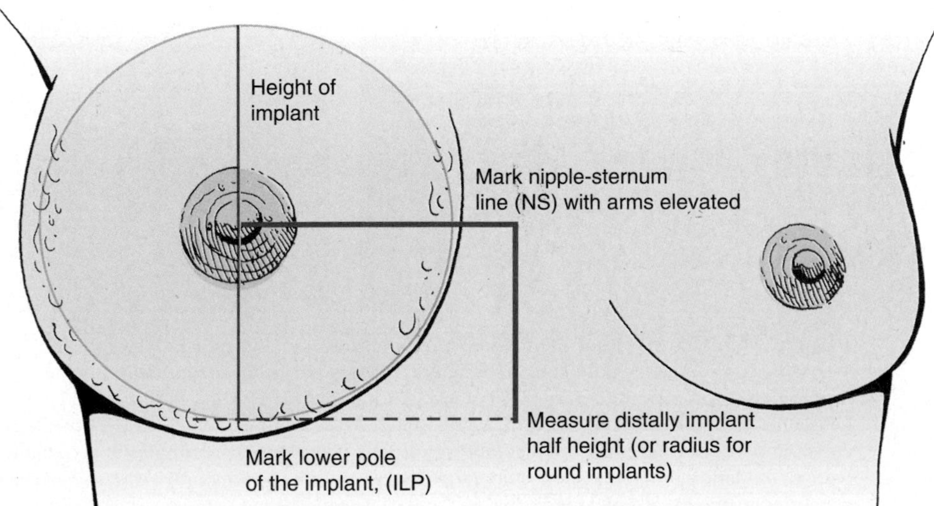

Figure 115.14. The Akademikliniken method for calculating the vertical positioning of the implant on the thoracic wall.

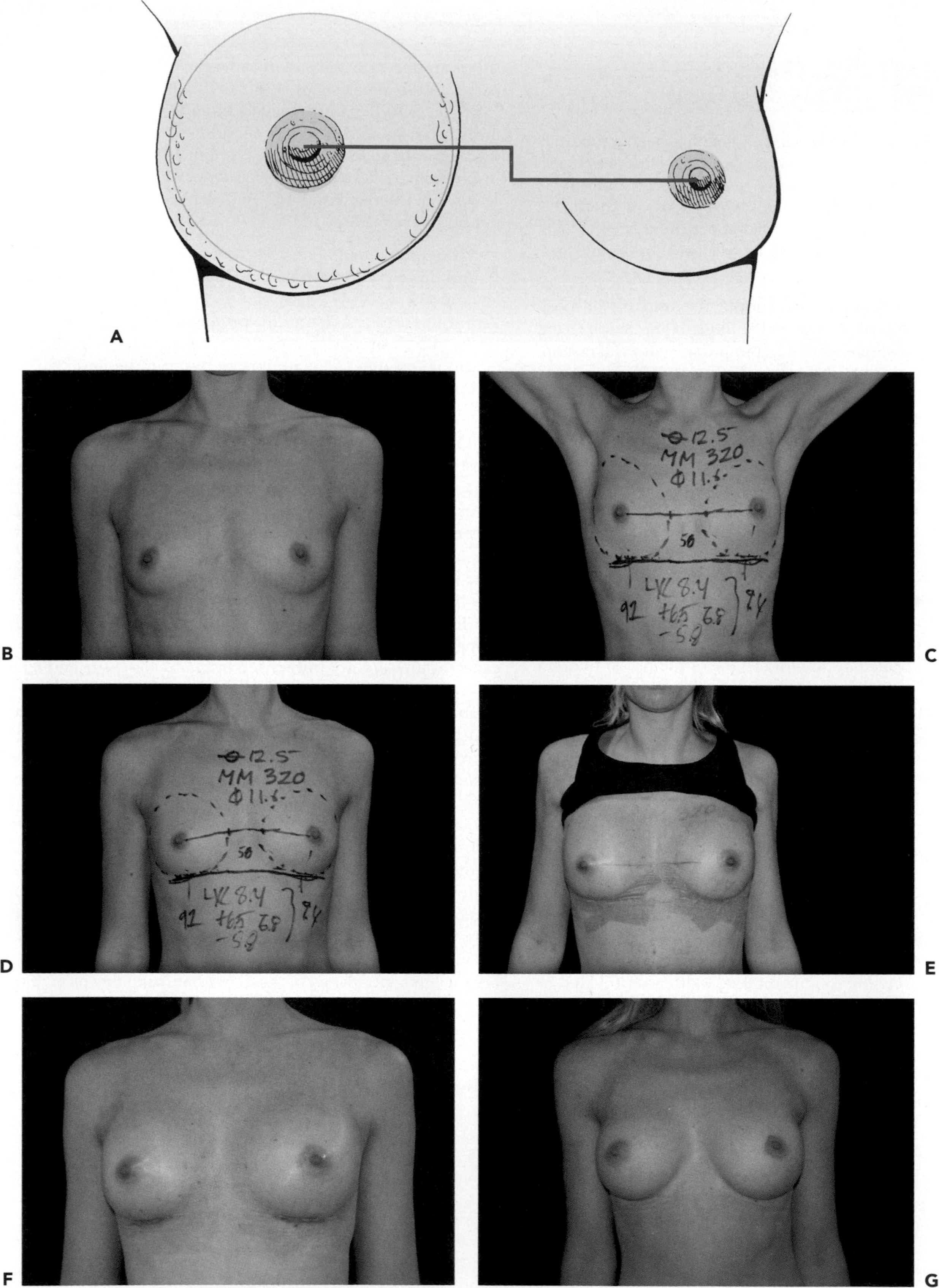

Figure 115.15. **A:** A fundamental step in nipple sternum-to-inframammary fold (NS-IMF) measurement according to the Akademikliniken (AK) method is the observation that a breast augmentation elevates the nipple-areola complex. **B:** Before preoperative markings, Style 410 MM implants, 320 g. **C:** The line drawn between the nipple and sternum with arms elevated. **D:** The appearance with the arms hanging. **E:** The appearance 4 hours after the augmentation (note the elevation of the nipples in accordance with the preoperative simulation. **F:** One week postoperative. **G:** Six months postoperative when tissues have relaxed and expanded in the lower pole.

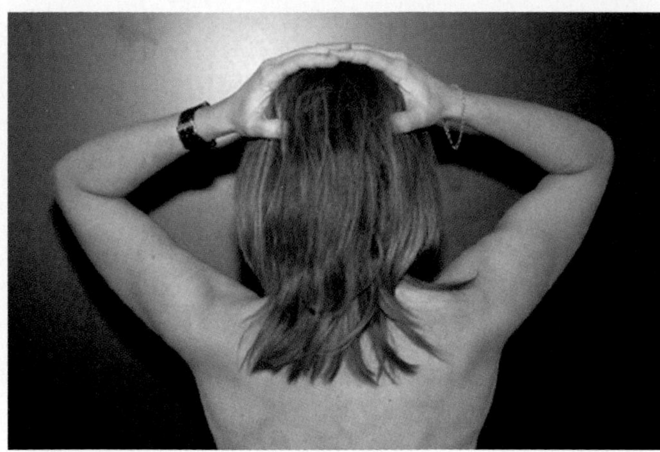

Figure 115.16. A simplified way to simulate the postoperative nipple position is to let the patient close her hands on top of her head.

implant is of great importance for calculating where the lower pole of the implant should be positioned on the operating table. With the patient's arms hanging and the patient in standing position, one half of the height of the implant or, in round implants, one half of the diameter (i.e., the radius) is measured distally along the sternal midline. In form-stable round implants 55% of the implant diameter may be favored. From the distal end of this measurement in the midline a horizontal ILP line extending laterally is drawn. This technique takes asymmetric heights of the nipple into consideration. During NS-IMF markings the NS line will be at different heights on the two breasts, and thus the lower pole positions of the implants will and should be placed at different heights to produce a natural appearance of the two asymmetric breasts, provided that the different nipple heights will not be corrected with a mastopexy.

The sequence of NS-IMF measurements and markings is summarized as follows:

1. Look up the implant base height or diameter in the manufacturer's charts.
2. Divide this number by 2, which provides the radius or half-height of the implant.
3. With the patient in standing or sitting position with the arms elevated to 45 deg above the horizontal plane (hands on the top of the head), draw a horizontal line between the nipple and the sternum (NS line).
4. After the patient lowers her arms, measure distally from the inner part of the NS line and one half the height of the implant inferiorly from this distal point along the sternum, extend a horizontal line (ILP) laterally under the breast. This line is then used to guide the surgeon where to position the lower pole of the implant on the operating table.

CALCULATION OF THE LENGTH OF LOWER BREAST POLE SKIN: NIPPLE–INFRAMAMMARY FOLD LENGTH

Marking of the distance of skin needed between the nipple and the new inframammary fold in the augmented breast depends on the following factors:

1. The base plate dimensions and the projection of the implant
2. The amount of covering glandular tissue
3. The envelope characteristics (loose or tight tissue)

Two different measurements have to be added to gain knowledge about ideal N-IMF distance, as follows (Fig. 115.17).

Length of the Lower Ventral Curvature of the Implant

It is surprising that we have been doing breast augmentation surgery for more than 40 years without clear attention to the obvious fact that a breast implant with a larger base plate and more projection needs considerably more and longer nipple–inframammary fold distance than a breast with much less projection and base plate dimensions. The amount of skin in relation to the implant is equal to the distance between the ideal projection point on the ventral surface of the implant measured to its lower border. This so-called lower ventral curvature (LVC) of the implant is a measurement that is not provided by the manufacturer. I have made all of these measurements for a number of different implants, however, and have also provided these to the manufacturers. Upon request the lower ventral curve dimensions of several implants can be obtained from some manufacturers (e.g., Allergan). For implants without the LVC value available a simple way for the surgeon to obtain knowledge about this important distance is to make a drawing on a piece of paper with the radius or half

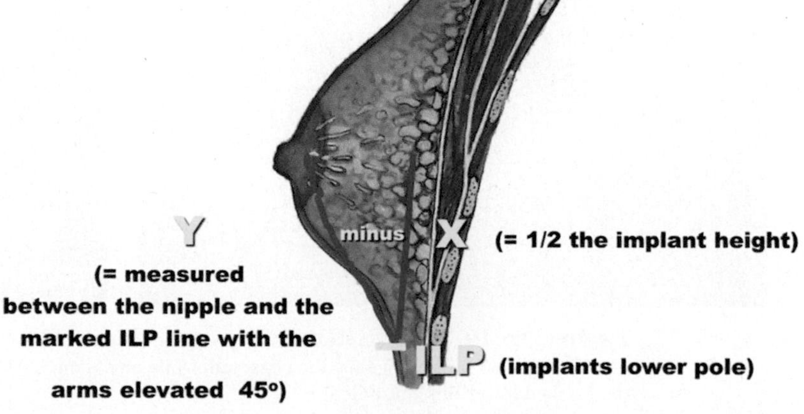

Figure 115.17. Cross section of the breast. The length of skin needed between the nipple and the new inframammary fold (N-IMF) in the augmented breast is equal to the lower ventral curvature (LVC) of the implant plus the distance that has to be added for the amount of covering glandular tissue.

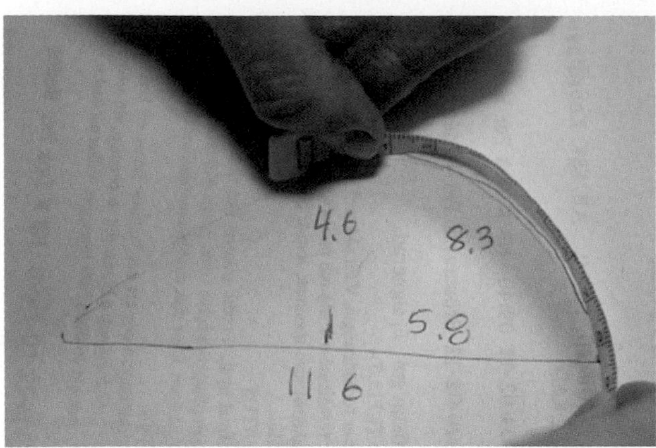

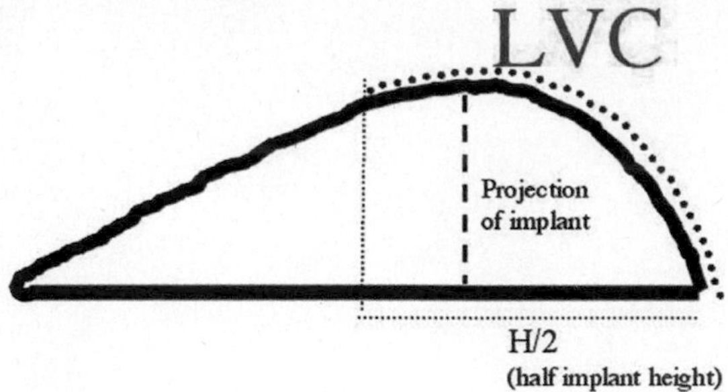

Figure 115.18. The lower ventral curvature (LVC) for an implant can be measured on a 1:1 sketch of the implants with a tape measure. This provides information on how long the nipple–inframammary fold (N-IMF) distance should be with respect to the implant's dimensions.

the height of the implant on the *X* axis and the projection of the implant on the *Y* axis. Measuring between these two points with a tape measure slightly curved similar to the surface of the implant provides information on how long the N-IMF distance should be with respect to the implant's lower ventral surface (Fig. 115.18 and Table 115.1). If the patient is completely flat, the ideal distance between the nipple and the new inframammary fold is equal to this LVC of the implant, but as most patients have a certain amount of covering glandular tissue, this also has to be taken into consideration when calculating ideal length between the nipple and the new inframammary fold and/or where to make a submammary fold incision.

Nipple–Inframammary Fold Distance in Relation to Amount of Covering Glandular Tissue

Calculating the amount of lengthening of the N-IMF distance in relation to the amount of glandular tissue can be done in three different ways.

1. The most accurate way is to measure the convex side of the breast and subtract the "inside." This can be done after marking of the NS-ILP lines according to the foregoing description. If the patient once again folds her hands on top of her head and a tape measure is used to measure the distance between the nipple and the ILP line marked as described earlier, the convex breast mold can be registered. From this figure the NS-ILP distance (= the radius of the implant for round implants or one-half the height of anatomic implants) should be subtracted. This NS-ILP distance is equal to the "inside" of the breast. This equation yields the distance that has to be added to the LVC of the implant as described previously. The resulting sum [LVC (lower venral curvature of the implant) + N-ILP (nipple to ILP line distance) − ½ the implant height] is equal to the ideal N-IMF distance after the augmentation. Observe that breast implants compress the glandular tissue when inserted into the breast, and thus the nipple should be slightly compressed while measuring the distance between the nipple and the marked ILP line (Fig. 115.19).
2. The second way to calculate how much distance has to be added to the LVC of the implant is to measure a pinch of the gland straight across the nipple areola complex and divide this by 2. This is slightly less accurate than the method just given, but the correlation is relatively good. This method is also favored in secondary augmentation.
3. The third way is not a true calculation but rather an estimation of how much skin that has to be added to the LVC measurement of the implant to gain information about the ideal distance between the nipple and the new inframammary fold. In very small breasts the added distance is 0 to 1 cm, in

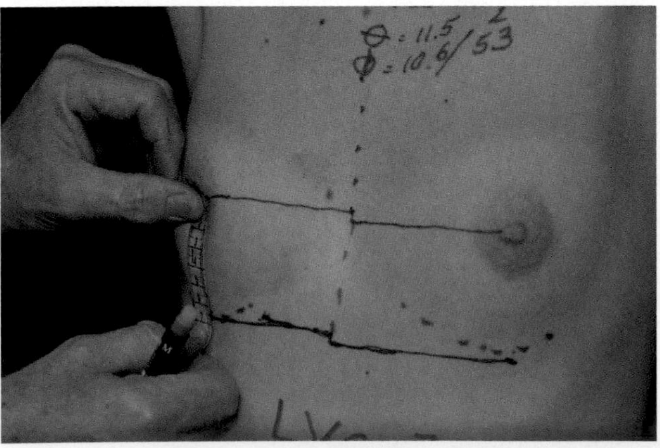

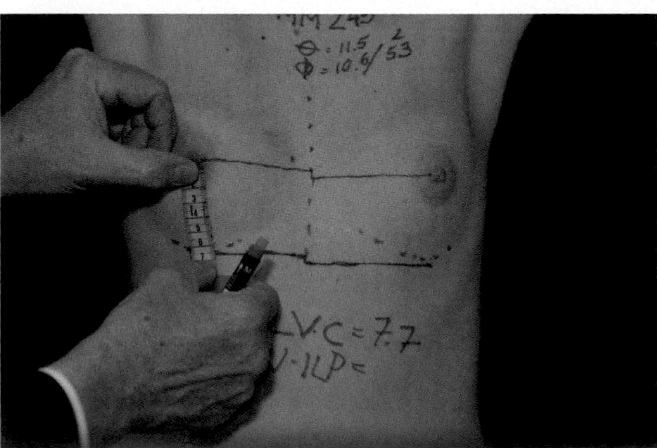

Figure 115.19. Breast implants compress the glandular tissue when inserted into the breast, and thus the nipple has to be pressed against the chest wall while one is measuring the distance between the nipple and the marked lower implant pole line.

TABLE 115.1 Akademikliniken (AK) preoperative marking system by Per Hedén© Allergan Style 410 implants
Implants LVC (lower ventral curvaure) measurment

Baseø	*FL*	*LVC*	*FM*	*LVC*	*FF*	*LVC*	*FX*	*LVC*	*ML*	*LVC*	*MM*	*LVC*	*MF*	*LVC*	*MX*	*LVC*	*LL*	*LVC*	*LM*	*LVC*	*LF*	*LVC*	*LX*	*LVC*
9,5			155	7,1	160	7,3	185	7,8					140	6,5	165	7,2					125	6,1	145	6,7
10	140	6,8	180	7,4	185	7,6	215	8,2	125	6	160	6,6	165	6,9	195	7,6			140	6,3	150	6,5	175	7,1
10,5			205	7,7	220	8	245	8,6			185	6,9	195	7,2	225	7,9	135	6,1			175	6,9	195	7,5
11	190	7,4	235	8	255	8,3	280	9	170	6,6	215	7,2	225	7,5	255	8,2			190	7	205	7,4	225	7,9
11,5	220	7,7	270	8,3	290	8,6	315	9,3	195	7	245	7,7	255	7,9	290	8,6	180	6,7	220	7,4	240	7,7	255	8,3
12	250	8,1	310	8,7	335	8,9	360	9,7	220	7.4	280	8	295	8,3	325	9	210	7	250	7,8	270	8	290	8,6
12,5			350	9	375	9,3	410	10			320	8,4	335	8,7	370	9,4	240	7,4					330	9
13	320	8,6	395	9,4	425	9,8	450	10,4	285	8,1	360	8,8	375	9,1	410	9,8			320	8,4	310	8,6	365	9,3
13,5			440	9,8	475	10,1	495	10,8			400	9,2	420	9,4	445	10,1	14	8,1			390	8,9	405	9,6
14			500	10,2	535	10,5	560	11-2			450	9,5	470	9,7	520	10,4					440	9,3	455	10
14,5			550	10,5	595	10,8	615	11-3					525	10	550	10,7					490	9,7	515	10,3
15			605	10,8	655	11,1	690	11,7					580	10,4	620	11					540	10	570	10,7
15,5			670	11,1	740	11,5	775	12,11					640	10,8	685	11,3					595	10,4	625	11,1

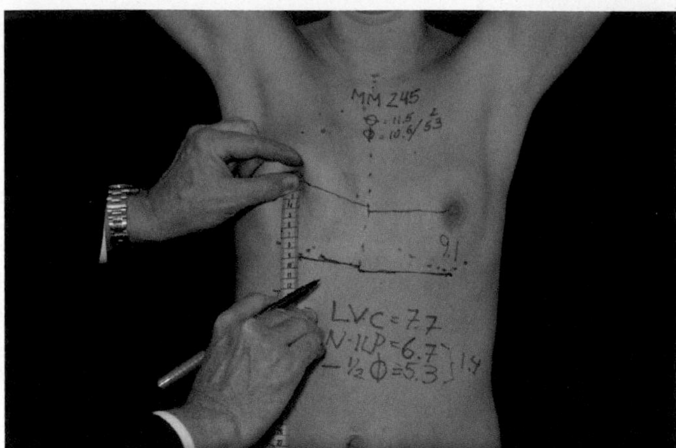

Figure 115.20. When marking the amount of skin between the nipple and the inframammary fold, the breast skin should be stretched so as to mimic the stretching effect of the implant.

the average-sized typical breast for augmentation it is between 1 and 1.5 cm, and only in the large breast is the distance added to the LVC greater than 2 cm.

When marking the ideal N-IMF distance (A + B), one should stretch the breast skin so as to mimic the stretching effect of the implant. This maneuver is recommended to compensate for the characteristics of the breast envelope. If an inframammary fold incision is planned, the NS-IMF distance calculated in this way provides information on where this incision should be positioned (Fig. 115.20). In a standard breast augmentation the IPL line and the marked ideal N-IMF fall into the one and same line. In patients with laxity of the breast the incision may end up above the ILP line, and thus dissection is done distal to the incision to provide space for lower positioning of the implant. In tight-skin individuals requesting large implants the marked incision may end up distal to the ILP line, and thus skin has to be recruited to the lower pole of the breast. If the distance between ILP line and the incision (N-ILP measurement) exceeds 2 cm, it may be difficult to line up these two lines with the sutures at the end of the procedure (see later discussion), and some faults in the implant selection or preoperative planning are likely. This way of performing submammary fold incisions is considerably different from the standard techniques, and I have thus named it "the new submammary fold" incision or the "AK" incision.

SURGICAL TECHNIQUE IN BIODIMENSIONAL BREAST AUGMENTATION

The importance of preoperative markings and measurements plus careful analysis cannot be stressed enough. Poor planning is usually the basis for a poor result. Although many different surgical techniques can provide excellent results, some techniques are prone to a higher incidence of postoperative malposition and complication. In my 30 years of experience in breast augmentation surgery it has been my observation that blind and blunt dissection, especially in combination with axillary incisions and round, smooth implants, has a significantly higher incidence of malposition and poorer long-term results than the techniques that I use today, which are described in what follows.

SUBGLANDULAR VERSUS SUBMUSCULAR IMPLANT POSITION

Both subglandular and submuscular implant positioning can provide excellent results. In the submuscular position, thicker soft-tissue cover over implant edges is provided. Thereby less implant visibility, especially in the most important part of the breast, the upper medial pole, is likely. Thicker soft-tissue cover also results in less visible rippling and irregularities of implants. Long term, submuscular implants may have less tendency to become ptotic due to capsular adhesion to the rigid ribcage. Because the implant is covered by the muscle, it is also likely that less glandular atrophy will develop. Contrary to common belief, the submuscular technique is a quicker surgical dissection. Subglandular positioning of the implant, on the other hand, results in less movement of the breast during pectoralis muscle activity. Division of the distal medial origin of the pectoralis muscle during submuscular implantation may produce indentation and irregularities during muscle activities. In subglandular placement this risk does not exist. It is also initially less painful to have an implant inserted in the subglandular position. In the ptotic and in the tuberous breast it is easier to achieve a natural appearance with subglandular implantation. Subglandular implant position also reduces the risk for double-bubble deformity in the lower pole of the breast. This risk is more pronounced if a contracted lower pole exists preoperatively.

Typical patients for submuscular implant positioning are thin with poor upper pole cover and no ptosis. A larger amount of glandular tissue and ptotic breast appearance are indications for subglandular placement. Submuscular and subglandular implant positionings produce different appearances with muscle tension. Even if the lower medial origin of the pectoralis muscle is divided, the breast will shift laterally and the intermammary distance will increase during muscle tension. In subglandular implant positioning more implant edge definition may become visible during pectoralis muscle tightening (Fig. 115.21). With dual-plane II-IV (see later discussion) dissection the aforementioned disadvantages with submuscular positioning has been minimized and animation during pectoralis tightening can be minimal (Fig. 115.22).

With the NS-IMF measurements described in this chapter the upper border of the implant can be located and marked on the chest wall prior to surgery. A pinch test in the glandular tissue in this area is a useful guideline for deciding whether submuscular or subglandular implant positioning should be selected. If the pinch test is less than 2 cm, then submuscular implant placement is always favorable. If the pinch is more than 2 to 3 cm (larger breasts), then subglandular placements is possible but frequently not advocated due to the benefits of dual-plane muscle dissection. However, clear indications for subglandular placement still exist.

INCISIONS

When using AHCSIs, it is possible to insert these through a periareolar, axillary, or submammary incision. Due to the more cohesive gel and firmer nature of the implant, a slightly longer incision is needed than when performing implantation with a less cohesive implant. Usually 5 to 5.5 cm is sufficient. In large implants, the incision may need to be extended to 6 or even 6.5 cm. Smaller form-stable implants (around 150 cc) may even safely be inserted through a 4-cm incision. Even if a different

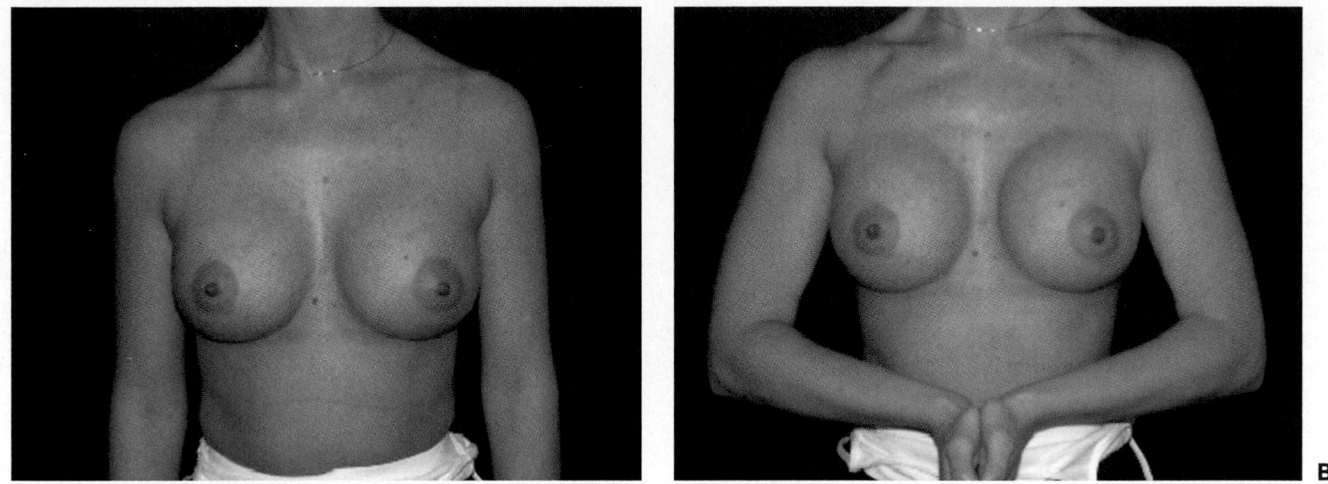

Figure 115.21. **A:** Subglandular high-cohesiveness silicon breast implant without capsular contraction. **B:** Implant edge definition and visibility increase during pectoralis muscle tightening.

type of incision could be used, I prefer the "new submammary fold" incision described in this chapter. When using AHCSIs, it is of great importance that the implant be positioned correctly and that no folds or buckles are present after implantation. This is much easier to control through an inframammary fold incision. Two longitudinal marking dots on the ventral surface of the lower pole of the Style 410 implants are easily palpated from this incision. Another advantage of the inframammary route is less sensory nerve loss compared to the periareolar and axillary incisions. There is also less contamination of the implant compared to these types of incisions. From the submammary fold it is also easy to inspect the whole implant pocket and have good control of the implant positioning, but perhaps most important is the superior control of the dual-plane

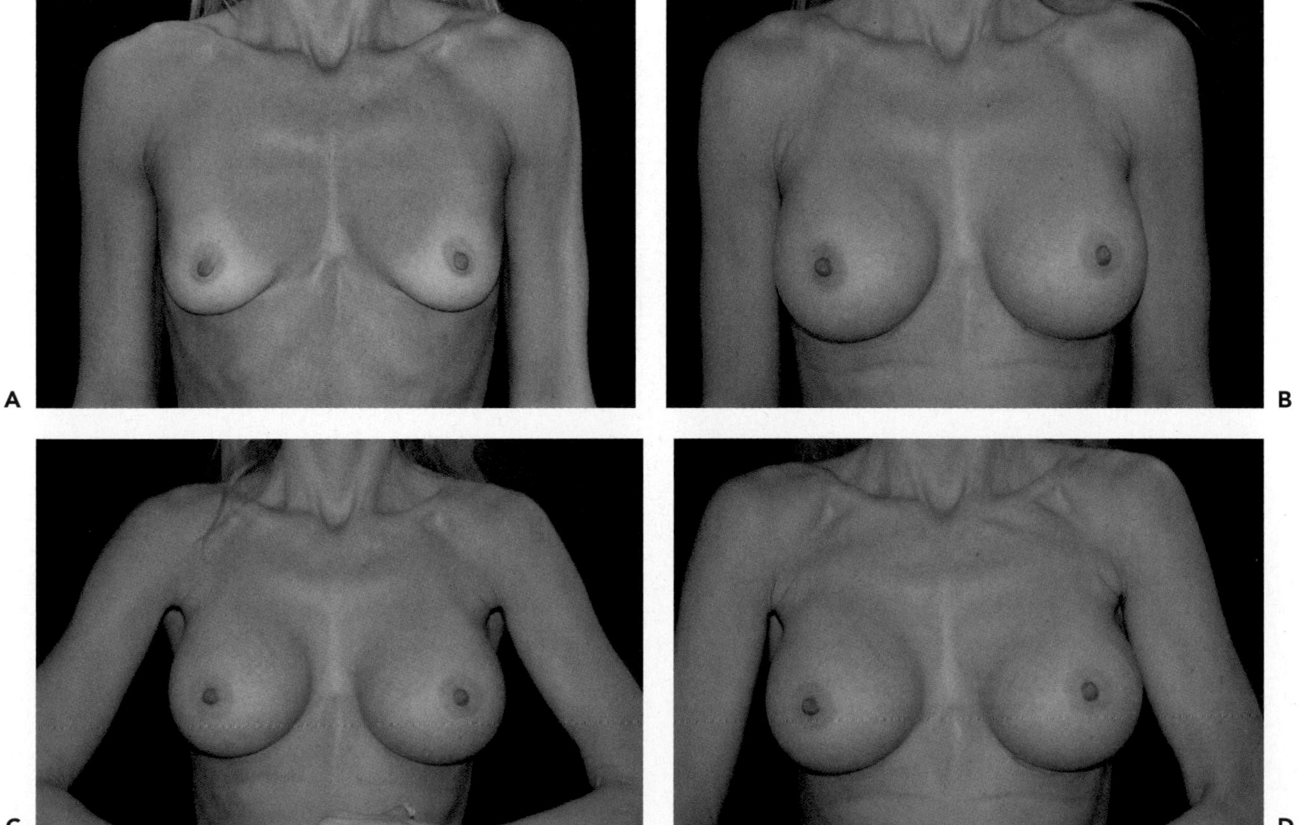

Figure 115.22. During dual plane II to IV dissection, the subglandular dissection allows the lateral pectoralis to retract and minimize animation. Note that the medial origin of the muscle should be preserved. The medial muscle division should always respect the previously marked nipple sternum (NS) line with at least 2 to 3 cm. **A:** Before dual-plane II-III submuscular breast augmentation with Style 410 MM 280-g implants. **B, C:** Three months later with relaxed pectoralis muscle. **D:** During tightening of the pectoralis muscle.

dissection and the division of the pectoralis major muscle origin. Inframammary fold scars are also improved if the suturing technique described in what follows is used.

There is only one disadvantage of the inframammary fold incision compared to other types of incisions—it results in a scar located in the fold. The main reason for the development of periareolar and axillary incisions was the desire to improve and hide the scar. The previous poor reputation of the inframammary fold incision was due to the fact that the final location of the incision was often suboptimal. It was common that the scars were placed on the lower pole of the breast instead of the fold. With the AK measuring technique described earlier the ideal location of the incision can be calculated and the incision based on the new submammary fold position. To improve the appearance of the scar, a specific suturing technique described later is also included in this technique. A series of 30 patients with breast augmentation scars in two locations has been evaluated. On one hand, these patients had a previous scar located either periareolar or axillary, and, on the other hand, they also had the new submammary fold scar. More than 70% of the patients perceived the new submammary fold scar as better than their previous scar, 20% that there was no difference, and only 10% that the periareolar or axillary scar was better than this new way of making a submammary fold incision (Fig. 115.23).

Submammary fold incisions resulting in scars located in the lower pole of the breast are much more visible than scars located exactly in the new submammary fold. The AK measuring technique described in this chapter is a tool for locating the scar exactly in the new submammary fold. If pronounced capsular contraction develops, it is common that scars located on the lower pole of the breast may develop indentation due to fibrous bands between the skin and the implant capsule (Fig. 115.24). In contrast, a scar located in the fold may even be improved if it is pulled deeper into the fold.

OPERATIVE PROCEDURE

It is recommended that the procedure be commenced with a liberal injection of local anesthesia along the planned dissection borders. Infiltration is given into muscle and fascia. Up to 100 cc of 0.25% Xylocaine with epinephrine (5 μg/mL) can be used. This minimizes anesthesia depth and perioperative bleeding. It has not been found to increase postoperative bleeding and adds significantly to postoperative pain relief. It has even been shown that the effect of pain relief is longer lasting than that with local anesthesia itself (22). Local anesthesia also speeds up the recovery time significantly, and the majority of patients can be ambulatory within 2 to 5 hours after surgery.

Useful equipment and instrumentation for the surgical procedure are fiberoptic retractors and xenon forehead lights. Use of Colorado-tip tungsten needles with cutting cautery speeds up the surgical procedure considerably. A large variation in cautery equipment quality and capacity exists. My preference is the Valleylab Force FX cautery equipment with spray blend mode. This reduces intraoperative bleeding to a minimum. Other useful tools include different retractors such as those designed by Tebbetts (Karl Storz, Culver City, CA) and insulated cauterizing forceps.

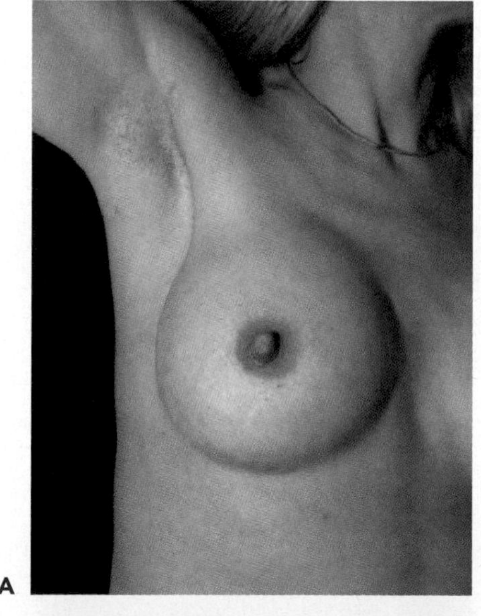
A

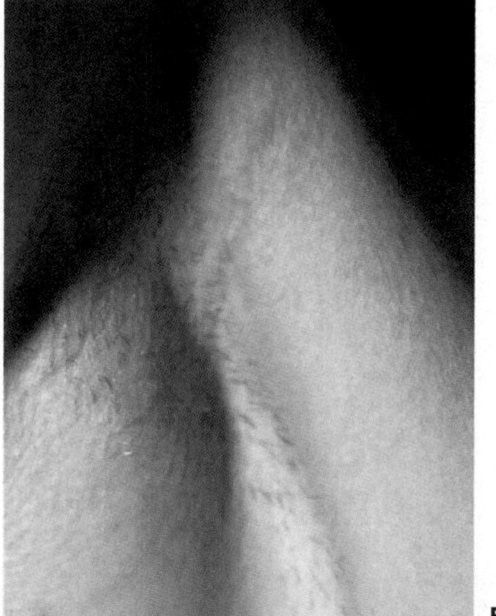
B

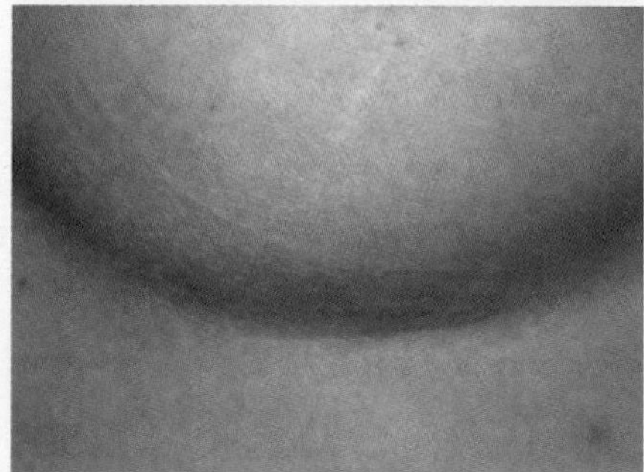
C

Figure 115.23. **A:** Patient with both an old axillary scar (**B**) and a newer submammary scar (**C**) who experienced a much better cosmetic appearance of the submammary scar made with the dimensional calculation according to the Akademikliniken method.

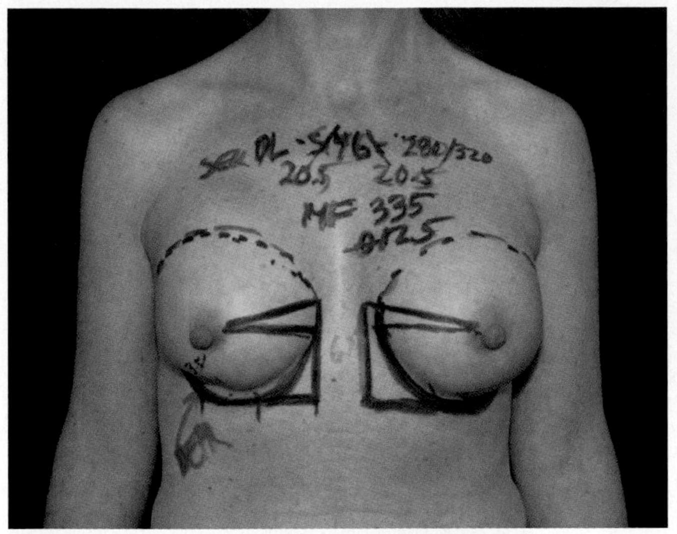

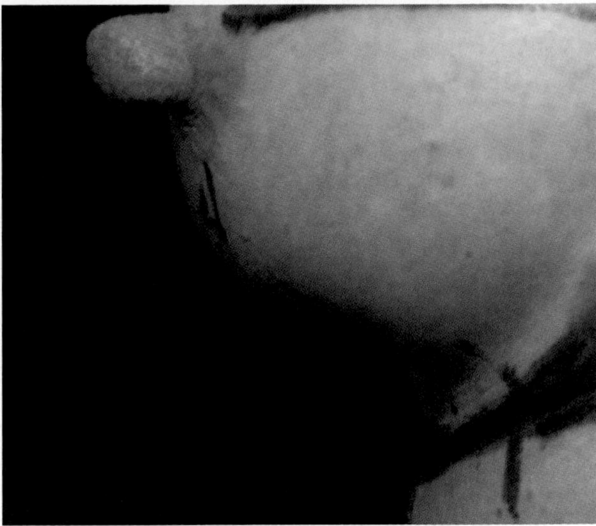

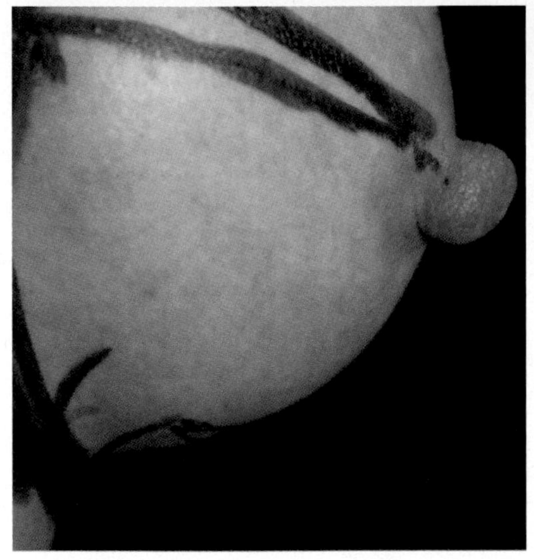

Figure 115.24. Scars should be mathematically located in the new submammary fold location. **A:** If the incision is more arbitrary, it tends to be located on the lower pole of the breast. **B:** If capsular contraction occurs as in the right breast, indentation due to fibrous bands between the skin and the implant capsule may occur. **C:** Compare to the even skin surface on the noncontracted left breast.

After incision of the skin with a scalpel blade, the rest of the dissection is done with the cutting cautery using the Colorado tip. The initial dissection is vertical down to the superficial thoracic fascia, which is followed cranially past the border of the pectoralis major muscle. If a submuscular implant position is planned, the amount of dissection superiorly along the anterior surface of the pectoralis muscle depends on the type of dual-plane dissection that will be undertaken. In youthful, well-shaped breasts without ptosis, dual-plane II dissection is favored. The lower border of the pectoralis muscle is exposed and freed up to the level of the nipple-areola complex. A simple way to identify the border between pectoralis and serratus anterior is to percutaneously pinch the pectoralis muscle in the axilla and stimulate the muscle fibers with the cautery. Twitching of muscles fibers in the axilla clearly illustrates which fibers are pectoralis major and which are serratus anterior. The pectoralis muscle is then divided horizontally a couple of centimeters above the level of the ILP line (see earlier discussion). This leaves a rigid structure on the chest wall for later suturing of the fold (Fig. 115.25). Dual-plane dissection permits the lateral small pectoralis muscle flap to retract and eliminates the risk for visible banding and irregularities during muscle animation. The division of the muscle is slightly oblique and while pulling the muscle ventrally with a forceps. Thus muscle division is more parallel to the ribcage than perpendicular. This weakens the lower border of the muscle and permits better transition between the subglandular and the submuscular parts of the implant pocket. When entering the submuscular plane a loose connective tissue layer is entered. This tissue should be left intact on top of the ribs in an attempt to help to reduce the risk of postoperative seroma, hematoma, and pain. Thus the dissection should not be blunt. Instead, it is carried out with a cutting cautery directly below the deep side of the pectoralis muscle. The distal medial origin of the pectoralis muscle is divided from the deep side with cutting cautery. The muscle division is carried on until the fat is seen on top of the muscle. Medially, the muscle division is curved slightly cranially, but it should be noted that the preoperatively marked NS line always should be respected. To minimize irregularities along the sternal border, it is important that muscle division be stopped 2 to 3 cm distal to the NS line.

In a tuberous and/or ptotic breast the subglandular dissection is carried on further superiorly along the surface of the pectoralis muscle. In dual-plane III dissection the muscle division is similar to what is described for dual-plane II dissection but the subglandular dissection goes past the level of the nipple-areola complex. In dual-plane IV dissection the pectoralis muscle is

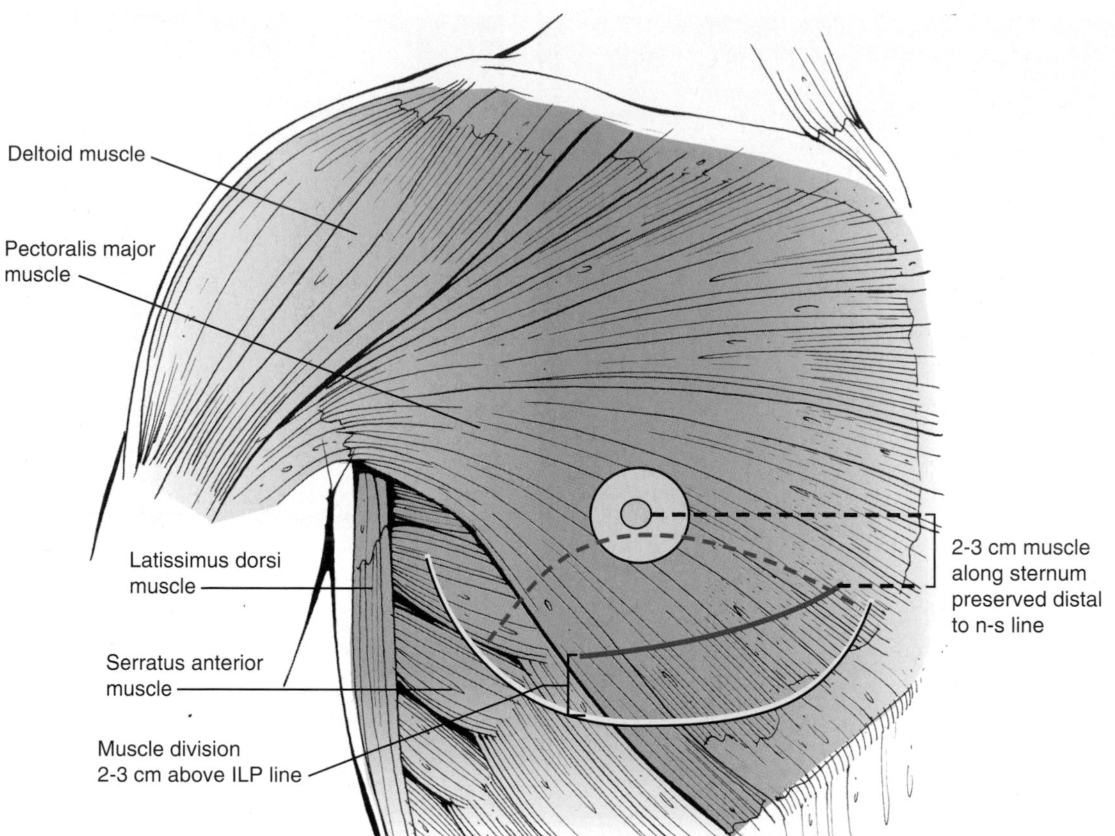

Figure 115.25. Performing the dual-plane II and III procedure is the most common technique in naturally shaped youthful breasts. The subglandular or subfascial dissection on top of the pectoralis muscle is done to the level of the nipple-areola complex (II) or slightly above it (III). The muscle is then divided distally but well above the lower pole of the implant (ILP) line to provide a rigid structure for the later anchoring of the incision to the inframammary fold. The weakened lateral pectoralis flap retracts and minimizes animation during pectoralis activity. The nipple-sternum line in the midline is respected, and usually division of the muscle should be kept well below this level (2 to 3 cm).

divided laterally higher up on the chest wall and the muscle division is more parallel to the fibers but still respecting the N-S line at the sternum as mentioned previously. In this dual-plane IV dissection the subglandular dissection is 2 to 3 cm higher than in dual-plane III dissection. This technique provides the benefit of the subglandular position without adhesion of the implant capsule to the ribcage in the lower pole of the breast. Dual-plane IV dissection is favored in tuberous and the more pronounced ptotic breasts (Fig. 115.26). This new type of dual-plane dissection is different than previous descriptions (23,24).

In all submuscular dissections the space between pectoralis major and minor muscles is entered, and thus the pectoralis minor should be left intact on top of the ribs. A safe way to minimize the risk for elevation of this muscle is to first dissect in the direction of the sternal notch when the submuscular level has been entered as described. From the upper part of the implant pocket the dissection is carried out laterally, thus easily entering between the two pectoralis muscles. The most lateral part of the dissection should be careful, and this is the only part of the dissection that could be blunt to minimize the risk for sensory nerve injury. When the dissection is complete the implant pocket dimensions can be measured with a steel ruler. The width of the pocket should only exceed that of the implant by about 0.5 cm on each side, and thus, in contrast to when using smooth, non–form-stable implants, a snug-fitting implant pocket should be created.

If a subglandular or subfascial implant position is planned, the dissection is carried along as described previously but only along the anterior surface of the pectoralis major muscle. Similar to the submuscular implant positioning, the lateral part of the pocket may be extended bluntly. When using AHCSIs in the subglandular position it is very important not to underdissect the pocket cranially. It is easy to underestimate the height of the pocket, and it is mandatory to check this with a steel ruler. If the height of the pocket is too short, an AHCSI implant may bend in the weaker upper pole and produce a buckle as the capsule develops (16). The height of the implant pocket should exceed the implant height by approximately 1 to 2 cm, thus allowing draping of the gland without risk of buckling of the upper pole. As for submuscular implants, however, the pocket width should not exceed the base width of the implant by more than 0.5 cm on each side.

In a breast with a constricted lower pole, subglandular implant positioning or dual-plane dissection with only upper pole muscle cover is recommended. In these tuberous breasts, it is also important to divide the glandular tissue in the lower pole. This could be done as a flap or radial from the center of the breast to the new submammary fold. Spreading of the constricted gland on top of the implant reduces the risk for a double-bubble deformity in the lower pole. Dividing the gland is also easiest done with the cutting cautery. A smooth and naturally transitioning zone between implant lower border and

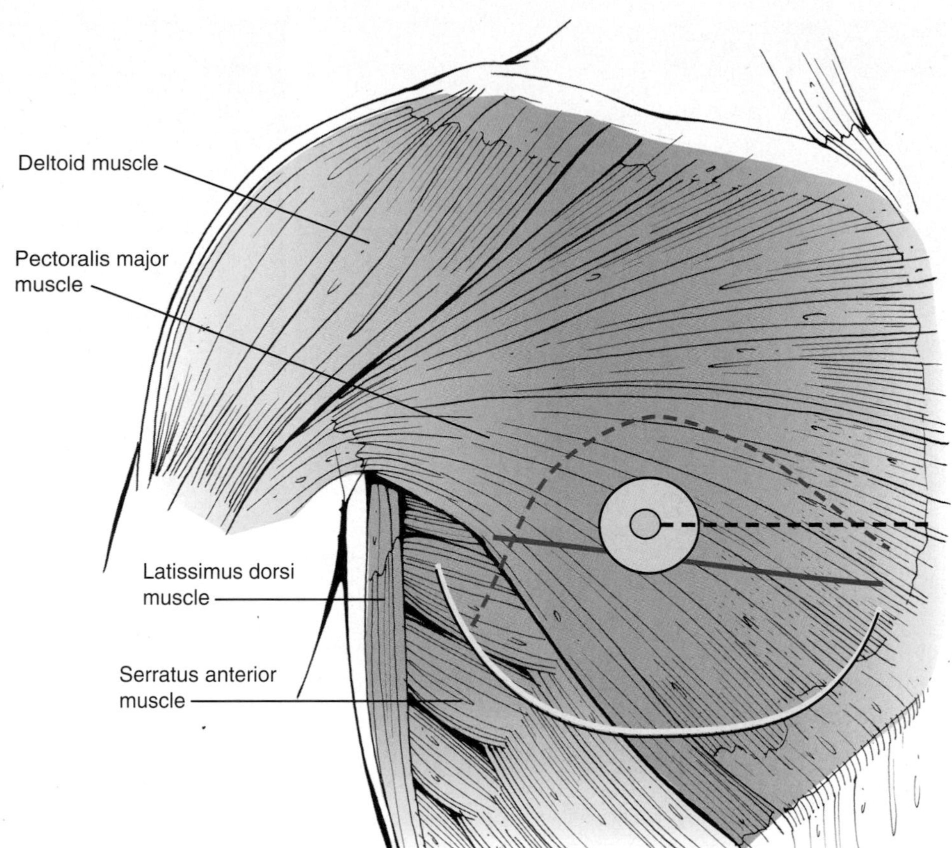

Figure 115.26. Dual-plane IV techniques are useful in patients with severe ptosis or in tuberous breasts. The subglandular or subfascial dissections in these cases are more extensive, going well above the nipple-areola complex, and the muscle division is higher laterally (close to the nipple level). The dissection of the pectoralis muscle is more parallel to the muscle fibers, but in the midline the nipple-sternum line is still respected by at least 2 to 3 cm. This creates a true subglandular position of the lower pole of the implant without attachment to the ribs.

glandular tissue should be seen at completion of the procedure.

IMPLANTATION

It is important not to force AHCSI implants through too small a hole, which may produce a fracture in the high-cohesiveness gel and result in irregularities of the breast surface. Lubrication of the implant can facilitate implantation. Soaking of the implant in saline is usually sufficient. Other options are Betadine solution or sterile Xylocaine gel. Betadine is prohibited in many countries.

A simplified way to insert the implant is to hold the implant at a 90-deg angle below the retractor. Usually the implant slides easily into place if the upper pole of the implant first is rotated into the pocket followed by alternating pushing of the right and left sides of the implant. After implantation, it is mandatory to control implant rotation. Most AHCSIs have indicator dots or lines to illustrate the vertical axis of the implant. The axis of these should be carefully aligned along the desired vertical line before closure of the pocket. Implant edges should be palpated and lie flat on the thoracic wall. No implant folds or buckling should be accepted. If this is noted, the implant should be taken out and the pocket adjusted. After hemostasis and correct implant position are ensured, the wound is closed. With the cutting cautery technique describe earlier, bleeding is usually insignificant and drains are not necessary. To improve submammary fold scars, the suturing technique is very important. Scarpa's fascia should be fixed to the thoracic fascia. Before doing this, the lower pole of the implant should be adjusted to the ILP line as described earlier. Usually three stitches are placed along this line with a strong bite in the thoracic fascia and muscle. The middle one is first inserted and left untied until the lateral and medial ones have been closed. By suturing the supra Scarpa's fascia layer to thoracic wall, the scar is usually confined to the fold even during arm elevation postoperatively (Fig. 115.27). This deep suturing is than followed by deep dermal stitching. A ridge suturing technique is recommended in the deep dermal layer (Fig. 115.28). This is followed by a subcuticular running suture. Usually the only suture material used is Monocryl or Monosyn 3/0. Other suture material may produce equally good results. Selection depends on the surgeon's preferences.

RESULTS

From 1995 to 2009 we implanted close to 12,000 AHCSI (Style 410) implants. Previous review (19) of 1,676 of these implants revealed a low frequency of capsular contraction problems (4.2%). Other complications included seroma (0.7%) and postoperative hematoma (0.6%). These were treated without further healing problems. Infections were seen in 14 patients (1.7%) mainly in the combined mastopexy augmentations. Only 3 patients with pure augmentation had infections. Two patients had implants removed due to infections. Since prophylactic antibiotics were introduced in the second half of the 1990s, no further infection has been noted in primary augmentations. Rotations have been seen but have been uncommon (0.42%). These implants should not be inserted into old implant pockets, especially if these are the result of previously used smooth implants. I described the creation of a neo-submuscular pocket in the late 1990s, and this is a very safe and good way to also treat complications such as rotation, descent, poor animation during pectoralis activity, and so on. The

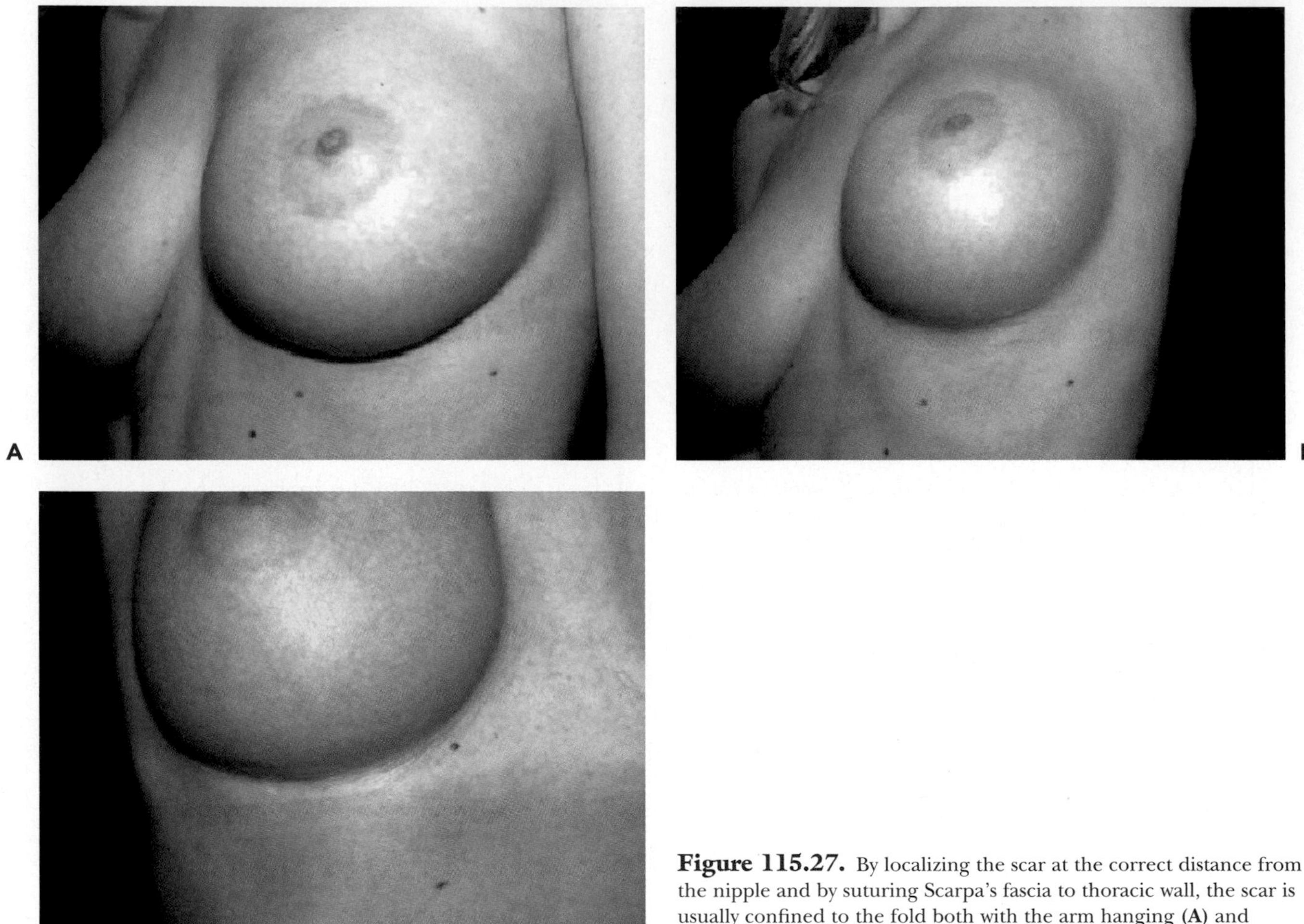

Figure 115.27. By localizing the scar at the correct distance from the nipple and by suturing Scarpa's fascia to thoracic wall, the scar is usually confined to the fold both with the arm hanging **(A)** and elevated **(B)**. **C:** Close-up 6 months after meticulous ridge suturing.

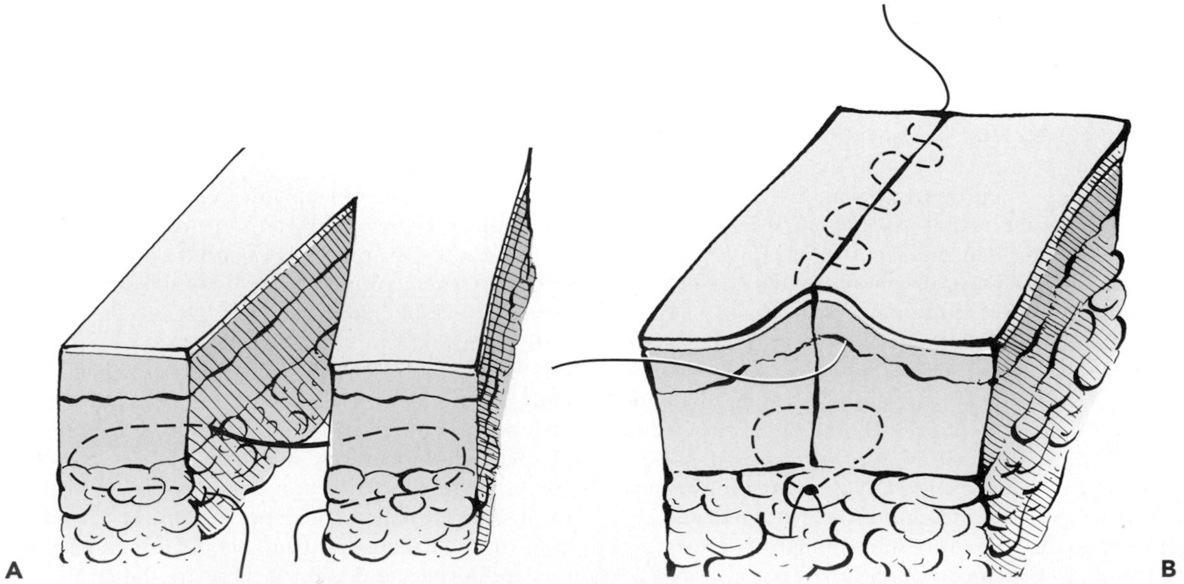

A B

Figure 115.28. Deep dermal suture relaxation and long postoperative surgical taping (Micropore) prevents scar widening and counteracts scar hyperactivity. **A, B:** The ridge suture is placed deeper at the wound edge and more superficial far away from the wound edge. (*continued*)

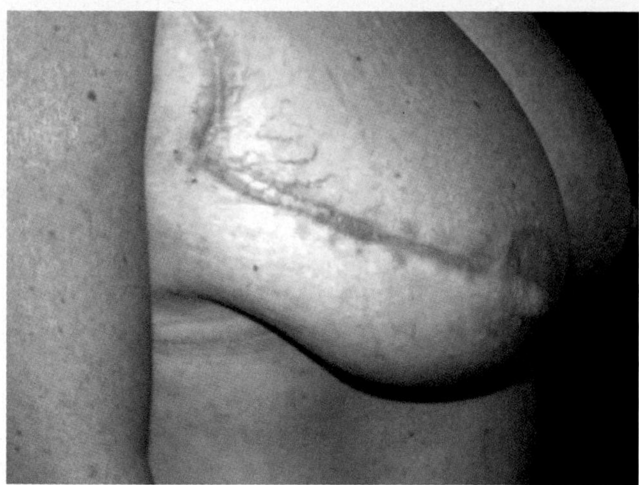

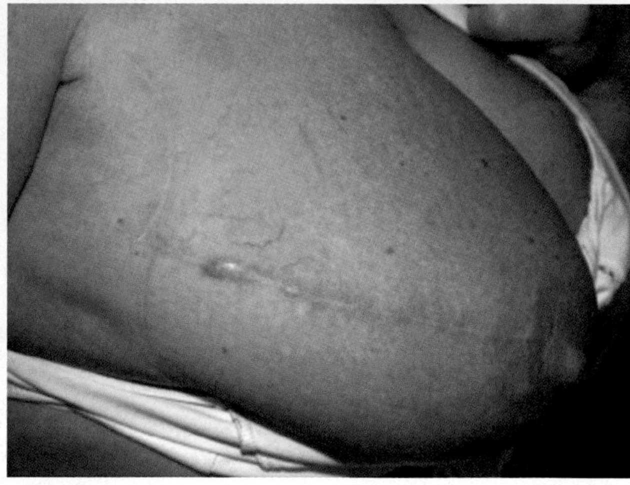

Figure 115.28. (*Continued*) **C:** Example of primary healed hypertrophic scar 2 years after partial mastectomy. Result only 6 months after ridged suturing. Note the small hypertrophy in the only area of the scar that as a test was injected with corticosteroids at the time of scar correction.

capsule is then exposed and followed proximally without removal of the old implant. The dissection is carried on as far a possible until it becomes technically difficult. The implant is then removed and the capsule stretched distally with vessel clamps, and the dissection is carried on between the capsule and the muscle until the appropriate pocket is created. The incision in the capsule is closed and left behind as a posterior wall in the new implant pocket. Secondary cases should always be drained when using form-stable implants. To minimize the risk for rotation, new pocket dissection is recommended in secondary cases, and careful surgical technique as described earlier is a prerequisite for avoiding rotation. A review of the present larger series of Style 410 implants is in progress.

In conclusion, AHCSI implants provide a high degree of patient satisfaction with a low frequency of complication.

EDITORIAL COMMENTS

Dr. Hedén's extensive knowledge with regard to silicone gel breast implants is clearly evident when reading this chapter. It is no surprise that he is one of the world's leading authorities on this subject. He thoroughly reviews the evolution of these devices over the last 20 years. There are many benefits the reader will obtain by reading this chapter. It is particularly helpful in reviewing the history of how dimensional planning and advanced dimensional planning have evolved. Dr. Hedén's review on the various cohesive devices is useful and provides clarity on the topic. He nicely reviews the importance of proper texturing of these contoured gel devices, as well as the importance of proper placement to prevent malrotation. Dr. Hedén also presents his perspective on how to select patients, select implants, and plan the surgery. His discussion in particular about how to site the lowermost part of the dissection and to pick the site of the inframammary fold is very useful. Overall, this is a very comprehensive chapter that is geared toward the advanced user but will also be useful for students and residents of plastic surgery.

M.Y.N.

REFERENCES

1. Czerny V. Plasischer ersatz der brustdruse durch ein lipoma. *Chir Kong Verhandl* 1895;2:126.
2. Cronin TD, Greenberg RL. Our experiences with the silastic gel breast prosthesis. *Plast Reconstr Surg* 1970;46(1):1–7.
3. Burkhardt BR, Eades E. The effect of Biocell texturing and povidone-iodine irrigation on capsular contracture around saline-inflatable breast implants. *Plast Reconstr Surg* 1995;96(6):1317–1325.
4. Hakelius L, Ohlsen LA. clinical comparison of the tendency to capsular contracture between smooth and textured gel-filled silicone mammary implants. *Plast Reconstr Surg* 1992;90(2):247–254.
5. Maxwell GP, Falcone PA. Eighty-four consecutive breast reconstructions using a textured silicone tissue expander. *Plast Reconstr Surg* 1992;89(6):1022–1034; discussion, 1035–1026.
6. McCurdy JA. Relationships between spherical fibrous capsular contracture and mammary prosthesis type: a comparison of smooth and textured implants. *Am J Cosmet Surg* 1990;7(4):235–238.
7. Danino AM, Basmacioglu P, Saito S, et al. Comparison of the capsular response to the Biocell RTV and Mentor 1600 Siltex breast implant surface texturing: a scanning electron microscopic study. *Plast Reconstr Surg* 2001;108(7):2047–2052.
8. Deapen DM, Pike MC, Casagrande JT, et al. The relationship between breast cancer and augmentation mammaplasty: an epidemiologic study. *Plast Reconstr Surg* 1986;77(3):361–368.
9. Nelson NJ. Silicone breast implants not linked to breast cancer risk. *J Natl Cancer Inst* 2000;92(21):1714–1715.
10. Berkel H, Birdsell DC, Jenkins H. Breast augmentation: a risk factor for breast cancer? *N Engl J Med* 1992;326(25):1649–1653.
11. Brinton LA, Malone KE, Coates RJ, et al. Breast enlargement and reduction: results from a breast cancer case-control study. *Plast Reconstr Surg* 1996;97(2):269–275.
12. Gabriel SE, O'Fallon WM, Kurland LT, et al. Risk of connective-tissue diseases and other disorders after breast implantation. *N Engl J Med* 1994;330(24):1697–702.
13. Sanchez-Guerrero J, Schur PH, Sergent JS, et al. Silicone breast implants and rheumatic disease. Clinical, immunological and epidemiological studies. *Arthritis Rheum* 1994;37:158.
14. Perkins KK, Clark BD, Klein PJ, et al. A meta-analysis of breast implants and connective tissue disease. *Ann Plast Surg* 1995;35(6):561–570.
15. Wong O. A critical assessment of the relationship between silicone breast implants and connective tissue diseases. *Regul Toxicol Pharmacol* 1996;23:74–85.
16. Hedén P, Boné B, Murphy DK, et al. Style 410 cohesive silicone breast implants: safety and effectiveness at 5 to 9 years after implantation. *Plast Reconstr Surg* 2006;118(6):1281–1287.
17. Hodgkinson DJ. Buckled upper pole breast style 410 implant presenting as a manifestation of capsular contraction. *Aesthet Plast Surg* 1999;23(4):279–281.
18. Hamas R. The postoperative shape of round and teardrop saline-filled breast implants. *Aesthet Surg J* 2000;20:4.
19. Hedén P, Jernbeck J, Hober M. Breast augmentation with anatomical cohesive gel implants: the world's largest current experience. *Clin Plast Surg* 2001;28(3):531–552.
20. Tebbetts JB. Use of anatomic breast implants: ten essentials. *Aesthet Surg J* 1998;18(5):377–384.
21. Hedén P. *Plastic Surgery and You.* Stockholm: Silander and Fromholtz; 2003.
22. Metaxotos NG, Asplund O, Hayes M. The efficacy of bupivacaine with adrenaline in reducing pain and bleeding associated with breast reduction: a prospective trial. *Br J Plast Surg* 1999;52(4):290–293.
23. Tebbetts JB. Dual plane breast augmentation: optimizing implant–soft-tissue relationships in a wide range of breast types. *Plast Reconstr Surg* 2001;107(5):1255–1272.
24. Spear SL, Carter ME, Ganz JC. The correction of capsular contracture by conversion to "dual-plane" positioning: technique and outcomes. *Plast Reconstr Surg* 2003;112(2):456–466.

CHAPTER

116

Bradley P. Bengtson

The Highly Cohesive, Style 410 Form-stable Gel Implant for Primary Breast Augmentation

The Natrelle 410 highly cohesive, form-stable gel breast Implant was developed in the early 1990s in conjunction with McGhan Medical Corporation as part of the search for a more optimal filler for a shaped breast implant (1) (also, J. B. Tebbetts, private communication). It was first released in Europe in 1993, secondary to the Food and Drug Administration (FDA) moratorium placed on silicone gel devices in the United States in 1992 and has been described as a fifth-generation device (2). This delay has placed plastic surgeons in the United States at a distinct disadvantage: Even though we have been the innovators in conjunction with industry and developed these devices, we have been unable to use them clinically in an unrestricted manner. In February 2001, a premarket approval study monitored by the FDA was initiated at approximately 80 sites in the United States by surgeons with shaped-implant experience. To date, more than 12,000 patients have been enrolled, and as of this writing, we are beginning the ninth year of enrollment. This chapter discusses the specific characteristics of the Style 410 device, its disadvantages and advantages, tissue-based planning principles specific to it, patient and implant selection, differences in surgical techniques when using this device, personal, national, and global experience along with published results with the 410, and some pearls of wisdom and caveats when using this device.

CHARACTERISTICS

FORM STABILITY

Form stability may be defined clinically as the ability of a device to hold its shape in all positions. In the upright position such an implant is unique in that it has no collapse or bending of the upper pole whatsoever (Fig. 116.1). Secondarily, it has no inherent wrinkling or rippling when held in various positions and maintains shape retention and memory. In the absence of any capsular contracture forces, the implant itself defines the shape of the breast, in contrast to a standard gel implant, for which the breast defines the shape of the implant.

COHESIVITY

Form stability is slightly different than cohesivity. Form stability describes the device as a whole—the shell and filler characteristics—whereas cohesivity describes the physical characteristics of the internal gel filler. Silicone gel breast implants have various degrees of internal gel cohesivity. Cohesivity is measured as a stiffness coefficient, which has somewhat of a negative connotation, but in fact measures the degree of cohesivity of the filler. The 410 has the greatest degree of cohesivity of any implant. There is a softer, less cohesive filler called the Soft Touch, which is similar in stiffness/cohesivity to the Mentor CPG device. These two devices are in turn more cohesive than the standard Responsive gel or MemoryGel devices on the market. This increase in cohesivity also provides a less fluid filler and less likelihood of gel to exude from the shell if it is cut or damaged (Fig. 116.2). This increase in cohesivity does create a slightly increased degree of firmness in the hand at room temperature; however, there is a common misconception among patients and surgeons that the 410 is overly firm following implantation. This is in fact not the case. The 410 creates a "one-breast feel" after augmentation and will be further explored in this chapter (3) (Fig. 116.3).

BIOCELL TEXTURING

The 410 has an extremely coarse, heavily textured surface of irregular pores in the range of 300 μm (Fig. 116.4). This texturing facilitates holding the implant in position along with a tight hand-in-a-glove pocket dissection discussed later. This texturing and the 410's form stability are likely contributing factors to its low reported capsular contracture, rotation, and malposition rates (4–6).

MATRIX OF OPTIONS

There are approximately 200 different shapes of the 410 in 12 separate cells varying in height, projection, and width (Fig. 116.5). These options provide a wide and unique range of implant selections that can be dialed in to accommodate any patient's measurements and breast tissue characteristics. These devices are described first by their height— full (F), moderate (M), and low (L)—then by their projection—extra (X), full (F), moderate (M), and low (L)—and finally by their base width in 0.5-cm increments. The available of these options, however, represents a bit of a double-edged sword: The great thing about the 410 is there are so many options available, but the challenge of the 410 is that there are so many options available! There is a method in the works to help simplify implant selection with the 410, and this overall process will be described in detail.

ADVANTAGES AND DISADVANTAGES

These myriad unique factors also create a number of advantages and disadvantages or trade-offs when considering using the 410 device. Although there is not one implant that is best

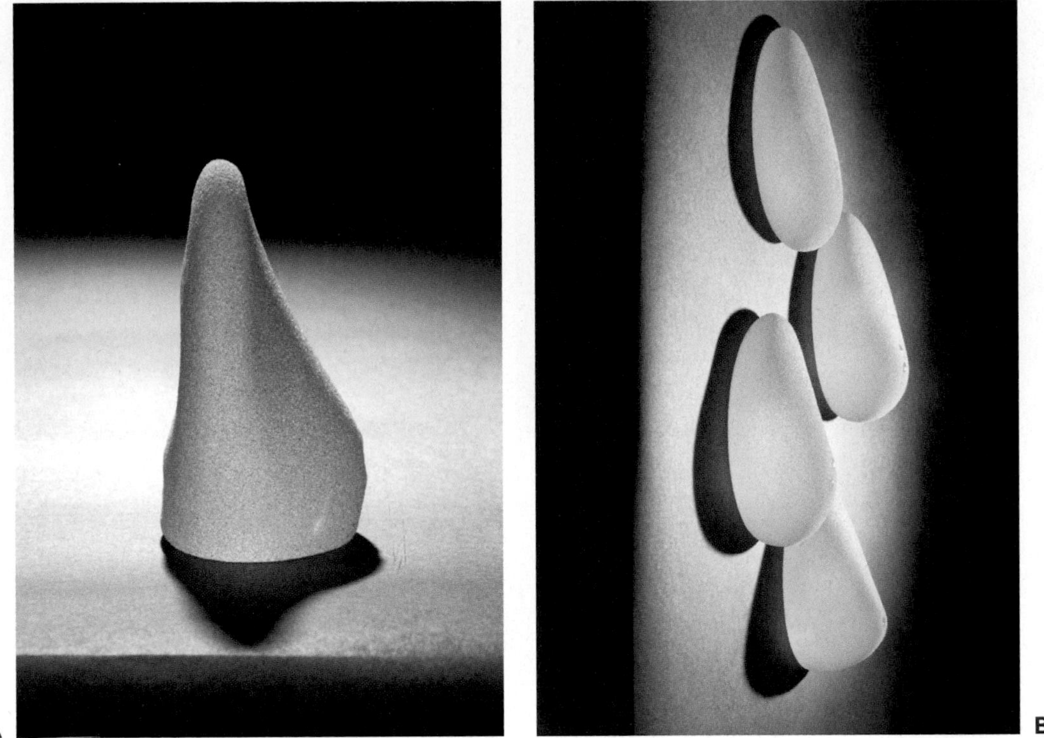

Figure 116.1. **A:** The Natrelle Style 410 gel implant has the highest degree of cohesivity of any current breast implant, creating clinical form stability. When the device is held upright, the increased internal gel cross-linking in conjunction with its shell dynamics helps to holds its position in all dimensions without collapse of the upper pole and without any inherent wrinkling or rippling. **B:** Style 410 FL, FM, FF, and FX projections.

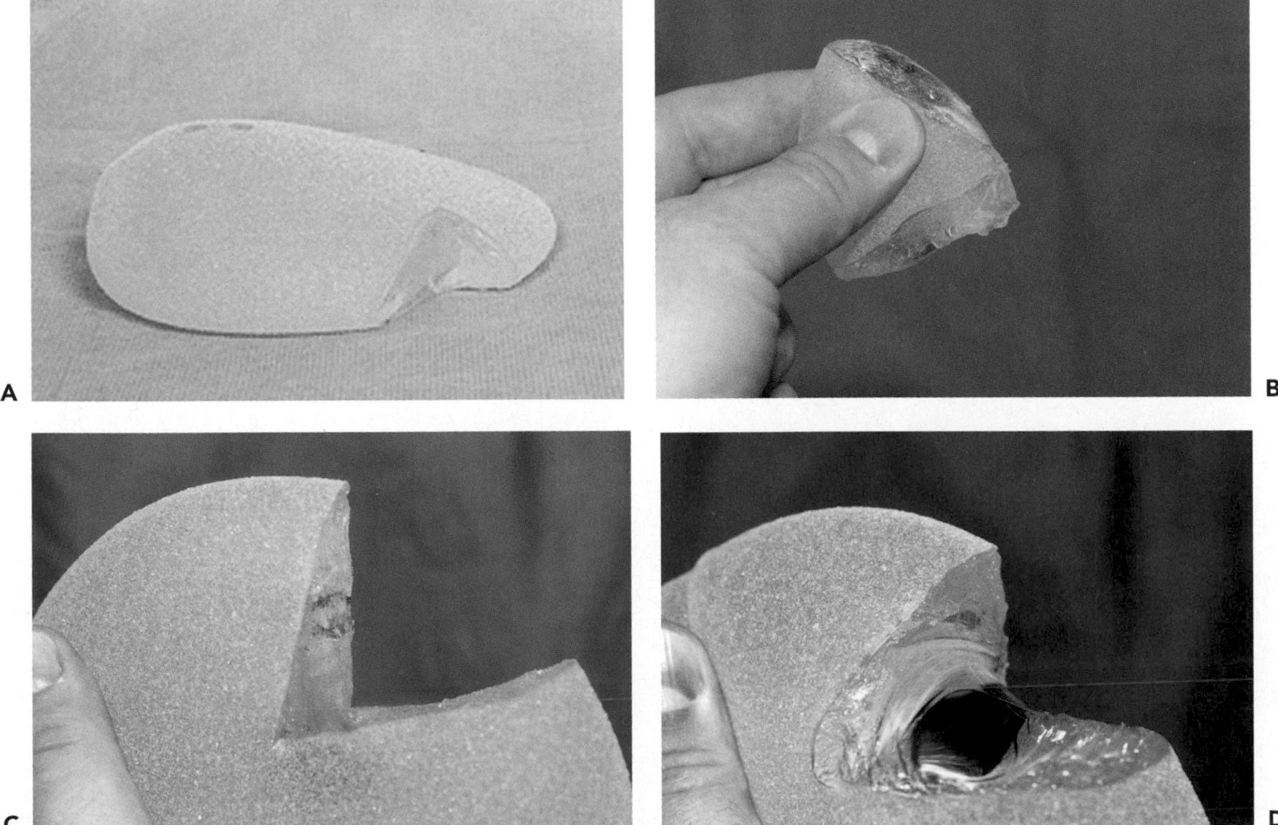

Figure 116.2. **A, B:** When a Style 410 is cut, the high internal gel cohesiveness keeps the gel inside the device shell. **C, D:** Even with firm pressure, the gel may bulge out, but when the pressure is released, the gel returns into the confines of the shell.

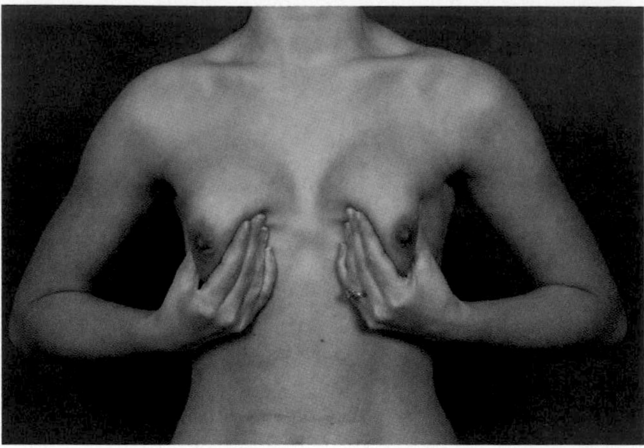

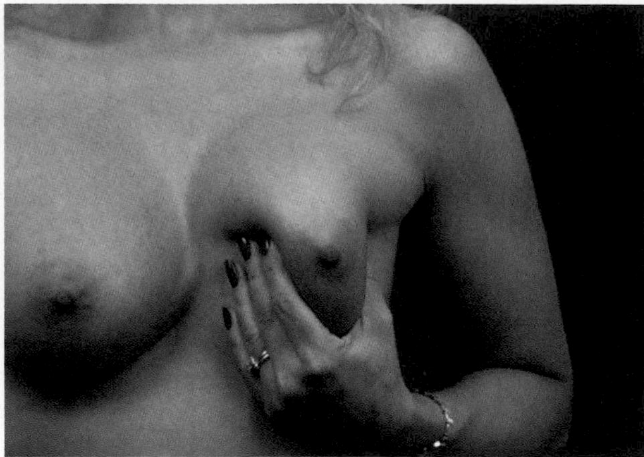

Figure 116.3. In the absence of any capsular contracture (less than 2%), breast augmentation patients with Natrelle 410 devices have a slightly firmer feel than a standard gel device but still maintain a soft, "one-breast feel."

for every patient or in every circumstance, the 410 certainly increases the palate of options for the breast augmentation patient.

General **Dis**advantages include the following:

- The implant is more expensive initially (but early results increased longevity at 9 years) (7).
- It has the potential to rotate, being a shaped device (full height in particular).
- The implant is more technically demanding to use surgically.

Figure 116.4. Photomicrograph of the BioCell, irregularly shaped pore size, which allows for a higher degree of implant–soft tissue fusion, helping to hold the 410 in position along with a hand-in-a-glove pocket dissection. (From Maxwell GP, Baker MR. Augmentation mammaplasty: general considerations. In: Spear SL, ed. *Surgery of the Breast. Principles and Art.* 2nd ed. Baltimore: Lippincott Williams & Wilkins; 2006:1237.)

- The implant is more difficult to use in secondary or revision cases, requires a new or virgin pocket for placement, and does not fill the envelope like a responsive gel or low-cohesive filler.
- It creates less of an ideal result in patients with loose skin and inability to fill the breast envelope.
- There is some increase in edge palpability secondary to form stability and cohesivity.
- Implant selection is more challenging.
- Tissue-based planning principles are an absolute.
- Its use requires a new mindset and should be considered as a new technique (further discussed in Precise Surgical Technique section).

General **Ad**vantages include the following:

- The implant provides form stability with no inherent wrinkling, rippling, or implant collapse.
- It comes in a wide variety of shapes, including different widths, heights, and projections (410 Matrix), providing a huge range of options.
- It is less likely to "leak" with a more highly cohesive filler.
- The Biocell surface encourages adherence and less mobility with softness.
- The implant performs well in challenging, thin patients with less soft tissue coverage and in particular constricted breasts.
- It has the ability to "shape the breast" versus having the "breast shape the implant."
- The 410 has the lowest capsular contracture rates reported in the literature.
- There is very low visible and palpable wrinkling and rippling.
- Lower shell failure rates have been reported with the 410 versus standard gel devices,

In addition, Heden lists some of the specific additional advantages of the 410 implant's form stability (7,8):

- It imparts shape to the breast.
- It resists deforming forces from a capsular contraction.
- It resists implant collapse and has no inherent wrinkling or rippling or implant irregularities.
- It limits gel content motion and may increase implant longevity by decreasing wear on the envelope.

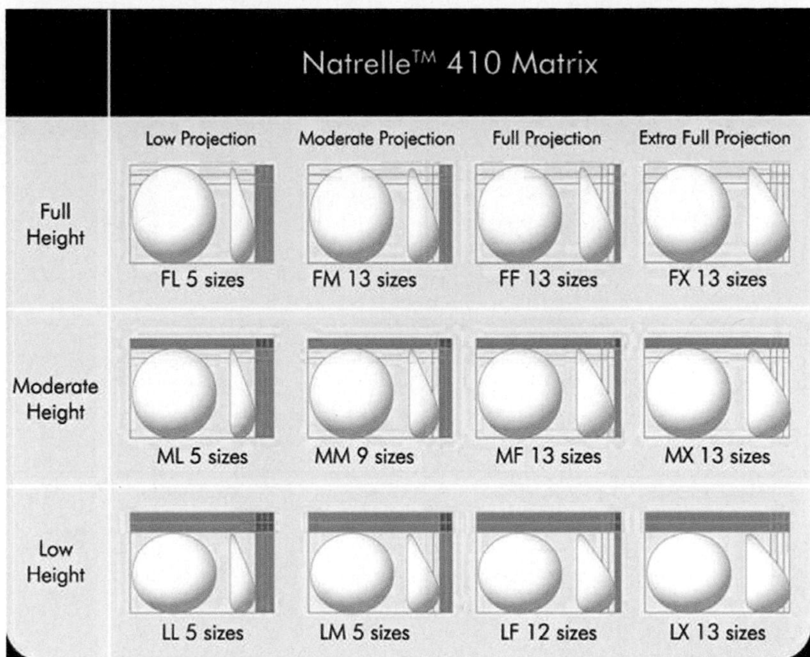

Figure 116.5. The Natrelle 410 Matrix gives nearly 200 different implants, in 12 cells comprising three separate heights (L, low; M, moderate; F, full) and four projections (L, low; M, moderate; F, full; X, extra). The four core cells recommended for use in a surgeon's first 20 primary augmentation patients are MM, MF, FM, and FF.

- It allows for easier explantation with minimal to no gel extravasations and no implant changes even after many years, except for occasional yellow-serous discoloration.
- It may be a major advantage particularly in breast asymmetry cases and in constricted breasts as well as in breast reconstruction and patients with thoracic or chest wall deformity.

The disadvantages of form stability include the following:

- It imparts a slightly firmer consistency to the breast.
- It decreases deformation, and thus it is difficult to insert through a small incision; a larger incision is required or the gel may fracture (5.5 cm or greater).
- Incision is not limited to, but is preferential to, the inframammary fold (IMF).
- By imparting a certain shape, form stability is not for patients desiring a "non-proportional or exaggerated breast augmentation" (7,8).

TISSUE-BASED PLANNING PRINCIPLES

In the past, breast augmentation was viewed as a procedure or technical exercise. However, more recently this procedure has been more properly recognized as a series of processes that are important for a consistent, quality results. These biodimensional principles have been redefined and expanded into a complete *process* of breast augmentation (9). This process includes patient education/informed consent, tissue-based preoperative planning, refined surgical technique, fast-track recovery, and defined postoperative care.

One of the first critical aspects when using this implant is that the 410 requires a transition from a purely volumetric method to a defined, measurable, planned, dimension-based approach for breast augmentation to include specific patient measurements and breast soft tissue characteristics. A much more detailed planning system and patient evaluation is also required when using this device when adding a third dimension of height into the equation. Because the use of the 410 is much less forgiving, if prior subjective, volume-only evaluation techniques are applied to the use of this implant, results will be less than optimal and lead to higher complication rates and dissatisfied patients. Stated another way, if tissue-based planning principles and processes are not an integral part of the planning, I would recommend not using this device.

STYLE 410 PATIENT SELECTION AND EDUCATION

There is not one best implant for every patient. Each implant has advantages and disadvantages, or trade-offs, that must be weighed and discussed with each patient preoperatively. Figure 116.6 gives a basic algorithm with general guidelines for patient selection. Patients encouraged to select a standard gel device include, first and foremost, patients with a loose skin envelope where the breast dimensions cannot be filled. This is the main patient dissuaded from the 410: the patient with an envelope-to-implant mismatch. Also in this category are patients with significant ptosis where a vertical to full mastopexy or lifting the nipple more than 4 cm above the transposed inframammary fold is called for. In addition, in patients with significant chest wall deformities such as pectus carinatum or excavatum, I prefer a standard gel device that blends into the chest wall defect to a greater degree. When a form-stable device is used in these types of patients the implant becomes an extension of the chest, and instead of molding into the rib/sternal deformities, it tends to accentuate them. Mild to moderate asymmetry may be improved with this device, but marked breast asymmetry greater than 150 to 200 cc is difficult to judge. Style 410 sizers and in particular three-dimensional imaging and simulation are creating major strides in improving more predictable outcomes with the 410 in patients with significant asymmetry. Although this chapter deals with primary augmentation, unless one is revising a small subglandular augmentation with a partial submuscular device or performing a neo-subpectoral pocket

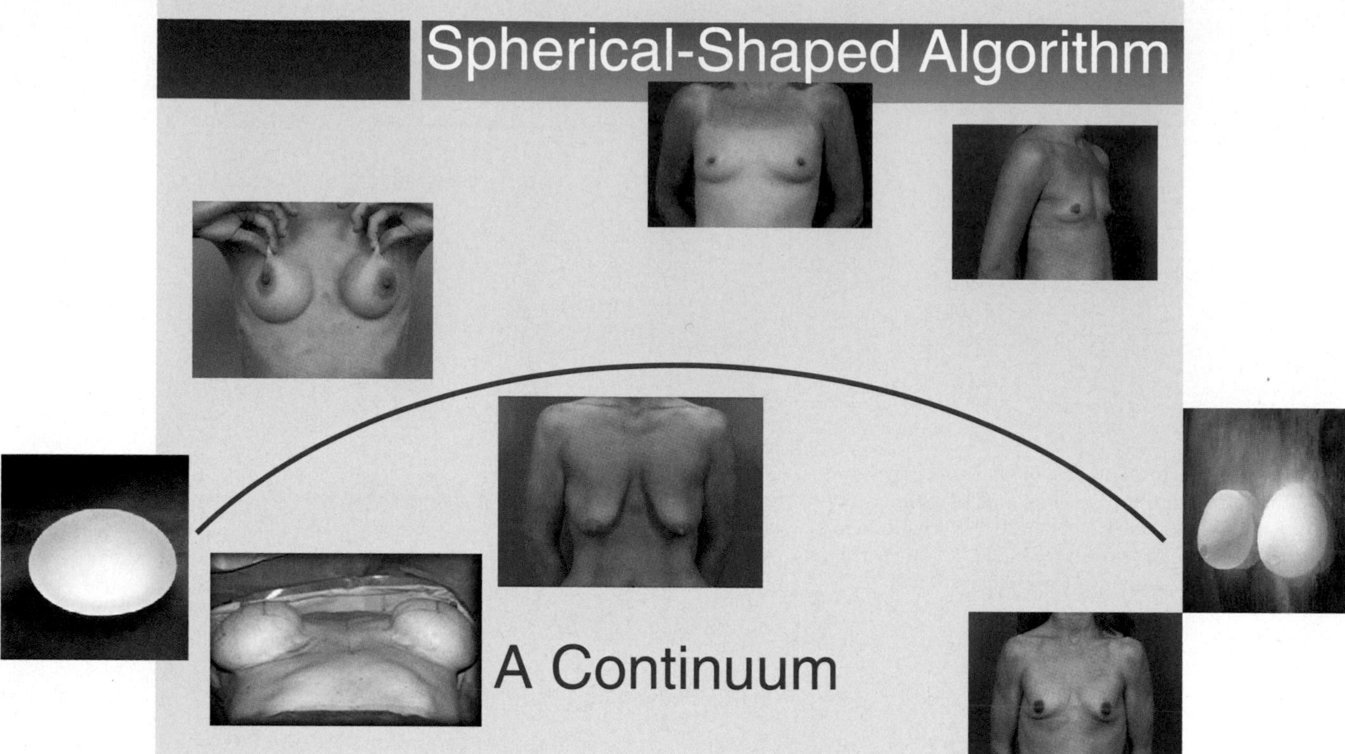

Figure 116.6. Shown here is not an absolute but instead my current algorithm of breast types and presentations to consider for standard gel on one end of the spectrum and Natrelle 410 on the other end. Many patients are candidates for both styles; however, patients with high degrees of ptosis or a loose skin envelope have higher complication rates and surgical revision rates when using the 410 versus round/elliptical devices.

and using a significantly larger device, the surgeon should consider a standard gel implant or a round/elliptical device with a more form-stable filler when available. However, patients preferring this implant and having a relatively normal to tight skin envelope with less than 3 cm of skin stretch, patients who are extremely safety conscious, patients without ptosis, and younger patients are encouraged to consider the Style 410 device. In addition, patients with a constricted breast deformity and high fold are excellent candidates for a 410 with results that are difficult to match with standard devices, particularly in one stage (Fig. 116.7).

TISSUE-BASED PLANNING PRINCIPLES

Careful assessments of a patient's tissues including some basic measurements are important in determining the range of implants that will fit and match each patient's breast and body. These tissue-based planning principles are important in all breast augmentation procedures, but they are absolutely critical when using shaped, form-stable devices. First, one evaluates the chest wall architecture, breast soft tissue volume, and skin stretch, noting the degree of asymmetry and whether any ptosis is present. These are important to document and show the patient. There are potentially more than 20 specific measurements of the breast; however, there are just a few that are vital in determining an implant range for each patient. This part of the process is both art and a science. We tend to be in an either-or society; however, the plastic surgeon must take into account all of these factors, including patient desires, in choosing a breast implant. I believe that the patient should decide the final implant size but that the plastic surgeon should set the range of what will fit each patient's breast. There are consequences in going too large and creating malposition, symmastia, or other complications and also too small and not achieving an optimal fill or breast shape. The constant goal should be to continue to minimize surgical revisions for patients.

There are many current implant selection methods available; however, there are no current implant selector systems that take a patient and a plastic surgeon from an examination and evaluation through the selection of a specific range of devices that will fit each individual patient's breast in a simple, straightforward, uncomplicated manner. Current systems are either extremely complicated or too overly subjective and not based on objective long-term deliverable data or results.

The key measurements and principles are as follows: determining base width of the breast, the breast tissue type, including stretch, and then using the sternal notch-to-nipple (SN-N)

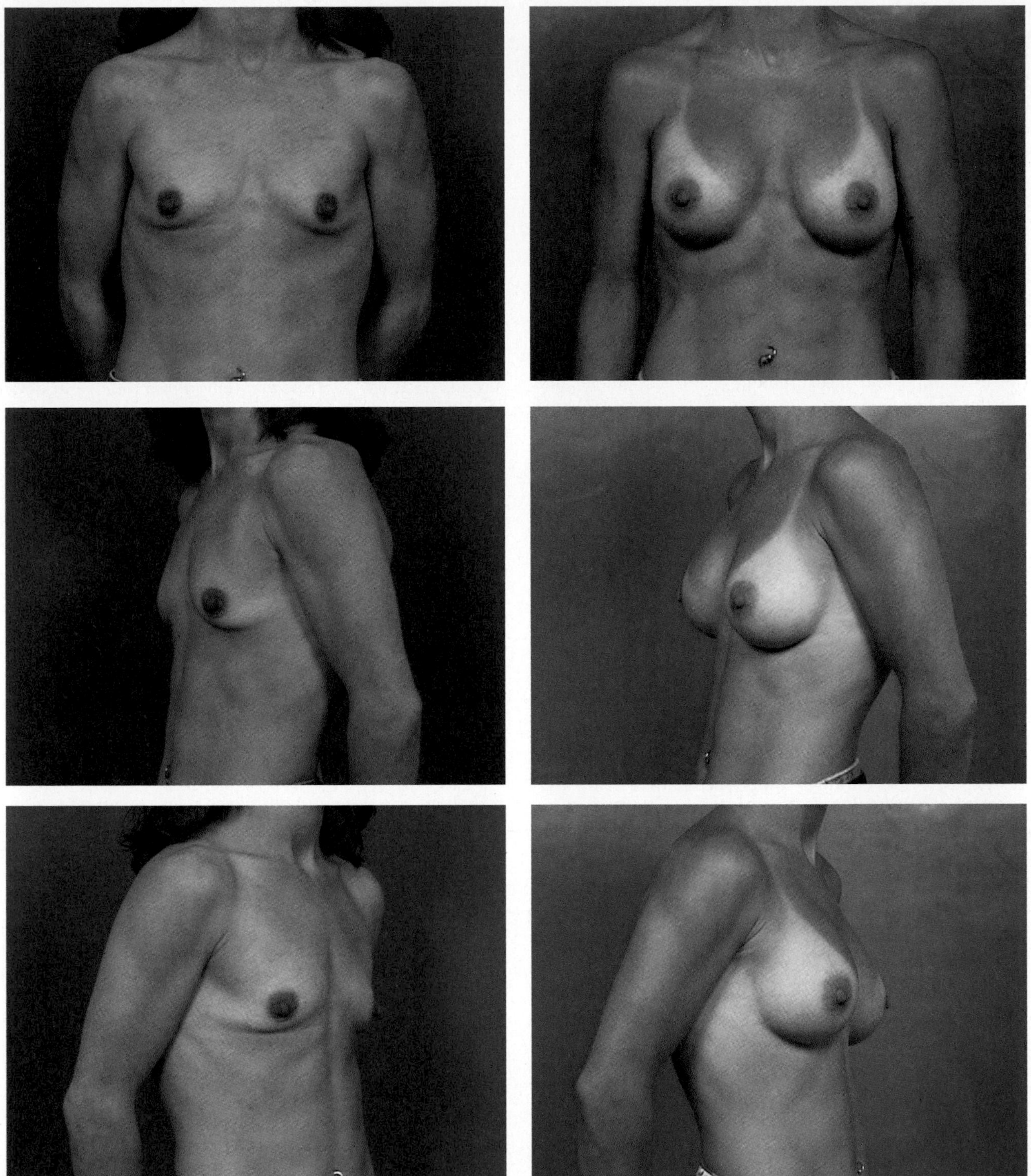

Figure 116.7. Patients with a constricted breast and or a high-riding inframammary fold, particularly thin patients with minimal coverage, are among the most difficult breast augmentation candidates. Results in this subset of patients with the Style 410 are very difficult to match up against any other device. The Style 410, with its increased form stability, has the ability to *shape* the breast versus standard gel devices, which are shaped *by* the breast (nipple-to-inframammary fold distance 4.0 cm preoperative and 8.0 cm postoperative).

measurement and nipple-to-inframammary fold (N-IMF) distance to help define the implant height. The breast base width is the keystone of the breast and the first critical measurement (Fig. 116.8). This measurement is best performed with calipers or a clear ruler, but is also very accurately measured with new three-dimensional camera systems. The breast base width determines the range of the breast implant width. In general, in the absence of a constricted or unusual situation, the breast implant should not exceed the breast width by more than 5 mm to less than 1 cm.

- Main principle: The base diameter of the device should generally not exceed the base diameter of the breast.
- Base width is a key measurement: One should choose an implant generally within a range not 1 cm less or 5 mm more than the existing breast base width.

The next important measurement is the assessment and type of the breast, including the elasticity or stretch. This is generally determined objectively, but there is a subjective aspect as well. The standard breasts presenting for breast augmentation may be generally divided into five breast types, recognizing that there is an obvious continuum. This classification ranges from minimal breast tissue and a very tight and full skin envelope (skin stretch less than 1 cm), to tight with a minimal glandular component (skin stretch 1 to 2 cm), to average/normal amount of laxity and fullness (skin stretch 2 to 3 cm), to a loose skin envelope (skin stretch 3 to 4 cm, N-IMF distance less than 9 cm), to very loose skin envelope with fatty breast tissue (N-IMF distance of 9 of 10 cm, skin stretch 3 to 4 cm) (Fig. 116.9A).

In general, the degree of stretch helps to determine the projection of the implant chosen. In tighter skin envelopes with less stretch, moderate projection implants—either MM or FM devices—are selected, although low-projection devices are also options. With average amounts of stretch and type III breasts, moderate- to full-projection implants are best suited to fill the envelope, so selection of MF and FF devices are typical. When dealing with loose breasts and a greater degree of laxity, full- or extra-projection devices are prioritized: MF, MX, FF, and FX (Fig. 116.9B, C).

SN-N distance is another key measurement for determining the potential implant height. Although there are multiple variables in choosing the implant height and certainly no absolutes, the SN-N measurement is critical (Fig. 117.10). SN-N measurement is recorded to document asymmetry and degree of ptosis. In general, again in the absence of any significant constriction or other deformities, if the patient has a short distance from the sternal notch/clavicle to the nipple (<18 cm), a moderate-height device is chosen. If there is an average distance of 18 to 21 cm, then either a moderate- or a full-height device may be used, depending on the IMF location and volume and shape desires of the patient and the surgeon. If a patient is tall or has a relatively longer SN-N distance and low-set breasts (>21 cm), a preferred option of a full-height device is usually chosen (Table 116.1).

Nipple to Inframammary Fold (N-IMF) Distance and the New IMF

The N-IMF fold measurement is the next core critical measurement. If the breast base width is the *keystone* of the breast, then the inframammary fold is the *foundation*. There is a great deal of renewed interest and deserved attention to the IMF clinically and in the literature. The IMF deserves a great deal of respect, and understanding its unique anatomic features is important. I discuss the differences in the IMF position—the resting versus the actual fold—in Chapter 130 of this text. The oblique orientation of the fascial fibers allows for the implant even if the IMF is undisturbed surgically to sit 1 to 2 cm lower than its transposed position on the skin. This is very important in helping the surgeon both select a device and set and determine the final implant position. After a specific volume of implant is chosen based on its width, projection, and height, the final implant volume and style may be used to determine very accurately the new IMF position. On the basis of working with and documenting thousands of Natrelle Style 410 patients and in collaboration with shaped-implant pioneers such as John Tebbetts, Per Heden, Charles Randquist, Bill Adams, Steve Teitelbaum, Pat Maxwell, Mitch Brown, and others and careful analysis of their work and other published work (8,10,11), very accurate nipple-to-fold measurements have been determined. In general, as a starting point, for example,

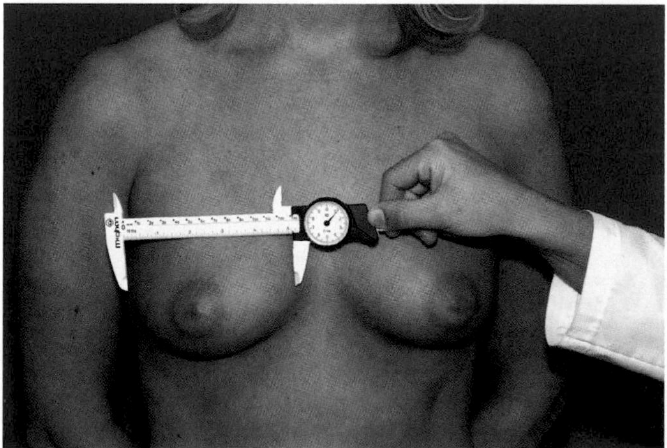

Figure 116.8. Breast base width is the key measurement of the breast and may be measured with calipers, a clear ruler, or new three-dimensional imaging systems at the maximum base diameter. Implant width is then matched to the breast base width, choosing a device in a typical range 1 cm smaller to 5 mm larger than the existing breast base width.

TABLE 116.1 Determining Height Selection of Style 410 Implant Using Sternal Notch-to-Nipple (SN-N) Distance

SN-N < 18 cm: consider moderate-height devices
SN-N = 18–21 cm: consider moderate- or full-height devices, depending on nipple-to-inframammary fold distance measurements and patient/surgeon desires
SN-N > 21 cm: consider full-height device, particularly in a patient without true ptosis or pseudoptosi

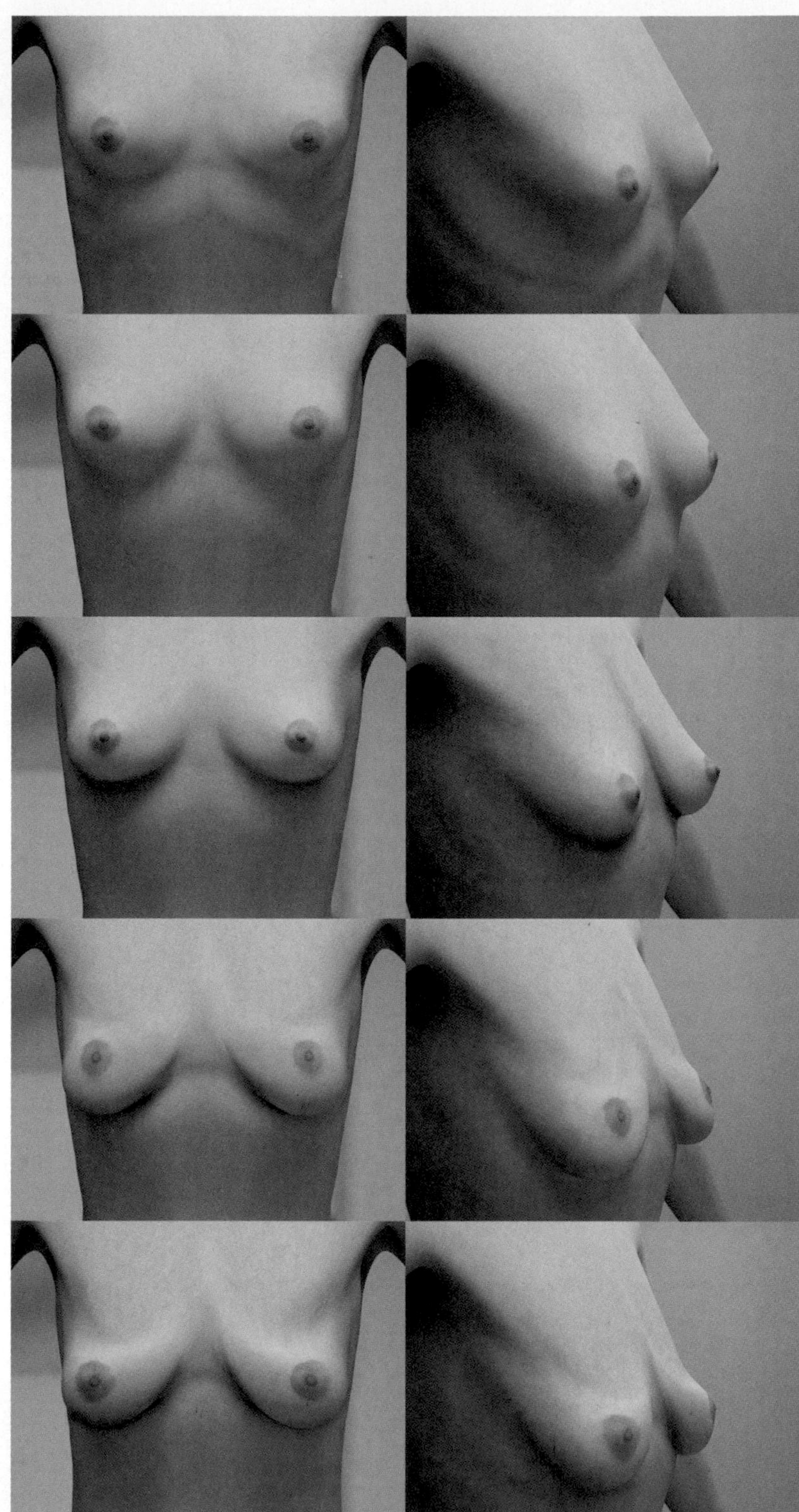

Figure 116.9. **A:** The full spectrum of breast types encountered in augmentation patients may be categorized for the purpose of simplifying and demystifying implant selection with the 410 and divided into the five breast types shown with varying degrees of skin elasticity and skin stretch. (*continued*)

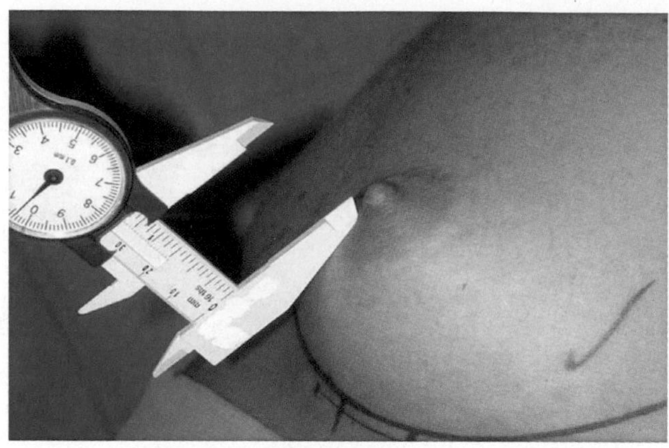

B

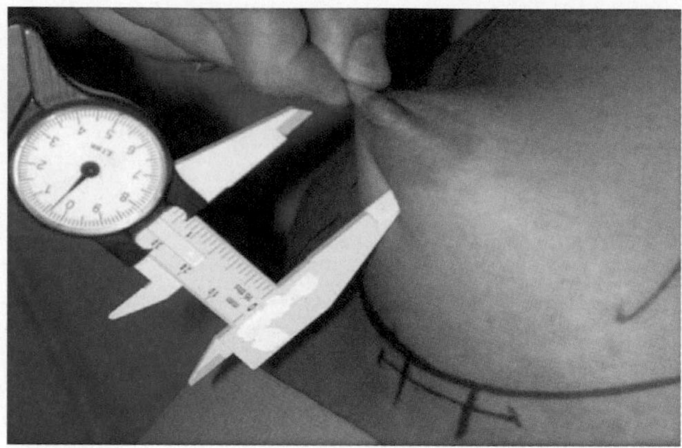

C

Figure 116.9. (*Continued*) **B, C:** Skin stretch and elasticity is also combined into the breast type and may be measured preferably objectively but also subjectively. (Images courtesy of William P. Adams)

if a 300-cc implant is chosen, the N-IMF incision should be 8 cm on maximal stretch. There is a 1-mm increase or decrease for every 10-cc, or a 5-mm increase or decrease for every 50 cc. Thus, when using a 250-cc implant, the N-IMF distance on maximum stretch should be 7.5 cm, and for a 400-cc implant, it should be 9.0 cm. In type I and type II breasts with tighter skin envelopes, 5 to 10 mm is added, otherwise the incision will ride up on the lower pole of the breast. In type IV and type V breasts with more laxity, 5 to 10 mm is subtracted because the skin is already loose and the implant will load and stretch the skin postoperatively. This 1 cm of extra distance added or subtracted is well within the difference between the resting and actual IMF, so there is some degree of variability and wiggle room for the surgeon. The goal again is to have the final IMF incision end up in the IMF itself as closely as possible (Table 116.2).

Why is this so critical? Although not relegated to the IMF incision alone, it is the preferred incisional approach when placing this device. It is very important to know where to make the incision in the IMF and place the final incision as close to the new IMF as possible. It is very daunting to place a 5.0- to 5.5-cm incision on the chest wall of a small, thin patient, particularly with a constricted breast, and lower the IMF 4 cm. The IMF and incision location will be based on what implant specifically is chosen—both its volume and its style (Fig. 116.11).

Figure 116.10. The sternal notch-to-nipple distance is another key measurement to take when assessing tissue-based planning dimensions and will help in determining implant height.

Implant Selection Example for a 410 Patient

Let us go through a sample 410 implant selection on an actual patient. This patient (Fig. 116.12) is a very typical breast augmentation patient who would benefit from a Style 410 implant. She has a breast base width of 12.5 cm, is a type II patient with average skin stretch of 2 cm. Her SN-N distance is 20 cm, and her N-IMF is 7.5 cm on stretch. She is looking for a natural but full proportional breast to her body. Walking her through the implant selection process, with a 12.5-cm breast base width, her implant range is from 320 to 375 g in the four core cells (MM, MF, FM, and FF) (Table 116.3). Her N-IMF distance is not too short or long, and she has minimal asymmetry and no constriction. Her SN-N distance is average at 20 cm (18 to 21 cm), so either a medium- or a full-height device will work well. In accord with her desire for a full and proportional augmentation, a full-height device with moderate projection is chosen, and her result at 3 years is shown (Fig. 116.13).

TABLE 116.2 Determining the Approximate Nipple-to-Inframammary Fold (N-IMF) Distance on Maximal Stretch

Size of Implant (g/cc)[a]	*N-IMF on Maximal Stretch (cm)*
250	7.5
300	8
400	9.0

Tight envelope, add 5 mm; extra tight, add 10 mm. Loose envelope, subtract 5 mm; extra loose, subtract 10 mm.
[a]When it comes to the Style 410 device, g/g and g/cc are very close. Saline is actually slightly more dense than gel, but this accounts for less than 10 cc in difference in an average-size device.

TABLE 116.3 410 Matrix Size Options

Implant Width	*FM Size*	*FF Size*	*MM Size*	*MF Size*
10.0 cm	180	185	160	165
10.5 cm	205	220	185	195
11.0 cm	235	255	215	225
11.5 cm	270	290	245	255
12.0 cm	310	335	280	295
12.5 cm	350	375	320	335
13.0 cm	395	425	360	375
13.5 cm	440	475	400	420
14.0 cm	500	535	450	470

There are obviously many variables involved in breast implant selection. Because of its additional height dimension and projection options, the range of choices of a Style 410 device is a double-edged sword. It provides a huge matrix of options for selection, but this can also be overwhelming and potentially confusing, particularly when one is just starting implant selection with this implant matrix. A simplified approach is presented that will be useful as starting point. The base width helps to determine the *range* of breast implants that will fit each patient's body. The breast type and skin stretch help determine the *projection* of the device used, and the sternal notch-to-nipple and nipple-to-fold measurements aid in determining the 410 *height* selected. Making these choices on the basis of art, science, and ongoing experience with shaped devices will allow the patient and surgeon to come to a predictable and consistent implant range and optimal breast fill for each patient.

THREE-DIMENSIONAL IMAGING AND SIMULATION

One of the most exciting and potentially significant additions to tissue-based planning is the introduction of three-dimensional imaging into the consultation and tissue-based planning process of breast augmentation. This technology has very dramatically affected my practice in a very positive way from both an educational and a marketing standpoint. After breaking down the barriers of cost and safety of silicone gel, the next barrier blocking a patient from scheduling surgery is outcome: What am I going to look like following surgery? I don't want to look too big, but also too small is not good either. This new three-dimensional imaging and simulation software helps to break through this barrier. It is prudent for a surgeon not to promise too much or set the patient or himself or herself up for disappointment or any medicolegal risk. Simulated or manipulated images should not be given to a patient in such as way as make any implied warranty or promise, but simply to say, "This is the range that can be achieved barring any complications. I use this as an educational tool. Has this simulation been helpful?" I still discuss honestly with all patients that there are no guarantees. No surgeon can say, "This is what you will look like postoperatively." On the other hand, in patients without significant ptosis, it is remarkable how close the simulated image and the actual postoperative images are (Fig. 116.14). This new technology is just ramping up, and we are continuing to improve and modify these systems and software, but it is easy to predict that these units will be in every plastic surgeon's office in the near future. Lower-resolution simulation methods are already available online. I also predict that standard two-dimensional photography will soon be replaced with three-dimensional imaging, which will be increasingly used for standard archiving and presentations. We are completing studies now comparing computer-scored measurements and surgeon/staff-based measurements, and they are very accurate. The current challenges are in patients with ptosis and also measuring the N-IMF on stretch. This measurement can be estimated with maximal reach of the arms above the head, but to accurately record this, it will still need to be physically measured at this point. This technology is also very good at helping to determine volume differences between breasts, and it dramatically helps in implant selection when different sizes and projections are used, improving the symmetry of patients postoperatively.

A

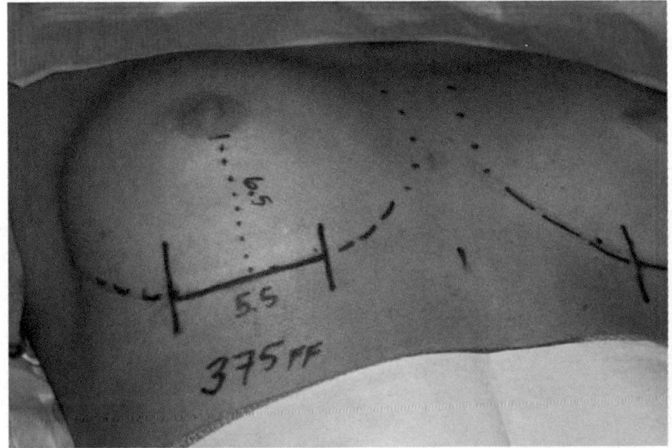

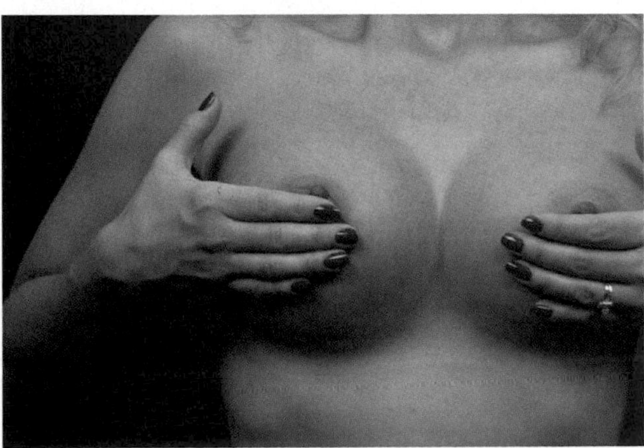

B

Figure 116.11. **A:** Base width helps to determine the implant volume range, the breast type including skin stretch helps to determine the 410 implant projection, and the sternal notch-to-nipple distance helps to determine the 410 implant height. Once the specific implant is chosen, its final volume and style determine where to set the inframammary fold (IMF) by measuring the nipple-to-inframammary fold on maximum stretch. The IMF incision is then placed directly in the fold. **B:** If measured and sized correctly, the IMF incision should be aligned directly in the new IMF.

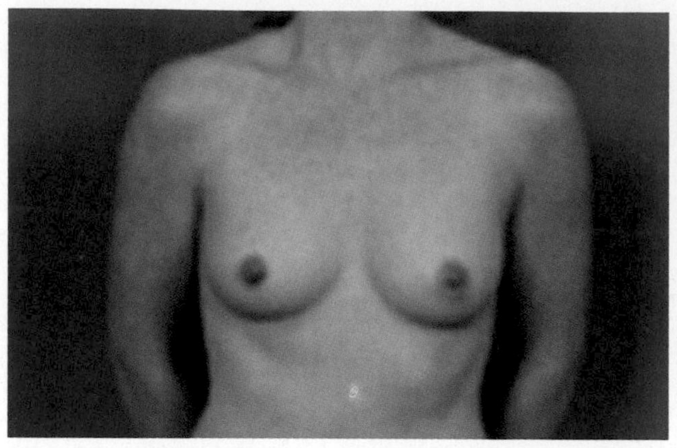

A

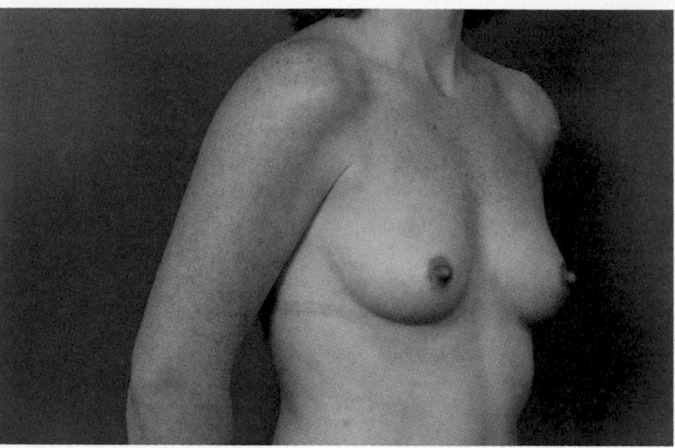

B

Figure 116.12. Going through a patient selection with these tissue-based planning principles, this patient has a breast base width of 12.5 and is a breast type II patient with firm glandular tissue and 2 cm of skin stretch. Her sternal notch-to-nipple distance is 20 cm, and her preoperative nipple-to-inframammary fold distance is 7.5 cm preoperatively.

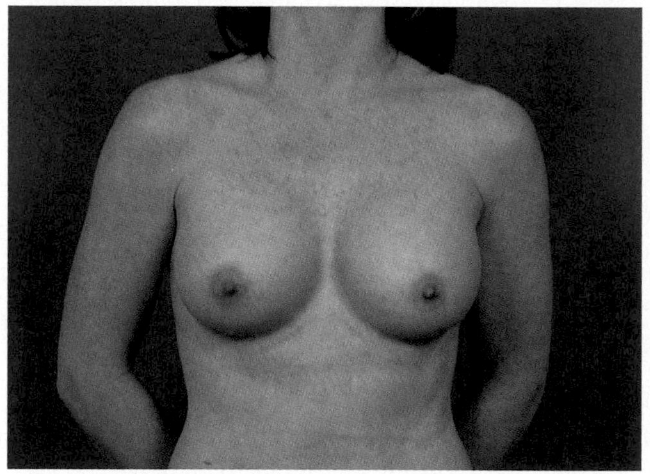

A

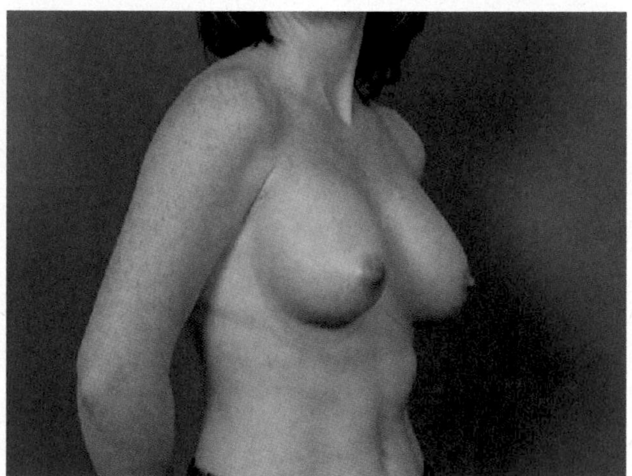

B

Figure 116.13. The patient desired a proportional result to her body but also a very full breast **(A)**, so in conjunction with the patient, a 350-g FM implant was chosen. Her postoperative results are shown at 3 years **(B)**. The base width is 12 to 12.5 cm, the sternal notch-to-nipple distance is 20 cm, and the nipple-to-inframammary fold distance is set at 8.5 cm.

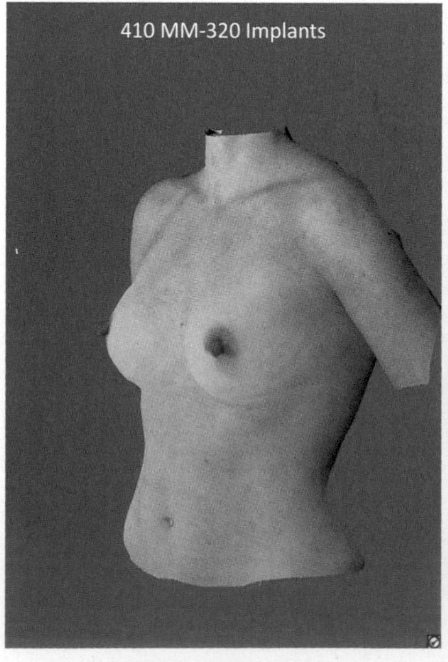

A

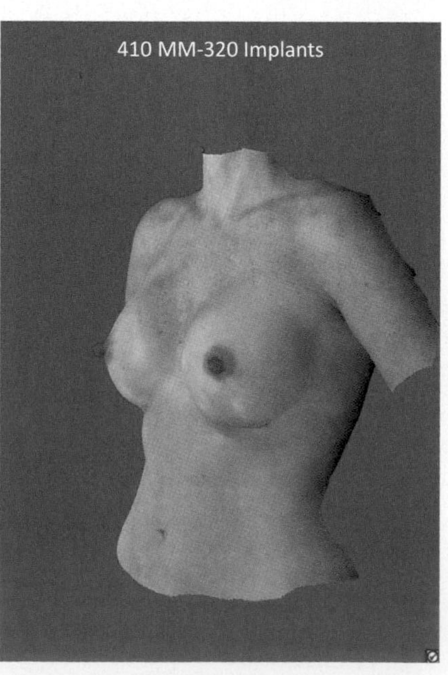

Figure 116.14. This series of images depicts a patient preoperatively, then simulated with the specific implant size used intraoperatively, and then compared to her actual postoperative result. The simulated and actual images are then ghosted and show near-complete overlap. (*continued*)

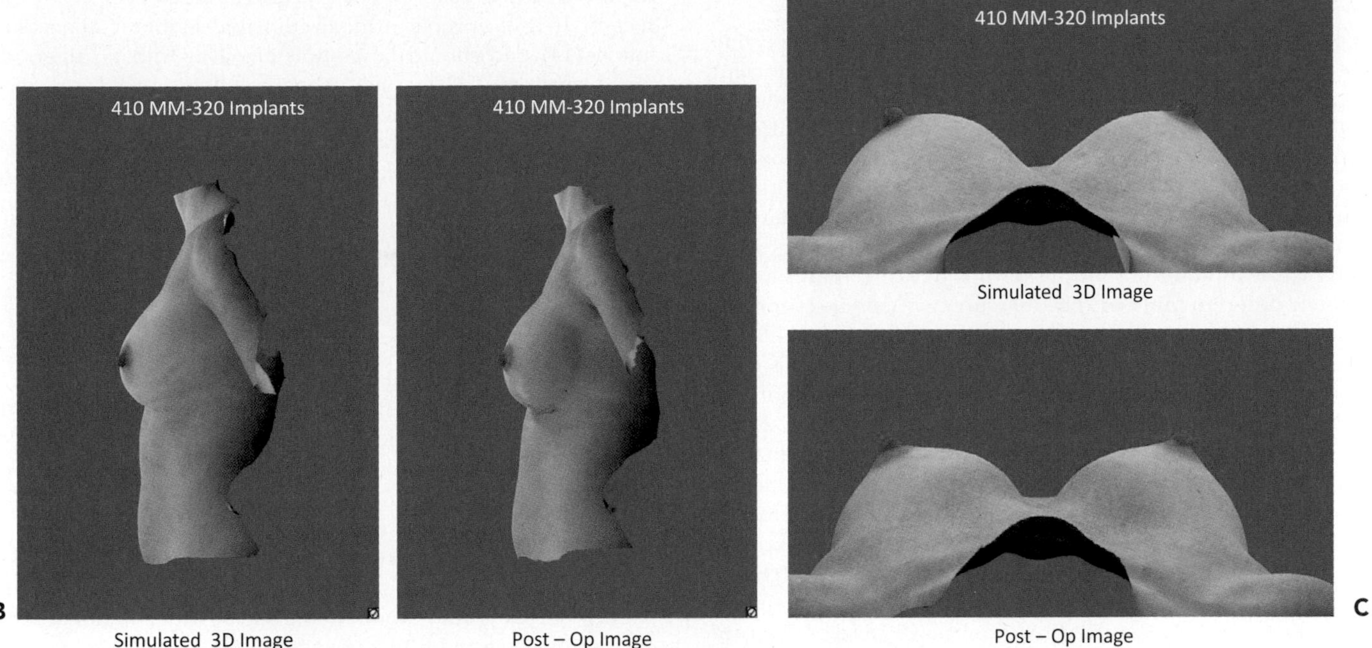

Actual Post-operative results compared to the Simulated 3D Image

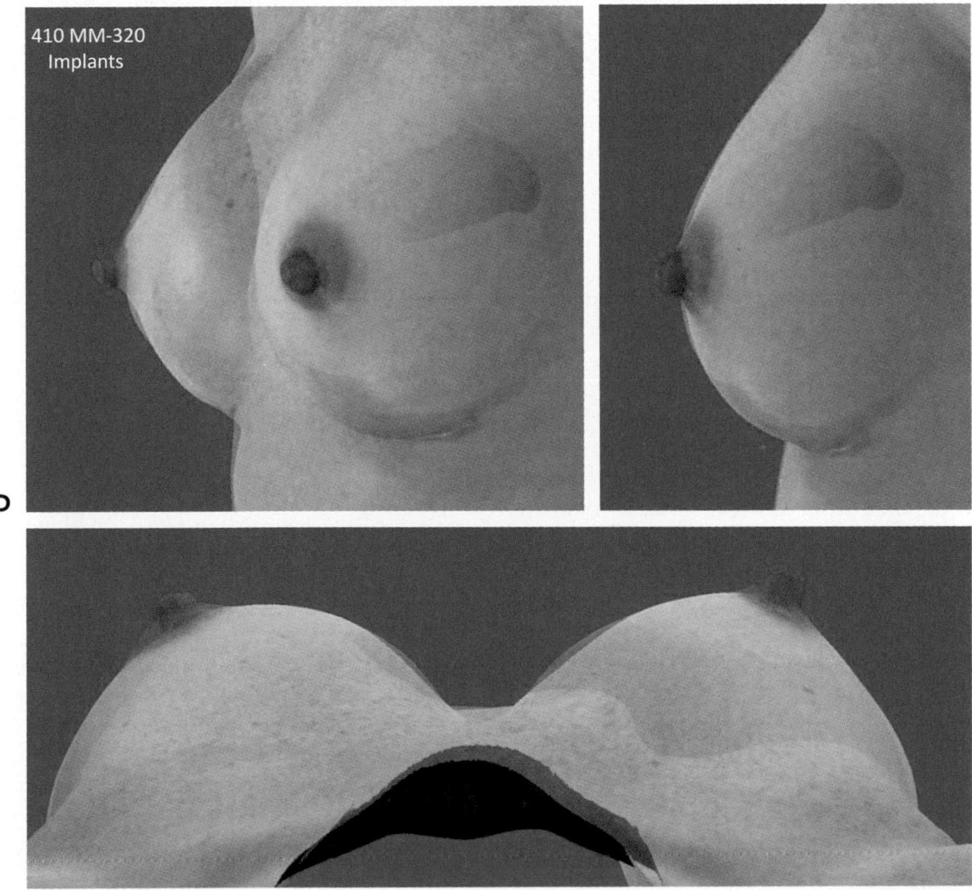

Figure 116.14. (*Continued*)

PRECISE SURGICAL TECHNIQUE

Following patient education and selection and implant selection, it is time to deliver a surgical result in a consistent, efficient, reproducible, and high-quality way that is defined, atraumatic, bloodless, and accurate. There are obviously many different approaches to breast augmentation surgery, but here I focus on principles that will produce consistent results and also on how surgical placement of the 410 varies from that of a standard round implant. First, as described above, and not just for the surgical technique portion, using this device requires a completely different mindset. The measurement and assessment of the patient are as critical as the surgery itself.

Following the patient assessment given earlier in this chapter, an implant of one specific size and style is brought into the operating room and rarely changed intraoperatively. I do not routinely use intraoperative sizers in primary augmentation. This dramatically decreases the time in surgery while increasing efficiency, and it also decreases potential contamination and tissue trauma. Knowing the specific implant size and style chosen, the patient's breast type, chest wall, and breast characteristics, one knows and marks the N-IMF on maximal stretch. This distance is then reconfirmed intraoperatively. When the nipple is in the meridian of the breast, a perpendicular approximately 1 cm medial to the areola is marked directly in the planned incision in the IMF. As an example, if a 350-g implant is chosen with a type III average-stretch breast, the incision is planned 8.5 cm from the midnipple to the fold on maximal stretch (see Fig. 116.13). If the nipple-to-fold distance is greater than 8.5—say 9.0 cm—then the incision is placed in the current fold; if less than 8.5 cm, it is lowered to 8.5 cm. The procedure is optimally performed with very few instruments, with a monopolar coagulating forceps, double-handle retractor, and lighted retractor with suction being essential. A minimum incision of a 5.5 cm is then marked laterally from this point so the main incision is located in the central breast and least visible. A barrier drape such as Ioban is placed over the breast, or at a minimum a Tegaderm dressing is placed over the nipple (12,13). Marcaine 0.25% with epinephrine is placed in the incision line, and after time for local setup, an incision is made with a 15 blade. Dissection then begins directly in a cranial or superior direction at a minimum 60-deg angle. A double-handle retractor is then positioned with constant upward retraction and repositioning, lifting the pectoralis major off the chest. Only the pectoralis can be distracted off the chest versus the intercostals. As confirmation, the pectoralis will contract in the axilla during muscle division. The muscle is divided approximately 1 cm anterior to the rib insertion, with any perforators cauterized with monopolar forceps. After entry into the subpectoral space, dissection is continued cranially and centrally in the pocket. The upper position of the implant is marked on the skin based on the implant height with dissection performed to that point. Minimal dissection is performed laterally and may be performed with the cautery tip in the off position, being careful near the lateral intercostal nerves and vessels. Dissection then proceeds medially along the fold, dissecting the muscle from the ribs from above, carefully locating and cauterizing prospectively any perforators that are inserting on the deep surface of pectoralis major. Dissection continues to the sternal margin with care not to disinsert the muscle off the sternum. Maintaining a fascial shelf medially helps to support the device in position, and a dual-plane procedure is performed if required. Care is taken not to overdissect the pocket in any direction. Irrigation is performed with triple-antibiotic Adams solution (14) and should be completely clear with no tinge of blood whatsoever. Gloves are changed following pocket dissection bilaterally, and the implants are placed in triple-antibiotic solution. If a complete barrier drape is not used, I prefer a sleeve, which facilitates placement and positioning of the 410, avoids overt trauma to the shell, and minimizes gel disruption distributing the forces. The implant is placed, and a twist tie is placed at the 6 o'clock position (Fig. 116.15). The implant is positioned at 90 deg and then rotated back and forth into position versus any side-to-side motion. Bacitracin in the irrigant is slippery and foamy and facilitates the insertion. The sleeve facilitates positioning the implant in the pocket with the twist tie at the 6 o'clock position. If the hand-in-glove pocket dissection is done correctly, it is difficult to reposition the 410 after sleeve removal. Fingers are introduced inside the sleeve, lifting the back of the implant off the chest, and the sleeve is withdrawn on the back side first and then the front.

Following implant placement and positioning in both pockets, the patient is sat up on the operating table and final implant positioning and symmetry checked. Any additional leftover Marcaine may be placed in the pocket. Surgeon fingers are placed in triple-antibiotic solution prior to coming into contact with the device as needed for positioning. Closure is initiated by placing a 2-0 Vicryl setting the IMF (Fig. 116.16) from the chest wall to the superior edge of the upper portion of the incision, creating mild flattening in the lower pole of the breast in some cases. Currently I run the fascia with a 3-0 Vicryl and following three deep dermal sutures run a 3-0 Monoderm Quill suture or 4-0 Monocryl. Longitudinal Steri-Strips are placed, or a small silicone sheet and a supportive garment are used.

FAST-TRACK RECOVERY AND DEFINED POSTOPERATIVE INSTRUCTIONS

Postoperatively, the patient is instructed to gently lift her arms above her head beginning in recovery. Current postoperative bras tend to pull up or put pressure on the IMF and incision. New garments have been designed to place a mild downward pressure on the upper pole of the breast that may be helpful with postsurgical edema. The patient is encouraged to return to all routine activities of daily living as quickly as possible with minimal routine restrictions. In contrast to standard devices, implant massage or implant displacement exercises are *not* recommended, to allow for proper soft tissue integration of the heavily textured device. Patients are discouraged from submerging their incisions for 2 weeks, although they may shower immediately, avoiding direct water pressure to the incision. Typical return to full exercise, including running, high-impact aerobics, and bouncing activity, is 4 to 6 weeks. Patients are informed that they will have a heavy pressure sensation in the upper chest. Ibuprofen is prescribed for postoperative pain, 800 mg three times daily with food. Occasionally Darvocet is given for breakthrough pain, but it is rarely required.

NATRELLE 410 RESULTS AND DATA

Data at 3 years are available for the 410, with 6-year data pending. The results are favorable when compared to standard gel

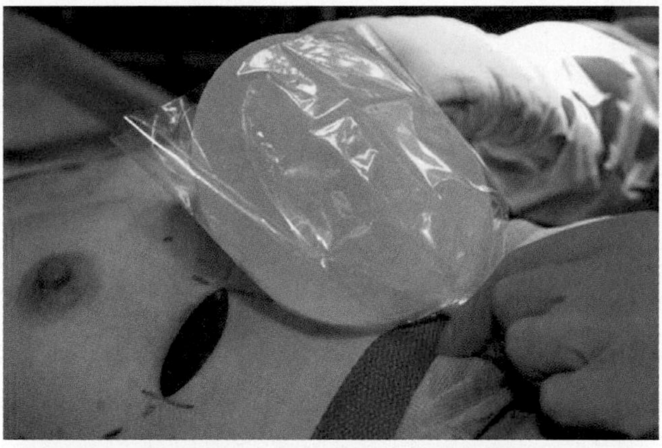

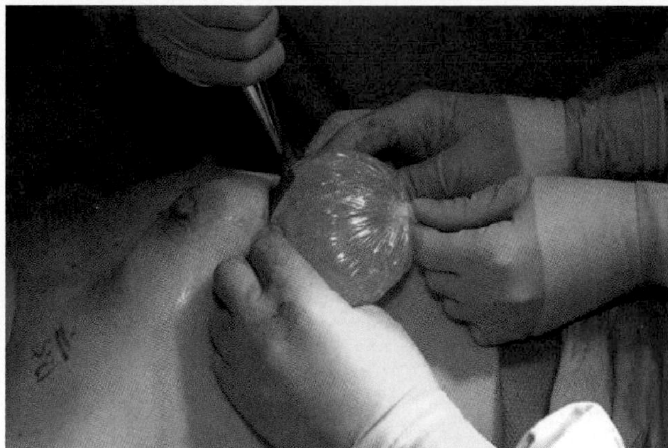

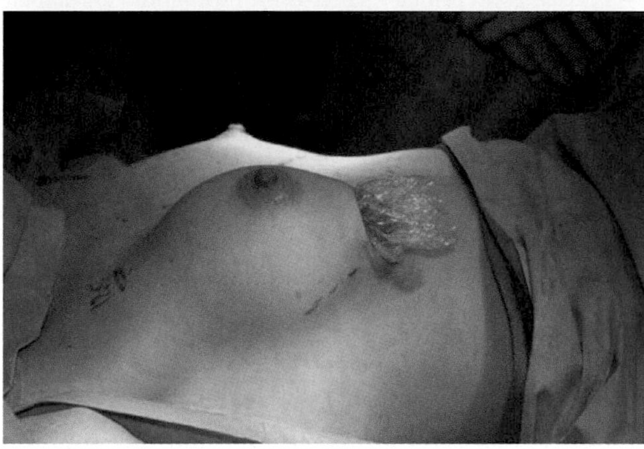

Figure 116.15. An insertion sleeve is very helpful in placing a 410 implant. It helps to avoid skin contamination of the device into the BioCell implant surface on insertion, distributes the forces to minimize gel fracture or shell damage, and positions the implant into the tight pocket when a twist-tie maneuver is performed at the 6 o'clock position.

devices in nearly every area except rotation, given that they are shaped versus elliptical devices (Tables 116.4 and 116.5). In particular, capsular contracture rates remain low, as do implant shell failure rates.

INDIVIDUAL PATIENT RESULTS AND EXAMPLES

Results in properly selected patients are among the most consistent and long-lasting of any implant used clinically. We are completing a study following the N-IMF distance over time and with a mean follow-up of 5 years. The average distance increase from 1 year to up to 8 years is 2 cm on maximal skin stretch and 1 cm at rest in more than 400 patients. I believe that this is due to the tight pocket and submuscular positioning, leaving a medial fascial shelf, the form stability of the gel and the heavily textured BioCell surface all acting in concert to provide position stability. I include here a series of 410 patients with a variety of breast types, implant sizes, and styles (Figs. 116.17–116.20).

No implants are complication free. Results including complications and revision for my first 300 primary augmentations are being submitted, and the results have been presented (16). To date, with an average 5-year follow-up, I have a 5% surgical revision rate. Eighty percent of the revisions occurred in the first 60 patients, showing a significant learning curve. Two percent of the surgical revisions were elective size-change requests. The remaining 3% of patient revisions were for recurrent ptosis, capsular contracture, small lateral skin dehiscence, and unilateral fold malposition.

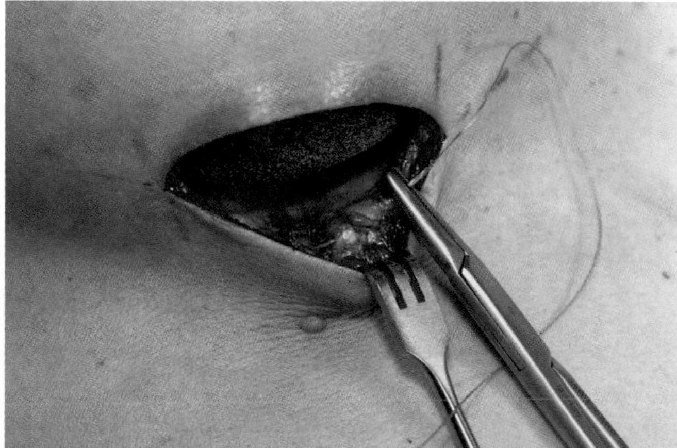

Figure 116.16. To help set the inframammary fold, a 2-0 Vicryl suture is placed from the chest wall at the base of the implant pocket and triangulated through the superficial breast fascia. This may produce some short-term lower pole flattening that if present will resolve in a few weeks. This also helps to hold the device in position and promote adherence.

TABLE 116.4 Kaplan-Meier Key Risk Rates Through Three Years

Complication	Augmentation (n = 492)
Key risk rates	
Reoperation	12.5 (9.5–15.4)
Implant removal with replacement	4.7 (2.8–6.6)
Implant removal without replacement	0.7 (0.0–1.4)
Implant rupture	0.7 (0.0–2.1)
Capsular contracture: Baker grade III/IV	1.9 (1.0–3.7)
Additional risk rates occurring in ≥2.0% of patients	
Implant malposition	2.6 (1.5–4.5)
Swelling	1.8 (1.0–3.5)
Infection	1.3 (0.6–2.8)
Breast pain	1.2 (0.6–2.7)
Delayed wound healing	1.0 (0.4–2.5)
Hypertrophic/abnormal scarring	0.9 (0.3–2.4)
Asymmetry	0.8 (0.3–2.2)
Hematoma	0.8 (0.3–2.2)
Seroma/fluid accumulation	0.8 (0.3–2.2)
Wrinkling/rippling	0.5 (0.1–1.8)
Upper pole fullness	0

From Bengtson BP, VanNatta BW, Murphy DK, et al. Style 410 highly cohesive silicone breast implant core study results at 3 years. *Plast Reconstr Surg* 2007;120(7):40S–48S.

SOME MYTHS AND MISCONCEPTIONS CONCERNING THE 410

There is always myth surrounding new techniques or devices. Contrary to some beliefs, although these devices feel slightly firmer in the hand at room temperature, they are soft in the body. This is likely due to a combination of factors, including the low capsular contracture rate, a "one-breast feel," and possibly a different stiffness/firmness coefficient at body temperature versus room temperature (see Fig. 116.3). This increased degree of form stability and position stability in the partial submuscular position also helps to resist motion artifact and hyperanimation. With proper muscle release off of the rib insertions and dual-plane approach, the vector is changed from an upward oblique to a transverse direction, creating intermammary cleavage widening (Fig. 116.21).

The 410 is not leak-proof or immune to shell failure, but it does have low reported shell failure rates long term (7). The increased form stability of the gel also helps to limit the extension of gel outside of the shell versus less-form-stable fillers.

RECOMMENDATIONS FOR EARLY USE AND SUMMARY

Recommendations for early use include the following:

- Use preferably in primary augmentation patients versus revision patients.
- Choose good primary patients with straightforward anatomy, not extremely difficult breasts: constriction, asymmetry, and revision patients.
- Avoid in patients with significant ptosis.
- Use tissue-based planning principles with basic measurements, including, at a minimum, breast base width, SN-N, N-IMF, and skin stretch.
- Use atraumatic, bloodless, prospective hemostasis with hand-in-glove pocket dissection.
- Consider Ioban or Tegaderm protection and also insertion sleeves.
- Use moderate-height, moderate-projection (MM) 410 implants for the first 10 to 20 patients.
- Education is key! Visit surgeons with 410 experience.

The Natrelle 410 is beginning its ninth year of premarket approval in the United States and is pending approval by the FDA at the time of this writing. There is a great deal of enthusiasm growing concerning the 410's upcoming launch. This device will add a great deal to the list of options for breast augmentation. It also brings with it some challenges. It is best to look at this device as a brand-new procedure. Many aspects are completely different or counterintuitive to using round gel devices, such as pocket dissection: tight versus a larger loose pocket, no massage or implant displacement exercises with the 410, and the need for a much higher degree of tissue-based planning than many U.S. surgeons are using in their practices. Surgeons can make the transition, just as we have for open versus closed rhinoplasty, subcutaneous musculoaponeurotic system techniques for facial rejuvenation, and endoscopic techniques.

TABLE 116.5 Comparison of Kaplan-Meier By-Patient Risk Rates

Complication	Augmentation with Style 410 Highly Cohesive Gel Implants Through 3 Years (n = 492) (%)	Augmentation with Current Standard Silicone Gel Implants Through 4 Years (n = 455) (%)	Augmentation with Current Saline Implants Through 3 Years (n = 901) (%)
Reoperation	12.5	23.5	21.1
Implant removal with replacement	1.7	7.5	7.6 (combined)
Implant removal without replacement	0.7	2.3	
Implant rupture/deflation	0.7	2.7	5.0
Capsular contracture: Baker grade III/IV	1.9	13.2	8.7

From Bengtson BP, VanNatta BW, Murphy DK, et al. Style 410 highly cohesive silicone breast implant core study results at 3 years. *Plast Reconstr Surg* 2007;120(7):40S–48S.

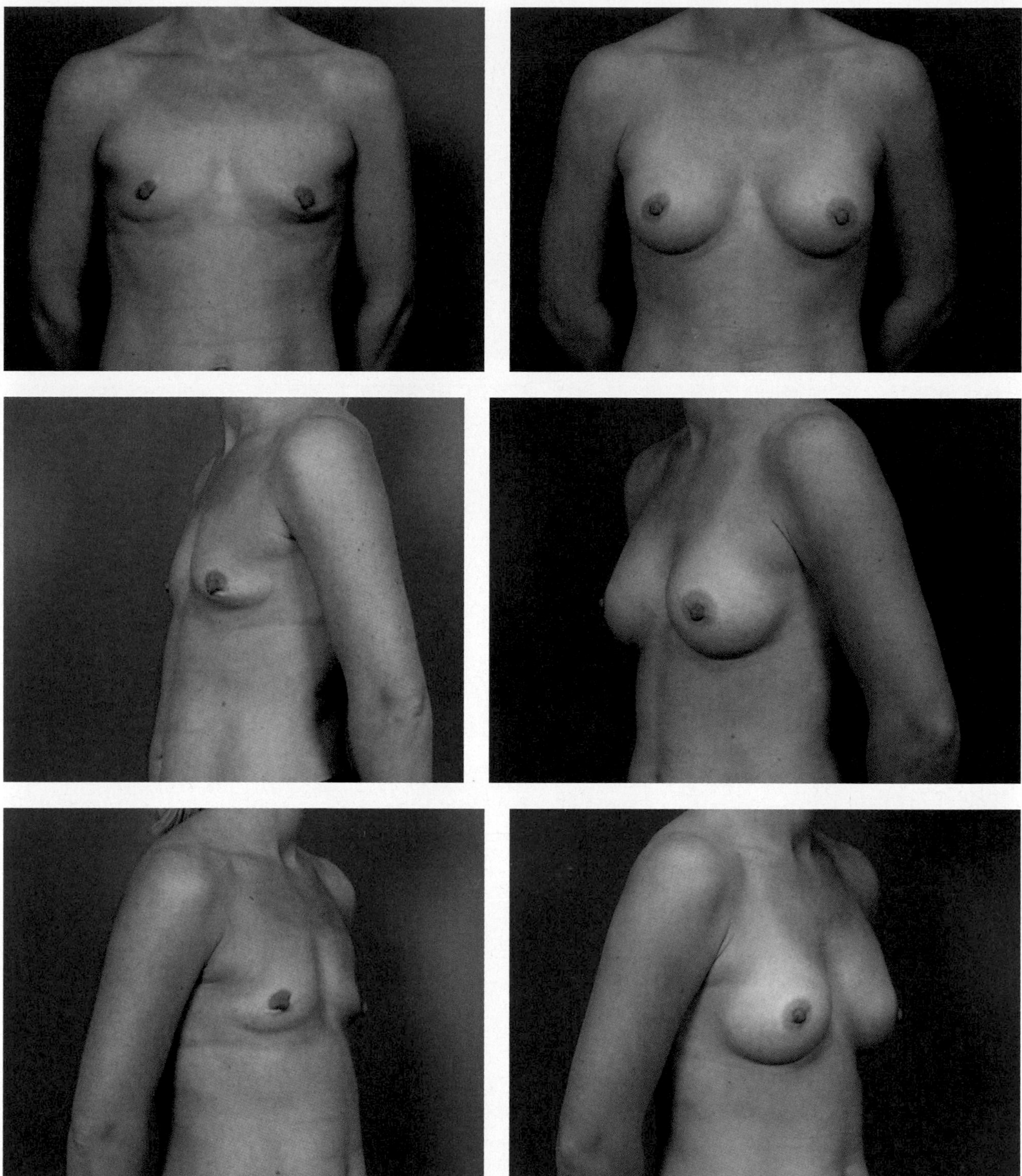

Figure 116.17. This patient's tissue-based planning measurements include a 12-cm breast base width, breast type III with an average amount of skin stretch of 2 cm ,and a 19-cm sternal notch-to-nipple distance. A 310-g FM implant was placed in a partial subpectoral position, and her postoperative result at 3 years is shown.

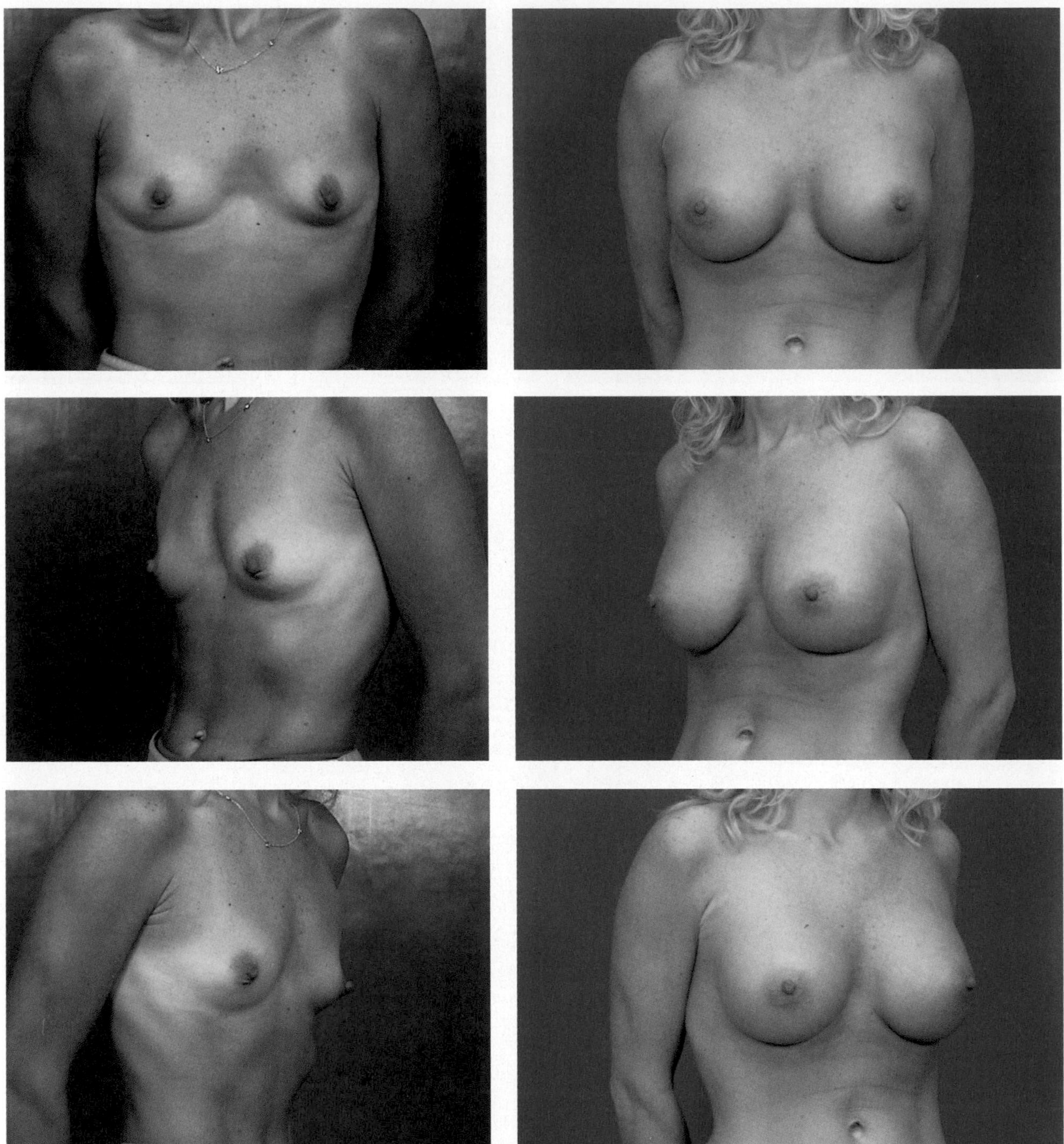

Figure 116.18. This is a 30-year-old patient with tissue-based planning measurements, including a 12.5-cm breast base width, breast type III with an average amount of skin stretch of 2 cm, and a 20-cm sternal notch-to-nipple distance. A 350-g FM implant was placed in a dual-plane pocket position, and her result at 6 years postoperatively is shown.

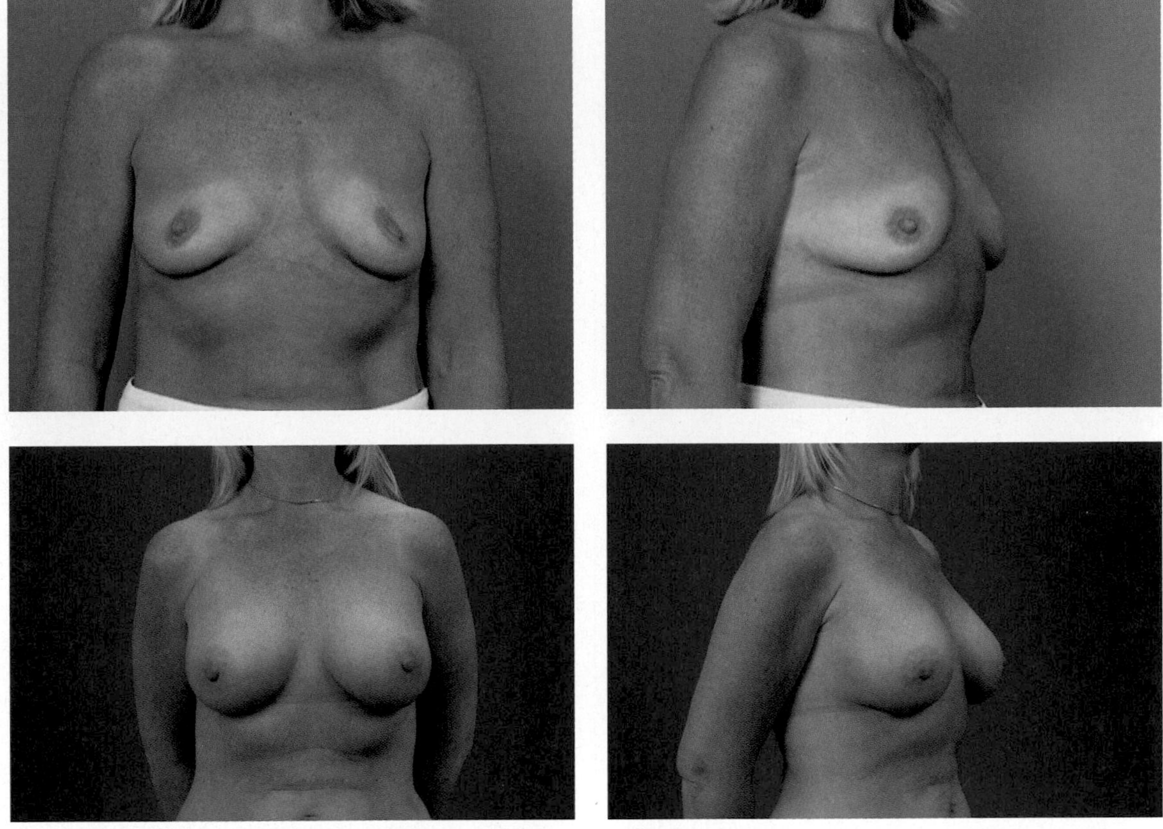

Figure 116.19. This patient has a type V breast with a loose skin envelope and 4 cm of skin stretch, a 21-cm distance from her sternal notch to nipple, and a 14-cm breast base width. A 375-g MF Style 410 was placed in a dual-plane pocket, and her result at 4 years is shown.

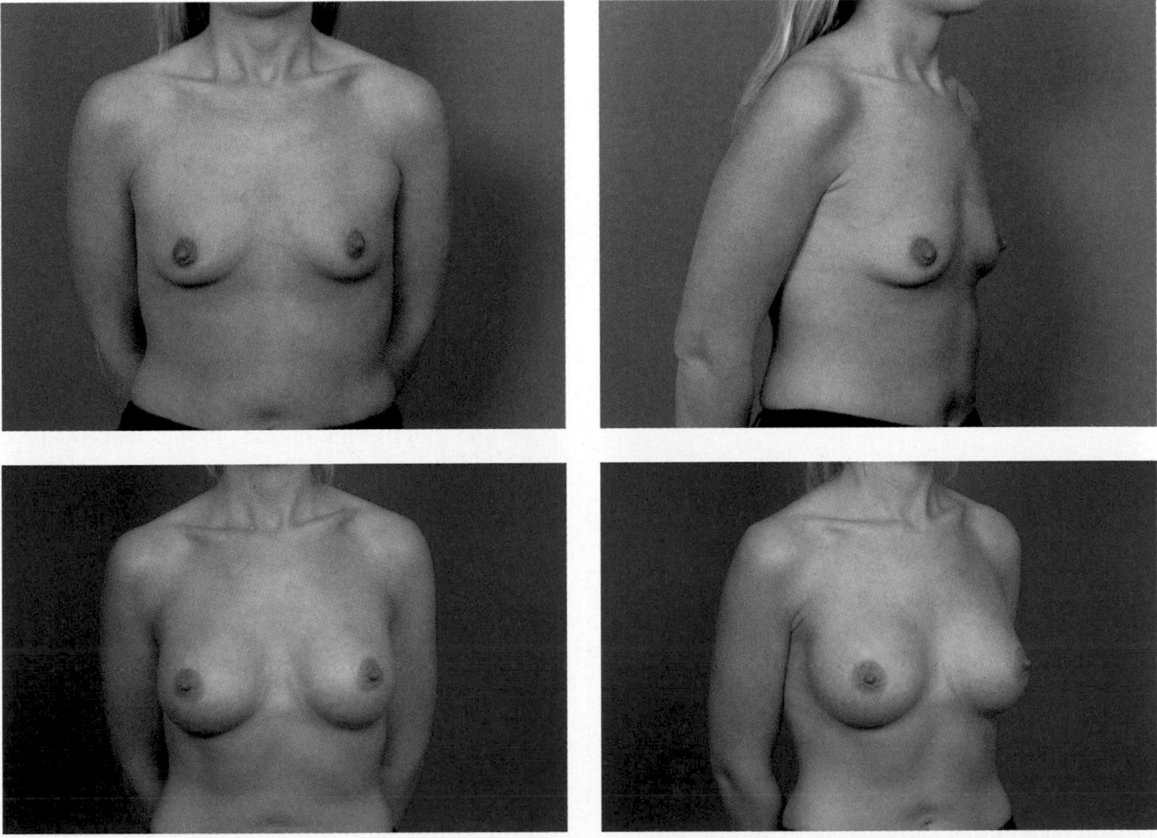

Figure 116.20. This patient with postinvolutional breast changes is a breast type IV with 3 cm of skin stretch, a 20-cm sternal notch-to-nipple distance, and a 12.5-cm breast base width. A Style 410 375-g FF implant was used, and her result at 3 years is shown.

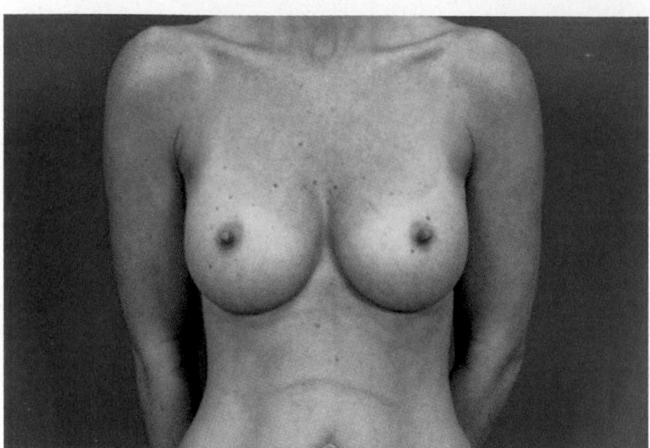

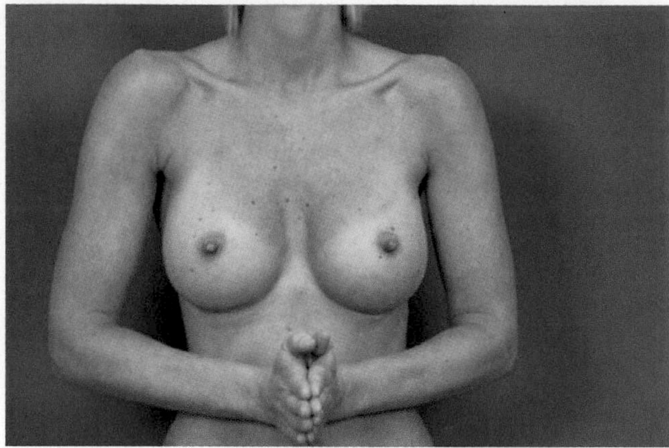

Figure 116.21. It is often preferable to obtain maximum soft tissue coverage and place Style 410 implants in a partial retropectoral, dual-plane position. This also helps to minimize any edge palpability. The main disadvantage is the potential for hyperanimation deformity. However, if adequate pectoral muscle releases off of the rib insertions and dual-plane release are used as needed, the form-stable 410 help to resist muscle contraction, and the upward oblique pull is translated into more of a transverse vector, creating some cleavage/intermammary widening, which is rarely a complaint.

However, the specific implant selection and use of the 410 are markedly different than current approaches with elliptical, round devices. Patient demand for this new device will be high, but the 410's ultimate success will be largely determined by its proper use, including patient selection, implant selection, precise surgical technique, and defined postoperative care. Plastic surgeons should take advantage of the educational opportunities offered surrounding the launch of this implant above and beyond the general certification process, including any additional face-to-face training and courses, taking time to visit surgeons with 410 experience, and other interactive educational events.

EDITORIAL COMMENTS

Dr. Bengtson provides an excellent review on the Style 410 form-stable silicone gel implant for breast augmentation. The chapter is introduced with a nice review and comparison of the characteristics of the various gel devices currently on the market. A listing of the advantages and disadvantages is presented. The importance of proper patient selection is emphasized. Poor candidates include those with significant breast ptosis or those with chest wall deformities. Good candidates include those with mild to moderate asymmetry, tight skin, and no ptosis. Dr. Bengtson states that the 410 device is not for everyone. In patients who are good candidates, dimensional planning and measurements are critical. The important measurements include base width, skin stretch, sternal notch-to-nipple distance, and nipple-to-inframammary fold distance. Precise surgical technique is mandatory. Only the inframammary approach is recommended. My main concern with this chapter is that it describes the use of a device that is not available to the majority of plastic surgeon in the United States (at least at the time of this preparation). Its distribution and use are restricted to surgeons in the Allergan clinical trials. It is therefore difficult to prepare a commentary on a device that I have never used. I am, however, very interested in using this device when it does become available, for all of the aforementioned reasons. As an outside onlooker, I do have some concerns. Will the device be too firm? Will the edges be palpable? I think that the BioCell texturing is excellent, but if there is any rotational deformity, the breast will distort. The mechanics of implant insertion are complicated. Extensive planning is necessary, and a precise pocket dissection is required. The myriad of implant choices may be exhausting and confusing for even the experienced surgeon. I wonder if we are taking a relatively straightforward operation and making it a bit more complicated. The reality is that from 1992 to 2007, plastic surgeons in the United States had a single option for breast augmentation: the saline implant. The option of silicone gel devices became available after the FDA approved the use of round silicone gel devices in 2007. The majority of us have become quite skilled, adept, and comfortable using the devices currently available. Although many of us are curious about this device based on the experiences of surgeons such as Drs. Bengtson, Maxwell, and Spear, questions remain as to the predictability and reproducibility of this device, given its meticulous characteristics. Perhaps in the near future, the Style 410 device will become available for widespread use in the United States. I suspect that a mandatory instructional session will be necessary prior to using the device. Overall, I appreciate Dr. Bengtson's enthusiasm about this device, as well as his excellent outcomes.

M.Y.N.

REFERENCES

1. Tebbetts JB. *Augmentation Mammaplasty: Redefining the Patient and Surgeon Experience.* St. Louis, MO: Mosby; 2009.
2. Maxwell GP, Baker MR. Augmentation mammaplasty: general considerations. In: Spear SL, ed. *Surgery of the Breast. Principles and Art.* 2nd ed. Baltimore: Lippincott Williams & Wilkins; 2006:1237.

3. Brown MH, Shenker R, Silver SA. Cohesive silicone gel breast implants in aesthetic and reconstructive breast surgery. *Plast Reconstr Surg* 2005;116(3):768.
4. Bengtson BP, VanNatta BW, Murphy DK, et al. Style 410 highly cohesive silicone breast implant core study results at 3 years. *Plast Reconstr Surg* 2007;120(7 suppl 1):40S–48S.
5. Heden P, Jernbeck J, Hober M. Breast augmentation with anatomical cohesive gel implants: the world's largest current experience. *Clin Plast Surg* 2001;28(3):531–552.
6. Inamed. Directions for use: Inamed style 410 silicone-filled breast implants. 2006. Available at: http://www.allergan.ca/assets/pdf/L037-02_410_DFU.pdf. Accessed July 27, 2010.
7. Heden P, Bone B, Murphy DK, et al. Style 410 cohesive silicone breast implants: safety and effectiveness at 5 to 9 years after implantation. *Plast Reconstr Surg* 2006;118(6):1281.
8. Heden P. Breast augmentation with anatomic high-cohesiveness silicone gel implants. In: Spear SL, ed. *Surgery of the Breast. Principles and Art.* 2nd ed. Baltimore: Lippincott Williams & Wilkins; 2006:1344.
9. Ad ams WP. The process of breast augmentation: four sequential steps for optimizing outcomes for patients. *Plast Reconstr Surg* 2008;122(6):1892.
10. Tebbetts JB, Adams WP. Five critical decisions in breast augmentation using five measurements in 5 minutes: the high five decision support process. *Plast Reconstr Surg* 2005;116:2005.
11. Adams WP, Bengtson BP, Jewell M, et al. Optimizing results in breast augmentation. Presented at Instructional Course S8 at the American Society for Aesthetic Plastic Surgery Meeting, New Orleans, Louisiana, 2005.
12. Shestak KC, Askari M. A simple barrier drape for breast implant placement. *Plast Reconstr Surg* 2006;117:1722.
13. Bengtson BP. Additional uses for a barrier drape in breast implant surgery: barrier protection for suspected silicone implant rupture. *Plast Reconstr Surg* 2009;123(2):76.
14. Adams WP, Rios JL, Smith SJ. Enhancing patient outcomes in aesthetic and reconstructive breast surgery using triple antibiotic breast irrigation: six year prospective clinical study. *Plast Reconstr Surg* 2006;117(1):30.
15. Bengtson BP. Style 410 cohesive gel implants: clinical data and follow-up of the largest current cohort in the United States. Presented at the Workshop in Plastic Surgery, U.S. Virgin Islands, 2004; Canadian Society of Plastic Surgery, Banff, Alberta, Canada, June 2007; Atlanta Breast Symposium, February 2009.

CHAPTER

117

Sydney R. Coleman
Alesia P. Saboeiro

Lipoaugmentation

INTRODUCTION AND HISTORY OF FAT GRAFTING TO THE BREASTS

The concept of transplanting autologous fat to the breasts is not new. In 1895 Czerny published a paper describing the successful transfer of a fist-sized lipoma from the buttock to the breast of a patient who had undergone glandular excision for mastitis (1). In 1910 Hollander was the first to describe fat injections to the breast for correction of mastectomy defects (2). Numerous publications followed as the idea of fat grafting for the correction of both cosmetic and functional problems developed. Many of the early attempts at fat grafting, however, were not successful, primarily due to the tendency of the fatty tissue to resorb, making the results unpredictable (3–7). Thus, fat grafting fell out of favor for many years. With the advent of liposuction by Fournier (8) and Illouz (9) in the 1980s there was renewed interest in the use of autologous fat for reinjection. Chajchir and Benzaquen (10) reported their experience of transplanting fat over a 4-year period and noted 86% favorable results, while Ersek reported disappointing results in a 3-year follow-up (11). Thus, fat grafting in general was still thought to be unpredictable.

In 1985, Mel Bircoll presented the first modern-day paper on breast augmentation using fat grafting at the California Society of Plastic Surgeons (12). This paper, as well as another paper describing fat grafting after transverse rectus abdominis musculocutaneous flap reconstruction (13), led to a position paper by the Ad-Hoc Committee on New Procedures of the American Society of Plastic Surgeons (ASPS) "deploring the use of autologous fat injection in breast augmentation." The committee made no reference to any scientific findings, but it was their opinion only that the scarring and calcifications that would develop would make mammography difficult and that breast disease might go undetected. Coincidentally, in the same issue of *Plastic and Reconstructive Surgery*, an article by Brown was published reporting calcifications in 50% of mammograms performed 2 years after breast reduction surgery (14). There was no suggestion that breast reduction surgery was "deplorable" despite mammographic findings similar to those after fat grafting. Nonetheless, fat grafting to the breast again fell out of favor and was not performed, or at least not discussed, at any plastic surgery meetings.

In the 1990s, after several years of refining the technique, Coleman published his first of many papers using the successful, reproducible technique of lipostructure (15,16). Encouraged by positive results with fat grafting to the face, hands, and body, Coleman began to experiment with fat grafting to the breasts. From 1995 to 2000, he performed breast fat grafting to 17 patients. Some of these patients were primary augmentations, while others were patients with tuberous breasts, visible implants, or tissue defects secondary to breast cancer. These results in 2007 showed a lasting volume correction and soft, natural breasts. Postoperative mammography revealed a few oil cysts and a few calcifications, which were changes typically seen after any breast procedure (17). There was no interference with breast cancer detection, and 1 patient was diagnosed with a breast cancer in an area other than that which was grafted. As more plastic surgeons around the world have begun to successfully perform breast fat grafting procedures and have published their work, the ASPS and the American Society for Aesthetic Plastic Surgery have reversed their earlier moratorium. They now state that "Fat grafting may be considered for breast augmentation and correction of defects associated with medical conditions and previous breast surgeries; however, results are dependent on technique and surgeon expertise" (18, p.10). Thus, fat grafting has returned to the surgeon's armamentarium for both breast augmentation and for the correction of a multitude of breast problems.

PATIENT SELECTION

Fat grafting may be performed to correct or improve a wide variety of breast problems. These problems may be small, such as residual defects after flap reconstruction or lumpectomy defects, or large, such as the creation of an entire breast after mastectomy or implant removal. Other uses include disguising breast implants in thin patients or in patients with visible capsular contractures, correction of tuberous breasts, correction of Poland syndrome, creation of breast cleavage, correction of pectus excavatum, and covering of a bony sternum. Because the fat can be placed in the exact areas where the deficiency exists, the uses are endless. Specific shaping of the breast or chest can be accomplished with fat, whereas an implant is not as versatile.

The primary limitation of fat grafting to the breast is associated with the availability of donor sites and the volume that can be obtained. In patients with a paucity of excess fat, fat grafting may not be an option. The volume of fat that needs to be grafted to make a significant change is considerably more than one would expect based on experience with breast implant volumes. Because the fat is integrated into the tissues and not placed behind the gland or muscle in one unit as with implants, the change is not as dramatic. In general, the addition of approximately 300 cc of fat per breast will result in an increase of approximately one cup size. The addition of much more than that during one procedure is not usually possible due to tissue compliance and the potential of fat necrosis due to a lack of blood supply. Additional volume may be added during subsequent procedures if the patient still has available donor sites. To be appropriate candidates, patients must have realistic expectations for a modest change in size. A change in cup size from an A to a C, for example, is not realistic in one procedure. If that is the patient's desire, then silicone or saline implants should be considered. It is unlikely that fat grafting to the breast will ever replace the need for implants in patients who desire significant volume changes or in patients with a very low body mass index (19,20).

PLANNING

The design for the surgery is different for each patient, depending on the goal to be achieved. Preoperative photos are taken of each patient with hands at the sides, with hands on the hips, and with hands placed on top of the head. In addition, photos are often taken in those positions with the patient also bending 45 deg at the waist and with the patient standing and the photographer sitting. Having patients with implants squeeze the implants with their hands demonstrates the degree of capsular contracture, and squeezing the implants with their pectoralis muscles often demonstrates defects that cannot otherwise be appreciated. This gives an excellent opportunity to really study the breasts and to identify subtle asymmetries. From those photos, a tracing is done, and the procedure is mapped out specifically for that patient. We use a color-coded system to indicate where fat will be placed (green for significant volume changes and yellow for feathering), where fat will *not* be placed/borders of fat placement (orange), where the incisions will be made (red), and where the fat will be harvested (purple). The plan is made in consultation with the patient so that she will have a thorough understanding of where fat will be added and where it will be removed (19,20).

OPERATIVE TECHNIQUE

General anesthesia is the preferred type of anesthesia for fat grafting to the breasts due to the length of time required to harvest the fat using 10-cc syringes, process it, and reinsert it (usually a total of 4.5 hours). Fat-harvesting sites are chosen based on the patient's desire for volume reduction and to improve contours. When excess fat is limited, small amounts will be removed from multiple areas, often including the calves and ankles. The donor areas are infiltrated with lactated Ringer with lidocaine 0.5% and epinephrine 1:200,000 in a volume equal to the anticipated fat removal.

Fat is then hand suctioned using a Coleman harvesting cannula attached to a 10-cc syringe. The fat is then centrifuged for 3 minutes at 3,000 rpm and then separated, discarding the upper oil layer and the lower local anesthetic/blood layer. The middle fat layer is then transferred to 3-cc syringes for placement into the breasts. Fat is grafted into the breasts via 4-mm incisions in the inframammary crease and within the areola. Occasionally an additional incision may be made in the axillary fold.

A blunt 17-gauge infiltration cannula of 9 or 15 cm in length is used for placement of fat into all levels of the breast, often including the pectoralis major muscle. One of the advantages of fat grafting to the breast is the ability to selectively contour the area depending on the specific needs of each patient. Placement of tissue deep against the chest wall will provide volume, but more controlled shaping of the breast occurs at the more superficial levels.

The key to survival of the fat grafts and the minimization of fat necrosis is placement of the fat in very small aliquots. In general, with each pass of the cannula, only approximately 0.2 cc of fat is deposited (during the withdrawal of the cannula), thus making the procedure very time consuming. *If large volumes of fat are injected with each pass of the cannula, the likely outcome will be fat necrosis, oil cysts, lumps, and calcifications.* For this reason, great care should be taken when considering fat grafting to the breasts, and surgeons inexperienced in fat grafting should ideally start in a more forgiving area of the body, such as the hands.

The amount of fat to graft is entirely dependent on the problem or the desired outcome. For a small depression secondary to a biopsy, as little as 25 to 50 cc of fat may be needed to smooth the contours. However, for an average augmentation, 250 to 400 cc of fat per breast is usually needed. The yield of graftable fat after processing is usually about 50%; therefore, to obtain 800 cc of graftable fat, approximately 1,600 cc of hand-suctioned fat must be removed (19,20).

POSTOPERATIVE CARE

Similar to standard liposuction, compression garments or Reston foam may be used on the donor sites. The breast dressing usually consists of Reston foam along the inframammary fold and occasionally over the sternum, followed by Tegaderm over the breasts, cotton "fluffs," and a surgical brassiere. No cold therapy is used, and dressings are removed 3 to 5 days postoperatively (19,20).

COMPLICATIONS AND LIMITATIONS

Short-term complications, such as bleeding and infection, are extremely rare with fat grafting. We have patients wash with Hibiclens soap the night before and the morning of the surgery and give one dose of intravenous Ancef prior to surgery. Postoperative antibiotics are not prescribed unless signs of infection are present. More common early issues are bruising, swelling, and discomfort in both the donor sites and the grafted sites. In the donor sites, this is similar to what is seen with standard liposuction. In the breasts, the discomfort is usually less; however, the swelling will make the breasts appear considerably larger than they will ultimately be.

Late complications may include contour deformities in the donor sites, unacceptable scarring in the incision sites, lack of adequate volume or correction, and fat necrosis resulting in oil cysts, lumps, and calcifications in the breasts. Contour deformities that arise can be corrected using the same techniques described. Scarring is minimized using the oil that is removed after centrifugation to lubricate the harvesting cannula. Despite using the oil, incisions are sometimes unacceptable secondary to the friction created during the suctioning and may need to be revised. One of the main limitations of this procedure for the breasts is the degree of volume change that can be made. This may be due to a paucity of fat in the donor sites, as well as to a tight skin envelope, but it is also due to a limitation in the amount of fat that can be placed next to existing tissue to ensure the grafted fat gets a blood supply. After approximately 4 months, when the grafted fat has "taken," it is possible to perform a second fat grafting procedure to further augment the breast.

The problem of fat necrosis may become evident as a palpable lump in the breast or may be seen on mammogram as an oil cyst or calcification. The calcifications that occur with fat grafting, or with any form of trauma or surgical intervention to the breast, have a benign appearance as compared with microcalcifications that are typical of breast cancer. If there were any question as to the nature of any finding in the breast postoperatively, a biopsy for confirmation would be recommended.

Finally, the issue of time is a major limitation to this procedure. Hand suctioning of the fat is necessary for preservation of the fat cells and, ultimately, the longevity of the results. The centrifugation, separation, and preparation of the fat for grafting is very labor intensive, but this does not add time to the overall

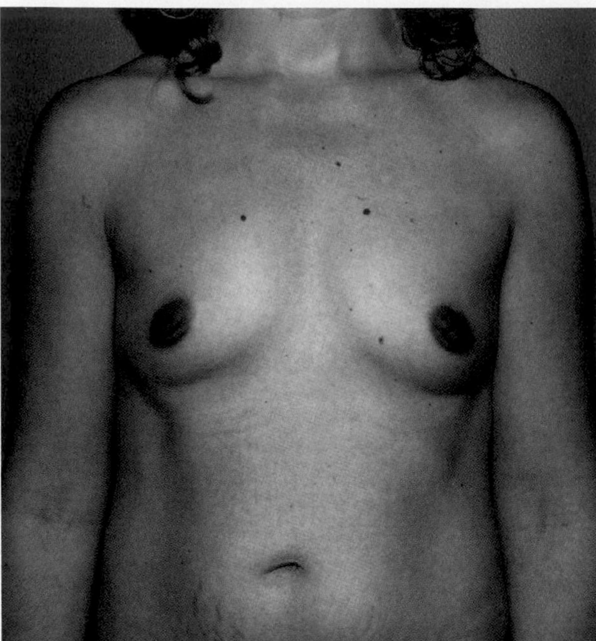
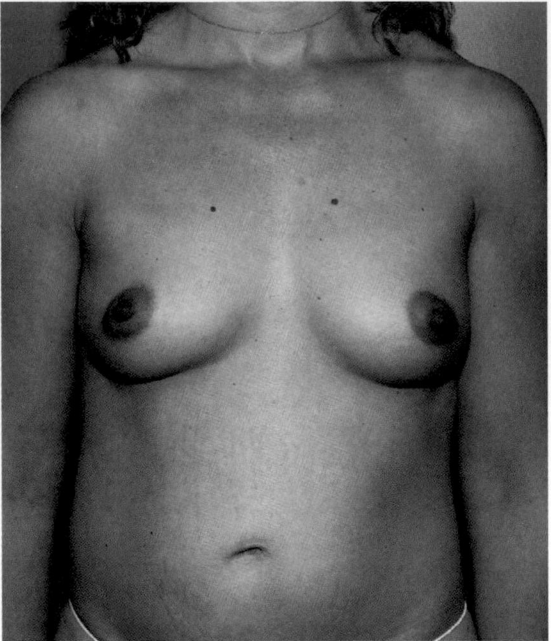

Figure 117.1. A 34-year-old woman presented with micromastia for a primary augmentation. The following volumes were placed: left breast 315 cc, right breast 342.5 cc. Postoperative photographs were taken at 8 months.

procedure. Meticulous placement of the fat to ensure its survival does add time to the procedure. This step is probably the most important, however, as this is where the shaping of the breasts takes place and where more significant problems of fat necrosis can arise (19,20).

RESULTS

After fat grafting to the breasts, there is bruising that takes several weeks to resolve, as well as a few months of swelling during which the breasts appear larger and more firm than they will be ultimately. The photos show examples of three patients who underwent one fat grafting procedure. Each patient had a nice change in size and shape of the breasts but is planning a second procedure to increase the volume even further. With difficult tuberous breast abnormalities, it is expected that more than one procedure will be necessary to adequately improve the breast shape. Postoperatively, none of the patients had any palpable masses, and there were no mammographic abnormalities on the patient with the 19-month follow-up (Figs. 117.1 to 117.9).

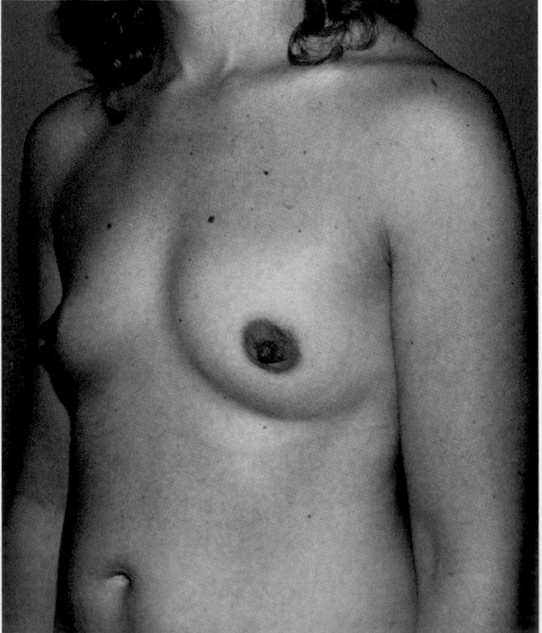
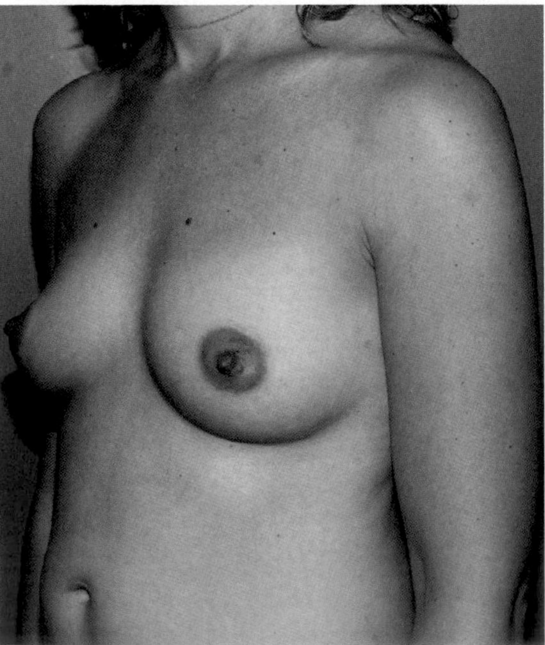

Figure 117.2. See legend to Figure 117.1.

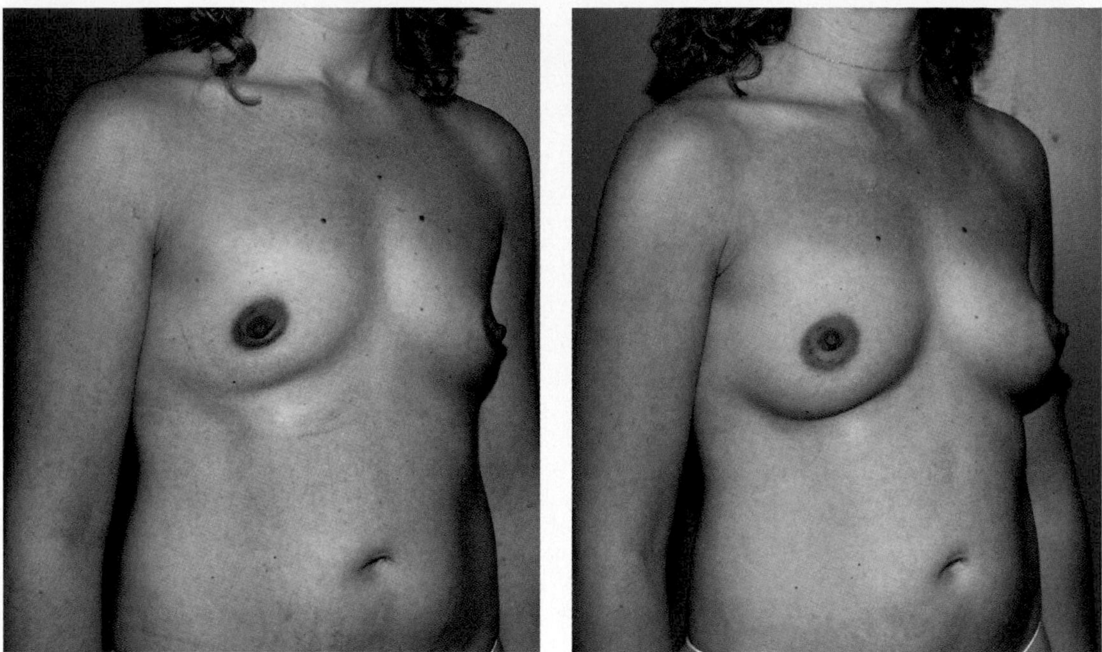

Figure 117.3. See legend to Figure 117.1.

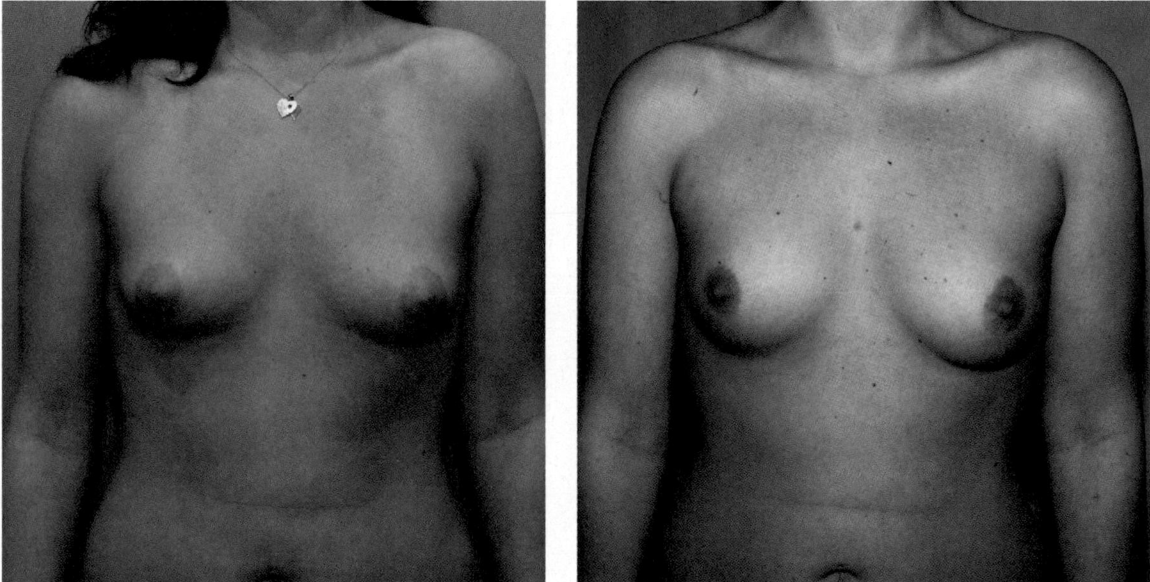

Figure 117.4. A 28-year-old woman presented with micromastia for a primary augmentation. The following volumes were placed: left breast 267.5 cc, right breast 195 cc. Postoperative photographs were taken at 19 months.

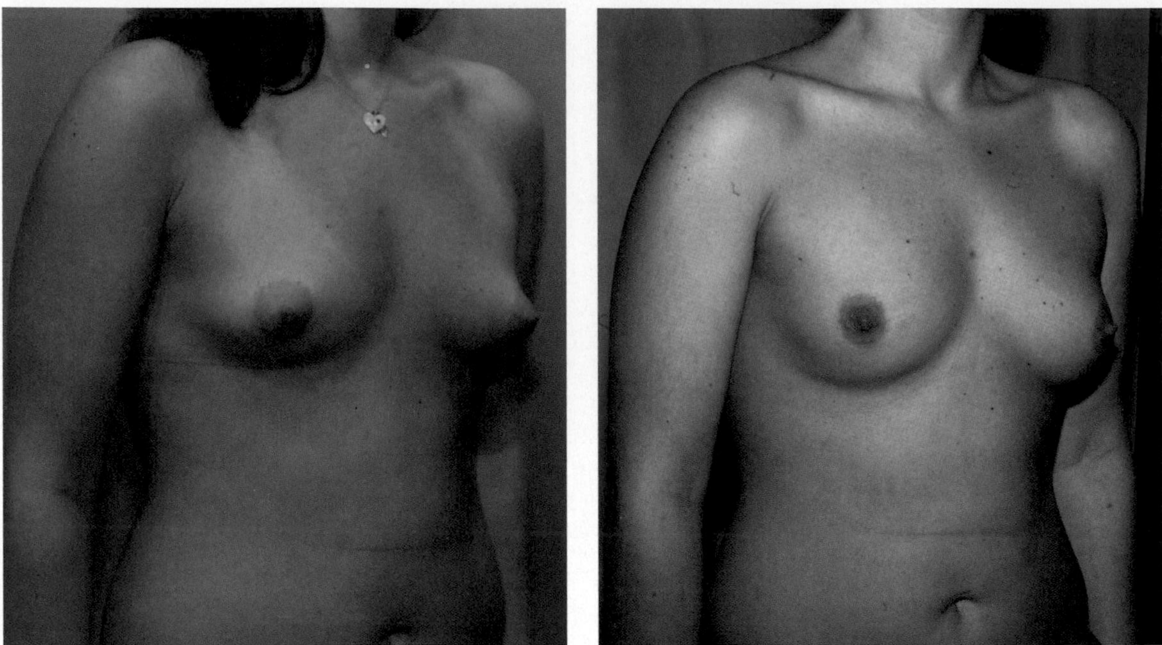

Figure 117.5. See legend to Figure 117.4.

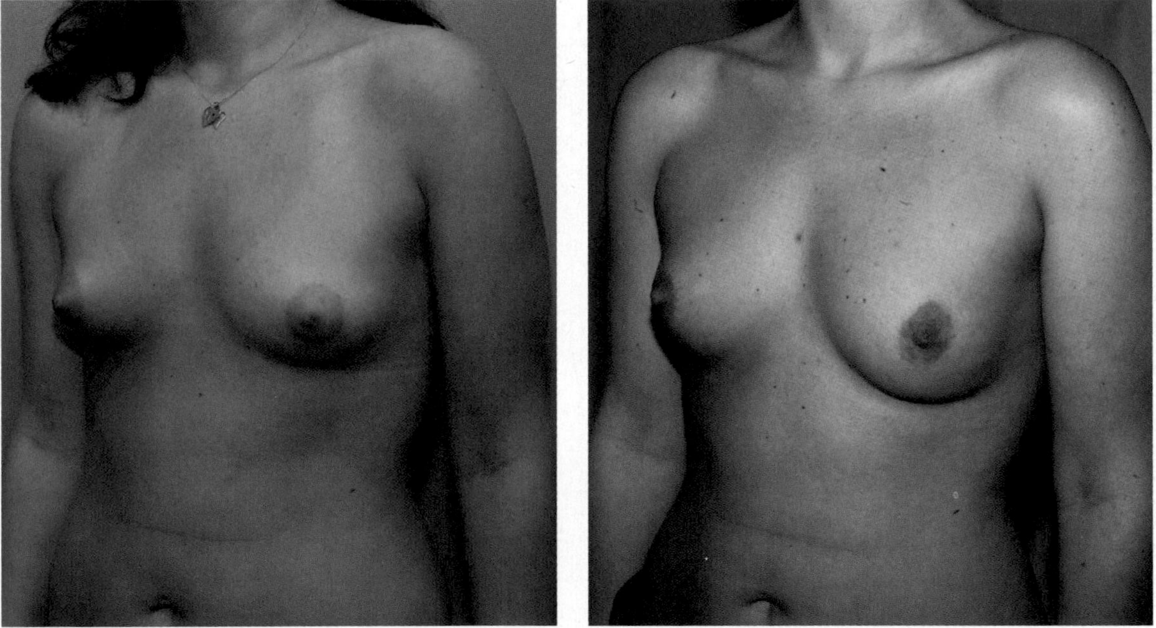

Figure 117.6. See legend to Figure 117.4.

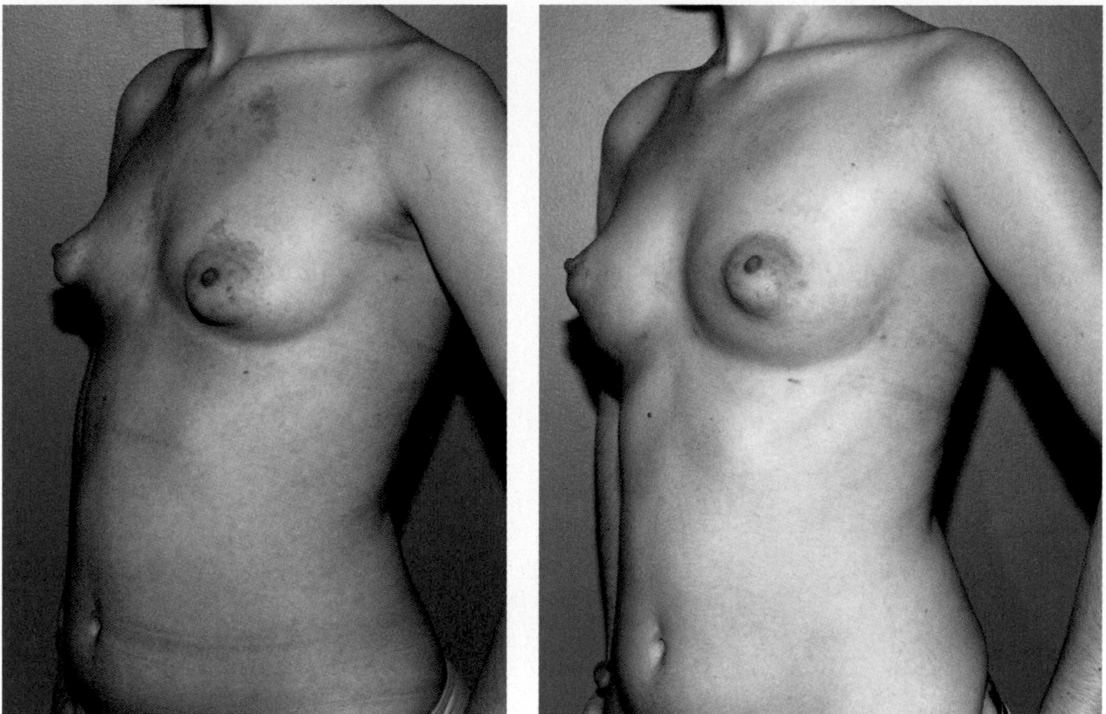

Figure 117.7. A 24-year-old woman presented with tuberous breasts for correction. The following volumes were placed: left breast 202.5 cc, right breast 245 cc. Postoperative photographs were taken at 3.5 months.

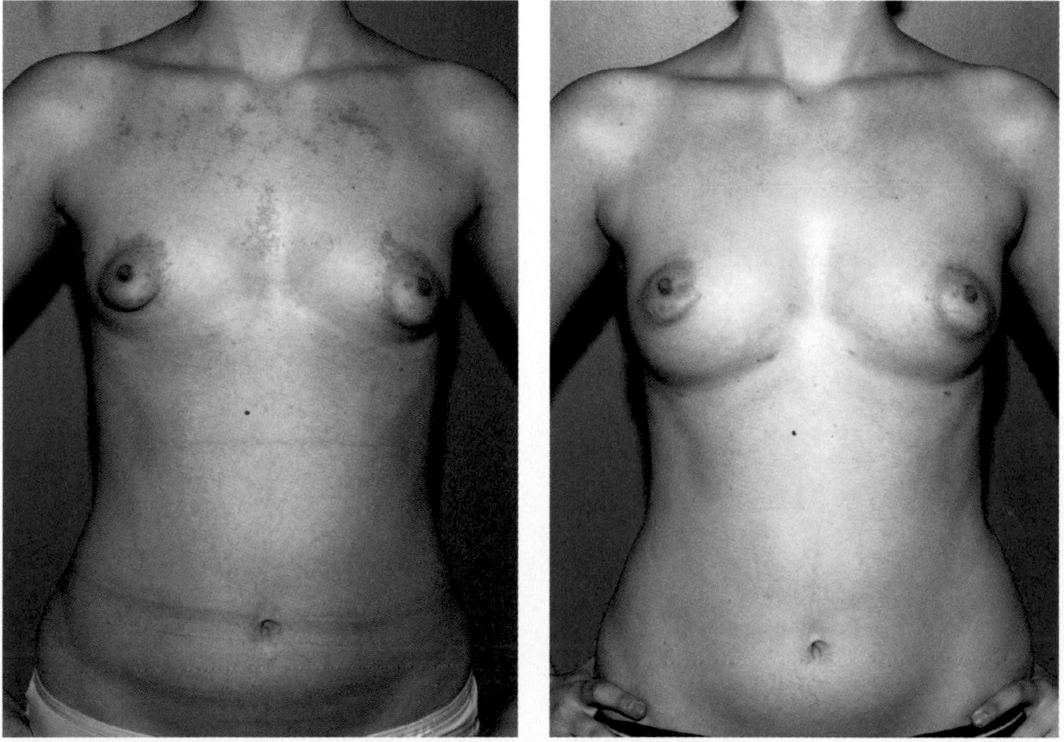

Figure 117.8. See legend to Figure 117.7.

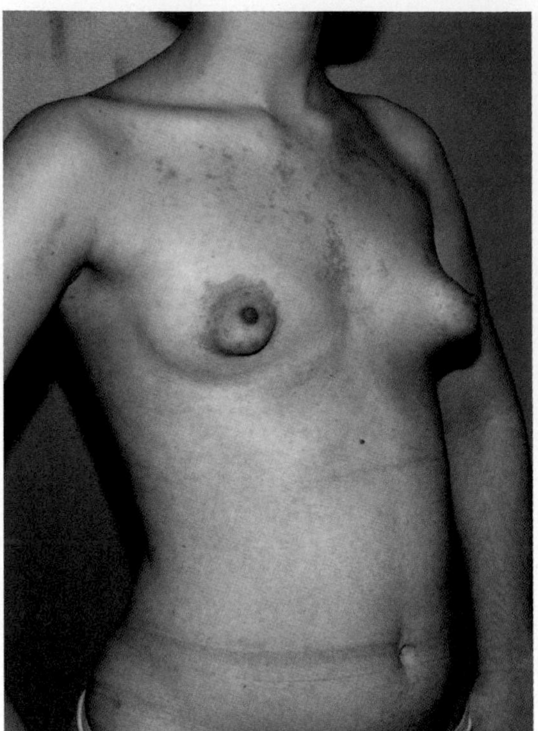

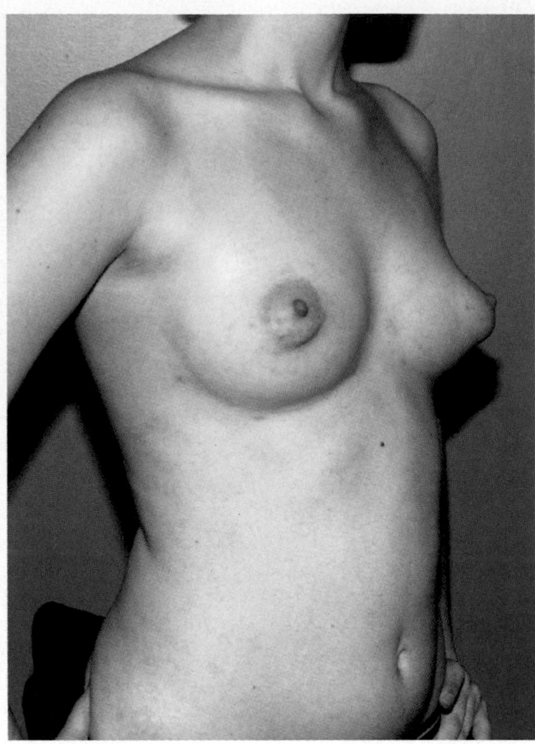

Figure 117.9. See legend to Figure 117.7.

CONCLUSION

Fat grafting to the breasts once again offers the plastic surgeon a valuable tool for augmentation of the breast. It can be not only helpful, but also often the only solution, to small residual defects after biopsies, lumpectomies, reconstruction, or visible implant edges after traditional breast augmentation techniques. Selective expansion of the breast envelope with fat is particularly useful in difficult breast problems such as tuberous breasts. Modest augmentations are possible in the average patient with reasonable donor sites. Technique is particularly important to ensure survival of the grafted fat and to minimize complications.

EDITORIAL COMMENTS

The authors have provided an excellent synopsis of the current state of fat grafting for breast augmentation. Acceptance of this technique for this indication is increasing as we learn more about its safety and efficacy. Dr. Coleman has certainly been one of the central figures in this debate, and the authors have provided valuable insight into how this technique should be performed in order to obtain predictable and reproducible results. The authors stress the importance of proper patient selection and the need to ensure realistic expectations. They review the salient aspects related to proper technique in order to ensure maximal graft survival and take. The excellent results are clearly demonstrated by the photographs in the chapter.

My thoughts related to aesthetic fat grafting for lipoaugmentation are based on my experience using fat grafting in the setting of breast reconstruction following mastectomy. I feel that the technique for both settings is safe and effective, but we have not yet proved it in a scientific manner. The scientific evidence for this is mounting every month as new studies are being published. That said, I believe that we are headed in the right direction and that fat grafting for lipoaugmentation may soon be an accepted modality much like it is for contour deformities following breast reconstruction. Currently, there are surgeons who believe that definitive and conclusive data demonstrating the safety of this technique for lipoaugmentation are lacking and that controlled, prospective, level 1 studies are necessary. Many feel that the questions and controversies related to tumor promotion and induction using fat grafts in an estrogen-rich environment such as the breast in a young woman should be answered and resolved. Surgeons and patients need to know that frequent and unnecessary biopsies for postoperative changes that occur following this procedure will not be necessary.

In summary, we should remember the controversy surrounding silicone gel breast implants and all of the issues related to a lack of data. Prior to 1990, there were only 8 indexed papers that were related to silicone gel breast implants. Since 1990, there have been nearly 900. As a specialty, we need to be cognizant of this and not duplicate the mistakes of the past as we continue to move forward. I look forward to the day when all plastic surgeons will feel comfortable with lipoaugmentation as we attempt to duplicate the beautiful results that Dr. Coleman has been able to achieve. Dr. Coleman deserves special thanks for all of his efforts in this arena.

M.Y.N.

REFERENCES

1. Czerny V. Plastischer Erzats de Brustdruse durch ein Lipom. *Zentralbl Chir* 1895;27:72.
2. Hollander E. Uber einen Fall von fortschreitenden Schwund des Fettgewebes und seinen kosmetischen Ersatz durch Menschenfett. *Munch Med Wochenschr* 1910;57:1794–1795.
3. Pennisi A. *Trapianti di Tessuto Adiposo a Scopo Chirurgico.* Rome: Tipografia Operaia; 1920: 37–58.
4. Wederhake K. Uber die Verwendung des menschlichen Fettes in der Chirurgie. *Berl Klin Wochenschr* 1918;55:47.
5. Tiemann W. The use of human oil (melted human fat) in surgery [in German]. *Berl Klin Wochenschr* 1918;55:343.
6. Brunning P. Contribution a l'etude des greffes adipeuses. *Bull Mem Acad R Med Belg* 1919; 28:440.
7. Lexer E. Fettgewebsverpflanzung. In: Lexer E, ed. *Die freien Transplantationen.* I. Teil. Stuttgart: Enke; 1919:264–547.
8. Fournier PF. Microlipoextraction et microlipoinjection. *Rev Chir Esthet Lang Fr* 1985; 10:36–40.
9. Illouz YG. The fat cell "graft": a new technique to fill depressions. *Plast Reconstr Surg* 1986;78:122–123.
10. Chajchir A, Benzaquen I. Fat-grafting injection for soft-tissue augmentation. *Plast Reconstr Surg* 1989;84:921–934.
11. Ersek RA. Transplantation of autologous fat: a 3-year follow-up is disappointing. *Plast Reconstr Surg* 1991;87:219–228.
12. Bircoll M. Cosmetic breast augmentation utilizing autologous fat and liposuction techniques. *Plast Reconstr Surg* 1987;79:267–271.
13. Bircoll M, Novak BH. Autologous fat transplantation employing liposuction techniques. *Ann Plast Surg* 1987;18:327–329.
14. Brown FE, Sargent SK, Cohen SR, et al. Mammographic changes following reduction mammaplasty. *Plast Reconstr Surg* 1987;80:691–698.
15. Coleman SR. The technique of periorbital lipoinfiltration. *Oper Tech Plast Surg* 1994; 1:120–126.
16. Coleman SR. Long-term survival of fat transplants: controlled demonstrations. *Aesthet Plast Surg* 1995;19:421–425.
17. Coleman SR, Saboeiro AP. Fat grafting to the breast revisited: safety and efficacy. *Plast Reconstr Surg* 2007;119:775–786; discussion, 786–787.
18. Gutowski KA; and ASPS Fat Graft Task Force. Current applications and safety of autologous fat grafts: a report of the ASPS Fat Graft Task Force. February 2009. Available at: http://www.plasticsurgery.org/Documents/Medical_Profesionals/Health_Policy/guiding_principles/Fat-Grafting-Task-Force-Report.pdf. Accessed July 16, 2010.
19. Coleman SR. *Structural Fat Grafting.* St. Louis, MO: Quality Medical Publishing; 2004.
20. Coleman SR, Mazzola RF, eds. *Fat Injection from Filling to Regeneration.* 1st ed. St. Louis, MO: Quality Medical Publishing; 2009.

CHAPTER

118

Roger K. Khouri
Daniel Del Vecchio

Breast Augmentation and Reconstruction Using BRAVA External Breast Expansion and Autologous Fat Grafting

INTRODUCTION

In plastic surgery few topics warrants as much controversy, excitement, and curiosity as fat grafting to the breasts. Although the solution to the "fat puzzle" is far from solved, results from a variety of independent investigators suggest that fat grafting to the breast is a legitimate procedure that warrants careful study. In January 2009 the American Society of Plastic Surgeons (ASPS) reversed their previous position on fat grafting to the breasts, stating, "studies provide consistent evidence for…fat grafting for breast augmentation…as a safe method" but cautioned "results of fat transfer remain dependent on a surgeon's technique and expertise" (1). This chapter we outline our rationale, collective techniques, and clinical experience in more than 100 cases and describe our current process from initial patient selection to postoperative care.

HISTORY

In 1983 Illouz (2) showed that fat can be removed from small port incisions using a cannula connected to vacuum. This offered surgeons an opportunity to use liposuctioned fat as an autologous filler. However, because many of the variables so important to fat grafting were not well understood, early results were disappointing as related to volume maintenance. At the same time, the success of the silicone breast implants reduced the interest in fat grafting for breast augmentation.

In 1987, Bircoll published his experience with the autologous grafting of liposuctioned fat for breast augmentation (3,4). This was followed by a series of opinion letters to the editor that culminated in the American Society of Plastic Surgeons issuing a position statement questioning the safety of fat grafting to the breast (5). This opinion statement suggested that fat grafting would compromise breast cancer detection and should be prohibited. Because of this unprecedented strong ban and because early results were neither impressive nor reproducible, this position statement stood, and the technique was largely abandoned for more than 20 years.

Some Europeans, undeterred by the ASPS position, persisted and continued to push for the technique, although not for cosmetic augmentation. Emmanuel Delay in Lyon, France, presented a series at the French Society of Plastic Surgery in 2001 and Gino Rigotti in Verona, Italy, also had a large series that he presented at the American Association of Plastic Surgeons in 2005.

At the 2006 meeting of the American Society for Aesthetic Plastic Surgery (ASAPS), Baker et al. presented a series of 20 patients augmented with a combination of external expansion and fat grafting (6). Using serial breast magnetic resonance imaging (MRI) and three-dimensional (3D) volumetric analysis, they described a 180-mL augmentation with documented volumetric survival of the grafts. None of the women had difficult-to-interpret findings on the mammogram. At the latest update of this prospective clinical trial, with more than 40 women followed up for at least 6 months and for an average of 30 months, there were still no issues with breast imaging or difficult-to-interpret masses (7).

In 2007, Coleman and Saboeiro published a review of 17 patients who were grafted using autologous fat and were followed up with serial photography (8). The results were overall successful, with maintenance of volume over 7 to 12 years of follow-up. They used serial grafting sessions instead of injecting large volumes in a single session in a preexpanded recipient breast like Baker et al.

With the growing realization that with optimal technique, fat grafts to the breast have potential to survive long term and that the radiographic arguments behind the ASPS-imposed ban were no longer valid (9–15), many surgeons across the world have started publishing their previously unpublished work (16–21).

LARGE-VOLUME FAT GRAFTING

SCIENTIFIC VARIABLES AND THEIR RELATIVE IMPORTANCE

Large-volume fat grafting required for effective breast augmentation and reconstruction has to be distinguished from the relatively smaller volume fat grafting needed to improve contour defects or to restore age-related fat atrophy in the face. Because of the large volume of donor necessary, it represents greater technical challenge. The first step in understanding the science and optimizing patient safety and results in fat grafting is to understand the many variables involved. Applying what is known from skin grafting and solid organ transplantation can provide a starting point. A more basic science approach to variables in fat grafting might employ tissue transplantation as a benchmark as suggested in Table 118.1.

A more challenging step is quantifying the relative *weights* of these variables. Determining the relative importance of each variable helps to guide priorities in patient selection, surgical management, and technique.

Percentage graft survival is a frequently referred to outcome measure that has to be put in proper perspective. It would be relatively easy to get a 10-mL graft volume to survive completely

TABLE 118.1 Variables in 3-D Fat Transplantation

Donor ←—— ——→ Transplantation Event	←—— ——→ Recipient
Patient age	Centrifugation vs. sedimentation vs. filtration
Age of graft/graft preservation	Centrifugation effects
Adipocyte concentration	Cell protectants
Stem cell concentration	Effect of washing
Cell size	Degree of 3D pre-expansion
Total extracorporeal time	Degree of angiogenesis
Negative pressure on aspiration	Dispersion technique of graft
Exposure to air, desiccation	Percutaneous 3D meshing
Tumescent medication effects	Maximum interstitial pressure
Graft to recipient volume ratio	Growth factors
Cannula size	Post operative graft care & immobilization

if evenly dispersed, one cell at a time, in a 100-mL recipient, while it would be rather impossible to squeeze 100-mL grafts into a 10-mL recipient site. Therefore percentage graft survival is critically dependent on the ratio of graft to recipient volume. This is illustrated in Figure 118.1.

THEORETICAL CONCEPTS IN LARGE-VOLUME, THREE-DIMENSIONAL FAT GRAFTING

Fat grafting is 3D grafting, a novel concept for surgeons more familiar with the two-dimensional skin grafting. Large-volume fat grafting can be compared to sowing seeds in a 3D field. To harvest the best crop possible, one needs to optimize the following four critical components:

1. The *seeds* (e.g., the graft, its quality, viability, stem cell content)
2. The *planting method* (e.g., the surgical technique of diffusely, evenly, and atraumatically sowing to avoid clumps)
3. The *field* (e.g., the recipient tissue, its size, its vascularity, the presence or absence of growth-promoting factors)
4. The *nurturing* postplanting (e.g., postoperative care, immobilization, stimulation of growth)

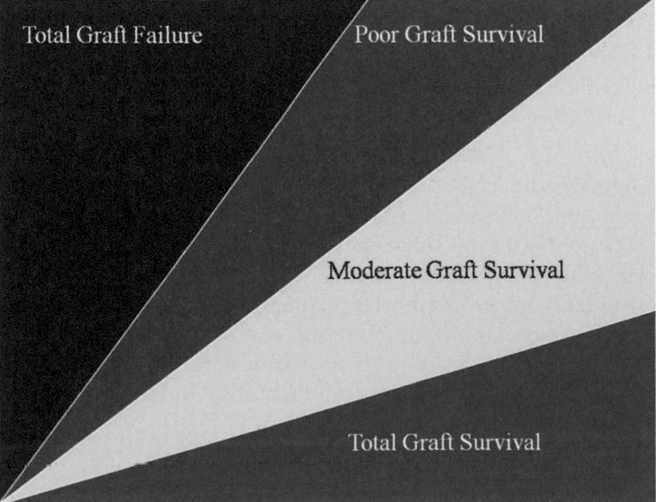

Figure 118.1. The fallacy of percentage graft survival. Graft survival is critically dependent on the graft-to-recipient volume ratio. Most experimental studies that investigate graft harvesting and processing techniques or the effect of the recipient site measure "percentage graft survival" as the main outcome while failing to take into account the much more important factor of volume ratios.

It does not matter whether three of these components are maximally optimized; if one component is poor, the yield will be poor. It is the least optimized of these four components, the bottleneck factor, that becomes rate limiting and determines the overall result. To illustrate this, consider that poor seeds planted in a large, fertile field will not yield much, and, conversely, excellent seeds squeezed and crowded in a small, rocky soil will not yield much either. Moreover, while the best possible seeds poorly planted in the best fertile soil will yield a poor crop, even the best seeds optimally planted in the best fertile soil will not yield a good crop if after planting the soil is stirred or the field is left to dry out.

Some surgeons have shown acceptable results using a variety of fat harvesting and preparation methods, some often diametrically opposite to each other. This is because methods of fat harvest and preparation are not bottleneck rate-limiting factors in large-volume fat grafting. Our experience points to the fact that the major limiting factor in large-volume fat grafting is *the recipient site*, not management of the graft material.

MANAGING THEORY AND SCIENCE IN FAT GRAFTING

As surgeons seeking to optimize the results of autologous fat grafting, we have to manage the technical variables over which we have some degree of control:

1. Donor material: fat harvesting and fat processing
2. Fat grafting technique: mapping technique and reverse liposuction technique
3. Recipient-site management: pregraft and postgraft

Donor Material

Fat Harvesting

Harvesting: Role of the Cannula. Using smaller cannula sizes during harvesting creates less donor-site trauma and allows for removal of smaller lobules of fat, which may improve flow characteristics during reinjection. However, the smaller the cannula size, the slower is the fat removal process, and for fat-grafting breast augmentation to be a viable technique, one must be conscious of operative time. For the procedure to gain adoption in breast augmentation, for example, it must be performed in 2 hours or less. These opposing incentives—harvesting time and quality of donor graft—represent one pair of several diametrically opposed variables in fat grafting.

As important as cannula size are *cannula hole size* and *number of holes*. We have studied the effect of varying the number of side holes on the efficiency of liposuction and confirmed the intuitive assumption that the larger the number of side holes, the more efficient is the liposuction at less traumatic pressures (Fig. 118.2). A 12-gauge (2.7-mm-diameter) cannula with 9 to 12 side holes of size 2 × 1 mm can extract a significant amount of fat despite its small caliber.

Harvesting: Role of Suction Negative Pressure. Although it is not well documented, some studies demonstrate that the lower the absolute value of the negative pressure used at harvest, the better is the graft viability (22). However, studies

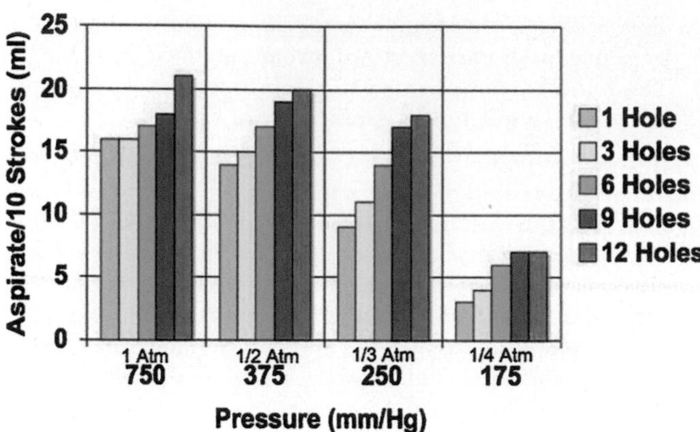

Figure 118.2. Effect of aspiration pressure and number of cannula side holes on harvesting efficiency.

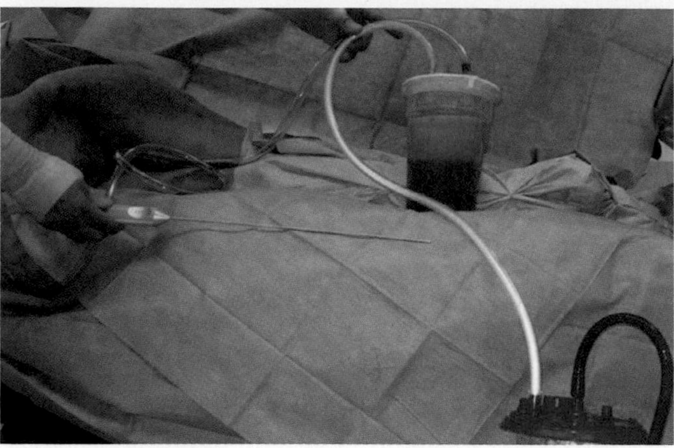

Figure 118.4. "In-line" mechanical system for fat collection.

that use clinical volume maintenance as endpoints may not be as accurate as those using adipocyte integrity immediately postharvest. Until this is studied in a well-controlled setting with quantitative data, it is best to assume that the lower the absolute value of the negative pressure needed to obtain the graft, the less is the trauma to the adipocyte. Figure 118.3 shows that our choice of a 12-hole cannula set at 1/3 atm (250 mm Hg) is a more efficient harvesting instrument than a single-hole cannula operating at 1 atm.

Harvesting: Syringe Versus Liposuction Aspirator. Harvesting the fat for grafting can be accomplished at the recommended low pressures either with a mechanical liposuction aspirator vacuum source or with a handheld syringe. Mechanical aspiration is more efficient, but it presents potential problems. The fat collection reservoir needs to be in series with the vacuum source and has to remain vertical, lest the collected fat continues toward the pump. The reservoir also has to be rigid to stay open and hold the vacuum, and it also has to remain sterile (Fig. 118.4.)

This arrangement requires long connection tubes that generate potential dead space losses. At every instance of vacuum loss, whenever one of the holes of the liposuction cannula comes close to the surface, air can flow through the tubing to desiccate the adipocytes trapped in the long tubing, and the air gush splashes the collection bottle. We found this to be more difficult in patients with low body mass index who only have small amounts of fat.

The concern over air exposure is not well quantified. It has been reported in one communication that greater than 50% of adipocytes undergo cytoplasmic lysis on exposure to air (23). This potential concern led us to develop a two-way tissue routing valve that separates the syringe vacuum source from the collection receptacle and directs the aspirate toward a collection bag when the syringe is full (Fig. 118.5.)

Harvesting: Graft Harvest Site. Although it has been suggested that there are specific donor areas that allow for a higher survival of fat grafting, we, like others (24), have not found the anatomic location of the donor site to be of significance to outcomes. It may turn out that that adipocyte cellular size, which varies in different body regions and also among different patients, may be the more important variable. Larger cells have a higher likelihood of mechanical cell membrane damage during extraction, and it may be this variable of cell size relative to cannula hole size that is more important than the area on the body used for harvest per se.

Fat Processing

Air Exposure During Processing. As stated earlier, a variable of unknown weight in fat harvesting and processing remains the negative impact of air exposure (23). Fat concentration techniques range from drying the fat on Telfa rolls (high air exposure, high likelihood of cell damage and contamination), to completely closed systems that keep the fat inside intravenous (IV) tubing, two-way routing valves, and IV bags. Washing harvested graft with saline-buffered solutions and adding growth factors or cell preservatives (25) has been described and may show promise in the future. We believe that there are already many potential factors (stem cells, growth factors) in the lipoaspirate that should be preserved in the graft. This is one of the reasons we do not favor washing or filtration and prefer not to completely remove fluid by high-speed centrifugation.

Role of Stem Cell–Enriched Graft. Concentrating adipocyte stem cells and remixing them with mature adipocytes to increase cell viability has been described (26). The theoretical benefit of a stem cell–enriched graft is that the smaller stem cells improve volume yield. The smaller graft volumes will differentiate and grow into larger mature adipocytes to yield a larger augmentation. Although this may be an effective strategy in the future, this technique is not proven, nor is it approved by the Food and Drug Administration, and we do not employ it.

The Fallacy of "Percentage Yields". One of the most confusing metrics in fat grafting is a lack of standardization regarding "percentage yields." Once fat is lipoaspirated as donor graft

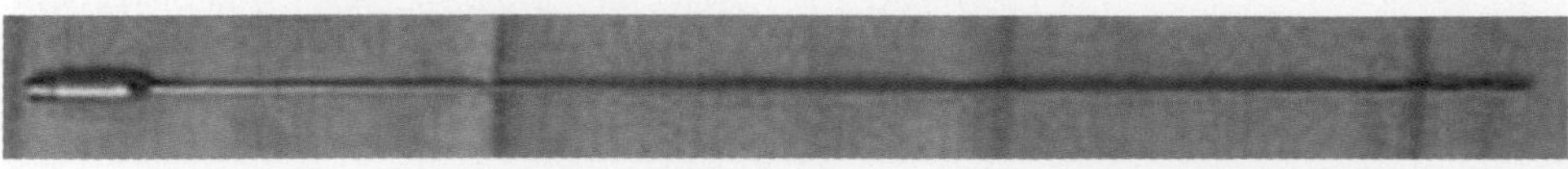

Figure 118.3. The 12-hole cannula currently used with the syringe aspiration system.

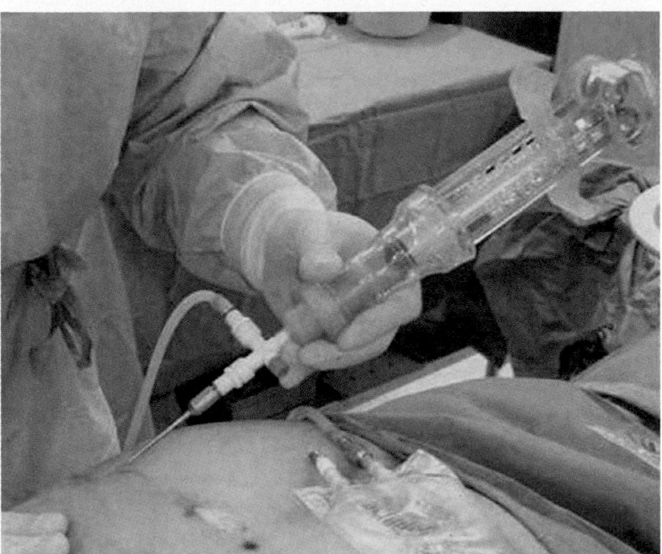

Figure 118.5. The lipografter closed technique for fat harvesting and grafting allows little or no air exposure. Fat is passively drawn up into the syringe under the effect of a constant-force spring that pulls the plunger up with a steady 300–mm Hg vacuum pressure throughout its excursion. When the syringe plunger is all the way up, the surgeon pushes it back down, purging the lipoaspirate from the syringe to the collection bag and cocking back the spring for the next cycle of suction. An atraumatic, nonclogging, two-way valve system directs the flow from the syringe toward a sterile collection bag on the field. The bag is then gently centrifuged to rid the excess fluid and used as a reservoir for reinjection using the same tubing and the routing valves in reverse mode.

there is an infinite number of different concentrations of fat relative to crystalloid that can be reached prior to grafting the recipient site. Unless we know this percentage, or "fatocrit," we can never really know what percentage of fat survived grafting. Another reason is there is no standardization regarding how to measure percentage yields. Are we measuring percentage volume retention? Are we measuring percentage increase in volume of the recipient site? Are we measuring the actual proportion of grafted cells that survived? Recent animal models may help to standardize attempts at cellular percentage survival (27) and may help to describe methods to better quantify volume retention pre and post grafting. We believe that careful documentation of the following should be done in fat-grafting patients, in order to better understand the yield in each case:

1. Document the preexpansion volume of the breast (MRI, 3D imaging, or both).
2. Document the method of crystalloid separation (double decanting, low-speed centrifugation, high-speed centrifugation).
3. Document the volume of material grafted.
4. Document the postgraft volume of the breast at 6 months or more (MRI, 3D imaging, or both).

High-speed Centrifugation. Centrifuging the lipoaspirate at 1,000 × *g* for 3 minutes is the method of fat processing that had been popularized as a strategy for effective fat grafting. Historically, the penchant for centrifugation arose from the need to graft as much adipocyte biomass as possible into a limited space. Although centrifugation can yield highly concentrated fat, there are four potential problems with centrifugation (Fig. 118.6):

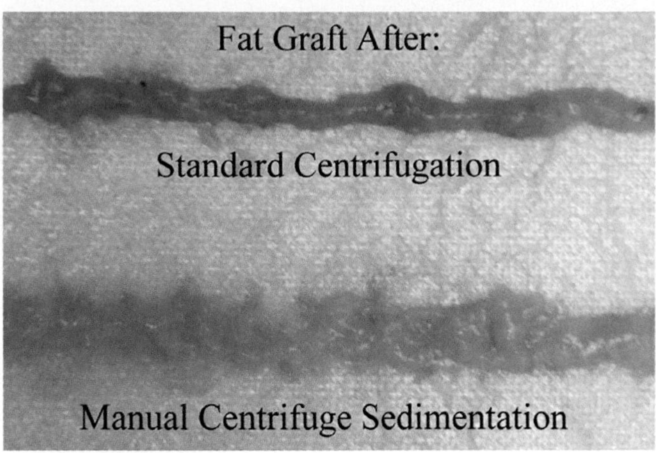

Figure 118.6. Comparison between high-speed centrifuged fat and low-speed, hand-centrifuged sedimented fat. Loosely packed fat droplets interface better with the recipient bed and have a higher likelihood of engraftment and survival.

1. The cells may be damaged with high *g*-forces, although studies have shown that the standard centrifugation protocol has no significant deleterious effect on survival.
2. It is a time- and labor-consuming process and one that exposes the graft to potential contamination.
3. High fat concentrations may cause clumping and more difficult flow during reinjection.
4. Clumped cells have less-than-optimal graft-to-recipient interface and thus lower engraftment potential for the individual cells at the center of the clump.

Low–g-Force Centrifugation. Use of the BRAVA system of preexpansion of the recipient site has emancipated fat grafting from the need for centrifugation and its potential disadvantages. The BRAVA-expanded breast has the advantage of space and thus reduces the deleterious effect of crowding. In the expanded space, a larger amount of loose fat slurry can be more diffusely dispersed and survive better. Through use of an external centrifuge with bags in the closed technique (Fig. 118.7), fat cells are still separated from crystalloid with little trauma at 1.5 to 2 × *g*.

The "Double-decanting" Technique: "One g" of Separation. If effective preexpansion of the recipient site can generate a hyperexpanded recipient parenchymal space, it means that the more expanded the breast is, the less concentrated does the harvested adipocytes need to be. At some expansion volume, there may be no need to centrifuge the fat. Simply decanting the crystalloid off in the collection canister (step 1) and then transferring the decanted fat into a 60-cc syringe (step 2) can process fat at a suitable concentration for grafting (Fig. 118.8) This is called the "double-decanting" technique.

Fat Grafting Technique

There are two popular methods of fat grafting: the "mapping" technique and the "reverse liposuction" technique. There is no

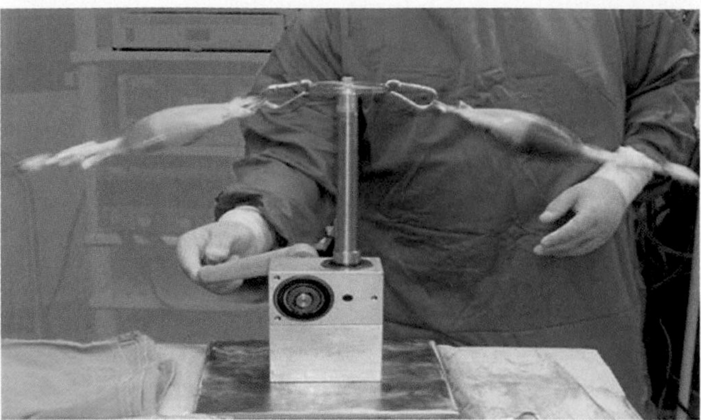

Figure 118.7. Bag centrifugation technique. The bags are already filled with fat and are simply spun at low revolutions per minute by a hand-cranked device on a sterile side table. This takes minutes to prepare, as compared to hours for high-speed centrifugation.

strong data to prove which technique is better or yields better results. As stated earlier, the overall technique must take into consideration the relative time and manpower demands of each variable discussed to render an "optimized" operation, not a "maximized" variable per se.

The Mapping Technique. Donor cells have the highest chance of survival with the technique that best ensures an even, three-dimensional dispersion of the fat. The higher the surface-to-volume contact with the recipient-site tissue for each fat lobule transplanted, the higher is the likelihood of sufficient oxygen diffusion and survival of the graft. The mapping technique involves the use of small (3 to 5 cc) syringes handheld and connected directly to a 14-gauge blunt side-hole cannula. Markings are made in the recipient areas to aid in a systematic, diffuse, and even injection of the entire recipient. From 8 to 10 circummammary and 4 circumareolar entry points are usually made with a 14-gauge hypodermic needle. Through each entry point the 15- to 20-cm-long cannula makes multiple tunnels that fan out radially and inject 2 to 3 cc of fat upon withdrawal. The cannula is then inserted into another adjacent entry point, and the process is repeated to yield a 3D weave that evenly crisscross covers the recipient space (Fig. 118.9). Multiple levels of graft are deposited, deep from the base of the breast just above the pectoralis fascia, to the subcutaneous space immediately subjacent to the dermis. Direct injection of fat into the dense parenchyma of the breast is never performed. This technique is deliberate and exact but does take time. In addition, it requires the operator to deploy the plunger and withdraw the needle at the same time.

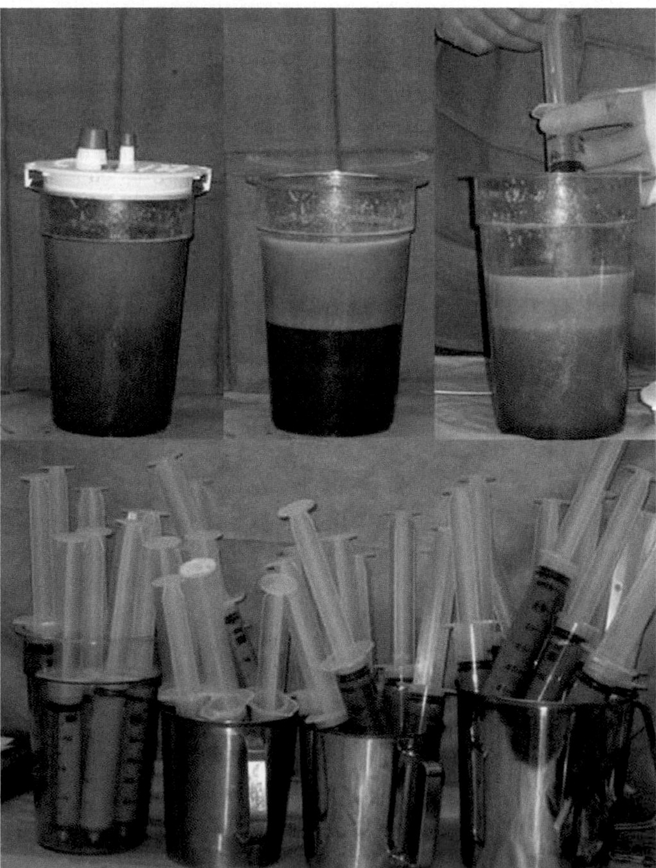

Figure 118.8. Double-decanting technique. In this technique, fat simply rises to the top and crystalloid settles in two canisters: the collection canister and then the 60-cc syringe.

Reverse Liposuction Technique. The reverse liposuction technique uses three to five insertions on the breast, two or three in the inframammary fold (IMF), and several laterally and toward the axilla. The IMF insertions are made below the native IMF, as this will descend 1 to 2 cm, similar to the effect seen in augmentation with breast prostheses. The "décolletage" or "social" part of the breast is avoided in the event hyperpigmentation of the needle sites occurs. With a 15- to 20-cm side-hole, 14-gauge needle loaded directly onto 60-cc syringes, the fat is injected using a controlled and deliberate liposuction movement of the plunger along a fanning pattern of vectors at

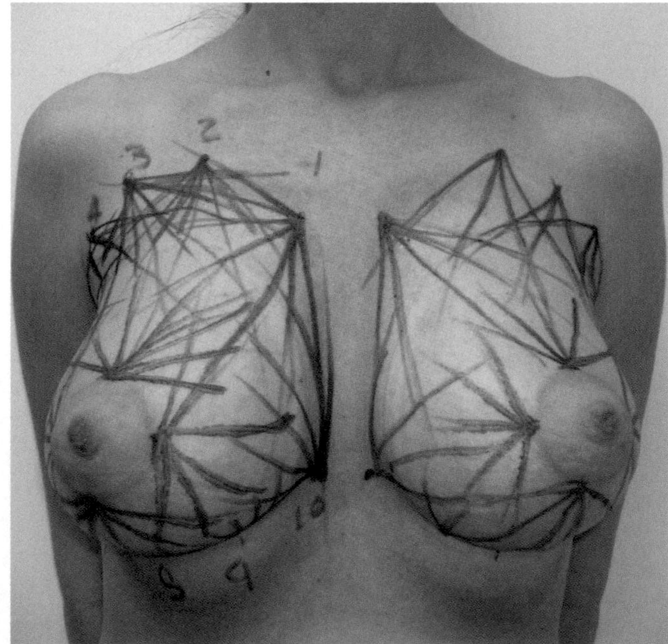

Figure 118.9. Markings for the mapping technique of fat injection on the expanded breasts. Eight circummammary and four circumareolar needle puncture entry sites with radially fanning tunnels from each site provide a well-diversified insertion of the grafts.

multiple planar levels from the base of the breast. The axillary insertion is also used to place the graft in the submuscular position. The rate of insertion in this technique should be 2 to 4 seconds per cc, which results in a rate of 2 to 3 minutes/60 cc of fat, or a grafting session of 300 cc per breast performed in 10 to 15 minutes on each breast.

An example of optimizing a technique versus maximizing a variable, the reverse liposuction technique strives to reduce grafting time and the number of insertion sites. There is a higher potential for less diversified dispersion if this technique is not effectively performed. Another potential benefit of the reverse liposuction technique is that 60-cc syringes used from double decanting can be immediately loaded, decreasing fat handling. The 60-cc syringes generate *lower* maximum pressures than do 5-cc syringes, which are used in other techniques. Therefore, if there is a blockage of flow along the insertion needle due to clumping, this will occur at a lower pressure level using a 60-cc syringe, with less potential damage to the grafted cells.

A summary of the three commonly used techniques is outlined in Table 118.2.

Recipient-site Management

No other variable in fat grafting has been less studied or appreciated than the recipient site. To better appreciate the role of the recipient site in fat grafting, consider the history of fat grafting compared to those of skin grafting. Descriptions in Sanskrit indicate that small skin grafts were employed in India by 3000 BC (28). Eventually, improvements in instrumentation afforded more uniform donor thicknesses. Only during the last 60 or so years have more advanced wound care, debridement, antibiotics, and methods of graft immobilization helped to improve graft take. In recent years the introduction of vacuum-assisted closure (VAC) has further revolutionized skin grafting by a variety of postulated effects, including bacterial clearance, neovascularization, and reduction in edema of the wound bed. When we consider the recent introduction of fat grafting relative to skin grafting, it is clear that we have just begun. Recipient-site management has only recently been suggested as an important variable in fat grafting that could be potentially manipulated and improved. The size, vascularity, and pressure compliance of the recipient site are the most prominent components.

Recipient-site Size. In the familiar 2D skin grafting of wounds, the surface of the wound determines the upper limit of skin graft that survives, and overgrafting more skin does not help. Similarly, in 3D grafting, the volume of the recipient bed sets the maximal limit to the volume of graft that can survive, and overgrafting with more fat will lead to necrosis and oil cysts.

We devised a geometric model of 3D grafting of tissue droplets that assumes the following:

1. Evenly diversified 3D dispersion of the grafted droplets
2. A similar size range for graft droplets and recipient stromal cells
3. Preservation of the recipient matrix 3D vascular stromal interconnections
4. Infinite compliance of the recipient stroma as it is stretched to accommodate the graft droplets

This model suggests that even with the most perfect technique and the most even graft distribution, graft volume cannot exceed two thirds of the recipient volume. Filling above this limit will lead to overcrowding, and by worsening the graft-to-recipient contact and the diffusion gradient, drastically decrease cell survival.

Using the previously described "seeds in a field" analogy, the size of the field, not the number of seeds, ultimately sets the upper limit of the crop size. "Overcorrection" or overgrafting is definitely counterproductive; the reasonable approach is to try to match the graft volume to the recipient volume. With the understanding that we can modulate the recipient site in fat grafting, the overcorrection and overgrafting of yesterday become the overexpansion of today.

This opens up an opportunity for positive intervention. For megavolume grafting in a tight space, temporary expansion of the recipient loosens the extracellular matrix and creates many more interstices where many more individual fat droplets can optimize their graft to recipient interface and survive (see Fig. 118.10).

Recipient-site Vascularity. It is well established that muscle tissue with its high capillary density is an excellent graft recipient, and that the more vascular the recipient, the better is the graft survival (29,30).

TABLE 118.2

	Standard Coleman Method	*Lipografter and Mapping Method*	*Mechanical and Reverse Liposuction Method*
Aspiration Cannula	12 G Single Hole Coleman Cannula	12 Gauge 12 Holes Luer Lock Cannula	12 Gauge 12 Holes Ergonomic Handle
Aspiration Force	Manually Activated Syringe	Spring Activated Syringe	Vacuum Pump Motorized pump
Ease of Use	Hard on Fingers	Easy, Spring Loaded	Easy, Vacuum Unit
Air Exposure	Mild to Moderate	Minimal to none	Moderate
Pressure	Erratic	Constant Low	Potentially Excessive
Collection Chamber	Multiple Syringes, Syringe Racks	100 cc IV bag	1200 cc Rigid Canister
Crystalloid Separation	1000 g Centrifuge Individual Syringes	Low Speed Centrifuge	Double Decanting
Injection Cannula	14 G Single Hole	14 G Single Hole	14G Single Hole
Injection Force	1–3 cc Syringe (Highest)	3 cc syringe (higher)	60 cc syringe (low)
Injection Technique	Switch individual Syringes & Cannulas	Mapping	Reverse Liposuction
Op. time for Breast Augmentation	Long (4–6 hrs)	Short (2hrs)	Shortest (1–2 hr)

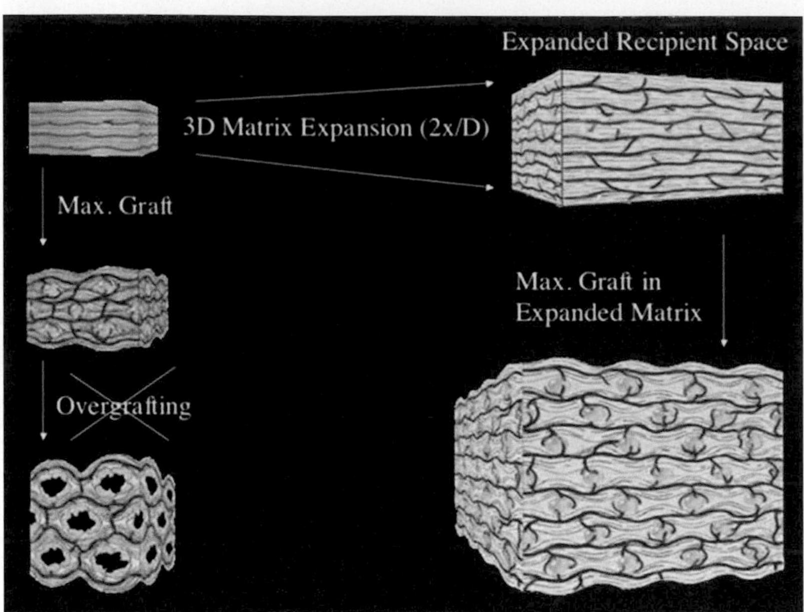

Figure 118.10. Hypothetical block of tissue maximally filled with fat grafts, then overfilled to crowding; next, temporary three-dimensional stretching of that block of tissue showing how many more grafts can be placed without crowding in the expanded and hypervascular space.

Furthermore, a number of cytokines and growth factors can accelerate the process of graft angiogenesis and improve survival. Future attempts at priming the recipient site by increasing its vascularity and endogenously stimulating angiogenic cytokine production may potentially improve engraftment.

Recipient-site Filling Pressure. From the general surgery trauma literature and from consideration of hand and upper extremity trauma, the importance of compartment pressure and the grave consequences of high interstitial pressure are well understood. If it were possible to preexpand the recipient space prior to fat grafting, it would make it more compliant and allow the injection of larger volumes of graft into the recipient site before reaching physiologically excessive interstitial pressures.

RECIPIENT-SITE MODULATION: BRAVA EXTERNAL BREAST EXPANSION

The BRAVA bra was initially developed in the 1990s as an external soft tissue expander to enlarge the breast. The device consists of a pair of semirigid domes with silicone gel rim cushion that interfaces with the skin and that are worn around the breasts like a bra. A small battery-operated "sport" pump maintains a low negative pressure inside the domes that does not interrupt capillary flow and imparts on the breast surface a constant gentle isotropic distraction force (Fig. 118.11). Studies have shown that when the device is worn in an uninterrupted fashion for 10 to 12 hours/day, true and long-lasting breast augmentation ensues over a period of weeks to months (31–35).

A total of 40,000 women have used nonsurgical breast expansion with BRAVA over the last 7 years, but compliance with the cumbersome treatment and the slow pace of real tissue growth have limited its popularity. However, within a few weeks of use, substantial temporary swelling of the breast develops. This was found to be an ideal way to prepare the breast for large volumes of fat grafts. The threefold to fourfold increase in volume that can be attained over 4 weeks of use allows a proportionate increase in fat graft amount without crowding. The expansion effect also appears to be angiogenic, as documented by MRI (Fig. 118.12).

Experience with the VAC as a means of wound management has proven that microangiogenesis is a direct result of negative mechanical pressure (Fig. 118.13) (36). The extensive VAC data on vascular in-growth and improvement in skin graft take coupled with the MRI findings from BRAVA preexpanded breasts support our thesis that increased microcirculation, combined with the larger interstitial space created by the expansion, may contribute to the potential for increased graft volumes and increased diffusion gradients.

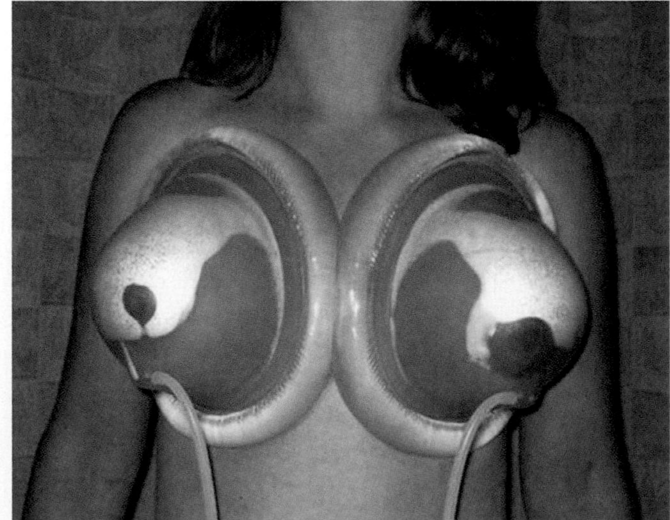

Figure 118.11. The BRAVA external tissue expander worn by a patient just prior to the fat grafting procedure. Note that the expanded breast tissue is almost in contact with the domes. Fogging of the domes due to evaporative water loss is normal.

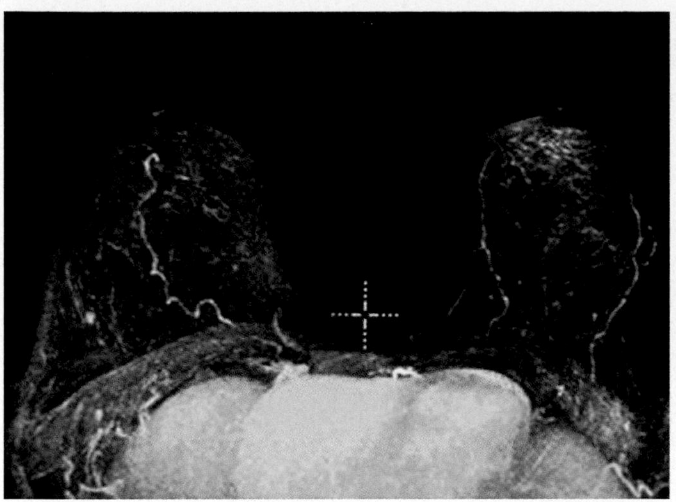
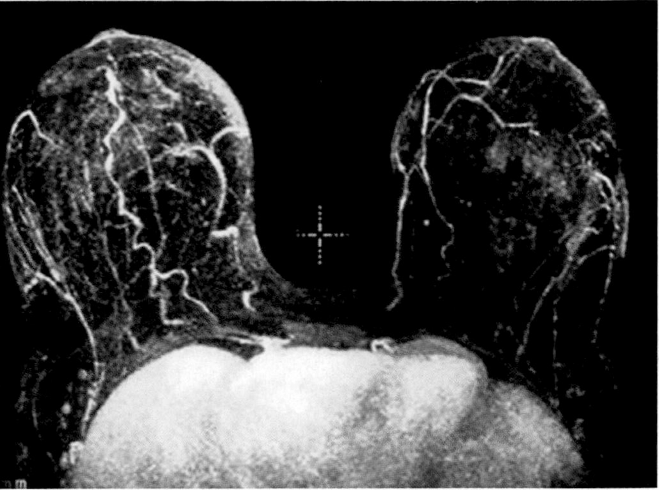

Figure 118.12. Magnetic resonance imaging of the breasts with contrast in a patient before and after 3 weeks of 10 hours per day of BRAVA use. There is significant expansion of the breasts with the creation of a larger and more fertile recipient matrix, which will allow more fat grafts to be placed. Note the marked angiogenic effect of expansion with increase in number and size of blood vessels.

BRAVA NONOPERATIVE PREEXPANSION: PARALLELS TO VACUUM-ASSISTED CLOSURE

Negative pressure on the breast draws in fluid that expands the parenchyma and increases the size and caliber of the endogenous blood vessels to generate a fertile recipient scaffold that can be seeded with fat grafts (Fig. 118.14).

We postulate that BRAVA enhances fat grafting results by five main effects:

1. **B**igger potential spaces are available for overall volume of graft.
2. **R**educed demand on adipocytes creates the expansion, which may kill them.
3. **A**ugments tension on internal constrictions and scars, so breast *shape* can be addressed
4. **V**ariables that are time consuming (e.g., centrifugation) become less demanding.
5. **A**ngiogenesis effect may increase recipient-site oxygen tension and better graft take.

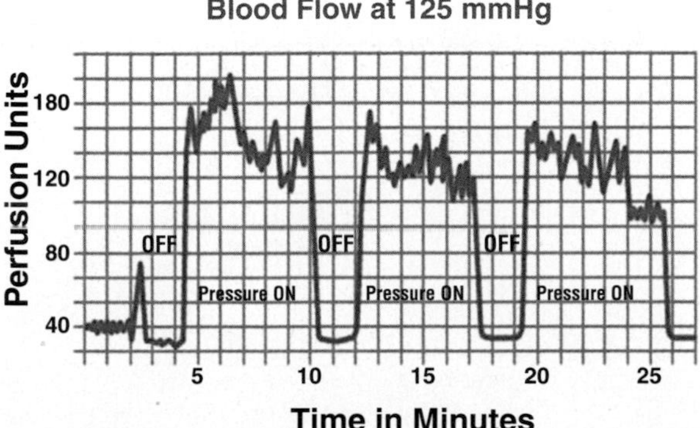

Figure 118.13. Increased capillary blood flow with cyclical negative pressure. (Data from KCI Incorporated, San Antonio, Texas.)

The increased parenchymal space created by BRAVA preexpansion allows more volume of graft to be inserted before high subcutaneous interstitial pressures are reached. It is this high interstitial pressure that often limits the graft volume that can be achieved in more conventional grafting techniques. By increasing the recipient-site space, there is less dependence on concentrating the donor fat, which may reduce the need for time-consuming, high-speed centrifugation and syringe transfer of fat. With BRAVA preexpansion, the patient performs the size expansion, not the injected fat. In conventional fat grafting techniques, we require the fat to act in four key ways:

1. As an internal positive pressure expander
2. To survive by oxygen diffusion for 5 to 7 days
3. To eventually receive a blood supply from the recipient site
4. To remain viable and to act as a spacer

This first demand—the internal positive pressure expansion—likely works against the other three demands and probably leads to adipocyte necrosis. BRAVA potentially relieves the adipocyte from this first burden.

Our experience with more than 50 breast augmentations using nonsurgical expansion followed by fat grafting has allowed us to establish a significant dose-response curve of preoperative expansion to final augmentation volume. The most important determinant of final augmentation volume was *the degree of preoperative expansion.*

Many breasts demonstrate a range of deformities, from subtle, often underappreciated internal ligamentous constrictions to tuberous or severely constricted breasts. Some of the more subtle effects, such as occult "double-bubble" deformities, are only appreciated at the time of prosthetic breast augmentation when internal tension and volume changes exacerbate these underlying deformities. Using BRAVA for external preexpansion prior to the fat grafting serves two valuable roles in reshaping breasts: (a) deformities, even subtle deformities, can be demonstrated to the patient *before* any surgical intervention is performed, and (b) during fat grafting, internal scar ligaments can be selectively lysed using a "percutaneous 3D meshing"

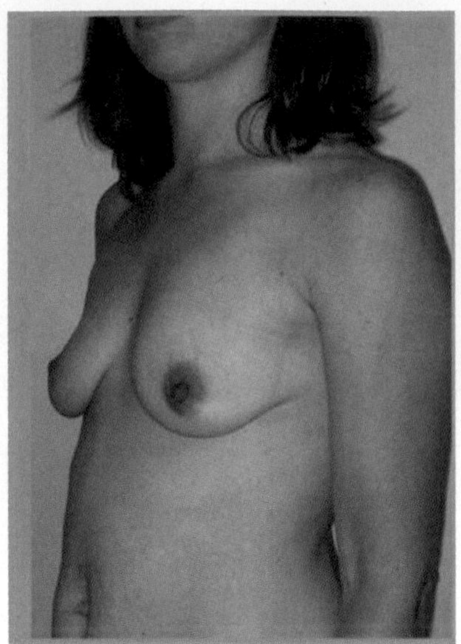

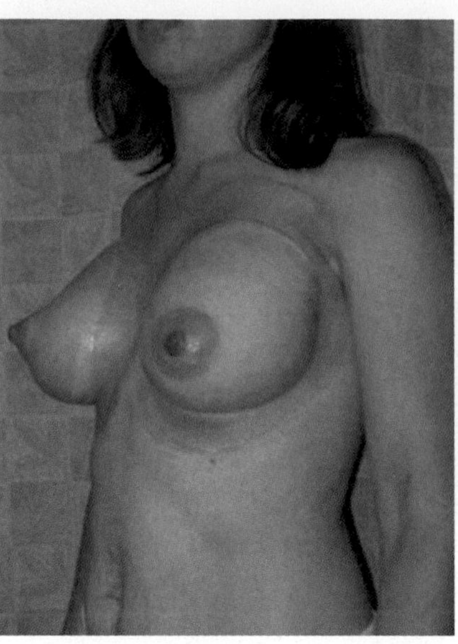

Figure 118.14. Patient before BRAVA Expansion and 3 weeks after BRAVA expansion, immediately prior to grafting. Note that the volumetric increase is three to four times that of the preexpansion state. A total of 480 cc of fat was injected in this case into each breast.

technique to reshape the breast immediately after grafting the fat.

From the collective experience in facial fat grafting, it is well known that fat grafts in the mobile perioral region are not as successful as grafts placed in less mobile areas such as the periorbital region. At the very least, immediate postgraft immobilization is crucial. Using BRAVA postoperatively at low steady pressure helps to stabilize the graft by immobilizing it as a stent and also by keeping open millions of tiny "Morrison growth chambers," which have been proven experimentally to stimulate fat graft growth (37).

BRAVA EXTERNAL BREAST EXPANSION AND MEGAVOLUME FAT GRAFTING DIFFERS FROM CLASSIC AUTOLOGOUS FAT GRAFTING

The case of no expansion whatsoever represents the classic technique of fat grafting. It is important to appreciate in how many ways nonsurgical preoperative expansion followed by fat grafting differs from the classic technique (Table 118.3). In conventional fat grafting, the fat is injected into a nonexpanded breast. Therefore, any expansion of the parenchymal space occurs as a result of the internal pressure created by the fat graft itself. This, in turn, limits the volume of fat that can be injected before interstitial hypertension occurs. At some limiting interstitial pressure (greater than 25 to 30 mm Hg), fat cells will not survive by oxygen diffusion in the initial days postgrafting. Therefore, in conventional fat grafting, smaller volumes are placed before reaching a high interstitial pressure. Such a technique therefore requires concentrated or hyperconcentrated fat cells, as available volume is limited. This hyperconcentration of fat cells, in turn, requires a high-speed centrifuge, which increases fat handling, transfer, and operating room time. In addition, hyperconcentrated fat flows less easily, clogs needles and syringes, and requires injection through a smaller syringe (1 to 3 cc), which can generate higher pounds per square inches of pressure than a larger syringe (10 to 60 cc). The demand on smaller syringes and increased pressure may lead to increased trauma to fat cells and definitely increases procedure times.

By adequately expanding the recipient site prior to fat grafting, the BRAVA system eliminates the need for many of the aforementioned constraints. The larger available space puts less pressure on the cells in the recipient site. The larger recipient space also puts less pressure on the surgeon to hyperconcentrate fat cells by centrifugation. This less-concentrated fat

TABLE 118.3

	C-AFG	*BEBE-AFG*
The Expander	Injected adipocytes	The BRAVA expander
Role of Fat in Expansion	Internal pressure expander	"Backfills" Expansion in Place
Apparent interstitial pressure*	High	Lower
Use of Centrifuge	Dependent	Not Necessary
Syringe Size	5 cc	5–60 cc
Av. Safe Graft Volumes for an A cup breast or a mastectomy defect	150 cc	300–600 cc
Estimated operating time	6 hrs	2 hrs
Number of Assistants	2 to 3	0–1
Ecchymoses	Significant	Minimal

flows more easily and can be inserted using lower-pressure, larger syringes. Overall, the liberation of these constraints reduces this procedure from 6 to 2 hours, increases volumes grafted from 150 to up to 700 cc, and increases the viability of this approach as a "user-friendly" technique.

Eliminating high-speed centrifugation from our procedure has resulted in the following advantages:

1. The operation can be performed with no "back table" assistants.
2. There is less transfer to smaller syringes, less air exposure, and less potential contamination.
3. Less concentrated fat can be injected because there is more space in the recipient site.
4. Less concentrated fat disperses better and leads to less clumping of graft.
5. Less concentrated fat flows better, resulting in less clogging and less trauma to cells.
6. Less fat concentration retains potentially vital high-density elements (stem cells).
7. Less concentrated fat allows us to perform the procedure on patients who have less body fat. As a matter of fact, some of our best results are in thinner patients.
8. The operation can be performed in 2 hours or less.

MAXIMIZING VARIABLES VERSUS OPTIMIZING A PROCEDURE

If it is true that concentrating fat cells is an important variable but requires 3 to 4 hours to maximally perform, and if after 3 to 4 hours outside of an oxygen-rich environment fat cell survival drops to low levels, the two variables also have opposing effects. In this simplistic example, trying to maximize one variable may negatively impact another variable, which could lead to a failed procedure as a whole. *In megavolume fat grafting, the choice of the overall technique must take into consideration the relative time and manpower demands of each variable discussed to render an "optimized" operation, not a "maximized" variable per se.*

FAT GRAFTING IN PRACTICE: AESTHETIC AND ANATOMIC CONSIDERATIONS

From the diffuse enhancement of an existing perfectly shaped breast to the multistage creation of a breast mound in a mastectomy patient, the technique of nonsurgical preexpansion and autologous fat grafting exhibits a spectrum of fill effects that can be achieved.

BREAST AUGMENTATION: CONSIDERATIONS

In augmentation patients the main variables are breast density and size. A key consideration in the preoperative evaluation, as in the case of reconstruction, is the overall starting volume of the breast. Assume the following simple function between preexpansion and postgrafting volumes: $y = 2x$, where y is the final volume 4 to 6 months after grafting and x is the initial breast volume preexpansion. Then it becomes clear that smaller breasts require on average more sessions to achieve the same final volume, or, stated differently, that smaller breasts cannot expand in a nominal amount as much as larger breasts (Figs. 118.15 and 118.16).

Dense parenchymal breasts will also expand with more difficulty than soft, multiparous breasts. Patients with dense parenchymal breasts must be encouraged to increase the negative pressure on the domes to achieve an adequate expansion preoperatively. Often, the dense parenchymal breast will expand more in some areas, like the periareolar region, than in others. This will result in a "double-bubble" constriction deformity that must be released at the time of surgery (Fig. 118.17). Constricted or tuberous breasts require aggressive expansion, and following this, the residual constrictions can be released mechanically using the percutaneous 3D mesh release technique (Fig. 118.18).

Even more difficult to expand and graft are patients whose breast tissue has been removed (mastectomy) or removed and irradiated (mastectomy + XRT). These patients require the highest number of grafting sessions (Fig. 118.19).

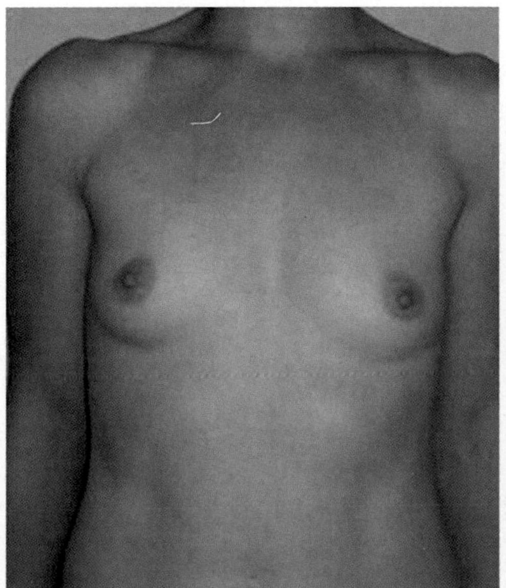

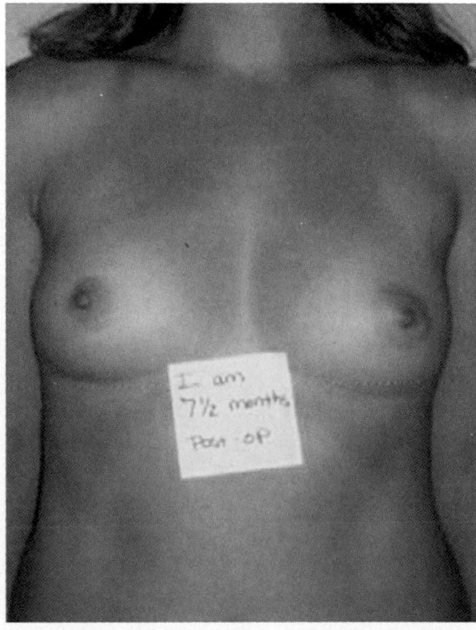

Figure 118.15. Smaller breasts, even if doubled in volume, are still not very large.

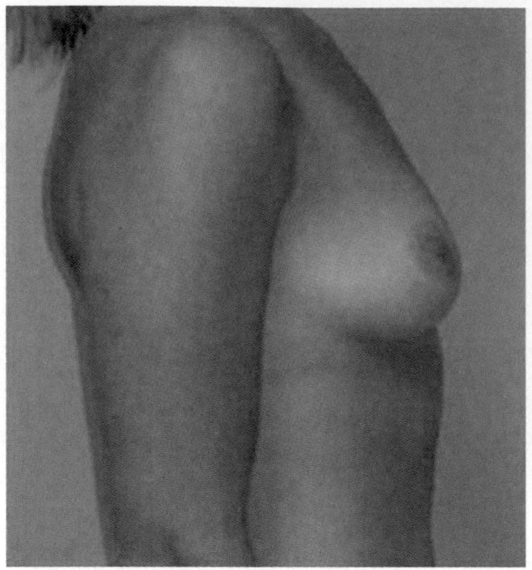
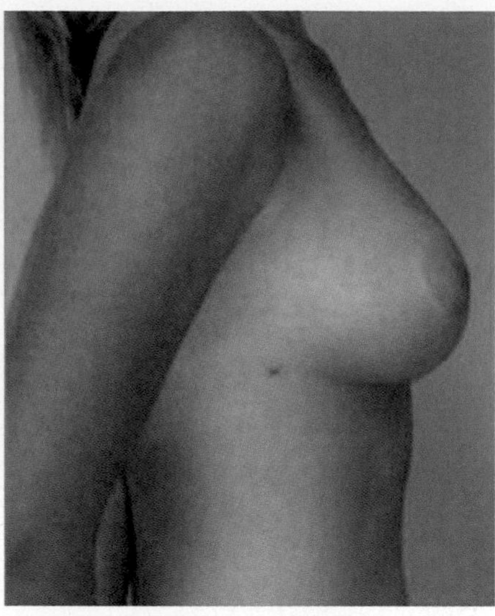

Figure 118.16. Breasts with larger initial volume, if doubled in size, can achieve higher final volumes with just one session of BRAVA expansion and fat grafting.

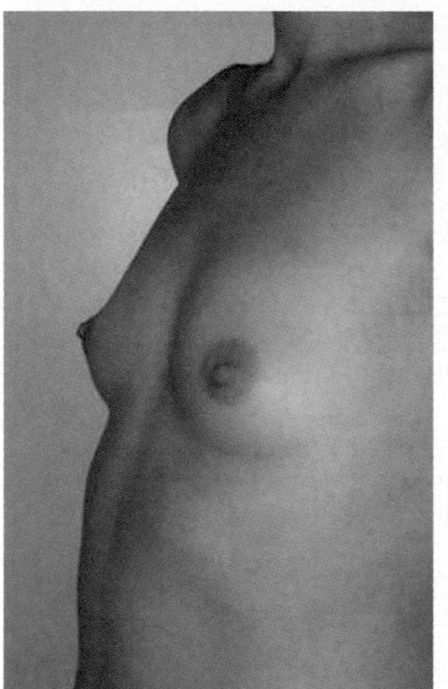
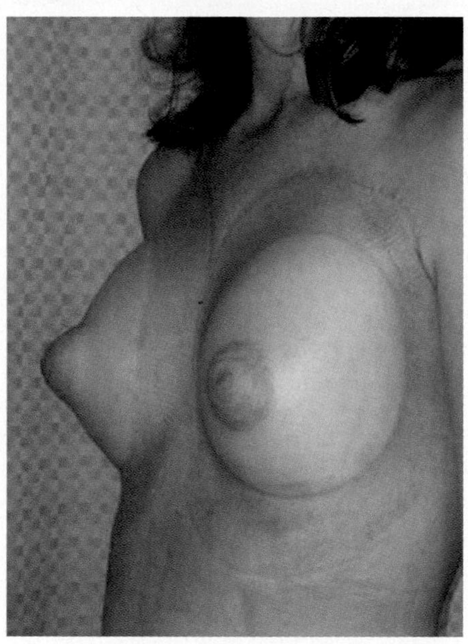

Figure 118.17. Smaller, dense breasts. After expansion, there is a step-off deformity at the breast–areolar junction due to lower resistance of the areolar tissue compared to the breast tissue. This patient will require percutaneous three-dimensional mesh release intraoperatively to address this deformity.

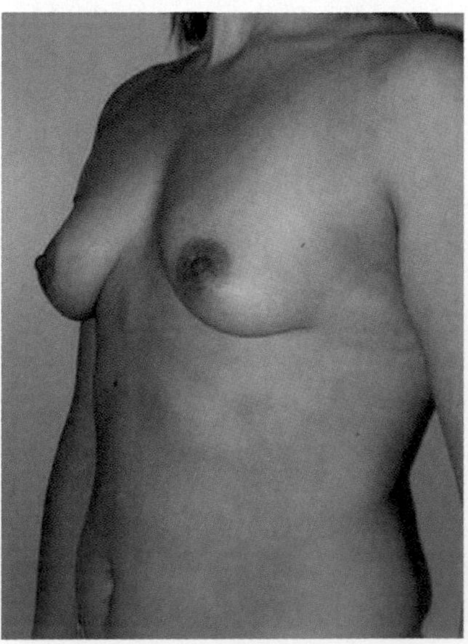
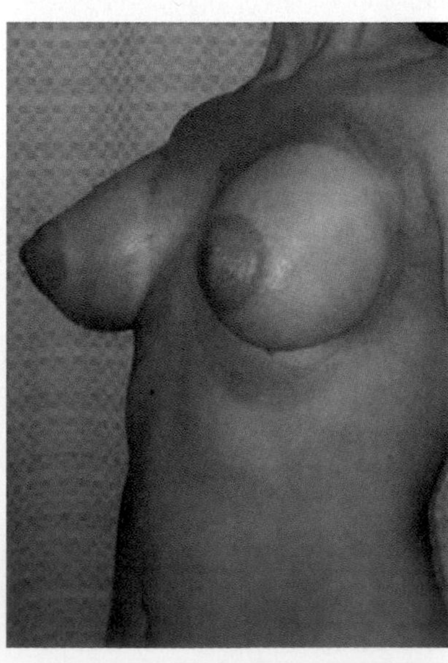

Figure 118.18. Constricted breasts preexpansion and postexpansion with BRAVA (no fat grafting has been performed yet). This patient will require aggressive release of the inferior mammary fold using percutaneous three-dimensional meshing at the time of fat grafting.

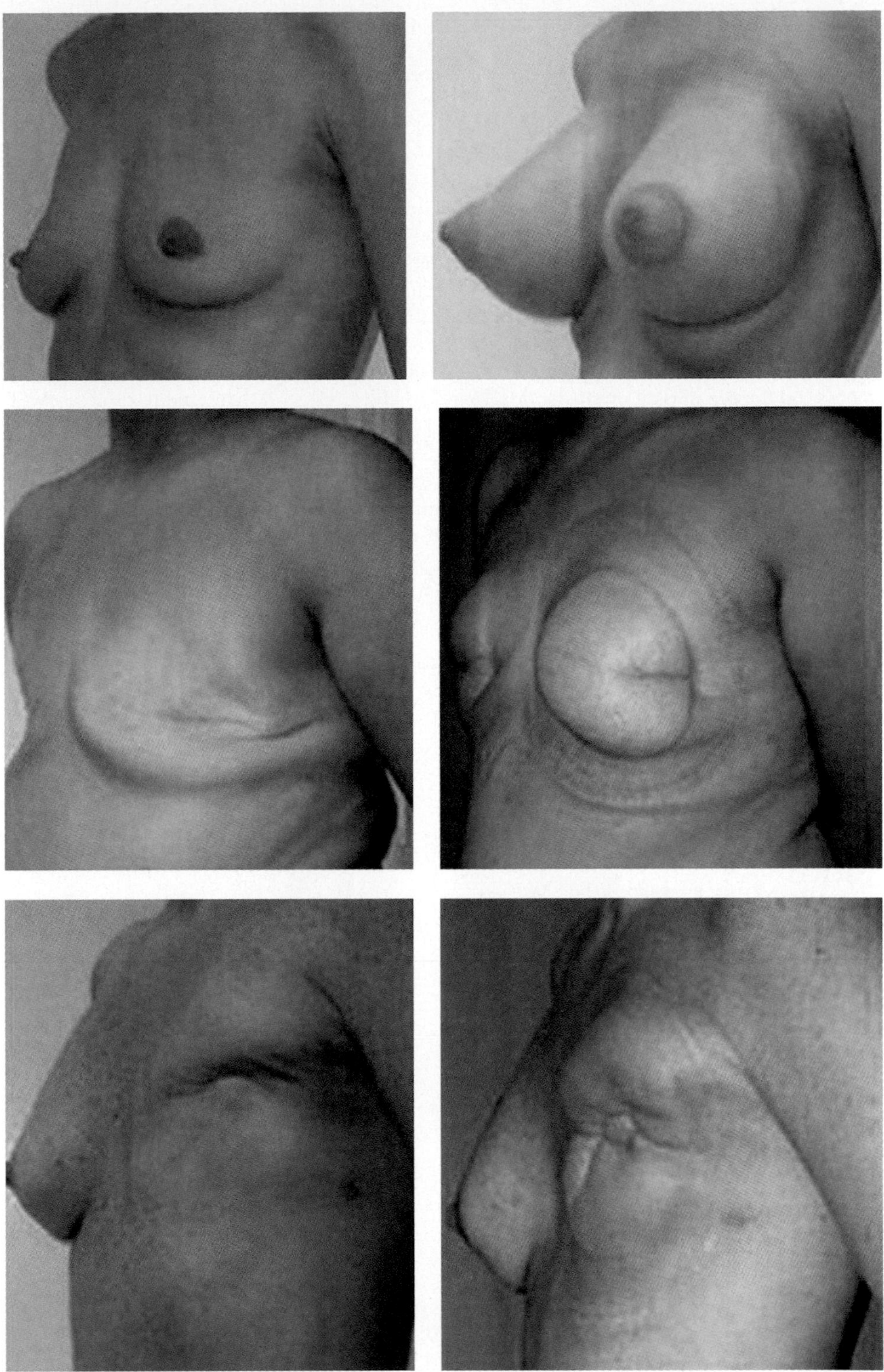

Figure 118.19. Spectrum of tissue compliance: simple augmentation **(top)**, simple mastectomy **(middle)**, irradiated mastectomy **(bottom)** sites with preexpansion. Note the varying range of expansion possible in each category.

NONSURGICAL PREEXPANSION AND FAT GRAFTING IN BREAST RECONSTRUCTION

THE MINIMALLY INVASIVE AUTOLOGOUS MASTECTOMY INCISIONLESS RECONSTRUCTION

Breast reconstruction with BRAVA external expansion and liposuctioned fat grafts is a paradigm shift poised to become a viable method of breast reconstruction. Instead of surgically implanting conventional internal expanders that are serially filled with saline to only expand an envelope and leave behind a dead space eventually replaced by a prosthetic implant, minimally invasive autologous mastectomy incisionless (MIAMI) reconstruction offers a gradually expanded parenchyma seeded with natural fat. Expansion of the skin envelope occurs from the outside, without any surgical intervention, while generating a recipient scaffold that is serially filled with fat graft, eventually yielding a live tissue–engineered breast mound. The result is the equivalent of an autologous flap reconstruction achieved by a series of minimally invasive minor outpatient procedures performed over a period of months. As for the donor-site defects, the patients appreciate the body contour improvement offered by the serial liposuction, and they appreciate the fact that there are no incisions in the donor or in the recipient site. Furthermore, because the cutaneous sensory nerve endings expand with the mound, it is endogenously innervated and the new breast mound feels like "self" to the patients.

The procedure restores a breast mound that is minimally invasive, requires no implants, and has a donor-site bonus. By lowering the threshold of acceptance, the procedure is attractive to many "orphaned" patients who would have otherwise elected not to undergo a breast reconstruction. In the segment of our breast reconstruction patients treated we have observed an unparalleled degree of patient satisfaction (Fig. 118.20).

In the case of mastectomy, the first session of grafting will obviously allow fewer planes of grafting, and, depending on the preoperative assessment of the expanded recipient volume, the graft volume during the first session should be planned depending on the amount of expansion and the size of the "edema" breast created. For subsequent sessions, there are more potential planes, as a thicker recipient space exists. Generally, the more parenchyma one has to begin with, the larger are the volumes of fat that can be grafted. In subsequent grafting sessions in reconstruction, 200 to greater than 300 cc can be planned. For irradiated cases, one should be extremely careful not to overgraft and should expect a minimum of four or five sessions (Figs. 118.21 to 118.26).

COMPARISON OF TRANSVERSE RECTUS ABDOMINIS MUSCULOCUTANEOUS AND MINIMALLY INVASIVE AUTOLOGOUS MASTECTOMY INCISIONLESS TECHNIQUES

We have performed more than 100 fat grafting procedures to the breast over the last 5 years, including reconstruction and augmentation cases (Table 118.4). There were no difficult-to interpret masses in any of the patients. About 20% of the grafted women had small foci of fat necrosis identifiable by MRI and readily recognized as benign calcifications at the 1-year postgrafting mammography. One patient suffered an episode of delayed mastitis 4 months postgrafting. All patients noted that the size of their breasts changed with fluctuations in their body weight.

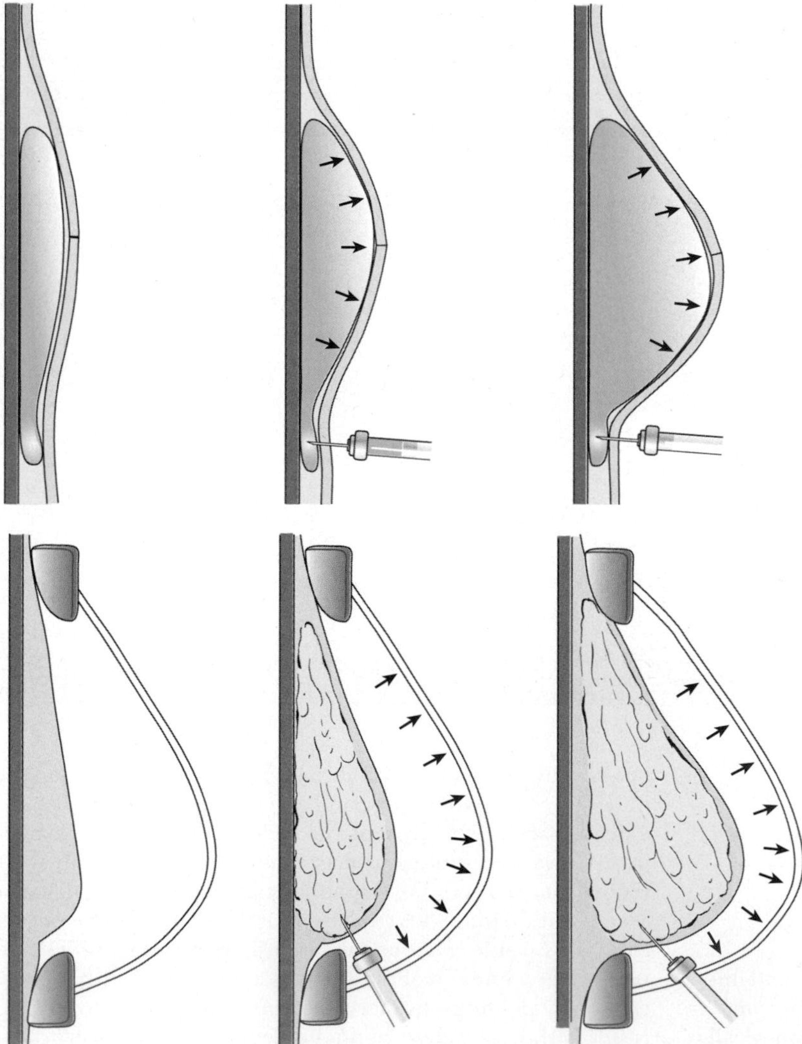

Figure 118.20. The minimally invasive autologous mastectomy incisionless (MIAMI) technique of engineering a breast mound represents a paradigm shift in breast reconstruction. **Top:** conventional expander-implant breast reconstruction method. A surgically implanted expander serially filled with saline creates a skin envelope and a dead space to be replaced by an implant. **Bottom:** MIAMI technique. A nonsurgical external expander creates both a skin envelope and a vascularized recipient scaffold that is serially seeded with fat grafts to create a live-tissue engineered breast mound.

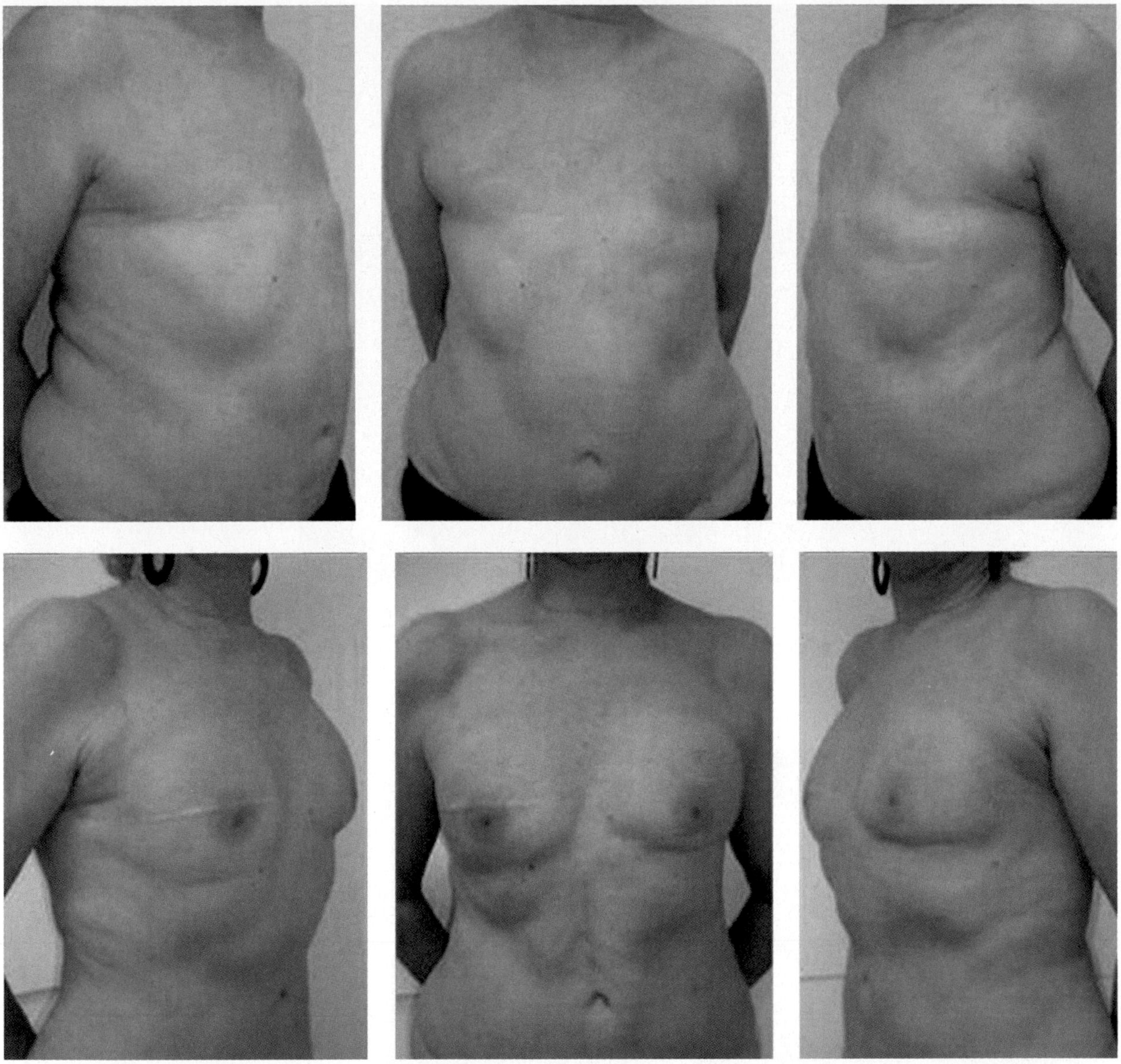

Figure 118.21. Technique of fat grafting in the early stages of postmastectomy reconstruction. (Patient of Dr. Roger Khouri.)

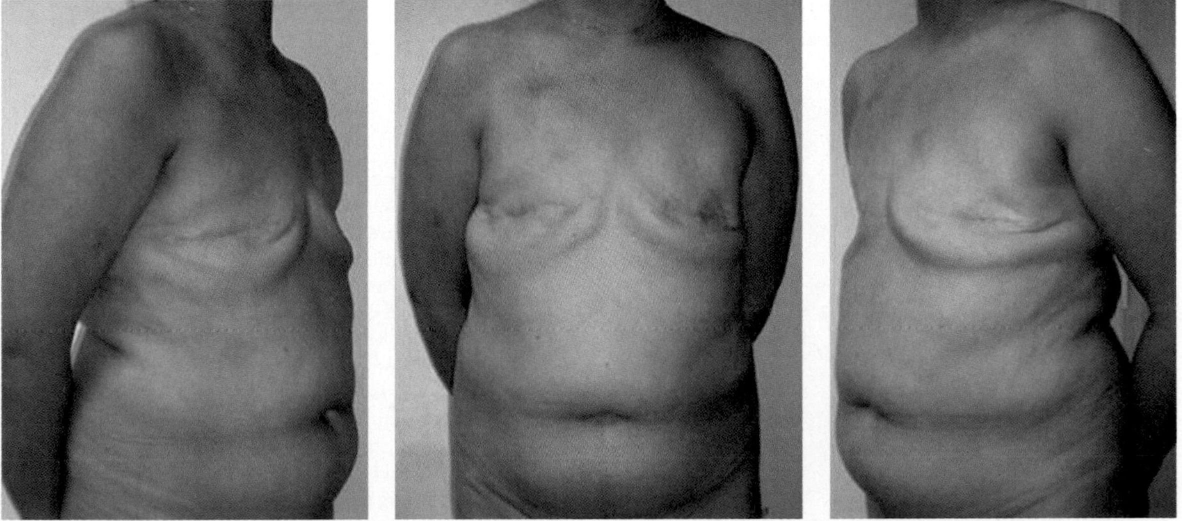

Figure 118.22. Pretreatment baseline of a 42-year-old patient 9 months after bilateral mastectomies and lymph node dissection and no radiation. (Patient of Dr. Roger Khouri.)

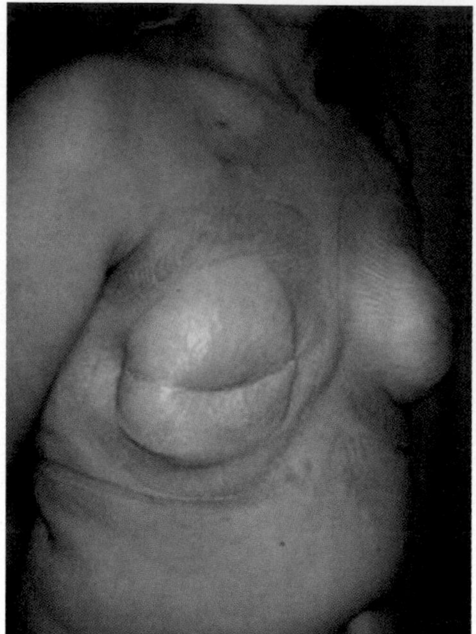

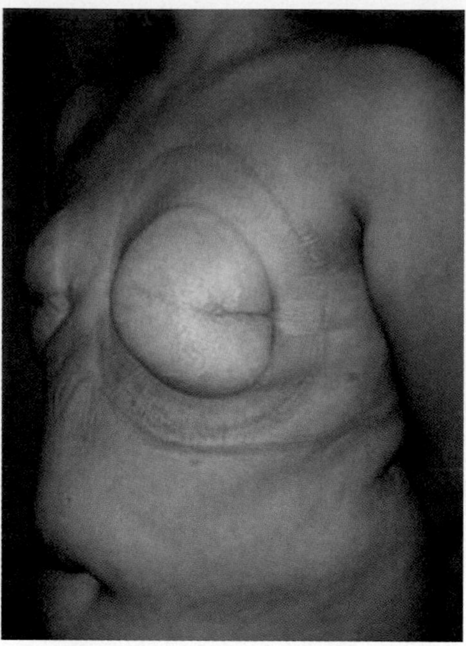

Figure 118.23. Four weeks of BRAVA preexpansion at the time of the first grafting session. Note that the mastectomy scar is released and the breast matrix is well expanded and ready to be seeded with megavolume fat grafts.

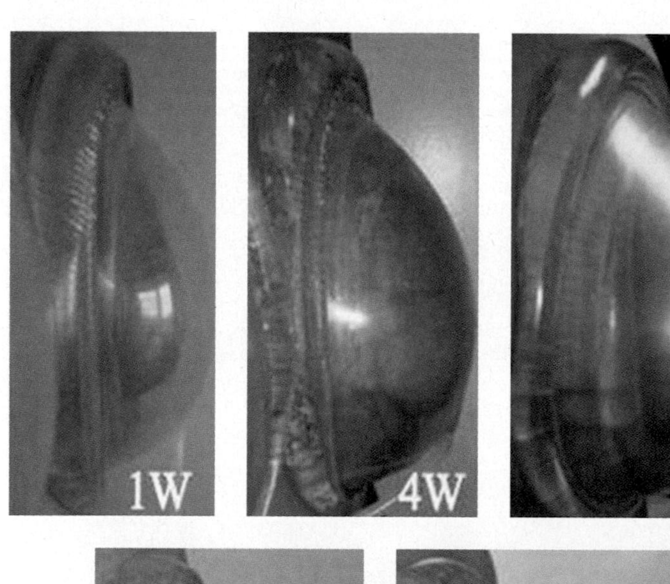

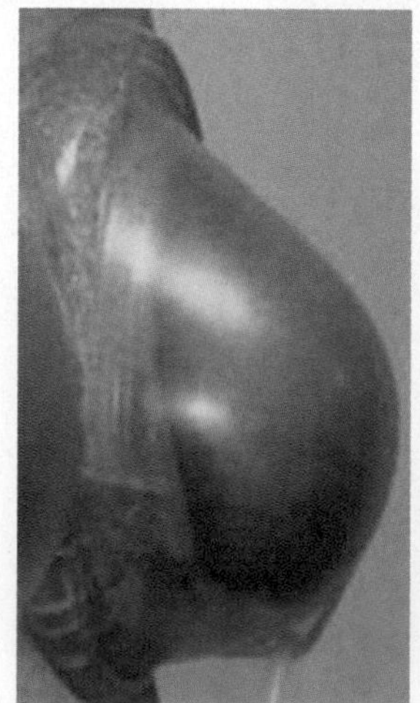

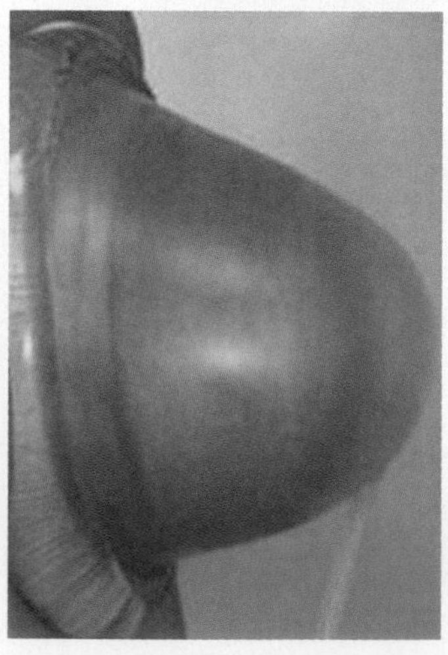

Figure 118.24. View of the left breast inside the BRAVA expander illustrates the gradual external expansion through the stages of the reconstruction process. **A:** At the first week ("1W") of expansion there is a small breast mound. **B:** This gradually fills up the small BRAVA dome at the fourth ("4W") week. **C:** At the time of the first grafting session, a deeper (medium size) BRAVA dome is required to accommodate the expanded breast, and 180 cc of lipoaspirate could be grafted. **D:** At the time of the second grafting session 6 weeks later, the breast fills the medium-size dome, and there is a parenchymal recipient site available for grafting of 240 cc. **E:** At the time of the third session 6 weeks later a large dome is required, and 320 cc of graft could be added.

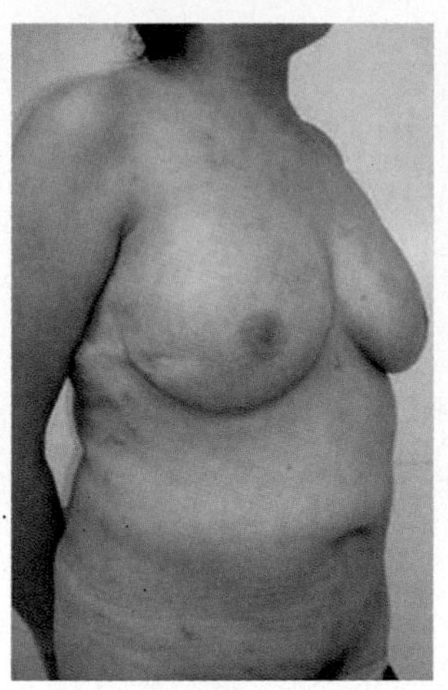
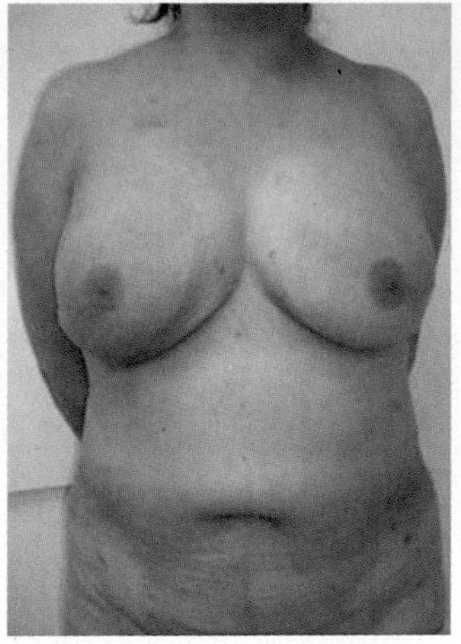
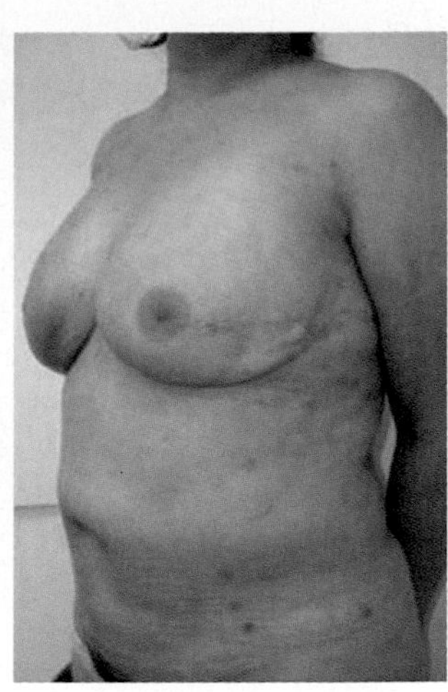

Figure 118.25. Final result 6 months after the last grafting session using the minimally invasive autologous mastectomy incisionless reconstruction. By all parameters, including "feel" to the patient and to the examiner, magnetic resonance imaging, mammography, and histology, the reconstructed breasts in this method are equivalent to those with a vascularized flap transfer.

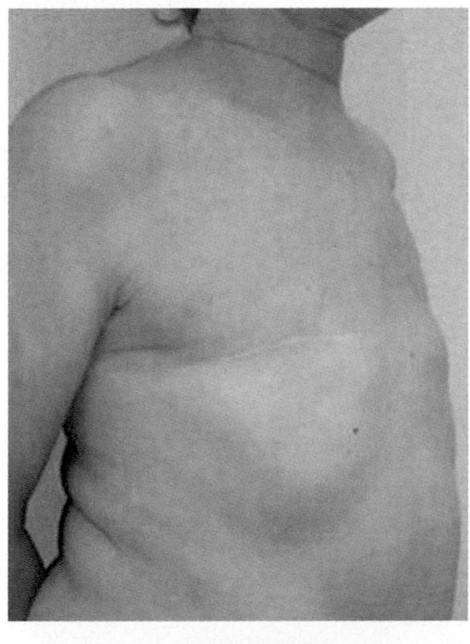
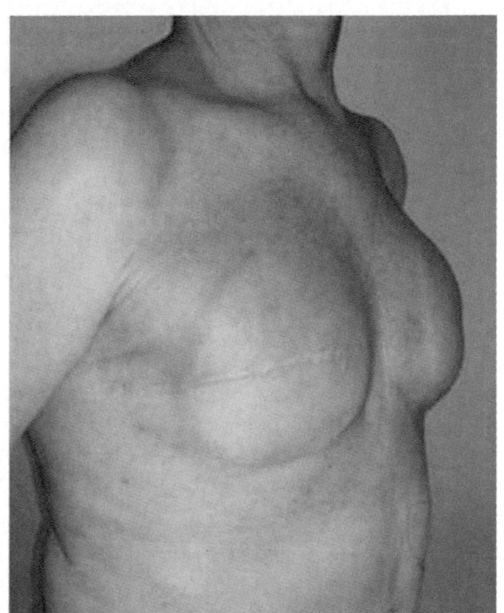
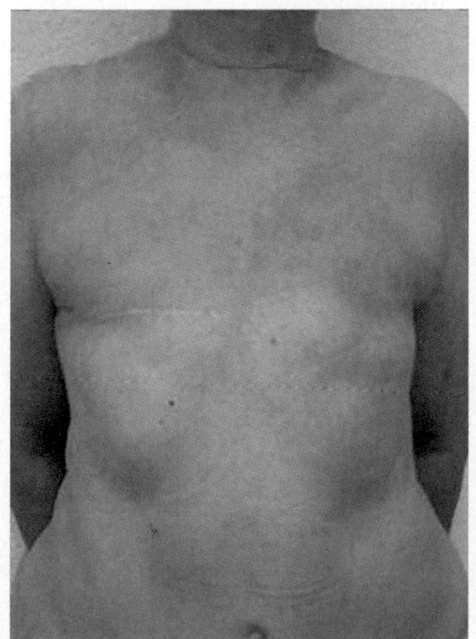
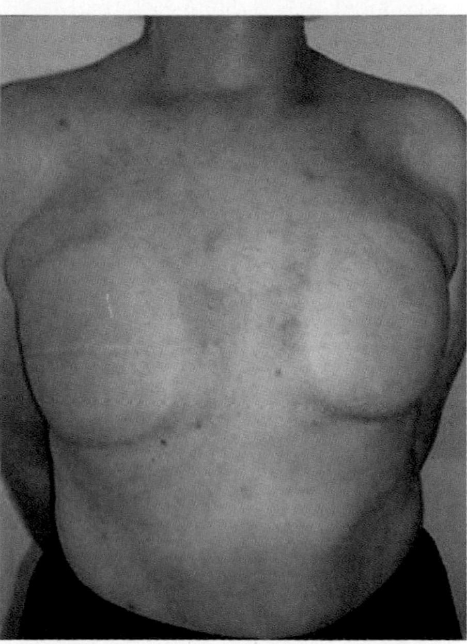

Figure 118.26. Another case example. For 30 years, a 72-year-old patient was unwilling to undergo breast reconstructions. She was offered the minimally invasive autologous mastectomy incisionless reconstruction. She underwent three small outpatient grafting sessions over a period of 4 months. Note the body contour improvement bonus at 1 year follow-up. Her follow-up mammogram was read as "fatty breasts." Magnetic resonance imaging showed several small oil cysts and normal fatty tissue in the breast mound. (Patient of Dr. Roger Khouri.)

TABLE 118.4

	TRAM	*MIAMI*
Pain Level	High	Low
# Procedures	1–2	2–5
General Anesthesia	2	Local + Sedation
Invasiveness/morbidity of the Surgery	Significant	Minimal
New Scars	Significant	None
Donor Site Morbidity	Significant	Bonus-Improvement Liposuction
Cosmetic Result & pt. Satisfaction with "Feel of Reconstruction Breast"	3–4	5–6
Applicable after Radiation	Yes	Yes
Hospital Days	3–5	None
Patient Compliance	N/A	Compliance is KEY
Reoperation Tolerance	Unlikely	Simple
Cost to System	High	Low

NONOPERATIVE PREEXPANSION AND FAT GRAFTING: PROGNOSTIC CLASSIFICATION OF BREAST TYPES

Based on our experience with many breast types, we have developed a hierarchy of preoperative breast morphologies, as follows (Table 118.5). This classification takes into account the compliance of the patient's parenchymal tissue and the starting volume of tissue available for expansion. In this way, patients can be counseled as to the effort required for the expansion and the realistic number of sessions required to achieve the desired result.

In an existing average-sized breast, combining BRAVA external expansion and fat grafting can predictably yield a 200- to 300-mL breast augmentation per grafting session. The better the preoperative expansion, the greater is the amount of fat that can successfully be grafted, and the larger is the augmentation. Multiparous patients with excess body weight are obvious candidates. However, some of the most impressive results on a percentage increase basis are also seen in very small breasted women (less than 100 mL), where the 200-mL breast augmentation can make a real difference compared to the woman who already has breasts greater than 500 mL.

Preexpansion and autologous fat grafting should *not* be considered in cases of severe breast ptosis, in patients with a low likelihood of compliance with preexpansion, in patients with a history of severe skin sensitivity or open wounds on the chest wall, or in cases of active breast lactation. This procedure is effective in a responsible, compliant patient who can understand the concept of fat grafting and can take ownership of her result by adhering to the expansion protocol. Our absolute contraindications for the procedure are smoking, in the case of cosmetic augmentation, a strong positive family history of breast cancer, and failure to successfully expand.

TABLE 118.5 Preoperative Classification of BRAVA Breast Morphology

Type	*Description of Breasts*	*Sessions*
1	Multiparous, Soft	1
II	Nulliparous, Dense	1–2
III	Constricted or tuberous	2–3
IV	Mastectomy, Non Radiated	2–5
V	Mastectomy, Radiated	4–6

PRACTICAL PATIENT MANAGEMENT: THE FOUR P'S

We divide the technique of breast augmentation using BRAVA preexpansion and fat grafting into four important clinical phases:

Patient evaluation and selection
Preparation of the recipient site
Procedure of harvesting and grating
Postoperative management

Each of these phases is vital to the success of the result. Excellence in any one phase cannot compensate for a defect in any other phase.

PATIENT EVALUATION AND SELECTION

MEDICAL EVALUATION

Like breast augmentation with implants, it is important to obtain a baseline evaluation of the recipient breasts before any iatrogenic intervention. Our routine protocol calls for a baseline MRI for all women requesting augmentation with fat grafting. In young women with dense breasts this is the most sensitive test. It also provides a 3D image analysis of the breast unattainable with conventional biplanar mammography. In the near term, sophisticated 3D imaging units may be able to accurately determine preexpansion and postgrafting volumes, but these do not asses the breast parenchyma for lesions. Until such time as the safety of this technique can be absolutely assured, MRI is probably a good standard to adhere to.

Patients should be evaluated for associated medical conditions that might otherwise exclude them from safely undergoing a liposuction procedure. We believe that this is the aspect of the intervention that is actually higher in short-term morbidity than the breast fat grafting. Smokers with their impaired microcirculation are not candidates for fat grafting. Potential fat donor sites are evaluated for their availability. In patients who would not otherwise come forward for liposuction in whom there is little localized excess fat, an adequate amount of fat can still be harvested.

We have treated irradiated patients with BRAVA preexpansion, and there is evidence that negative pressure and fat grafting improve the cyclical process of postirradiation fibrosis and chronic ischemia (38). External expansion of irradiated tissue does not appear to be fraught with the same risk of complications as internal conventional tissue expansion. The main difference is that the external expander can be removed nonsurgically at any time, allowing potential trauma to be circumvented, whereas an internal expander is an "all-or-nothing," binary intervention. Irradiated tissue is more edematous and fibrotic and expands more slowly, necessitating serial expansion/injection sessions. It is generally advised to begin breast reconstruction in nonirradiated mastectomy patients and to first become familiar with these techniques before embarking on the more complex irradiated defects. The assessment of the opposite breast is addressed with the same principles as for any breast reconstruction.

PHYSICAL EVALUATION

The ideal patient for BRAVA is a patient who has had one or more children, in whom there is breast deflation but not frank ptosis, and in whom there is an adequate amount of donor fat (Fig. 118.27).

Multiparous breasts have already been expanded and are the best breasts for BRAVA. Patients who have had children have already undergone one or more episodes of parenchymal expansion with breast milk. Engorgement of the breasts creates a natural stretching and loosening of the parenchymal ligaments. Although this may have occurred years prior to the BRAVA expansion, this prior expansion allows an easier, more rapid expansion when BRAVA is applied, given the same degree of negative pressure and time used.

Often, the breast deflation seen in multiparous patients is low-grade ptosis or pseudoptosis. Patients with frank ptosis requiring a breast lift can also benefit from BRAVA, but the timing of the mastopexy surgery is best performed at the completion of the grafting process.

Thin patients with small breasts often do not desire a major volume increase; therefore, even thin patients may be candidates for BRAVA fat grafting, as long as realistic expectations are discussed preoperatively.

EVALUATION FOR COMPLIANCE

There are two compliances—the patient and her tissues. Breasts prestretched by pregnancy or weight loss are more compliant than the younger nulliparous ones, especially if they are also constricted or tuberous. The postmastectomy, densely scarred and radiated chest is also much less compliant than the softer, loose, and nonradiated defects. Compliance of the breasts determines how effectively they will respond to external expansion.

With regard to the patient's compliance, there is no substitute for sustained moderate-to-high negative-pressure preexpansion to maximize the pre–fat grafting volume of the recipient site. Indeed, the earliest versions of the negative-pressure pumps were low-voltage, battery-operated suction devices that exerted a low negative pressure. These patients exhibited less dramatic pregrafting expansion compared to patients using the more powerful vacuum pumps currently used. These pumps are similar in negative pressure and in terms of size and portability as the VAC pump and have demonstrated a "dose-response curve" between the preexpansion volume increase and overall fat graft survival volume results postgrafting.

We have established a dose-response curve on the basis of results from more than 100 women augmented with expansion and fat grafting; the better the pregrafting expansion, the greater is the amount of fat that can be diffusely grafted without crowding and without increasing the injection pressure. We believe that there is no substitute for adequate preexpansion. Last minute "cramming" on part of the patient has been

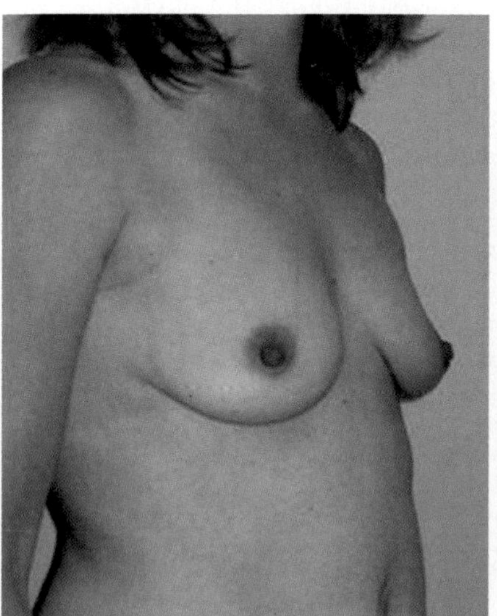
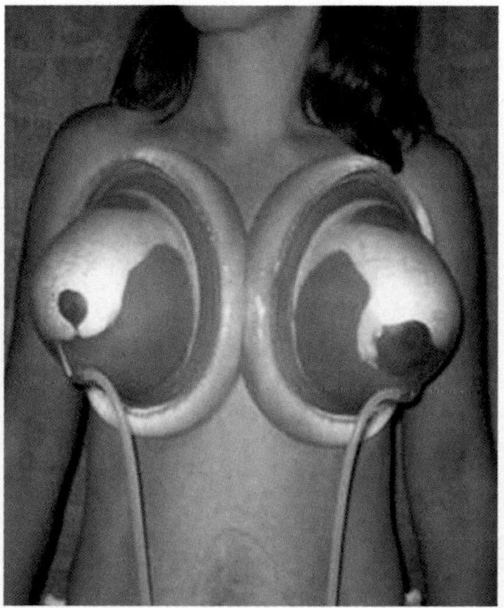
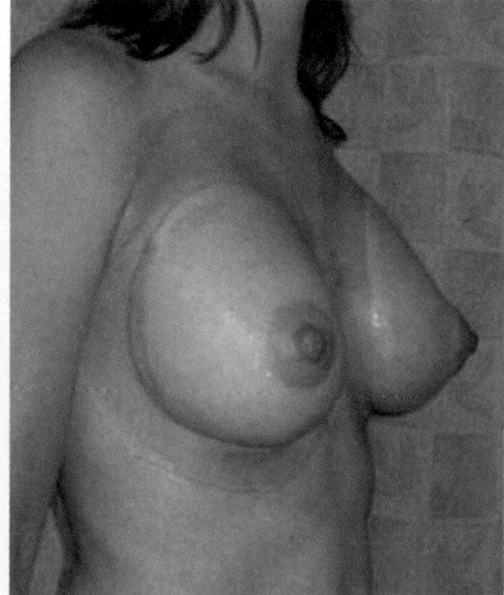

Figure 118.27. The ideal BRAVA candidate is multiparous, exhibiting previously expanded breasts. These patients expand the best.

experienced and does not result in successful preparation. It is ultimately the responsibility of the surgeon to adequately select, educate, coach, and trouble shoot patients to ensure adequate and optimal preexpansion.

Patient education is crucial. Patients must fully understand the "sowing seeds in a field" analogy. Prospective patients are shown pictures of the expected BRAVA expansion effect, and it is explained that the larger they get by the time of grafting, the greater is the number of grafts that can be injected and the larger they will end up. The educated informed patient then becomes responsible for her result. In our practice, patients sign a contract before expansion begins stating that they will follow the expansion guidelines but that surgery is not guaranteed to be performed unless the expansion is adequate. Our patients are seen weekly in the office to monitor compliance and expansion progress and to make necessary corrections to the program. Although this process is budgeted to take 3 weeks, it is really not as much a matter of time as it is a matter of adequate expansion. In our practice, we have seen patients expand to three times initial volumes in 2 weeks, while in other cases, we have seen patients who had little or no expansion after "months" of use. The duration of use and the negative pressure during use are the two variables that can be modified (usually up) to achieve the desired expansion. On occasion, we have postponed the surgery to get more expansion time.

"*No expansion = no surgery*": Despite adequate screening for compliant behavior, some patients who initially intend to proceed with BRAVA preexpansion and grafting will simply fail to expand. Device non-use is the most common cause. In these patients, fat grafting is not performed. The patient is encouraged to continue to expand until a satisfactory expansion is obtained. *It is far better to cancel a procedure after a failed expansion than it is to move forward and perform a failed operation.*

Without adequate preexpansion, the results of fat grafting to the breast are limited to small graft (100 cc or less) volumes that do not exceed high interstitial pressures. In breast augmentation, such volumes are rarely adequate to achieve a significant or desired result. Therefore, if a surgeon grafts a patient who has failed to expand, it is a near certainty that the patient will not be satisfied with one procedure and that repeat procedures will be necessary. Inevitably, this may be interpreted by the patient and by the surgeon as a failure of the procedure, whereas it is really a failure to appreciate the importance of the process as a whole.

LESSONS FROM HAIR TRANSPLANTATION

In plastic surgery we already perform an aesthetic procedure in which a micrografting technique is employed that involves specialized cells—hair transplantation. What began as the installation of "plugs" has evolved over the last 50 years to tedious yet effective microfollicular grafting, with spectacular results. Nonetheless, microfollicular hair transplantation is not a popular technique among plastic surgeons, and the rate of hair transplantations performed by plastic surgeons has declined 57% over the last 5 years (39). The explanation for this is unknown, but several important observations emerge.

First, technique- and result-oriented plastic surgeons believe that outcomes are mainly dependent on what is performed in the operating room. In microfollicular hair transplantation, patient selection, preparation, and expectation management are equally vital if not more vital than the surgical technique. Second, because plastic surgeons elected to not perform this relatively tedious procedure, it was adopted by dermatologists and other providers.

Microfat grafting is a relatively simple technique that does not require the high-tech instrumentation, ancillary nursing services, and expensive postoperative monitoring that some procedures in plastic surgery demand. Microfat grafting has been and can be performed in an office setting under local anesthesia with sedation in selected cases.

If plastic surgeons approach microfat grafting to the breast in the same manner they approached hair transplantation, microfat grafting, a relatively simple technique, may be adopted by other surgical and nonsurgical colleagues in medicine. As experts on breast augmentation and reconstruction, plastic surgeons have an obligation to promote the science and to perfect the technique of microfat grafting to the breast.

PREOPERATIVE PREPARATION

At the time of this writing, all patients having megavolume fat grafting to the breast, on signing their initial contract, have a preexpansion breast MRI and photographs before BRAVA expansion begins. The BRAVA bra is then fitted on the patient by the nurse or by the surgeon, who makes certain that the patient can apply the bra and the suction on her own. The BRAVA bra comes in several dome sizes and in several base diameter sizes. Patients are encouraged to consult directly with the manufacturer to select the best-fitting bra for their body type. It is important to educate patients on how to apply the bra so that there is no room for error or lack of compliance during the expansion process.

Using a postoperative questionnaire, we have found that our patients reported difficulties in compliance with the BRAVA bra as follows, in decreasing order:

1. Appearance of the domes prohibiting use outside the home (used less often)
2. Difficulty applying a suction (less often and less pressure)
3. Skin irritation at the base of the dome (less pressure)
4. Breast pain (less pressure)

Because the bra's dome size must be larger than the breast to obtain expansion, there is not much that can be improved in this regard to allow patients to wear the bra outside the home. The base of the domes rest on a two-dimensional plane, and the chest wall is rarely two dimensional. It appears that a lack of compliance could often stem from a lack of achieving adequate suction. Design improvements to the BRAVA bra in the future may help to address these issues.

During the initial evaluation and throughout the preexpansion process it is often important to coach and to motivate the patient. We often use the " 3 vs. 30" rule: "Would you rather spend 3 weeks in a BRAVA bra 8 to 12 hours a day or spend 30 years with breast implants?"

ENDPOINTS FOR EXPANSION

It is also important to educate the patient as to the extent of the desired expansion. All too often, patients expand to their desired breast size and then stop. This is a mistake. The BRAVA

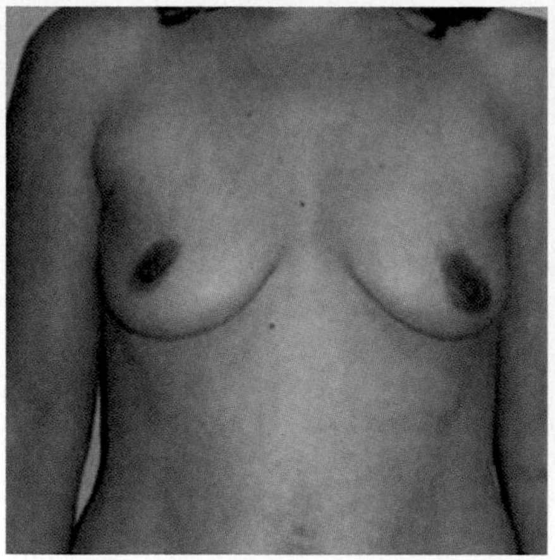

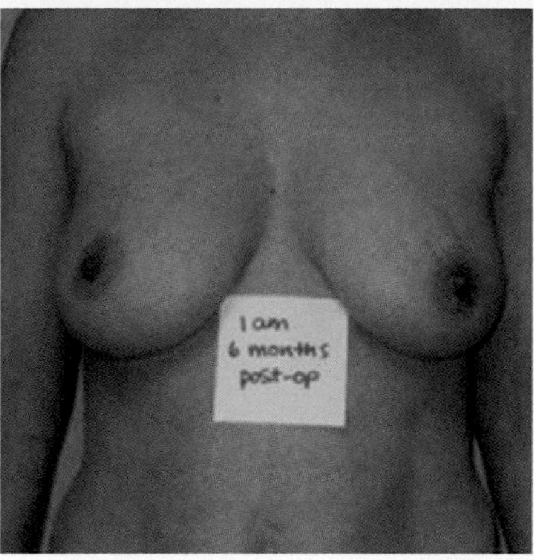

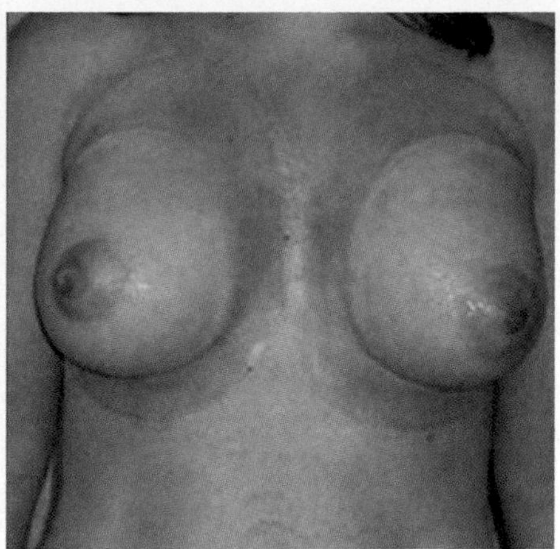

Figure 118.28. The "1-2-3 rule": A patient **(left)** who wants to double final volume **(center)** must triple in expansion **(right)**. Patients should not expand to their desired breast volume but must hyperexpand and surpass their desired size to achieve optimal results.

expansion should be greater than the desired volume so that there is a much larger potential space created by BRAVA compared to the desired volume of fat to be grafted. We have developed the "1-2-3 rule" for our patients so they can easily understand the endpoints of expansion in preparation:

"1-2-3 Rule": If you are a "1" and you want to be a "2," you must expand to a "3" (Fig. 118.28).

At the beginning of the expansion process, the patient is given a target date; however, this date is not guaranteed. The surgery, as stated previously, should only be performed if there has been adequate documented preexpansion by follow-up office evaluation or by examination of intraexpansion photos sent to the office in the case of patients coming from long distances. Once a physician offers an operative date, the physician takes all the risk that noncompliant patient behavior and inadequate breast expansion might occur, over which the physician has no control. An operative date may be construed as an implied guarantee that surgery will be performed, and this may set up a difficult situation in the event of inadequate preoperative preparation.

PROCEDURE: TECHNICAL GUIDELINES

THE DAY OF SURGERY

Patients arrive in the operating room on the day of surgery wearing their BRAVA bra. Preoperatively, the patient is initially marked for areas to be suctioned, and the breasts are marked circumferentially for areas of proposed needle insertions. Any constricted areas are outlined for planned percutaneous three-dimensional meshing. Markings are placed at 8 to 12 proposed sites, circumferentially around the breast. Once markings are completed, the BRAVA bra is reapplied. Once in the operating room under general anesthesia, the patient is positioned supine with the domes still in place and under manual bulb suction. The anesthesiologist monitors the suction intermittently during the liposuction phase of the procedure so that the negative pressure can still be applied to maximize the recipient-site space.

The specific techniques that have evolved over the last several years have taken into consideration the relative time and manpower demands of each of the fat grafting variables discussed, as well as the variables themselves. The emphasis on rendering an "optimized" operation that can be completed in 2 to 3 hours and not a "maximized" series of independent variables with no time limit serves as the basis for the slight variations in some of the techniques between the authors.

HARVESTING

Liposuction is performed using a 12-gauge multihole cannula. Use of smaller cannula sizes leads to less subcutaneous tissue trauma, faster recovery, and smaller fat lobules, which result in better fat flow and less clumping. Multiple holes lead to more efficient and faster fat removal. One of the two aforementioned collection techniques is used:

1. Syringe collection method (Fig. 118.29)
2. Machine "in-line" method (Figs. 118.30 and 118.31)

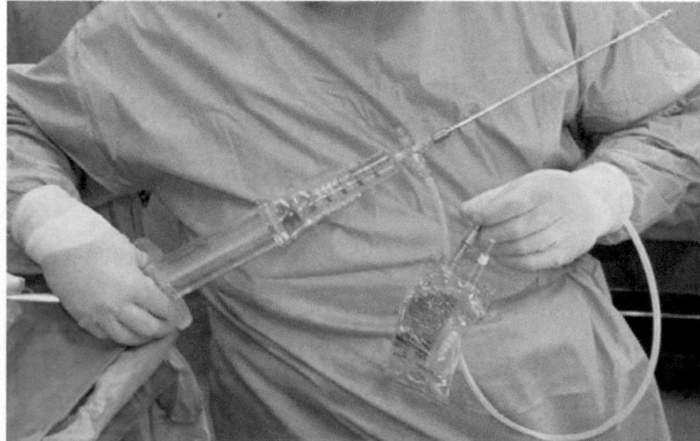

Figure 118.29. Syringe collection method of fat harvesting. Via a specialized stopcock, fat is transferred via intravenous tubing to a 100-cc sterile intravenous collection bag on the field with minimal or no air exposure.

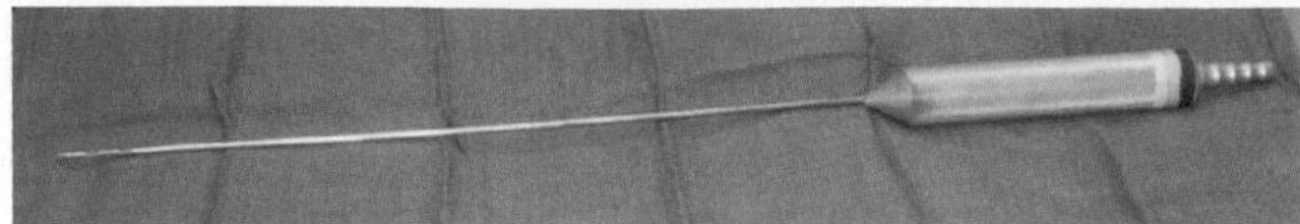

Figure 118.30. A 12-gauge multihole cannula fused to an ergonomic handle can be used in the machine "in-line" method. This cannula reduces operator fatigue and reduces instrument breakdown at the handle–tubing interface.

TABLE 118.6

Collection Method	*Separation Method*
Syringe	Bag Centrifugation
Machine "In Line"	Double Decanting

Once the fat is collected, two general methods for removing unwanted crystalloid are employed:

1. "Bag centrifugation" method: The previously mentioned 100-cc IV bags are hung on a hand-spun 5-1 gear-ratio spinner and centrifuged at low revolutions per minute (approximately 2 × *g*) for several minutes. The resultant crystalloid is tapped off, and the fat is ready for reinjection. (See Fig. 118.5.)
2. "Double-decanting" method: By changing several in-line collection canisters during the machine liposuction, the canisters are allowed to stand for 10 minutes, allowing fat to separate from crystalloid. This fat is then drawn up into 60-cc syringes directly from the collection canister and placed tip down in a graduate for an additional 10 minutes, allowing a second decanting process. Centrifugation of these 60-cc syringes is possible and is optional.

In general, when the syringe collection method is employed it is done do in conjunction with low-speed bag centrifugation. When the machine "in-line" method of collection is used, it is done in conjunction with double decanting, reflecting the two authors' preferred techniques (Table 118.6). What is probably the most powerful fact of all is that both techniques yield reproducible results because we agree on the supreme importance on preparation of the recipient site with proper expansion.

As stated previously, the emphasis on ultraconcentrated fat is less important the greater the overexpansion is of the recipient-site space using BRAVA. Overexpansion of the recipient site affords us the opportunity to inject less-concentrated fat. This less-concentrated fat is theoretically less traumatized, flows better, disperses better because it is less concentrated, and finally takes less operative time and manpower to process. As stated earlier, the emphasis on "overcorrection" of fat grafting in the past with resultant overcrowding, interstitial hypertension, and fat necrosis can now be applied to "overexpansion" of the recipient site before fat grafting.

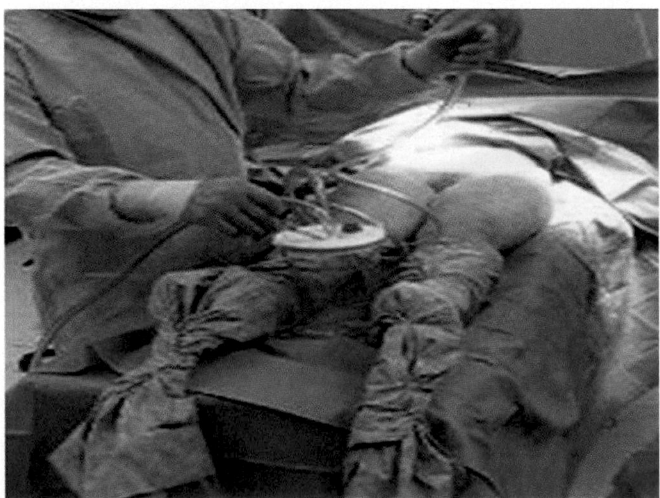

Figure 118.31. Depiction of the machine "in -line" system with the left-hand tubing going to the cannula and the right-hand tubing headed off the field to a liposuction machine. The sterile canister on the field collects the fat.

Once the fat is separated from unwanted crystalloid, injection into the breast begins. Injections are performed using a 15-cm Coleman side-hole needle.

GRAFTING TECHNIQUES

Injection techniques also vary and play a major role in fat grafting survival. Injections into a cavity or a lake and bolus injections are to be avoided. They usually result in fat liquefaction, necrosis, and oil cysts. The most reliable method of creating a diversified injection of adipocytes into a recipient site with the highest surface-to-volume transplant-to- recipient site contact is probably the previously described mapping technique. Although it takes longer than the previously described reverse liposuction technique, it should probably be used by those becoming familiar with megavolume fat grafting (Fig. 118.32).

PERCUTANEOUS THREE-DIMENSIONAL MESHING

Tuberous breast correction and other cases of constricted breasts can be treated with selective percutaneous release of constriction bands immediately after grafting, which we term percutaneous 3D meshing. In these types of deformities exhibiting internal parenchymal constriction and aesthetic breast disharmony, volume enhancement alone will not adequately address the problem. An internal release of the constriction bands has historically been performed at the time of open surgery for tubular breasts by means of "scoring." In contrast to classic techniques, the external negative pressure placed on the tuberous breast by the BRAVA bra, followed by the insertion of fat into the non–surgically expanded parenchymal spaces, offers the opportunity for surgeons to manually release persistent bands under tension internally, using a percutaneous needle. Once released, the already injected fat immediately fills the newly created spaces and keeps the release open. This technique can be performed using a percutaneous needle. Just as a skin graft is meshed in two dimensions to increase its cover in two dimensions, percutaneous 3D meshing is a method of further expanding the breast parenchyma in three dimensions above and beyond what the preoperative external expansion has already accomplished (Fig. 118.33).

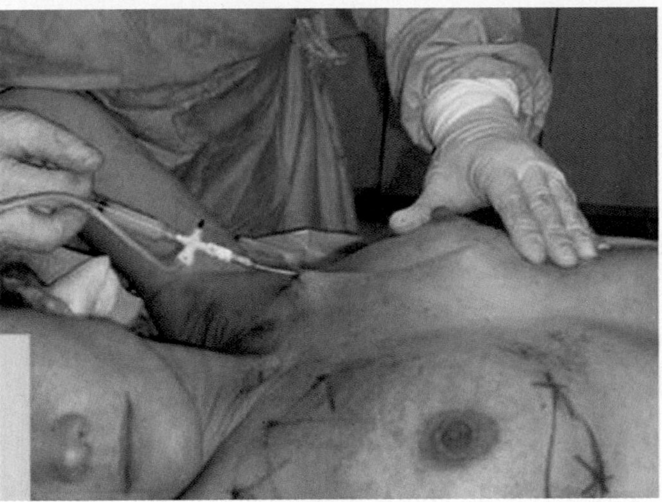
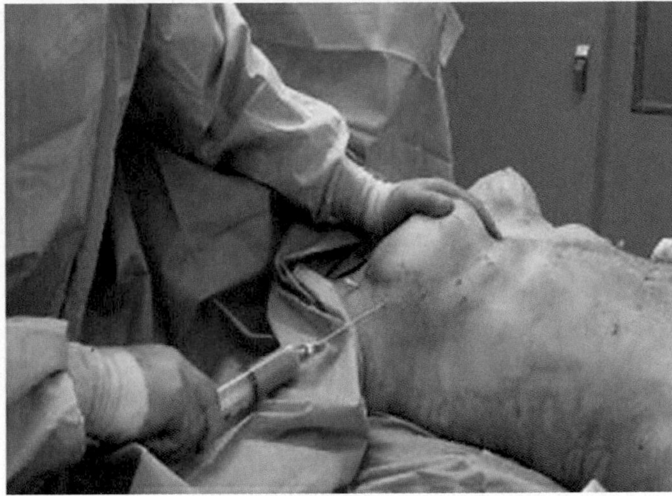

Figure 118.32. Mapping technique **(left)** and reverse liposuction technique **(right)**. In the mapping technique, injection only occurs on withdrawal of needle. In reverse liposuction, a steady flow is achieved with deliberate liposuction-like movement of the needle.

PREFERENTIAL FILL

Unlike the spherical limitations imposed by breast implants, fat grafting allows for the insertion of complex 3D shapes and "preferential fill" of the ptotic breast, especially in the lower pole in cases of Baker I and II breast ptosis. In cases of breast asymmetry the patient often desires an increase in both breasts. In these cases, it is possible to preferentially fill the smaller breast with more graft material at the time of grafting, but preoperative expansion of the breast should be performed as usual. Finally, small defects following breast reconstruction such as zone II fat necrosis in transverse rectus abdominis musculocutaneous (TRAM) and inferior gluteal artery perforator flaps and rippling in saline augmentations can be addressed with preferential localized external expansion and subsequent grafting.

SUBCUTANEOUS FILL DURING REMOVAL OF IMPLANTS

In treating breast implant "cripples" who have or will undergo explantation, full obliteration and collapse of the implant pocket is optimal after prosthesis explantation. However, most patients do not want to wait 6 to 12 months for this to occur. At the time of explantation, the subcutaneous space is quite redundant immediately upon removal of the breast prosthesis. Therefore, there is an opportunity for an initial modest (100 to 150 cc per breast) session of fat grafting to be performed, which is beneficial for the patient *prior* to external expansion for two reasons: (a) the patient will exhibit *some volume* after explantation, and (b) the expansion process will *begin at a higher initial starting volume* than it otherwise would have had the fat not been grafted at the time of explantation.

AESTHETIC ENDPOINTS OF BREAST SIZE AND SHAPE POSTGRAFTING: A PARADIGM SHIFT

There is a major paradigm shift between what a surgeon should expect from an aesthetic perspective following prosthetic breast augmentation and augmentation using megavolume fat grafting. While the "on-table" aesthetics with prostheses can be critically examined for size, symmetry and position and are more "WYSIWYG" (what you see is what you get). The immediate on-table result with megavolume fat grafting represents the

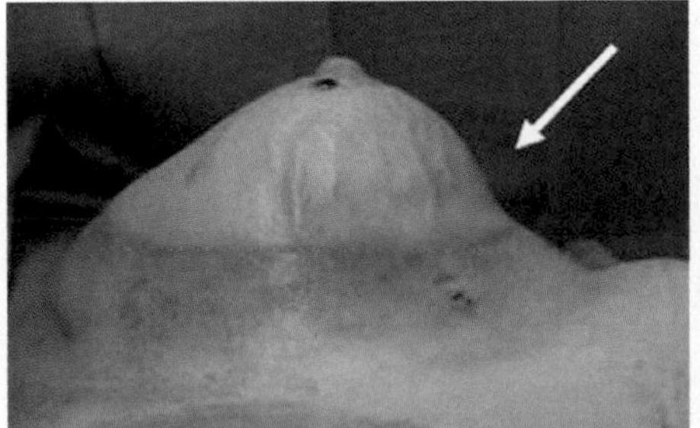
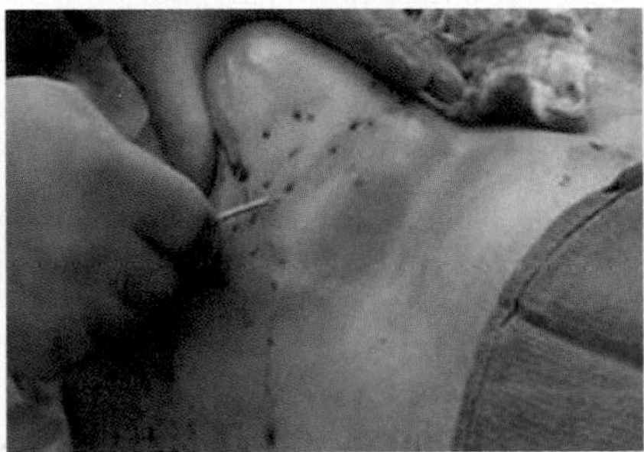
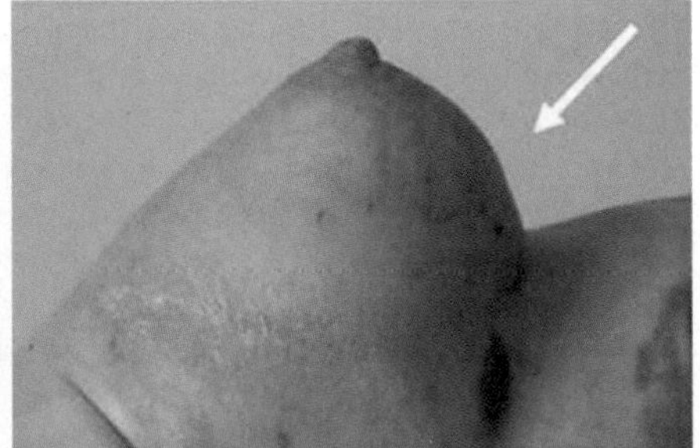

Figure 118.33. Immediately after fat grafting, the injected fat provides an internal traction effect to help identify specific areas of deforming scar or ligamentous bands, as seen in this patient with a "double bubble" immediately after grafting 600 cc of fat into the right breast **(left)**. After insertion of a 14-gauge needle into multiple sites and release of the constriction bands **(center)**, the irregularity is released and the fat immediately fills the space created, changing the shape to a more aesthetic result, seen 5 days postoperatively **(right)**.

first stage of a dynamic process. First, there is a volume of fluid represented by the expansion itself and by the liposuction fat that will reabsorb in the first 5 to 10 days postgrafting. The surgeon should not get too concerned with the appearance of breasts that look too "large" on the table but should be reassured by focusing on the volume of material that was injected. Second, because the augmentation is intraparenchymal as opposed to a single-cavity volume enhancement seen in implants, there are more on-table surface irregularities that resolve in the early postoperative period and require no additional manipulation.

POSTOPERATIVE MANAGEMENT

In the first 24 hours postgrafting there is no external compression or negative pressure used. Patients are placed in standard girdles as for routine liposuction. Beginning at 24 to 48 hours after grafting, patients are placed into BRAVA domes, which are placed under low suction for a period of 10 to 14 days. The use if BRAVA in the postoperative period may act as a splint. The importance of immobilizing a split-thickness skin graft postoperatively is well recognized. Conversely, the low negative pressure exerted by the BRAVA bra may help to immobilize the fat cells and aid in neovascularization to the graft. In any event, application of the domes in the postoperative period certainly protects the breast from external trauma, which could serve to shift the graft and potentially disturb neovascularization.

It has been postulated that the negative-pressure environment created by the BRAVA bra used in the postgrafting phase may draw more interstitial fluid into the recipient site, which may serve as an impediment to neovascularization (James W. May, Jr., MD, personal communication). We have not seen edema in the breasts postoperatively, but instead, a gradual shrinkage of the breast as interstitial fluid diminishes from the recipient site. We suggest that BRAVA used postoperatively using a battery-operated sport pump exerts suction that is probably too low to draw in excessive fluid. The positive effects of immobilization and external protection probably outweigh the potential negative effects of fluid accumulation postulated.

CASE EXAMPLES: AUGMENTATION

CASE 1. ONE-STAGE BREAST AUGMENTATION

A 28-year-old nulliparous female desired increased breast size. She was pleased with the overall shape. She demonstrated relatively symmetric, well-developed soft breasts with no constrictions or severe density. She did not desire breast implants. She was initially expanded with a BRAVA handheld pump for 10 hours per day for 3 weeks. She was a very compliant patient, and her expansion proceeded well over serial office visits. After 3 weeks of expansion she underwent 400 cc of fat injected into each breast, harvested during liposuction of the thighs. At 6 months postgrafting her result is stable. Even in patients in whom liposuction alone would not likely be entertained, it is possible to obtain a sufficient amount of fat. This case also demonstrates that not all nulliparous patients expand poorly. The anatomic compliance of the breast and the nonanatomic compliance of the patient are equally vital to successful preexpansion (Fig. 118.34).

CASE 2. BREAST AUGMENTATION FOR DEFLATED BREASTS FOLLOWING IMPLANT REMOVAL

A 59-year-old woman had previously had silicone breast implants, which had been removed 15 years prior due to implant complications. At the time of her implant removal her breast tissue had atrophied and thinned, and her surgeon had performed a Wise-pattern breast lift to remove excess skin. The patient was never happy with the size reduction and with the deflated appearance but did not wish to go back to prosthesis.

When she presented for a thighplasty involving an initial thigh liposuction followed 6 to 8 months later by a medial thigh lift, the possibility of using the liposuction fat for her breasts was discussed with her. The patient wore the BRAVA bra, using the higher-pressure hand pump, for 3 weeks preoperatively during the late afternoon/early evening for approximately 8 hours per day. This patient, a practicing physician, had a busy schedule, and compliance was a challenge. Despite her less-than-ideal compliance, she had enough parenchymal and skin laxity to expand well and to receive 600 cc of fat in each breast during her thigh liposuction. After 6 months, she demonstrated significant volume increase and maintenance of volume. Patients who have removal of breast implants already have experienced significant skin expansion as well as subcutaneous parenchymal redundancy once the implants are removed. This is an opportunity to backfill this space with fat (Fig. 118.35).

CASE 3. TWO-STAGE BREAST AUGMENTATION FOR CONSTRICTED TUBEROUS BREASTS

A 32-year-old woman with tuberous breast deformity desired increased breast size and improved shape. She demonstrated constricted inframammary folds and herniation of the nipple-areolar parenchyma. She did not desire breast implants. She was initially expanded with a BRAVA sport pump, a low-pressure, battery-operated pump, for 3 weeks prior to her first fat grafting procedure, in which 300 cc of fat was injected into each breast and she underwent needle band release and periareolar reduction. It was felt that the low negative pressure created by the sport pump was not optimal and that additional expansion could have been achieved with a more-negative-pressure handheld pump.

After 4 months, she underwent a second round of BRAVA preexpansion using a hand pump and had a second round of grafting with 350 cc of additional fat per breast. Her results by photography and by MRI preoperatively and 8 months after her second procedure demonstrate a significant increase in volume and in breast aesthetics (Figs. 118.36 and 118.37).

THE SCIENCE, THE SURGERY, AND THE CONSUMER: THE FUTURE OF FAT GRAFTING TO THE BREAST FOR AUGMENTATION

Scientifically, what we do not know about fat grafting to the breast is staggering. Unknown effects of stem cells, aromatase, potential carcinogenic effects, cysts, fat necrosis, and difficulty reading mammograms and breast cancer detection have all been raised as concerns in fat grafting to the breasts. Over the next several decades, these issues and the relative safety of the procedure will be better understood. A body of evidence is

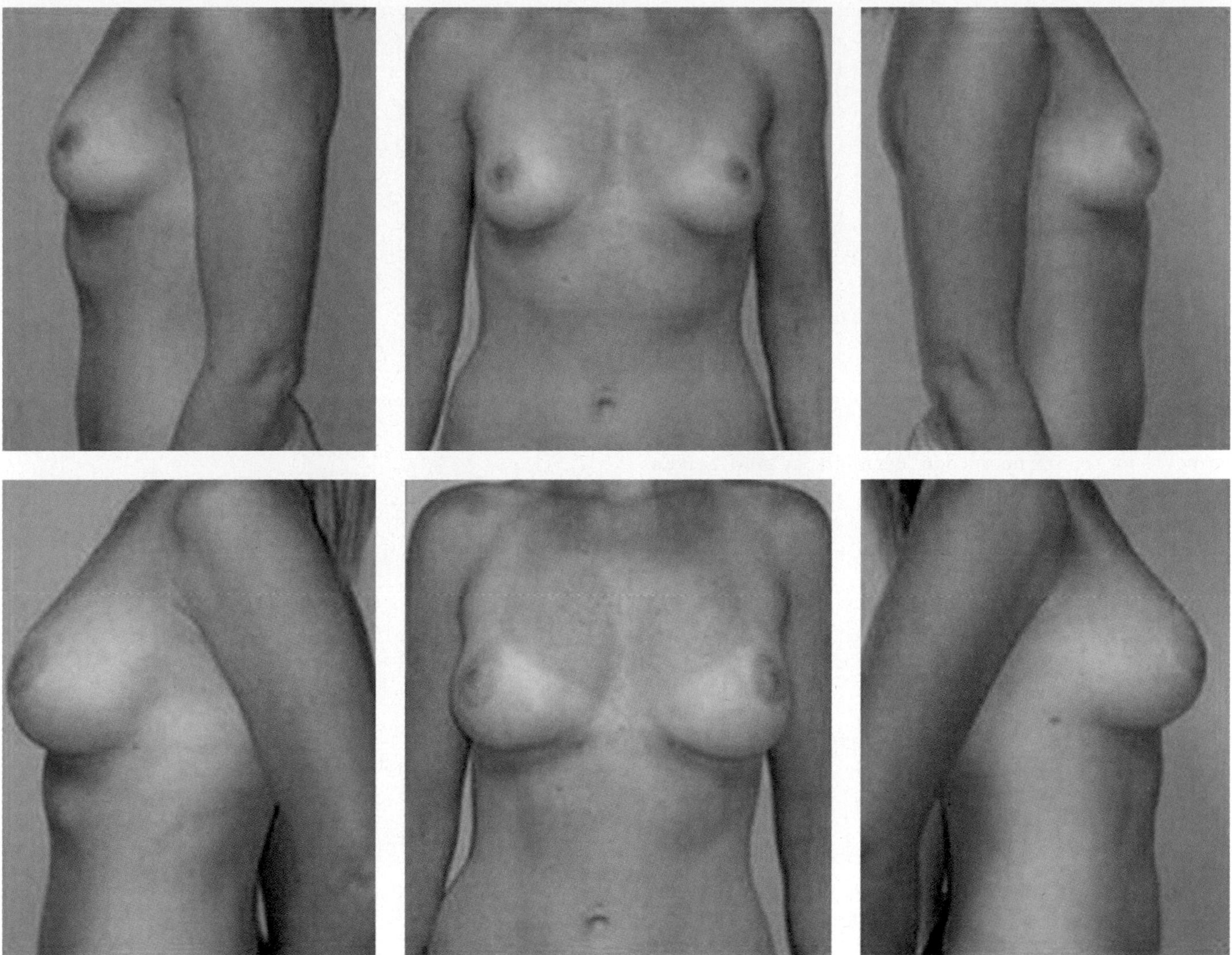

Figure 118.34. Nulliparous patient with soft breasts and very good preoperative expansion. Postoperative views at the bottom are at 6 months postgrafting. (Patient of Dr. Daniel Del Vecchio.)

emerging that suggests that transplanted fat has a regenerative effect (38). Fat grafting to lumpectomy defects is being evaluated in a multinational, multicenter study (40). Some day we may know whether fat grafting to the breasts imparts a detrimental or a beneficial effect as it relates to cancer.

Clinically, based on case reports, small clinical series, and limited experience, we know that today it is not outside the standard of care in the United States to perform breast augmentation utilizing autologous fat grafting. We also know that the procedure can be performed in a reasonable (2 to 3 hours) period of time with stable results at 1 year as documented by MRI and by physical examination (41). We also know that the complication rate in the near term is extremely low. Standardization, clinical improvements in technique, and standards for preoperative breast radiologic documentation are necessary for patient safety and for the examination of outcomes on a go-forward basis.

Of the approximately 300 million people in the United States in 2007, 150 million were female. A total of 347,000 breast augmentation procedures were performed in the United States that year (13). This results in a rate of 0.23% of women each year in the United States who currently undergo breast augmentation. These numbers do not appear large enough to get excited about fat grafting using BRAVA and megavolume fat grafting unless we consider that this procedure *probably will not compete* with breast augmentation on a result basis. Patients who desire breast augmentation are willing to undergo a surgical procedure in which incisions are made, are willing to accept prosthesis with a 10-year or less quoted life, and accept the certainty of additional procedures in their lifetimes.

The percentage of women who may eventually wish to undergo a procedure that does not involve incisions, does not involve an artificial implant, and in which unwanted fat is transferred may be considerably higher. Approximately 30% of bras sold in the United States are padded bras (42). This equates to 17 million women in the United States who, based on their purchasing behavior, wish to give the appearance that their breast size is larger than it is.

What these facts suggest is that for every woman who actually undergoes a breast augmentation, there are at least 100 women who wish their breasts were larger. The desire to undergo breast augmentation by fat grafting to the breasts using one's unwanted fat may lie somewhere between that of undergoing surgical breast augmentation with prostheses and using a padded bra.

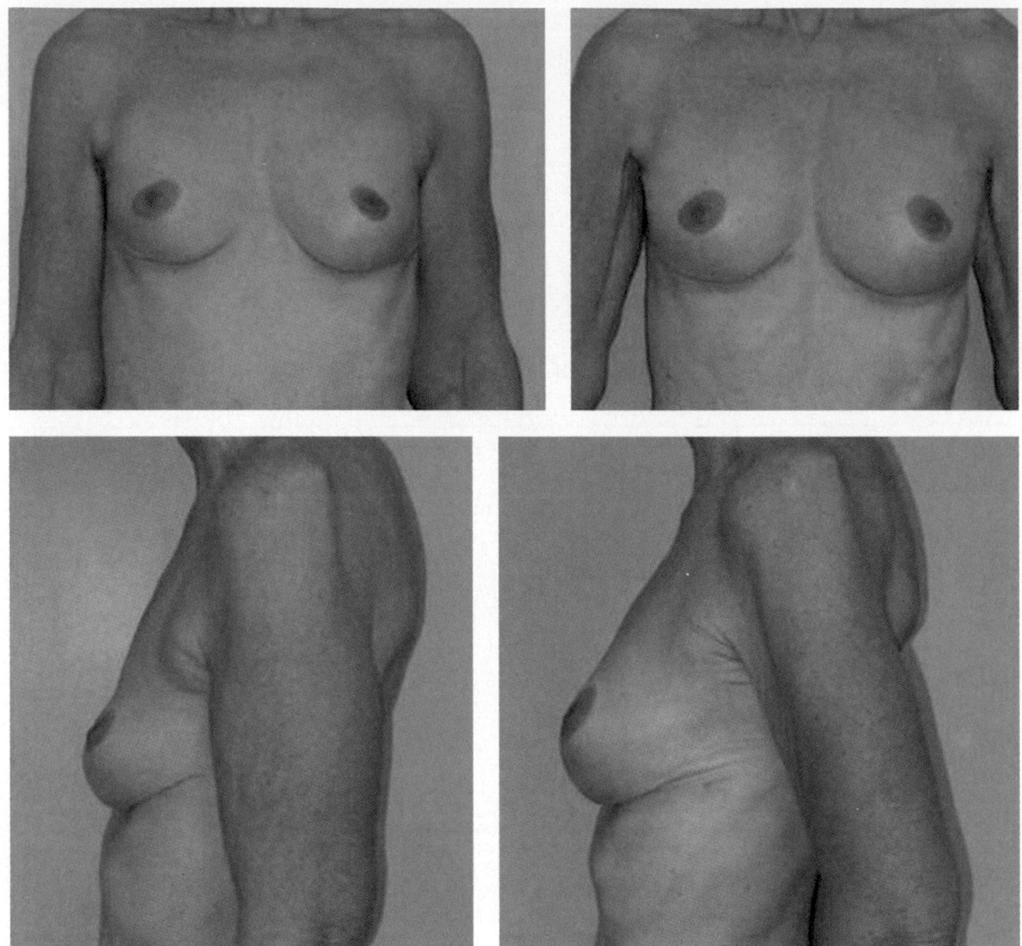

Figure 118.35. Patients after implant removal are candidates for augmentation with BRAVA and fat grafting. (Patient of Dr. Daniel Del Vecchio.)

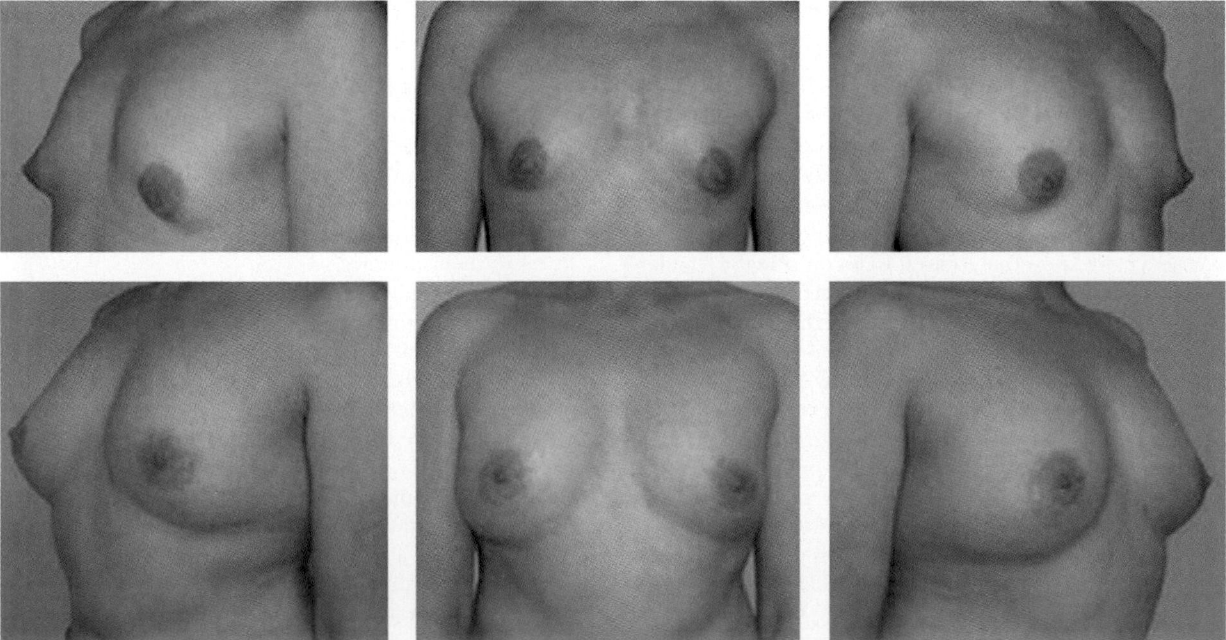

Figure 118.36. Constricted tuberous breasts can be augmented and reshaped, usually in two stages. (Patient of Dr. Daniel Del Vecchio.)

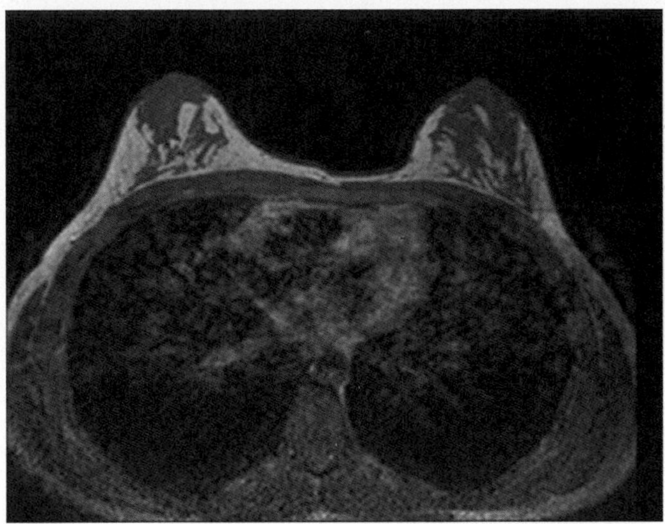
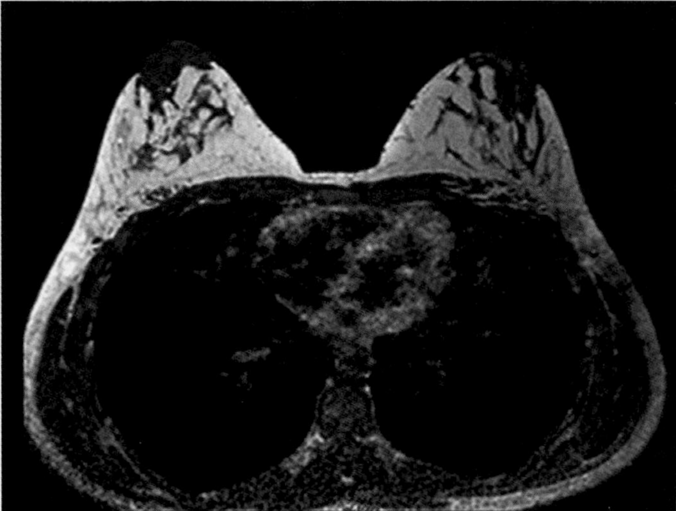

Figure 118.37. **Left:** Preexpansion magnetic resonance imaging (MRI) of the patient in case 3. **Right:** MRI 6 months after second fat grafting.

CONTROVERSIAL TOPICS

We are still in the early days of breast augmentation and reconstruction using fat transplantation. There are more questions than there are answers, and it is easier to ask the questions than it is to answer them. The following represent some of the biggest controversies and challenges facing this technique in the near, medium, and long term.

IMAGING AND DETECTION OF BREAST CANCER

In 1987, an American Society of Plastic Surgeons position paper strongly condemned fat grafting to the breast, suggesting fat grafting would distort the efficacy of breast cancer detection. Breast fat grafting has been demonstrated to sometimes result in microcalcifications. However, these microcalcifications have been classified as Bio RAD 1 and are generally felt to be distinguishable from calcifications of higher grade that are suggestive of malignancy.

CANCER RISK

The breast will undergo malignant transformation in one in nine women, and a great deal of clinical and basic science work is needed to clarify the effect of fat grafting on breast imaging and breast cancer detection. While fat grafting to the breast is still in its infancy, it is important to establish safety standards that will serve patients and clinicians in the future. While this chapter helps to define the current standards in fat grafting to the breast, we expect that the clinical and basic science knowledge base will grow rapidly and will improve on our present understanding.

Besides a few recognized predisposing factors, the etiology of breast cancer is believed to be multifactorial. A question, however, has been raised that since aromatase activity is present in adipose tissue, more fat in the breast might be detrimental (43). (Aromatase is a key enzyme in estrogen synthesis, and its inhibition is an effective treatment of estrogen-positive breast cancer.) The validity of this hypothesis is unproven at the time of this writing. Theoretically, one could also posit that since the fat infiltrated caused a lower ratio of breast tissue to breast volume, the risk could be lower, since less-dense breasts are known to be less cancer prone. Furthermore, it would take a nearly impossible study size to prove any statistical association, whether positive or negative. Of interest, studies have found that the silicone of breast implants is a very potent stimulant of aromatase activity. Despite this fact, breast implants are now well proven to be noncarcinogenic. After hundreds of thousands of fat flap transfers and TRAM flaps invariably performed in residual cancer-prone tissues, there is no evidence, retrospective or prospective, that the fat added with these procedures is associated with a higher recurrence of breast cancer (44).

Furthermore, if fat necrosis is a potential culprit, surgeons have performed thousands of reduction mammoplasty procedures with 50% incidence of fat necrosis with no evidence of any increase in breast cancer. In fact, the incidence of breast cancer is decreased after reduction mammoplasty (45).

There is nothing at all in the experimental and clinical literature and in experiments of nature to suggest that fat grafting the breast is carcinogenic. Over the next decade, the increased popularity of this technique should shed more light on the science of fat grafting, on optimizing volume yields through standardization of the technique, and, most important, on patient safety in this procedure.

EDITORIAL COMMENTS

The authors have provided an excellent review of the BRAVA system and its role in lipoaugmentation of the breast. The BRAVA system has been available for several years, and although its use as a sole modality for breast augmentation was limited to about a 100-cc increase, its role in preparing the recipient site for fat grafting is becoming increasingly appreciated. This is principally related to the parenchymal proliferation and angiogenic effect of the negative-pressure system elicited by the

BRAVA apparatus. These in turn result in a greater volume or capacity of the breast parenchyma, subcutaneous fat, and pectoralis major muscle to facilitate revascularization of the injected fat.

The authors have stressed the importance of proper technique for this procedure. Strict attention to the injected volume is critical. Large-volume injection is fraught with the potential for failure, and small-volume injection is relatively ineffective. The art is based on knowing what constitutes just the right amount to maximize graft take and minimize graft resorption. It is interesting that Drs. Coleman and Khouri differ in some aspects related to fat harvest and preparation. Dr. Coleman is a strict believer in fat centrifugation, whereas Dr. Khouri is not. His main objection to centrifugation is fat clumping and damage induced by the high speed. Dr. Khouri emphasizes that fat is never injected directly into breast parenchyma. It is injected into the subcutaneous fat and pectoralis major layers.

Another application of the BRAVA system that the authors have presented is in regard to breast reconstruction following mastectomy. The principles and concepts for this application are much like those for breast augmentation, namely, preexpansion with BRAVA followed by serial fat grafting. Although I feel that this is a potentially useful technique, my concern is that it will have limited application. It has been my observation that most women will prefer an option that provides immediate results. When adipose tissue is desired, the use of musculocutaneous and adipocutaneous flaps has performed very well. The limitation of this technique will be the time required to obtain desired results and the donor-site considerations, especially in thin women.

Overall, I feel that this is a very important chapter. The reader will appreciate the nuances related to fat grafting and understand the factors that may lead to success. Having heard Dr. Khouri speak on this topic and been witness to his results, it is clear that he is on to something and that some day this may represent an option that many surgeons and patients will consider.

M.Y.N.

REFERENCES

1. American Society of Plastic Surgeons. Fat transfer/fat graft and fat injection. ASPS guiding principles. January 2009. Available at: http://www.plasticsurgery.org/Documents/Medical_Profesionals/Health_Policy/guiding_principles/ASPS-Fat-Transfer-Graft-Guiding-Principles.pdf. Accessed July 16, 2010.
2. Illouz YG. Body contouring by lipolysis: a five year experience with over 3000 cases. *Plast Reconstr Surg* 1983;72(5):591–597.
3. Bircoll M, Novack, BH. Autologous fat transplantation employing liposuction techniques. *Ann Plast Surg* 1987;18(4):327–329.
4. Bircoll M. Cosmetic breast augmentation utilizing autologous fat and liposuction techniques. *Plast Reconstr Surg* 1987;79(2):267–271.
5. ASPS Ad-Hoc Committee on New Procedures. Report on autologous fat transplantation. *Plast Surg Nurs* 1987;7:140–141.
6. Baker T. Presentation on BRAVA nonsurgical breast expansion, American Society for Aesthetic Plastic Surgery Annual Meeting, Orlando, Florida, 2006.
7. Khouri R. Follow up presentation on BRAVA nonsurgical breast expansion, American Society for Aesthetic Plastic Surgery Annual Meeting, San Diego, California, 2008.
8. Coleman SR, Saboeiro AP. Fat grafting to the breast revisited: safety and efficacy. *Plast Reconstr Surg* 2007;119(3):775–785.
9. Tse GM, Tan PH, Pang AL, et al. Calcification in breast lesions: pathologists' perspective. *J Clin Pathol* 2008;61(2):145–151.
10. Esserman LE, Da Costa D, d'Almeida M, et al. Imaging findings after breast brachytherapy. *Am J Roentgenol* 2006;187(1):57–64.
11. Pui MH, Movson IJ. Fatty tissue breast lesions. *Clin Imaging* 2003;27(3):150–155.
12. Bilgen IG, Ustun EE, Memis A. Fat necrosis of the breast: clinical, mammographic and sonographic features. *Eur J Radiol* 2001;39(2):92–99.
13. Missana MC, Laurent I, Barreau L, et al. Autologous fat transfer in reconstructive breast surgery: indications, technique and results. *Eur J Surg Oncol* 2007;33(6):685–690.
14. Gosset J, Guerin N, Toussoun G, et al. Radiological evaluation after lipomodelling for correction of breast conservative treatment sequelae. *Ann Chir Plast Esthet* 2008;53(2):178–189.
15. Pierrefeu-Lagrange AC, Delay E, Guerin N, et al. Radiological evaluation of breasts reconstructed with lipomodeling. *Ann Chir Plast Esthet* 2006;51(1):18–28.
16. Spear SL, Wilson HB, Lockwood MD. Fat injection to correct contour deformities in the reconstructed breast. *Plast Reconstr Surg* 2005;116(5):1300–1305.
17. Delay E, Gosset J, Toussoun G, et al. Efficacy of lipomodelling for the management of sequelae of breast cancer conservative treatment. *Ann Chir Plast Esthet* 2008;53(2):153–168.
18. Zocchi ML, Zuliani F. Bicompartmental breast lipostructuring. *Aesthet Plast Surg* 2008; 32(2):313–328.
19. Moseley TA, Zhu M, Hedrick MH. Adipose-derived stem and progenitor cells as fillers in plastic and reconstructive surgery. *Plast Reconstr Surg* 2006;118(3S) (suppl 1):121S–128S.
20. Zheng DN, Li QF, Lei H, et al. Autologous fat grafting to the breast for cosmetic enhancement: experience in 66 patients with long-term follow up. *J Plast Reconstr Aesthet Surg* 2008;61(7):792–798.
21. Kanchwala SK, Glatt BS, Conant EF, et al. Autologous fat grafting to the reconstructed breast: the management of acquired contour deformities. *Plast Reconstr Surg* 2009; 124(2):409–418.
22. Shiffman MA, Mirrafati S. Fat transfer techniques: the effect of harvest and transfer methods on adipocyte viability and review of the literature. *Dermatol Surg* 201;27(9):819–826.
23. Kaufman MR, Miller TA, Huang C, et al. Autologous fat transfer for facial recontouring: is there science behind the art? *Plast Reconstr Surg* 2007;119(7):2287–2296.
24. Toledo LS, Mauad R. Fat injection: a 20-year revision. *Clin Plast Surg* 2006;33:47–53.
25. Nguyen J, Medina MA, McCormack MC, et al. Enhanced fat protection and survival in fat transplantation via treatment with poloxamer 188. *J Surg Res* 2009;151(2):210–211.
26. Cytori Therapeutics. Adipose-derived stem and regenerative cells improve fat graft retention in preclinical study. Press Release. December 15, 2007.
27. Medina MA, Nguyen J, McCormack M, et al. High-throughput model for adipocyte preservation. Presented at the 26th Annual Meeting, Northeastern Society of Plastic Surgeons, Philadelphia, Pennsylvania, October 2008.
28. Herman AR. The history of skin grafts. *J Drugs Dermatol* 2002;1(3):298–301.
29. Bucky LP, Godek CP. Discussion of "The behavior of fat grafts in recipient areas with enhanced vascularity" by Baran CN, et al. *Plast Reconstr Surg* 2002;109(5):1652.
30. Karacaoglu E, Kizilkaya E, Cermik H, et al. The role of recipient sites in fat-graft survival: experimental study. *Ann Plast Surg* 2005;55(1):63–68.
31. Schlenz I, Kaider A. The BRAVA external tissue expander: is breast enlargement without surgery a reality? *Plast Reconstr Surg* 2007;120(6):1680–1689.
32. Khouri RK, Schlenz I, Murphy BJ, et al. Nonsurgical breast enlargement using an external soft-tissue expansion system. *Plast Reconstr Surg* 2000;105(7):2513–2514.
33. Khouri RK, Baker TJ. Initial experience with the BRAVA nonsurgical system of breast enhancement. *Plast Reconstr Surg* 2002;110(6):1593–1595.
34. Smith CJ. Initial experience with the BRAVA nonsurgical system of breast enhancement: reply. *Plast Reconstr Surg* 2002;110(6):1595–1598.
35. Greco RJ. Nonsurgical breast enhancement: fact or fiction? *Plast Reconstr Surg* 2002;110(1):337–339.
36. Morykwas MJ, Argenta LC, Shelton-Brown EI, et al. Vacuum assisted closure: a new method for wound control and treatment: animal studies and basic foundation. *Ann Plast Surg* 1997;38(6):553–562.
37. Hofer SOP, Knight KM, Cooper-White JJ, et al. Increasing the volume of vascularized tissue formation in engineered constructs: an experimental study in rats. *Plast Reconstr Surg* 2003;111(3):1186–1192.
38. Rigotti G, Marchi A, Galiè M, et al. Clinical treatment of radiotherapy tissue damage by lipoaspirate transplant: a healing process mediated by adipose-derived adult stem cells. *Plast Reconstr Surg* 2007;119(5):1409–1422.
39. American Society of Plastic Surgeons. 2009 Plastic surgery procedural statistics. Available at: http://www.plasticsurgery.org/x9972.xml. Accessed July 16, 2010.
40. ClinicalTrials.gov. Study of Autologous Fat Enhanced w/Regenerative Cells Transplanted to Reconstruct Breast Deformities After Lumpectomy (RESTORE-2). Available at: http://clinicaltrials.gov/ct2/show/NCT00616135. Accessed July 16, 2010.
41. Del Vecchio D, Bucky L. Breast reconstruction and breast augmentation using non-operative pre expansion and mega-volume fat grafting. A clinical and radiological study. Presented at the Northeastern Society of Plastic Surgeons Annual Meeting, Charleston, South Carolina, September 2009.
42. Roger K. US bra sales statistics, 1960–1982. Available at: www.corsetiere.net/Spirella/Roger_Bra_Sales.htm. Accessed July 16, 2010.
43. Purohit A, Ghilchik MW, Duncan L, et al. Aromatase activity and interleukin-6 production by normal and malignant breast tissues. *J Clin Endocrinol Metab* 1995;80(10):3052–3058.
44. Slavin SA, Love SM, Goldwyn RM. Recurrent breast cancer following immediate reconstruction with myocutaneous flaps. *Plast Reconstr Surg* 1994;93(6):1191–1204.
45. Boice JD Jr, Persson I, Brinton LA, et al. Breast cancer following breast reduction surgery in Sweden. *Plast Reconstr Surg* 2000;106(4):755–762.

CHAPTER

119

Dennis C. Hammond

Augmentation Mammaplasty in the Patient With Tuberous Breasts and Other Complex Anomalies

INTRODUCTION

Perhaps no other condition of the breast presents the same type of surgical challenge as the tuberous breast deformity. Although a wide spectrum of clinical presentations can be encountered, in the most severe of cases, the degree of deformity is significant. Typically all of the elements of the breast are present in that there is a variable amount of breast tissue with a nipple and areola. However, the deranged relationships these structures have with each other and the degree of asymmetry they often demonstrate can create to the inexperienced eye a bizarre breast appearance. Truly the emotional sequelae of dealing with this condition can be devastating to the young women afflicted with any degree of tuberous breast deformity.

DEFORMITY

The clinical findings associated with the tuberous breast typically include a reduced breast base diameter, a high and variably constricted inframammary fold, breast hypoplasia, and "herniation" or preferential expansion of the growing breast bud through the area of the areola. It is not uncommon for a significant asymmetry to be present with a small and more severely involved breast present on one side, and a larger, more ptotic breast with a tight inframammary fold being present on the other (Fig. 119.1).

SURGICAL MANAGEMENT

Surgical management of the tuberous breast is dictated by the severity of the deformity. Options for treatment range from simple augmentation to reconstruction of the breast skin envelope with tissue expansion. Soft-tissue manipulation invariably includes periareolar mastopexy to manage the herniated areola with or without various internal flaps to reshape the breast. Choosing the most appropriate technique for a given patient requires a considered evaluation of all the elements that describe the preoperative deformity. Once these elements are defined, methods of surgical correction can be identified and a final surgical plan developed.

Perhaps the most important preoperative surgical decision to be made involves whether to use an implant or a tissue expander to manage the lower pole of the breast. In cases of mild constriction of the base of the breast, soft-tissue release with incisions that extend radially away from the nipple toward the breast periphery can result in enough of a release that the implant can smoothly recontour the inferior pole of the breast without any residual clefting being visible. This soft-tissue release typically extends all the way through the breast parenchyma to the level of the dermis (Fig. 119.2). If, however, any residual tightness is present in the lower pole, even after soft tissue release, then placement of a tissue expander may be a better option. In severe cases, the lower pole skin does not physiologically expand, and thus a tissue expander is required to create the smooth, rounded contour of an attractive breast. Determining preoperatively whether a tissue expander will be required can be difficult, and at times this only becomes obvious after a full soft-tissue release does not allow proper recontouring of the lower pole. This decision also has social implications. Unfortunately, some insurance plans do not consider correction of the tuberous breast deformity to be a covered benefit. For this reason, many patients are forced to cover the cost of surgical correction privately and are eager to hold down potential costs as much as possible. This tends to place the plastic surgeon in a difficult position as an emotionally distraught patient and family with high expectations present with a significant deformity and the ability to afford only one operation. Under these circumstances, it is tempting to choose an implant over a tissue expander to avoid a second procedure with the attendant associated additional costs. It is highly advisable to discuss with the patient and family the limitations simple implant placement can have on the ultimate result to avoid postoperative disappointment and allow patients to make informed planning decisions (Fig. 119.3).

MILD CONSTRICTION

A very mild form of the tuberous breast deformity presents as a hypoplastic breast with a subtle constriction of the medial inframammary fold area on one or both sides. If this is not recognized preoperatively, a disappointing flatness to the medial breast after simple breast augmentation will be noted which detracts from the overall shape of the breast. To prevent this deformity from occurring, it is necessary to fully release the soft-tissue attachments in this area with radial incisions extending through the parenchyma to the dermis. It is helpful if the subglandular or partial subpectoral pocket is used because this will prevent the intact muscle in the lower medial corner of the breast from tethering the breast shape. This also will allow access to the breast to facilitate the parenchymal scoring. Usually, with this type of soft-tissue release, a breast implant can then provide the needed volume to fill out the lower pole, and in particular the lower medial pole of the breast, and quality results can be obtained (Fig. 119.4).

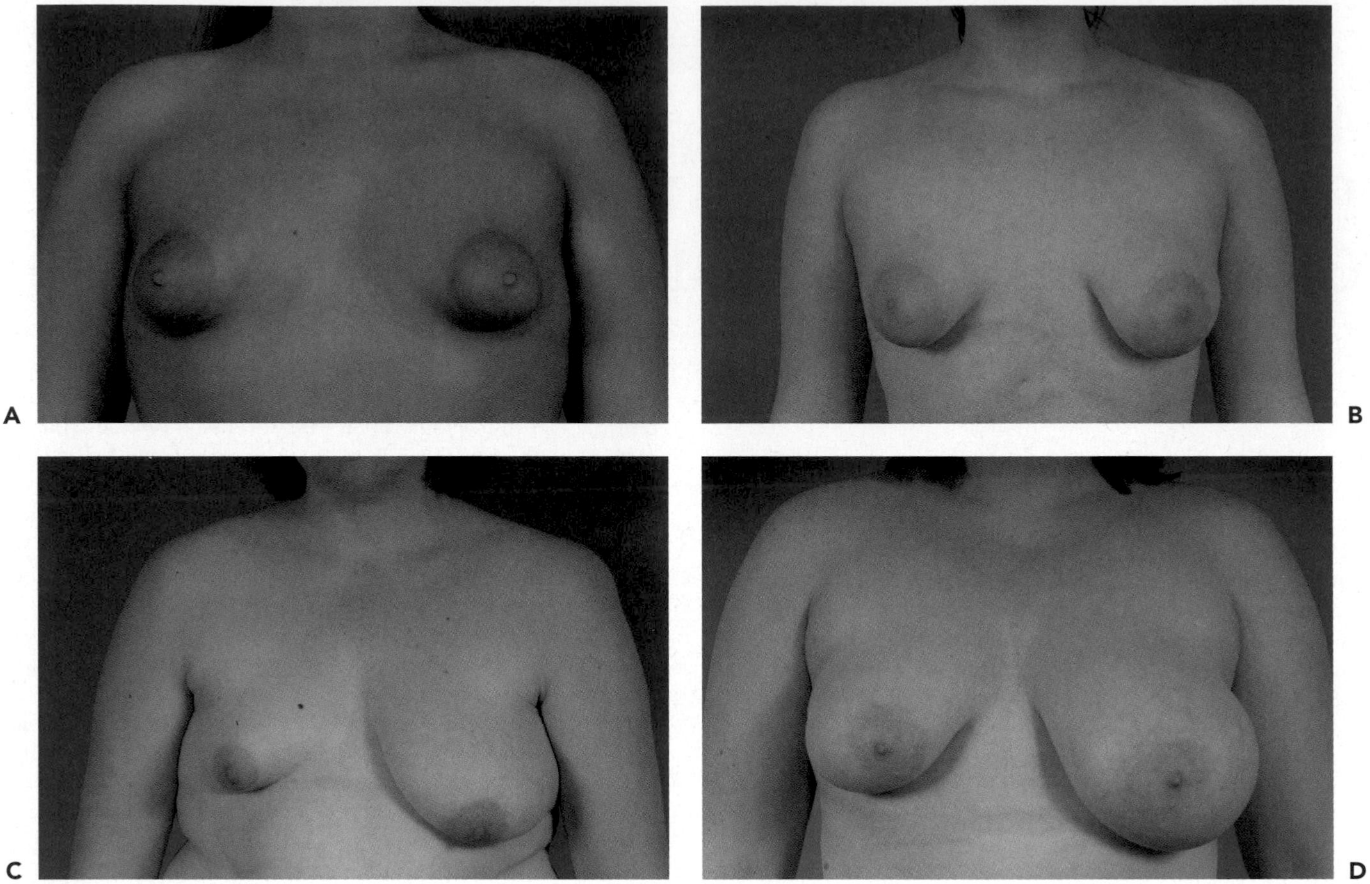

Figure 119.1. The spectrum of clinical presentations seen in patients with the tuberous breast deformity.

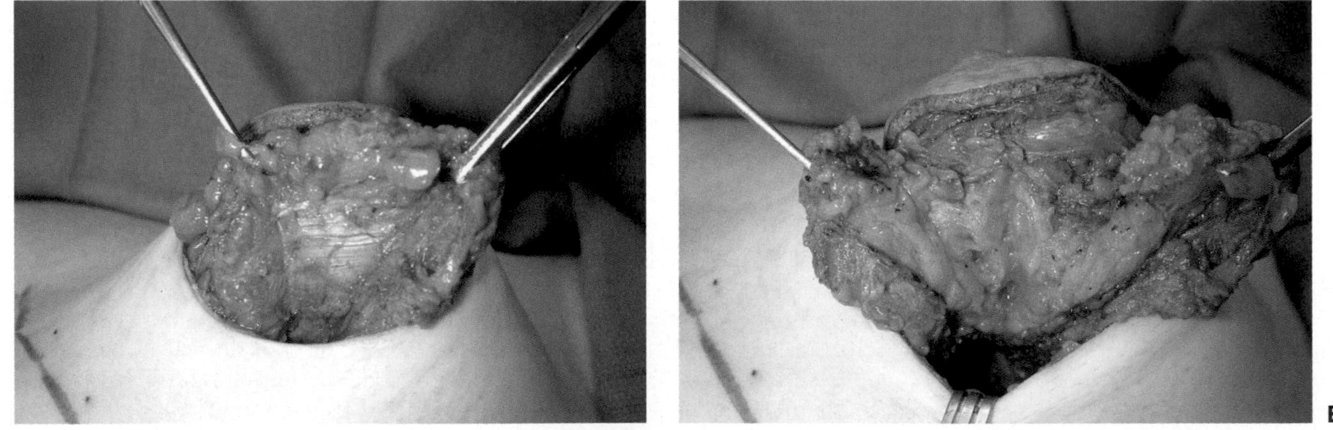

Figure 119.2. **A:** The base of the breast in patients with tuberous breast deformity can often be seen to have constricting bands tethering the parenchyma and preventing normal breast expansion. **B:** By incising through these tethering bands, the constriction through the base of the breast can be released, allowing the breast to re-expand.

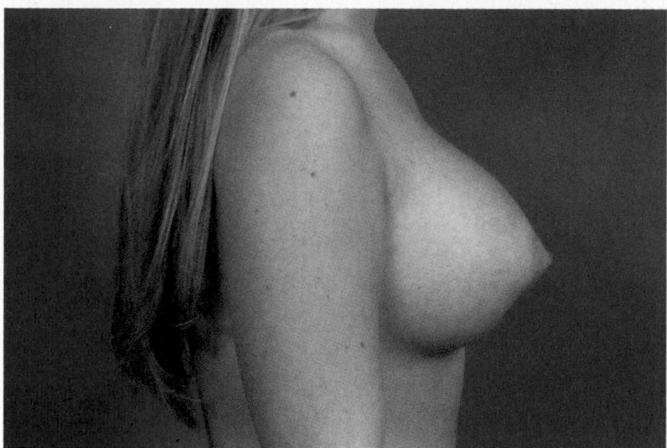

Figure 119.3. Postoperative appearance of a young woman with a tuberous breast deformity with persistent deformity of the lower pole contour despite aggressive soft-tissue release followed by placement of a breast implant.

CONSTRICTION WITH HYPERPLASIA

A relatively common presentation of the tuberous breast variant is the patient with macromastia associated with a high and relatively constricted inframammary fold. In these cases the breast volume is excessive and the nipple and areola tends to "bend" over the constricted fold to create a very ptotic appearance. In addition, the areola tends to be enlarged. Treatment of these patients is quite straightforward, and any of several breast reductions techniques can be used to correct the misshapen breast along with the macromastia. My preference is the SPAIR (short-scar periareolar inferior pedical reduction) mammaplasty. Here, the internal base constriction is released during the development of the inferior pedicle, the breast reshaped with internal sutures, the breast skin envelope retailored using a circumvertical pattern, and the areolar diameter reduced with a periareolar purse string suture. Taken together, these surgical maneuvers provide particular advantage in this type of tuberous breast patient, and excellent results can be obtained with complete correction of the preoperative deformity (Fig. 119.5).

UNILATERAL HYPOPLASIA

Another common presentation of the tuberous breast deformity is unilateral hypoplasia with constriction of the base in the presence of a normal opposite breast. Here, it is not only the deformity that causes concern, but the asymmetry as well. As these typically younger girls develop, the asymmetry becomes more noticeable, and at age 14 or 15 years they will commonly present for consultation. A particularly attractive operative strategy to use in these patients is to place a tissue expander in the subcutaneous plane for maximal soft-tissue effect, and then expand the device as the breasts develop. An attempt to catch up with the larger breast is made early in the expansion process to restore symmetry. Once the desired volume and shape have been provided, the expander can be left in place until full development has been achieved. At that point it is a straightforward procedure to remove the expander and replace it with a permanent prosthesis. Another alternative is to use a combination gel/saline expander/implant with a removable valve at the first procedure. Later, all that is required is removal of the valve. Both strategies provide an excellent option for these younger girls to achieve symmetry at a very important time in their lives, and then provide the opportunity to maintain that symmetry with ease as they develop. Using this strategy, one can obtain excellent long-term results (Fig. 119.6).

HYPOPLASIA, CONSTRICTION, AND AREOLAR HERNIATION

The full manifestation of the tuberous breast deformity includes a breast that is hypoplastic, has a constricted and elevated inframammary fold, and most distressingly has a variable herniation of a small developing breast bud through the areola. It is commonly the herniation through the areola that creates the greatest and most distressing deformity for the patient. In these cases, the

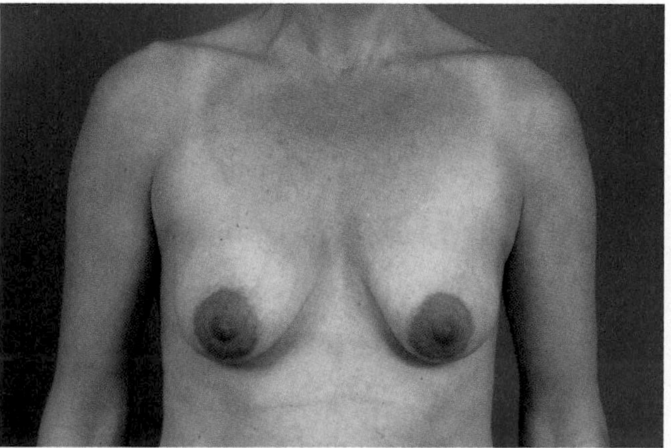

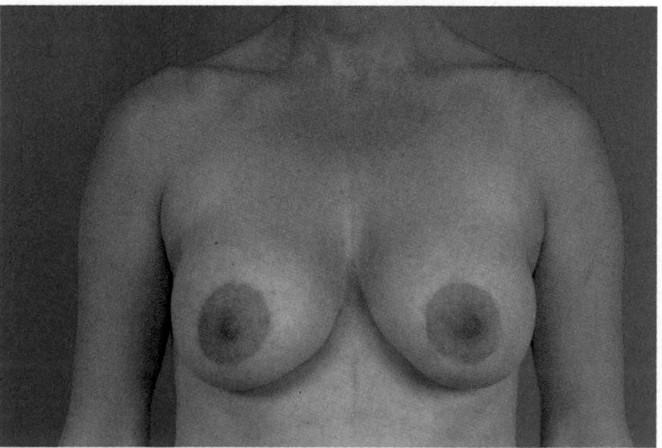

Figure 119.4. **A:** Preoperative appearance of a 43-year-old woman with a mild tuberous breast deformity. She lost breast volume after breast-feeding but still demonstrates a mild tethering of the medial inframammary fold. It is important to recognize this tethering preoperatively to allow appropriate release of the parenchyma in this area. **B:** Postoperative result after breast augmentation with associated release of the inferomedial inframammary fold.

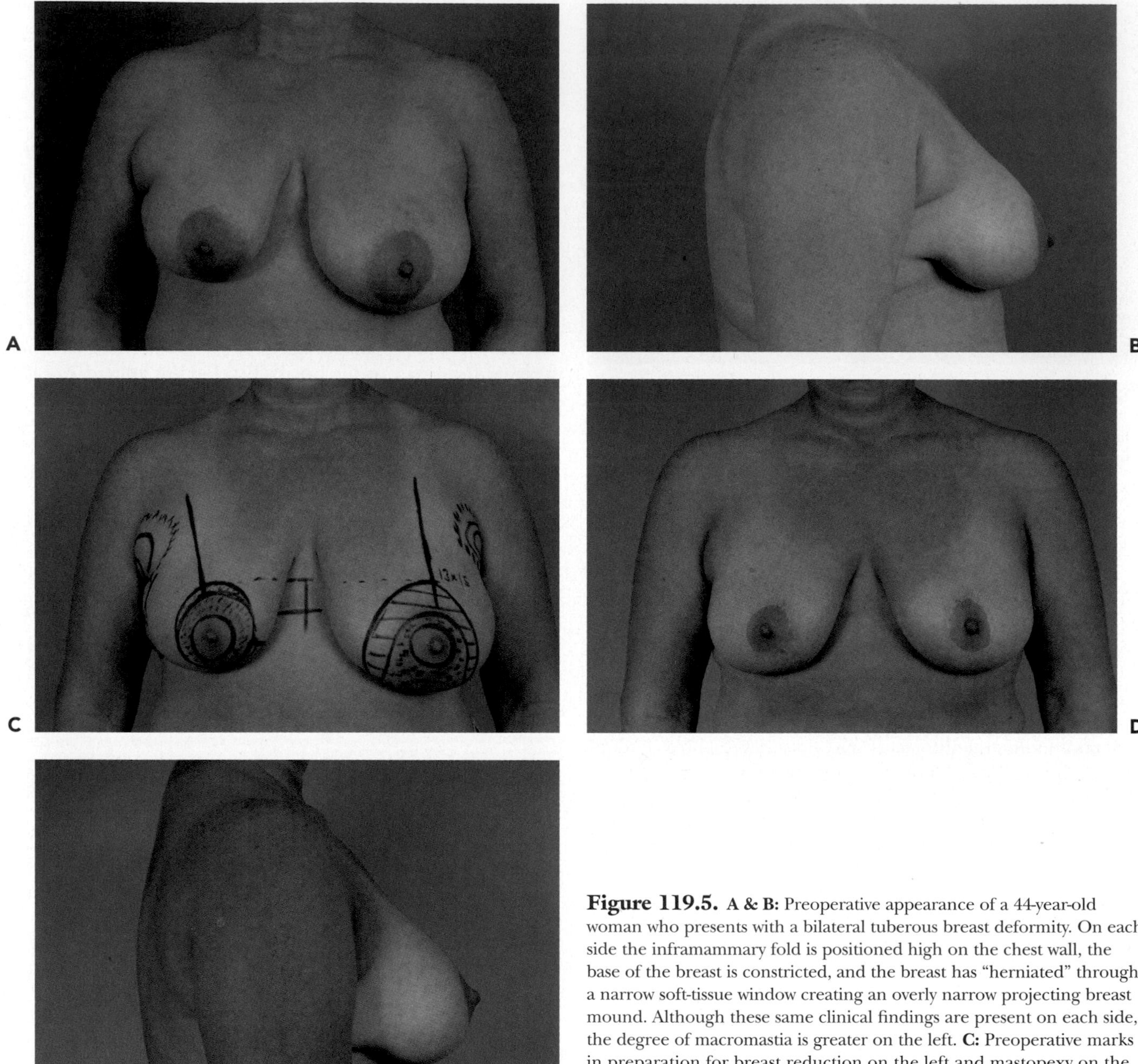

Figure 119.5. **A & B:** Preoperative appearance of a 44-year-old woman who presents with a bilateral tuberous breast deformity. On each side the inframammary fold is positioned high on the chest wall, the base of the breast is constricted, and the breast has "herniated" through a narrow soft-tissue window creating an overly narrow projecting breast mound. Although these same clinical findings are present on each side, the degree of macromastia is greater on the left. **C:** Preoperative marks in preparation for breast reduction on the left and mastopexy on the right using the SPAIR technique. **D & E:** One-year postoperative appearance after removal of 540 g of tissue on the left and 10 g on the right.

placement of a tissue expander is required to provide the most consistent and aesthetic long-term results. As the breast skin envelope is expanded, the lower pole constriction is relieved and a pocket of sufficient dimension is created to allow subsequent placement of an appropriately sized implant to provide symmetry with the opposite breast. In addition, periareolar mastopexy with soft-tissue release reduces the herniated breast parenchyma and relieves the pressure on the areola, and restores a more proportional areolar diameter for a breast of a given volume. Although it is a two-stage surgical approach, this operative strategy can provide remarkable correction of severe preoperative deformities and can restore the breasts to an aesthetic shape and proportional size (Fig. 119.7).

POLAND'S SYNDROME

Patients presenting with Poland's syndrome have a hypoplastic breast with absence of the sternal head of the pectoralis major muscle. Associated maldevelopment of the associated upper limb has also been noted. In these patients, operative correction of the deformity is geared toward restoring volume to the hypoplastic breast and, in some instances, restoring the anterior axillary fold contour by transposing the latissimus dorsi muscle anteriorly and reinserting the insertion of the muscle into the humerus. The volume provided by the muscle can also serve to soften the contours of the reconstructed breast mound. In mild cases, simple placement of an implant may

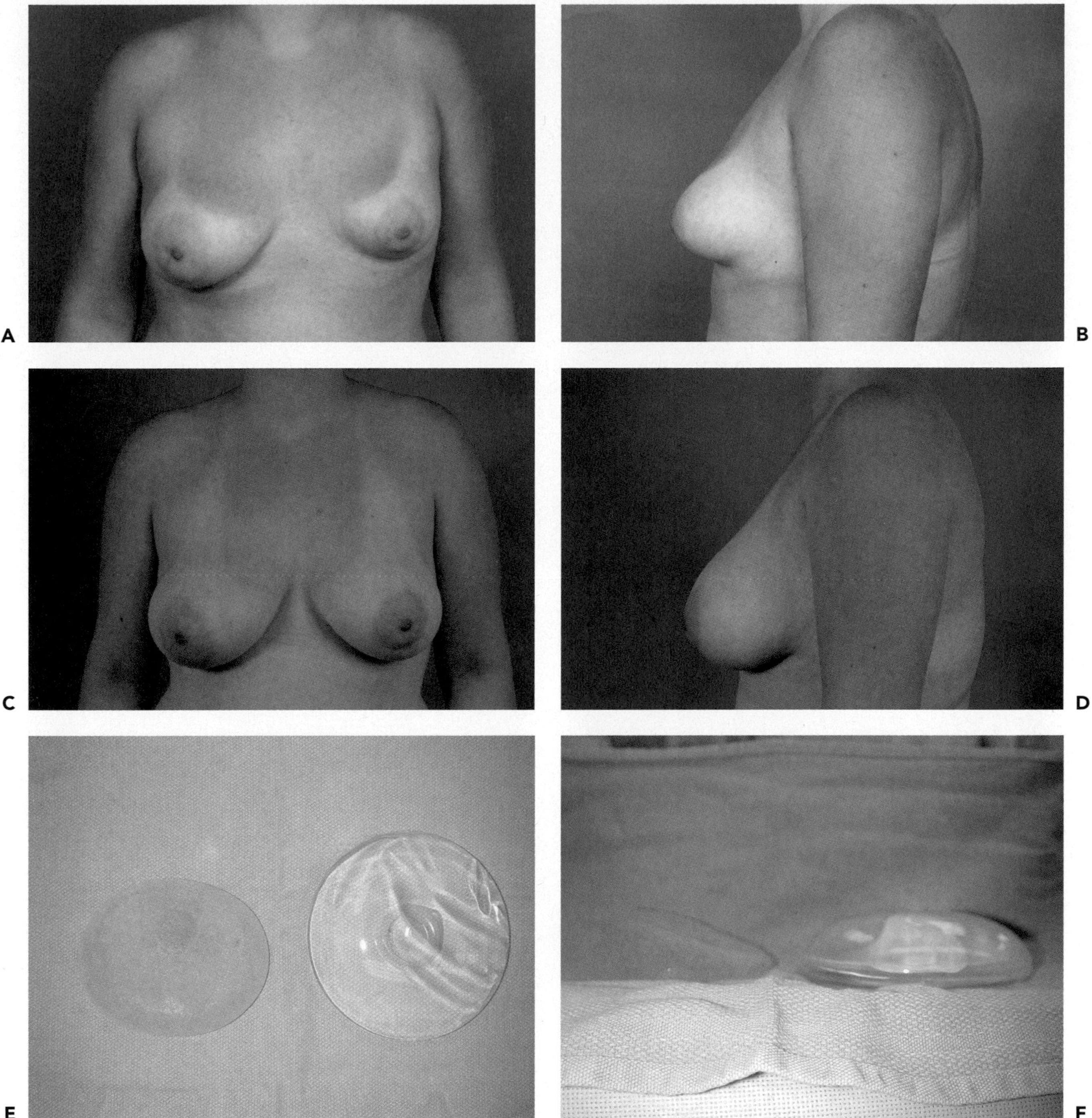

Figure 119.6. **A & B:** Preoperative appearance of a 15-year-old girl with a mild tuberous breast deformity on the left with asymmetry. The right breast is uninvolved. The preoperative plan includes placement of a shaped anatomic tissue expander in the subcutaneous plane on the left to fill out the skin envelope and provide volume to the hypoplastic breast. The expander will be left in place and inflated as needed over the next few years until full breast development is complete. **C & D:** Appearance after 3 years with the eventual addition of 200 cc to the left subcutaneous tissue expander. **E & F:** At the second-stage procedure performed when the patient was 18 years old, the tissue expander was removed and replaced with a 400-cc moderate profile plus smooth round silicone gel implant. (*continued*)

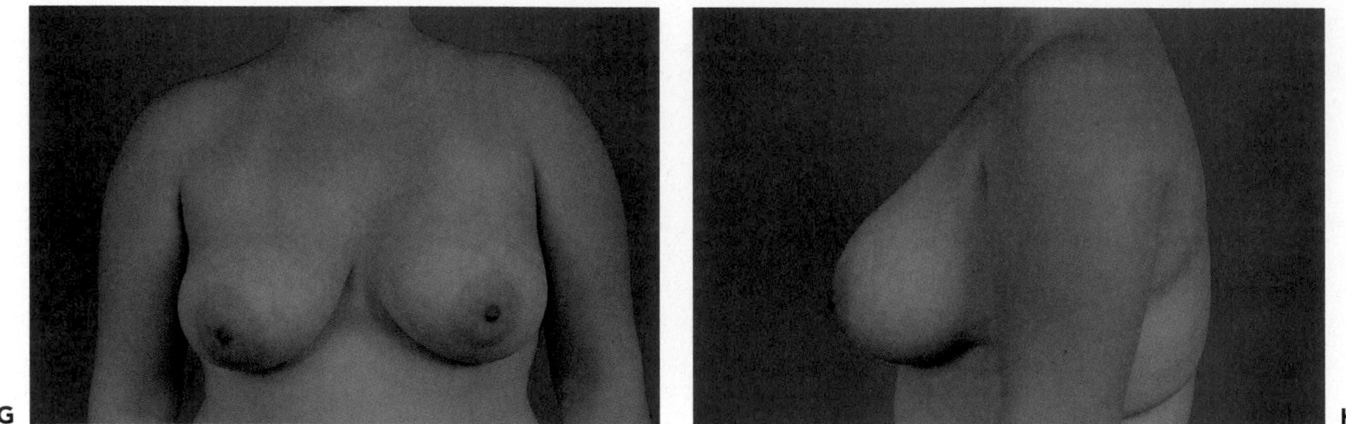

Figure 119.6. (*Continued*) **G & H:** Postoperatively the left breast has been filled out, there is no constriction of the lower pole skin envelope, and the patient demonstrates improved overall aesthetics and symmetry.

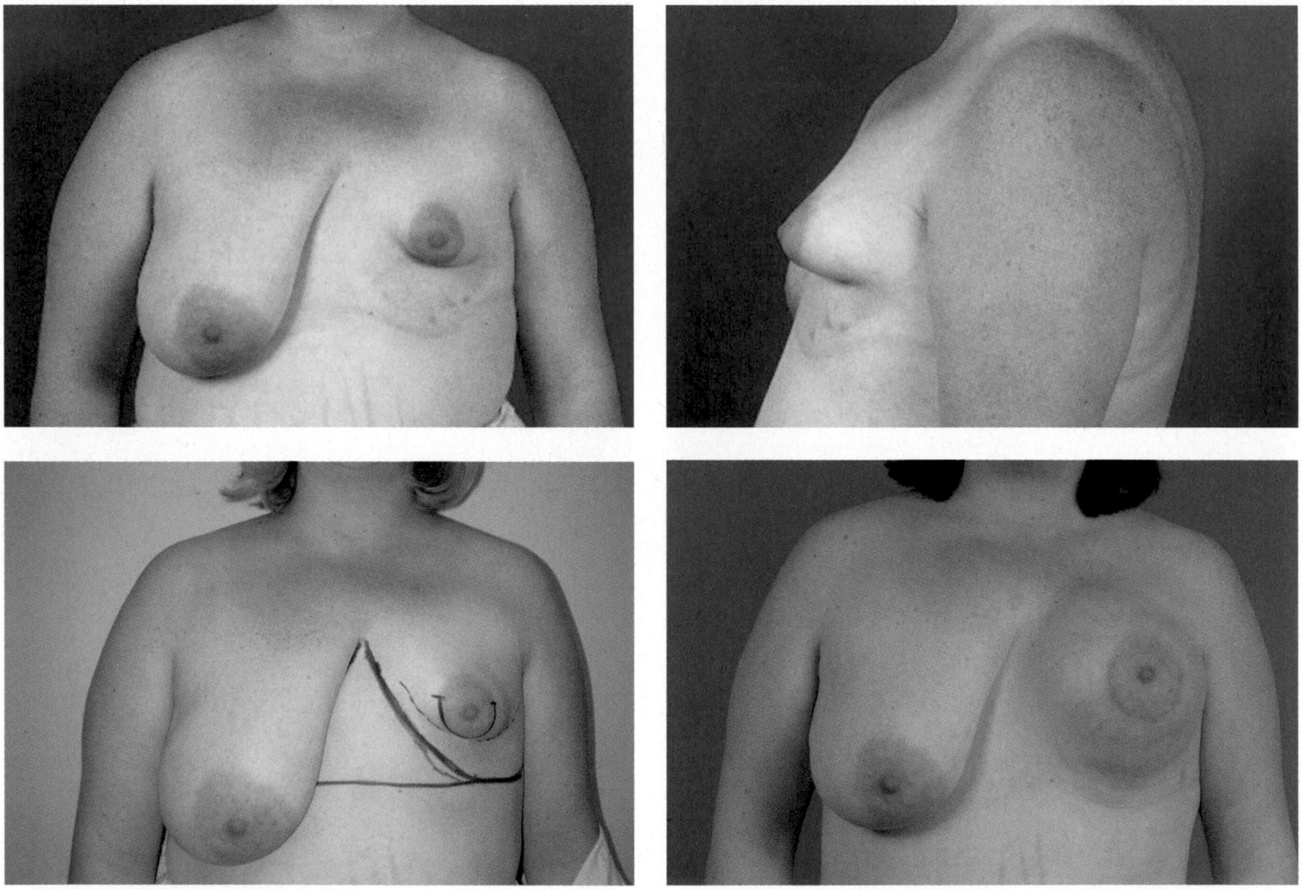

Figure 119.7. **A & B:** Preoperative appearance of a 30-year-old woman with a severe tuberous breast deformity on the left and associated macromastia on the right. **C:** Preoperative marks in preparation for subcutaneous placement of a textured anatomic tissue expander with associated aggressive parenchymal scoring. **D & E:** Appearance of the left breast after bringing the volume in the tissue expander to 1,120 cc. (*continued*)

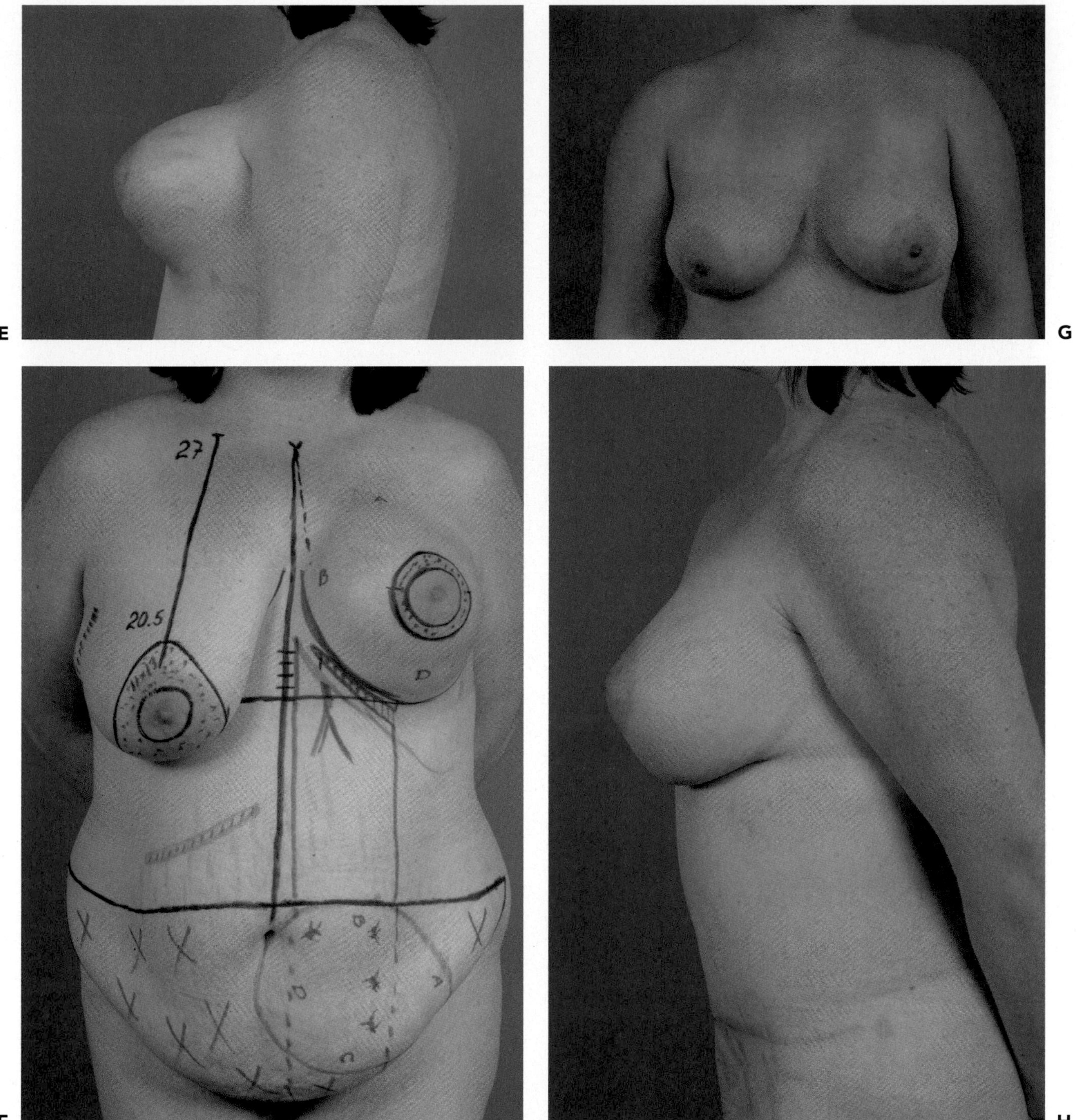

Figure 119.7. (*Continued*) **F:** Preoperative marks in preparation for removal of the left tissue expander, left periareolar mastopexy, right breast reduction, and replacement of the tissue expander with a de-epithelialized TRAM flap. **G & H:** Postoperatively the skin envelope of the left breast has been filled out, the constriction has been released, and the patient demonstrates improved overall aesthetics and symmetry.

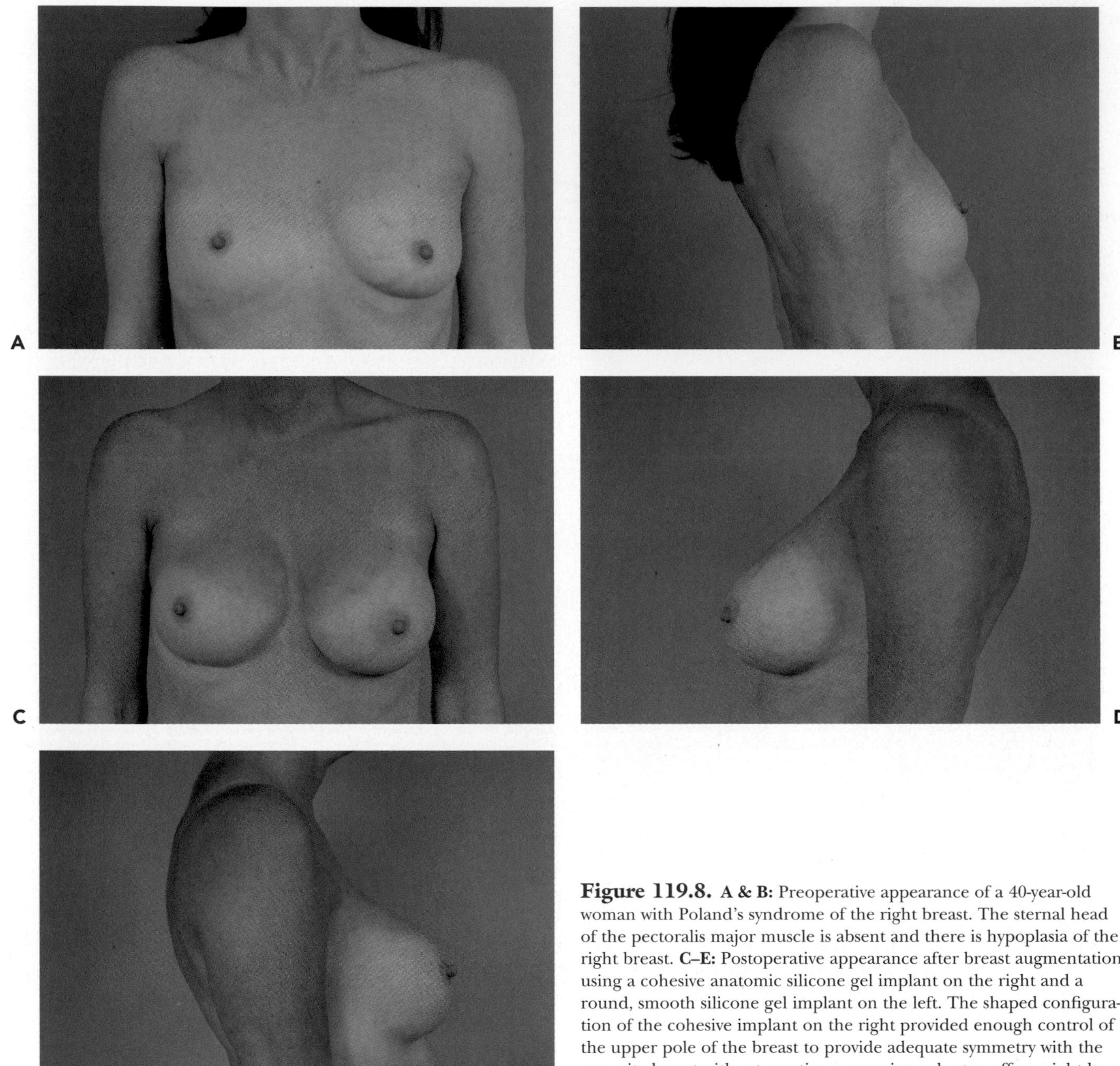

Figure 119.8. **A & B:** Preoperative appearance of a 40-year-old woman with Poland's syndrome of the right breast. The sternal head of the pectoralis major muscle is absent and there is hypoplasia of the right breast. **C–E:** Postoperative appearance after breast augmentation using a cohesive anatomic silicone gel implant on the right and a round, smooth silicone gel implant on the left. The shaped configuration of the cohesive implant on the right provided enough control of the upper pole of the breast to provide adequate symmetry with the opposite breast without creating a superior pole step-off as might have occurred if a round implant had been used.

provide the missing volume without the need for latissimus muscle transposition. In these patients, due to the variable absence of the pectoralis major muscle, the soft-tissue envelope of the breast may be thin. Here, anatomically shaped cohesive silicone gel implants may be indicated to provide better control of the upper pole of the breast and allow a filling out of the soft-tissue envelope without creating a sharp, unnatural step-off superiorly. The opposite breast can be augmented as needed to provide symmetry. Often, significant improvement in the appearance of the breasts can be obtained with just this simple approach, (Fig. 119.8).

SUMMARY

Although difficult, it can be very gratifying for both the patient and the surgeon to successfully correct the tuberous breast deformity. These patients can be severely affected from a psychological standpoint, and the effect that successful surgery can have is often life altering. Using standard principles of aesthetic and reconstructive breast surgery, one can correct the clinical features of the deformity in all its various presentations with the end result being a breast with normal aesthetics and symmetry.

EDITORIAL COMMENTS

In this chapter, Dr. Hammond details the physical characteristics of the tuberous breast deformity and the options for management. It is well recognized that correction of the tuberous breast deformity is one of the most challenging operations that plastic surgeons encounter. What has been lacking is a suitable algorithm for management based on the degree of the deformity. Dr. Hammond has provided such an algorithm that will facilitate the planning and execution of these procedures. He categorizes the deformity into five groups that include mild constriction, constriction with hyperplasia, unilateral hypoplasia, Poland's syndrome, and the most severe form, which includes hypoplasia, constriction, and areolar herniation. For each of these variants, a strategy for management is provided.

The use of a permanent implant versus a temporary tissue expander during the initial operation has always been controversial. Dr. Hammond provides the option of either a one- or two-stage correction based on the individual characteristic of the breast. In a woman with mild constriction, a permanent implant should correct the deformity. If asymmetry is present, different-size implants can be used to obtain symmetry. However, in a woman with the more severe variants, a tissue expander may be necessary to achieve adequate volume, contour, and positional symmetry. I too have found that the use of a Becker implant as a single-stage and postoperatively expandable device can be effective in these situations. The use of breast volume measurements using three-dimensional imaging techniques can be useful when there are questions regarding the difference in volume between the breasts or when deciding on the size of the implant.

Finally, I would like to comment of the possible etiologies of the tuberous breast deformity. The characteristic of the deformity are well described; however, the reasons for its occurrence have not been adequately studied. Is this condition due to an abnormality of the glandular, cutaneous, or muscular components of the breast and chest wall? My opinion is that the tuberous breast deformity is due to an abnormality of the investing fascia of the breast that for unknown reasons is triggered to constrict, resulting in the classic appearance. This is certainly an area for future investigation.

M.Y.N.

SUGGESTED READINGS

Atiyeh BS, Hashim HA, El-Douaihy Y, et al. Pernipple round-block technique for correction of tuberous/tubular breast deformity. *Aesthetic Plast Surg* 1998;22(4):284–288.

Bass CB. Herniated areolar complex. *Ann Plast Surg* 1978;1:402.

Choupina M, Malheiro E. Tuberous breast: a surgical challenge. *Aesthetic Plast Surg* 2002;26(1): 50–53.

Grolleau JL, Lanfrey E, Lavigne B. Breast base anomalies: treatment strategy for tuberous breasts, minor deformities, and asymmetry. *Plast Reconstr Surg* 1999;104(7):2040–2048.

Hodgkinson DJ. Re: tuberous breast deformity: principles and practice. *Ann Plast Surg* 2001; 47(1):97–98.

Hoffman S. Two-stage correction of tuberous breasts. *Plast Reconstr Surg* 1982; 69(1): 169.

Hoffman S. Correction of tuberous breasts. *Plast Reconstr Surg* 1998;102(3):920–921.

Mandrekas AD, Zambacos GJ. Aesthetic reconstruction of the tuberous breast deformity. *Plast Reconstr Surg* 2004;113(7):2231–2232.

Meara JG, Kolker A, Bartlett G. Tuberous breast deformity: principles and practice. *Ann Plast Surg* 2000;45(6):607–611.

Mira JA. Anatomic asymmetric prostheses: shaping the breast. *Aesthetic Plast Surg* 2003;27(2): 94–99.

Rees TD, Aston SJ. The tuberous breast. *Clin Plast Surg* 1976;3:339–347.

Ribeiro L, Accorsi A Jr, Buss A. Short scar correction of the tuberous breast. *Clin Plast Surg* 2002; 29(3):423–431.

Ribiero L, Canzi W, Buss A Jr, et al. *Plast Reconstr Surg* 1998;101(1):42–50.

Sadove AM, van Aalst JA. Congenital and acquired pediatric breast anomalies: a review of 20 years' experience. *Plast Reconstr Surg* 2005;115(4):1039–1050.

Sheepers JH. Tissue expansion in the treatment of tubular breast deformity. *Br J Plast Surg* 1992; 45:529.

Spear SL, Kassan M, Little JW. Guidelines in concentric mastopexy. *Plast Reconstr Surg* 1990; 85(6):961–966.

Spear SL, Pelletiere CV, Menon N. One-stage augmentation combined with mastopexy: aesthetic results and patient satisfaction. *Aesthetic Plast Surg* 2004;28(5):259–267.

Toranto IR. Two-stage correction of tuberous breasts. *Plast Reconstr Surg* 1981;67(5):642–646.

Vecchione TR. A method for recontouring the domed nipple. *Plast Reconstr Surg* 1976;57:30.

von Heimburg D. Refined version of the tuberous breast classification. *Plast Reconstr Surg* 2000; 105(6):2269–2270.

von Heimburg D, Exner K, Kruft S, et al. The tuberous breast deformity: classification and treatment. *Br J Plast Surg* 1996;49(6):339–345.

Williams G, Hoffman S. Mammaplasty for tubular breasts. *Aesthetic Plast Surg* 1981;5:51.

CHAPTER

120

Scott L. Spear
Jesse A. Goldstein
Christopher V. Pelletiere

Augmentation Mammaplasty in Women With Thoracic Hypoplasia

INTRODUCTION

Since the original accounts by Froriep in 1839 and Poland in 1841, congenital chest wall deformities have long challenged surgeons in both diagnosis and treatment (1–14). In the past, these deformities were classified into five categories: Poland syndrome, pectus excavatum, pectus carinatum, sternal clefts, and generic skeletal and cartilage dysplasias (e.g., absent ribs, vertebral anomalies, chondroglandiolar depressions) (11). Of these, Poland syndrome, pectus excavatum, and skeletal dysplasias cause a depression in the anterior thoracic skeletal or soft tissue that results in a variety of chest wall deformities. Such deformities can be very disfiguring, especially when concomitant breast anomalies increase asymmetry and exaggerate chest wall depressions (7,10,11,14). Recently, however, an additional syndrome has been identified that falls into the subset of chest wall depressions, a syndrome called anterior thoracic hypoplasia (14).

Anterior thoracic hypoplasia consists of posteriorly displaced ribs resulting in a unilateral sunken anterior chest wall, hypoplasia of the ipsilateral breast, and a superiorly placed nipple-areola complex (Fig. 120.1). In these patients, the chest wall depression corresponds with posterior displacement of ribs 3 to 7 unilaterally and an average chest wall depression volume of 160 mL. There is no involvement of the pectoralis muscle, and the sternum is in normal position (14). This separates it from Poland syndrome, which is defined by the partial or complete aplasia of the sternal head of the pectoralis muscle, variable ipsilateral limb deformities, and variable breast hypoplasia (2,4–6,11–13). In contrast, anterior thoracic hypoplasia is associated with normal upper extremities and hypoplasia of the breast (which is always present to some degree).

Unfortunately, women presenting with an anterior thoracic depression, breast hypoplasia, and subsequent breast asymmetry are often diagnosed with Poland syndrome, regardless of pectoralis involvement. This is an important distinction because women presenting for augmentation mammaplasty and/or correction of chest wall deformities with Poland syndrome often require autologous tissue reconstruction to replace the missing pectoralis, whereas anterior thoracic hypoplasia can often be corrected with augmentation mammaplasty techniques when proper preoperative planning has been used.

PREOPERATIVE EVALUATION

Women presenting with anterior thoracic hypoplasia should be evaluated initially with a history to identify any confounding factors that may be contributing to or associated with breast asymmetry and unilateral anterior thoracic hypoplasia. A clinical examination, including evaluation of the patient's anterior and posterior thorax, breasts, and extremities, should be performed on all patients. The chest wall should be observed from multiple views and both sides palpated for lack or excess of the soft tissues and bony structures. The sternum should also be evaluated for degree of anterior projection, depression, or rotation in relation to the ribcage. The breasts should be evaluated for size and fullness with base width measurements of both sides, cup size as measured by patient's bra size, and size and position of both nipple-areola complexes by visual inspection. The posterior thorax should be examined for any degree of scoliosis and the extremities examined for any congenital malformations.

Radiographic evaluation after physical examination further enhances the diagnosis and assists in planning the operative strategy. Computed tomography (CT) scans, with three-dimensional reconstruction when available, allow for visualization of the anterior chest wall depression and accurate volume measurements (Fig. 120.2) (5). CT scans not only provide more precise measurements of breast volume and chest wall deformity, but also allow for evaluation of the surrounding thorax, which may not be visible with preoperative or intraoperative visual inspection. Unfortunately, these may add additional costs to the patient because the nature of the surgery may be viewed as cosmetic by insurance companies.

After completion of the patient assessment, reconstruction options should be discussed with the patient. Although there are a number of different ways that the chest wall depression can be camouflaged, one effective technique is augmentation mammaplasty.

TECHNIQUES FOR CORRECTION

Augmentation mammaplasty is a powerful tool, when used correctly, for correction of both the unilateral chest wall depression and the ipsilateral hypoplastic breast (14). Implants for the hypoplastic side should be chosen based on preoperative base width and height measurements from the physical examination and CT scan. Using manufacturer measurement and volume tables for available implants, one should first augment the hypoplastic side with an implant that closely fits each patient's specific measurements. Anatomic implants are used not only to provide increased breast volume and projection, but also to provide increased volume in the depressed subpectoral space. Because of the overlying hypoplastic breast tissue, we recommend dual-plane subpectoral placement. Because of the increased volume requirement to fill the chest wall depression, contralateral implants are then chosen based on the final volume of the hypoplastic implant minus the chest wall volume deficit. In a study by Spear et al. (14), the average chest wall volume deficit was 160 cc. Sizers can be used to determine the best fit for the contralateral breast based on the apparent volume

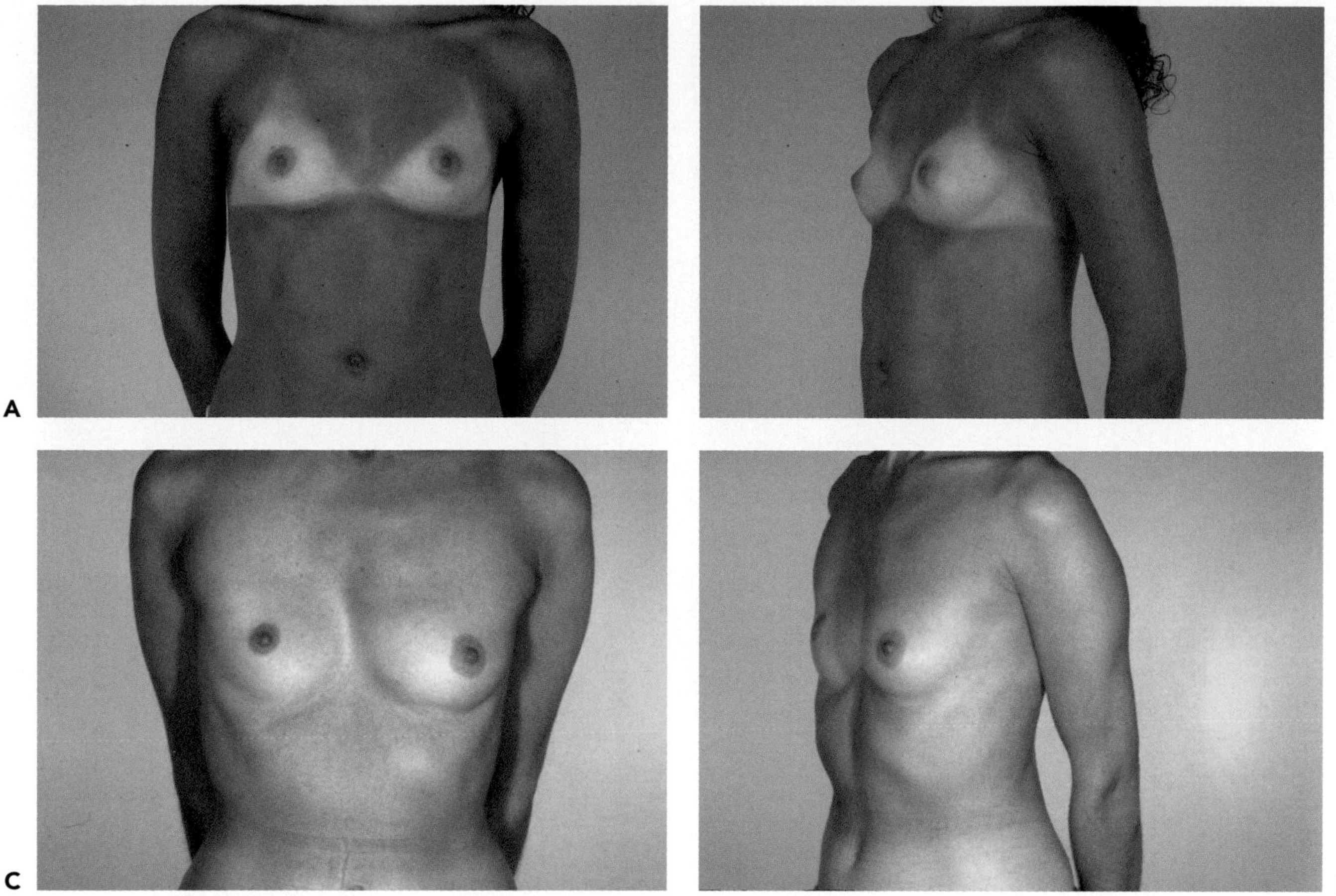

Figure 120.1. Mild and severe forms of anterior thoracic hypoplasia. **A:** A 26-year-old woman with thoracic hypoplasia on the right side. Chest wall depression volume on the right side is 50 cc. **B:** Oblique view. **C:** A 38-year-old woman with anterior thoracic hypoplasia on the right side. Note the depressed thoracic wall and hypoplastic breast, resulting in marked asymmetry. Chest wall depression volume on the right side is 240 cc. **D:** Oblique view.

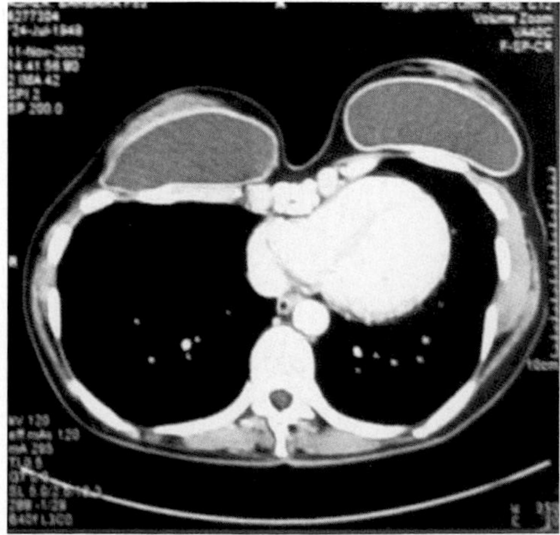

Figure 120.2. Computed tomography scan of a patient with anterior thoracic hypoplasia on the right side. The patient had previous augmentation mammaplasty with round, subglandular implants at another institution. Note the asymmetry in chest wall projection compared with the left side and continued discrepancy with implants of the same size and fill volumes on each side.

needed. Volume adjustments are then tailored to match the size and projection of the hypoplastic side. Intraoperative examination of the pectoralis muscle should be performed to establish the presence and quality of the sternal head of the pectoralis major muscle and thus definitively rule out Poland syndrome as a diagnosis. The ribcage should also be examined intraoperatively to fully assess the deformity and depression of the underlying ribs.

Although augmentation mammaplasty techniques yield excellent results in most cases, additional chest wall augmentation may be necessary in some cases. Customized silicone implants as a chest wall onlay have been used extensively in the correction of Poland syndrome as well as other chest wall deformities and may have a role here (4,7,8,11–13). Placing a customized implant allows for precise filling of the rib depression and provides a platform on which an implant might be placed for correction of the breast hypoplasia. However, this necessitates that the breast implant be placed in a subglandular position because placement subpectorally would result in contact friction between the silicone onlay and the breast prosthesis. This can lead to weakening of the implant shell and shortening of the implant lifespan. Depending on the degree of breast hypoplasia present in the

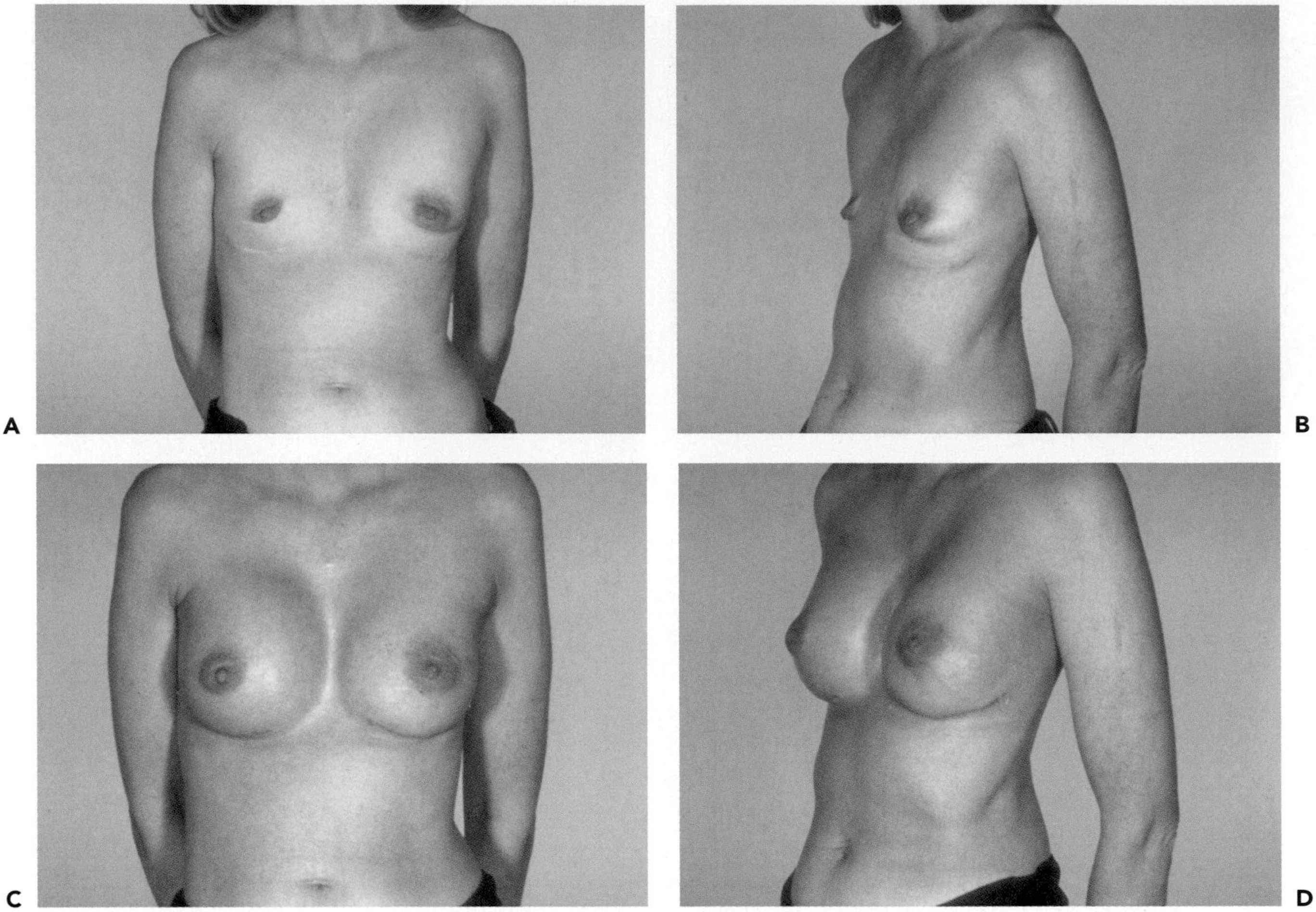

Figure 120.3. **A:** A 40-year-old woman with anterior thoracic hypoplasia on the right side. The patient previously had placement of bilateral subglandular implants and subsequent removal. However, preoperatively before original surgery, the breast size was 34B on the left and 34 A on the right. **B:** Preoperative oblique view. Note the right chest wall depression. **C:** Postoperative view after bilateral inframammary approaches, subpectoral dual-plane augmentation with a McGhan 68 implant filled with 190 cc of saline on the left, and a McGhan 468 implant filled to 430 cc of saline on the right. **D:** Postoperative oblique view.

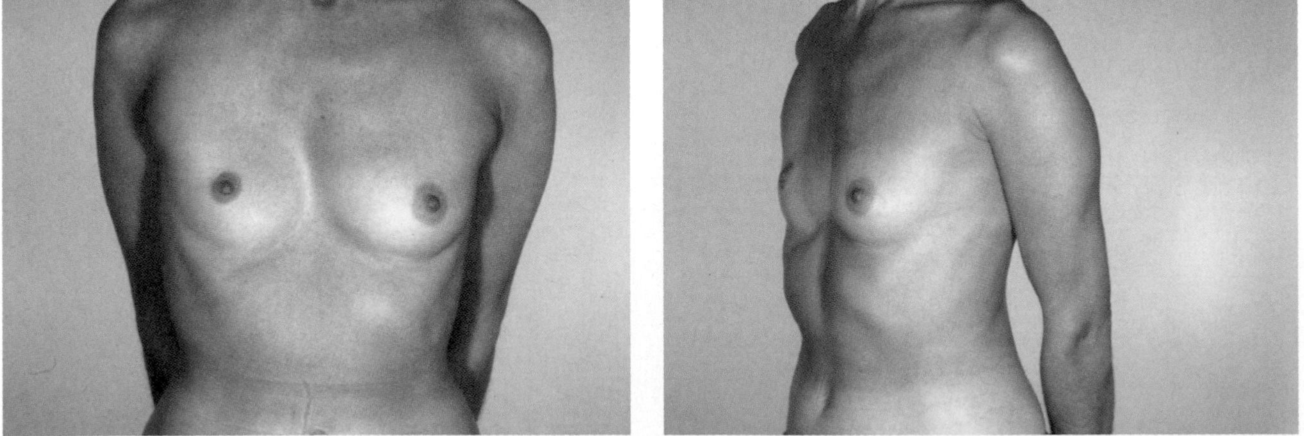

Figure 120.4. **A:** A 38-year-old woman with anterior thoracic hypoplasia on the right side. Preoperative breast size was 34B on the left and 34A on the right. **B:** Preoperative oblique view. (*continued*)

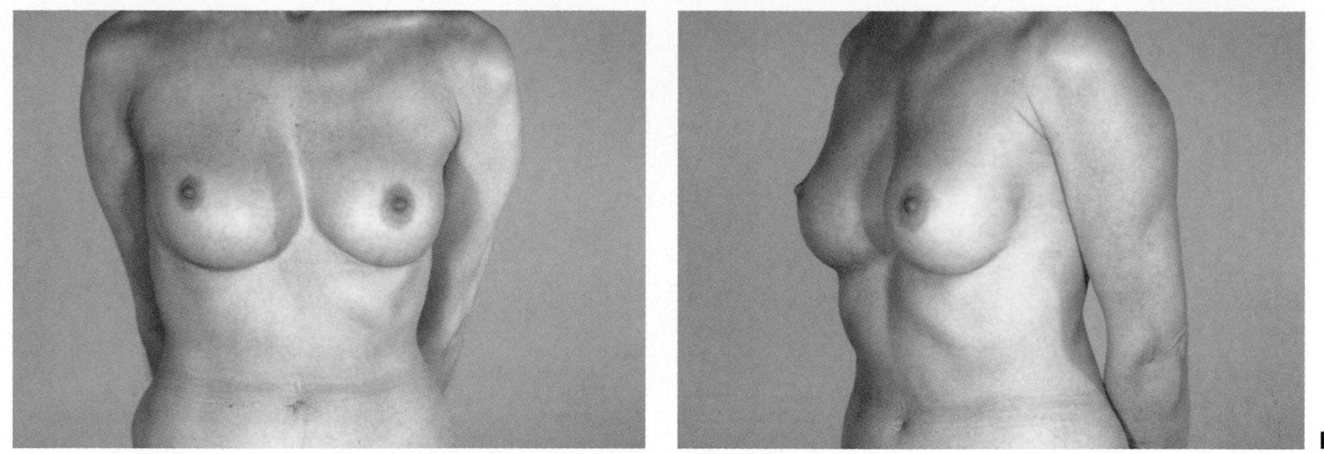

C D

Figure 120.4. (*Continued*) **C:** Postoperative view after bilateral inframammary approaches, subpectoral dual-plane augmentation with a McGhan 68 implant filled with 265 cc of saline on the left, and a McGhan 468 implant filled to 505 cc on the right. **D:** Postoperative oblique view.

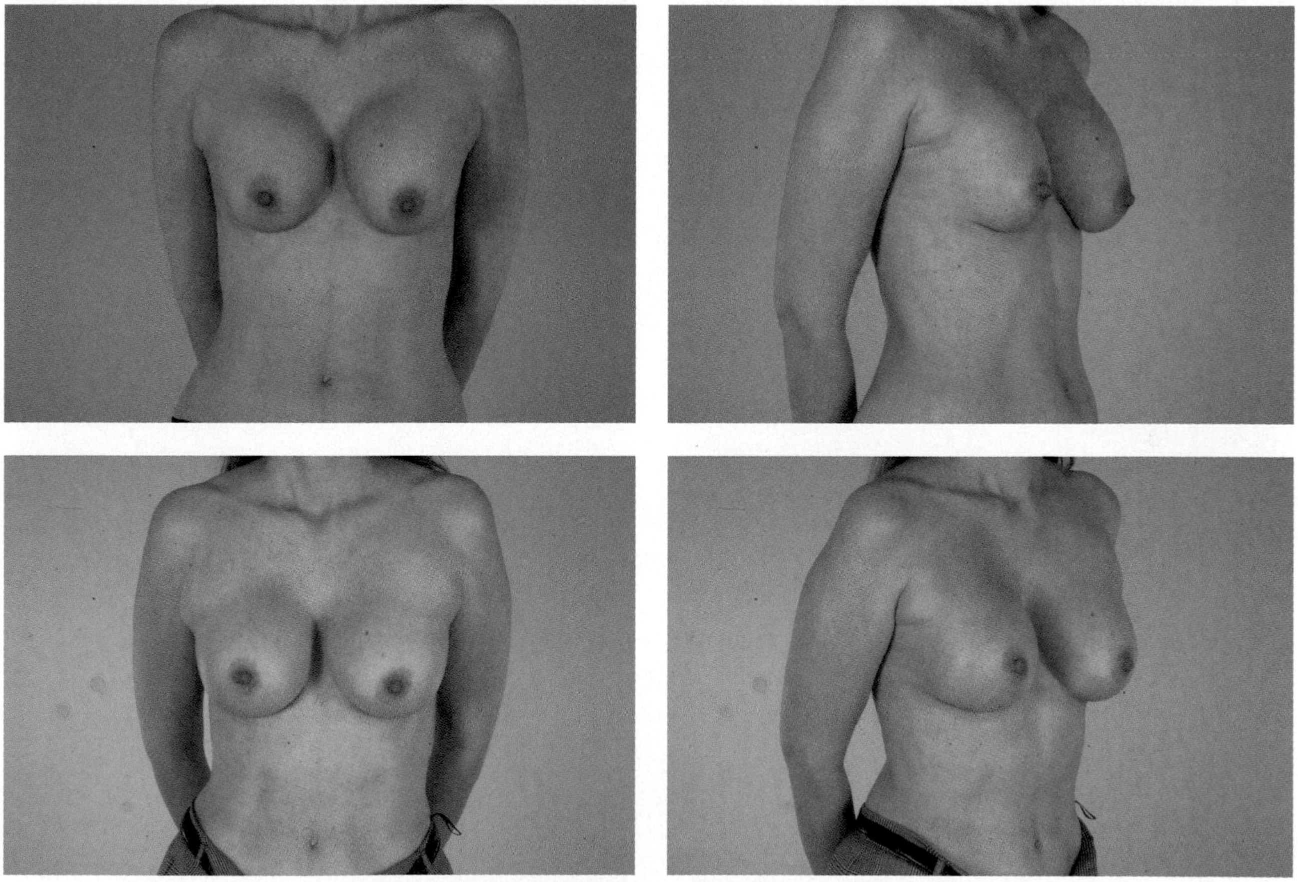

A B

C D

Figure 120.5. **A:** A 43-year-old woman with anterior thoracic hypoplasia on the right side. The patient underwent bilateral subglandular breast augmentation 10 years prior. **B:** Preoperative oblique view. **C:** Postoperative view after removal of subglandular implants, capsulectomies, and subpectoral dual-plane reaugmentation using inframammary approaches. On the right, a McGhan 20 375-cc device was used. On the left, a McGhan 10 270-cc device was used. **D:** Postoperative oblique view.

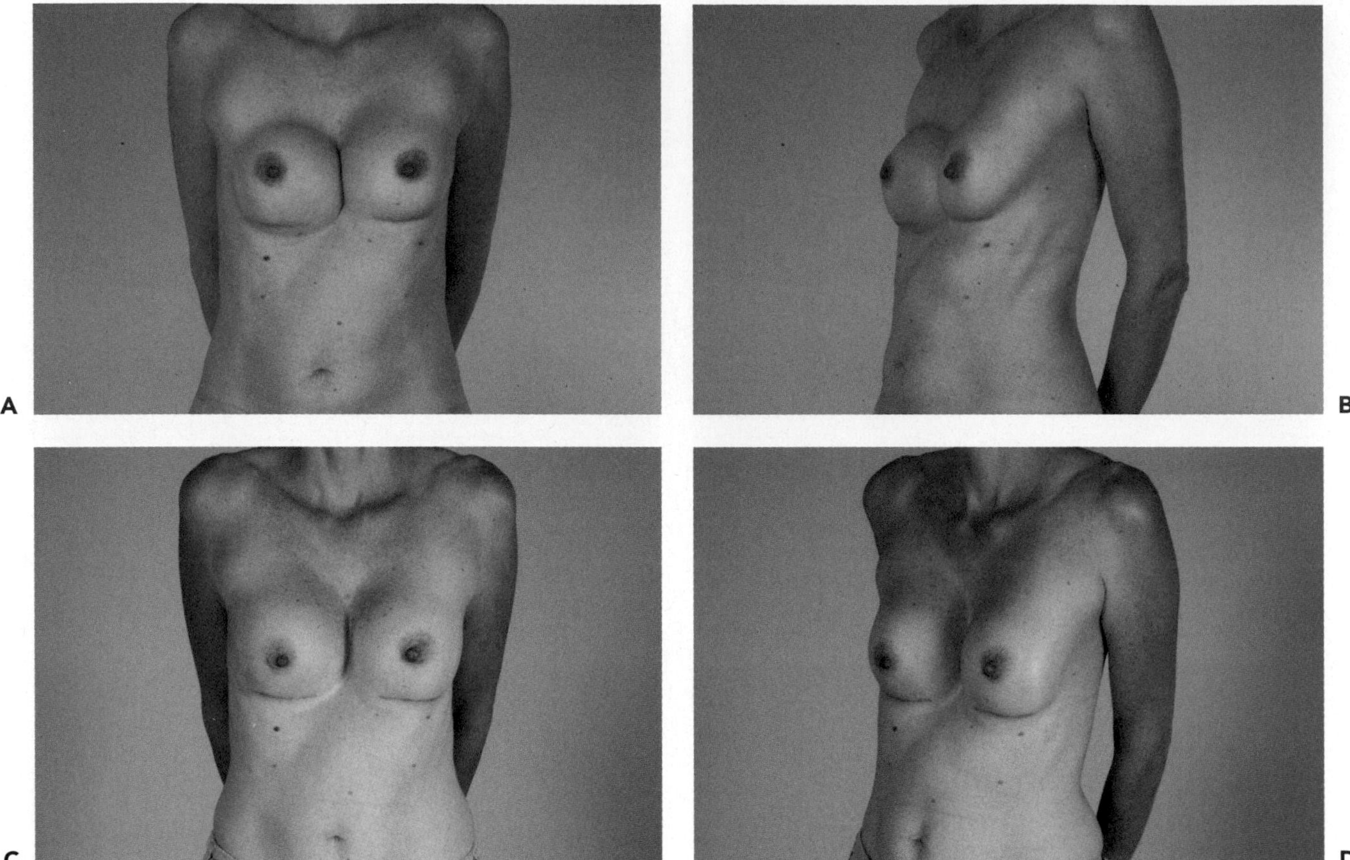

Figure 120.6. **A:** A 42-year-old woman with anterior thoracic hypoplasia on the right side. The patient underwent several augmentation procedures in an attempt to achieve symmetry, most recently 6 years prior. Most recent augmentations were a McGhan textured 330-cc saline device filled to 395 cc on the right and a McGhan textured 300-cc saline device filled to 255 cc on the left. **B:** Preoperative oblique view. **C:** Postoperative view after removal of subglandular implants, capsulectomies, and subpectoral dual-plane reaugmentation utilizing inframammary approaches. On the right, a McGhan 20 425-cc device was used. On the left, a McGhan 15 286-cc device was used. **D:** Postoperative oblique view.

ipsilateral breast, subglandular implant placement could lead to increased visibility, palpability, and capsular contracture, and these factors should be considered before onlay reconstruction is attempted. Fortunately, with the available anatomic implants, a customized silicone onlay usually is not necessary. However, this is an option in women who have mild breast hypoplasia and asymmetry and who do not desire breast augmentation but want correction of their underlying chest wall depression.

Another option for filling of the chest wall depression is the use of autologous tissue, a technique that has also been used extensively in Poland syndrome (15). However, in thoracic hypoplasia, where the pectoralis muscle is normal, the autologous tissue would fill the volume deficit of the posteriorly displaced anterior chest wall. With the advent of endoscopic flap harvest, the latissimus dorsi pedicled flap is an ideal muscle for augmentation of the thoracic depression with minimal donor-site morbidity. However, this does add a level of complexity, cost, and morbidity to the operation that is often not necessary if proper preoperative measurements and implant selection have occurred.

We have treated a number of patients with thoracic hypoplasia and have been able to achieve good results with augmentation mammaplasty techniques alone (Figs. 120.3 to 120.6) (14). Only one of our patients had a volume deficit that would have been better suited for a customized silicone onlay and breast implant, and none opted for or needed autologous tissue augmentation.

EDITORIAL COMMENTS

The topic of thoracic hypoplasia is important because it is often overlooked as a source or etiology of breast asymmetry. Dr. Spear and colleagues have provided a systematic approach to the evaluation and management of women with thoracic hypoplasia. It is differentiated from the pectus excavatum condition because the position of the sternum relative to the costochondral junction is normal in the patient with thoracic hypoplasia. When suspected, imaging studies are useful for the preoperative planning. The authors mention the utility of implants in the correction of this deformity but also mention the occasional need to recontour the hypoplastic chest wall with autologous tissue in some cases. This chapter provides useful tips and pearls from a highly experienced breast surgeon that will certainly facilitate the ability to correct these complex conditions.

M.Y.N.

REFERENCES

1. Froriep R. Beobachtung eines Falles von Mangel der Brustdruse. *Notizen Gebiete Natur Heilkund* 1839;10:9.
2. Clarkson P. Poland's syndactyly. *Guy's Hosp Rep* 1962;111:335.
3. Spear SL, Romm S, Hakki A, et al. Costal cartilage sculpturing as an adjunct to augmentation mammaplasty. *Plast Reconstr Surg* 1987;9:921.
4. Marks MW, Argenta LC, Izenberg PH, et al. Management of the chest-wall deformity in male patients with Poland's syndrome. *Plast Reconstr Surg* 1990;87:674.
5. Bainbridge LC, Wright AR, Kanthan R. Computed tomography in the preoperative assessment of Poland's syndrome. *Br J Plast Surg* 1991;44:604.
6. Samuels TH, Haider MA, Kirkbride P. Poland's syndrome: a mammographic presentation. *Am J Radiol* 1996;166:347.
7. Hodgkinson DJ. Chest wall implants: their use for pectus excavatum, pectoralis muscle tears, Poland's syndrome, and muscular insufficiency. *Aesthet Plast Surg* 1997;21:7.
8. Gatti JE. Poland's deformity reconstruction with a customized, extrasoft silicone prosthesis. *Ann Plast Surg* 1997;39:122.
9. Hoffman S. Augmentation mammaplasty for tuberous breasts and other complex anomalies. In: Spear SL, ed. *Surgery of the Breast: Principles and Art.* Philadelphia: Lippincott-Raven; 1998:907.
10. Wieslander JB. Congenital breast deformity is a serious handicap; an important indication for breast reconstruction with silicone implants [in Swedish]. *Lakartidningen* 1999;96:1703.
11. Marks MW, Iacobucci J. Reconstruction of congenital chest wall deformities using solid silicone onlay prostheses. *Chest Surg Clin North Am* 2000;10:341.
12. Urschel HC. Poland's syndrome. *Chest Surg Clin North Am* 2000;10:393.
13. Hodgkinson DJ. The management of anterior chest wall deformity in patients presenting for breast augmentation. *Plast Reconstr Surg* 2002;109:1714.
14. Spear SL, Pelletiere CV, Lee E, et al. Anterior thoracic hypoplasia: a separate entity from Poland's syndrome. *Plast Reconstr Surg* 2004;13:69.
15. Bains RD, Riaz M, Stanley P. Superior gluteal artery perforator flap reconstruction for anterior thoracic hypoplasia. *Plast Reconstr Surg* 2007;120:7.

CHAPTER

121

James D. Namnoum

Breast Reconstruction in Patients With Poland Syndrome

INTRODUCTION

In 1841, while completing a preceptorship in anatomy at Guy's Hospital in London, Alfred Poland described the characteristics of a cadaver with notable unilateral chest wall and upper extremity deformities involving the pectoralis major and minor, serratus, and external oblique muscles (1). This syndrome, later named after him by Clarkson (2)—although, according to Ravitch (3), it had been described earlier in separate reports by Lallemand and Foriep—includes a variety of findings of varying combinations and degrees of severity. Classically, the deficiency or absence of the sternocostal portion of the pectoralis major muscle with some degree of breast involvement is the hallmark feature of Poland syndrome. However, other muscles of the thorax and abdomen and underlying bony skeleton may also be affected in the thoracic component of this syndrome. The various hand and upper extremity anomalies found in frequent association are beyond the scope of this discussion (4).

ETIOLOGY AND INCIDENCE

Most cases of Poland syndrome occur spontaneously; however, a familial form of inheritance has been described, as well as a case of bilateral involvement (5,6). The incidence ranges from 1 to 20,000 to about 1 to 30,000 births (7,8). Poland syndrome has been observed primarily in males and appears to generally affect the right side (9). Several theories abound regarding possible etiologies, but no causation has been established (10–14).

CLASSIFICATION

Conceptually, patients with Poland syndrome can be organized into three categories based on their physical findings (Table 121.1).

MILD POLAND DEFORMITY

These patients demonstrate the mildest form of the Poland deformity (Fig. 121.1). Typically, these patients show hypoplasia of the breast, nipple-areolar complex, and pectoralis major muscle that may only be appreciated radiographically (15). In this respect it may be a different entity than the anterior thoracic syndrome described by Spear et al. (16).

MODERATE POLAND DEFORMITY

The classic deformity seen in Poland patients includes hypoplasia of the affected breast and nipple-areolar complex, as well as absence of the sternocostal portion of the pectoralis major muscle (Fig. 121.2). Some portion of the sternoclavicular portion of the pectoralis muscle is present in most cases, although it may be rudimentary. On frontal view, the patients demonstrate marked breast asymmetry, with a small, elevated nipple-areolar complex. Absence of the anterior axillary fold and deficient soft tissue "fill" in the infraclavicular region are common features (Fig. 121.3).

SEVERE POLAND DEFORMITY

The most challenging deformity to reconstruct is characterized by absence of the breast and at times nipple-areolar complex, absence of the pectoralis muscle, and absence or marked deformities of the ribs and sternum. Tight skin of the chest and axillary webbing may be seen (Fig. 121.4).

TREATMENT

Treatment of the Poland patient is indexed to the severity of the deformity. The goal, as in all breast surgery, is to create a breast that is symmetric with the opposite side. Options for treatment include tissue expanders, permanent breast implants, and autologous tissues, free and pedicled, with or without implants (17–27). Adjunctive procedures such as the use of fat transfer to the breast and chest or acellular dermal matrix help to refine the results and may extend the application of certain treatment options.

The timing of surgery is a sensitive topic that requires judiciousness on the part of the surgeon. It is difficult to underestimate the profound insecurities of the early teenage years for patients and their families. Feelings of extreme self-consciousness regarding body image coupled with an overlay of parental guilt create a charged atmosphere in which "something must be done" may be the overriding sentiment. In general, it is best to delay surgery until the early teenage years when the breasts have changed sufficiently to create a noticeable degree of asymmetry. Ideally, an adjustable implant can be placed to permit the affected breast to keep up with the opposite side. Patients and their families should be counseled that a series of procedures will be needed over the years to make volume and symmetry adjustments as the breasts develop .

TISSUE EXPANDER AND IMPLANT RECONSTRUCTION

Patients with mild deformities are ideally treated with the placement of an adjustable implant during adolescence. These may be exchanged after maturation is completed or left in place following removal of the port, during which time any adjustments of the opposite breast are made (Fig. 121.5).

TABLE 121.1 Classification of Poland Syndrome

Type	*Breast*	*Nipple-Areola*	*Pectoralis Major*	*Thoracic Skeleton*
Mild	Hypoplastic	Small and elevated	Hypoplastic	Not affected
Moderate	Hypoplastic	Small and elevated	Absent sternocostal	Not affected
Severe	Hypoplastic or absent	Hypoplastic or absent	Absent	Absent, deformed or hypoplastic ribs and sternum

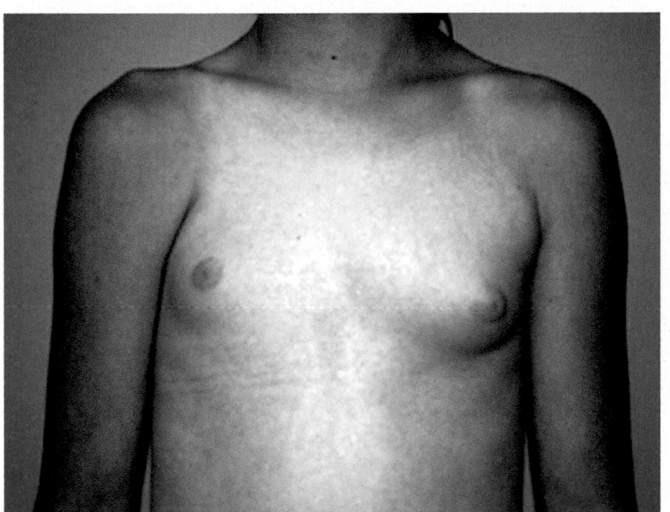

Figure 121.1. Mild Poland deformity. Hypoplastic breast and nipple-areolar complex, resulting in marked breast and nipple asymmetry.

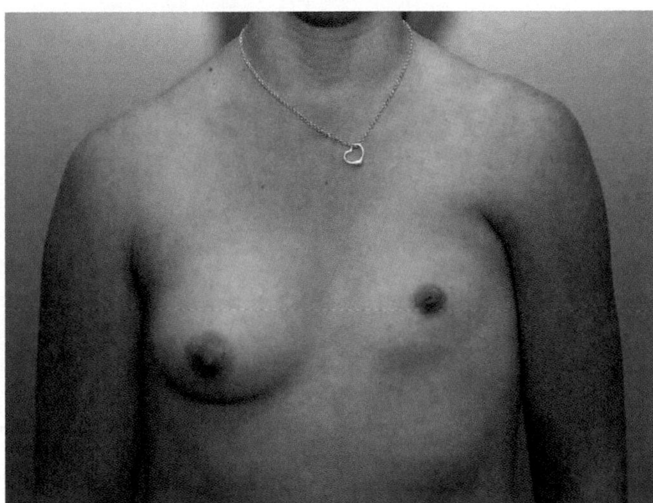

Figure 121.2. Moderate Poland deformity. Hypoplasia of the breast and nipple-areolar complex with more severe asymmetry. Sternocostal pectoralis muscle is absent. Loss of anterior axillary fold.

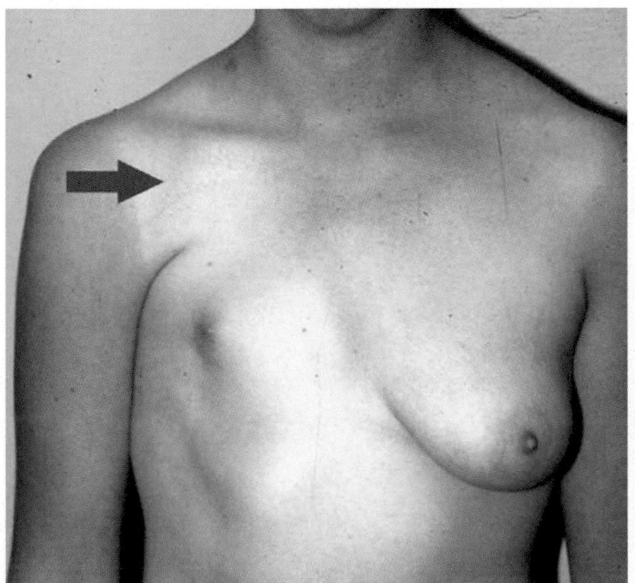

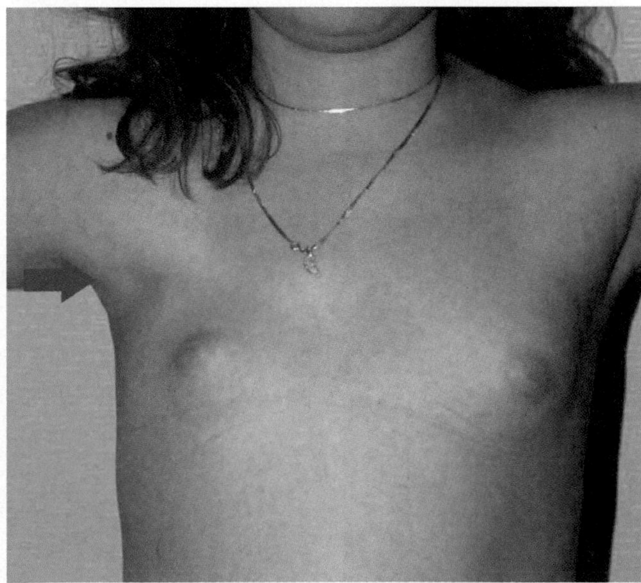

Figure 121.3. A: Absence of the anterior axillary fold in a patient with a moderate deformity. **B:** Deficient infraclavicular soft tissue "fill" in a patient with a more severe deformity.

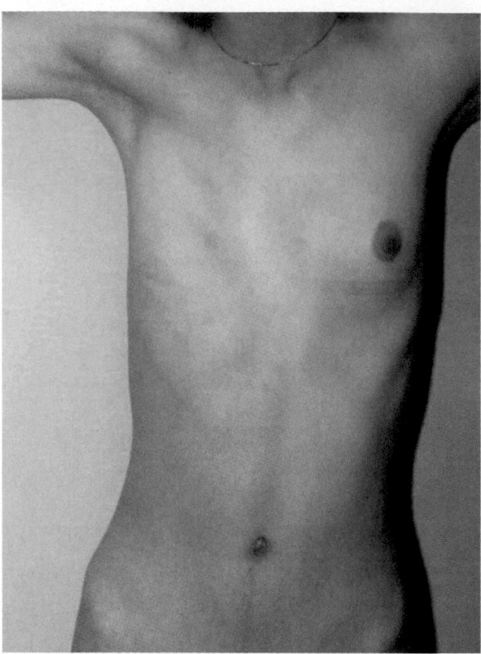

Figure 121.4. Severe Poland deformity. Absence of the breast, nipple-areolar complex, and pectoralis muscle in a patient with underlying rib abnormalities. Tight skin and deficient subcutaneous fat.

A

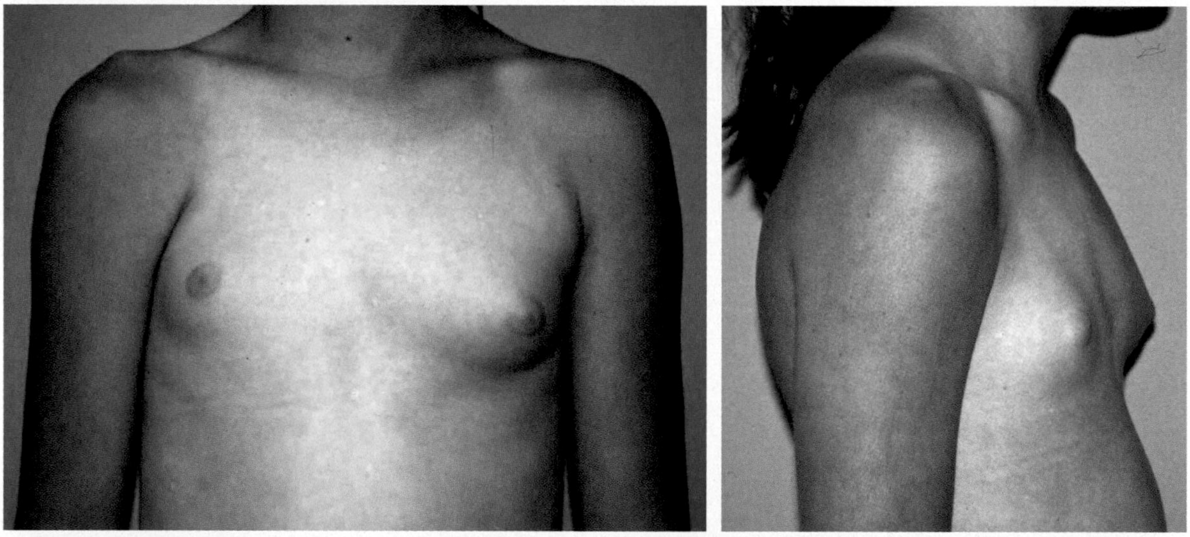

B

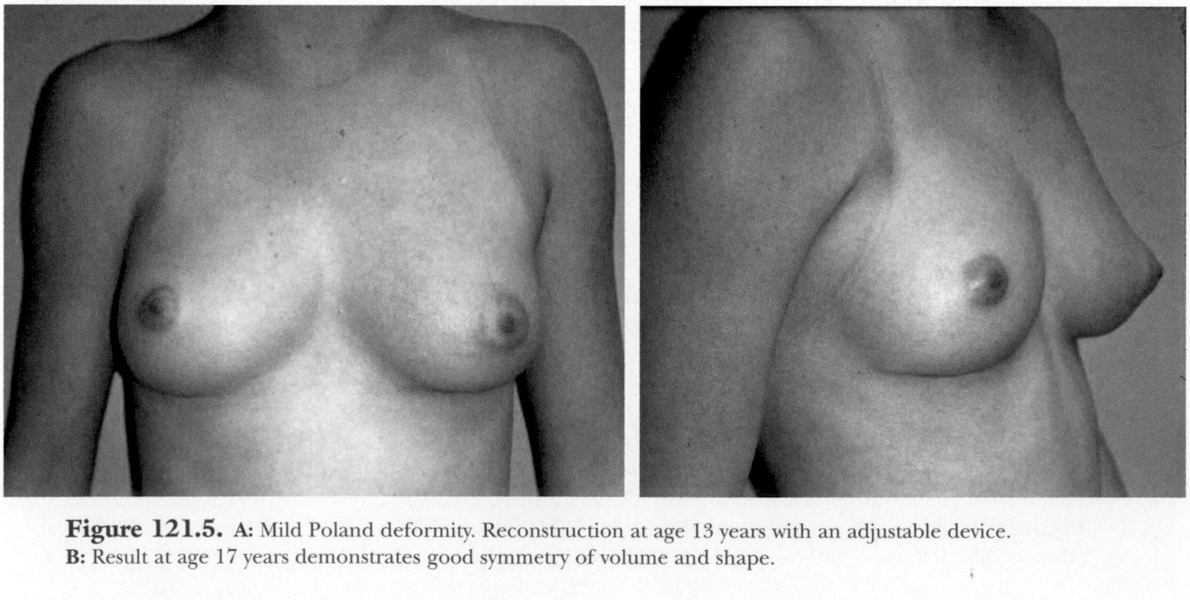

Figure 121.5. **A:** Mild Poland deformity. Reconstruction at age 13 years with an adjustable device. **B:** Result at age 17 years demonstrates good symmetry of volume and shape.

Moderate deformities may also be treated with placement of adjustable devices during the early teenage years. Fat transfer to the breast and chest wall is a useful adjunctive procedure in these patients and offers promise in treating the soft tissue deficit of the upper chest, as well as aiding in the creation of the axillary fold (Fig. 121.6). Form-stable, shaped devices may well offer significant advantages in these patients owing to the many options available for devices of different heights, volumes, and projections.

AUTOLOGOUS TISSUE RECONSTRUCTION

Autologous tissue transfer is most often reserved for patients who have completed development, have an ample source of donor material, have moderate or severe deformities, or have failed implant reconstructions. Historically, the latissimus flap was preferred in combination with implants in the Poland patient; it is now reserved as a secondary option. Patients with a moderate or severe deformity involving absence of the pectoralis are hesitant to sacrifice another thoracic muscle on the affected side. The latissimus itself is occasionally involved in the deformity; preoperative scans may be needed to determine whether it is suitable for use (28–30).

In contrast, the transverse rectus abdominis musculocutaneous (TRAM) flap is an excellent option for autologous reconstruction in the more seriously affected patient. The potentially large amount of soft, pliable fat available from the lower abdomen permits excellent camouflage of the underlying chest wall deformity, reconstruction of the axillary fold, and balancing of the breast mound (Fig. 121.7).

The TRAM flap is particularly useful in cases of failed implant reconstruction. In the past, more severely affected patients were treated with a combination of chest wall implants for the upper chest and breast implants for the creation of the breast mound. While this may have offered reasonable short-term correction, over time, the devices invariably shift and contractures form around the implants. Performance of capsulectomy, device removal, and TRAM flap reconstruction is ideal for restoring balance and achieving a symmetric result (Fig. 121.8). Often, patients who have had device reconstructions

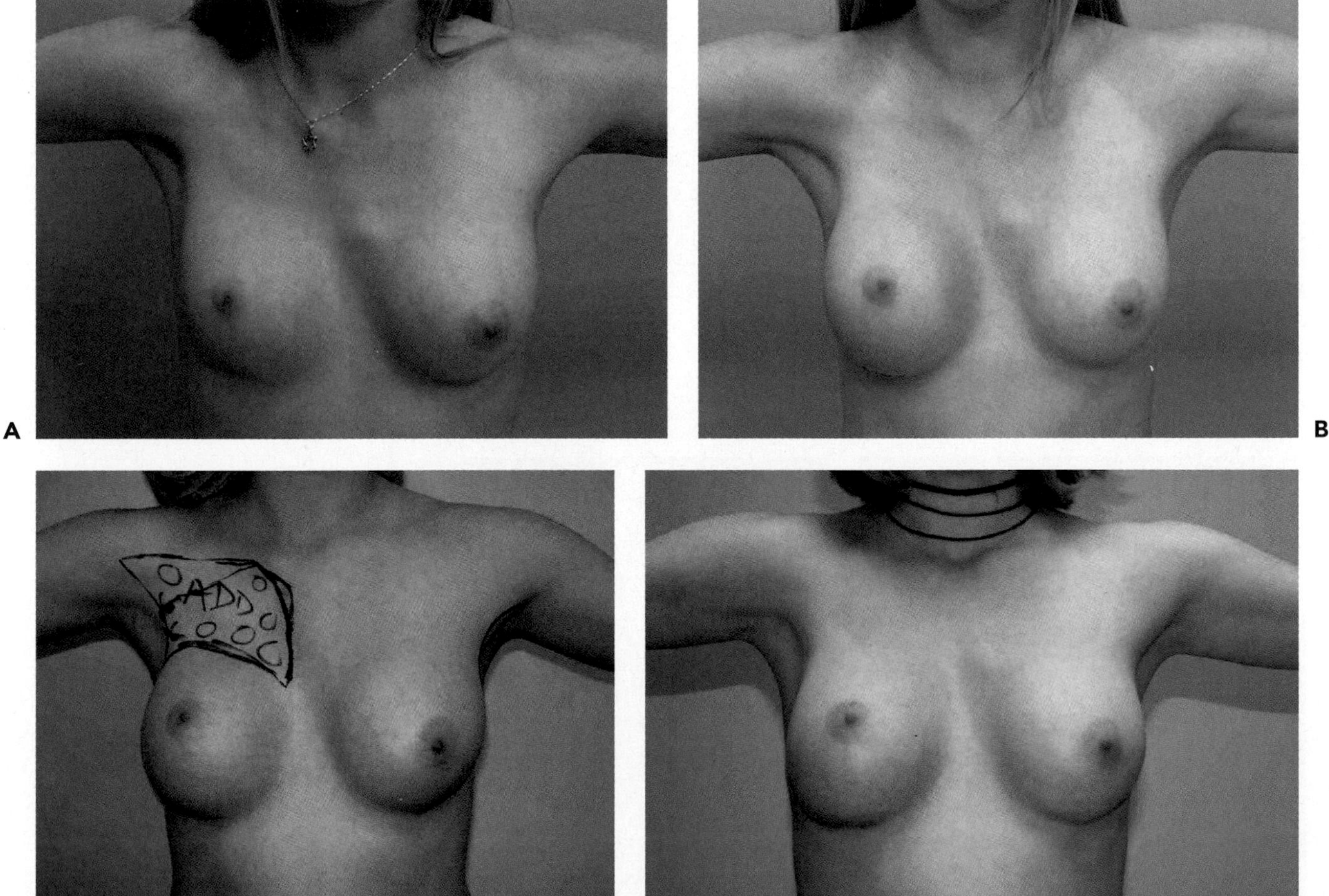

Figure 121.6. **A:** Moderate Poland deformity; Asymmetry with deficient soft tissue of upper chest and absent anterior axillary fold. **B:** Appearance after reconstruction with round, adjustable device; symmetry is improved but still lacking soft tissue. **C:** Appearance prior to fat grafting of chest and anterior axillary fold. **D:** Result following two transfers of 60 cc each; significant improvement in soft tissue fill of chest and anterior axillary fold. (*continued*)

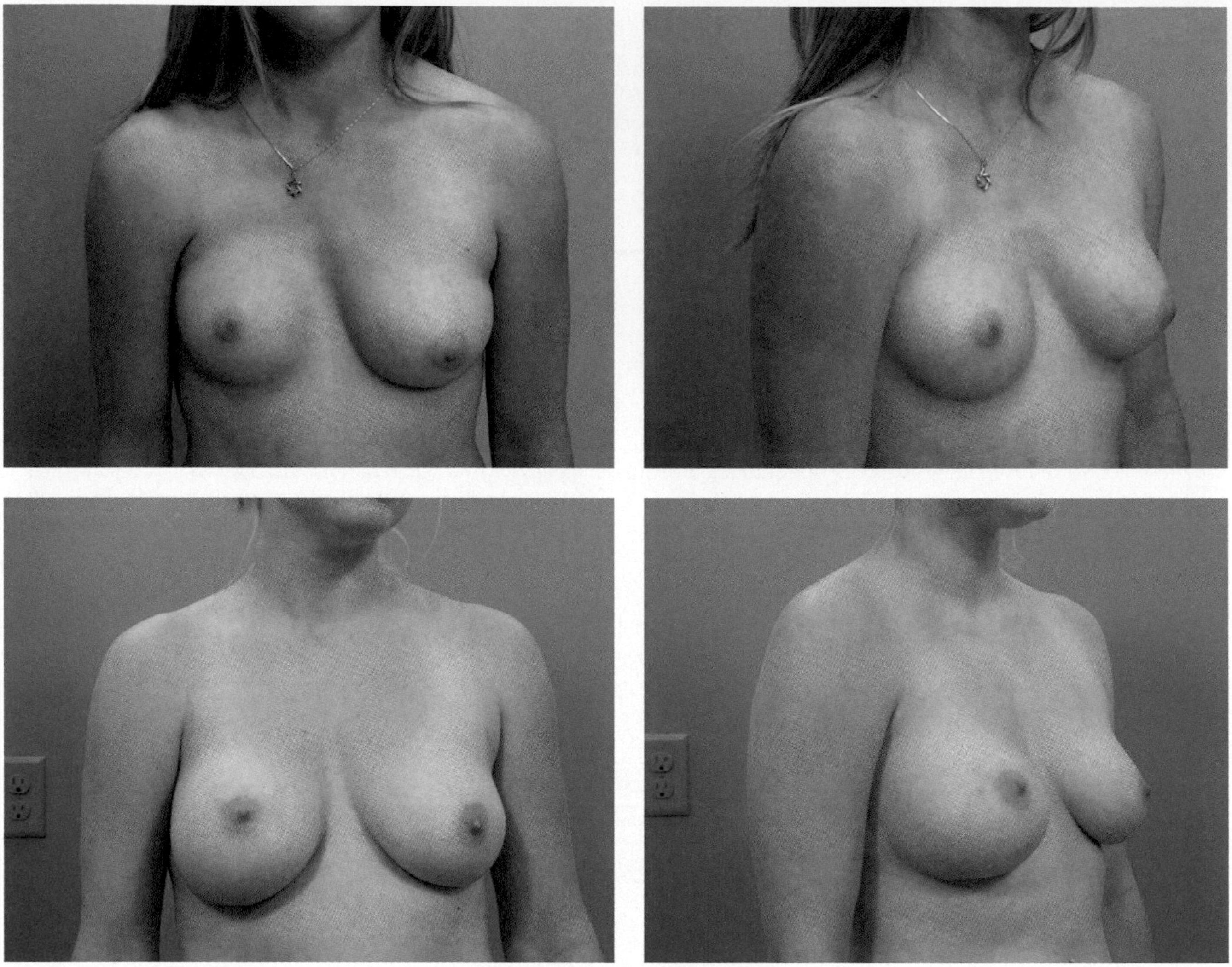

Figure 121.6. (*Continued*) **E:** Preoperative view and 5-year postoperative view.

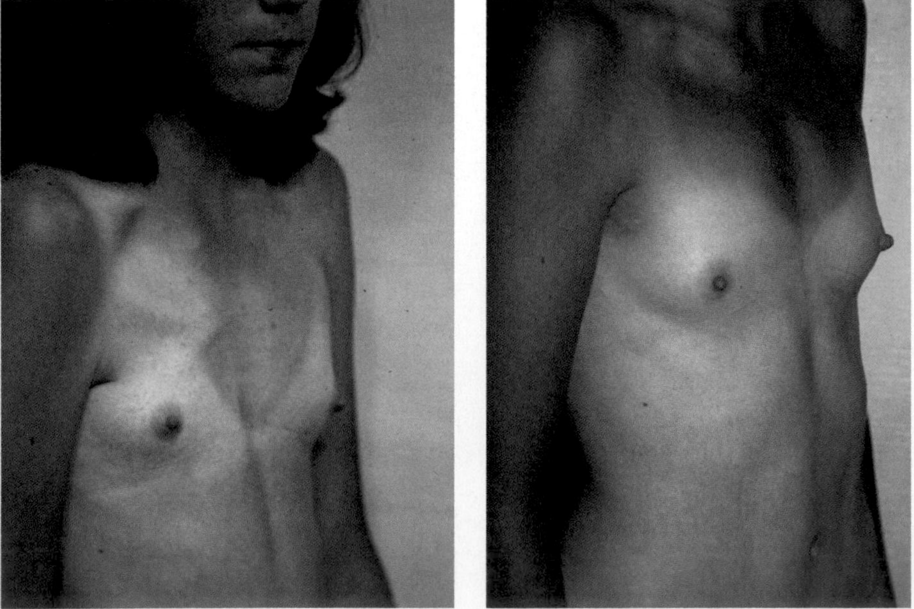

Figure 121.7. **A:** Moderate to severe Poland deformity with significant bony deformity especially in area of upper chest. **B**: Appearance 2 years following single-stage reconstruction with a pedicled transverse rectus abdominis musculocutaneous flap.

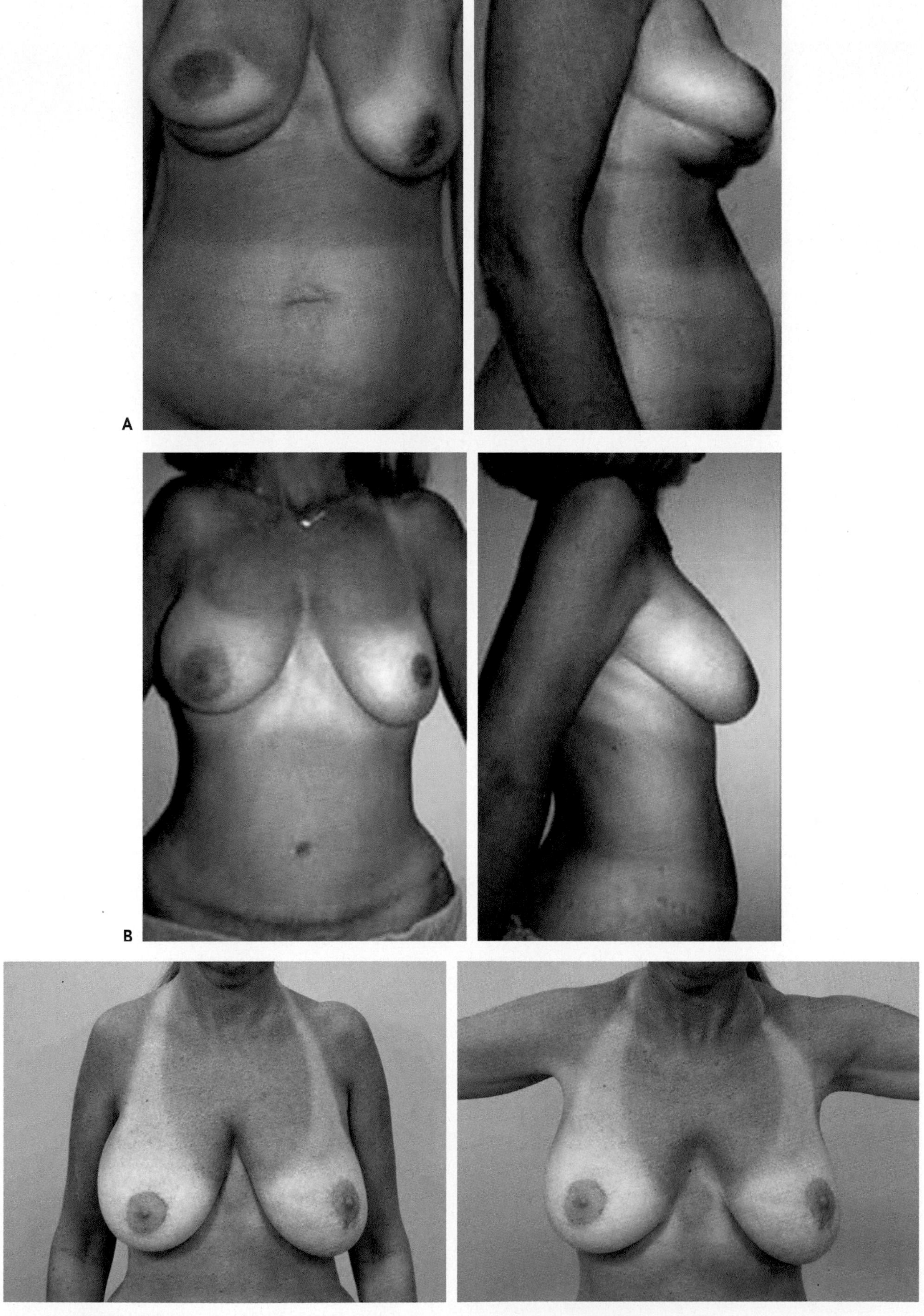

Figure 121.8. **A:** Inferior malposition of an implant in a patient 12 years following placement of a stacked chest wall and breast implant. **B:** Two-year result following implant removal, capsulectomy, and transverse rectus abdominis musculocutaneous flap reconstruction; contralateral mastopexy for balancing. **C:** Seven-year postoperative result.

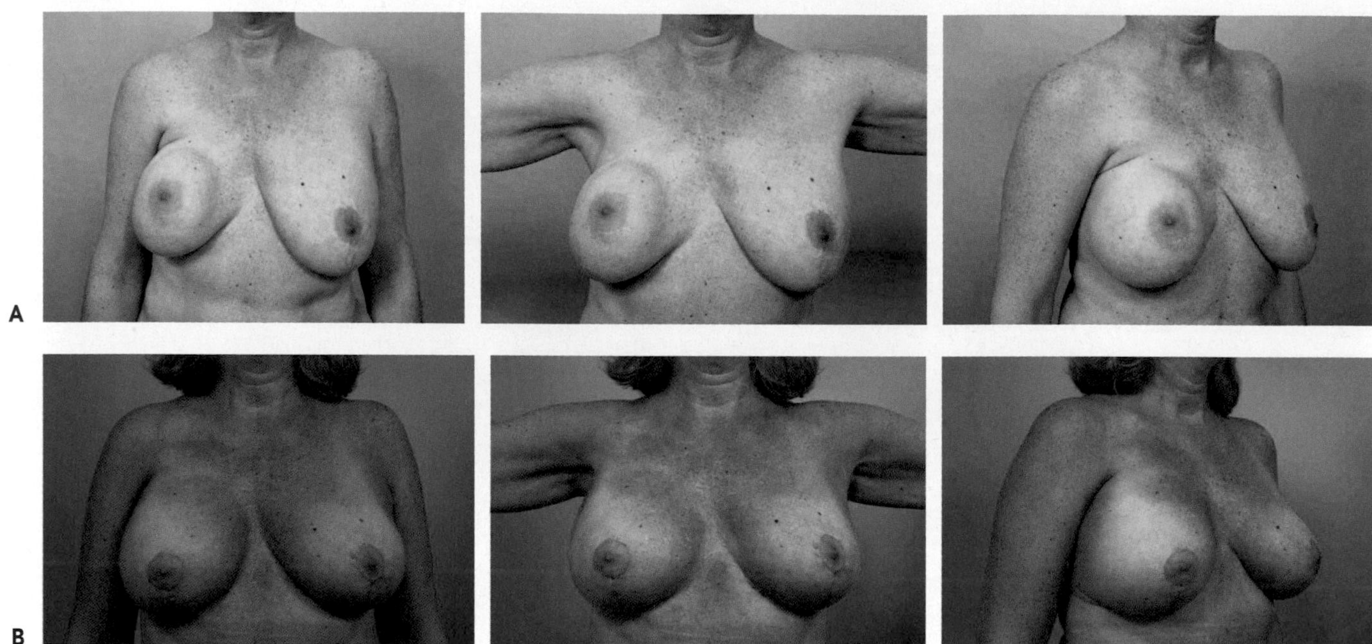

Figure 121.9. **A:** Asymmetry, capsular contracture, and thinning of tissues in a patient with moderate Poland deformity following multiple attempts at implant reconstruction. **B:** Appearance following capsulectomy, explantation, and free transverse rectus abdominis musculocutaneous flap reconstruction; contralateral augmentation/mastopexy.

have undergone several exchanges over the years, with thinning of their tissues. They may also be good candidates for explantation, capsulectomy, and TRAM reconstruction (Fig. 121.9).

RECONSTRUCTION WITH ACELLULAR DERMAL MATRIX

Male patients with Poland syndrome have historically undergone reconstruction of the chest wall deformity with either customized implants or latissimus flaps (Fig. 121.10). Neither is truly ideal. Chest wall implants often become displaced over time, form a seroma, or become infected. They are stiff, unyielding, and unaesthetic. Even more than their female counterparts, male patients with Poland syndrome are extremely reluctant to sacrifice the latissimus muscle for chest wall reconstruction. They want neither the attendant posterior thoracic deformity nor any potential reduction in athletic performance.

Acellular dermal matrix can be used to correct the chest wall deformity in male patients with Poland syndrome. Acellular dermal matrix becomes revascularized over time and incorporated into host tissues; this avoids the pitfalls of chest wall reconstruction with prosthetic devices, while creating no donor-site morbidity (Fig. 121.11).

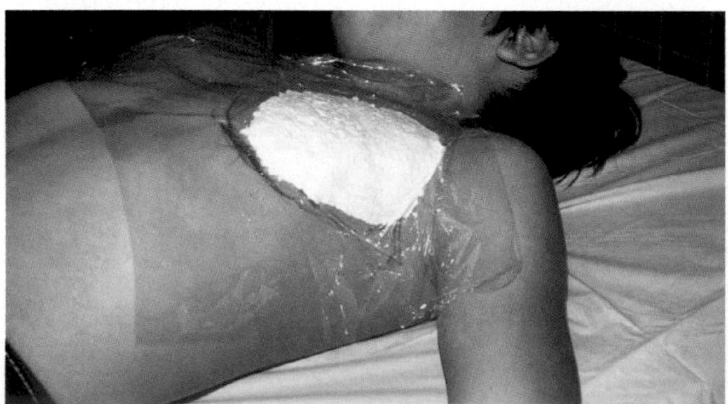

Figure 121.10. Creation of a plaster moulage of the chest in a patient with a moderate Poland deformity.

CONCLUSION

Patients with Poland syndrome demonstrate a variety of breast, nipple, and chest wall deformities of different degrees of severity. Milder deformities can be successfully treated with adjustable implants placed in the early teen years and adjusted with development of the opposite breast. More significant deformities may be treated using adjustable implants in conjunction with fat transfer until development is completed. Deformities of greater severity and failed implant reconstructions are best treated with autologous reconstruction with either free or pedicled TRAM flaps. Acellular dermal matrix reconstruction can be successfully used in male patients as an alternative to traditional prosthetic devices or latissimus flaps.

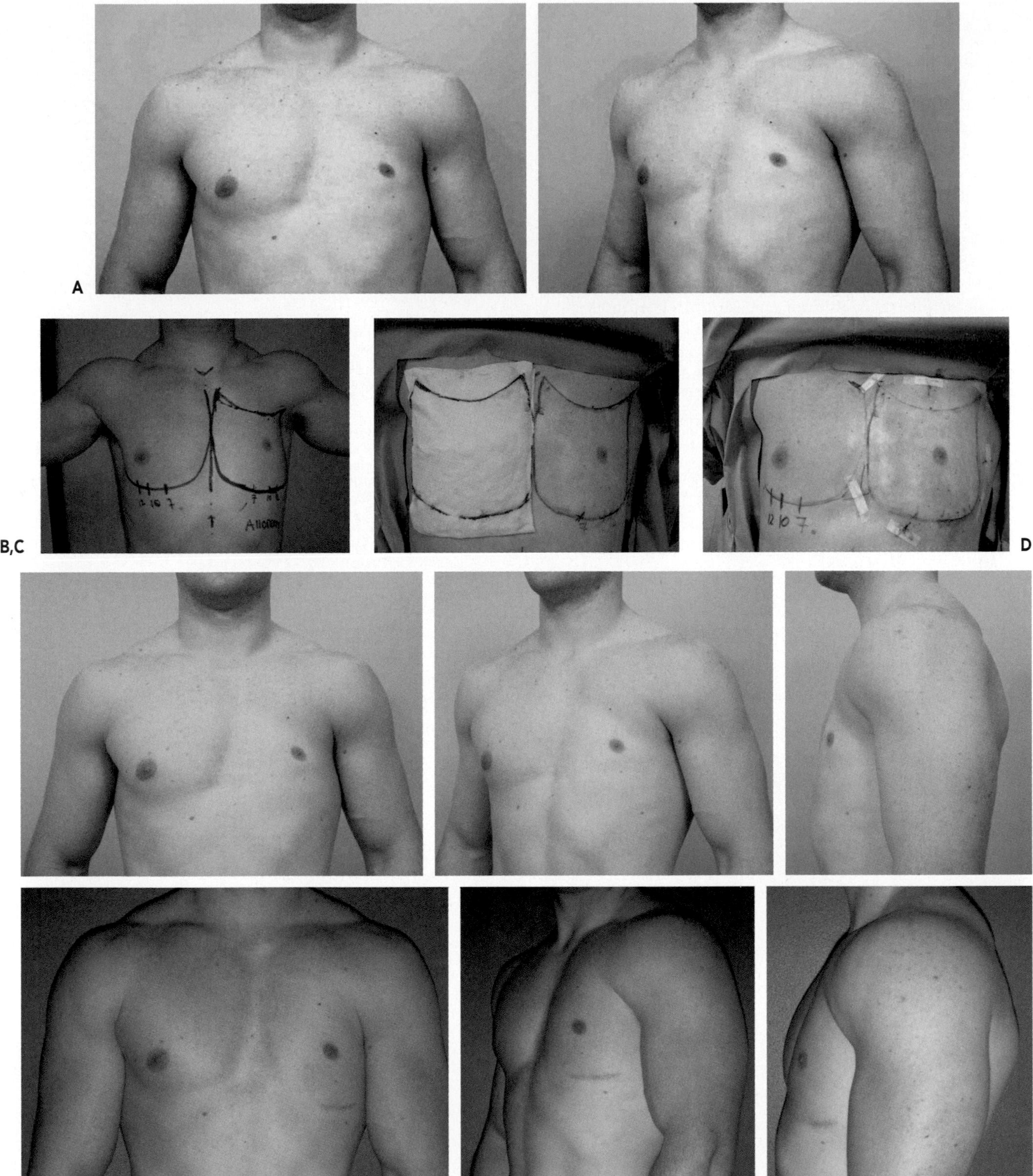

Figure 121.11. **A:** Chest wall reconstruction in muscular male patient with moderate Poland deformity of the chest. **B:** Preoperative plan. **C:** Stacked sheets of ultrathick acellular dermal matrix (18 × 20 cm) tailored to the deformity. **D:** Intraoperative appearance. **E:** Appearance at 8 months postoperatively.

EDITORIAL COMMENTS

Dr. Namnoum has prepared a nice synopsis of the etiology, physical characteristics, and management options for the patient with Poland syndrome. As he states, the optimal management will depend on the degree of breast deformity. For mild deformities, a prosthetic device will usually be effective. For moderately severe deformities, a latissimus dorsi flap with or without a prosthetic device may be effective. For the more severe deformities, autologous reconstruction using the abdominal donor site can be performed. This can be performed as a pedicle TRAM flap or a free tissue transfer (TRAM, deep inferior epigastric artery perforator, or superficial inferior epigastric artery). Another reconstructive option that is gaining in popularity is autologous fat grafting. Coleman and Saboeiro have demonstrated the feasibility of this technique for this indication by serial grafting (31). Overall, this chapter provides a useful overview and provides clinical correlation in the management of Poland syndrome.

M.Y.N.

REFERENCES

1. Poland A. Deficiency of the pectoral muscles. *Guy's Hosp Rep* 1841;6:191–193.
2. Clarkson P. Poland's syndactyly. *Guy's Hosp Rep* 1962;111:335.
3. Ravitch MM. Poland's syndrome: a study of an eponym. *Plast Reconstr Surg* 1977;59:508–512.
4. Namnoum JD. Breast reconstruction in patients with Poland's syndrome. In: Spear SL, ed. *Surgery of the Breast. Principles and Art.* 2nd ed. Philadelphia: Lippincott Williams & Wilkins; 2006:1383–1394.
5. Darian VB, Argenta LC, Pasyk KA. Familial Poland's syndrome. *Ann Plast Surg* 1989;23: 531–537.
6. Franzoni R, Scalercio A. Poland's syndrome: case contribution and critical review of the literature. *Minerva Pediatr* 1985;37:691–695.
7. Baban A, Torre M, Bianca S, et al. Poland syndrome with bilateral features: case description with review of the literature. *Am J Genet A* 2009;149A(7):1597–1602.
8. Freire-Maia N, Chautard EA, Opitz JM, et al. The Poland syndrome: clinical and genealogical data, dermatoglyphic analysis, and incidence. *Hum Hered* 1973;23:97–104.
9. McGillivray BC, Lowry RE. Poland syndrome in British Colombia: incidence and reproductive experience of affected persons. *Am J Med Genet* 1977;1:65–74.
10. Mace JW, Kaplan JM, Schanberger JE, et al. Poland's syndrome: report of seven cases and review of the literature. *Clin Pediatr* 1972;11:98–102.
11. Bouvet JP, Leveque O, Bernetieres F, et al. Vascular origin of Poland syndrome. *Eur J Pediatr* 1978;125:17–26.
12. Bavinck JN, Weaver DD. Subclavian artery disruption sequence: hypothesis of a vascular etiology for Poland, Klippel-Feil, and Möbius anomalies. *Am J Med Genet* 1986;23:903–918.
13. Pisteljic DT, Vranjesevic O, Apostolski S, et al. Poland syndrome associated with "Morning Glory" syndrome. *J Med Genet* 1986;23:364–366.
14. Sackey K, Odone V, George SL, et al. Poland's syndrome associated with childhood non-Hodgkins lymphoma. *Am J Dis Child* 1984;138:600–601.
15. David TJ. Nature and etiology of the Poland anomaly. *N Engl J Med* 1972;287:487–489.
16. Perez AJM, Urbano J, Garcia Laborda E, et al. Breast and pectoralis muscle hypoplasia. A mild degree of Poland's syndrome. *Acta Radiol* 1996;37(5):759–762.
17. Spear SL, Pelletiere CV, Lee ES, et al. Anterior thoracic hypoplasia: a separate entity from Poland syndrome. *Plast Reconstr Surg* 2004;113:69–77.
18. Baker JL, Mara JE. Simultaneous correction of the chest wall deformity and prosthetic augmentation mammoplasty in a case of Poland's syndrome. *Br J Plast Surg* 1976;29:347–351.
19. Hodgkinson OJ. Chest wall implants: their use for pectus excavatum, pectoralis muscle tears, Poland's syndrome, and muscular insufficiency. *Aesthet Plast Surg* 1997;21:7–15.
20. Argenta LC, VanderKolk C, Friedman R, et al. Refinements in reconstruction of congenital breast deformities. *Plast Reconstr Surg* 1985;76:73–80.
21. Berrino P, Santi PL. The permanent expandable implant in breast aesthetic, corrective, and reconstructive surgery. *Eur J Plast Surg* 1991;14:63–68.
22. Ohmori K Takada H. Correction of Poland's pectoralis major muscle anomaly with latissimus dorsi musculocutaneous flaps. *Plast Reconstr Surg* 1980;65:400–404.
23. Hester TR, Bostwick J. Poland's syndrome: correction with latissimus muscle transposition. *Plast Reconstr Surg* 1982;69:226–233.
24. Urschel He, Byrd HS, Sethi SM, et al. Poland's syndrome: improved surgical management. *Ann Thorac Surg* 1984;37:204–211.
25. Santi P, Berrino P, Galli A. Poland's syndrome: correction of thoracic anomaly through minimal incisions. *Plast Reconstr Surg* 1985;76:639–641.
26. Garcia VF, Seyfer AE, Graeber GM. Reconstruction of congenital chest-wall deformities. *Surg Clin North Am* 1989;69(5):1103–1118.
27. Fujino T, Harashina T, Aoyagi F. Reconstruction for aplasia of the breast and pectoral region by microvascular transfer of a free flap from the buttock. *Plast Reconstr Surg* 1975;56:178–181.
28. Longaker MT, Glat PM, Colen LB, et al. Reconstruction of breast asymmetry in Poland's chest wall deformity using microvascular free flaps. *Plast Reconstr Surg* 1996;99(2):429–436.
29. Versaci A. Refinements in reconstruction of congenital breast deformities [Discussion]. *Plast Reconstr Surg* 1985;76:81–82.
30. Cochran JH Jr, Pauly TJ, Edstrom LE, et al. Hypoplasia of the latissimus dorsi muscle complicating breast reconstruction in Poland's syndrome. *Ann Plast Surg* 1981;6:402–404.
31. Coleman SR, Saboeiro AP. Fat grafting to the breast revisited: safety and efficacy. *Plast Reconstr Surg* 2007;119(3):775–785; discussion 786–787.

CHAPTER

122

Scott L. Spear
Mark L. Venturi

Augmentation With Periareolar Mastopexy

Despite decades of use, breast augmentation with periareolar mastopexy remains a complex and controversial subject. According to some, augmentation with periareolar mastopexy represents a disproportionate number of legal problems in plastic surgery. Whether this is because it is a commonly performed procedure or because it is a procedure prone to mischief is hard to tell. This operation comes into play because many women who seek breast augmentation, in fact, would benefit from a mastopexy to achieve a reasonable result without the use of an overly large implant. Certainly one of the difficulties with augmentation with periareolar mastopexy has been its use either when it was not required or, on the other hand, when it was of insufficient power to solve the problem. This chapter, therefore, will focus on the indications for augmentation with periareolar mastopexy as well as the techniques of marking and surgical execution. We finish up with a discussion of complications, revision surgery, and medical legal issues.

The ideal indication for augmentation with periareolar mastopexy is the patient who seeks a breast augmentation but has too much ptosis on the one hand for augmentation alone but, on the other hand, too little ptosis to justify a more extended mastopexy. From the outset, part of the difficulty in picking the right patient for this operation has to do with inadequate tools for measuring breast ptosis.

Historically, breast ptosis was most commonly described according to Paula Regnault's classification of ptosis as: glandular ptosis, mild ptosis, moderate ptosis, and severe ptosis. Glandular ptosis, or pseudoptosis, was when the nipple was above the inframammary fold but the breast overhung the inframammary fold. Grade I (mild) ptosis was a nipple at the fold, grade II (moderate) was the nipple 1 to 3 cm below the fold but on the anterior surface of the breast, and grade III (severe) ptosis was the nipple more than 3 cm below the fold and pointing toward the patient's feet. This basic classification technique, however, did not take into account the size of the breast, the amount of skin on the breast, the position of the nipple in relationship to the breast gland, and, finally, the relationship of the breast gland to the chest wall. Depending on the size of the breasts and the amount of excess skin in the breast, it would be conceivable for a periareolar mastopexy to be satisfactory for a patient with moderate ptosis and the nipple below the fold, but be inadequate for a patient with mild ptosis and the nipple at the fold. The final decision regarding whether to perform a mastopexy and what kind of mastopexy to perform depends on the total surface area of breast skin and volume of the breast. Essentially, ultimately one must tailor the skin of the breast to fit the size of the newly enlarged breast, which includes both the current breast volume or parenchyma and the added volume from the implant. Thus, for a B-cup breast, 7 cm of skin between the nipple and inframammary fold may be sufficient, but for a D-cup breast, 10 cm of skin may be needed between the nipple and the inframammary fold.

As a general guideline, a mastopexy is not required when the nipple is above the inframammary fold or the areola is above the lower border of the breast such that there is unpigmented skin visible on the frontal view below the areola and there is no more than 2 to 3 cm of breast overhanging the inframammary crease. For a 4-cm-diameter nipple, this would mean that there would be approximately 6 cm of skin available between the nipple and the inframammary fold prior to the placement of an implant. Thus, there would be 6 cm of skin between the nipple and the fold to cover the surface of the newly enlarged breast including the current breast parenchyma and the breast implant volume.

A periareolar mastopexy is most appropriate for the patient where the nipple is near the inframammary fold, either just above, at, or slightly below the inframammary fold, the lower edge of the areola sits at the lower border of the breast when seen from the frontal view, and there is no more than 4 cm of breast overhanging the inframammary fold. This scenario would typically yield 6 to 8 cm of skin from the nipple to fold particularly when combined with a periareolar mastopexy.

Again, as a general guideline, when the nipple is at the bottom of the breast or pointing inferiorly, the nipple is below the inframammary fold by more than 2 cm, and the breast overhangs the inframammary fold by more than 4 cm, then either a vertical or a Wise pattern-type mastopexy would be appropriate and necessary to adequately tailor the breast skin to the new breast volume without distorting the nipple/areola shape.

It is one of the unique features of augmentation with a periareolar mastopexy that most often it does not make sense to do the mastopexy first in these patients because the mastopexy is part of a tailoring process to fit the breast skin and the nipple to the newly enlarged breasts. However, where there is doubt, it is acceptable to perform the augmentation first, preferably through a periareolar incision, and to hold off the mastopexy until a later date once the new breast has taken shape.

TECHNIQUE

One of the interesting features of augmentation with periareolar mastopexy is the marking and the positioning of the nipple. Almost all breast surgery begins with the same standardized marks including drawing the midline, marking the inframammary folds, and drawing the meridian of the breast through the nipple and across the inframammary fold (Fig. 122.1A). A good way to check the appropriate height of the nipple is to pinch the upper edge of the areola on the patient who is sitting in the upright position and then lifting that skin up onto the breast itself to determine visually where the upper edge of the areola would best fit (Fig. 122.1B). This should be done at the same time as pulling down gently on the upper breast skin because when the nipple is sutured to the upper breast skin, it will tend to pull that skin down slightly. Again, in many patients, the nipple will need to be located 4 to 6 cm above the existing inframammary fold, which means that the upper edge of the areola will ultimately be 6 to 8 cm above the inframammary fold.

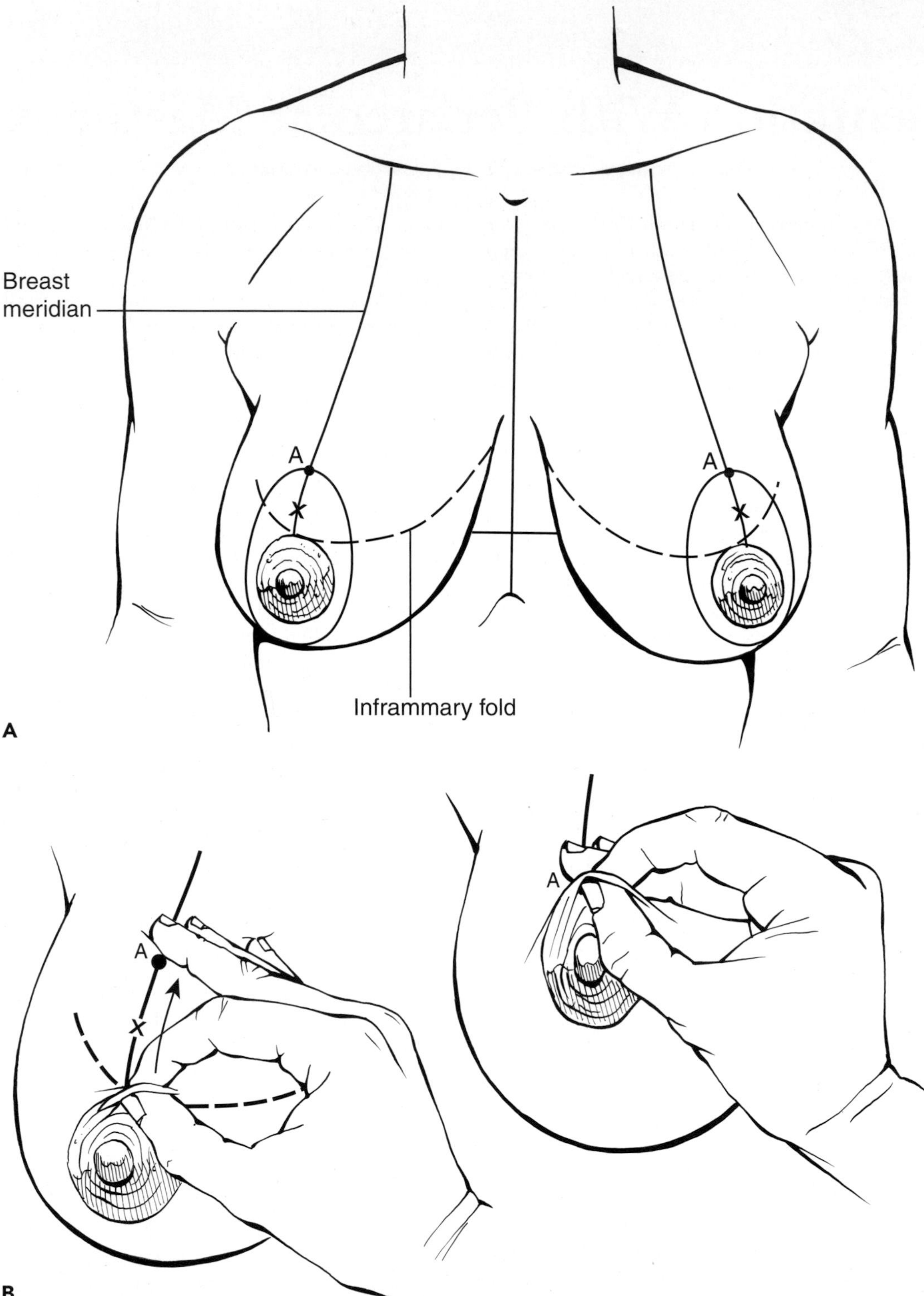

Figure 122.1. **A:** Marking the patient. The inframammary fold (IMF) and breast meridian are marked first. Point X represents the new nipple position. It is often marked 4 to 6 cm above the IMF. Point A represents the top of the areola located 6 to 8 cm above the IMF. **B:** Tailor-tacking. The desired upper border of the areola can be defined by lifting the edge of the areola between the thumb and index finger and pinning it on the upper breast.

Although in breast reduction, siting the nipple at the inframammary fold or just above is often appropriate, in augmentation with periareolar mastopexy, the nipple should be located a minimum of 4 cm above the inframammary fold to allow adequate distance between the nipple and the fold once the implant has been placed. In some cases, the nipple may actually be located at as much as 5 cm or even 6 cm above the inframammary fold when performing augmentation with periareolar mastopexy. The sites of the new nipple location and the new upper edge of the areola are marked on the breast meridian. Medially and laterally, as a rule, minimal excess skin is removed and the lines are drawn so they diverge just around the areolar borders. Inferiorly, one must assess how much skin is desirable between the lower edge of the areola and the inframammary fold. Often this mark is just at the lower border of the old areola, but in some cases it may be slightly lower. After this point is drawn, an oval or somewhat circular pattern can be drawn around the existing areola. These marks are made indelibly on both sides with the patient in the upright position, and then the rest of the operation proceeds under either general anesthesia or sedation.

When there is doubt about whether to proceed with the mastopexy, the operation can begin with an augmentation done either through a periareolar incision (my preference) or through an inframammary or axillary incision. My preference is to perform these operations in the dual plane. That means that the pocket that is ultimately created is beneath the pectoralis major muscle in its uppermost portions but is subglandular in the lower 20% to 30% of the implant space. Going through the periareolar incision, dissection is carried out obliquely through the breast down toward the inframammary fold to damage as little of the breast parenchyma as possible (Figs. 122.2 and 122.3). After the plane between the breast and the chest wall muscles is encountered, the subglandular portion of the dissection is performed in the lowermost 20% to 30% of the anticipated pocket (Fig. 122.4). This always exposes the lower edge of the pectoralis major muscle, which is then grasped with an Allis clamp, and a subpectoral dissection is carried out superiorly, medially, and laterally. Particular attention must be paid to avoid getting beneath the pectoralis minor or serratus muscles laterally. Likewise, care should be taken not to overdissect the pectoralis major muscle medially. The pectoralis major muscle is released entirely across its lower portion but is not released along the sternal border (Fig. 122.5).

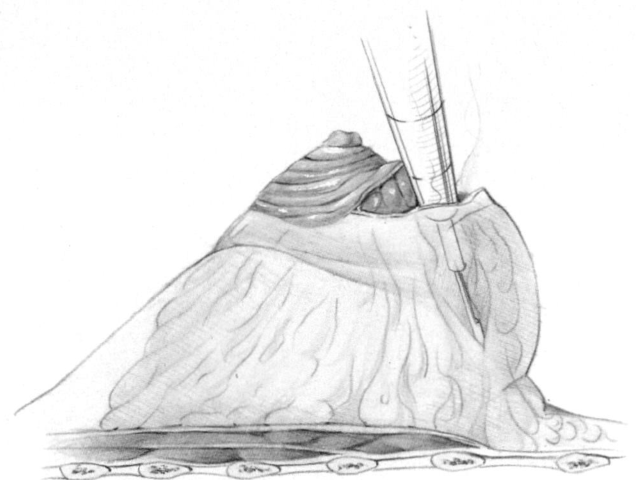

Figure 122.3. An oblique dissection is performed through the breast parenchyma to the lateral pectoral border. An adequate inferior flap thickness is essential to cover the implant.

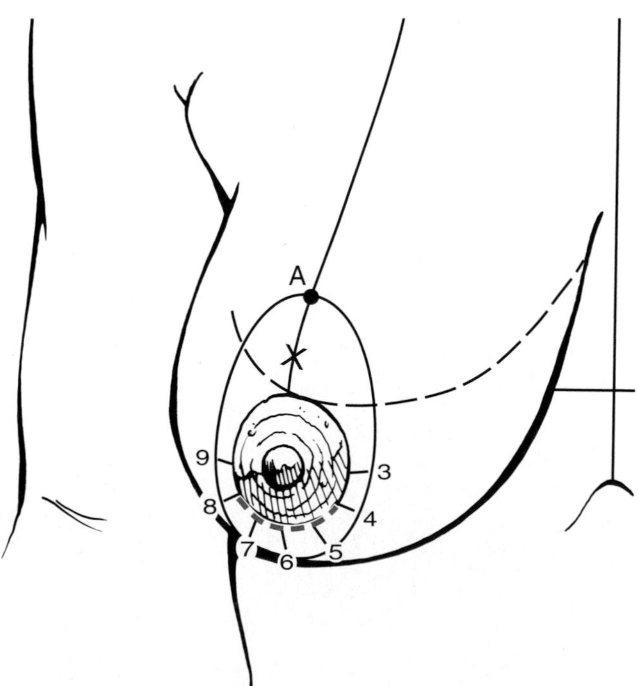

Figure 122.2. The periareolar incision for the augmentation is made from 4 to 8 o'clock on the lower border of the areola. This hides the incision for the augmentation while maximizing surgical access if the mastopexy is not completed.

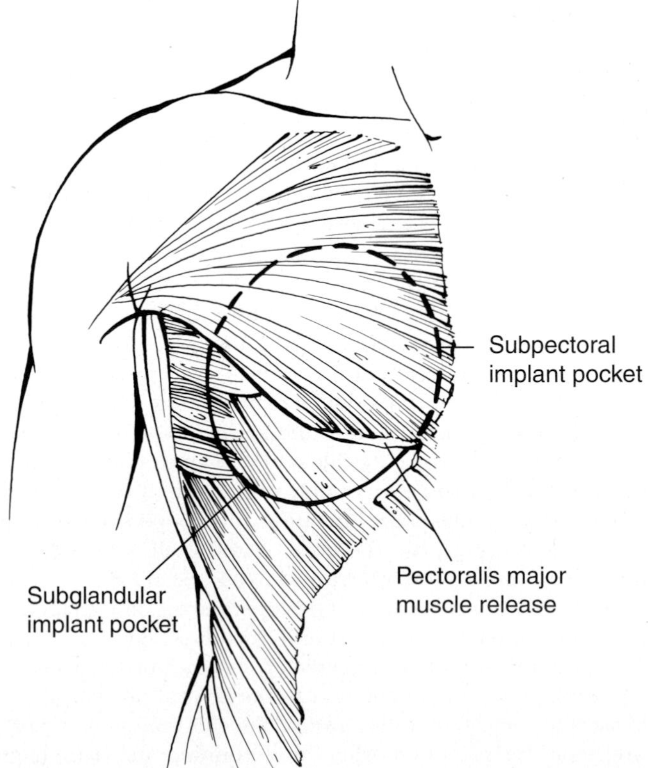

Figure 122.4. The dual-plane implant pocket is outlined.

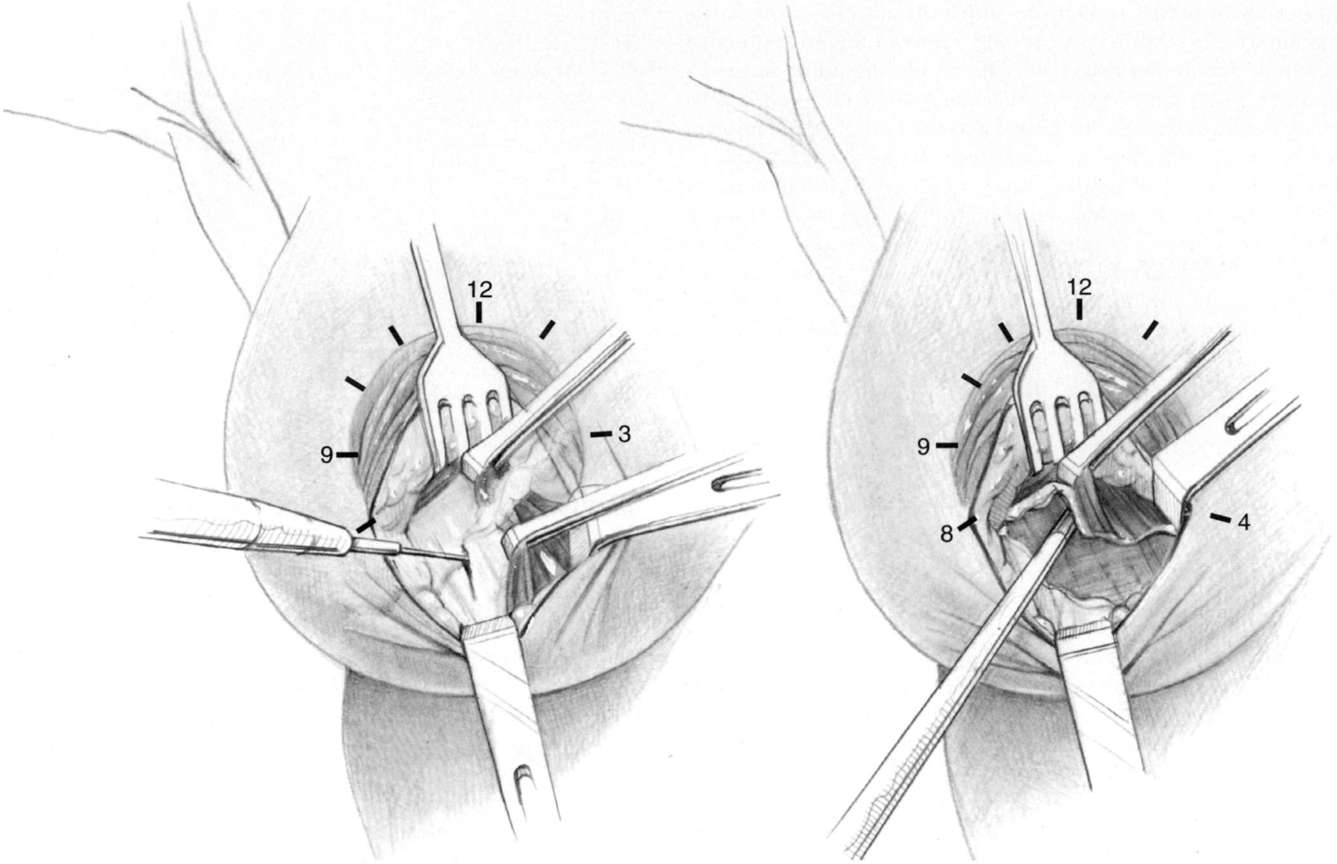

Figure 122.5. The subpectoral dissection commences along the lateral pectoral border and extends across the entire lower edge.

Ultimately, a confluent pocket is made which joins the pectoralis major dissection superiorly and a subglandular dissection inferiorly. The definitive implant or a sizer is then placed through the periareolar incision or through whichever incision was used. In those cases when proceeding with the mastopexy was uncertain, the patient can then be sat upright and the nipple-areola tailor tacked into the previously marked locations to assess their validity or to check whether any adjustments need to be done. In patients with whom one is more confident about the marking, the de-epithelialization can be performed first, reducing the areola down to a diameter of 38 to 42 mm.

As a rule, one should be conservative in the initial de-epithelializing and skin excision until the implant is placed. Thus, it is possible that one would mark out a conservative and less conservative option in the original plan and not commit to the most aggressive plan until after the implant was in. Assuming there is sufficient skin laxity, the final implant is placed and either filled, if it is saline, or simply positioned, if it is silicone. When doing the dual-plane operation, it is not possible to close the muscle or fascia, but the breast gland itself is closed over the implant with several interrupted 3–0 PDS sutures.

One of the critical aspects of this operation is understanding the blood supply to the breast and skin flaps. Because of the placement of an implant immediately beneath or subjacent to the breast gland, the circulation to the central portion of the breast is to some extent diminished. For this reason, particular care must be exercised when undermining the skin flaps around the areola so as not to further injure the blood supply to the nipple. Thus such undermining should be kept to a minimum and should not dive into the breast gland itself but stay quite superficial just beneath the skin of the surrounding breast (Fig. 122.6).

When performing periareolar mastopexy, in most cases a blocking suture or pursestring suture is used taking advantage of a permanent suture of Gore-Tex, Ethibond, Mersilene, or

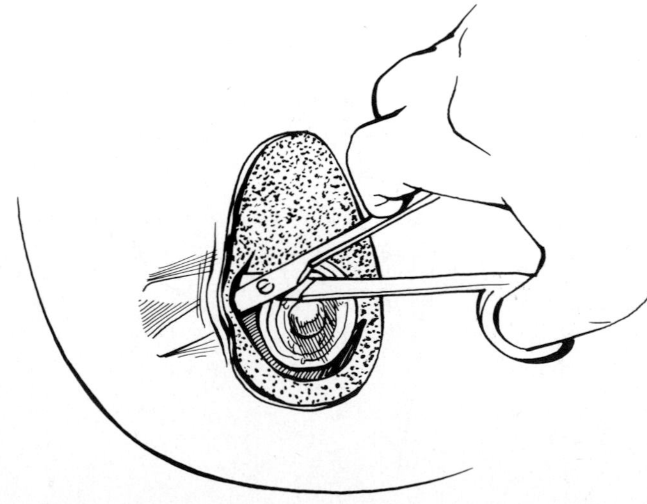

Figure 122.6. The periareolar skin is de-epithelialized and the breast skin is undermined minimally and superficially so as not to disturb the blood supply to the nipple.

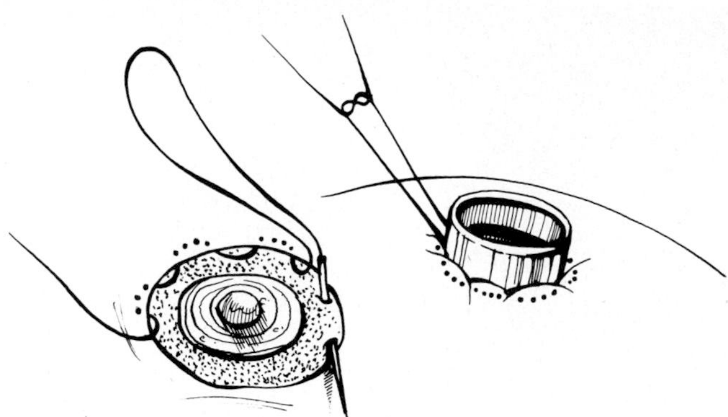

Figure 122.7. The periareolar mastopexy is closed with a pursestring closure using Gortex or Mersiline on a straight needle. The suture is cinched down around a cookie cutter. Use of the straight needle allows the suture to stay along the cut dermal edge, minimizing the scalloping of the breast skin edge.

other permanent material. To achieve the best result, a dermal fringe is left along the margins of the skin excision so that the pursestring suture is actually placed in that dermal fringe (Fig. 122.7). Thus, the pursestring suture is not placed at the skin edge, but 4 or 5 mm more central to the excision along the dermal fringe edge. This suture is placed with a straight needle to minimize scalloping and is then initially tied around a 38-mm cookie cutter so that the aperture that has been created is ultimately about 38 to 42 mm. The edge of the areola is then closed to the actual cut skin edge with interrupted and running intradermal 3–0 or 4–0 Monocryl sutures. If the procedure is performed technically correctly and if the patients are chosen appropriately, there should be minimal to no scalloping of the skin edges even at the time of primary closure. Thus, there is little reason to wait until such scalloping resolves over time because such scalloping is not allowed to occur even at the time of surgery (Figs. 122.8 and 122.9).

COMPLICATIONS

The most common complications with this operation include excessive widening of the areola, excessive flattening of the breast, poor scars around the areola, asymmetry of nipple position, undercorrection of nipple ptosis, overcorrection of nipple ptosis, asymmetry, total loss or partial loss of the nipple, and infection or extrusion of the implant. By prudent application of this operation to patients who have only moderate ptosis and who fit our criteria and by following our guidelines in terms of marking and picking patients, most of these complications should be minimal or avoidable. Poor planning or overzealous application of this technique in poor candidates is more likely to lead to severe complications.

REVISIONS

In our hands, most revisions from this operation deal with adjusting the height of the nipple (Fig. 122.10) on either side to achieve better symmetry, revising scars that are overly wide or thick, and adjusting the size of the areola on one or both sides to avoid an areola that is excessively widened (Figs. 122.11 and 122.12). Such scar revisions may in some cases even require converting the periareolar scar to a periareolar scar with a short dart on the inferior

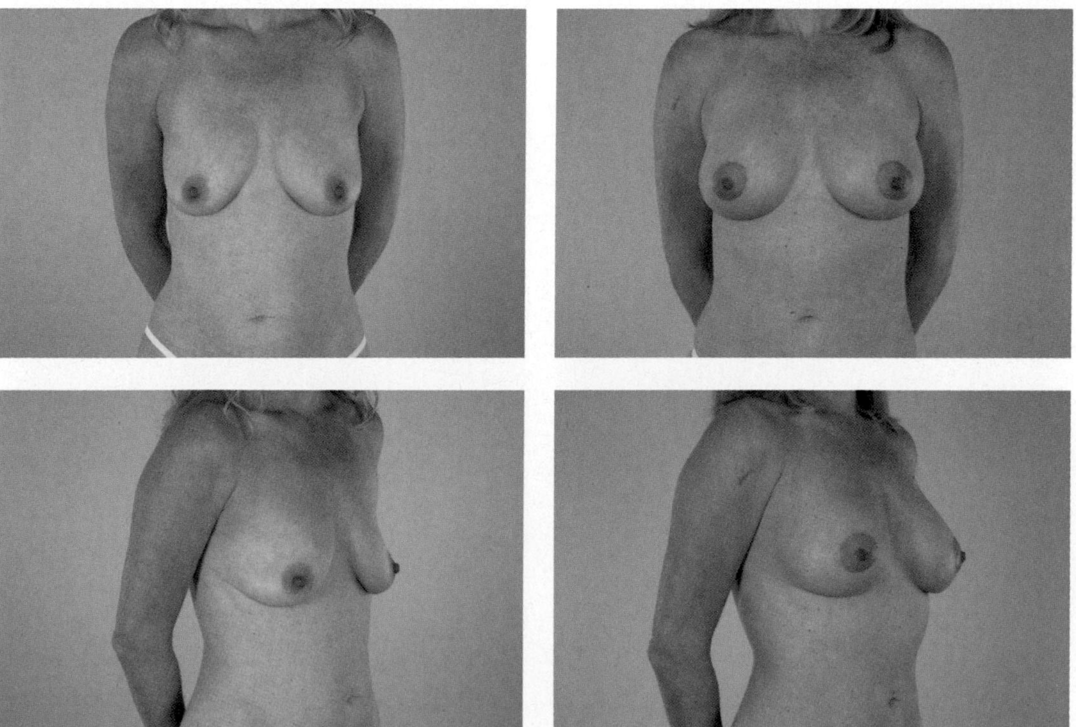

Figure 122.8. A 44-year-old woman who had first-degree breast ptosis with the nipple located at the inframammary fold. She underwent breast augmentation with 200-cc Inamed, McGhan Style 40 silicone gel–filled implants and periareolar mastopexy. Postoperative pictures were taken after 1 year.

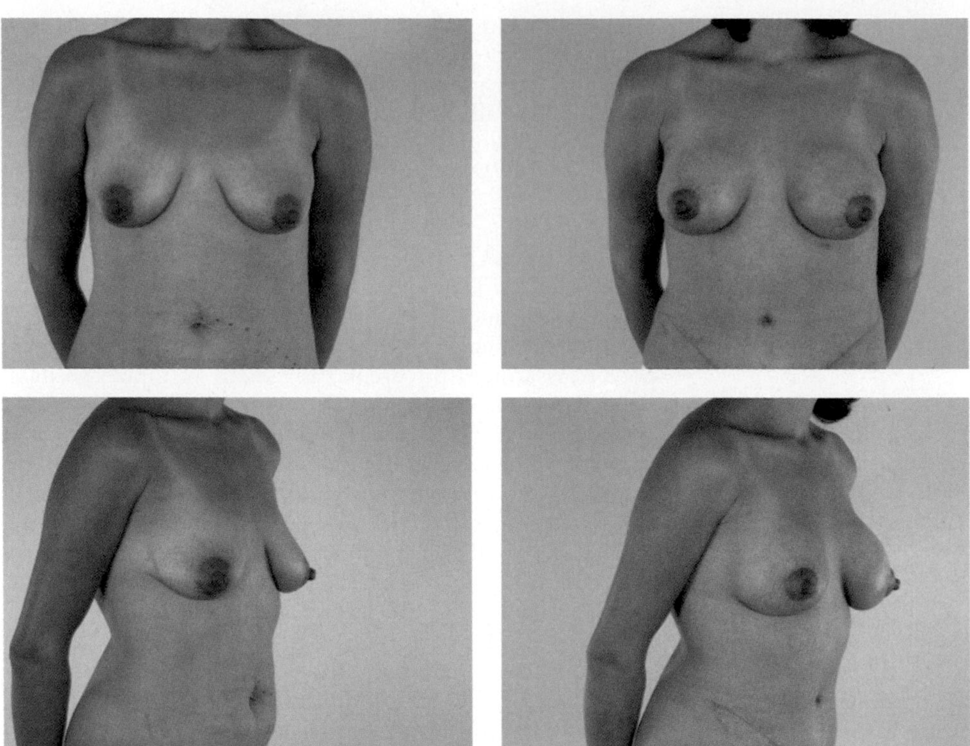

Figure 122.9. A 40-year-old woman who had second-degree breast ptosis with the nipple located 2 cm below the inframammary fold. She underwent breast augmentation with 210-cc Inamed, McGhan Style 68 round saline-filled implants and periareolar mastopexy. Both implants were filled to 230 cc. Postoperative pictures were taken after 1 year.

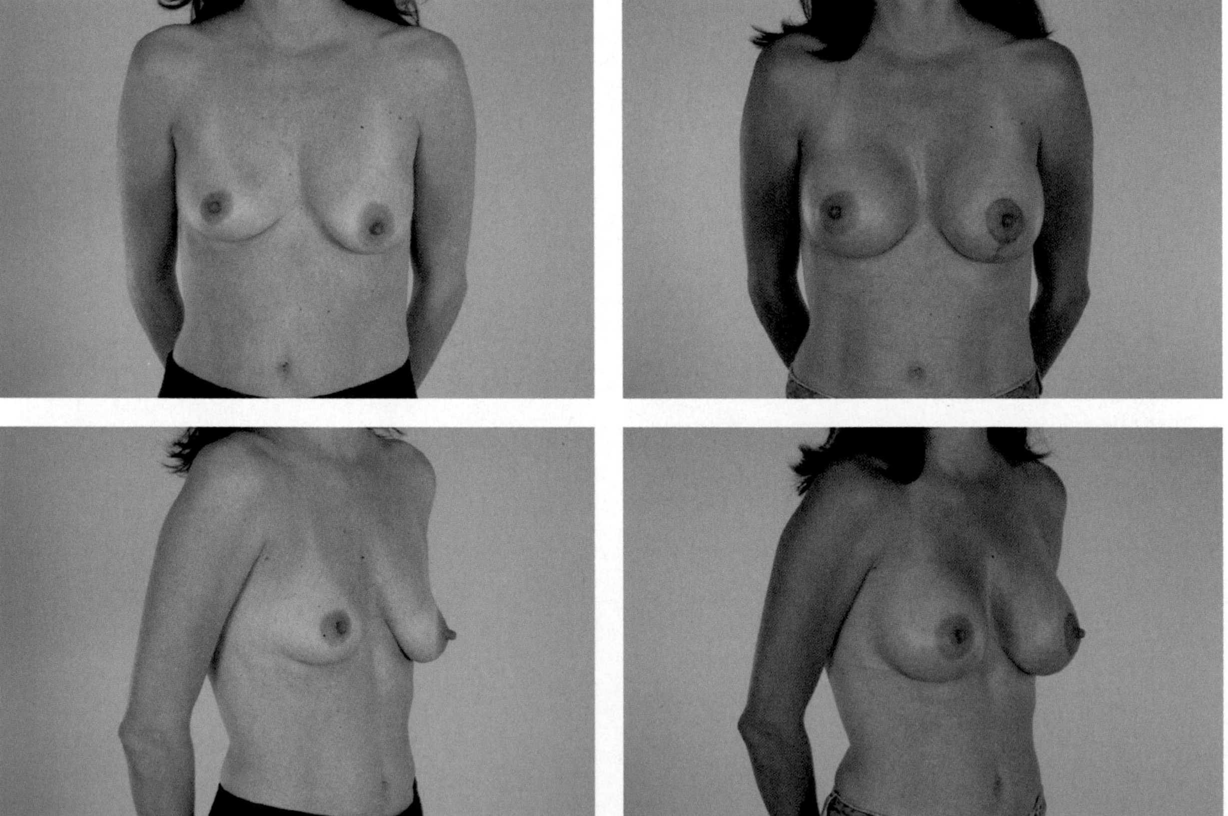

Figure 122.10. A 38-year-old woman who presented with breast asymmetry. The patient underwent breast augmentation with a 300-cc Inamed, McGhan Style 68 round saline-filled implant on the right filled to 305 cc and a 250-cc Inamed, McGhan Style 68 round, low-profile saline-filled implant on the left filled to 245 cc. On the left, a vertical mastopexy was performed to correct her excess skin envelope and nipple height. In this case, a short vertical scar helped to control the size and width of the areola. Postoperative photos were taken after 3 months.

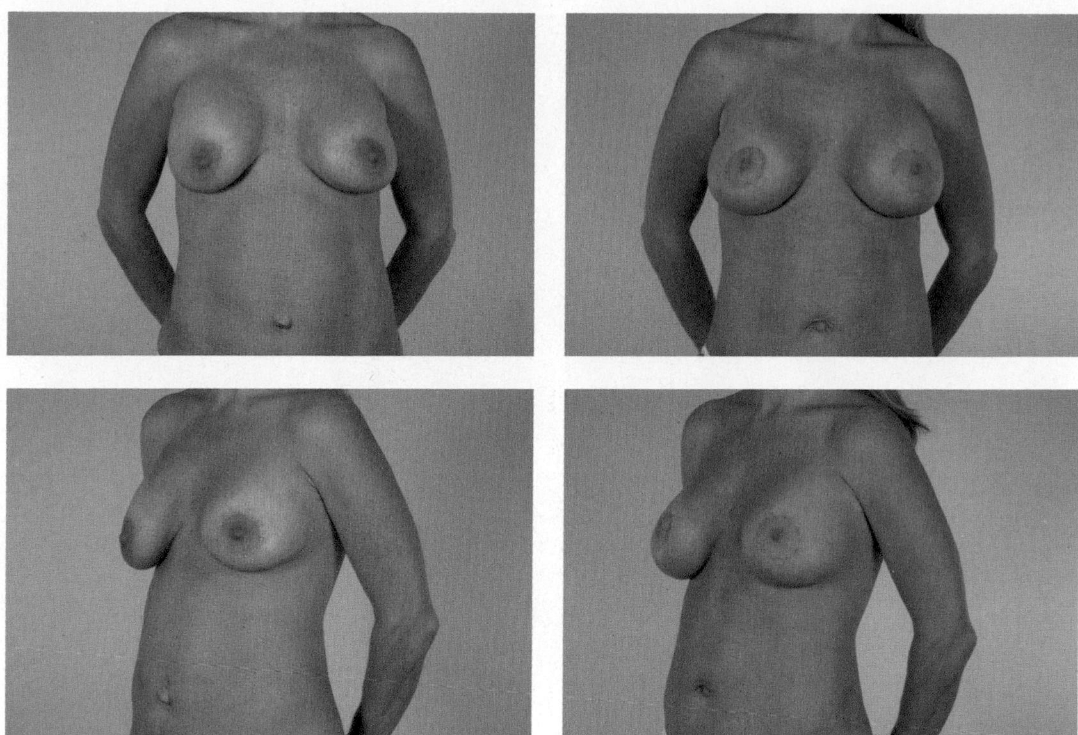

Figure 122.11. A 32-year-old woman who had a previous breast augmentation elsewhere with periareolar mastopexy presented with residual ptosis. This patient underwent reaugmentation with 420- to 450-cc Inamed, McGhan Style 68 round saline-filled implants and repeat periareolar mastopexy. Both implants were filled to 450 cc. Postoperative pictures were taken after 3 months.

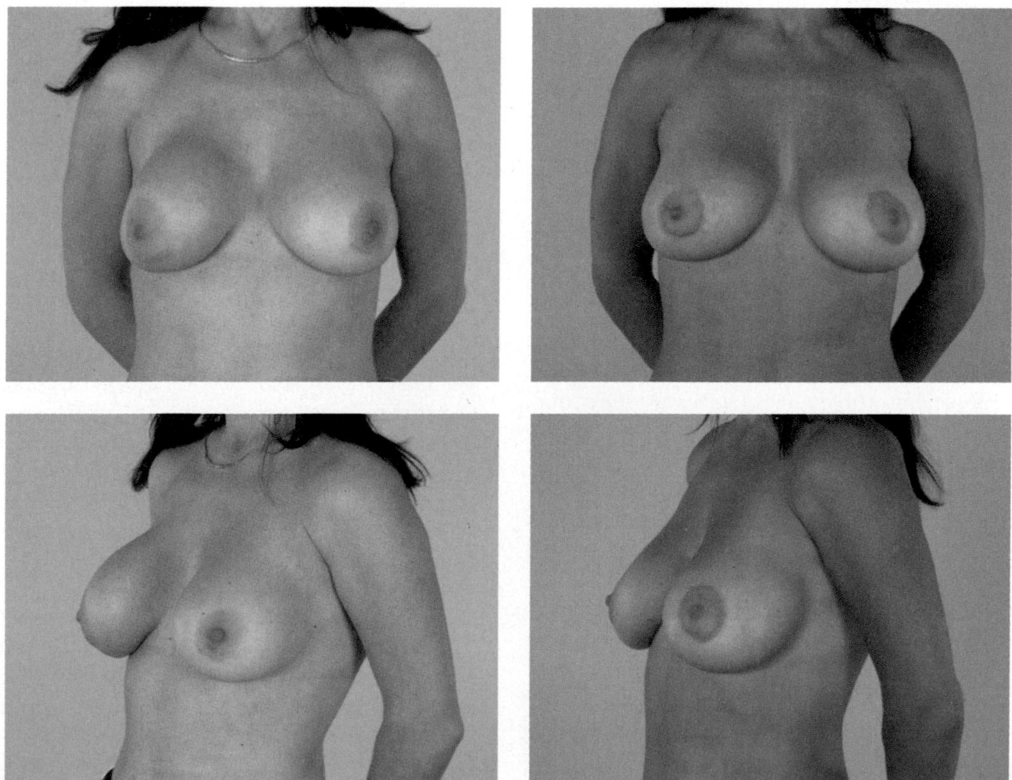

Figure 122.12. A 45-year-old woman who had previously undergone two subglandular breast augmentations elsewhere presented with capsular contracture and nipple asymmetry. This patient underwent bilateral capsulectomy, reaugmentation in a "dual-plane" subpectoral pocket using her existing implants, and periareolar mastopexy. Postoperative photos were taken after 1 year.

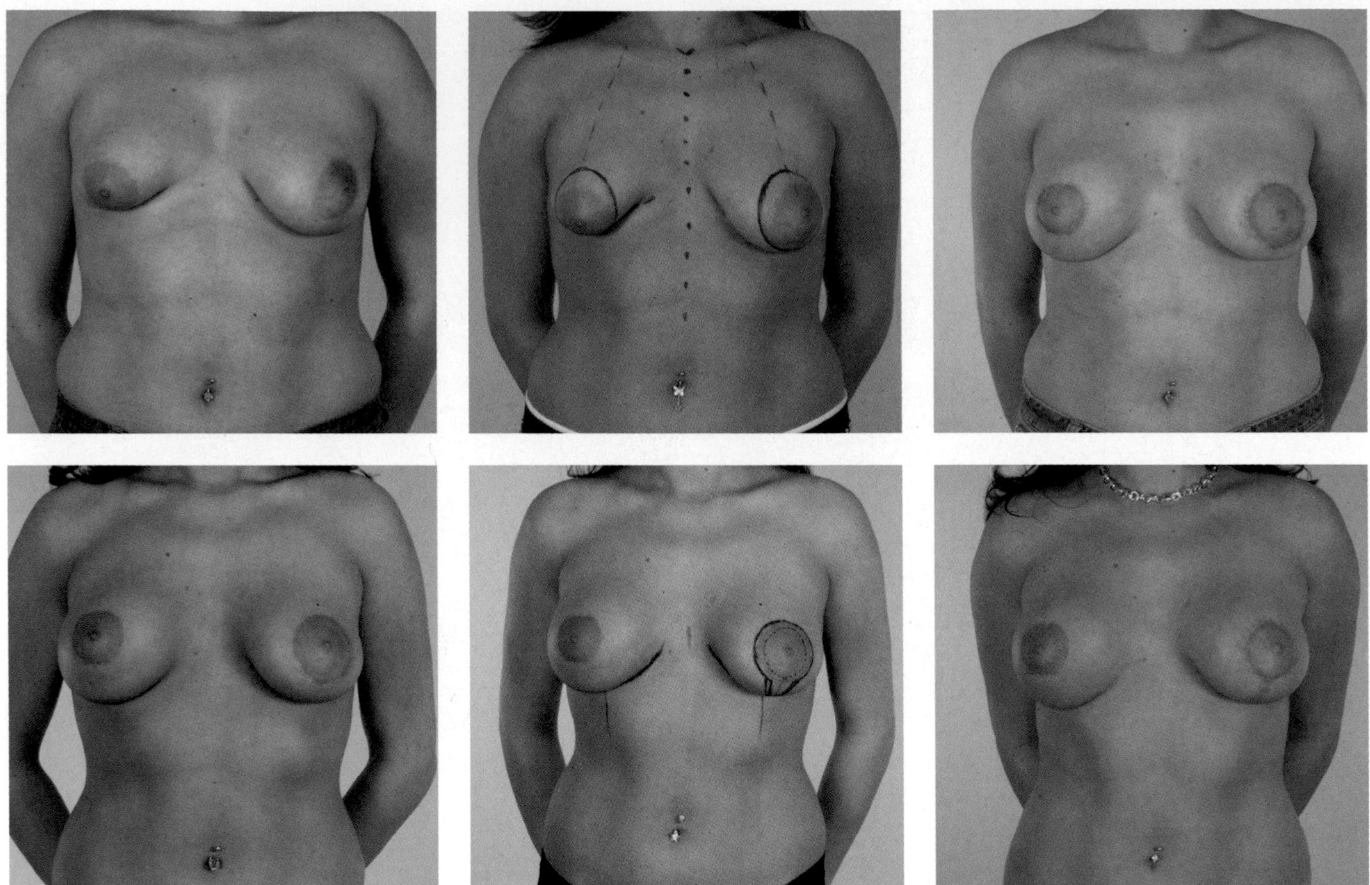

Figure 122.13. A 19-year-old woman who presented with a tuberous breast deformity on the right and an estimated 60-g-larger left breast with second-degree ptosis with the nipple located 2 cm below the inframammary fold. The upper row demonstrates the patient's initial surgery consisting of breast augmentation with Mentor, Spectrum Style 1400, 350- to 1450-cc adjustable saline-filled implants and periareolar mastopexy. The right implant was filled to 325 cc and the left implant was filled to 260 cc. Postoperatively the patient developed widening of the left areola and required a left vertical mastopexy to correct the asymmetry. The stages of the second procedure are shown in the bottom row. Final postoperative pictures were taken after 3 months.

vertical axis. The addition of the short dart along the inferior axis helps to control the width of the areola and avoids excessive widening of the pigmented areolar skin (Fig. 122.13).

From the legal perspective, we can only encourage surgeons to be careful about patient selection and not to, on the one hand, use this operation in patients who do not need a mastopexy, and, on the other hand, rely on this operation in patients who need a more aggressive procedure. In terms of operative technique, proper respect for the blood supply to the nipple-areola is critical. Conservative skin excision without excessive tension on the skin closure should help avoid overflattening of the nipple, a widened areola, or bad scars. Finally, it would be helpful for physicians performing this operation to provide suitable informed consent to patients about the important legal aspects.

EDITORIAL COMMENTS

Drs. Venturi and Spear nicely review the indications and technique for breast augmentation with periareolar mastopexy. They correctly highlight the complexities of this operation and the risk for poor outcomes when it is performed under suboptimal indications. Historically, this combination of procedures has been fraught with morbidity that has included complex scars, flattening of the point of maximal projection of the nipple-areolar complex, and irregular breast contour because of the circumareolar mastopexy. In fact, at one time, this operation was associated with a very high incidence of legal activity due to patient dissatisfaction. Despite these risks, the combination of breast augmentation and mastopexy is becoming more popular in certain geographic locations as a means of improving breast volume, projection, and contour. This increase in popularity is in part due to a better understanding of the indications and techniques that have reduced the morbidity and enhanced patient satisfaction. In this chapter, the authors provided critical information and various tips for avoiding the pitfalls associated with this operation.

Other points that merit note are that the mastopexy can be performed in a crescent or circumareolar fashion depending on the amount of lift that is necessary. In addition, the use of a silicone gel implant is permissible given the Food and Drug Administration guidelines that are currently in place. It is always recommended to insert and fill the implant prior to performing the mastopexy. It is important not to overresect the skin envelope because that will distort the contour and result in an unhappy patient. A tailor-tack approach will often keep one out of trouble.

M.Y.N.

SUGGESTED READINGS

Bartels RJ, Strickland DM, Douglas WM. A new mastopexy operation for mild or moderate breast ptosis. *Plast Reconstr Surg* 1976;57:687–691.

Benelli L. A new periareolar mammaplasty: the "round block" technique. *Aesthetic Plast Surg* 1990;14:93–100.

De la Fuente A, Martin del Yerro JL. Periareolar mastopexy with mammary implants. *Aesthetic Plast Surg* 1990;16:337–341.

Elliott LF. Circumareolar mastopexy with augmentation. *Clin Plast Surg* 2002;29:337–347.

Gonzales-Ulloa M. Correction of hypotrophy of the breast by exogenous material. *Plast Reconstr Surg* 1960;25:15–26.

Handel N. Augmentation mastopexy. In: Spear SL, ed. Surgery of the Breast: Principles and Art. Philadelphia, *PA: Lippincott-Raven*, 1998:921–937.

Karnes J, Morrison W, Salisbury M, et al. Simultaneous breast augmentation and lift. Aesthetic *Plast Surg* 2000;24:148–154.

Owsley JQ Jr. Simultaneous mastopexy and augmentation for correction of the small, ptotic breast. *Ann Plast Surg* 1975;2:195–201.

Persoff MM. Vertical mastopexy with expansion augmentation. *Aesthetic Plast Surg* 2003;27:13–19.

Puckett CL, Meyer VH, Reinisch JF. Crescent mastopexy and augmentation. *Plast Reconstr Surg* 1985;75:533–539.

Regnault P. The hypoplastic and ptotic breast: a combined operation with prosthetic augmentation. *Plast Reconstr Surg* 1966;37:31–37.

Spear SL. Augmentation/mastopexy: "surgeon, beware." *Plast Reconstr Surg* 2003;112:905–906.

Spear SL, Davison SP. Breast augmentation with periareolar mastopexy. *Oper Techn Plastic Reconstr Surg* 2000;7:131–136.

Spear SL, Giese SY. Simultaneous breast augmentation and mastopexy. *Aesthetic Surg J* 2000;20:155–165.

Spear SL, Giese SY, Ducic I. Concentric mastopexy revisited. *Plast Reconstr Surg* 2001;107:1294–1299.

Spear SL, Kassan M, Little JW. Guidelines in concentric mastopexy. *Plast Reconstr Surg* 1990;85:961–966.

CHAPTER

123

Dennis C. Hammond

Augmentation Mastopexy: General Considerations

INTRODUCTION

Augmentation mastopexy has proven to be one of the most difficult breast procedures plastic surgeons currently perform. There are several reasons for this. First is the fact that nearly every variable that determines the ultimate shape of the breast is being manipulated to some degree, including breast position, inframammary fold location, breast skin envelope surface area, position of the nipple-areola complex (NAC), and breast volume. All of this is performed through the most limited scar pattern possible, and it must all be done so as to create the same result on each side, despite the fact that more often than not there was preoperative asymmetry to start with. Second is that the procedure is an aesthetic operation, and patient expectations are generally exceedingly high and tolerance for complications low. Lastly, the procedure involves the use of breast implants in all their various sizes, shapes, compositions, and textures, and all of the potential complications associated with the use of breast implants also come into play. Given all of these variables, which must be managed to optimal effect, it would seem that augmentation mastopexy would be a daunting task. However, when each of the most common potential pitfalls associated with the procedure is analyzed, sound surgical solutions geared toward complication avoidance can be developed. The end result is a consistent, reliable approach that can be applied to any patient seeking an improved breast appearance via augmentation mastopexy.

PATIENT SELECTION

In most instances the decision to perform the augmentation is the most straightforward of all the decisions involved because a general size increase to the breast is desired by most patients. What becomes difficult to gauge is when a mastopexy will be required to obtain the most aesthetic result. Certainly a small degree of persistent ptosis may be tolerated by some patients, especially when the alternative is additional scars from mastopexy (Fig. 123.1). However, generally speaking, when the location of the nipple is at or below the level of the fold, some type of mastopexy will be required to achieve an acceptable result. All that needs to be determined at that point is what type of skin envelope procedure will be required to both lift the NAC and reshape the breast. This skin tightening can range from a simple periareolar procedure, to a circumvertical approach, and finally to a full inverted T-type procedure. One caveat to this approach relates to the inframammary fold. In patients who are just on the verge of needing a mastopexy, lowering the inframammary fold can position the breast implant lower on the chest wall just enough to restore harmony between the NAC and the breast mound, and thus avoid the need for additional scarring with the mastopexy. The effect of this strategy can be optimized when an anatomically shaped cohesive gel implant is used due to the fact that the upper pole of the breast can be reshaped without creating an excessive upper pole bulge (Fig. 123.2).

IMPLANT LOCATION

Where to place the breast implant with regard to the pectoralis major muscle remains a particular area of controversy in augmentation mastopexy. In evaluating how to best make this decision, it is helpful to ask, what is the breast implant designed to accomplish? The breast implant functions as a soft-tissue filler. The size, shape, consistency, and texture of the implant will all be chosen to help fill out the skin envelope to the best effect. To this end, any restricting force that prevents the breast implant from delivering the desired shape must be minimized. The pectoralis major is one such potential restricting force, along with previous scar in revisionary cases, and tight breast capsules in tuberous breast cases. To prevent such restriction, either the muscle is released along the inframammary fold when using a subpectoral pocket until no further lower pole tightness is present or a subglandular pocket can be used. Either strategy can be successful. It is advisable to use the partial subpectoral pocket in thin patients where the soft-tissue thickness of the upper pole is less than 2 cm because the muscle will help volumetrically to create a smooth contour in the superior pole of the breast and prevent an obvious step off between the implant and the chest wall. These patients must be informed, however, that there will be breast animation with pectoralis muscle contraction (Fig. 123.3). Although this is well tolerated by most patients, in many of the revisionary patients I see, this finding is a particular area of concern and a frequent source of overall dissatisfaction with their result. In patients who have adequate upper pole tissue thickness, it is my preference to use the subglandular pocket. With this strategy, the force of the implant is more directly delivered to the overlying soft tissue and a more effective lift effect is the result. Care must be taken to avoid injuring the medial intercostal perforators no matter which pocket is developed because these vessels are a vigorous source of vascularity for the breast (1). With the subglandular pocket, I have not observed any difference in the capsular contracture rate as compared to the partial subpectoral pocket, an observation that is likely due to improvements in implant construction over the last decade.

IMPLANT FILL AND SHAPE

As further evidence becomes available regarding the safety of silicone gel breast implants, restrictions on their use have

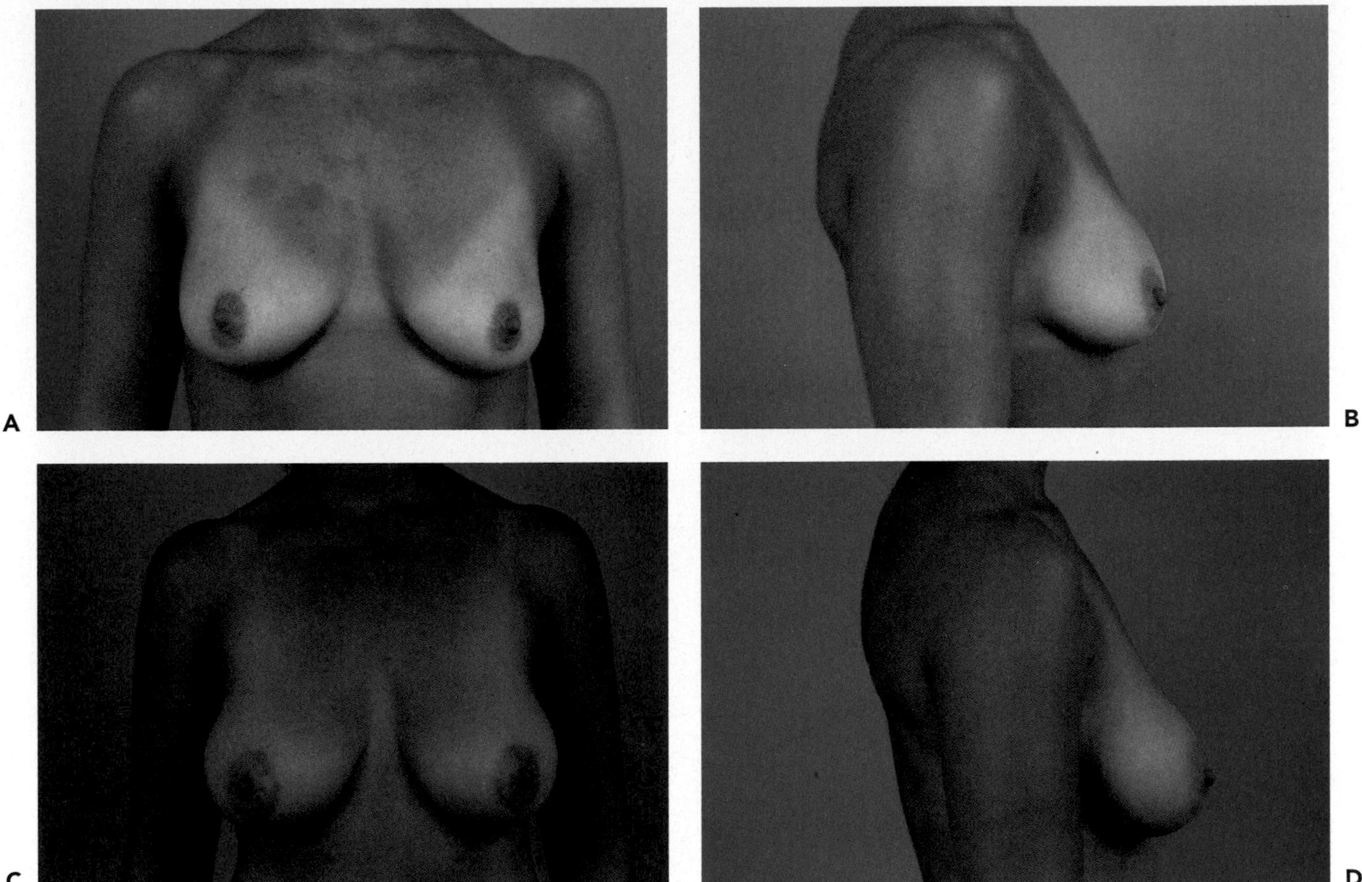

Figure 123.1. **A & B:** Preoperative appearance of a 35-year-old woman seeking breast augmentation. The patient declined any attempt at mastopexy due to concern over the cutaneous scars. Therefore the operative plan involved placing a smooth, round saline implant in the subglandular plane through an inframammary fold incision. **C & D:** Two-year postoperative appearance shows a pleasing breast contour with the nipple and areola centered at the most projecting point of the breast. Although the position of the breast is low on the chest wall, there is excellent breast fullness, and the overall aesthetics of the breast is good.

relaxed, and now gel implants can be used in conjunction with mastopexy according to the guidelines of several studies sponsored jointly by the Food and Drug Administration and the implant manufacturers. As a result, virtually any breast implant can reasonably be used in augmentation mastopexy. With such an assortment of available devices, experience has shown that certain observations can be made. For most patients, a smooth, round device, either saline or silicone, will provide an adequate shape to the breast (Fig. 123.4). Silicone gel, however, due to its increased cohesiveness and the ability to create "soft" wrinkles, can create a more natural-feeling result than saline. This difference will become more obvious in thinner patients where the implant makes up the major portion of the volume of the breast. In addition, in thinner patients, an anatomically shaped implant can create a more pleasing upper pole than a round implant. This difference between round and anatomic is more profoundly demonstrated in silicone gel devices as opposed to saline devices. Recent implant designs where a markedly cohesive gel is formed into an aggressive anatomic shape have produced outstanding results (Fig. 123.5). These types of devices are particularly useful in augmentation mastopexy where control of the upper pole of the breast can be difficult.

IMPLANT TEXTURE

Surface texturing of silicone gel breast implants was developed in an attempt to reproduce the outstanding results obtained with polyurethane-coated devices with regard to reducing the capsular contracture rate (2,3). The polyurethane effect was a biochemical one where gradual degradation of the foam lattice scaffold resulted in a chronic low-grade inflammatory response in the capsule. The net effect of this was to keep the capsule from contracting, although exactly how this occurred remains unknown. Unfortunately, surface texturing of silicone gel implants does not reproduce this same biochemical effect. This at least partly explains why clinical results with textured silicone gel implants have been mixed with regard to reducing the capsular contracture rate. Both textured and smooth devices can be used successfully in augmentation mastopexy depending on physician preference. What textured silicone surfaces do accomplish is a more active interface between the capsule and

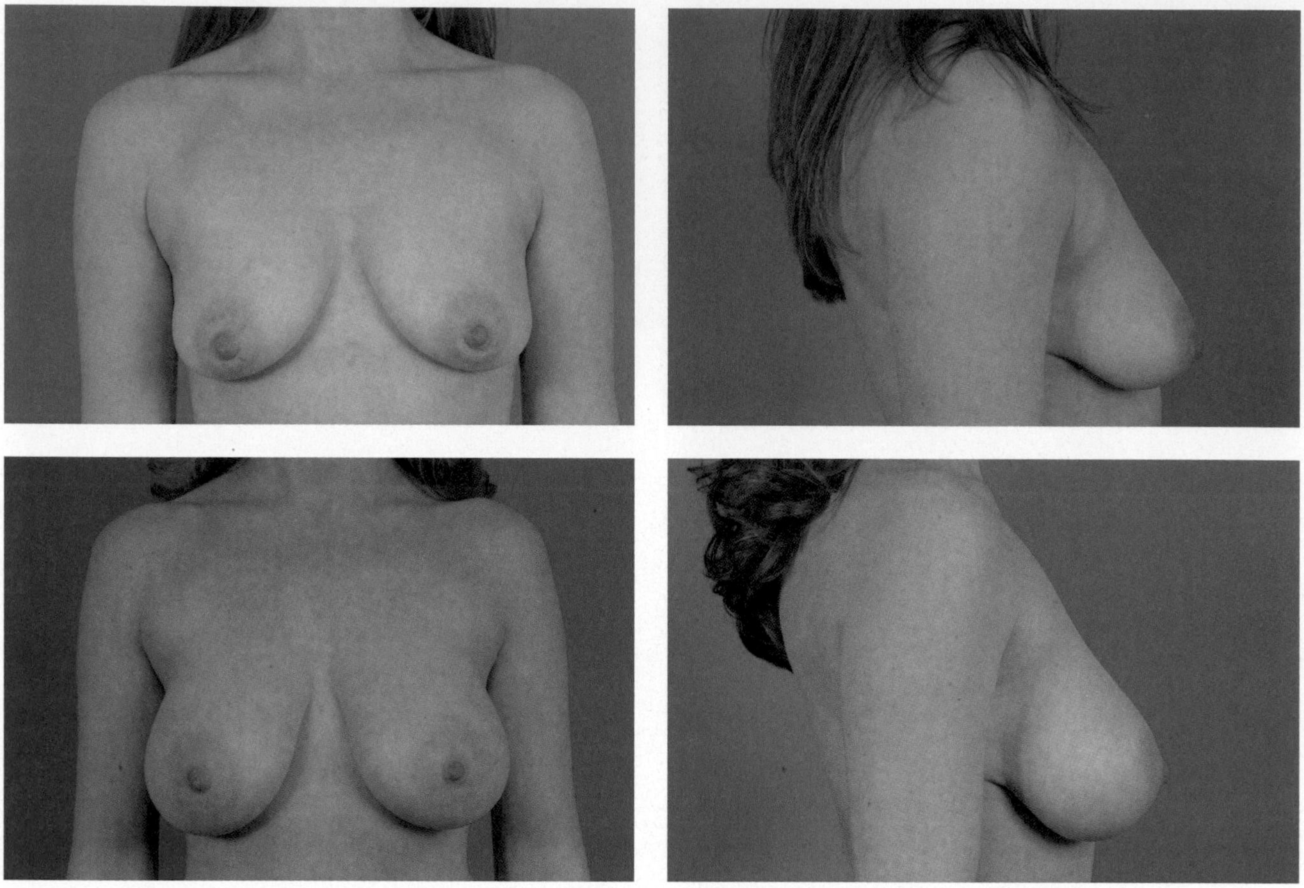

Figure 123.2. **A & B:** Preoperative appearance of a 35-year-old woman seeking breast augmentation. To avoid the need for mastopexy, the operative plan included placing a cohesive, shaped silicone gel implant in the subglandular space through an inframammary fold incision. During creation of the pocket, the inframammary fold was to be lowered to centralize the nipple and areola over the most projecting portion of the breast implant. **C & D:** One-year postoperative appearance after placement of a 395-cc implant shows a pleasing overall breast contour. The breast appears low on the chest wall; however, the nipple and areola are appropriately centered at the most projecting point of the breast due to judicious lowering of the fold. Using this strategy, one can avoid the cutaneous scars associated with mastopexy.

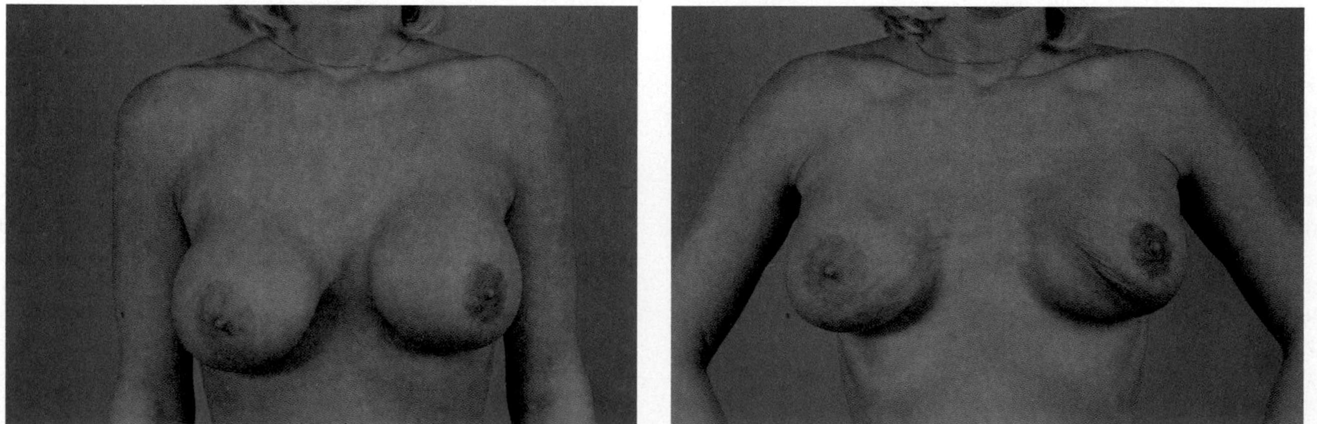

Figure 123.3. **A:** Postoperative appearance of a 27-year-old woman who underwent a previous periareolar augmentation mastopexy with a smooth, round saline implant in a partial subpectoral pocket. **B:** In addition to her overall dissatisfaction with the result, the animation present in the breast with contraction of the pectoralis major muscle was a particular area of concern.

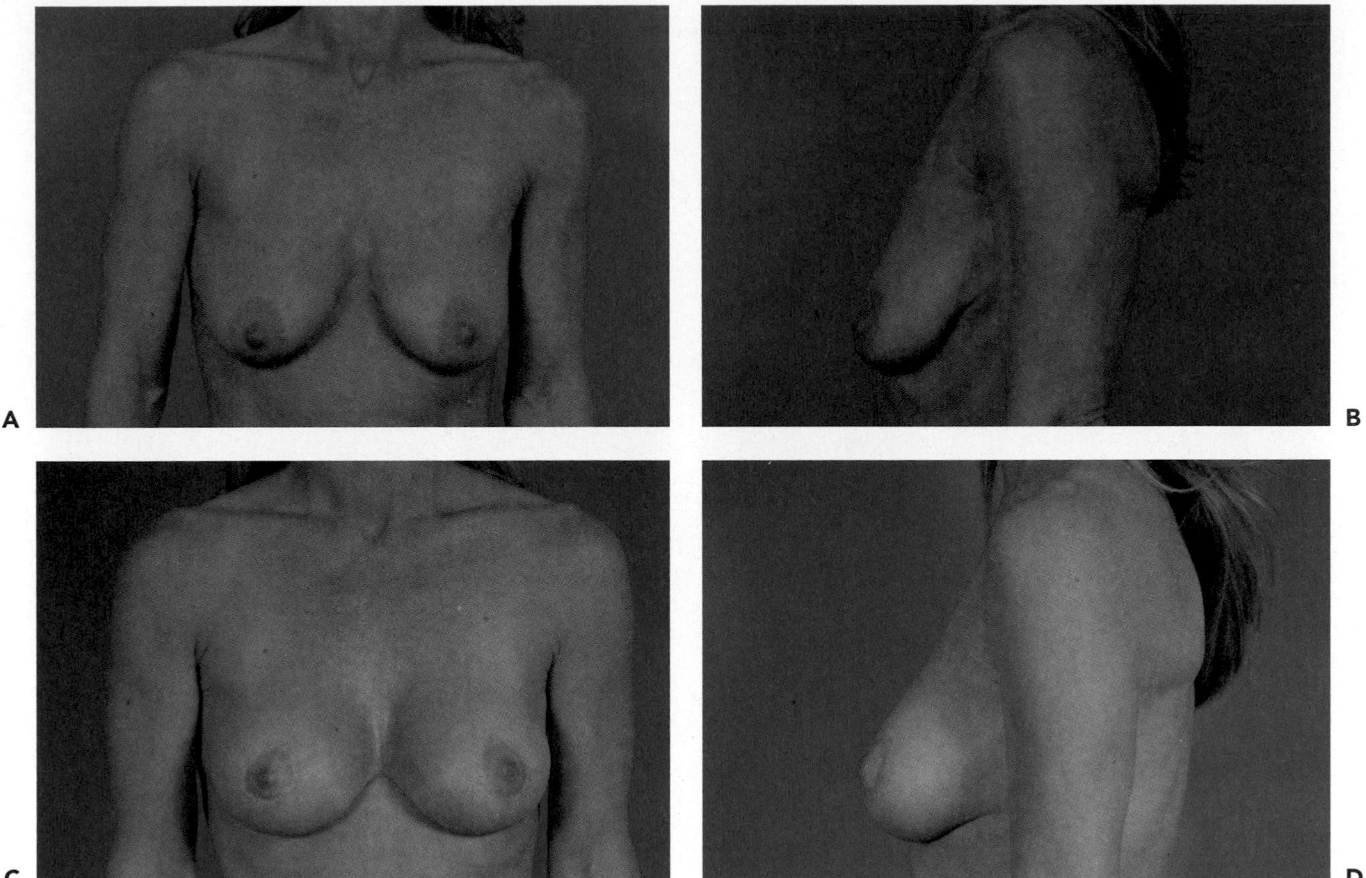

Figure 123.4. **A & B:** Preoperative appearance of a 40-year-old woman seeking mastopexy with breast augmentation. **C & D:** Six-month postoperative appearance after circumvertical mastopexy with the placement of a smooth, round gel implant in the subglandular space. Despite the significant degree of preoperative ptosis, the round implant has settled into the pocket to create an aesthetic upper pole without the creation of a sharp step-off.

the implant. At times, the capsule can actually "grow" into the more aggressively textured devices. Whether in-growth occurs or not, all textured surfaces provide increased friction between the implant and the capsule. This feature becomes important when using anatomically shaped devices because the interaction between the capsule and the implant surface can help to keep these asymmetric implants properly oriented and help resist rotation. For this reason, all anatomically shaped breast implants, whether saline or silicone, are manufactured with textured surfaces.

OPERATIVE SEQUENCE

When planning the operative sequence for performing augmentation mammaplasty, it is best to perform the augmentation first and then adjust the skin envelope to contour around the new breast volume. This strategy avoids the decidedly undesirable situation of overresecting skin such that the desired implant cannot be placed without tension, both on the breast skin envelope itself and more important on the areola. It is these circumstances, where excessive widening of the areola occurs, that can significantly detract from the ultimate overall result.

SKIN INCISION PATTERN

The various skin incision patterns used to manage the excessive skin envelopes in patients presenting for augmentation mastopexy are no different than in patients undergoing mastopexy alone. A gradual increase in the dimensions of the skin pattern design correlates with increasing ptosis of the breast and increasing breast skin envelope surface area. The major difference is that the added volume of the breast implant can change the requirements for skin management as opposed to mastopexy alone. This difference is critical to understanding how to avoid the unhappy circumstance of having resected too much skin when it is time to insert the implant.

The simplest mastopexy strategy involves using a periareolar approach where an asymmetric removal of skin above the NAC results in a lifting of the position of the NAC relative to the breast. The resulting periareolar scar usually heals well. In planning the procedure, care must be taken to adequately lift the NAC. The top of the periareolar pattern may be as high as 6 cm above the existing inframammary fold, depending on other factors that determine breast shape. When designing the oval it is best to limit the removal of medial and lateral skin to only that which is necessary to remove pigmented

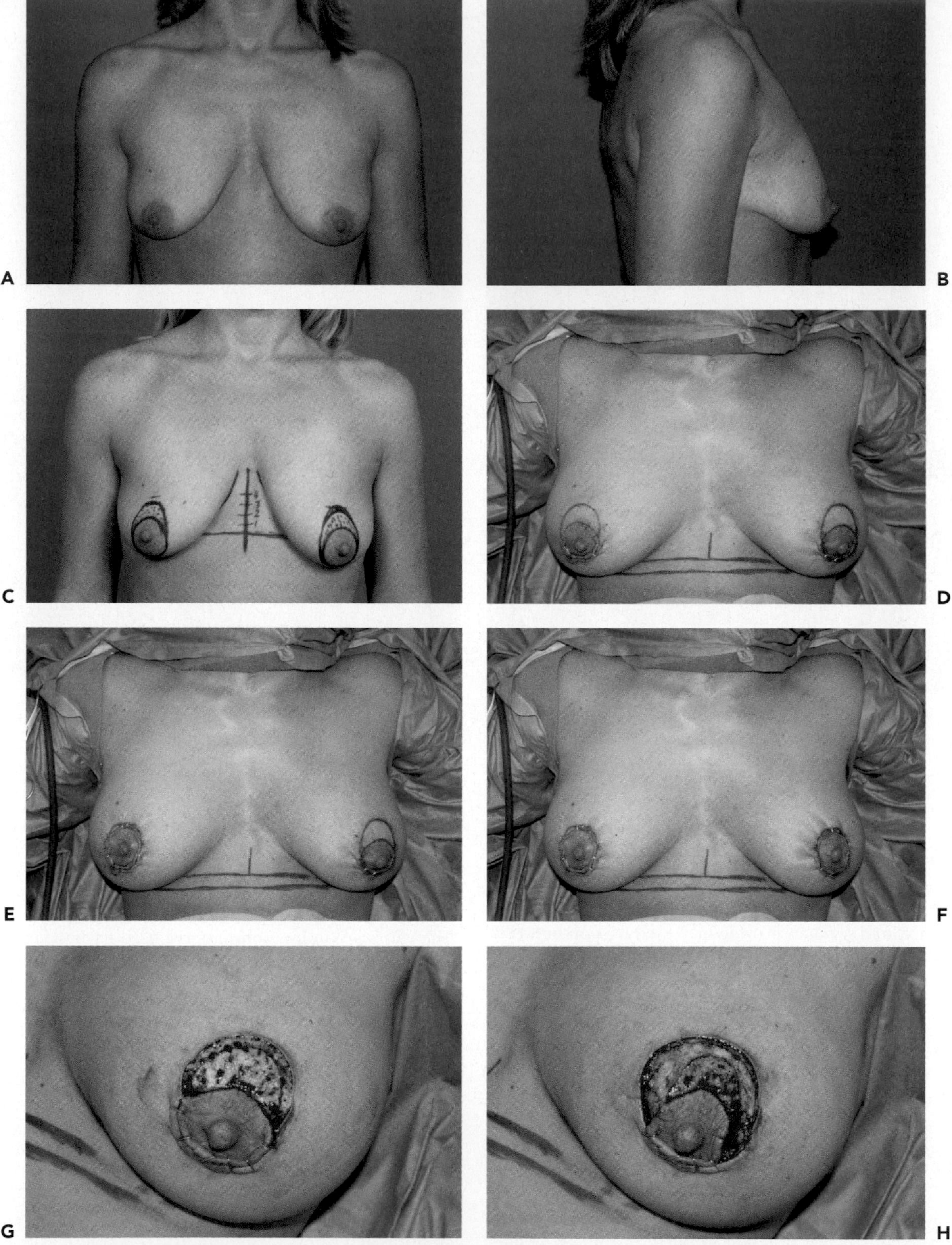

Figure 123.5. **A & B:** Preoperative anteroposterior and lateral views of a 28-year-old woman seeking augmentation mammaplasty. **C:** Preoperative marks demonstrate the degree of lift planned after placing a textured, cohesive gel anatomic implant in the subglandular plane. **D:** After placement of the implants, the position of the nipple and areola appears low. **E:** With the right areola temporarily stapled up into position, the degree of lift provided by the periareolar pattern can be estimated. **F:** After both sides have been plicated, an improvement in the appearance of the breast is evident. **G:** After confirming the degree of lift, the redundant areolar skin outside the areolar incision and inside the periareolar pattern is de-epithelialized. **H:** The dermis is then divided peripherally, leaving a small dermal shelf into which the purse string suture will be placed. (*continued*)

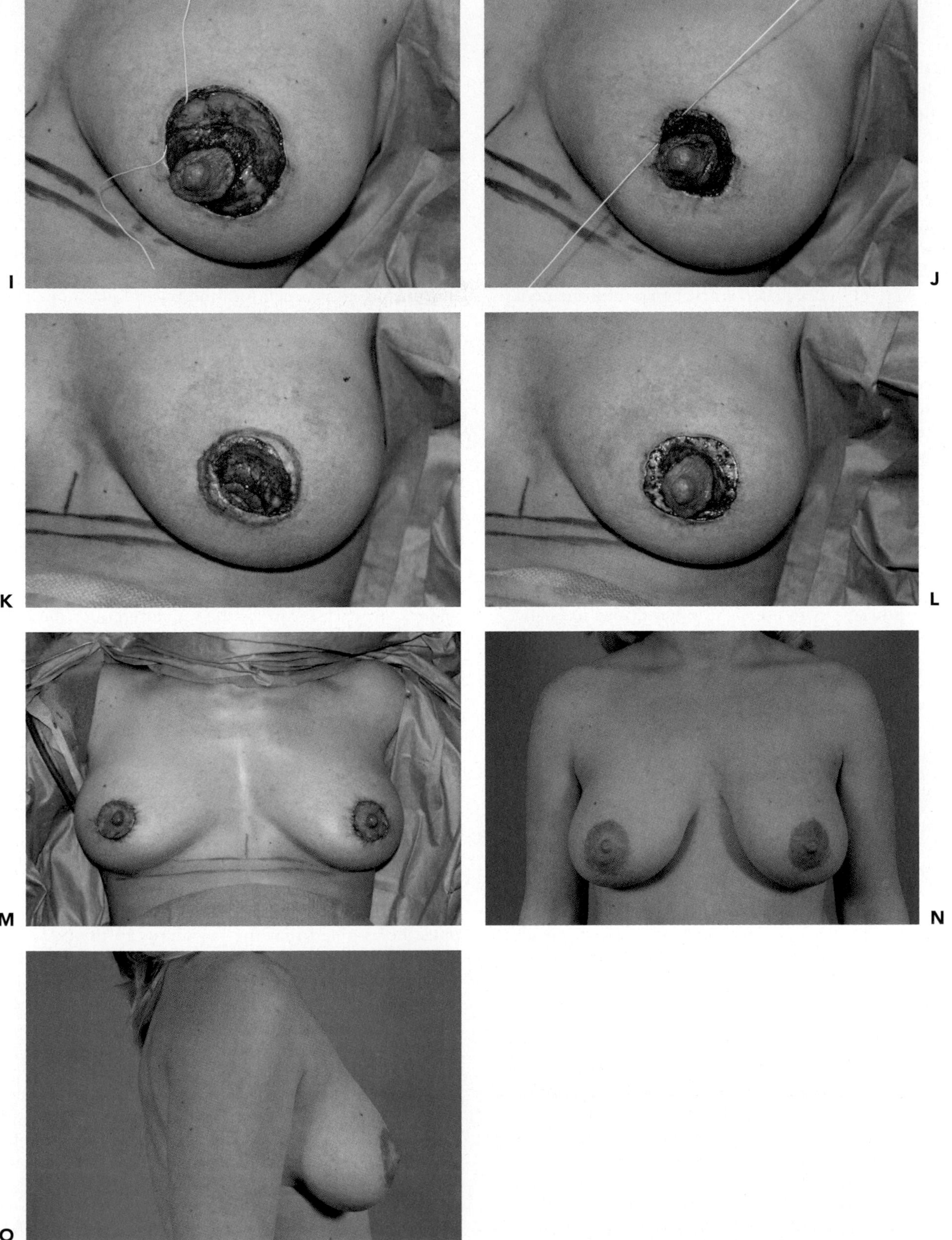

Figure 123.5. (*Continued*) **I:** A CV-3 Gore-Tex suture on a straight needle is passed within the dermal framework. **J:** The purse string suture is cinched down until the desired diameter is reached. **K:** The irregular defect is remarked as a circular pattern. **L:** The additional skin is de-epithelialized, with care being taken not to inadvertently cut the purse string suture. **M:** Immediate appearance after bilateral periareolar augmentation mastopexy. **N & O:** Result at 3 years postoperatively, and 6 months after delivering her first child. Despite the stress placed on the breasts postpartum due to lactation, no loss of breast shape is evident.

areolar skin (Fig. 123.5). This avoids skin overresection, which can create tension once the implant is inserted. An areolar diameter measuring 48 to 52 mm is diagrammed and incised centered on the existing areola, and the redundant skin between the areola and the periareolar incision is de-epithelialized. The dermis is divided circumferentially. leaving a 5-mm dermal shelf into which the eventual periareolar purse string suture will be placed. This shelf is undermined for 2 to 3 cm in all directions to allow the periareolar defect to be closed down by the periareolar purse string suture without tethering of the soft tissue. Access to the breast is easily made through this incision, usually through the lower half of the breast, and the implant is placed into the desired pocket. Although many different types of suture material may be used for the periareolar purse string, it is my preference to use a CV-3 Gore-Tex suture on a straight Keith needle. This suture material is strong and permanent and has excellent handling qualities. The smooth surface of the suture allows it to pass easily through the dermal shelf as the periareolar defect is cinched down, thereby allowing the dimension of the periareolar opening to be easily controlled. The guiding Keith needle is passed around the periareolar defect directly in the previously dissected dermal shelf. This suture is started by passing the needle from deep to superficial and ends by passing from superficial to deep. In this manner the knot will be buried deeply under the dermis, thereby reducing the risk of exposure. An opening diameter of 36 to 40 mm is created with this approach. It is necessary to use eight to ten throws to finally secure the knot and prevent it from slipping. Once the defect is controlled and the suture cinched down, the knot is buried under the medial breast flap. If the residual defect is not perfectly circular at this point, additional skin is marked for de-epithelialization to create a circular opening and the areola is inset. This determination must be made with the patient in the upright position to accurately assess areolar shape. Because the areola was incised at 48 to 52 mm and the subsequent opening cinched down to 36 to 40 mm, there should be no tension on the periareolar closure, which can assist in creating a more natural-looking areola.

Many patients will be inadequately treated with only a periareolar incision pattern because the breast will have a flattened appearance and a wide, compressed base diameter. In these patients, the addition of a vertical skin plication can dramatically improve the appearance of the breast. By taking out skin along the inferior pole of the breast, the base diameter can be narrowed and the projection increased. In addition, the dimensions of the periareolar closure can be reduced, which places less stress on the periareolar closure. This circumvertical-type approach is one of the most powerful shaping maneuvers that can be applied in any breast case where there is an element of ptosis. The addition of the vertical segment can be planned in obvious cases where there will be continued redundancy of the inferior skin envelope with only a periareolar skin pattern, or, in less obvious situations, the vertical segment can be added after the periareolar pattern has been developed and the implant inserted. In a planned circumvertical approach, access to the breast is made through the proposed midpoint of the vertical skin incision. The pocket is developed, the implant inserted, and the periareolar plication tacked into position with temporary staples. With the patient upright, the redundant skin envelope is then plicated together, again with temporary staples, until a pleasing breast shape is created. A slight flattening of the lower pole is ideal to allow for a modest degree of skin accommodation postoperatively. The edges of the plication are marked, the staples removed, and the involved skin de-epithelialized. The vertical incision is closed in layers and the periareolar defect managed as noted previously (Fig. 123.6). In periareolar cases, where the need for the vertical component is uncertain, the periareolar portion of the procedure is performed as described, with access to the breast made through the periareolar incision. Once the implant is positioned, the NAC is tacked into position and the patient placed upright to assess the shape of the breast. If it is noted that tightening the lower-pole skin envelope at all improves the shape of the breast, it is my practice to proceed with the vertical plication. The effect of adding this skin plication on the shape of the breast is so powerful that it far outweighs the disadvantage of the creation of an additional scar. Of all the scars routinely used in breast surgery, the vertical scar tends to heal in a very inconspicuous fashion, which only reinforces its potential as a shaping maneuver (Fig. 123.7).

Finally, in extreme cases of skin excess, the inverted-T pattern can be useful. Here, the flaps are elevated, the implant inserted, and the remaining flaps wrapped around the resulting breast mound to create the desired shape. It is recommended that the initial skin pattern be marked conservatively because the added volume of the implant will need additional skin cover as opposed to cases of inverted-T mastopexy alone. Any excess skin can be retailored once the implant is inserted.

AUGMENTATION/MASTOPEXY REVISION

Revising the unsatisfactory augmentation mastopexy can be one of the most challenging and yet one of the most rewarding procedures performed on the breast. In most instances, all of the surgical techniques described previously will be utilized to some degree. However, there are several important additional considerations that must be taken into account to avoid further difficulty. In the previously operated breast, it must be assumed that the vascularity to the NAC has been compromised to some degree by previous incisions. It is critical to note these incisions and identify the location of the vascular pedicle to the NAC when designing both access to the implant and further skin envelope manipulation. To this end, previous operative notes can provide useful information. Direct contact with the previous surgeon can also help in the understanding of the altered vascular anatomy of the breast. In cases of continued uncertainty, it is best to avoid wide incision patterns and excessive undermining of the breast. In this fashion, the disastrous complication of NAC ischemia and slough can be avoided.

Generally speaking, scar tends to be a common element in creating unsatisfactory results. This includes both scar in the skin and scar in the capsule in the form of capsular contracture. If there is any degree of capsular contracture noted in any case of breast revision after augmentation mastopexy, it is far preferable to perform a complete capsulectomy and remove all the tethering scar than to try some lesser procedure such as a simple capsulotomy. In selected cases, it can actually be advantageous to leave the

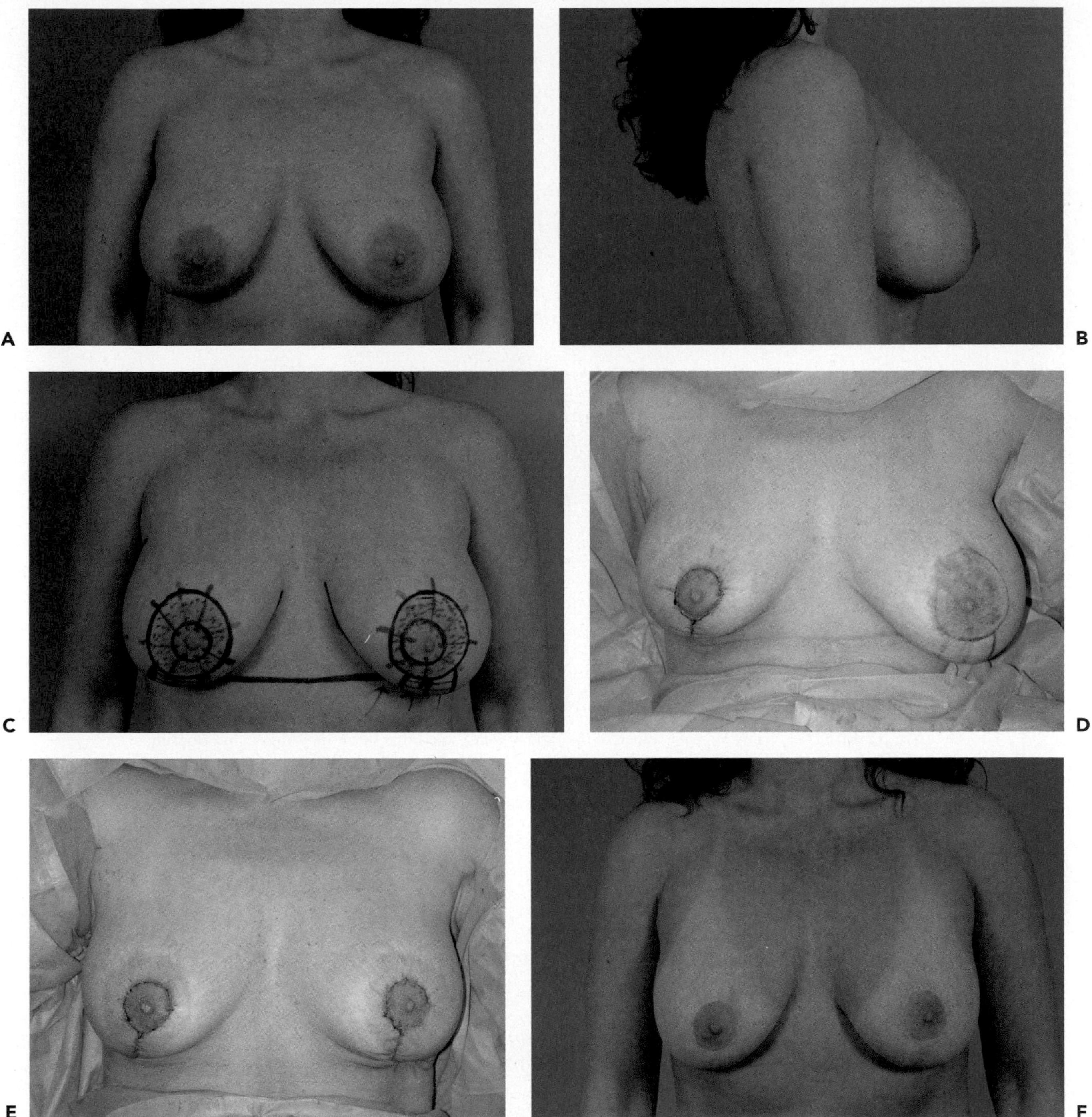

Figure 123.6. **A & B:** Anteroposterior and lateral appearance of a 34-year-old woman several years after prior breast augmentation with multiple implant exchanges. The patient is displeased with the size and shape of her breasts and the large diameter of her areolas. **C:** Preoperative marks showing the proposed circumvertical skin revision along with implant exchange. The areola diameter will be controlled with an interlocking Gore-Tex suture, and smaller, smooth, round saline breast implants will be inserted. **D:** The degree of reshaping can be seen after one side is completed as compared to the opposite breast. **E:** After both sides are completed, an immediate aesthetic result is obtained. **F & G:** Anteroposterior and lateral view of the completed result at 8 months postoperatively. A pleasing breast shape has been created, and the position of the nipple and areola is in harmony with the remainder of the breast. (*continued*)

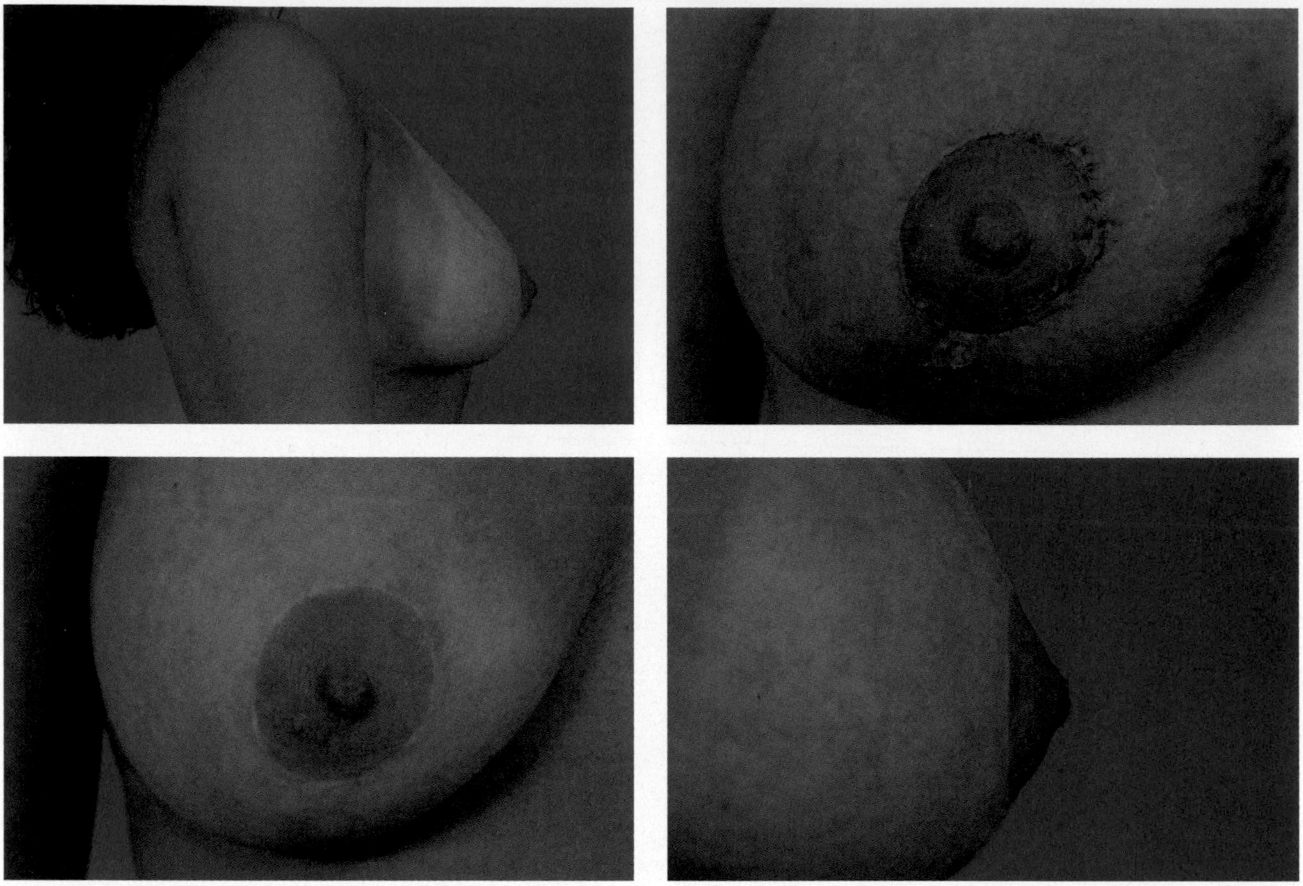

G H I J

Figure 123.6. (*Continued*) **H:** Appearance of the right areola 1 week after revision using the interlocking Gore-Tex technique. **I & J:** Appearance of the right areola 8 months after placement of the interlocking purse string suture. There has been minimal expansion of the areolar diameter, and the shape has been maintained due to the structural support of the suture locking the areola to the periareolar skin closure.

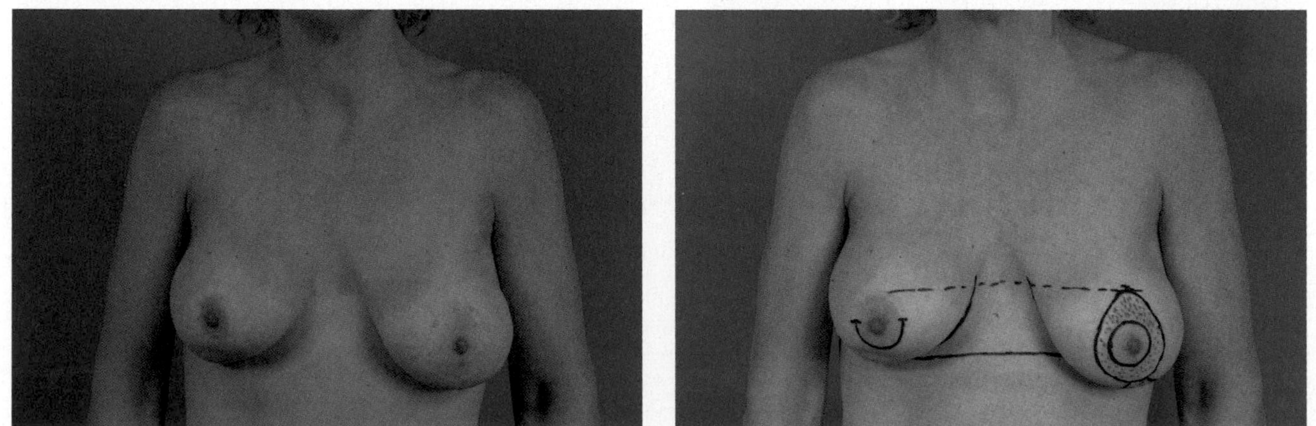

Figure 123.7. **A:** Preoperative appearance of a 42-year-old woman after previous periareolar augmentation mastopexy. Obvious asymmetry and recurrent ptosis on the left are evident. **B:** Preoperative markings showing the proposed periareolar revision. A circumvertical revision will likely be required on the left. (*continued*)

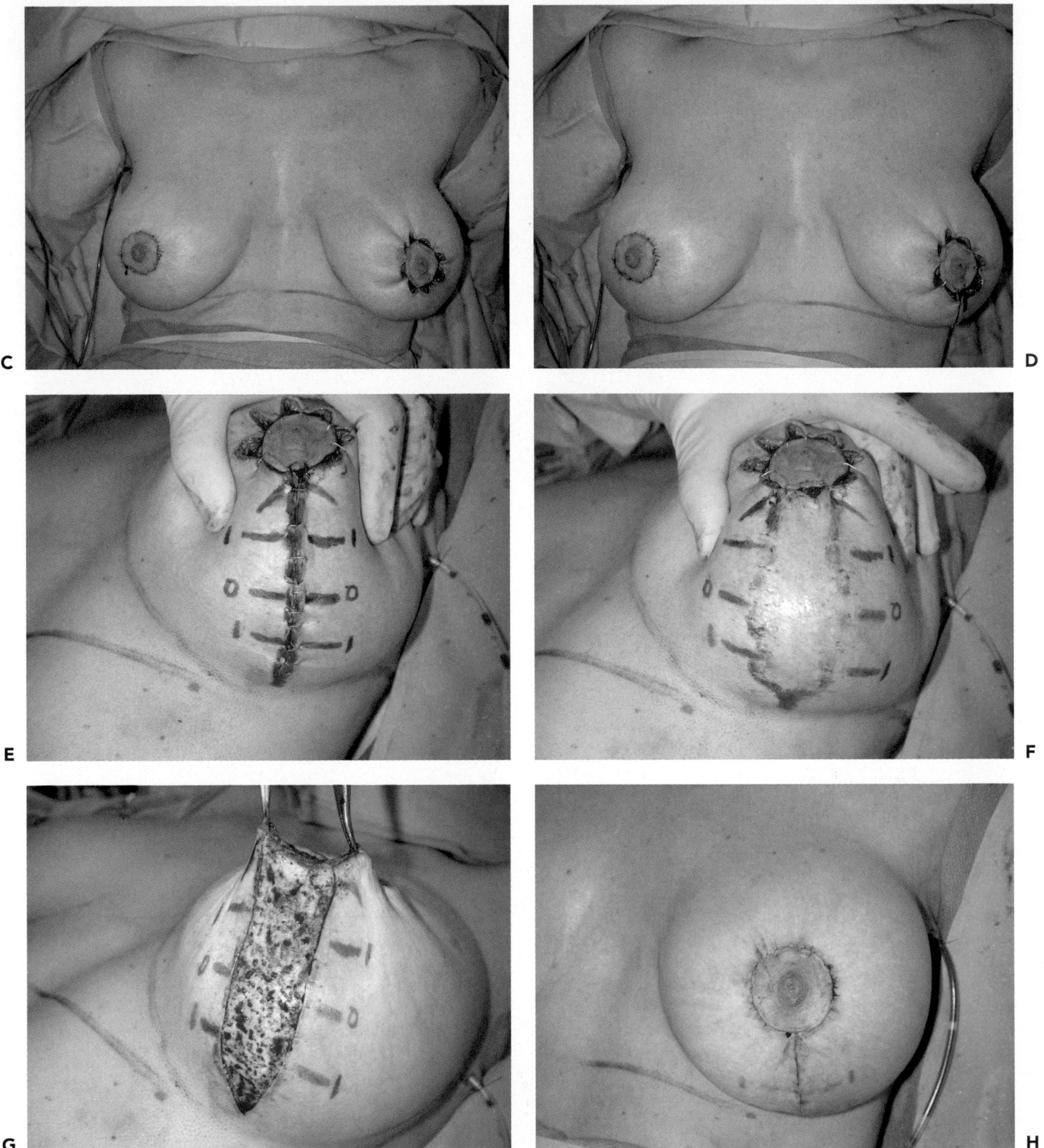

Figure 123.7. **C:** Appearance of the breast after periareolar revision alone. **D:** Appearance after the addition of a vertical plication on the left. The shape of the breast is improved. **E–G:** The plicated area is marked with a purple marker (**E**), the staples are removed showing the segment of redundant inferior pole skin (**F**), and the involved skin is deepithelialized (**G**). (*continued*)

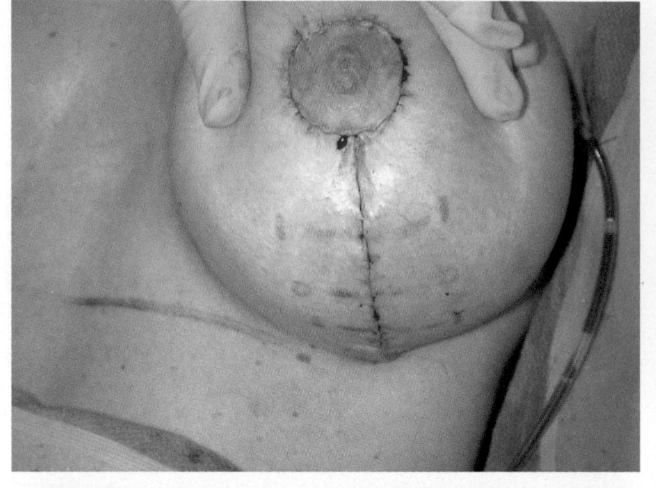

I

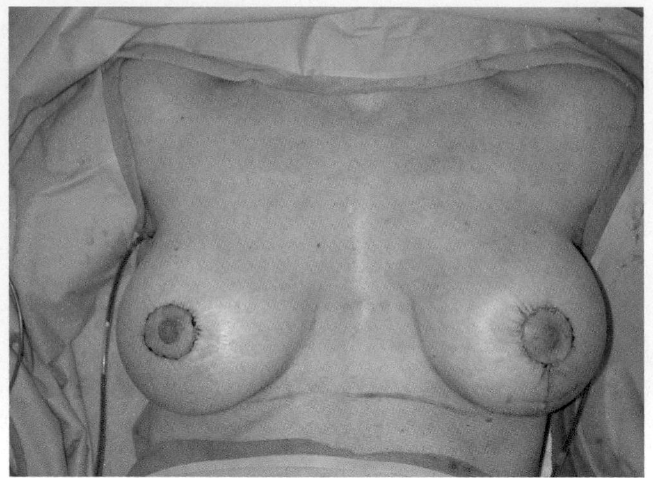

J

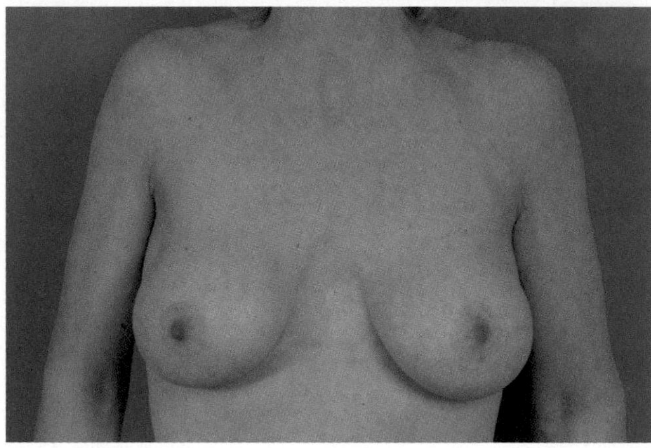

K

Figure 123.7. (*Continued*) **H & I** After completion of the circumvertical closure on the right, the improvement in breast shape can be seen. **J:** Appearance of both breasts immediately after revision showing improved symmetry and a pleasing aesthetic result. **K:** Appearance of the breasts 8 months after revision.

capsule along the inframammary fold intact if the fold is not displaced. This is because, in some cases, by removing the capsule along the fold, the position of the fold can actually be lowered, which then necessitates suture plication back up into position, a maneuver that can be quite tedious. In addition, if the capsule is closely adherent to the chest wall and ribs, it is best to leave it behind rather than risk inadvertent entry into the chest between the ribs with attempts at complete capsule removal. However, any scar attached to the breast is best removed to allow the soft tissues to redrape around the implant in an unrestricted fashion.

If undesirable muscle contraction occurs that animates the breast, it is very reasonable to change the pocket to the subglandular space. In these instances, the pectoralis muscle is easily sutured back into position and the implant placed on top of the muscle. This prevents the implant from inadvertently slipping back into the submuscular space. It is a prerequisite that the soft-tissue envelope be vigorous enough to cover the implant appropriately when a pocket change to the subglandular position is performed.

Choosing the appropriate implant in revisionary cases can dramatically improve the result. Generally speaking, moving from any type of round or anatomic saline device to a round, smooth silicone gel implant will significantly improve the overall result. As a result of the softer feel of the silicone implant and the tendency for these devices to form softer wrinkles, a marked improvement in shape and contour can be obtained. In cases where a wide dissection pocket is created, as after capsulectomy, anatomically shaped silicone gel devices should be used with caution because there can be a tendency for these devices to rotate.

Typically the last issue to be addressed relates to NAC aesthetics. Quite often the areola is dramatically enlarged and can have an irregular shape after augmentation mastopexy. Revision of the areolar diameter can be accomplished using any number of periareolar techniques. It is my strong preference to use the Gore-Tex suture described previously to stabilize the size and shape of the periareolar opening. One advanced technique that has given excellent results is to combine the periareolar Gore-Tex placement with evenly spaced "bites" in the areola. Again, because of the smooth handling characteristics of the suture, the purse string can be cinched down to the desired dimension without difficulty. Because the periareolar opening and the areola itself are linked together in the closure, the areolar diameter is locked into position and resists postoperative spreading. This technique is called the interlocking Gore-Tex and has given consistent and reliable control of the areolar diameter and shape in both primary and secondary augmentation mastopexy cases (Fig. 123.8).

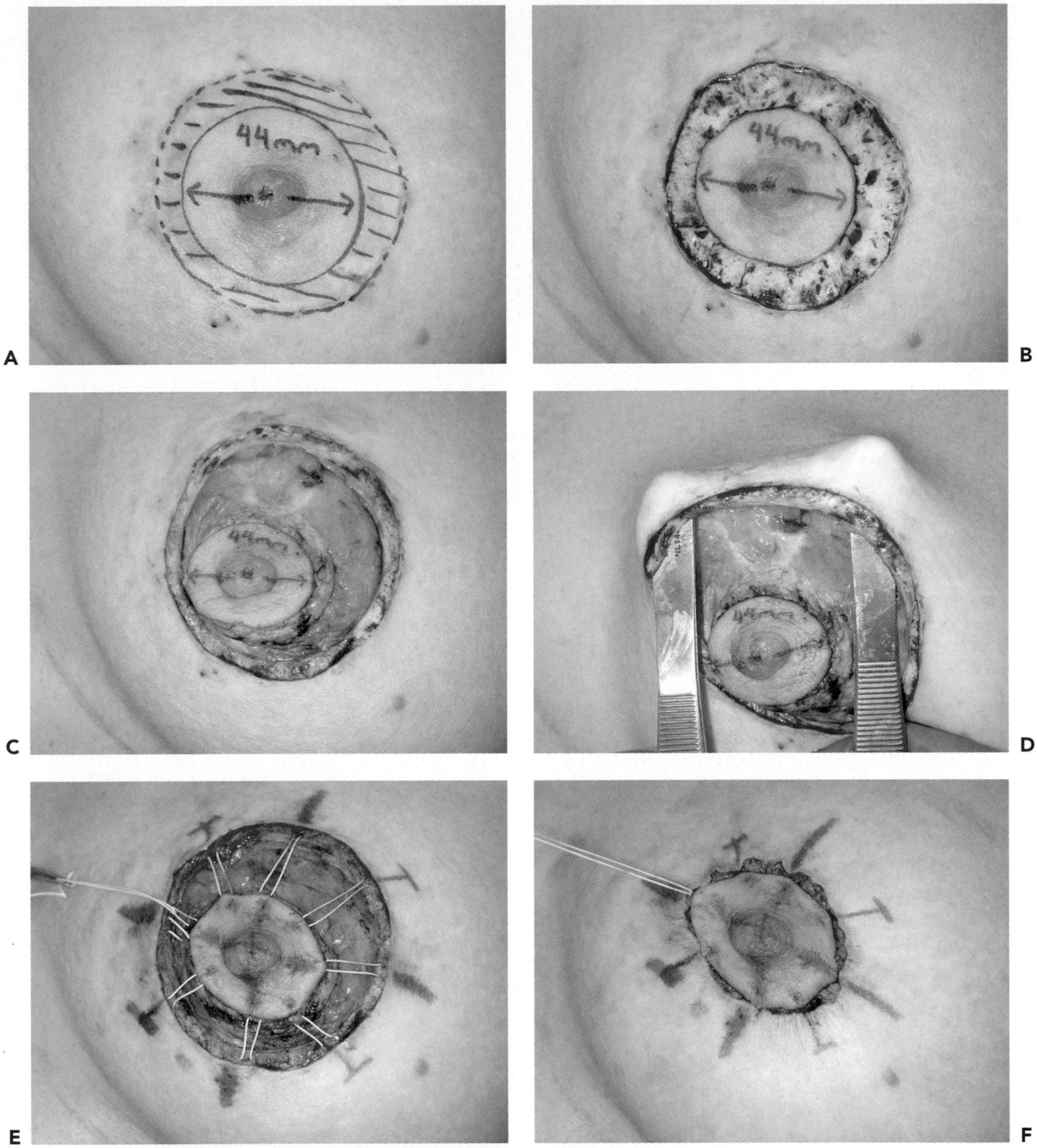

A B

C D

E F

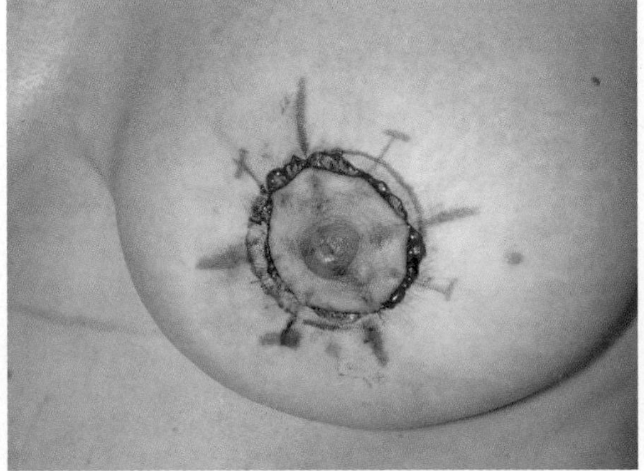

G

Figure 123.8. **A:** Marks in preparation for placement of the interlocking Gore-Tex suture. **B:** A 44-mm areolar diameter is measured, the incisions made, and the intervening skin de-epithelialized. **C:** The dermis is divided around the periareolar opening, leaving a small dermal shelf. **D:** The edges are slightly undermined to allow the purse string suture to close down the periareolar diameter without bunching. **E:** A CV-3 Gore-Tex suture on a straight needle is then passed around the periphery of the periareolar opening in the dermal shelf taking eight evenly interspersed bites in the dermis around the areola. This creates a "wagon wheel"-type pattern as the two incisions are locked together. **F:** The interlocking purse string suture is cinched down to the desired dimension. **G:** The opening, which often is slightly oval, is redrawn into a perfect circle. (*continued*)

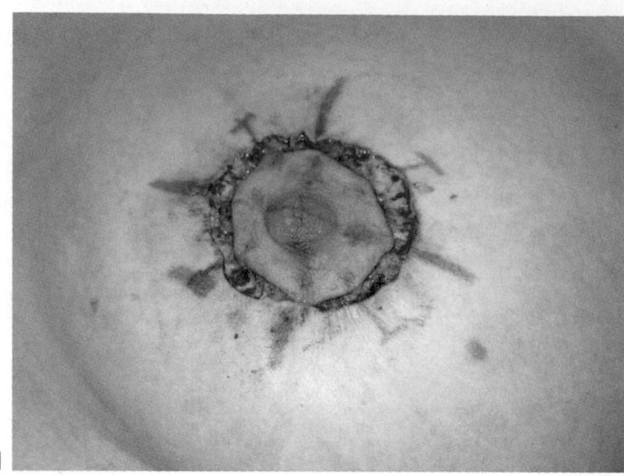

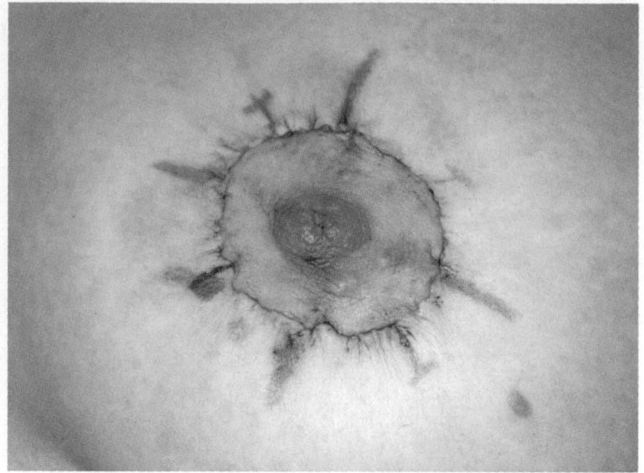

Figure 123.8. (*Continued*) **H:** The small additional amount of skin is rede-epithelialized. **I:** Appearance of the areola after final closure.

SUMMARY

Augmentation mastopexy can be one of the most difficult aesthetic procedures performed on the breast. However, with proper attention to the many variables involved in determining the ultimate shape of the breast, excellent results can be obtained.

EDITORIAL COMMENTS

Dr. Hammond has described the essential elements in the planning and execution of an augmentation/mastopexy. This clearly is one of the most challenging operations that the plastic surgeon performs because there are many variables that must be considered to optimize aesthetic outcome. With that in mind, this book includes several chapters that emphasize the indications and various techniques for the proper performance of an augmentation/mastopexy.

Dr. Hammond has reviewed the importance of patient selection, implant location, and features of the implants required to obtain a predictable and aesthetically acceptable result. He correctly emphasizes the importance of the inframammary fold in women with breast ptosis and that on some occasions simply lowering the fold will improve the position of the nipple-areolar complex (NAC) and avoid additional incisions. However, in many cases a mastopexy will be necessary. Although it seems intuitive that the breast implants be positioned before the mastopexy is performed, there are some who continue to challenge that principle. Performing the mastopexy before inserting the implant will increase the risk of developing complex scars, irregular contour, asymmetry, and patient dissatisfaction. Dr. Hammond reviews the three techniques by which a mastopexy can be performed in the setting of augmentation. These include the crescent or periareolar incision for mild ptosis, the addition of a vertical limb to the periareolar incision for mild to moderate ptosis, and the use of a Wise pattern for severe ptosis.

The final section of the chapter is focused on revising the previous augmentation/mastopexy patient. I agree with Dr. Hammond that when considering a revision, careful assessment of the previous incisions is critical to preserving the vascularity of the NAC. As mentioned, I also ask whether the previous operative report is obtainable so I can appreciate the specific mastopexy technique. In these cases, I have found that a conservative approach is safe and prudent. Usually, an implant exchange with capsulotomy and direct excision of excess skin along the previous incisions is all that is necessary. However, in the event extensive repositioning of the NAC is necessary and a capsulectomy has been performed, then caution must be exercised because of the possibility that the NAC depends on the capsular blood supply. In general, it is wise to avoid extensive mobilization of the NAC in this situation.

M.Y.N.

REFERENCES

1. van Deventer PV. The blood supply to the nipple-areola complex of the human mammary gland. Aesthetic Plast Surg 2004; 28: 393.
2. Hester TR Jr, Nahai F, Bostwick J, et al. A 5-year experience with polyurethane-covered mammary prostheses for treatment of capsular contracture, primary augmentation mammoplasty, and breast reconstruction. Clin Plast Surg 1988; 15: 569.
3. Maxwell GP, Hammond DC. Breast implants: smooth vs. textured. Adv Plast Surg 1993; 9:209.

CHAPTER

124

Neal Handel

Managing Complications of Augmentation Mammaplasty

Breast implants were first introduced in the United States nearly 50 years ago (1). Since that time they have been widely used for postmastectomy reconstruction, treatment of congenital anomalies, breast augmentation, and correction of ptosis. About two million American women currently have breast implants (2,3), the vast majority of which have been used for cosmetic purposes. The overall satisfaction rate among augmentation patients is high (4,5), but implants are associated with a significant incidence of risks and side effects (6). In spite of earlier concerns, it has now been proven that there is no relationship between implants and breast cancer, immune disorders, or systemic illnesses (7,8). However, recent studies of implant recipients have documented that local complications are relatively common and reoperation not infrequent (9,10). The Mentor Core Study of silicone implants used for primary breast augmentation revealed a reoperation rate of 15% within 3 years; the Allergan Breast Augmentation Core Study documented a reoperation rate of 24% at 4 years. Because of the significant incidence of local implant-related complications, plastic surgeons must be familiar with the diagnosis and management of these conditions.

Over the last five decades, a wide variety of implant types and styles have been introduced. There have been variations in shell thickness, filler materials, implant configuration, surface texture, and other characteristics. Some local complications arising from breast implants are specific to the particular type of device; most, however, are common to all breast implants.

Although there is some overlap, it is convenient to divide implant-related complications into those that generally occur "early" (within days or weeks of implantation) and those that typically occur "late" (months, years, or even decades later). Early postoperative complications include fluid accumulations such as seromas and hematomas, infections, galactorrhea, Mondor's disease, and breast asymmetry. Implant malposition (which may express itself in a variety of manifestations) and the "double-bubble" deformity can both occur either as early or as delayed phenomena. Late complications include palpability and rippling, capsular contracture, breast deformity and discomfort due to subpectoral positioning, implant exposure and extrusion, silicone gel bleed, shell disruption with gel extravasation, saline implant deflation, and interference with mammography.

EARLY COMPLICATIONS (DAYS OR WEEKS AFTER SURGERY)

SEROMA AND HEMATOMA

Excessive accumulation of blood or serum in the periprosthetic space during the early postoperative period is not unusual. The Allergan Core Study revealed a seroma rate of 1.3% following primary augmentation. If a breast becomes significantly more swollen than expected but is not painful, tender, or ecchymotic, it is usually due to a seroma. A fluid wave may be elicited on physical examination. Diagnosis can be confirmed by ultrasonography. Treatment is conservative: avoiding trauma to the breast and minimizing movement of the upper extremity on the affected side. This will hasten reabsorption of the fluid. A brassiere or elastic mammary support is worn day and night to immobilize the breast, and an arm sling may be employed to reduce movement of the upper extremity. The seroma will usually resolve spontaneously within a few weeks and does not appear to increase the risk of contracture or other complications. It is inadvisable to attempt needle aspiration of a seroma because of the risk of damaging the implant or introducing infection. In rare cases of a persistent or refractory seroma, it may be necessary to explore the pocket and insert a drain.

The reported frequency of hematomas after breast augmentation is in the range of 1% to 3% (11,12). In the Mentor Core Study the hematoma rate was 2.6%; in the Allergan Core Study it was 1.6%. Typically, hematomas are characterized by swelling of the affected breast, firmness, pain, tenderness, and excessive ecchymosis (Fig. 124.1). Treatment depends on the severity and anatomic location of the bleeding. If a small amount of blood has accumulated superficially, beneath the operative incision, it can easily be drained by opening a short segment of the wound. If there is minimal intraparenchymal bleeding and the breast is stable, conservative treatment, consisting of observation, immobilization, and application of moist heat, is indicated. If there has been accumulation of blood in the implant pocket (periprosthetic space), it is advisable to explore the breast and drain the hematoma. In the majority of cases a discreet bleeder is not identified due to clotting by tamponade. The blood is evacuated, the pocket thoroughly irrigated, and the implant reinserted. A surgical drain is optional. Patients with undrained hematomas after augmentation mammaplasty are at increased risk of developing capsular contracture (13) and infection.

INFECTION

Infection occurs following augmentation mammaplasty in 1% to 4% of cases (14–16). In the Mentor Core Study the infection rate was 1.5% after primary augmentation. Symptoms of infection usually manifest during the first postoperative week, but delayed infections have been reported months or even years after augmentation (17). The risk of infection does not appear to be related to the location of the operative incision, surface characteristics of the implant (smooth vs. textured) filler material (saline vs. gel), or implant position (submammary vs. subpectoral) (18). Local symptoms include excessive swelling, pain, tenderness, erythema, warmth of the breast,

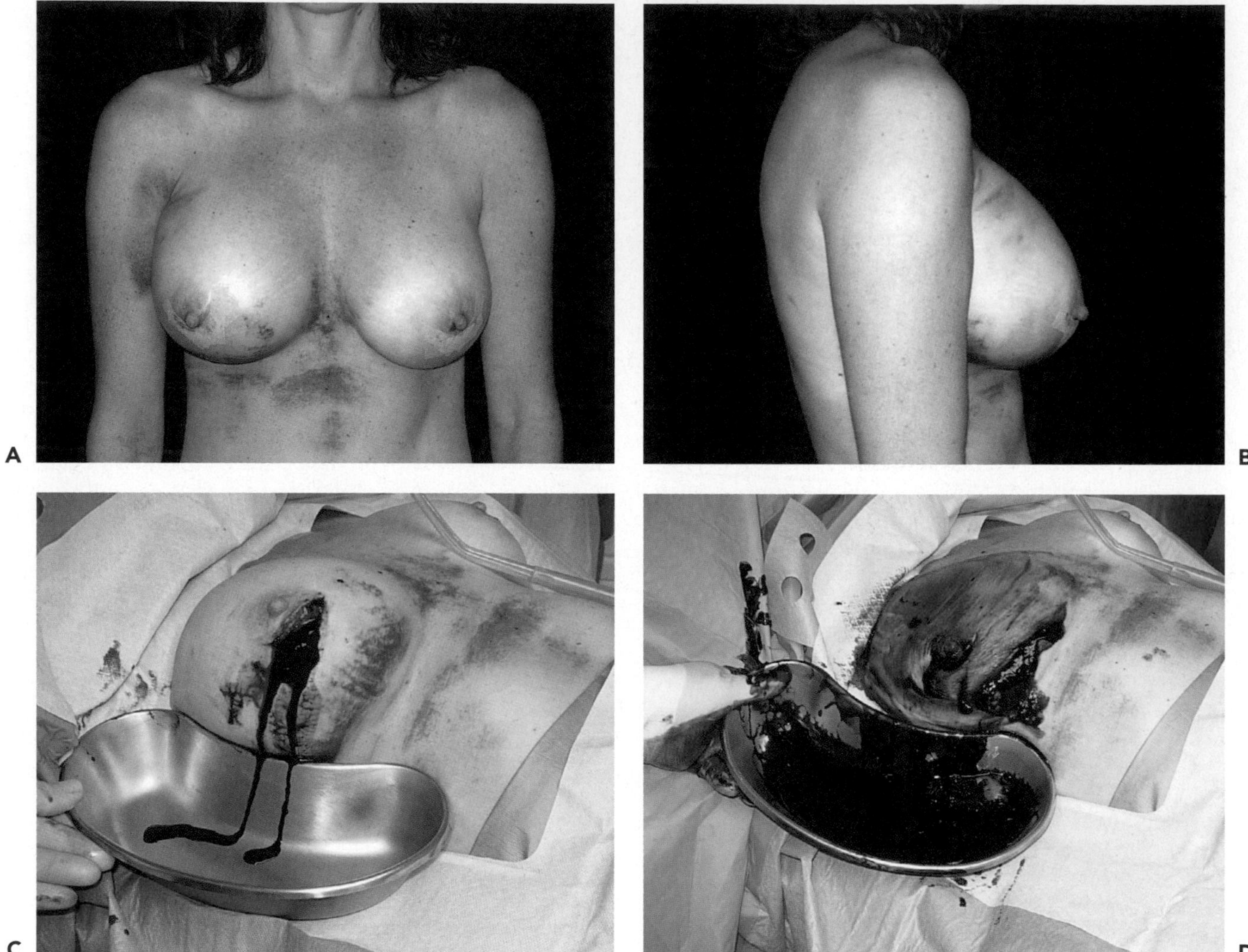

Figure 124.1. **A:** This 37-year-old patient is seen 3 days after augmentation; she has an obvious hematoma of the right breast **B:** Lateral view confirms massive enlargement of the breast. **C:** When incision is reopened there is immediate drainage of blood. **D:** Total volume of evacuated hematoma was approximately 200 cc.

and sometimes drainage from the incision (Fig. 124.2). The axillary lymph nodes may be enlarged and tender, and occasionally there are systemic manifestations such as fever or chills and an elevated leukocyte count. Diagnosis and treatment are usually based on clinical findings because wound exudate is rarely available for culture. In rare cases, infection may cause thinning of tissues and even erosion of the skin, resulting in a fistula that communicates with the periprosthetic space (Fig. 124.3).

Once infection is diagnosed, treatment should be initiated immediately. If the process is localized and superficial, such as a suture abscess, opening, irrigating, and packing the wound may be sufficient. If the process is more generalized, systemic antibiotics are indicated. When there is cellulitis without involvement of the periprosthetic space, oral antibiotics are often effective. Most infections are caused by gram-positive organisms, usually *Staphylococcus aureus*, *Staphylococcus epidermidis*, and *Streptococcus* types A and B. Less commonly, enteric bacteria, such as *Pseudomonas aeruginosa* or even atypical *Mycobacteria*, are the causative agents (19); when these are the responsible organisms onset of infection is usually delayed. In the absence of a specific culture diagnosis, broad-spectrum antibiotics are used empirically. In recent years the incidence of community-based methicillin-resistant *Staphylococcus aureus* (MRSA) infections has been steadily on the rise. For this reason, when treating breast implant infections empirically, many infectious disease specialists recommend a broader combination of antibiotic therapy (to cover the usual pathogens as well as MRSA). Ideally, "surveillance cultures" are obtained simultaneously with initiation of antibiotic coverage. The patient's armpit and nose may be swabbed for culture and sensitivity studies (with a single swab) to determine if the patient is an MRSA carrier. Pending the culture results, it is recommended administering amoxicillin/clavulanate (Augmentin) in non–penicillin-allergic patients to cover *Streptococcus* and sensitive *Staphylococcus* and sulfamethoxazole/trimethoprim (Bactrim) in non–sulfa-allergic patients to cover MRSA. In patients with a mild allergy to penicillin (e.g., skin rash), cephalexin (Keflex) may be substituted for Augmentin in conjunction with Bactrim. In sulfa-allergic patients, alternative drugs (e.g., clindamycin, doxycycline) may be substituted for Bactrim. In patients with more aggressive infections it may be prudent to start intravenous

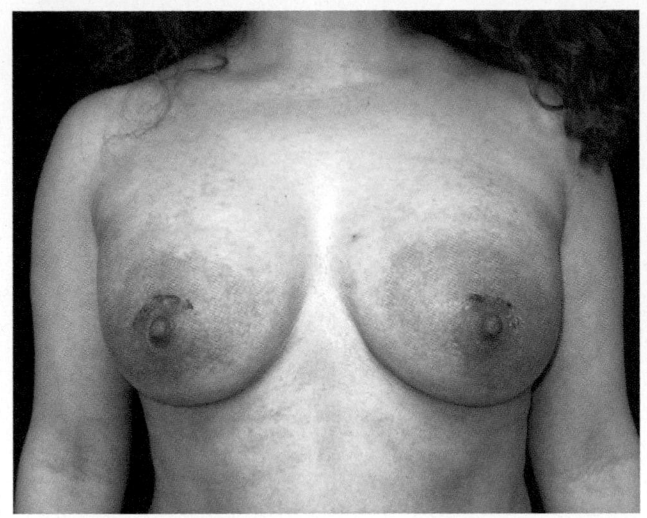

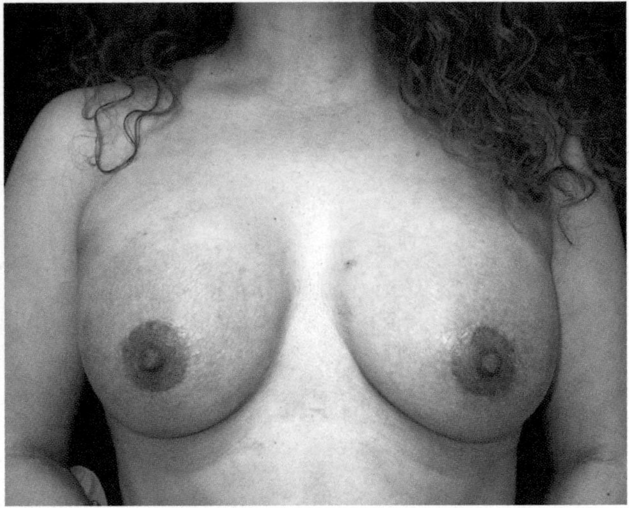

Figure 124.2. **A:** A 26-year-old patient 6 days after augmentation presented with erythema, tenderness, and increased warmth of the breasts bilaterally; she was treated with Augmentin and Bactrim for 10 days **B:** The patient is shown 2 weeks after completion of her antibiotic regimen with complete resolution of the infection.

therapy; one recommended regimen is vancomycin (administered for 1 to 3 days, depending on the clinical response) in conjunction with ceftriaxone (Rocephin). There is some evidence that infection, even when treated successfully, significantly increases the risk of subsequent contracture (14).

If the implant pocket (periprosthetic space) is involved, eradication of infection is difficult, if not impossible, unless the implant is removed. Sometimes symptoms are suppressed while the patient is on antibiotics but reappear when antibiotics are discontinued. In these cases, the most efficient approach is explantation and drainage of the pocket. The area is allowed to heal, and after about 3 months, when inflammation has subsided and tissues have softened, a new implant may be inserted (Fig. 124.4). Spear et al. (20) published specific guidelines for salvaging infected implants in selected cases; if implant exposure is threatened (or has actually occurred), local or distant flaps can be used for salvage. Sometimes such valiant efforts are justified. However, these extraordinary measures may be costly, time consuming, and extremely inconvenient to patients. In patients who develop severe infections after breast augmentation it is often more expedient simply to remove the implant and wait an adequate period of time before replacing it. If an implant is left in place and infection allowed to progress unabated, it could lead to a disastrous result, with extensive tissue loss and permanent deformity (Fig. 124.5).

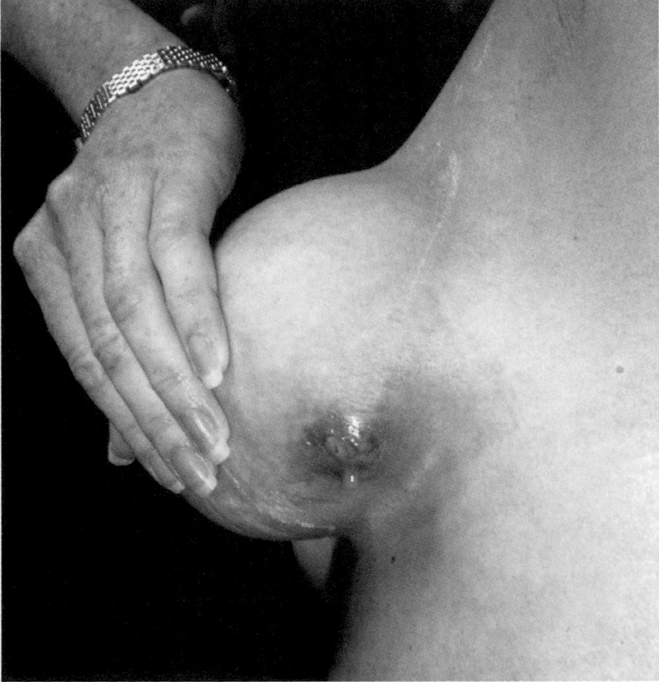

Figure 124.3. This patient was referred for a second opinion because of an infection following breast augmentation. Despite treatment with oral antibiotics, the infection progressed and she developed redness, thinning, and eventually skin erosion with purulent drainage from the inferior pole of the affected breast. The patient was advised to return to her surgeon for explantation.

MONDOR'S DISEASE

Mondor's disease, thrombophlebitis of the superficial superior epigastric vein, occurs postoperatively in less than 1% of augmentation mammaplasty patients (21). Usually this complication manifests during the first several weeks postoperatively. It is most common following an inframammary operative incision. Patients usually present with a slightly tender inflamed cordlike structure extending caudally from the inframammary fold (Fig. 124.6). The thrombus poses no risk of embolization. Patients are instructed to apply moist heat to the area. In very symptomatic cases, oral anti-inflammatory medications may be indicated. The condition is self-limited and usually resolves within 4 to 6 weeks (22). Mondor's disease has no permanent sequelae.

GALACTOCELE AND GALACTORRHEA

Galactocele (localized collection of milk) and galactorrhea (discharge of milk from the nipple or surgical incisions) after

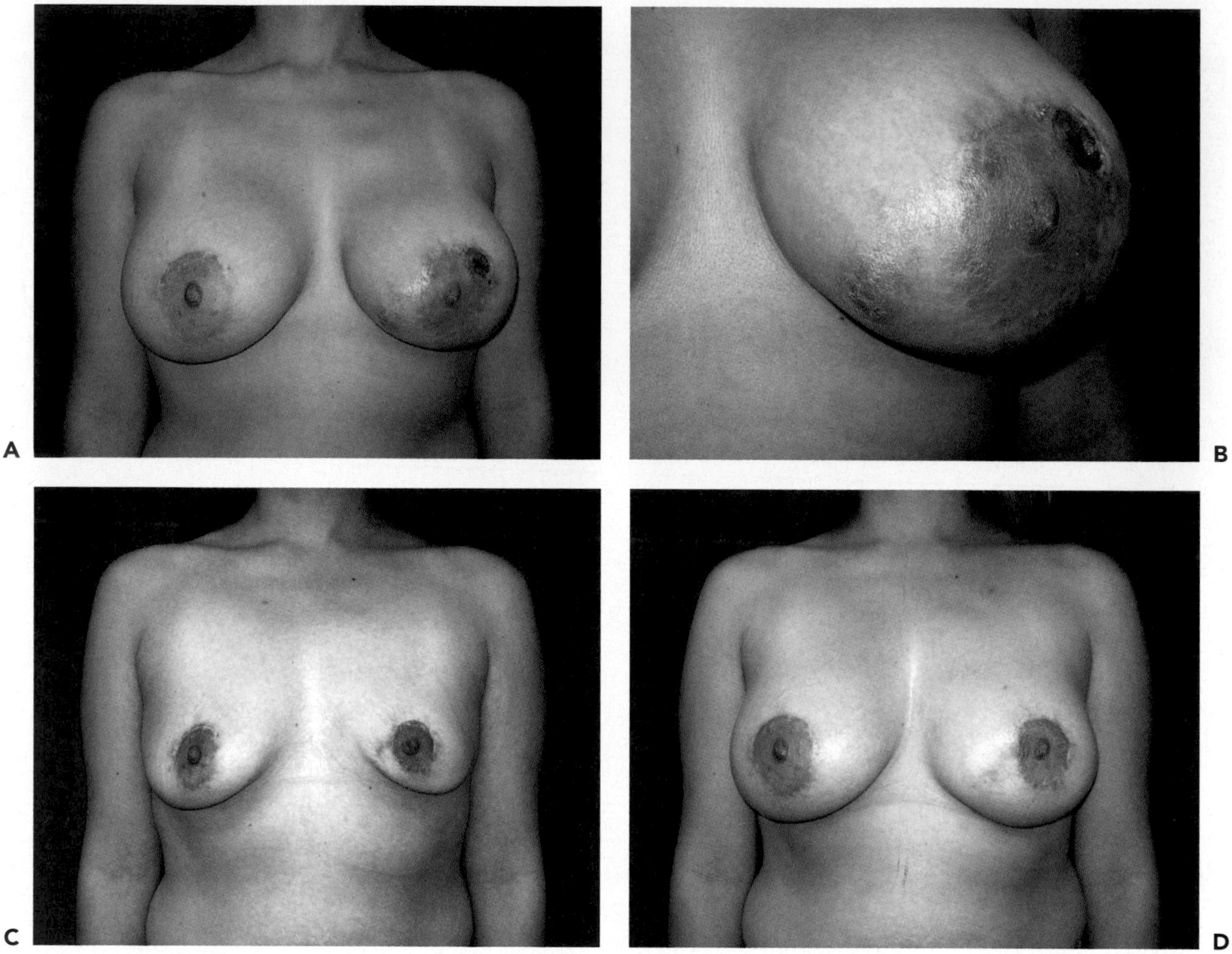

Figure 124.4. **A:** This 23-year-old patient had a breast augmentation and crescent "lift" 4 weeks earlier; she experienced wound separation and drainage on the left side. **B:** She was treated by her surgeon with oral antibiotics; however, the infection persisted, and she developed an area of thinning and impending implant exposure in the lower medial quadrant of the affected breast. **C:** The implants were removed bilaterally and the breasts allowed to heal for 4 months. **D:** A new pair of implants was inserted using a 25-cc-larger device on the left side to make up for tissue loss secondary to the infection.

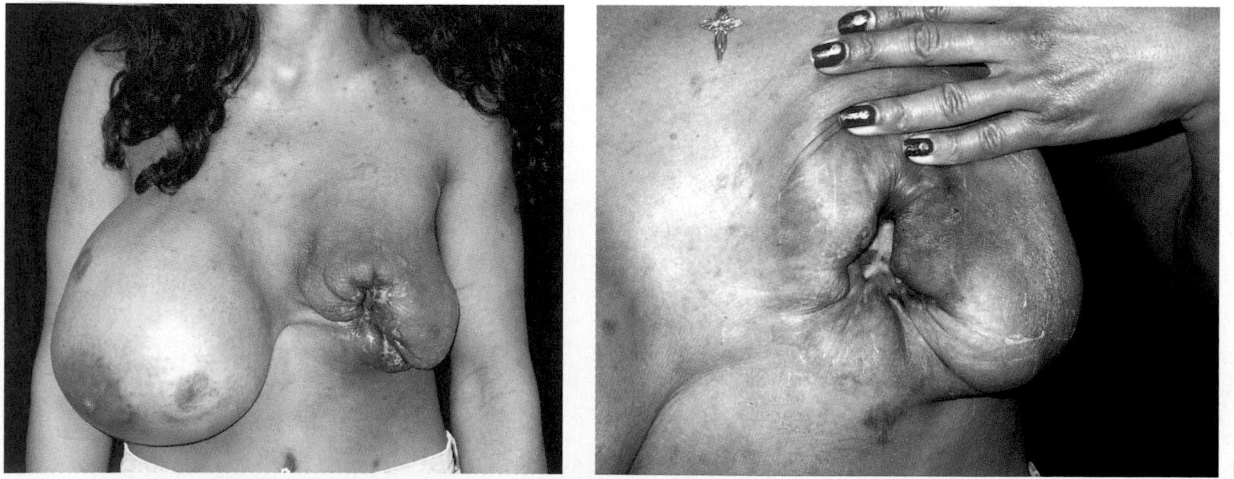

Figure 124.5. **A:** A 32-year-old patient who underwent multiple breast augmentation procedures with successively larger and larger implants developed an infection that was not adequately managed; this ultimately resulted in necrosis of breast tissue, implant exposure, and spontaneous extrusion. The patient was left with severe residual deformity. **B:** A close-up view reveals extensive tissue loss and chronic granulation tissue lining the periprosthetic space.

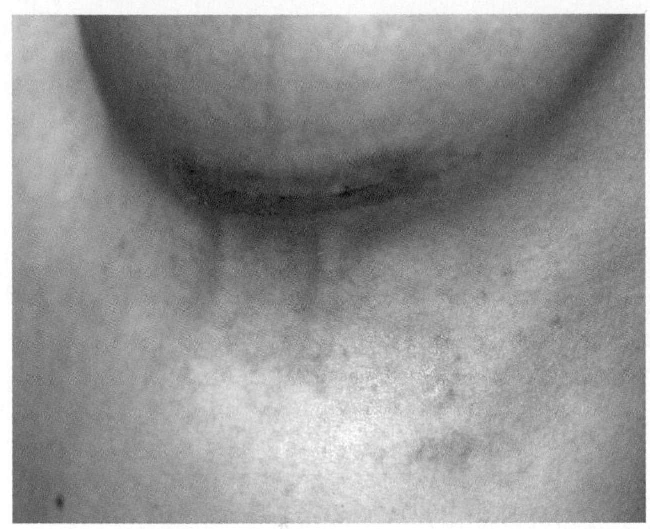

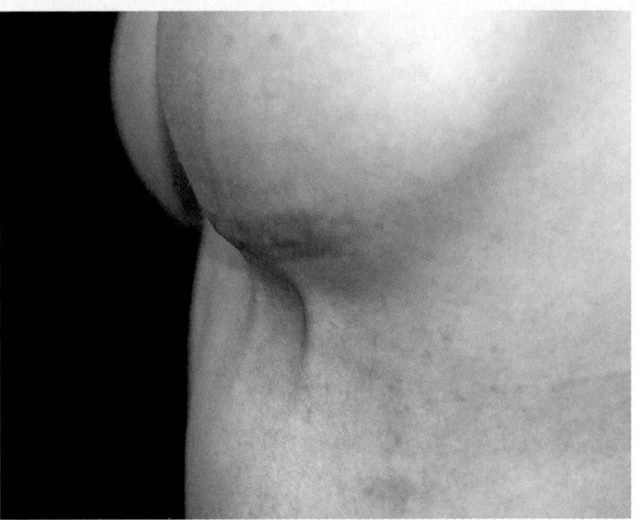

Figure 124.6. **A:** A 29-year-old woman 2 weeks following augmentation mammaplasty; tender, vertical bands beneath the breast are indicative of Mondor's disease. **B:** Oblique view of the same patient; Mondor's disease is seen most frequently in association with an inframammary incision (as in this case).

breast augmentation or other breast operations are infrequent (23,24). Drainage usually starts within several days of surgery and may be copious (25). Lactation is believed to occur secondary to prolactin elevation in the presence of falling estrogen and progesterone levels. Surgery may stimulate thoracic nerve endings, sending signals to the hypothalamus and pituitary, which cause increased prolactin secretion. Collections of milk may be significant enough to warrant aspiration or surgical drainage; antibiotics should be instituted. The process may last for only a few days, but, reportedly, can persist for months or even years (26). Administration of bromocriptine (Parlodel) or cabergoline (Dostinex), both of which suppress prolactin secretion, has proven helpful in managing postsurgical galactorrhea.

ASYMMETRY OF THE INFRAMAMMARY FOLD

Asymmetry of the inframammary fold is a distressing complication after augmentation mammaplasty. In the Allergan Core Study asymmetry was noted in 3.2% of patients. If asymmetry becomes apparent immediately after surgery, it probably results either from excessive or inadequate pocket dissection on one side. Early implant malposition sometimes responds to conservative measures. If the upper pole of the breast is too "high," patients are instructed to compress the implant downward. A circumferential elastic Velcro strap is applied around the upper pole of the breasts and worn continuously. Sometimes, these simple measures will enable the implant to "settle" into the correct position. If the implant is too "low," an effort may be made to immobilize the implant in the proper location so the flap can reattach to the chest wall and eliminate the potential space. This may be accomplished by having the patient wear a snug underwire bra continuously for 6 weeks. By that time, any fluid around the implant should reabsorb, and the tissue surfaces have time to adhere. Sometimes, these strategies fail and asymmetry persists, or patients present with asymmetry long after original augmentation. In these cases an open approach is necessary to achieve permanent correction.

If the inframammary fold is too high, surgical correction consists simply of inferior capsulotomy to deepen the pocket to the appropriate level (Fig. 124.7). If the fold is too low, surgical correction is a bit more involved. One well-established technique for raising the fold is "capsulorrhaphy" (27,28) (Fig. 124.8). Prior to surgery the difference between the levels of the inframammary folds is determined. This is accomplished with the patient in the standing position with the arms adducted. A horizontal line is drawn at the level of the lower fold across to the opposite side of the thorax. The distance between this line and the "normal" fold indicates how far the lower fold must be raised. Alternatively, the distance from the nipple to the fold may be measured on the two sides and the difference calculated.

Surgery is performed under general anesthesia; local anesthetic containing epinephrine is infiltrated into the area of the proposed incision. If the patient had prior augmentation through a transareolar, periareolar, or inframammary incision, the old scar can be used for access. If the patient was previously augmented through the axillary or umbilical approach, a new incision is made in the periareolar or inframammary location. The wound is deepened through the breast parenchyma with the electrocautery to minimize bleeding and prevent accidental puncture of the implant. The capsule is then opened with the electrocautery, exposing the implant. The prosthesis is carefully removed and set aside in a basin containing antibiotic solution or dilute Betadine (povidone-iodine) (Purdue Pharma L.P., Stamford, CT).

The inferior portion of the cavity is visualized and a marking pen used to draw an ellipse designating the area to be resected. The ellipse has a width twice the distance the fold is to be raised and extends the length of the inframammary crease. Excision of the elliptical segment of the capsule is accomplished with the electrocautery. When the anterior flap is allowed to fall into approximation with the chest wall, the raw surfaces will be crescent shaped and have a width equal to the distance the fold is being raised. After hemostasis is obtained, the cut edges of the anterior and posterior capsule are sutured

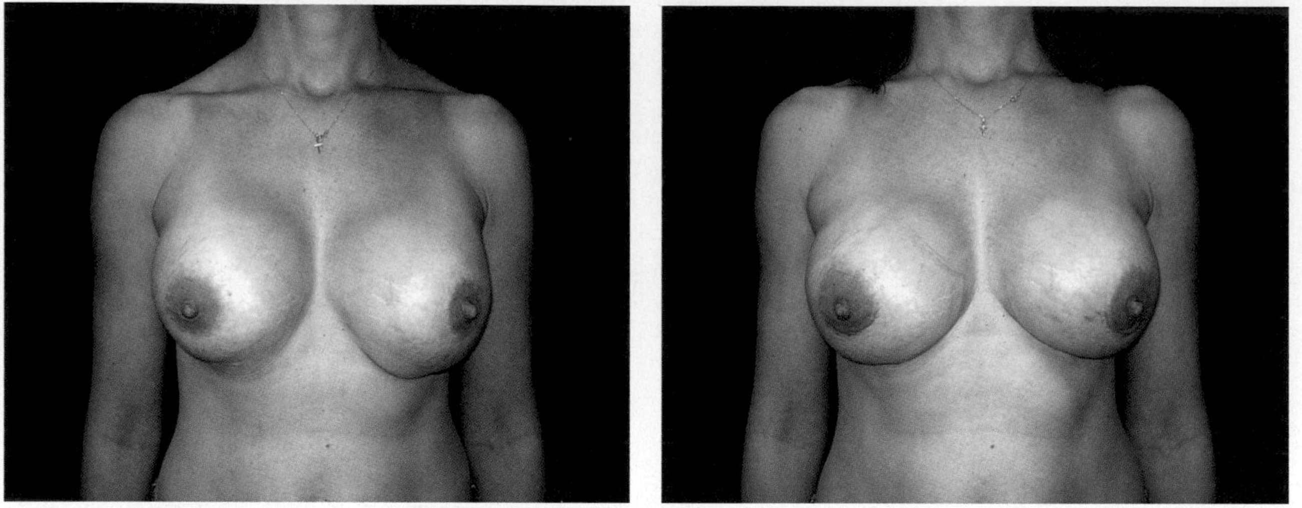

Figure 124.7. **A:** This 38-year-old patient had a breast augmentation 2 years earlier; she was dissatisfied because the breasts were asymmetric and the folds uneven; preoperative assessment revealed that the implant on her right side was "too high" and her fold "ill defined"; the inframammary fold on the left side was "irregular." **B:** Corrective surgery consisted of right capsulotomy to enlarge the pocket inferiorly; on the left side, a capsulorrhaphy was performed to reconfigure and better define the inframammary fold (result shown 4 weeks postoperatively).

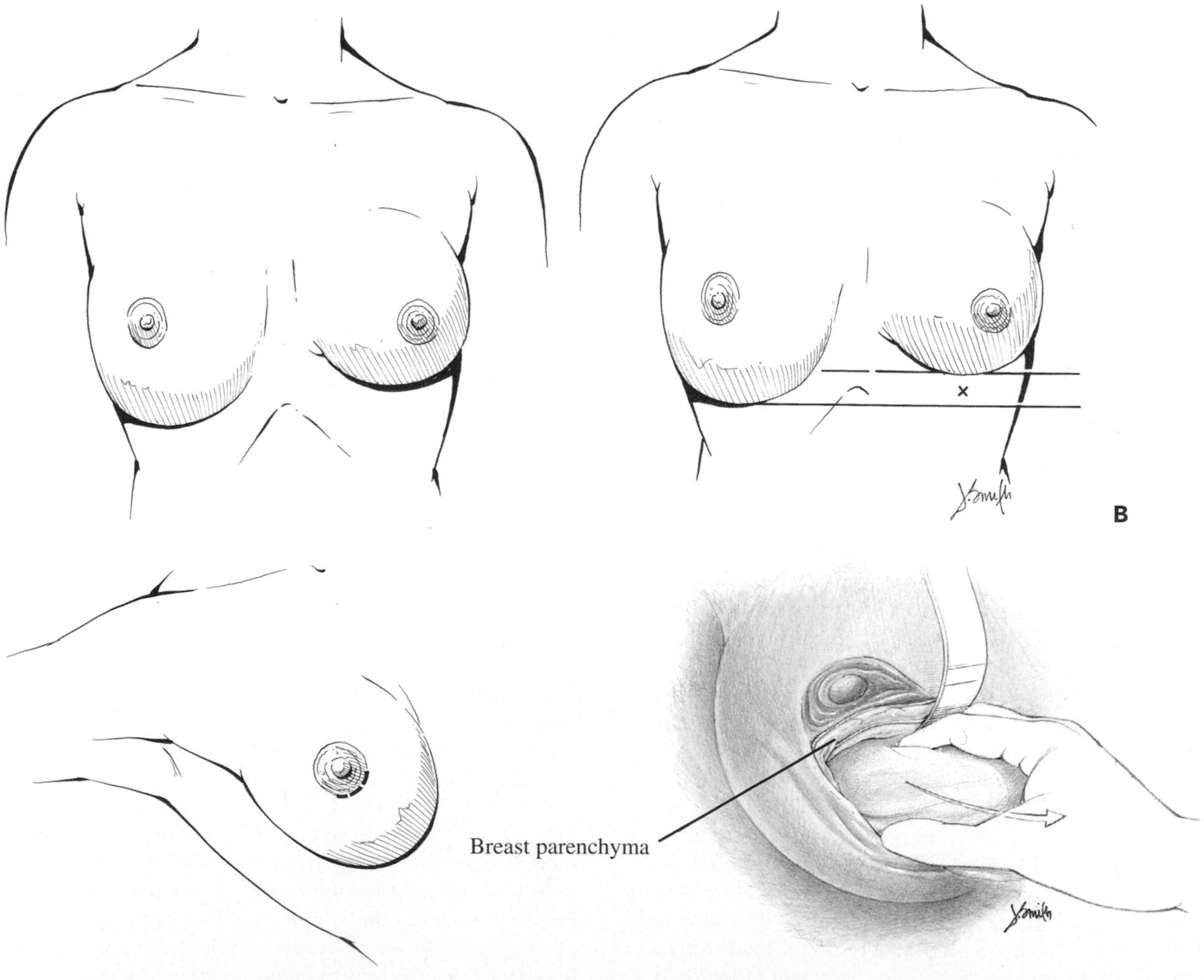

Figure 124.8. **A:** Asymmetry of the inframammary fold. **B:** Preoperative skin markings. Here X equals the distance the lower fold is to be raised. **C:** Location of inframammary operative incision. **D:** Breast implant being removed. (*continued*)

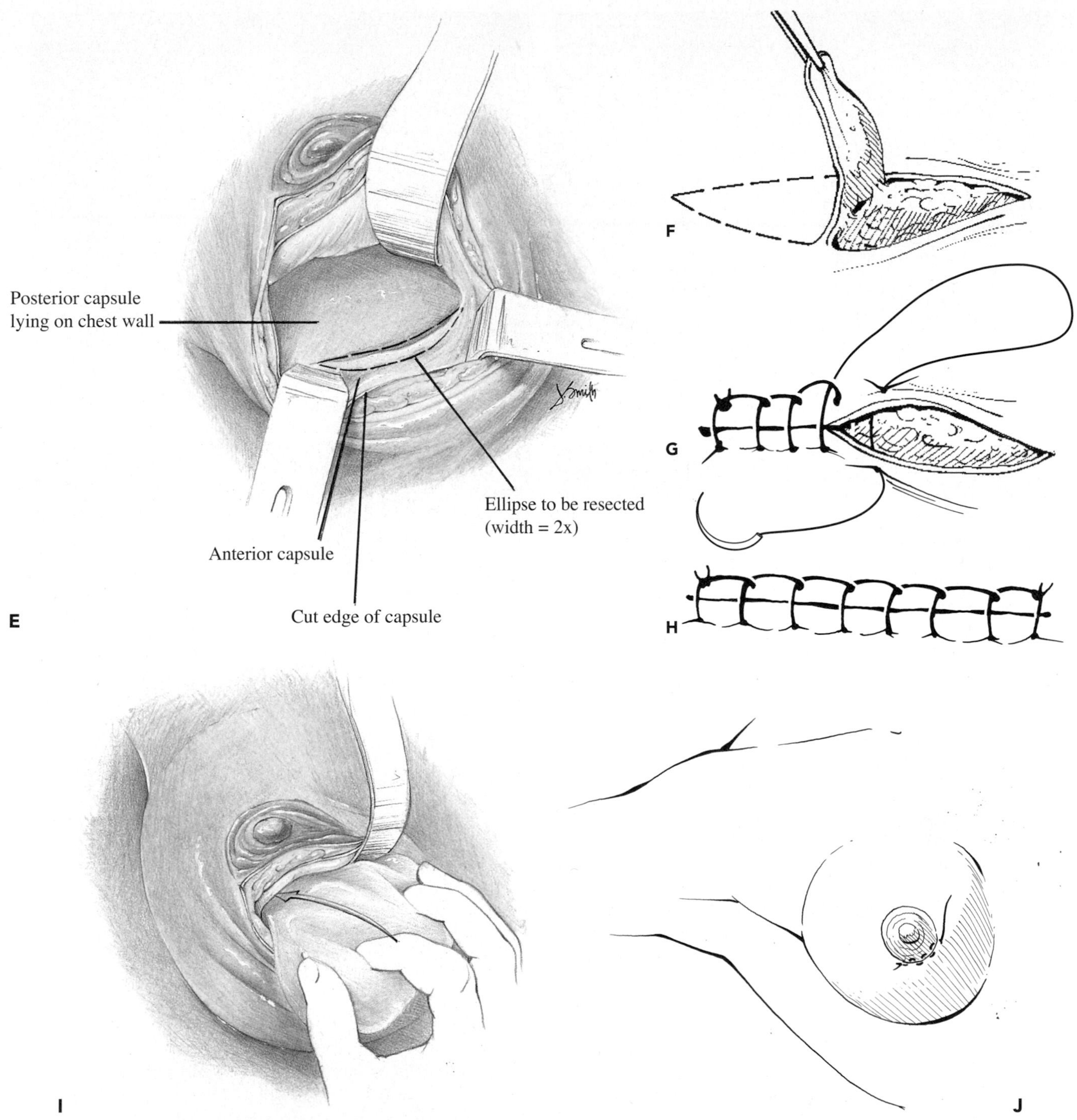

Figure 124.8. (*Continued*) **E:** Ellipse is marked with the long axis centered on the inframammary crease; the width of the ellipse equals 2X. **F:** Ellipse of scar tissue resected. **G:** Capsulorrhaphy performed. **H:** The sutured defect. **I:** Implant reinserted through operative incision. **J:** The final result.

together with a running locked nonabsorbable (nylon, Prolene, Ethibond) suture. The implant (or preferably a "sizer") is inserted and the patient elevated to the semi-sitting position to ascertain adequacy of correction and desired symmetry. If necessary, electrocautery dissection can be used to modify the fold as needed (by cutting through the anterior capsule adjacent to the suture line) to achieve the desired contour. In cases in which the implant is in the subpectoral position, conversion to a submammary pocket is also a useful adjunct when adjusting the level of the fold. With reintroduction of silicone gel implants, patients with an adequate layer of soft tissue (2 cm or greater pinch of upper pole of the breast) generally get excellent results with gel-filled implants in the submammary position. If the implant is left into the subpectoral position, the downward and lateral force vector applied to the prosthesis every time the pectoral is muscle is activated tends to displace the implant laterally and inferiorly. This sometimes disrupts a successful repair. Once the desired symmetry has

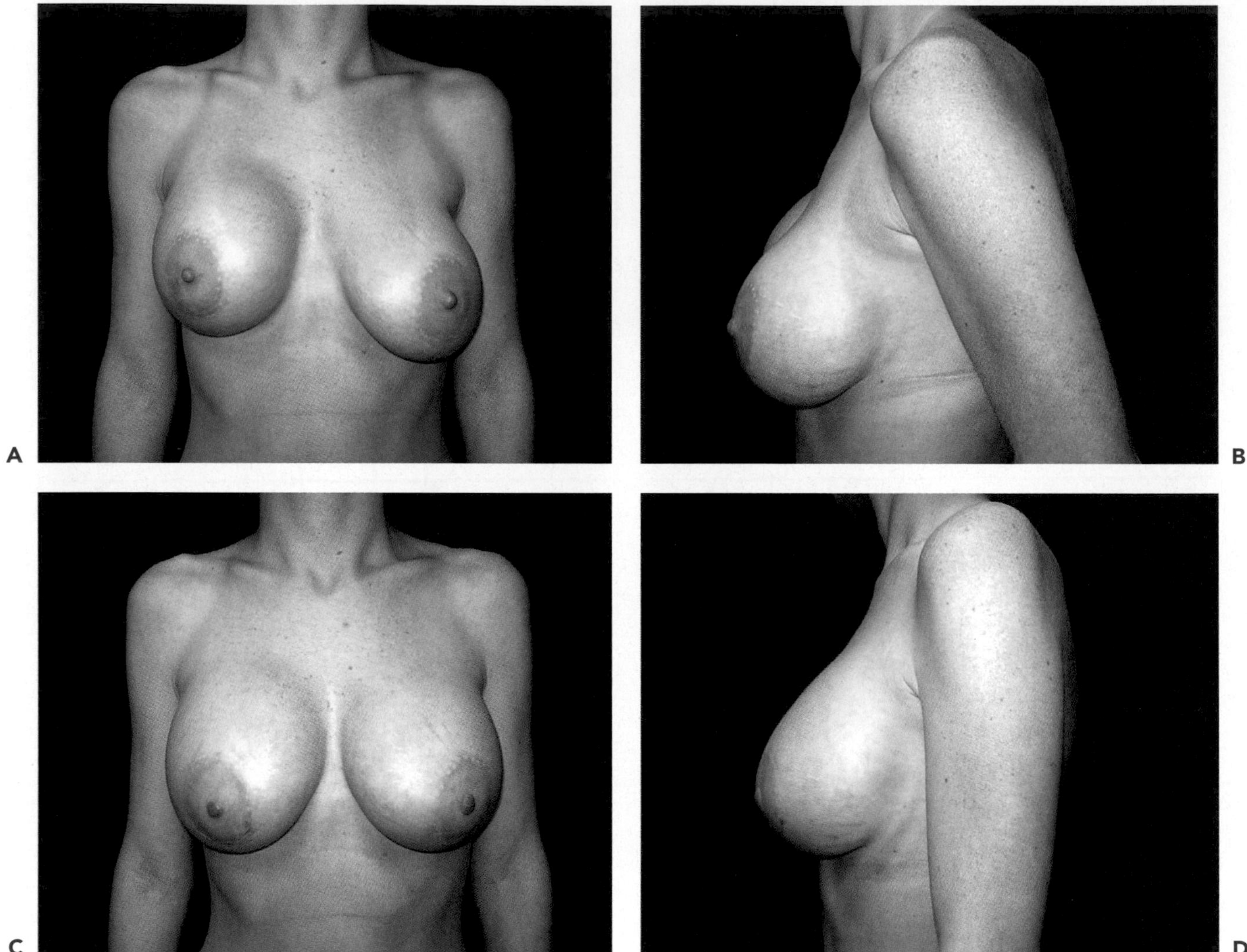

Figure 124.9. **A:** A 27-year-old patient 1 year after breast augmentation complained of asymmetry of inframammary folds; implants were in the subpectoral position. **B:** Lateral view demonstrates severe inferior displacement of the left implant **C:** The left inframammary fold was elevated with capsulorrhaphy and implants were converted bilaterally from subpectoral to submammary position. **D:** Lateral view after correction.

been achieved, the implant is reinserted and the operative incision is closed in the customary fashion. The newly defined inframammary fold can be reinforced by creating an "underwire bra" fabricated of strips of 0.5-inch paper tape secured by Mastisol. A light figure-of-eight pressure wrap is applied. Patients are instructed to wear snug-fitting underwire bras continually for 6 weeks after the repair to ensure proper healing (Fig. 124.9). The problem of a low inframammary fold may, of course, be only unilateral or may be bilateral (Fig. 124.10).

An alternative to capsulorrhaphy for correction of asymmetric folds or other manifestations of implant malposition is the use of capsular flaps. Such flaps can be elevated and advanced or transposed to reconfigure the pocket and reposition the implant (29).

IMPLANT MALPOSITION

The incidence of implant malposition is not precisely known. In the Allergan Core Study implant malposition was identified in 4.1% of breast augmentation patients by the end of 4 years. Implants of course may be malpositioned too far laterally or too far medially. When the pocket extends too far laterally, the implant can easily become displaced beyond the anterior axillary line, causing flatness of the breast in the parasternal region and excessive lateral fullness. This deformity is most apparent with the patient lying supine (Fig. 124.11) and may be more frequent after transaxillary augmentation. Conservative measures aimed at correcting lateral displacement are usually unsuccessful. The most direct approach is to explore the breast and reduce the dimensions of the pocket by capsulorrhaphy. Under direct visualization, the appropriate segment of scar tissue capsule is resected; the cut edges are approximated and sutured to one another to eliminate the lateral extension of the pocket. The technique is similar to that used to correct inferior malposition of an implant. Conversion from the subpectoral to the submammary plane (when there is adequate soft tissue coverage) helps to maintain the correction by eliminating lateral vector forces generated when the pectoral

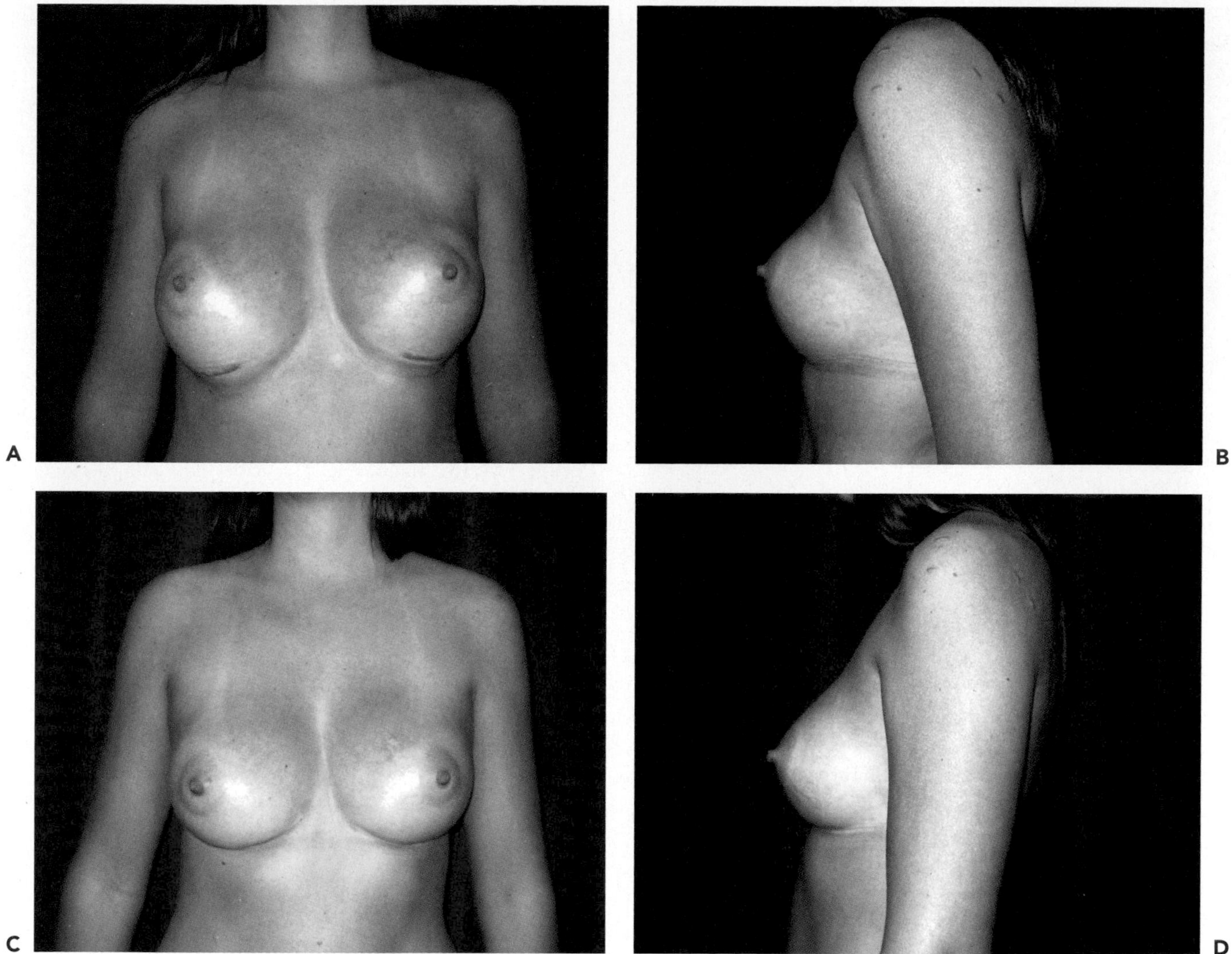

Figure 124.10. **A:** A 22-year-old patient 1 year postaugmentation who was dissatisfied with the appearance of her breasts and the visibility of inframammary scars. **B:** Lateral view demonstrates inferior displacement of the implants and lack of upper pole fullness **C:** Following bilateral capsulorrhaphy and implant conversion from subpectoral to submammary position. **D:** Lateral view after correction (postoperative views obtained 3 months after corrective surgery).

muscle contracts (Fig. 124.12). With the reintroduction of silicone gel implants into general use a much larger proportion of patients are candidates for submammary positioning of their implants.

If the implant pocket extends too far medially, it creates the disturbing condition known as synmastia (30). The term synmastia can be applied to any situation in which the breast implant crosses the midline, even if it is only on one side. Typically, patients present with confluence of the breasts at the midline and loss of normal cleavage (Fig. 124.13). Certain factors seem to contribute to the likelihood of this complication, including large implants, subpectoral placement, and multiple successive operations to increase implant size (31).

If the implants are submammary, one solution is to replace them in the subpectoral position (Fig. 124.14). The medial attachment of the pectoral muscle serves as a "restraining ligament" to prevent the implant from shifting too close to the midline. It is ordinarily necessary to divide partially the origins of the pectoral muscle to develop a submuscular pocket of adequate size. Care should be taken not to extend this dissection too far medially. The potential space superficial to the pectoral muscle (the preexisting submammary pocket) is eliminated by placing sutures between the lateral edge of the pectoral muscle and the overlying scar tissue capsule. This potential space must be permanently closed because if it is not, there is a chance the implant will migrate back into the submammary pocket. To ensure permanent eradication of this potential space, it is useful to roughen the capsular surfaces (both on the retromammary surface and the anterior pectoral surface) and to use permanent sutures for the repair (Prolene, nylon, or Ethibond).

In a patient with synmastia in whom the implants are already in the subpectoral position, conversion to the submammary plane may be effective. The implant is temporarily removed, and the lateral border of the pectoral muscle is identified beneath the capsule on the undersurface of the breast. Cautery is used to incise the capsule along the border of the muscle. Dissecting the breast parenchyma off the adjacent pectoral muscle creates a new submammary pocket. The pectoralis

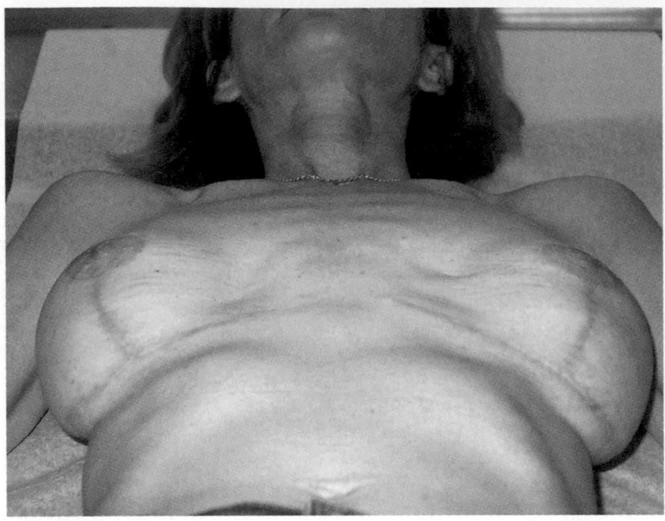

Figure 124.11. A woman with prior augmentation mastopexy presenting with lateral displacement of the implants, causing abnormally wide cleavage, flatness in the parasternal region, and excessive lateral breast fullness. These abnormalities are most evident with patients lying in the supine position.

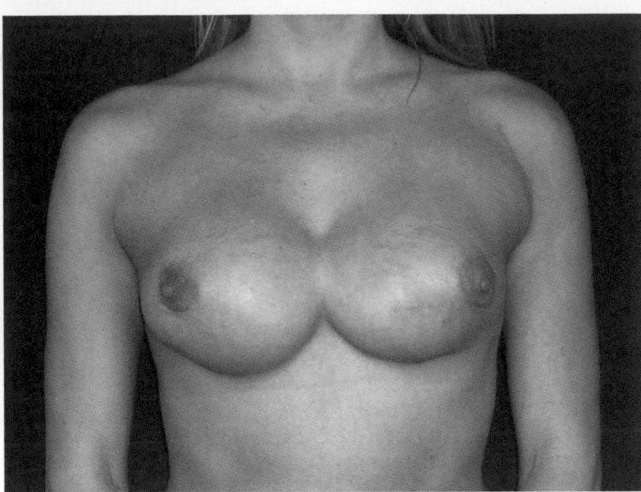

Figure 124.13. An example of synmastia with confluence of the breasts in the midline and loss of normal cleavage.

major is then reattached to the chest, with a series of nonabsorbable figure-of-eight stitches placed between the muscle and the adjacent capsule on the chest wall. As the new submammary space is created, extreme care is taken to avoid excessive medial dissection, which might detach the presternal skin and reproduce synmastia.

In some patients with synmastia, particularly those with abundant subcutaneous tissue and thick flaps, it is possible to correct the problem without changing the plane of the implant simply by performing an appropriate capsulorrhaphy. A partial capsulectomy is performed along the medial most extent of the pocket, and the aberrant extension of the pocket can be eradicated by placing sutures between the anterior flap and the chest wall. In many cases this is technically difficult because the skin flaps are thin and sutures are close to the epidermis, causing visible skin dimpling. It also may be difficult to place sutures in the thin posterior capsule or periosteum of the sternum. Under these circumstances, it is probably preferable to change the plane of the implant as previously described. Another useful strategy in patients with thin tissues is the interposition of allogeneic dermal grafts. Both AlloDerm (Life-Cell Corp., Branchburg, NJ) and NeoForm (Mentor Corp., Santa Barbara, CA) acellular dermal grafts have proven useful for treatment of synmastia (32).

When attempting to correct synmastia, it may also be helpful to replace smooth implants with textured prostheses; the roughened surface tends to secure the implant in place and discourage medial displacement. Surgical drains are useful for

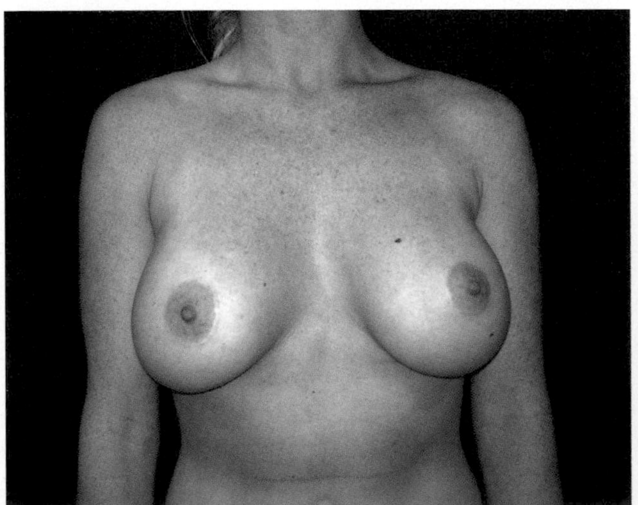

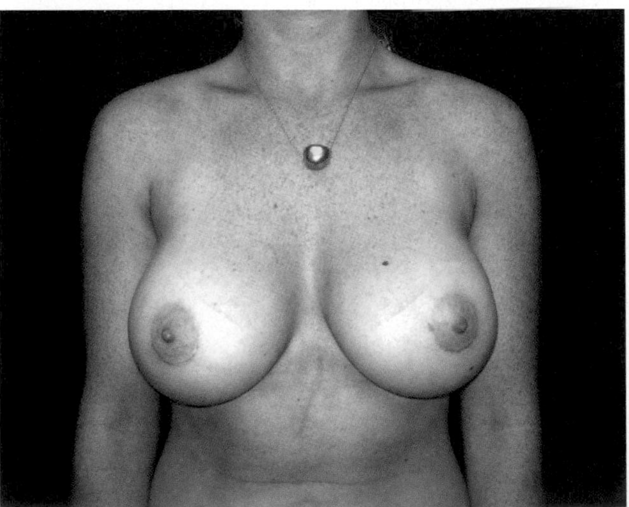

Figure 124.12. **A:** This 29-year-old patient with subpectoral saline implants felt that the area between her breasts was too wide and that the implants fell too far off to the side, particularly in the supine position. **B:** Correction consisted of lateral capsulorrhaphy in conjunction with substitution of silicone gel implants for the saline implants and conversion to the submammary plane (postoperative result at 4 months).

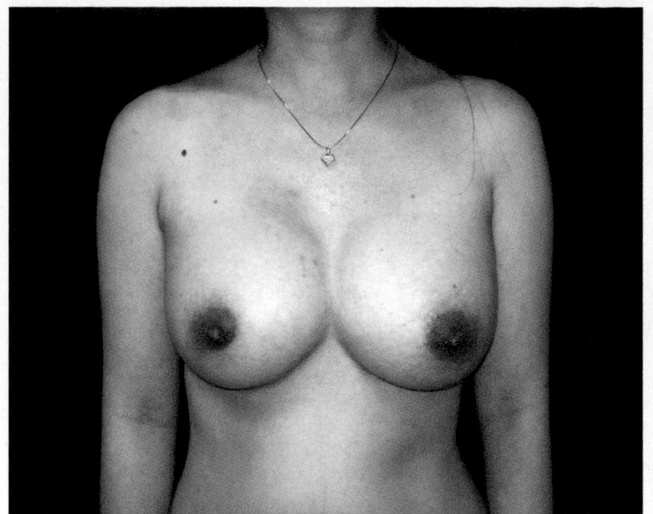

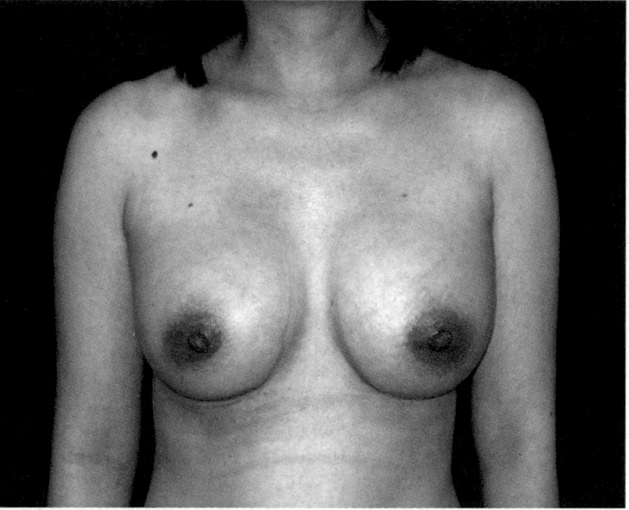

Figure 124.14. **A:** This 34-year-old patient with subglandular implants presented with synmastia; one prior attempt at repair had been unsuccessful. **B:** Her implants were replaced in the subpectoral plane with acceptable correction of synmastia (postoperative result at 6 weeks).

keeping raw tissue surfaces in approximation and promoting adherence. Lateral capsulotomy and placement of a smaller implant are additional measures that may help to ensure success.

In some patients with synmastia, particularly those who have had multiple prior breast operations, the tissues may be so thin and atrophic that it is preferable to perform repair in two stages. The first stage consists of explantation and partial capsulectomy or roughening of the capsular surfaces, to allow all tissue planes to reattach. At a secondary procedure, 3 to 6 months later, a new implant can be inserted, usually in the subpectoral plane.

While synmastia usually involves both implants, unilateral synmastia occurs when just one implant is positioned too far medially. In such a case, the contralateral implant need not be manipulated. The malpositioned implant is corrected by using one of the techniques described earlier (Fig. 124.15).

"DOUBLE-BUBBLE" DEFORMITY

Another anomaly that occasionally occurs after breast augmentation is the so-called "double-bubble" deformity. This manifests as a constriction or band extending transversely across the inferior pole of the augmented breast. It is caused by failure of the native inframammary fold to recontour over the lower portion of the implant. It is most frequently encountered in patients who have a tight or constricted inframammary fold, those with a short distance from the nipple to the fold, and those with "tuberous" breast deformity. In patients with these morphologic variations, it is important to fully release the ligamentous attachments that create the inframammary crease. Sometimes, a "double-bubble" occurs in patients without any predisposing factors. In these cases the pocket typically has been "overdissected" so that the inferior portion of the implant extends into the upper abdominal area. In this situation, the problem can be addressed by reconfiguring the pocket in the proper anatomic location either with capsulorrhaphy or a capsular advancement flap. In patients with a double-bubble in whom the pocket has not been over dissected, however, correction is directed at relieving the constriction. Sometimes this can be achieved by radial release, using cautery to make a series of cuts perpendicular to the band along the undersurface of the inferior breast flap. These "releasing" incisions are deepened to the level of the dermis. Intraoperative tissue expansion with an overinflated sizer or expander may also help stretch the tissues and release the constriction. In some cases, dissection of a new pocket, in a more superficial plane (just deep to the dermis), allows the tissues of the inferior pole of the breast to redrape in the desired fashion. In patients with subpectoral implants, conversion to the submammary plane, in conjunction with theses "releasing" maneuvers, is often helpful (Fig. 124.16). Use of a silicone gel–filled implant is recommended in such cases when the tissues of the inferior breast have been intentionally thinned or stretched, as there is less risk of undesirable palpability or waviness.

LATE COMPLICATIONS (MONTHS OR YEARS AFTER SURGERY)

Abnormal palpability of the implant and unsightly rippling or waviness of the breast are annoying complications that detract from patient satisfaction. Undesirable palpability is often secondary to an unusually thin layer of breast tissue covering the implant and, therefore, is more common in very small breasted women or thin patients with insufficient subcutaneous fat. In such individuals, submuscular positioning of the implant will provide a thicker layer of "padding," at least over the superior half of the implant (Fig. 124.17). The problem of a palpable implant edge along the inferolateral aspect of the breast is not helped by subpectoral placement because the muscle does not cover this portion of the prosthesis. Sometimes, a palpable saline implant edge is due to "underfilling" and can be corrected by adding more saline to the prosthesis. In other cases, replacement with a silicone gel–filled device will help.

Rippling or waviness of the breast is also more frequent in patients with thin tissue coverage. Therefore, they are often seen as a consequence of multiple successive operations, including capsulotomy, capsulectomy, and insertion of progressively

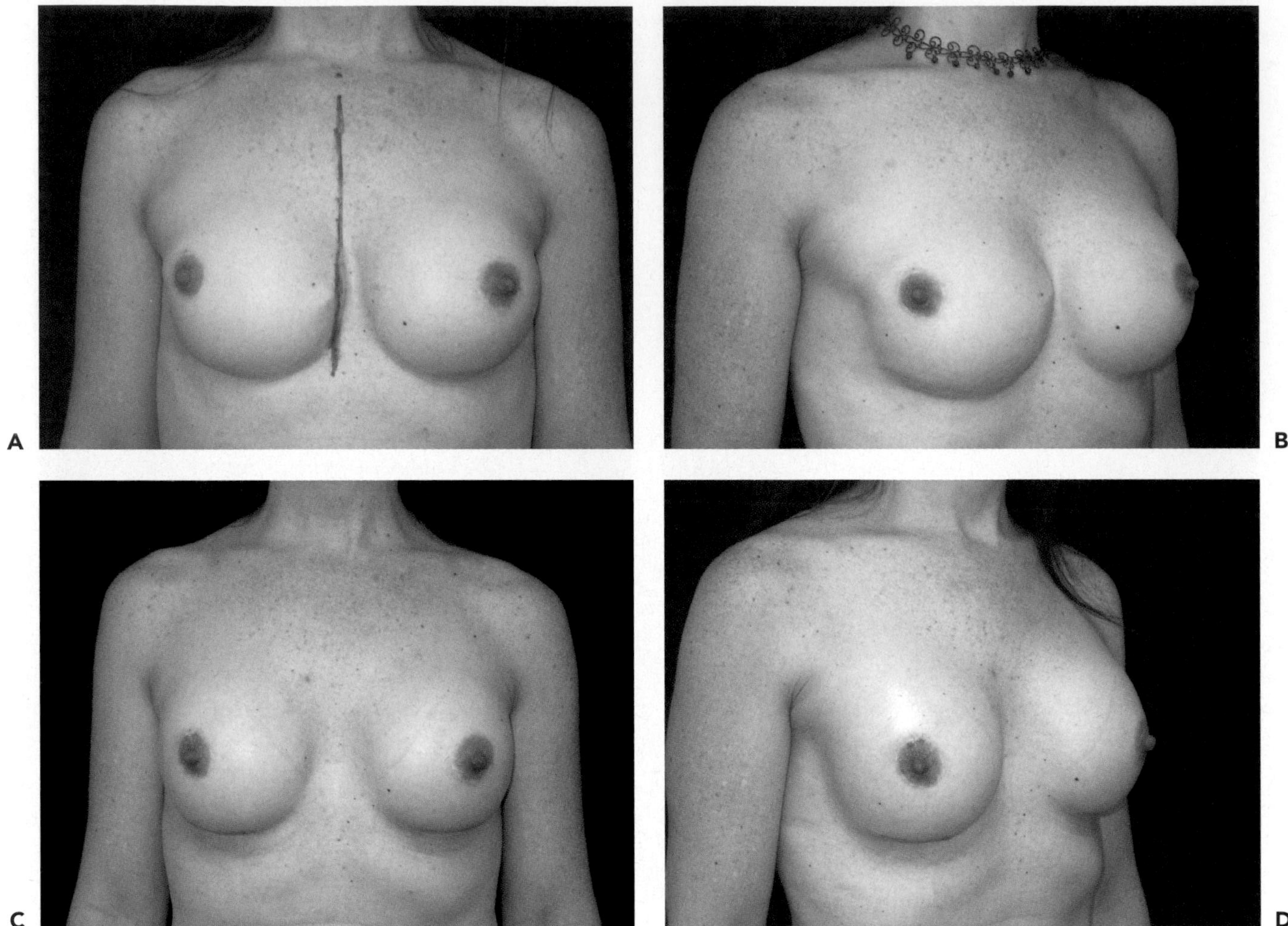

Figure 124.15. **A:** An example of a patient with unilateral synmastia due to malposition of the right implant (frontal view, true midline marked). **B:** Same patient with medial malposition of the right implant (oblique view); note that the nipple appears much too far lateral on the breast. **C:** Frontal view after surgical correction of medial malposition of the right implant. **D:** Oblique view after correction of malpositioned implant; the nipple now appears in the "correct" location on the breast.

larger implants, all of which may contribute to thinning of the flaps. Rippling is distinctly more common with textured implants than smooth ones and occurs more frequently with saline-filled than gel-filled devices (4). In a patient with a saline implant who complains of rippling or waviness, adding more saline may improve the appearance. Substituting textured implants with smooth surface devices often helps, and replacement of saline with a gel-filled implants is often effective. Other strategies are also available for correction of visible waviness of the breast. Recently fat grafting has been proposed as a technique to increase overlying tissue thickness and camouflage the waviness of the implant. This technique can be effective in patients who have suitable donor sites. The long-term consequences of fat grafting to the breast have not been fully determined, and it is important to explain this to patients as part of the informed-consent process (33).

Another technique that has effectively been used to correct waviness in patients with thin tissue is interposition or onlay of acellular dermal grafts (e.g., AlloDerm, NeoForm) (32,34). Such grafts may be used to reinforce a thin flap or to bridge the gap between the divided edge of the pectoralis muscle and the inframammary fold, in either case adding an additional layer of "soft tissue" over the prosthesis (Fig. 124.18).

CAPSULAR CONTRACTURE

Without a doubt, the complication that historically has caused the greatest morbidity for augmentation mammaplasty patients is capsular contracture (4,35,36). A scar tissue "capsule" inevitably forms around all breast implants. In most cases, this membrane remains soft and pliable and has little effect on the contour or texture of the breast. In some individuals, however, the scar tissue capsule undergoes progressive thickening and shrinkage, a phenomenon known as contracture or "encapsulation." When this occurs, the compressible implant is deformed, taking on an unnatural spherical configuration. Moreover, the breast may become undesirably firm.

The reported rate of symptomatic capsular contracture varies widely. It has been suggested that certain filler materials (saline) (37,38) and certain shell characteristics (low-bleed elastomeric shells, mechanically textured surfaces) (39,40) may reduce the incidence of contracture. Although some of these

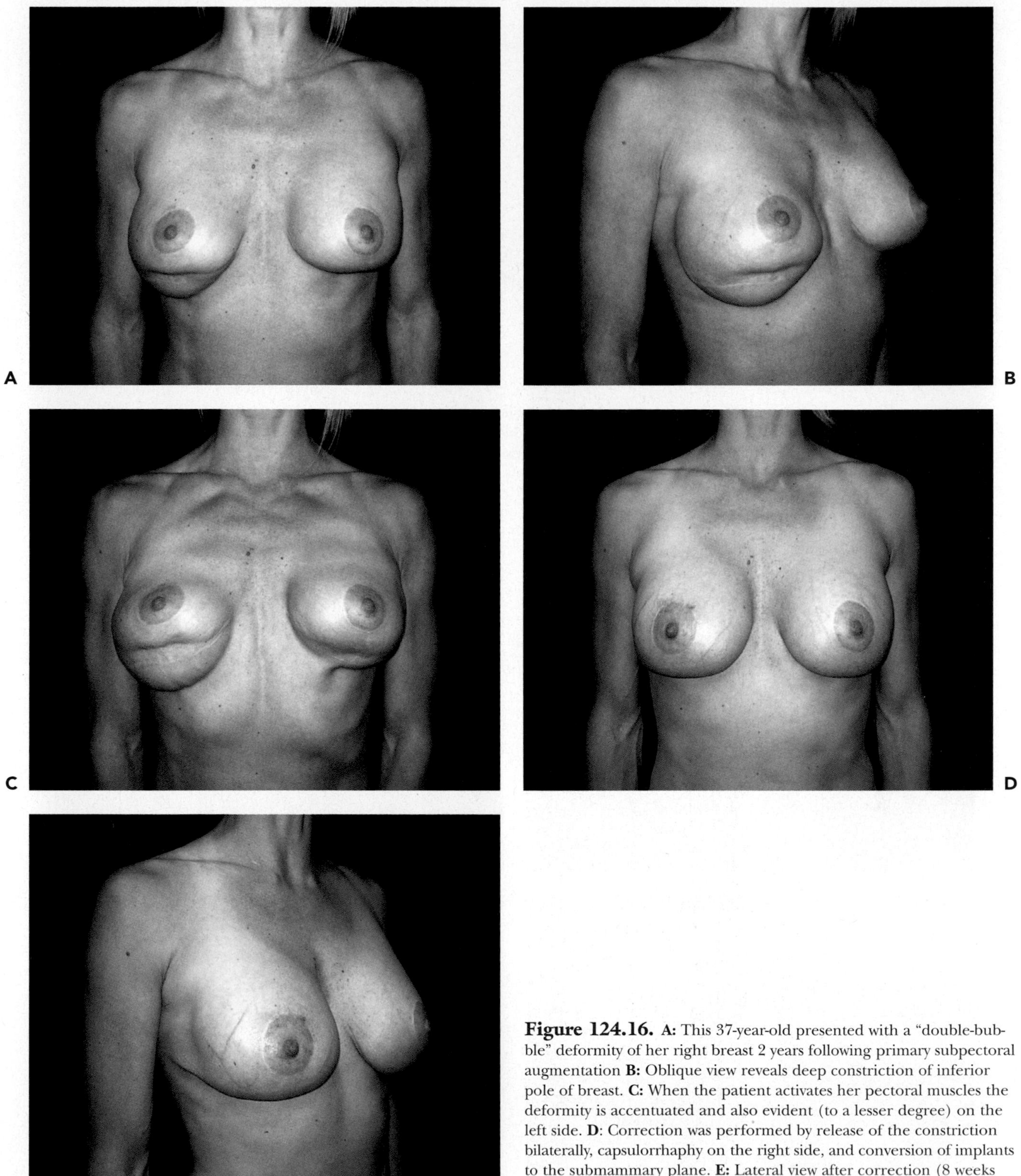

Figure 124.16. **A:** This 37-year-old presented with a "double-bubble" deformity of her right breast 2 years following primary subpectoral augmentation **B:** Oblique view reveals deep constriction of inferior pole of breast. **C:** When the patient activates her pectoral muscles the deformity is accentuated and also evident (to a lesser degree) on the left side. **D**: Correction was performed by release of the constriction bilaterally, capsulorrhaphy on the right side, and conversion of implants to the submammary plane. **E:** Lateral view after correction (8 weeks postoperatively).

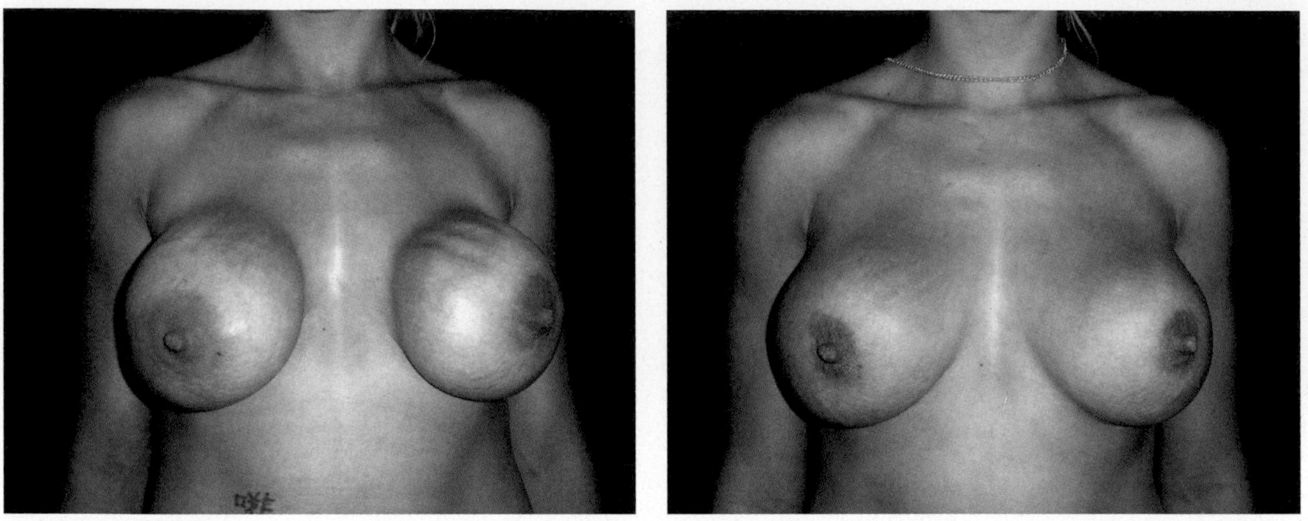

Figure 124.17. **A:** This 26-year-old patient with submammary, textured saline implants was displeased with the "unnatural" appearance of her breasts and troubled by visible rippling. **B:** The problem was corrected by converting to smooth-surfaced silicone gel implants in the subpectoral plane.

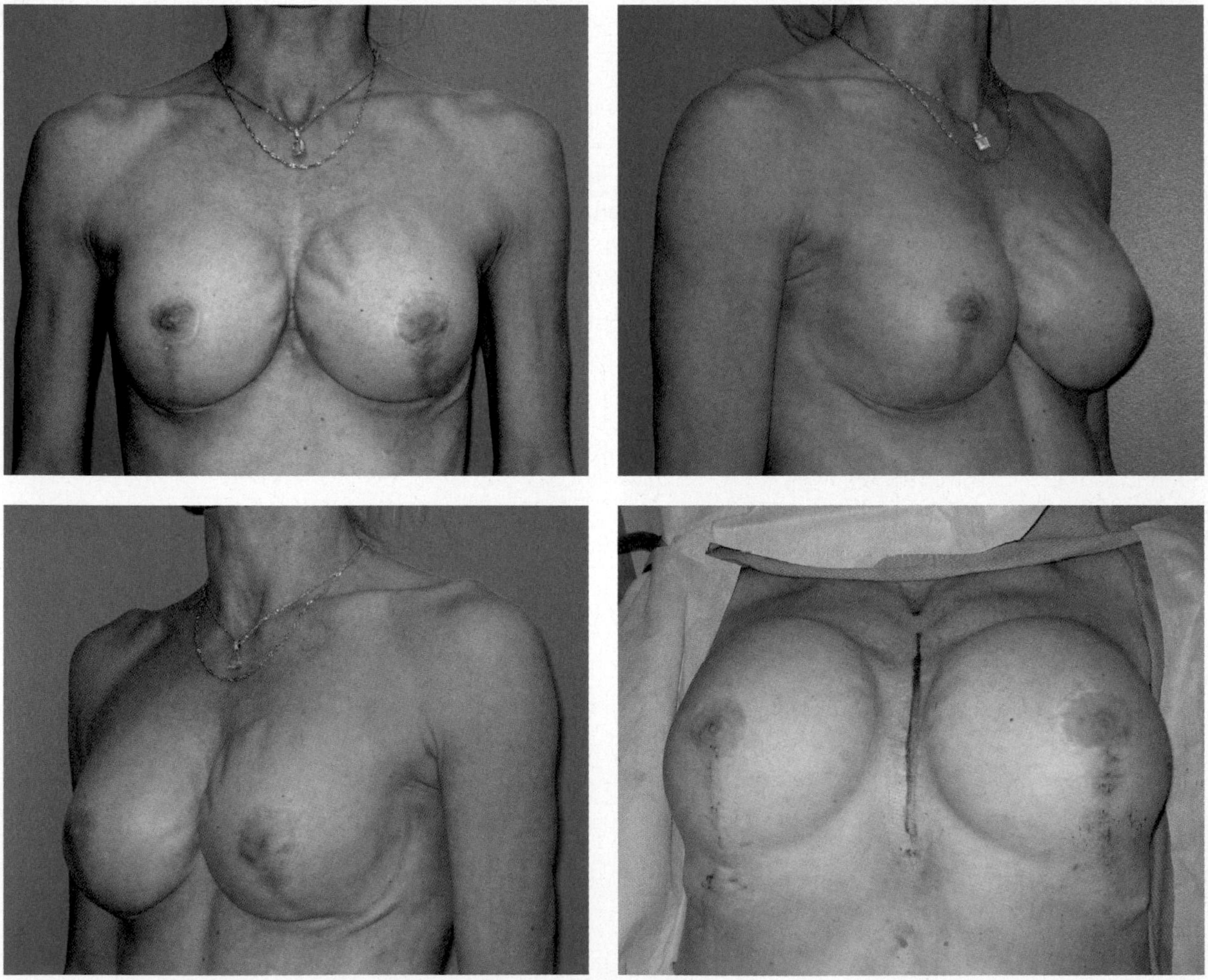

Figure 124.18. **A–C:** Preoperative views of a 46-year-old woman status post multiple procedures including breast augmentation, capsulectomies, and vertical mastopexy. She presented with textured silicone gel implants in the submammary position and was unhappy with visible waviness, synmastia, and wide scars from prior mastopexy. **D:** In the operating room with the "true" midline marked, demonstrating that the left implant is positioned too far medially. (*continued*)

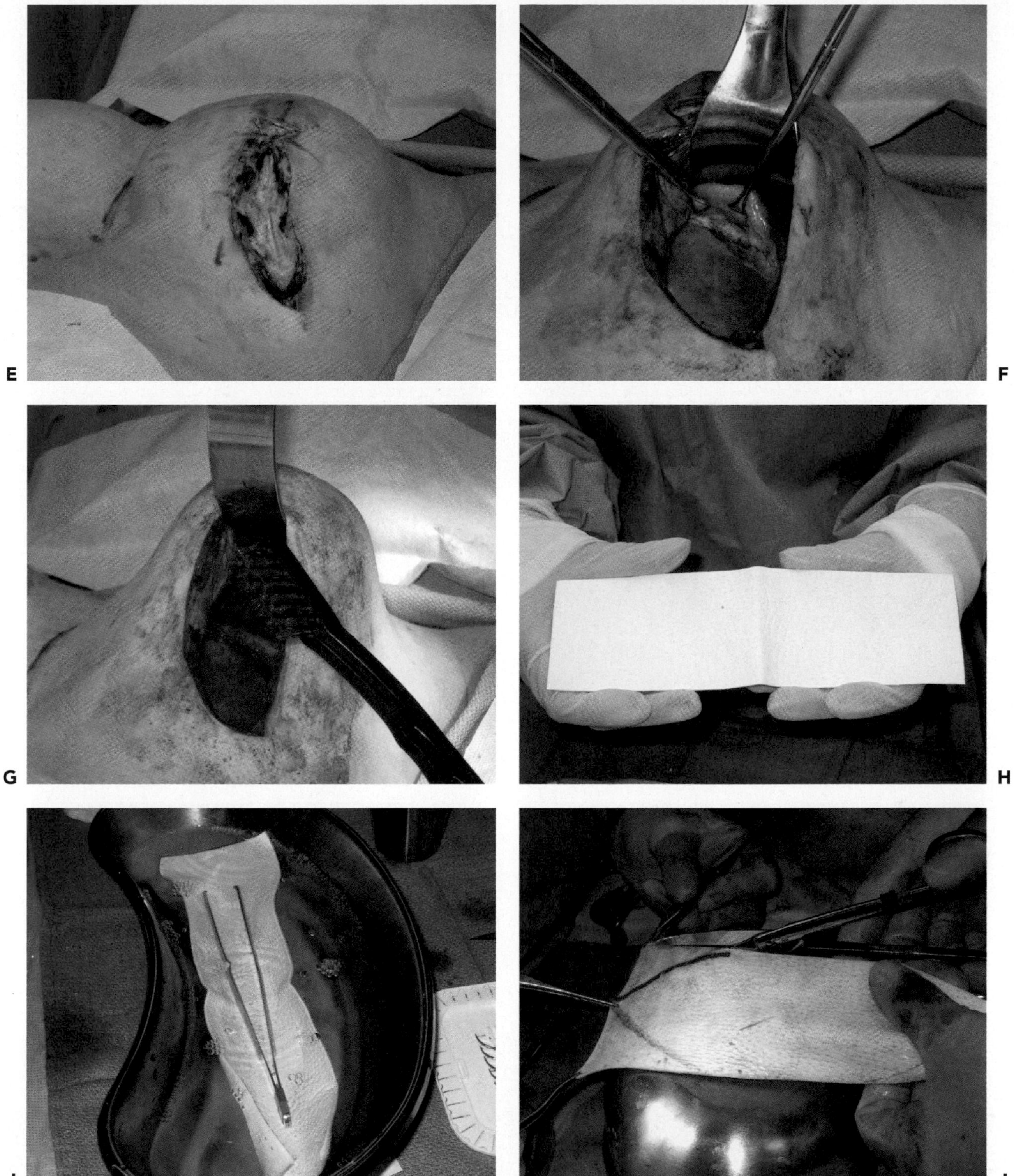

Figure 124.18. (*Continued*) **E:** The widened vertical scar is excised and the wound used to gain access to the periprosthetic space. **F:** The implant is removed from the submammary pocket, and the inferolateral border of the pectoralis major muscle is identified; dissection in the subpectoral plane is initiated to create a submuscular pocket. **G:** A stiff wire brush is used to roughen the smooth capsular surfaces; this is done on the anterior surface of the pectoral muscle, as well as over the entire anterior (submammary) capsule. The purpose of this maneuver is to promote adhesion of the pectoral muscle to the overlying breast and assure eradication of the old submammary pocket; it also promotes revascularization of the acellular dermal graft that will be applied to the undersurface of the breast flap. **H:** The NeoForm acellular dermal graft (Mentor Corp., Santa Barbara, CA) prior to rehydration. **I:** The acellular dermal graft immersed in saline (containing Bacitracin) for rehydration. **J:** The graft being trimmed to the desired shape and size. (*continued*)

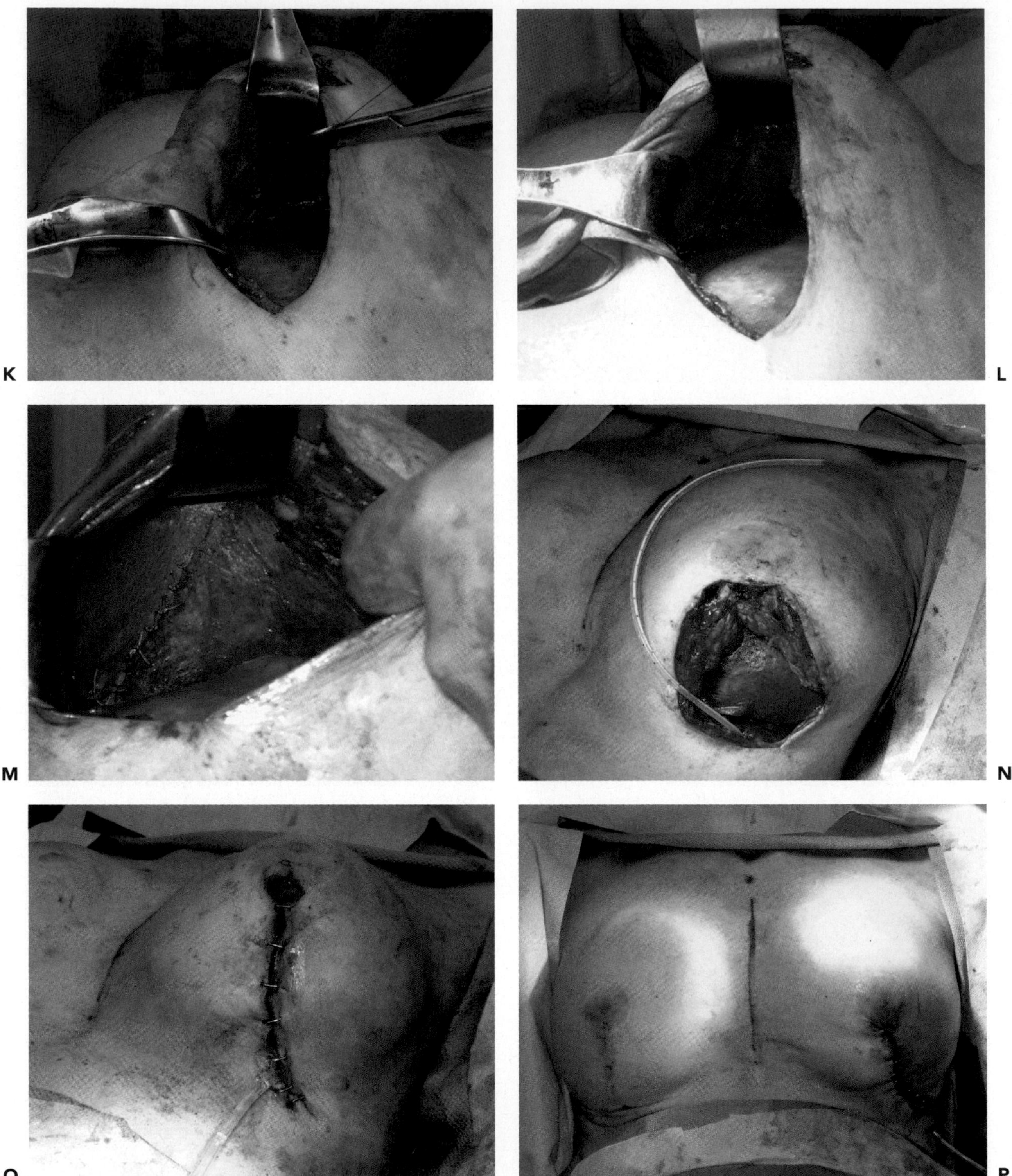

Figure 124.18. (*Continued*) **K:** The graft is sutured to the edge of the incised capsule medially, 1 cm lateral to the midline (to prevent recurrence of synmastia). **L:** The dermal graft has been sutured to the pectoral muscle superiorly (vertical suture line) and to the cut edge of the medial capsule (horizontal suture line). **M:** A close-up view of the suture line where the dermal graft has been secured to the edge of the pectoralis major muscle with interrupted Ethibond stitches. **N:** The implant has been reinserted into the subpectoral pocket and the dermal graft redraped over the inferior pole of the prosthesis; the inferior edge of the dermal graft will be sutured to the chest at the level of the inframammary fold. A silicone rubber drain is inserted beneath the breast tissue flap and atop the dermal graft and contiguous pectoral muscle to prevent fluid accumulation in this space. **O:** The wound edges are temporarily approximated to ensure that the desired breast contour and correct implant position have been achieved. **P:** Patient in the sitting position in the operating room demonstrating correction of synmastia and elimination of rippling. (*continued*)

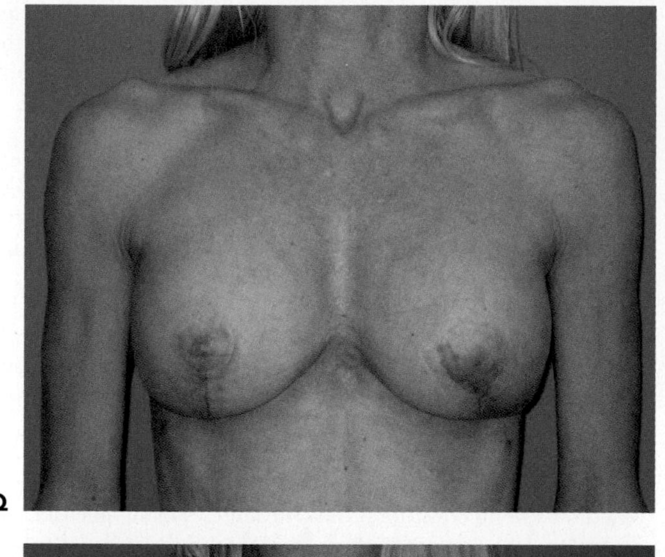
Q

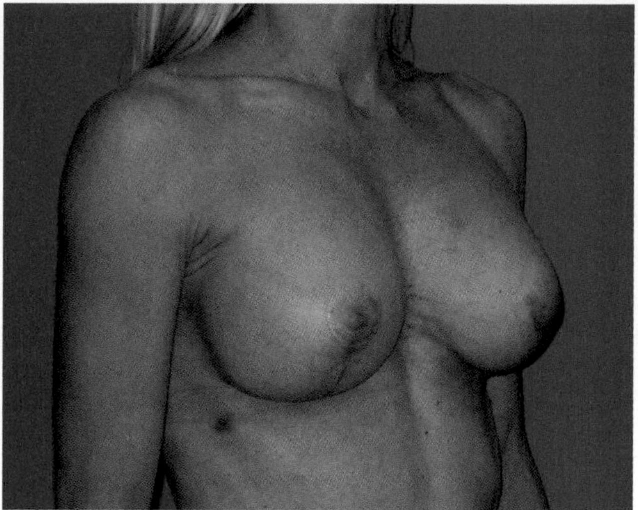
R

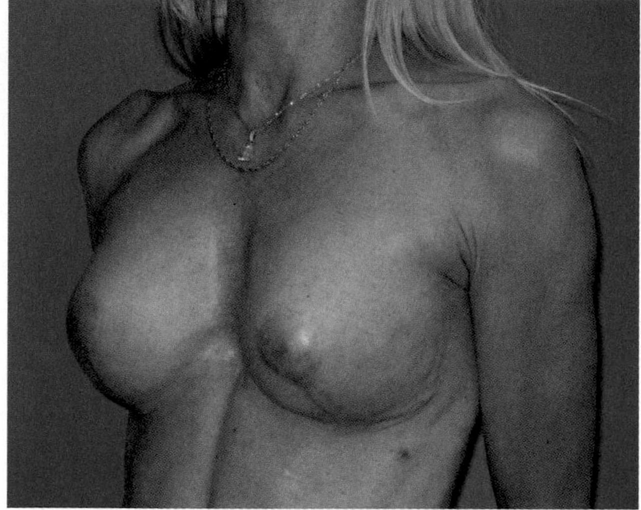
S

Figure 124.18. (*Continued*) **Q–S:** Postoperative frontal and oblique views 5 weeks after surgery.

measures reduce the incidence of the problem, none totally eliminates it. In some patients, contracture is mild and does not require treatment. In others, the condition can become extreme, causing marked distortion, extreme firmness, and even pain and tenderness of the breast.

Many attempts have been made to quantify capsular contracture. The most widely used system is a subjective one known as the Baker classification (41). In this system, grade I is assigned to breasts that are soft to palpation and easily compressible, a desirable result. Grade II is assigned to breasts having greater firmness than desired but no visible deformity. Grade III is applied when external deformity is apparent from contracture usually manifested as a spherical appearance; the breast may bulge superiorly because of upward displacement of the implant. Grade IV contracture is characterized by extreme firmness, marked deformity, pain or tenderness, and sometimes coolness to touch.

Mild degrees of contracture do not necessarily require treatment. Some patients actually prefer the slight firmness and greater projection associated with a grade II contracture. Typically, treatment is reserved for patients with Baker grade III or IV contracture. In the Mentor Core Study the rate of Baker grade III/IV contracture following breast augmentation was 8.1% by 3 years; in the Allergan Core Study the rate of Baker III/IV contracture was 13.2% at 4 years. Some noninvasive forms of therapy have been recommended, including high doses of oral vitamins A and E. No experimental evidence supports the efficacy of vitamins in the treatment of capsular contracture. Leukotriene receptor antagonists [Accolate (Zeneca Pharmaceuticals, Wilmington, DE) and Singulair (Merck & Company, Whitehouse Station, NJ)] have recently been advocated for amelioration of capsular contracture (42). These products have primary roles in asthma treatment. However, they have recently found clinical application in plastic surgery for their immunomodulation properties in the inflammatory cascade, with improvement in some women with Baker III or IV breast implant capsular contractures (43). Some surgeons are now using these medications prophylactically in "high-risk" women (those with prior capsular contracture or periprosthetic infection and those with a history of a tendency to form hypertrophic scars) in addition to treating already established contractures. Although clearly these are off-label uses of these products, they are not illegal (44).

For many years plastic surgeons performed a procedure known as closed capsulotomy, in which the breast was firmly grasped and manually compressed in an effort to rupture the scar tissue capsule. This technique was often effective, but sometimes the capsule tore eccentrically, creating an abnormally shaped breast due to "pseudoherniation" of the implant through the capsule. Closed capsulotomy also carried a risk of rupturing the elastomer shell (causing leakage of gel or saline), as well as a small risk of causing a hematoma. Because of heightened concern about the health risks of implants, especially about dissemination of silicone gel into adjacent tissues, the popularity of closed capsulotomy has diminished. At present, implant package inserts specifically advise against closed capsulotomy.

When contracture is severe enough to warrant intervention, surgical correction is usually indicated. Several options are available. Patients should be given the choice of having the implants removed without replacement. This is the only certain way to guarantee against further problems with contracture (or any other implant-related problems). When explantation without replacement is performed, complete or near-complete capsulectomy is indicated. It is advisable to resect the anterior scar tissue capsule to keep it from distorting the contour of the breast and to enable the potential space to heal. It may also be useful to resect the posterior scar tissue capsule to prevent accumulation of fluid and to promote reattachment of the breast to the chest wall. If complete resection of the capsule is impractical, scoring or roughening the smooth surface will help to promote tissue adherence. In many cases, satisfactory cosmetic results are obtained simply with explantation and capsulectomy, even when implants have been present for many years and there is some ptosis and atrophy. If the degree of ptosis is more dramatic, mastopexy may be indicated at the time of explantation (or as a delayed procedure) to improve breast contour.

Experience reveals that the vast majority of women with contracture will reject the option of explantation without replacement. Generally, augmented patients wish to continue having implants, despite any problems or inconveniences they have experienced. Treatment options for these women include open capsulotomy or capsulectomy (Fig. 124.19), often in conjunction with a "change of plane," either converting from retromammary to subpectoral or subpectoral to retromammary (if there is adequate tissue coverage) (Fig. 124.20). There is also recently published data to suggest that long-established capsular contracture can be reliably corrected by replacing the implants in a carefully created dual-plane, partly subpectoral position (45) (Fig. 124.21).

Often a new breast implant is inserted, especially if the existing implant has been present for a number of years and there is a possibility that a newer device will have less risk of recurrent contracture, gel bleed, or rupture. The exact nature of the treatment undertaken is individualized to meet the specific needs and desires of the particular patient.

Historically, a large proportion of women presenting for correction of capsular contracture have submammary, smooth-surface, single-lumen, gel-filled implants. In such cases, explantation, capsulectomy, and replacement are effective. The new implant may be reinserted into the submammary pocket or into a new space created beneath the pectoral muscle. The decision to transfer the implant to the subpectoral location is based on several considerations. Advantages of subpectoral (or dual plane) placement include the fact that there is more soft tissue padding over the implant (particularly superiorly) and that mammography is facilitated. There is also some evidence that subpectoral positioning of the implant reduces (but does not completely eliminate) the risk of recurrent contracture. Disadvantages of subpectoral placement include a more invasive surgical procedure, increased postoperative discomfort, and visible flattening or distortion of the breast when the pectoral muscle is contracted. This deformity is of particular concern to women who are very physically active. The decision about whether to replace the implant in the subpectoral or submammary position should be made in conjunction with the patient after fully informing her of the advantages and disadvantages of each approach.

Correction of contracture is best performed under general anesthesia. The patient is placed in the supine position with arms adducted to reduce tension on the pectoral muscle and allow relaxation of the soft tissues of the breast.

Once the skin incision is made at the appropriate site, the remaining dissection is performed with the coagulating current of

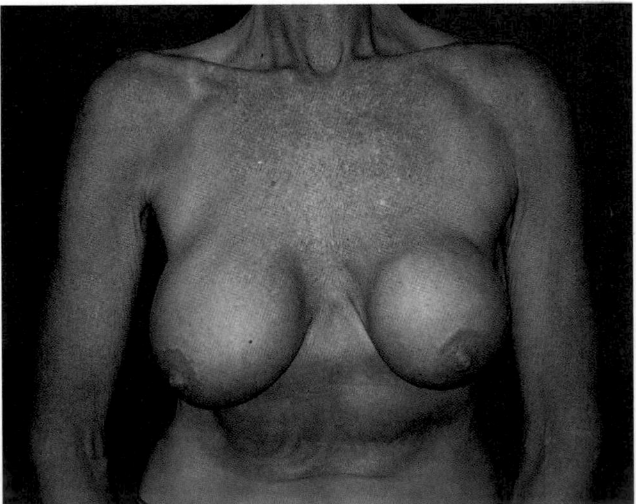
A

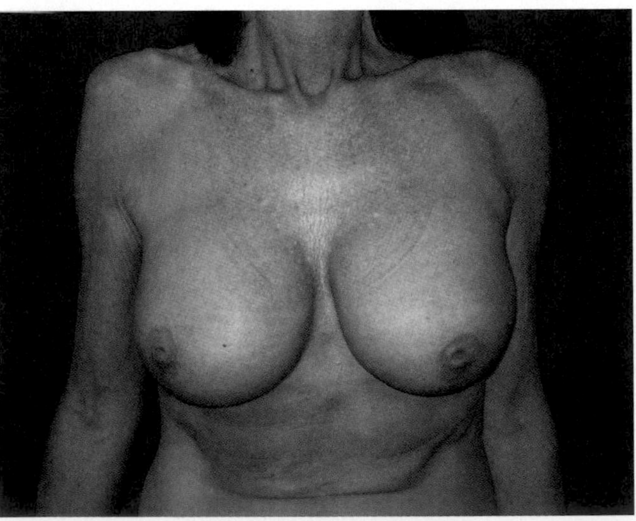
B

Figure 124.19. **A:** A 47-year-old patient with submammary silicone implants for more than 20 years with Baker III contracture on the right side and Baker IV contracture on the left side. **B:** After bilateral capsulotomy and subtotal capsulectomy with insertion of a new pair of silicone gel implants (submammary).

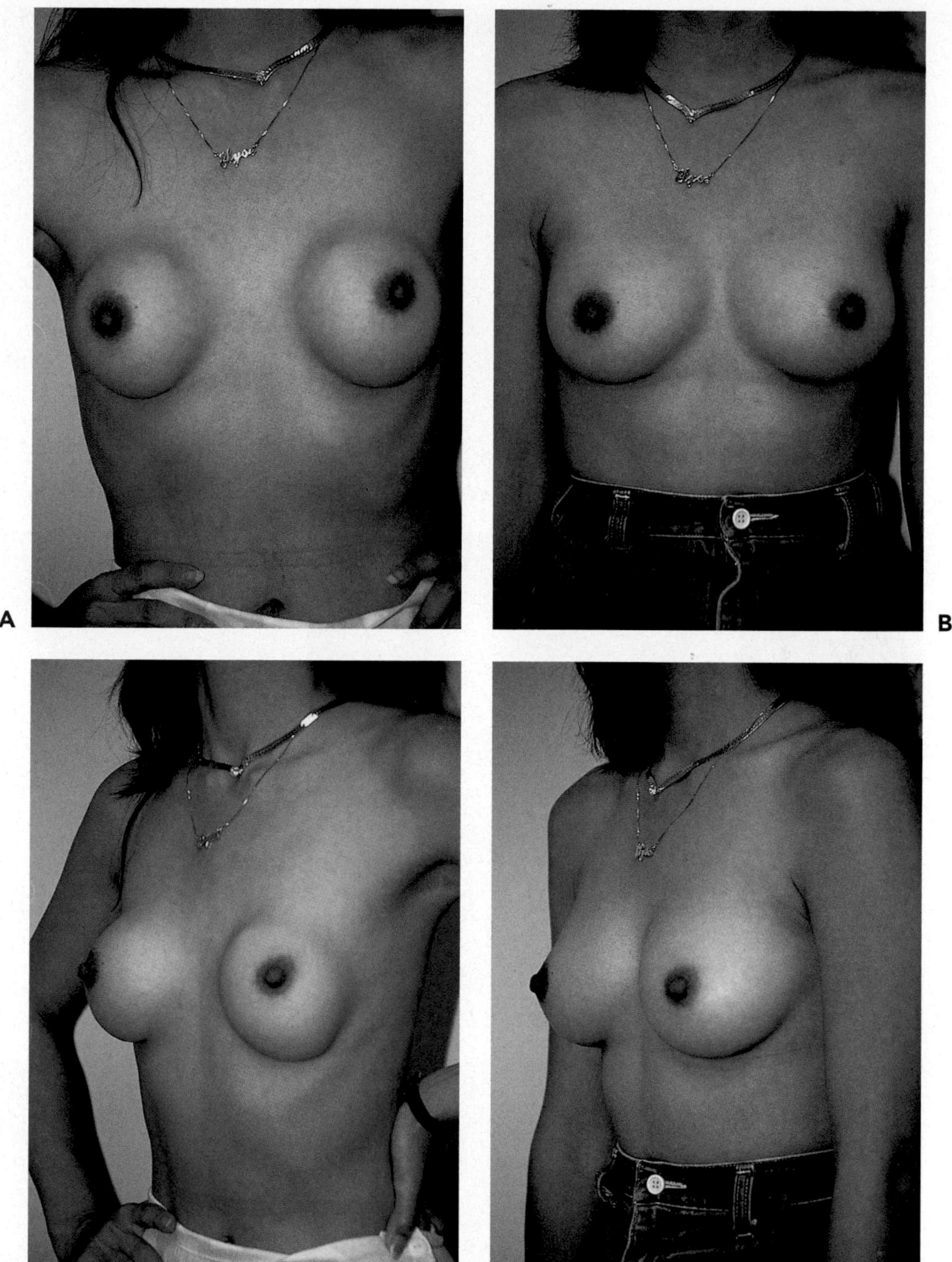

Figure 124.20. **A:** Frontal view of a 26-year-old augmented patient with Baker grade III capsular contracture. Note the abnormal hemispherical appearance of breasts and increased intermammary space. **B:** The same patient following explantation, capsulectomy, and replacement of the implants in the submuscular space. **C:** Three-quarter view before corrective surgery. **D:** Three-quarter view after surgical correction.

the electrocautery unit. This minimizes bleeding and prevents accidental puncture of the implant. After the wound is deepened to the level of the anterior capsule, it is often desirable to dissect between the capsule and the overlying breast tissue. Frequently, the entire anterior scar tissue capsule can be exposed without entering the periprosthetic space. It may even be possible to dissect the posterior capsule off the chest wall without exposing the prosthesis. In this case, the entire capsule and its contents can be removed in continuity. The advantage of staying outside the capsule is that many older gel implants have significant gel bleed and sometimes frank rupture. By keeping the entire dissection extracapsular, there is little chance of leakage and contamination of the wound with silicone.

Sometimes, it is not technically feasible to remove the implant and capsule as a single entity. In such cases, the cautery is used to make an incision through the capsule and the implant is removed. If the implant has bled or leaked, an effort is made to extract as much free gel as possible. Traction is applied to the scar tissue capsule as it is dissected off adjacent structures with the electrocautery. In most cases the entire scar-tissue capsule is removed. If the posterior capsule is densely adherent to the chest (particularly in cases where the pocket is in the subpectoral position), there may be a risk of penetrating the intercostal space and perforating the parietal pleura, resulting in pneumothorax. In such cases, a portion of or the entire posterior scar capsule may be left behind.

If the new implant is to be placed in the subpectoral position, it is not advisable to perform capsulectomy on the anterior pectoral surface. This will unnecessarily weaken the muscle, contributing to muscle dehiscence and retraction. The new

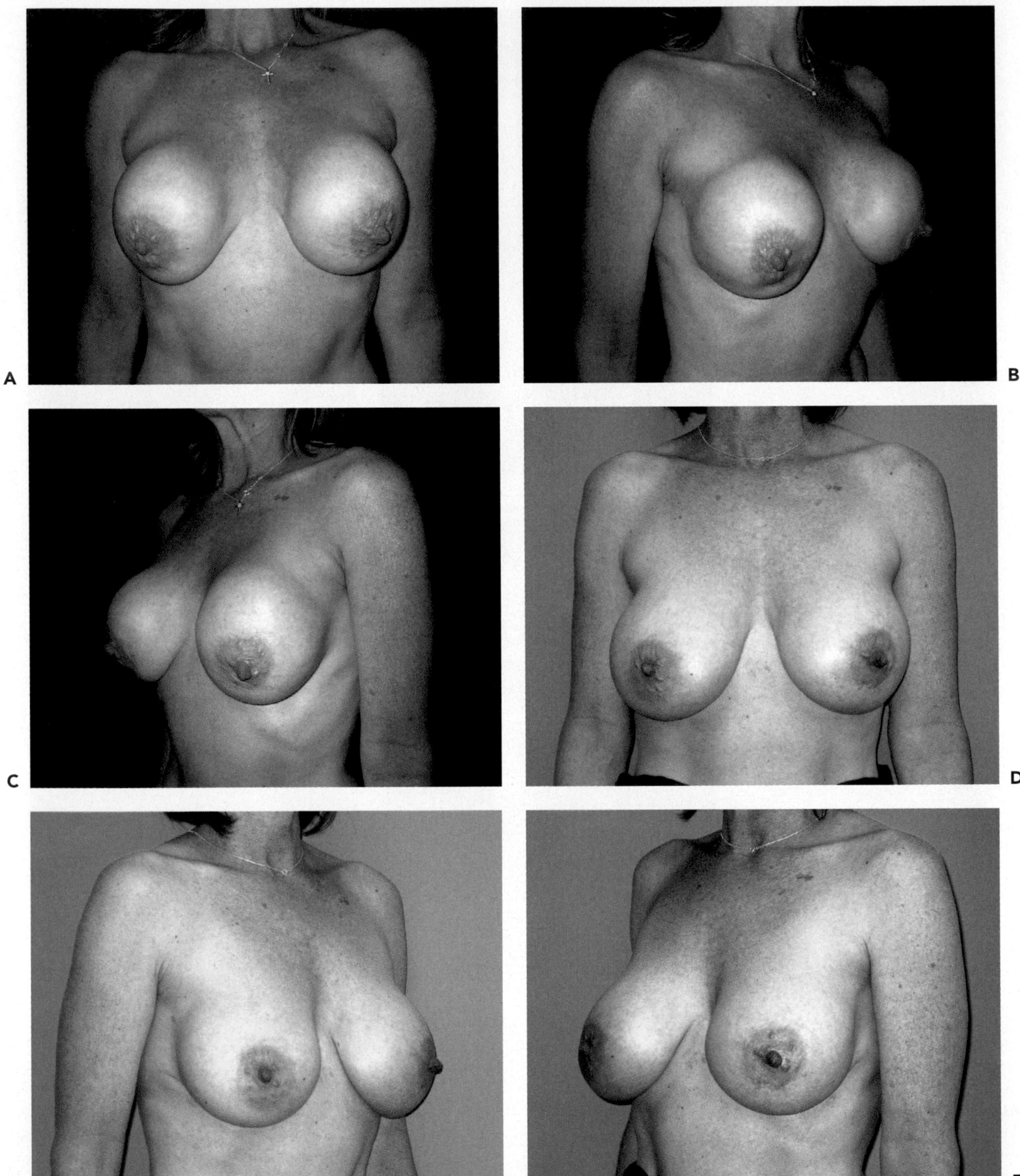

Figure 124.21. **A–C:** Preoperative frontal and oblique views of a 46-year-old woman with submammary saline implants that have been present for more than 15 years. She complained of firm, distorted, tender breasts and was also unhappy with her appearance due to upward malposition of the implants in conjunction with "drooping" of her breast tissues over the implants; she also complained of the wide space between her breasts. **D–F:** Postoperative views after removal of saline implants, eradication of the submammary pocket, and insertion of a new pair of moderate-plus-profile silicone gel implants in the dual-plane pocket; postoperative photos obtained 7 months after surgery.

submuscular pocket is created by elevating the pectoralis major muscle off the underlying pectoralis minor muscle. To create a pocket in the correct location and allow adequate breast projection, it is usually necessary to partially divide the origin of the pectoral muscle from the ribs and sternum. This is accomplished by placing anterior traction on the muscle and dividing the fibers of origin with the coagulating current of the electrocautery unit. Care must be taken not to carry this dissection too far medially, excessively dividing the muscle or detaching skin from the chest near the midline. If this occurs, it may disrupt medial cleavage, cause avulsion and retraction ("window shading") of the pectoral muscle, and increase the risk of synmastia. The risk of such complications is much greater in secondary cases because the pectoral muscle is no longer attached on its anterior surface to the overlying breast. Therefore, there are no attachments to keep it from retracting once it is divided. To prevent the implant from "herniating" from the subpectoral to the submammary space (preexisting implant pocket), it is necessary to eliminate the potential space between pectoral muscle and the posterior breast. This is accomplished by placing a series of interrupted figure-of-eight, nonabsorbable sutures between the anterolateral border of the muscle and the overlying breast parenchyma. Roughening the smooth capsular surfaces with the electrocautery will help promote tissue adherence.

Once an adequate subpectoral pocket has been created, "sizers" are temporarily inserted to determine the appropriate size implant for replacement. Frequently it is desirable to replace the old implant with a slightly larger prosthesis. When patients have capsular contracture, the breast may appear "larger" because of increased anterior projection due to spherical deformation. If the same size of implant is replaced, the breast may appear "smaller" to the patient, particularly as viewed from above. Replacing the implant with a prosthesis 25 to 50 cc larger than the original is recommended. Prior to wound closure, a 7-mm or 1-cm Jackson-Pratt or Blake silicone rubber drain is placed in the subpectoral pocket and brought out through a separate stab wound beneath the inframammary fold or in the axilla. After the wounds are closed, a figure-of-eight pressure dressing is applied for 48 hours; later the patient is placed in an elastic mammary support.

If a patient presenting with capsular contracture already has the implant in the subpectoral position, it can be reinserted into the same pocket or into the submammary space. If the new implant is going to be replaced in the submuscular location, the existing implant is exposed and removed as described earlier. Removal of the scar-tissue capsule on the undersurface of the pectoral muscle is technically difficult and may result in excessive bleeding. This area is adequately treated by scoring of the capsule (capsulotomy) rather than formal capsulectomy. In the remaining areas on the undersurface of the breast parenchyma, capsulectomy may be performed in conventional fashion using electrocautery. Another approach that has recently been described is to create a "neo-subpectoral" pocket by dissecting the plane between the anterior capsule and the overlying muscle; this is most easily done with the implant remaining in situ until the plane has been adequately developed. The implant can then be removed, the anterior and posterior capsular surface can be "tacked" together with several mattress sutures, and the new implant inserted into the "neo-subpectoral" pocket.

In some patients, it is appropriate to remove the implant from the subpectoral position and replace it in the submammary plane. This is acceptable if there is adequate breast tissue superiorly and medially to camouflage the prosthesis. In these cases, it is not necessary to completely extirpate the capsule. The pectoral muscle is dissected from its attachments to the overlying breast parenchyma to create a new submammary pocket. The muscle is then allowed to fall into its normal anatomic position adjacent to the chest wall. The pectoral muscle is sutured in place with a series of figure-of-eight stitches between the lateral border of the muscle and the chest wall (or cut edge of the posterior scar tissue capsule). The remaining exposed scar tissue lining the inferior portion of the periprosthetic space may be resected using the electrocautery.

Due to recent approval by the Food and Drug Administration, plastic surgeons now have unrestricted use of silicone gel–filled implants, so patients undergoing correction of capsular contracture have access to either saline-filled or silicone gel implants. There is some evidence that the risk of contracture is reduced with saline-filled implants (38,46); however, there is no doubt that the incidence of palpability, waviness, and rippling is greater, particularly in these secondary cases in which the tissues are thinned. In many capsulectomy patients, a gel-filled implant will yield a more normal-feeling and natural-appearing breast than a saline-filled device. When performing secondary surgery for contracture, it is reasonable to use either saline- or gel-filled implants, depending on local anatomic considerations and patient preference.

In addition to deciding about filler material, a choice must be made regarding surface texture. The silicone elastomeric shell comes with either a smooth or a mechanically roughened (textured) surface. The purpose of such outer surface texturing is to reduce the risk of contracture. Some studies indicate a reduction in contracture with textured implants (47,48), but there is still a question about the degree to which surface texturing is effective (18). In fact, studies of large numbers of women receiving silicone gel–filled implants (Mentor and Inamed Adjunct Clinical Trials) showed that there was no effect on the incidence of capsular contracture as a result of mechanical surface texturing (either with the Siltex or the Biocell surface texture). If a textured implant is used, it should be inserted into a pocket lined with fresh tissue (as opposed to mature scar tissue). Under these circumstances, the new capsule that forms will take on a textured morphology. For a textured implant to reduce the risk of contracture, it is necessary that a textured, scar-tissue capsule form adjacent to the shell. Textured implants have been associated with a higher incidence of waviness or rippling of the overlying skin, and this disadvantage must be weighed against the potential beneficial effect on recurrent contracture. Textured saline implants have also been associated with a significantly higher rate of spontaneous deflation than smooth saline implants.

In general, when a new implant is being inserted or an implant is being changed from a retromammary to a subpectoral position, surgery is performed bilaterally for the sake of symmetry even if significant contracture is present only on one side. Some recent theories about the etiology of capsular contracture invoke the hypothesis that a "biofilm" forms on the surface of the implant and provides an environment favorable to growth of microorganisms, and that this "subclinical" infection or contamination induces contracture (49,50). This provides the rationale for the use of povidone-iodine irrigation and various combinations of triple-antibiotic irrigation to reduce the incidence of contracture (51). At one time, the use of povidone-iodine in conjunction with breast implants was controversial; recent evidence suggests that contact between povidone-iodine and silicone implants is not deleterious to the implant and is an acceptable therapeutic intervention both to try to reduce the incidence of postoperative infection and to reduce the risk of contracture (52,53).

BREAST DEFORMITY ACCOMPANYING SUBPECTORAL IMPLANTATION

The advantages and disadvantages of subpectoral (or dual plane) positioning of implants were described earlier. Among the disadvantages of placing the implant subpectorally is a tendency for the breast to become flattened or distorted when the muscle is contracted (Fig. 124.22). The extent to which deformity occurs depends on a number of factors, including how aggressively the origin of the pectoral muscle was divided at the time of implantation, how well developed the muscle is, the degree of breast ptosis, and how much overlying breast tissue is present. The deformity is not apparent in most types of clothing but may be evident when the patient is undressed or wears form-fitting or revealing attire. Patients should be advised of this potential problem at the time of initial augmentation consultation. Most patients tolerate mild flattening or distortion of the breast and do not require treatment. Occasionally, a patient will be troubled by the appearance of the breast when the pectoral muscle is contracted or may even complain of discomfort. In such cases, surgical treatment is warranted.

At surgery, the submuscular implant is removed, and the lateral border of the pectoral muscle is identified beneath the anterior scar-tissue capsule. Electrocautery is used to make an incision through the capsule adjacent to the border of the muscle. The leading edge of the muscle is grasped with an Allis or a Lahey clamp. The overlying breast parenchyma is dissected off the anterior surface of the muscle using a combination of cautery and blunt finger dissection. When an adequate-sized submammary pocket has been developed, the pectoral muscle is released and allowed to fall back into its normal anatomic location on the chest wall and affixed with a series of interrupted figure-of-eight sutures (nonabsorbable suture material). This eliminates the potential subpectoral space. The implant is replaced in the submammary pocket and the operative incision closed in the usual fashion. Drains are usually unnecessary.

Patients who are disturbed by deformity or discomfort associated with subpectoral positioning of the implant are uniformly pleased with the improvement achieved by replacement in the retromammary plane. They must of course be willing to accept the limitations of retromammary placement, including a thinner layer of tissue covering the upper half of the implant and the possibility of greater interference with mammography. With the reintroduction of silicone gel implants into general use a much larger proportion of patients get excellent results with submammary positioning.

IMPLANT EXTRUSION

Augmentation mammaplasty patients occasionally present with impending or frank extrusion of an implant. This complication was more common when steroids were instilled into the surgical pocket or the outer lumen of bilumen implants. Steroid preparations caused atrophy of the soft tissues, and the skin and subcutaneous tissues overlying the implant sometimes became very thin, particularly in the dependent portion of the breast. Patients with impending implant extrusion commonly present with an area of bluish discoloration in the inferior pole of the breast. The skin overlying the implant may be tissue paper thin. In rare cases, ulceration or breakdown of the skin occurs with frank exposure of the implant (Fig. 124.23).

Whether the implant has actually eroded through the skin or is threatening to do so, treatment is necessary. If the area of thinning is discrete and localized, an effort may be made to excise the atrophic tissues and approximate the wound with a layered closure. Disadvantages of this approach include additional scarring on the breast, the possibility of subtle alteration of breast contour, potential dehiscence of the repair with resultant exposure of the implant, and recurrent thinning of the tissues. Techniques have also been described by which local capsular flaps can be configured to reinforce thin areas or additional soft tissue coverage can be achieved with local or distant flaps (20). A more conservative approach involves performing explantation and waiting several months to allow the tissues to heal. Later, if the patient desires reimplantation, a decision can be made whether to insert the implant in the submammary, subpectoral, or totally submuscular position.

A

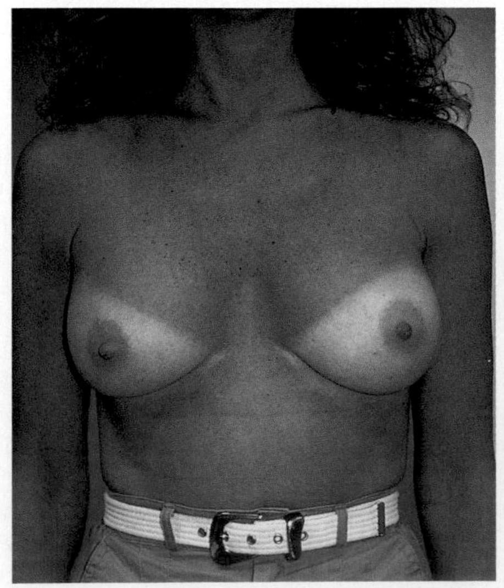

B

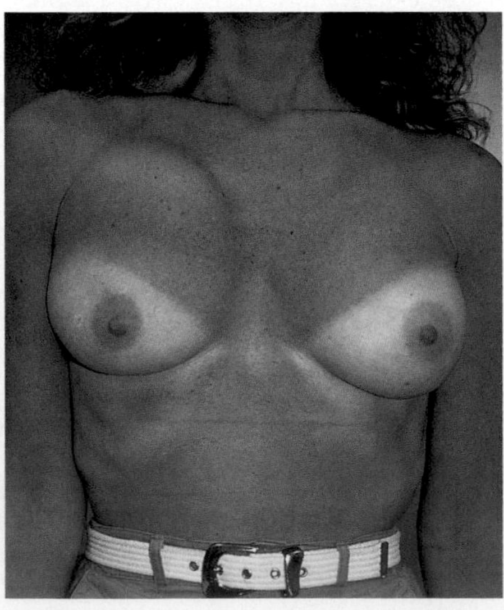

Figure 124.22. **A:** Augmented patient with subpectoral implants at rest. **B:** Same patient with the pectoral muscle activated. Note the flattening of the breast and the superior bulge.

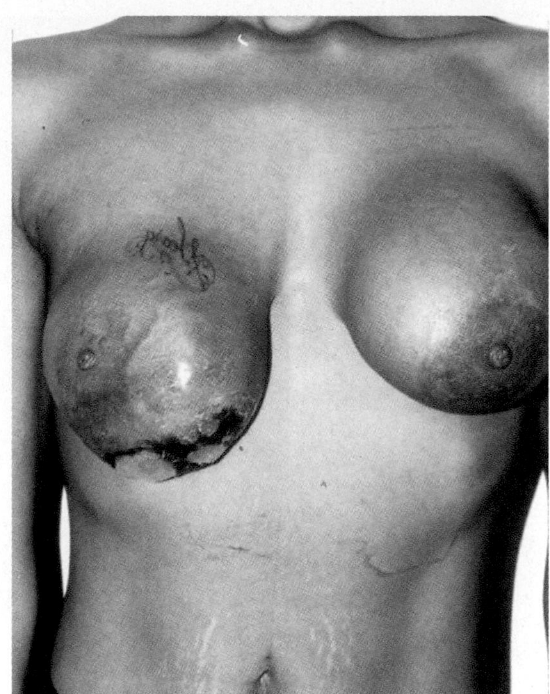

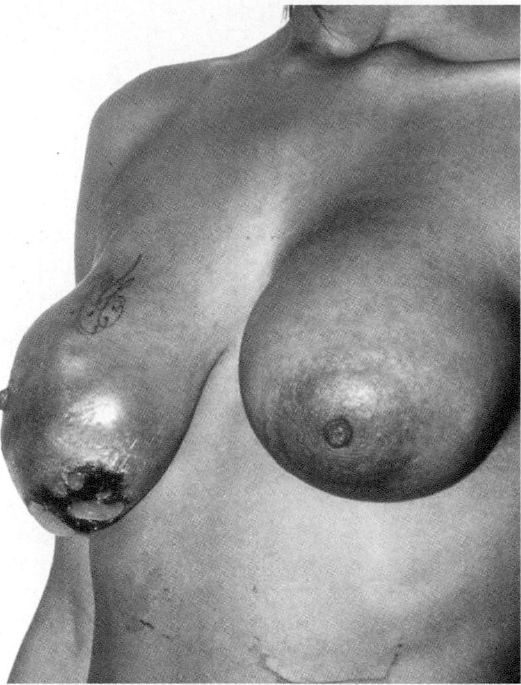

Figure 124.23. An augmented patient with severe atrophy and thinning of the tissues of the inferior pole of the right breast leading to implant exposure.

SILICONE GEL BLEED

A relatively common local problem associated with breast implants, particularly older-generation devices, is leakage of gel. Gel can escape even from intact implants by a phenomenon known as gel bleed. Molecules of silicone permeate the elastomeric shell, traversing back and forth from the adjacent capsule, until a state of equilibrium is achieved. Gel bleed was often dramatic with older-style, single-lumen implants that had a relatively thin shell and contained low-viscosity, non–cross-linked gel. Sometimes the scar-tissue capsule surrounding implants with significant gel bleed become densely calcified (Fig. 124.24). While such calcifications are readily apparent on mammograms, they have a distinct appearance and are readily differentiated from the microcalcifications sometimes associated with breast cancers. Modern implants (low-bleed shell, more cohesive gel) are associated with less bleed. Gel bleed usually is asymptomatic, although it sometimes can be identified on mammograms where the normally sharp border of the implant appears indistinct. Typically, gel bleed is diagnosed when a silicone implant is removed for some other reason (correction of capsular contracture, size change, malposition, or replacement with saline). The treatment of gel bleed is the same as (and usually incidental to) the treatment of capsular contracture.

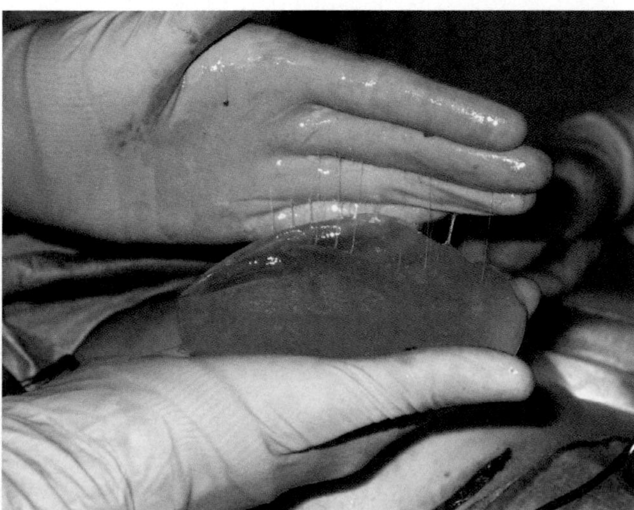

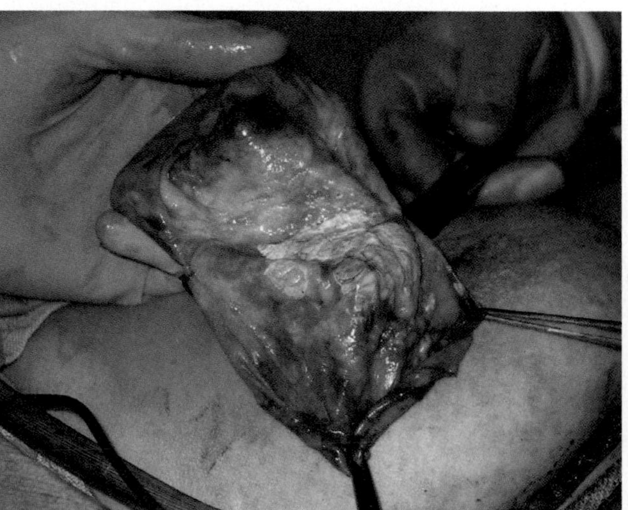

Figure 124.24. **A:** An example of diffuse silicone gel bleed, more common with earlier-generation implants. **B:** Eggshell calcifications within scar-tissue capsule surrounding an implant with extensive gel bleed.

RUPTURE AND EXTRAVASATION OF SILICONE GEL

Frank rupture of the silicone elastomeric shell sometimes occurs (Fig. 124.25). Implant failure rates differ greatly depending on the "generation" of the specific device (54). Rupture rates with "modern" silicone implants are much lower than with earlier devices. In the Mentor Core Study the rupture rate (as determined by magnetic resonance imaging [MRI]) was 0.5% at 3 years; in the Allergan Core Study the rupture rate (MRI cohort) was 2.7% at 4 years. One fact that has been established is that the longer an implant is in place, the greater is the likelihood of rupture (55). Often patients with ruptured implants are asymptomatic, particularly if the gel remains within the scar-tissue capsule (intracapsular rupture) (56). Usually, symptoms are apparent only if there is extracapsular spread of silicone. In these cases there may be a change in the shape of the breast, palpable lumps, axillary adenopathy, or inflammatory changes in the overlying skin due to silicone infiltration into the dermis (Fig. 124.26). Intracapsular or extracapsular rupture may be identified by ultrasonography or MRI. Extracapsular rupture is usually evident on mammography. Sometimes rupture is discovered only incidentally at the time of explantation for other reasons (contracture, size change, malposition, or saline replacement). In any case, when rupture of an implant is diagnosed either preoperatively or at the time of explantation, treatment is recommended. One option, of course, is explantation and capsulectomy without replacement. Most patients, however, request that the implant be replaced.

If rupture has occurred but the silicone gel that has leaked is confined within the capsule, capsulectomy is performed in the same manner as described for the treatment of contracture. If there is extracapsular leakage of silicone gel, it often will cause local areas of granuloma formation and inflammation (silicone mastitis) adjacent to the capsule. If such areas are small, they can be resected without compromising the final aesthetic result. If the silicone granulomata are large and extend to the skin or invade the underlying chest wall muscles, it may be difficult to remove them completely. In this case, subtotal resection is indicated. If the implant was in the retromammary space, it may be advisable to place the new implant in the submuscular position to "isolate" it from the field of gel contamination.

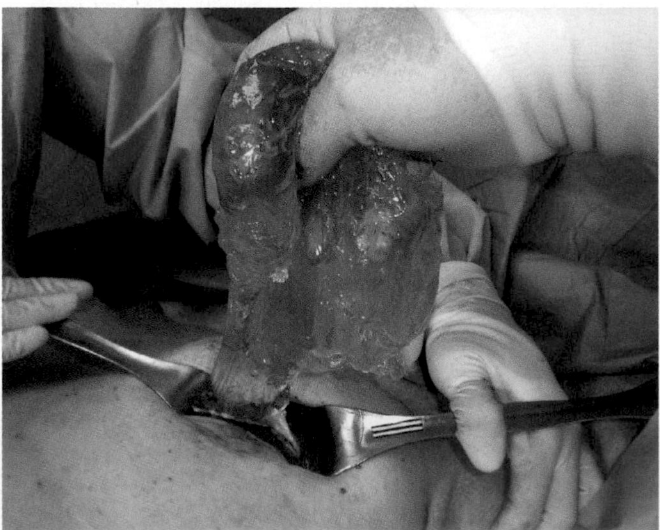

Figure 124.25. Free silicone gel resulting from frank rupture of implant shell.

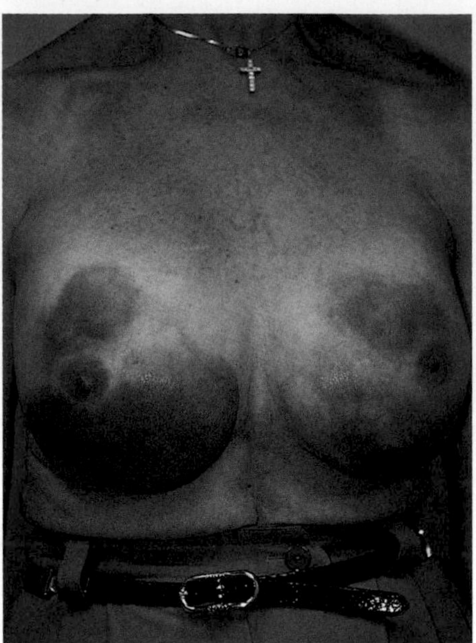

Figure 124.26. Extensive silicone dermatitis from extravasation of free silicone into the skin.

DEFLATION OF SALINE-FILLED IMPLANTS

Saline-filled breast implants comprise a silicone elastomeric shell inflated with normal saline at the time of implantation. Over time, some percentage of saline implants will leak, either from disruption of the integrity of the shell (fold-flaw failure) or incompetence of the valve. The exact "failure rate" of saline-filled implants varies among different brands and styles of inflatable implants. Recent data suggest that the deflation rate is significantly higher with textured implants than with smooth implants. Underfilling of saline implants also increases the risk of deflation. One thing is certain: The longer a saline-inflatable implant is in place, the greater is the likelihood of deflation. When saline-filled implants deflate, the patient is asymptomatic except for a decrease in breast volume. The diagnosis is easy to confirm on physical examination, which reveals an acute change in the size, shape, and consistency of the breast. There may be palpable or even visible wrinkles or folds in the shell (Fig. 124.27). Patients usually are eager to have the implant replaced. The surgery is straightforward and consists simply of explantation of the deflated device through the original incision and replacement with a new implant. In most cases, replacement can be performed under local anesthesia with intravenous sedation. Sometimes, even when the implant has been deflated for a relatively short period of time, the surrounding capsule begins to contract. If this has occurred, capsulotomy is indicated at the time of replacement to assure proper implant position and a soft breast.

INTERFERENCE WITH MAMMOGRAPHY

It has been recognized for some time that breast implants potentially may interfere with mammography (57). Both saline- and silicone gel–filled implants are radiopaque and, as such, cast a shadow on mammograms. Invariably, this shadow overlies

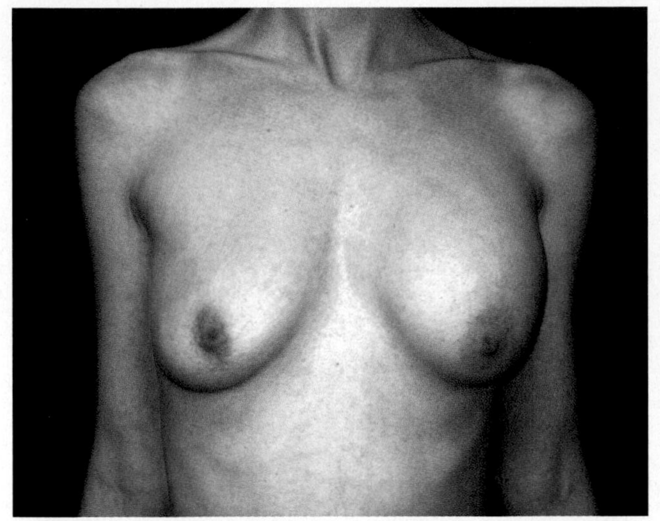

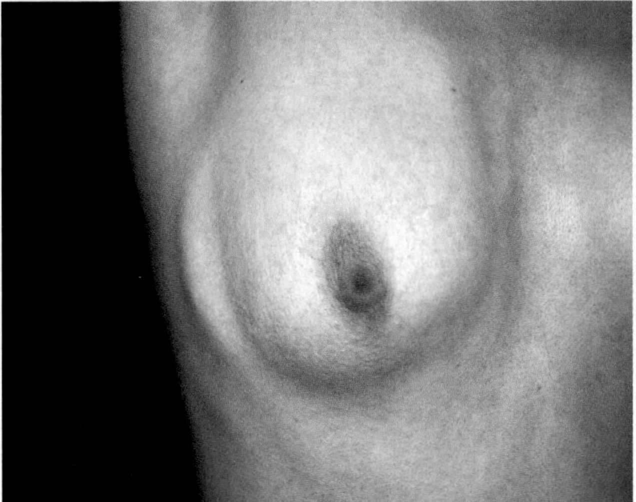

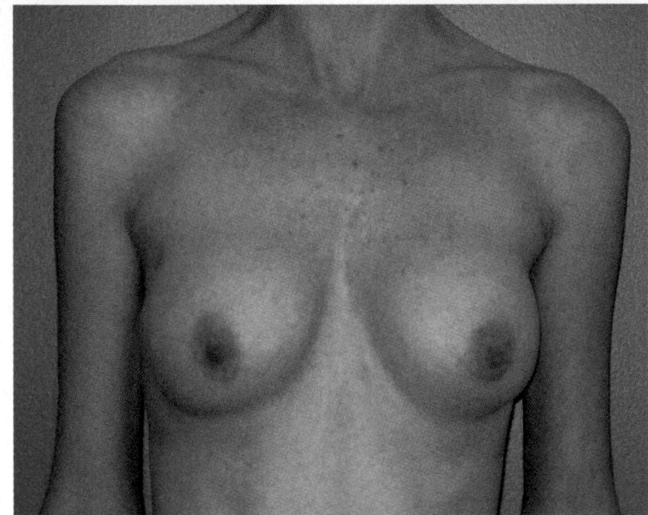

Figure 124.27. **A:** A 30-year-old patient with spontaneous deflation of a right saline implant. **B:** The edge of the deflated implant palpable and visible, especially with the arm abducted **C:** Following replacement of the deflated right implant (the left implant was repositioned inferiorly and medially and bilateral inverted nipples corrected at same operation).

part of the breast tissue and might obscure visualization of subtle lesions (small tumors, microcalcifications, parenchymal distortions, etc.) that could be the earliest indicators of breast cancer. Although numerous studies confirm that implants block visualization of breast tissue, clinical studies to determine the degree to which implants delay cancer detection have been equivocal. There is no definitive proof that augmented women are diagnosed with more-advanced cancers. In fact, recently published data suggest that augmented and nonaugmented breast cancer patients are diagnosed with the same stage of disease and have identical recurrence and survival rates (58). However, patients should be warned of the potential detrimental effect of implants on the accuracy of mammography. Factors that make mammography more difficult include capsular contracture and submammary positioning of the implant. Mammography is facilitated when the implant is in the subpectoral position, by obtaining both compression and displacement mammograms, by getting additional views when indicated, and by correlating mammography with physical examination (59).

CONCLUSION

Although local implant-related complications are relatively common after augmentation mammaplasty, most can be managed effectively while preserving the desired cosmetic result. It is important to advise augmentation candidates of possible complications; patients are more likely to tolerate complications (and the necessary corrective surgery) if they have been forewarned. Despite the shortcomings of breast implants and the frequent need for secondary surgery, the vast majority of patients are happy that they underwent breast augmentation. Most patients with implant-related complications choose treatment that enables them to keep their implants. It is distinctly uncommon for the augmented patient to elect explantation without replacement.

EDITORIAL COMMENTS

Dr. Handel does an excellent job of describing the diagnosis and management of problems that may occur following augmentation mammaplasty. He subdivides them into early and late. Early problems may include infection, hematoma, displacement or asymmetry of the inframammary fold, Mondor disease, galactocele, the "double-bubble" deformity, and implant malposition. Late problems may include rippling, capsular contracture, deformities of shape, implant extrusion, silicone gel bleed and rupture, saline deflation, and interference with mammography. Dr. Handel provides information on incidence, diagnosis, and management that is very useful, especially when consulting with patients.

Dr. Handel devotes a significant portion of this chapter to the management of capsular contracture. He thoroughly reviews the role of explantation, capsulotomy, capsulectomy, pocket conversion, and neo-subpectoral conversion. Another option that is currently being studied but not mentioned in this chapter is the role of human acellular dermal matrices (ADMs). Given the elastin content and observation of minimal fibrosis on the surface of the ADM, a potential benefit may be possible.

The concept of capsulectomy in the treatment of subglandular implants with capsular contracture or implant rupture is very useful. Leaving the periprosthetic capsule behind tends to encourage the formation of late seromas. In addition, the scar tissue can deform the breast and prevent it from resuming a natural position. On the other hand, when the implant has been previously placed in a subpectoral pocket, the removal of the capsule threatens significantly more morbidity, including bleeding, injury to the overlying pectoralis major muscle, and injury to the chest wall and even pneumothorax. For that reason, as a rule, the periprosthetic capsule in the submuscular pocket is usually left intact, and excision of the capsule is limited to when it is clinically necessary.

M.Y.N.

REFERENCES

1. Cronin TD, Gerow FJ. Augmentation mammaplasty: a new "natural feel" prosthesis. In: *Transactions of the Third International Congress of Plastic Surgery*. Amsterdam: Excerpta Medica; 1963:41–49.
2. Beisang AA, Geise MS, Ersek RA. Radiolucent prosthetic gel. *Plast Reconstr Surg* 1991; 87:885–892.
3. Bondurant S, Ernster V, Herdman R, eds. *Safety of Silicone Breast Implants*. Washington, DC: National Academy Press; 1999:28–32.
4. Hetter GP. Satisfactions and dissatisfactions of patients with augmentation mammaplasty. *Plast Reconstr Surg* 1979:64(2):151–155.
5. Handel N, Wellisch D, Silverstein MJ, et al. Knowledge, concern, and satisfaction among augmentation mammaplasty patients. *Ann Plast Surg* 1993;30:13–20.
6. McGrath MH, Burkhardt BR. The safety and efficacy of breast implants for augmentation mammaplasty. *Plast Reconstr Surg* 1984;74:550–560.
7. Schusterman MA, Kroll SS, Reece GP, et al. Incidence of autoimmune disease in patients after breast reconstruction with silicone gel implants versus autogenous tissue: a preliminary report. *Ann Plast Surg* 1993;31(1):1–6.
8. Gabriel SE, O'Fallon WM, Kurland LT, et al. Risk of connective-tissue diseases and other disorders after breast implantation. *N Engl J Med* 1994;330(24):1697–1702.
9. Gutowski KA, Mesna GT, Cunningham BL. Saline-filled breast implants: a Plastic Surgery Educational Foundation multicenter outcomes study. *Plast Reconstr Surg* 1997;100(4): 1019–1027.
10. Gabriel EE, Woods JE, O'Fallon M, et al. Complications leading to surgery after breast implantation. *N Engl J Med* 1997;336(10):677–682.
11. Rheingold LM, Yoo RP, Courtiss EH. Experience with 326 inflatable breast implants. *Plast Reconstr Surg* 1994;93(1):118–122.
12. Mladick RA. No-touch submuscular saline breast augmentation technique. *Aesthet Plast Surg* 1993;17:183–192.
13. Williams C, Aston S, Rees TD. The effect of hematoma on the thickness of pseudosheath around silicone implants. *Plast Reconstr Surg* 1975;56:194–198.
14. Courtiss EH, Goldwyn RM, Anastasi GW. The fate of breast implants with infections around them. *Plast Reconstr Surg* 1979;63:812–816.
15. Freedman A, Jackson I. Infections in breast implants. *Infect Dis Clin North Am* 1989;3: 275–287.
16. Cholnoky, T. Augmentation mammaplasty: survey of complications in 10,941 patients by 265 surgeons. *Plast Reconstr Surg* 1970;45(6):573–577.
17. Ablaza VJ, LaTrenta GS. Late infection of a breast prosthesis with *Enterococcus avium*. *Plast Reconstr Surg* 1998;102(1):227–230.
18. Handel N, Jensen JA, Black Q, et al. The fate of breast implants: a critical analysis of complications and outcomes. *Plast Reconstr Surg* 1995;96:1521–1533.
19. Brand KG. Infection of mammary prostheses: a survey and the question of prevention. *Ann Plast Surg* 1993;30:289–295.
20. Spear SL, Howard MA, Boehmler JH, et al. The infected or exposed breast implant: management and treatment strategies. *Plast Reconstr Surg* 2004;113(6):1634–1644.
21. fischl RA, Kahn S, Simon BE. Mondor's disease: an unusual complication of mammaplasty. *Plast Reconstr Surg* 1975;56(3):319–322.
22. Sahy NI. Recurrent Mondor's disease after augmentation mammaplasty. *Aesthet Plast Surg* 1983;7:259–263.
23. Deloach ED, Lord SA, Ruf LE. Unilateral galactocele following augmentation mammaplasty. *Ann Plast Surg* 1994;33:68–71.
24. Caputy GG, Flowers RS. Copious lactation following augmentation mammaplasty: an uncommon but not rare condition. *Aesthet Plast Surg* 1994;18:393–397.
25. Hartley JH, Schatten WE. Postoperative complication of lactation after augmentation mammaplasty. *Plast Reconstr Surg* 1971;47:150–153.
26. Rothkopf DM, Rosen HM. Case report: lactation as a complication of aesthetic breast surgery successfully treated with bromocriptine. *Br J Plast Surg* 1990;43:373–375.
27. Chasan PE. Breast capsulorrhaphy revisited: a simple technique for complex problems. *Plast Reconstr Surg* 2005;115:296–301.
28. Spear SL, Little JW III, Breast capsulorrhaphy. *Plast Reconstr Surg* 1988;81(2):274–279.
29. Voice SD, Carlsen LN. Using a capsular flap to correct breast implant malposition. *Aesthet Surg J* 2001;21:441–446.
30. Spence RJ, Feldman JJ, Ryan JJ. Synmastia: the problem of medial confluence of the breasts. *Plast Reconstr Surg* 1984;73(2):261–269.
31. Spear SL, Bogue DP, Thomassen JM. Synmastia after breast augmentation. *Plast Reconstr Surg* 2006;118(7 suppl) :168S–171S.
32. Baxter RA. Intracapsular allogenic dermal grafts for breast implant-related problems. *Plast Reconstr Surg* 2003;112(6):1692–1696.
33. Coleman SR, Saboeiro AP. Fat grafting to the breast revisited: safety and efficacy. *Plast Reconstr Surg* 2007;119(3):775–785.
34. Dowden DI. Correction of implant rippling using allograft dermis. *Aesthet Surg J* 2001;21:81–84.
35. Vinnik CA. Spherical contracture of fibrous capsules around breast implants. *Plast Reconstr Surg* 1976;58:555–560.
36. Caffee HH. The influence of silicone bleed on capsule contracture. *Ann Plast Surg* 1986;17:284–287.
37. Cairns TS, deVilliers W. Capsular contracture after breast augmentation: a comparison between gel- and saline-filled prostheses. *S Afr Med J* 1980;57(23):951–953.
38. McKinney P, Tresley G. Long-term comparison of patients with gel and saline mammary implants. *Plast Reconstr Surg* 1983;72(1):27–31.
39. Chang L, Caldwell E, Reading G, et al. A comparison of conventional and low-bleed implants in augmentation mammaplasty. *Plast Reconstr Surg* 1992;89(1):79–82.
40. Coleman DJ, Foo IT, Sharpe DT. Textured or smooth implants for breast augmentation? A prospective controlled trial. *Br J Plast Surg* 1991;44(6):444–448.
41. Little G, Baker JL Jr. Results of closed compression capsulotomy for treatment of contracted breast implant capsules. *Plast Reconstr Surg* 1980;65:30–33.
42. Rohrich RJ, Janis JE, Reisman NR. Use of off-label and non-approved drugs and devices in plastic surgery. *Plast Reconstr Surg* 2003;112(1):242–243.
43. Schlesinger SL, Ellenbogen R, Desvigne MN, et al. Zafirlukast (Accolate): a new treatment for capsular contracture. *Aesthet Surg J* 2002;22:329–331.
44. Dowden RV, Reisman NR, Gorney M. Going off-label with breast implants. *Plast Reconstr Surg* 2002;110(1):323–329.
45. Spear SL, Carter ME, Ganz JC. The correction of capsular contracture by conversion to "dual-plane" positioning: technique and outcomes. *Plast Reconstr Surg* 2006;118(7 suppl):103S–113S.
46. Reiffel RS, Rees TD, Guy CL, et al. A comparison of capsule formation following breast augmentation by saline-filled or gel-filled implants. *Aesthet Plast Surg* 1983;7:113–116.
47. Hakelius L, Ohlsen L. A clinical comparison of the tendency to capsular contracture between smooth and textured gel-filled silicone mammary implants. *Plast Reconstr Surg* 1992;90:247–254.
48. Burkhardt BR, Demas CP. The effect of Siltex texturing and povidone-iodine irrigation on capsular contracture around saline inflatable breast implants. *Plast Reconstr Surg* 1994;93: 123–128.
49. Pajkos A, Deva A, Vickery K, et al. Detection of subclinical infection in significant breast implant capsules. *Plast Reconstr Surg* 2003;111(5):1605–1611.
50. Prantl L, Schreml S, fichtner-Feigl S, et al. Clinical and morphological conditions in capsular contracture formed around silicone breast implants. *Plast Reconstr Surg* 2007;120 (1):275–284.
51. Adams WP Jr, Rios JL, Smith S. Enhancing patient outcomes in aesthetic and reconstructive breast surgery using triple antibiotic breast irrigation: six-year prospective clinical study. *Plast Reconstr Surg* 2006;118(7 suppl):46S–52S.
52. Wiener TC. The role of Betadine irrigation in breast augmentation. *Plast Reconstr Surg* 2007;119(1):12–15.
53. Becker HJ, Craig D. The effect of Betadine on silicone implants [Correspondence and brief communications]. *Plast Reconstr Surg* 2000;105(4):1570.
54. Peters W, Smith D, Lugowski S. Failure properties of 352 explanted silicone-gel breast implants. *Can J Plast Surg* 1996;4:1–7.
55. de Camara DL, Sheridan JM, Kammer BA. Rupture and aging of silicone gel breast implants. *Plast Reconstr Surg* 1993;9:828–834.
56. Holmich LR, Kjoller K, Vejborg I, et al. Prevalence of silicone breast implant rupture among Danish women. *Plast Reconstr Surg* 2001;108(4):848–858.
57. Silverstein MJ, Handel N, Steyskal R, et al. Breast cancer in women after augmentation mammoplasty. *Arch Surg* 1988;123:681–685.
58. Handel N. The effect of silicone implants on the diagnosis, prognosis, and treatment of breast cancer. *Plast Reconstr Surg* 2007;120(7) (suppl 1):81S–93S.
59. Handel N, Silverstein MJ, Gamagami P, et al. Factors affecting mammographic visualization of the breast after augmentation mammoplasty. *JAMA* 1992;286:1913–1917.

CHAPTER

125

Scott L. Spear
M. Renee Jespersen
Samir S. Rao

Neo-subpectoral Technique for Implant Malposition

It is generally accepted that revision breast augmentation is more complex and difficult than primary breast augmentation. The most common causes for secondary surgery in previously augmented patients are capsular contracture and implant malposition. In the case in which patients have a failed device or desire a different size, the surgery is straightforward. For the categories of capsular contracture and implant malposition, the implant capsule must be modified or removed, and the surgery becomes more complex. Several methods have been described to remove or modify a problematic implant capsule, and all have strengths and shortcomings (1–4).

Correcting a poorly positioned implant in a previously formed capsule is difficult. The simplest way to modify implant position is by capsulorrhaphy and/or capsulotomy. By tightening or releasing the existent capsule, the implant within it can be shifted into the new desired position. Efforts to tailor the previous capsule have been effective in the short term, but the malposition may recur once the sutures lose integrity. In addition, repositioning an implant with capsulorrhaphy requires finesse and can frustrate even the most experienced surgeon.

Alternatively, the position of an implant can be changed from subglandular to subpectoral and a new pocket created in that fashion. This offers the benefits of subpectoral positioning, as well as the advantage of a pristine tissue plane in which to work. For the surgeon, this is the near equivalent of a primary augmentation, as the limits of the uppermost portion of the implant pocket can be easily defined in the exact desired position. Should the patient already have a subpectoral implant, however, the change to a subglandular dissection may not be desirable due to local tissue characteristics. This may be the case where tissue is thin and likely to show implant edges or rippling, or in the case of a previous capsular contracture, where placing the implant subglandularly would increase the risk of recurrence (5).

Severe implant malposition in the subpectoral plane can also be addressed by removing the implant for a period of time and allowing the pocket to close. The augmentation is then performed at a later date. It is understandable that most patients dislike this method, and many surgeons choose it only as a last resort.

For capsular contracture the problems are similar. Simple capsulotomy may improve implant position, but it may lead to recurrence. Total capsulectomy is effective at removing the contracture but leaves the surgeon with a large implant pocket, which can lead to difficulty in controlling implant position precisely. This is even more troublesome with the newer generation of form-stable, textured silicone implants, which require a snug implant pocket for adherence and to avoid rotation.

The neo-subpectoral approach in secondary prosthetic breast augmentation combines the advantage of a new pocket dissection without the necessity of a total capsulectomy or a site change to the subglandular position (6). Using this method, the surgeon creates a new implant pocket using the pectoral muscle as the anterior component and the anterior leaflet of the previously existing capsule as the posterior component. Once the new space is dissected, the old capsule is collapsed and secured against the chest wall. This method allows the surgeon precise control over the parameters of the new implant pocket, regardless of the previous implant position. The technique is effective in correcting implant malposition and complex symmastia and may be appropriate in some cases of capsular contracture (Figs. 125.1 to 125.6). Recurrence of previous malposition is rare when the procedure is performed properly, and the surgeon has the ability to precisely control the implant pocket dimensions.

TECHNIQUE

Preoperative planning begins with evaluating the patient while she is standing or sitting upright. Sometimes the implant malposition is not obvious at rest (as is commonly the case with symmastia) and may be more evident when the patient flexes the pectoralis muscles or leans forward. The desired boundaries of the new breast implant position are then carefully marked. The ideal inframammary fold is marked as well. Proper positioning of the inframammary fold is dependent on the nipple-to-fold distance required for the particular volume and base width of the implant that is to be used. See Figure 125.7.

The choice of which incision to use is largely dependent on the anatomy and findings of the specific case. The "neo-subpectoral" pocket cannot be dissected with current instrumentation through the transaxillary or periumbilical approach. Therefore, if the previous implant was placed by the transaxillary or periumbilical approach, then either the periareolar or inframammary incision may be used for the correction. If the patient had a previous periareolar approach, then it may be desirable to correct the malposition using that same approach unless there is some specific local or technical reason not to. This may be the case if the areolar diameter and parenchymal thickness would not allow for direct visualization of the limits of the pocket, precise dissection, and atraumatic placement of the device. Located at the center of the breast, nearly equidistant from what will be the borders of the new pocket, the periareolar incision allows for clear, equal, and direct visualization of the entire perimeter of the pocket. By virtue of the areola's location near the "equator" of the implant, it allows visualization from "the high ground" down toward the limits of the pocket. If the patient has an inframammary scar, then the surgeon must evaluate whether or not to use this incision because it may not

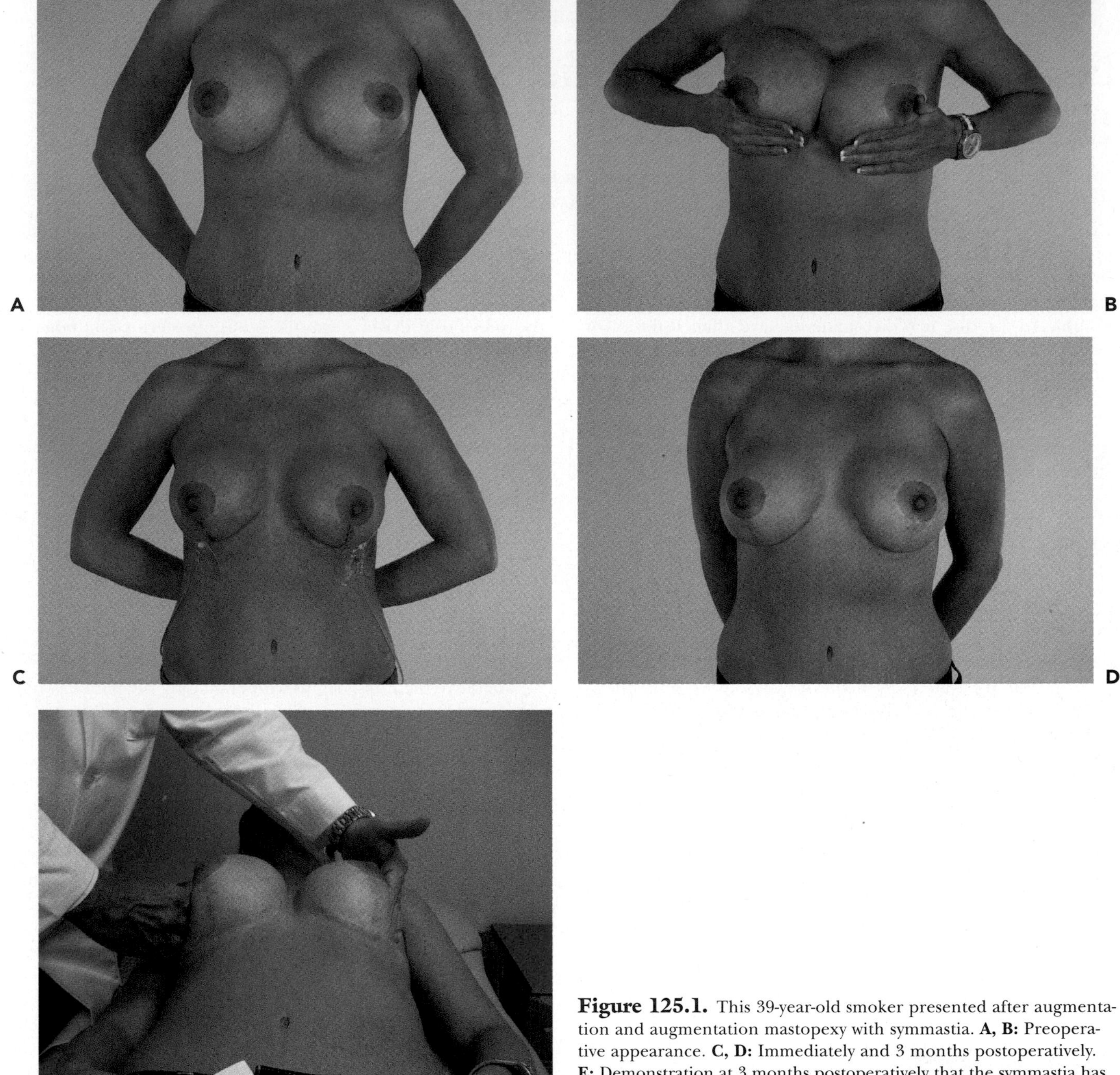

Figure 125.1. This 39-year-old smoker presented after augmentation and augmentation mastopexy with symmastia. **A, B:** Preoperative appearance. **C, D:** Immediately and 3 months postoperatively. **E:** Demonstration at 3 months postoperatively that the symmastia has been corrected.

provide adequate exposure to dissect the "neo-subpectoral" pocket up and over the implant, especially if the inframammary incision is low and the implant is large. In this case, a periareolar incision may still be preferable. In most cases, the previous incision will suffice.

Dissection is facilitated by leaving the implant in place as long as possible. While a projecting implant does not seriously handicap periareolar dissection, it can restrict visualization from the inframammary approach. In any case, dissection is continued with the implant in place as long as visualization is excellent, after which point the implant is removed and dissection continues without the implant providing countertension. The final choice of incision is a tactical one and should be based upon which method will allow the surgeon the best visualization in that particular patient.

Initially, dissection is identical to performing the anterior portion of a complete capsulectomy. After incision, dissection is carried down to the implant capsule and then proceeds along the anterior surface without entering it. Superomedially there will be muscle on the superficial surface of the pocket. Inferiorly and laterally there will be gland on the superficial surface of the new space. Thus, while this procedure is termed "neo-subpectoral," the surgeon should remember that there will not be pectoralis major muscle overlying the

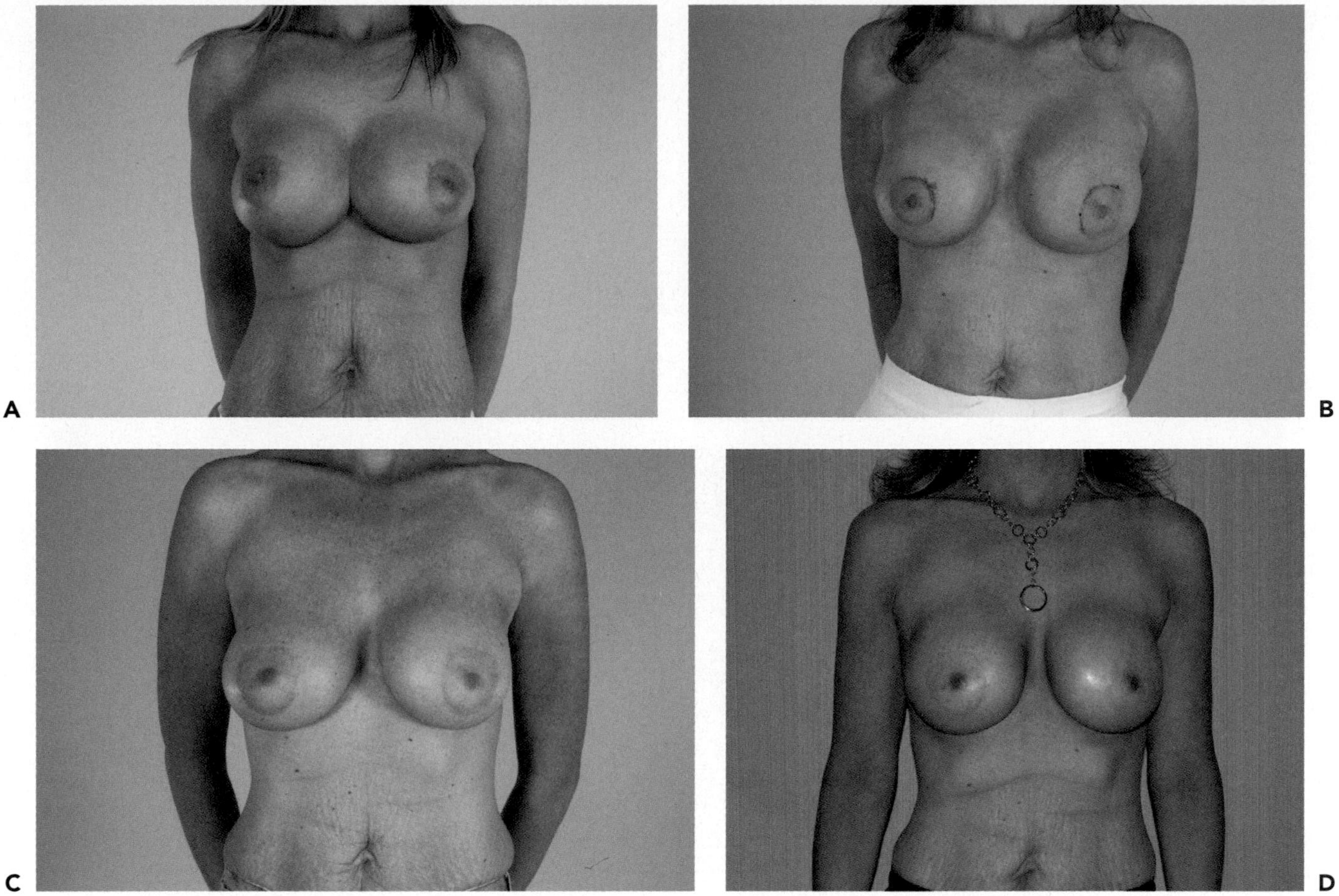

Figure 125.2. This 31-year-old woman developed symmastia after breast augmentation. She initially underwent capsulorrhaphy but had an early postoperative recurrence. **A:** Preoperative appearance. **B:** Immediate postoperative appearance after a neo-subpectoral symmastia repair. **C, D:** Five and 18 months postoperatively, respectively, showing enduring repair of the symmastia.

entire new pocket, just as there was not at the time of the initial augmentation.

Pocket dissection is always stopped short of the intended limits of the new pocket. Once the old implant is removed and stretch is removed from the pocket, the dissection has always gone farther than initially appreciated. It is better to underdissect and reassess the limits of the pocket with a sizer in place than to overdissect and compromise control of the implant position. Unlike a primary augmentation in which the dissection is mostly through a loose, areolar plane, this is a dissection

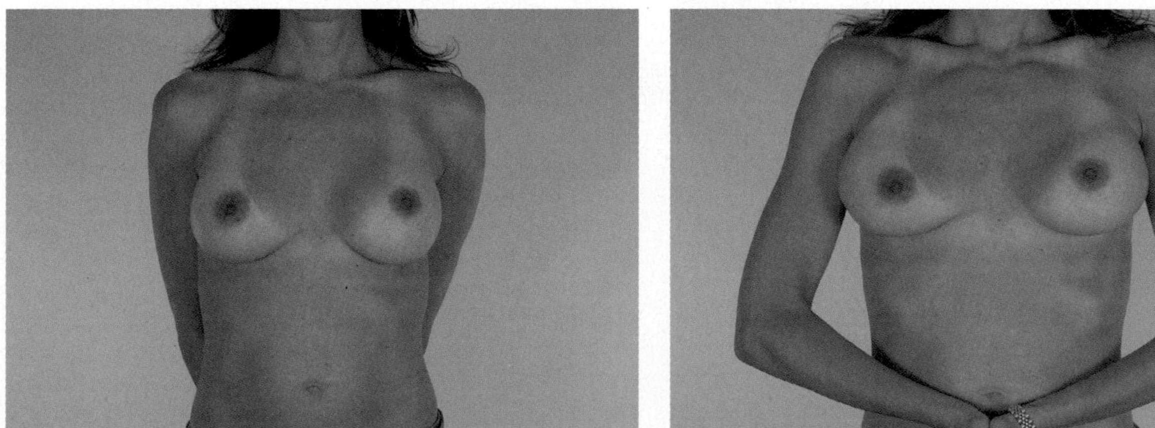

Figure 125.3. This 36-year-old woman presented with marked lateral malposition of her implants when contracting her pectoralis or lying supine after transaxillary augmentation. **A–D**: Preoperative photographs. Note the exaggerated animation deformity, as well as axillary implant displacement in the supine position. (*continued*)

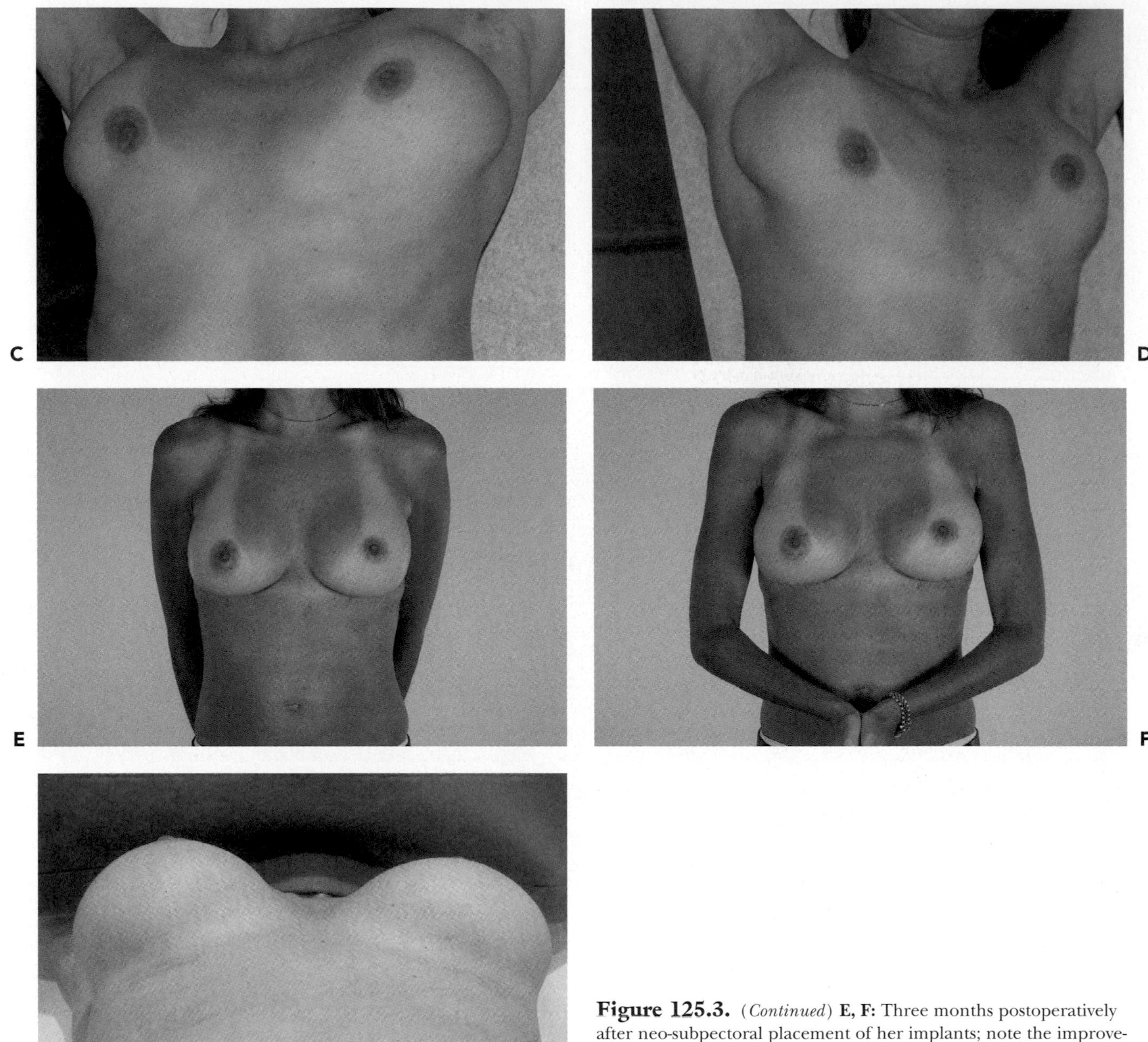

Figure 125.3. (*Continued*) **E, F:** Three months postoperatively after neo-subpectoral placement of her implants; note the improvement of the animation deformity. **G:** Ten months postoperatively; note that the lateral displacement has also been corrected.

through scar tissue. This typically allows for precise, stable borders of the new pocket once the dissection is complete.

The plane of dissection is most distinct between gland and capsule. As the dissection proceeds cephalad and under the muscle, the capsule often thins and can be very adherent to the deep surface of the pectoralis. The caudal edge of the pectoralis can be grasped with an Allis clamp and retracted inferiorly and anteriorly to facilitate this dissection, aided by downward pressure on the implant and capsule (Figs. 125.8 and 125.9).

The capsule is tightly bound to the underlying parenchyma and muscle. While blunt finger or instrument dissection can be used, in many cases the capsule itself is more delicate than the scar between it and the overlying tissues, thereby leading to inadvertent tearing of the capsule rather than dissection along the intended plane. The ease of this dissection is directly proportional to the thickness of the capsule. With translucent gossamer capsules, this dissection can be tedious, and tears are frequently made. With careful dissection, the operation can still be conducted, and none of our procedures needed to be abandoned for this or any other reason. When the capsule is thicker, the plane between it and the breast tissue becomes more distinct, allowing for more countertension and facilitating a speedier and easier dissection.

Dissection continues with the old implant in place until the new pocket is nearly complete or the presence of the implant impairs visualization, at which time the implant is removed via a convenient capsulotomy. Following the completion of the neo-subpectoral pocket dissection to the preoperatively marked borders, attention is turned to the old capsule. Internal

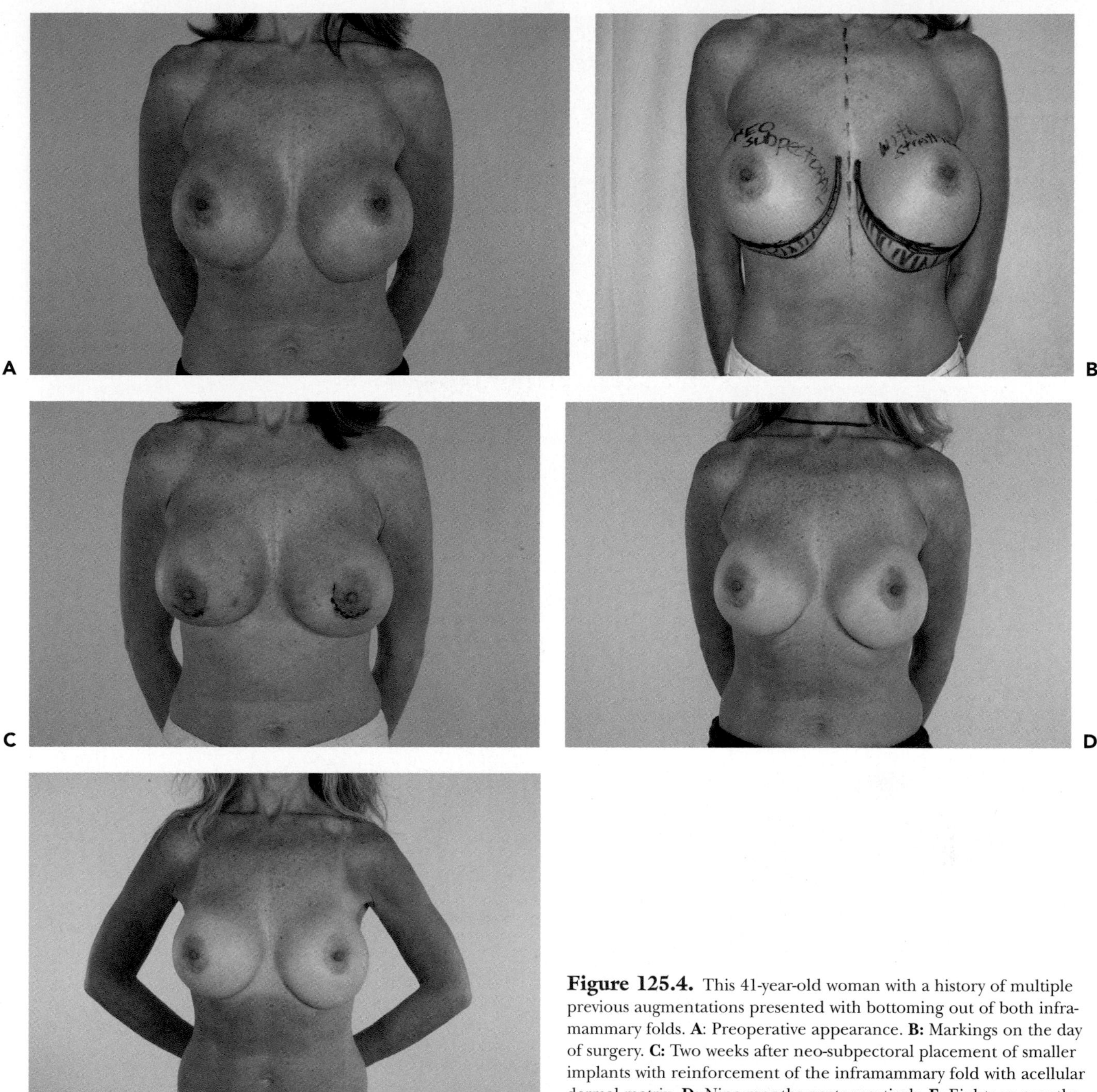

Figure 125.4. This 41-year-old woman with a history of multiple previous augmentations presented with bottoming out of both inframammary folds. **A**: Preoperative appearance. **B:** Markings on the day of surgery. **C:** Two weeks after neo-subpectoral placement of smaller implants with reinforcement of the inframammary fold with acellular dermal matrix. **D:** Nine months postoperatively. **E:** Eighteen months postoperatively, showing the implants remaining in good position.

suture repair is then performed to obliterate the old space. Following this, the two edges of the capsulotomy are approximated and tacked back down to the chest wall (Fig. 125.10). In some cases there may be excess capsule, which can be trimmed. It should be noted that obliterating this old space is not the key to repairing the actual malposition. It serves to stabilize the old capsule and prevent the implant from migrating back into it and keeps the anterior surface of the old capsule from sliding on the chest wall. The actual repositioning is a result of creating the "neo-subpectoral" pocket.

A sizer, the old implant, or a new implant is now placed anterior to the old capsule but behind the pectoralis major muscle in the newly created "neo-subpectoral" space (Fig. 125.10). Final pocket dissection should be reserved for this moment so as to avoid overdissection and potential malposition recurrence. Once the implant is in place, closure proceeds as in any other breast augmentation, including a layered closure of gland, superficial fascia, and dermis. Closed suction drains are placed in both the old capsule and the new space, and postoperative management includes instructing the patient to wear a comfortable support bra.

This procedure can be modified slightly to address only the inferior half of the breast (e.g., for a patient with bottoming out). To accomplish this, the old capsule is bisected horizontally. The superior half is left as is, and the inferior half is used as the posterior wall of a new space. By dissecting the new

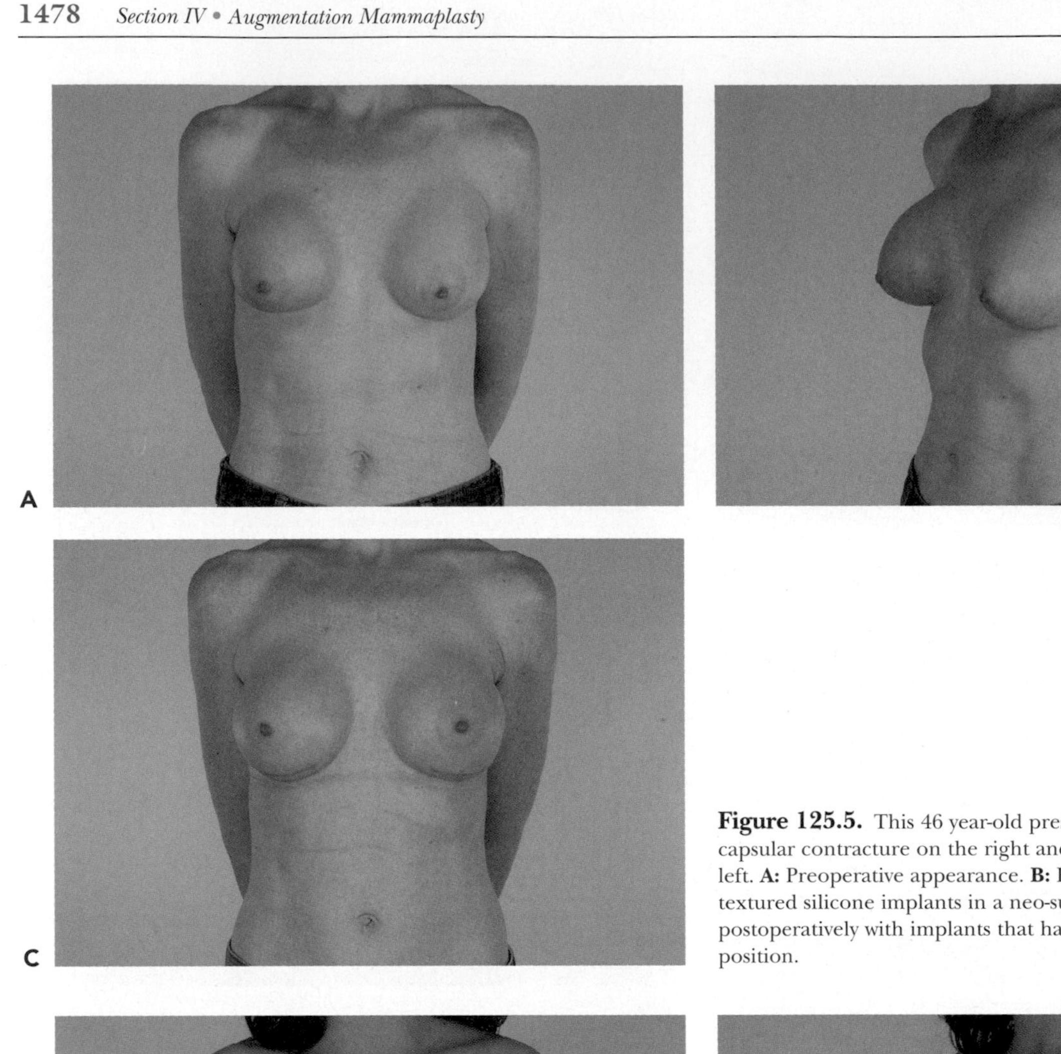

Figure 125.5. This 46 year-old presented with a Baker grade IV capsular contracture on the right and a grade IV contracture on the left. A: Preoperative appearance. B: Four months after placement of textured silicone implants in a neo-subpectoral space. C: Ten months postoperatively with implants that have remained soft and in good position.

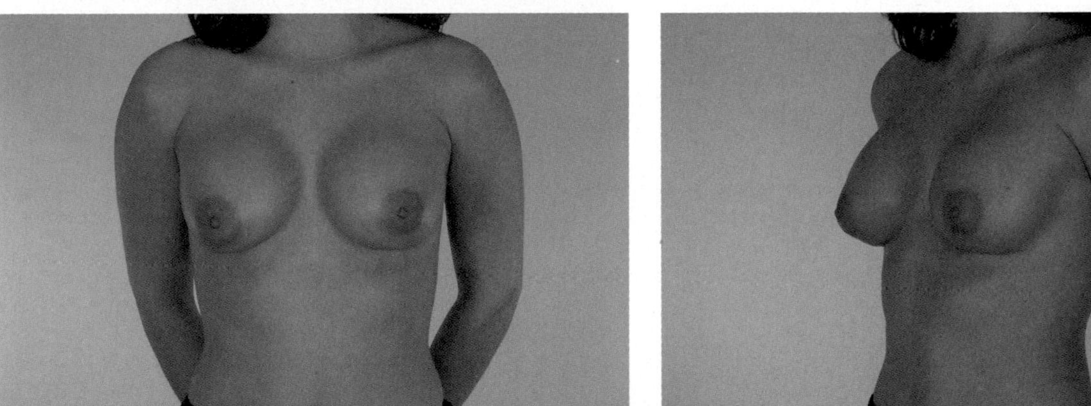

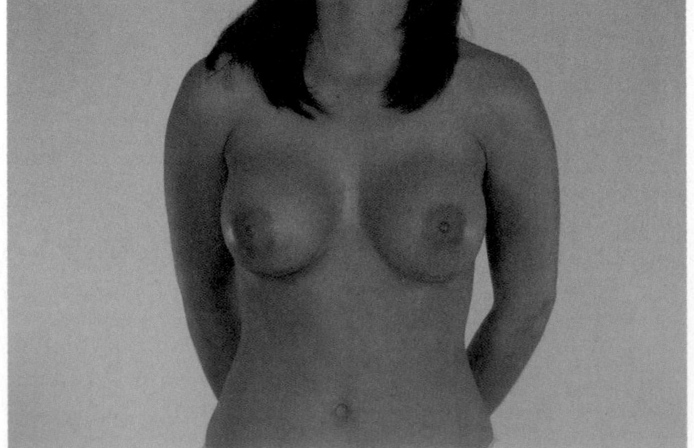

Figure 125.6. This 29 year-old woman had superior displacement of her breast implants and presented after an attempt to correct the malposition had failed. A: Preoperative appearance. B: Four months after dual-plane conversion and neo-subpectoral positioning of her implants. C: Eight months postoperatively, demonstrating a sustained good result.

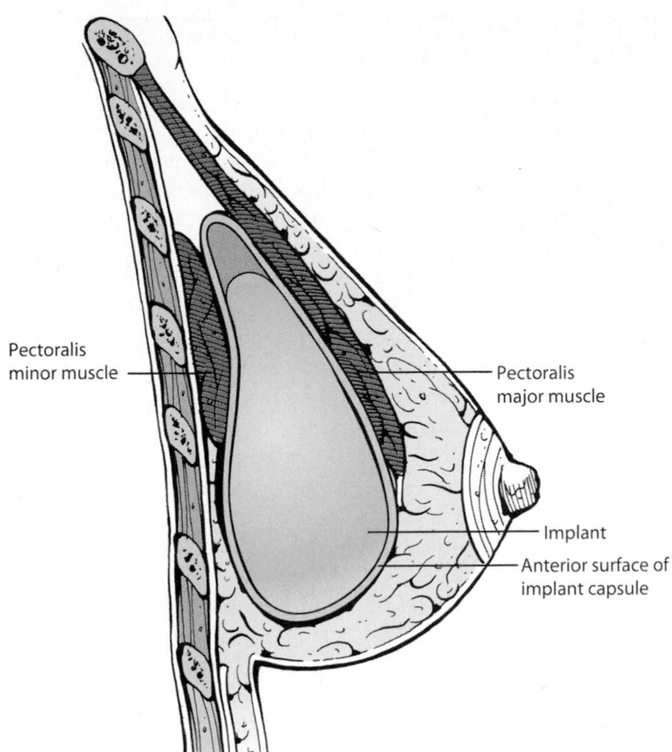

Figure 125.7. The relationship of the breast implant and the various layers of soft tissue as present preoperatively.

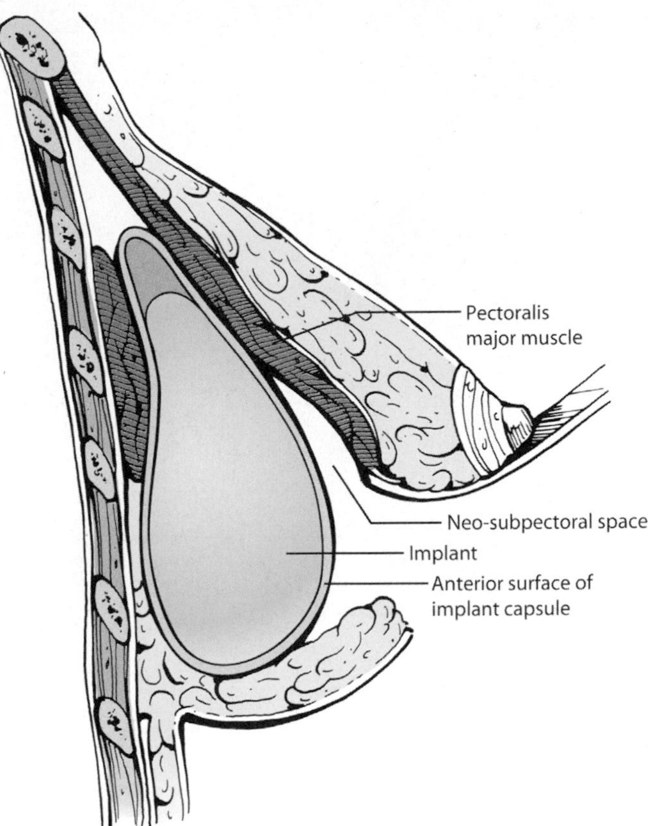

Figure 125.8. The neo-subpectoral plane is shown located between the anterior surface of the anterior implant capsule and the posterior surfaces of the pectoralis major muscle superiorly and breast parenchyma inferiorly. This dissection is performed, and the "neo-subpectoral" space is created using the dual-plane technique.

pocket between the gland and the anterior leaflet of the old capsule in the inferior half of the breast, the implant will rest on a new, higher inframammary fold and the superior neo-subpectoral dissection is unnecessary.

As an adjunct to the neo-subpectoral technique, acellular dermal matrix can be used to support the new implant position. Acellular dermal matrix can be tacked down at the level of an adjusted inframammary fold to prevent downward migration or placed medially to prevent medial migration of an implant. As long as there is a sufficiently thick capsule to work with and local tissue integrity is adequate, the neo-subpectoral dissection will likely hold the implant in position without buttressing. Should either of these factors be questionable, however, acellular dermal matrix is a useful safety net. For more details on the use of acellular dermal matrix, see Chapter 128 in this text.

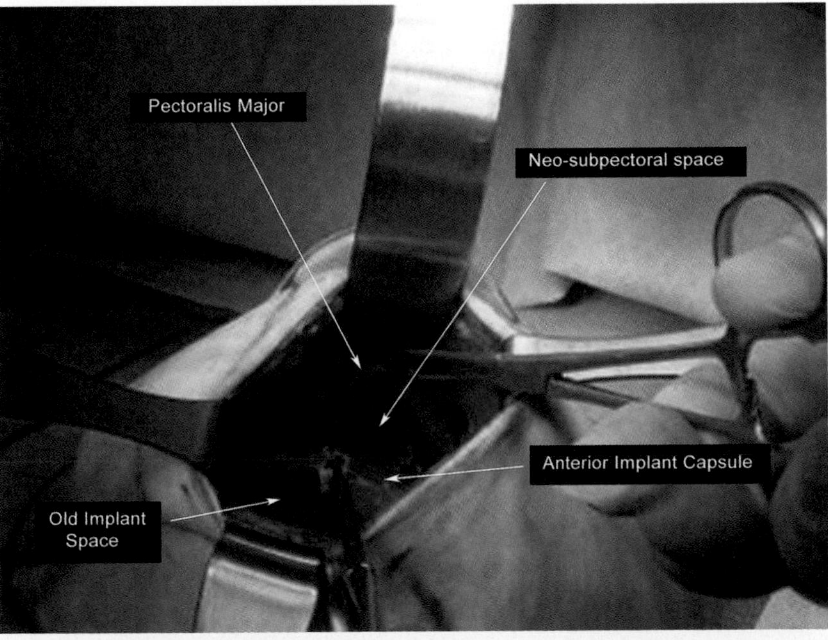

Figure 125.9. An intraoperative view of the plane of dissection between the pectoralis major muscle and the anterior leaflet of the implant capsule.

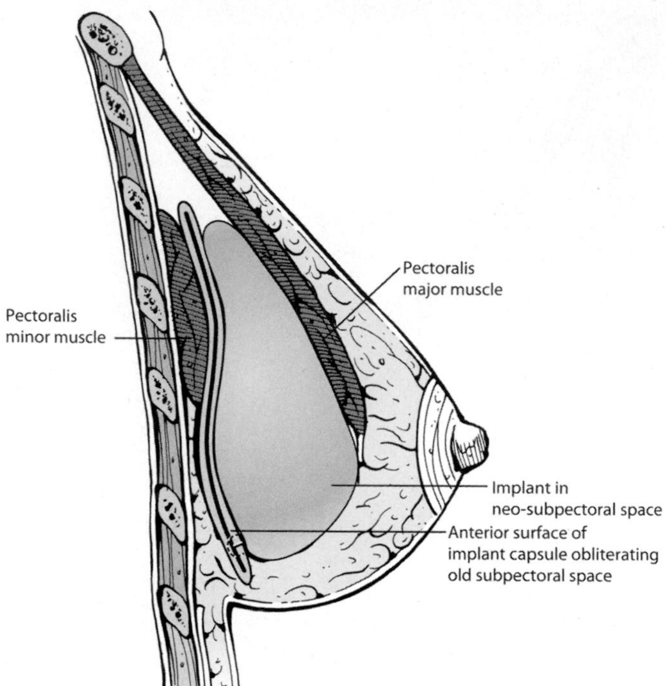

Figure 125.10. The implant is shown in the neo-subpectoral space on top of the obliterated old implant space.

CONCLUSION

The neo-subpectoral technique offers a powerful method of correcting implant malposition or capsular contracture with few limitations. The patient must have a mature capsule to facilitate the procedure, which commonly develops between 6 months and 1 year from the time of primary surgery. Obviously there can be no clinically evident infectious cause present and responsible for the initial capsular contracture, as this would clearly be transferred to the new space and cause an ongoing problem. Aside from these few requirements, the technique is flexible in most situations in which a subpectoral implant is malpositioned.

EDITORIAL COMMENT

The neo-subpectoral pocket has provided another option for the plastic surgeon faced with the situation of early capsular contracture, symmastia, or implant malposition. Prior to the description of the neo-subpectoral pocket, reconstructive options included capsulorrhaphy or pocket conversion. Capsulorrhaphy is often associated with relapse, and pocket conversions may result in breast distortions. The main requirement for successfully performing this operation is that there is moderate capsule formation. Capsules that are too thin or capsules that are too thick will be more difficult to work with. The orientation of the neo-subpectoral pocket will be based on the nature of the deformity. Lateral displacement can be corrected by medial release of the anterior capsule with enough undermining to create a lateral cul-de-sac. Symmastia can be corrected by lateral release of the capsule with enough undermining to create a medial border.

The authors have described the technique in detail. This operation is relatively easy to perform, and the benefits are noteworthy. It is clearly an option that plastic surgeons should consider when faced with a revision in the setting of breast augmentation.

M.Y.N.

REFERENCES

1. Esposito G, Gravante G, Marianetti M, et al. "Reverse" dual-plane mammaplasty. *Aesthet Plast Surg* 2006;30(5):521–526.
2. Spear SL, Carter ME, Ganz JC. The correction of capsular contracture by conversion to "dual-plane" positioning: technique and outcomes. *Plast Reconstr Surg* 2006;118(7 suppl): 103S–113S; discussion, 114S.
3. Tebbetts JB. Discussion: capsulorrhaphy revisited: a simple technique for complex problems. *Plast Reconstr Surg* 2005;1(115):302.
4. Tebbetts JB. Dual plane breast augmentation: optimizing implant-soft-tissue relationships in a wide range of breast types. *Plast Reconstr Surg* 2006;118(7 suppl):81S–98S; discussion, 99S–102S.
5. Spear SL, Bulan EJ, Venturi ML. Breast augmentation. *Plast Reconstr Surg* 2006;118 (7 suppl):188S–196S; discussion, 197S–198S.
6. Maxwell GP, Gabriel A. The neopectoral pocket in revisionary breast surgery. *Aesthet Surg J* 2008;28(4):463–467.

CHAPTER

126

Scott L. Spear
Jaime Schwartz

Outcome Assessment of Breast Distortion Following Submuscular Breast Augmentation

INTRODUCTION

Animation deformities or breast distortions during pectoralis muscle contraction following subpectoral breast augmentation are known entities, but their prevalence and significance are only beginning to be elucidated. There have been very few reports describing possible correction of such animation deformities, and, even more remarkably, there have been a few comprehensive reviews describing the frequency or severity of the problem (1–4).

While undoubtedly there are patients in whom distortion may be clinically significant, there is little information about how many patients are affected, how much the distortion bothers most patients, and with which specific activities the distortion is a problem. The purpose of this chapter is to review the frequency of animation deformities, how such deformities affect patients, how many patients have objective evidence of animation deformities, with the activities with which such deformities occur, and how to measure, quantify, or grade the degree of distortion.

TECHNIQUE FOR "DUAL-PLANE" SUBPECTORAL BREAST AUGMENTATION

Our preferred technique for breast augmentation involves a "dual-plane" approach in which the implant is placed beneath the pectoralis major muscle superiorly and in a subglandular plane inferiorly (4,5). This concept allows the parenchyma of the breast to redrape over the implant inferiorly and is particularly useful in patients with ptosis. It helps to avoid irregularities between the inferior border of the parenchyma and the inferior border of the implant, which can produce a "double-bubble" deformity. The procedure begins with an abbreviated subglandular dissection exposing the lower border of the pectoralis muscle. The amount of subglandular dissection is dependent on the degree of preexisting glandular ptosis and laxity. Patients with minimal or no breast ptosis may only require a couple of centimeters of dissection, while those with more significant ptosis may require a subglandular dissection up to the level of the nipple or as high as the superior border of the areola to allow for more redraping of the parenchyma over the implant. The subpectoral pocket is then developed by grasping the lower edge of the pectoralis major muscle with an Allis clamp and dividing its attachments along the inframammary fold under direct vision, leaving the sternal attachments largely intact. This prevents the pectoralis muscle from retracting superiorly while allowing the implant to fill out the lowermost portion of the breast parenchyma. The implant is placed in the subpectoral pocket but now lies in a "dual-plane" space, partly subglandular and partly subpectoral. The dual plane is particularly advantageous in thin patients with glandular ptosis or a constricted inferior pole, in whom purely subglandular placement would provide more control in the initial contour of the breast but at the expense of increased implant visibility and palpability. The dual-plane technique maintains the benefit of added soft tissue camouflage in the superior pole while providing greater contact between the implant and the lower aspects of the breast gland for better overall contour and redraping.

RESULTS

In order to gauge patient satisfaction with the procedure, a survey of a 195 consecutive patients operated on by the senior author who underwent primary subpectoral breast augmentation (without mastopexy) was conducted. The minimum time after breast augmentation for patients to be surveyed was 6 months. The questionnaire involved a self-evaluation of the degree of breast distortion, impact on various activities, and overall satisfaction.

There were 69 responses from the 195 questionnaires that were sent (35% response rate). Fifty-six patients (82%) rated their breast distortion as none to mild, 7 patients (10%) rated their distortion as moderate, and 5 patients (7%) felt that they had severe distortion (Table 126.1.) One patient did not answer the question regarding severity of breast distortion. When asked if the muscle-related breast distortion was a problem, the most common affected activities reported were weight lifting and exercising (24% and 19%, respectively). None of the respondents reported any interference from animation deformities with normal activities of daily living (Table 126.2.)

Overall, with subpectoral implant placement there was an 86% satisfaction rate, 3% of patients were neutral, and 10% felt somewhat unsatisfied, and one respondent was entirely unsatisfied. When asked if they would choose subpectoral implant placement again, 70% responded affirmatively, 28% were unsure, and 3% said they would not choose subpectoral implant placement. When asked if they would recommend subpectoral positioning, only one patient stated that she would not recommend subpectoral breast augmentation.

To improve the objective evaluation of breast distortion as seen in photographs in repose and actively flexing, a grading system was developed for breast distortion using a four-point scale (1): grade I, no distortion and unable to discern whether or not the implant lies in front of or behind the pectoralis muscle; grade II, one is able to tell that the implant is subpectoral, but there is minimal distortion, with an aesthetically pleasing result; grade III, moderate distortion but still an aesthetically acceptable result; and grade IV, severe distortion with an unattractive result during muscle contraction. Photographs of the

TABLE 126.1 Patient Self-assessment of Implant-Related Breast Distortion

Degree of Animation Deformity	*Number of Patients (N = 69)*	*Percentage of Patients (%)*
None	32	47
Minimal	16	24
Mild	8	12
Moderate	7	10
Severe	5	7
No answer	1	NA

TABLE 126.3 Objective Evaluation of Animation Deformities

Degree of Animation Deformity	*Number of Patients*	*Percentage of Patients (%)*
Grade I (none)	9	22.5
Grade II (mild)	25	62.5
Grade III (moderate)	4	10
Grade IV (severe)	2	5

patients are shown both at rest and with the pectoralis major muscles aggressively contracted (Figs. 126.1 to 126.4).

To quantify the data, 40 randomly selected primary subpectoral breast augmentation patients from our satisfaction survey were used. These patients had a minimum follow-up of 6 months and had preoperative and postoperative resting and animation photographs (Table 126.3). Out of the 40 patients' photographs that were evaluated, 85% were classified as grade I or II (none to mild distortion). The breakdown consisted of grade I (no distortion) 9 patients (22.5%), grade II (mild) 25 patients (62.5%), grade III (moderate) 4 patients (10%), and grade IV (severe) 2 patients (5%).

DISCUSSION

Animation deformities following subpectoral implant placement may be significant in certain patients, especially if they exercise frequently or lift weights. Overall patient satisfaction is high, but it is unclear whether those patients who were unsatisfied were unhappy because of animation problems or because of other factors such as dissatisfaction with their implant size or incision placement. Of note, the senior author has not performed any conversions from subpectoral to subglandular planes for animation deformities over the last 10 years in patients on whom he operated on primarily.

Ultimately, the patient's satisfaction with any procedure is the most important endpoint. Although there were some patients who felt that animation deformity was a problem during such activities as exercising (19%), the vast majority of patients were satisfied with their results, and only 3% of patients would choose not to undergo subpectoral implant placement if they could start over again. Only one patient said that she would not recommend subpectoral placement, and none of the patients have elected to reposition the implants in front of the muscle.

TABLE 126.2 Patient Evaluation of Animation Deformities With Various Activities

Activity Causing a Problem for Patient	*Number of Patients (N = 69)*	*Percentage of Patients (%)*
Activities of daily living	0	0
Lifting weights	16	24
Exercising	13	19
Yoga	6	9
Sex	3	4
Appearance in low-cut tops	2	3

To date, not much has been written on the subject of animation deformities. One study, by Pelle-Ceravolo et al., classified distortion into three categories—class I (mild), class II (moderate), and class III (severe)—and evaluated two groups totaling 348 patients (2). One group of patients underwent subpectoral implant placement, and the second group of patients underwent a modified subpectoral technique by which the inferior half of the pectoralis muscle was bisected vertically in an effort to avoid muscle-related distortion. With the modified technique, only 5.4% of patients were classified as class III, as opposed to 47.4% in the standard subpectoral group. However, the limited number and bias of the observers, who included only the surgeon, nurse, and patient, compromise the value of these results. Furthermore, only textured silicone and polyurethane-covered implants were used in that study. Although it has not been studied, it is possible that the type of implant used might have an effect on the degree of animation deformity. The unusually high incidence of class III deformities in the standard subpectoral group in Pelle-Ceravolo et al.'s study (47.4%) raises the question whether their technique, a textured silicone implant or polyurethane-coated implant, may exacerbate the incidence of animation deformities as opposed to our technique and the use of smooth implants, which were used almost exclusively in the study presented here. There may also be differences in the incidence of animation deformities between silicone and saline implants, as well as with the more or less cohesive gel implants.

Transecting the pectoralis major muscle would seem to be excessively destructive, especially given that most of the patients in our study did not complain of muscle-related animation deformities and this maneuver may cause secondary problems such as a depression or thinning in the inferior pole, especially if the patient is very thin. Other possible treatments for animation deformities include surgical or chemical pectoral nerve manipulation or change of the implant location (3). We believe that the only certain way to avoid or correct animation deformity is to place the implant in front of the muscle.

After investigating the incidence and significance of animation deformities, it is important to put the data into perspective. There are clearly some patients who might, from the perspective of animation deformities, be better served with a subglandular implant, namely those in whom rigorous exercise or weight lifting is central to their daily routine. The question ultimately

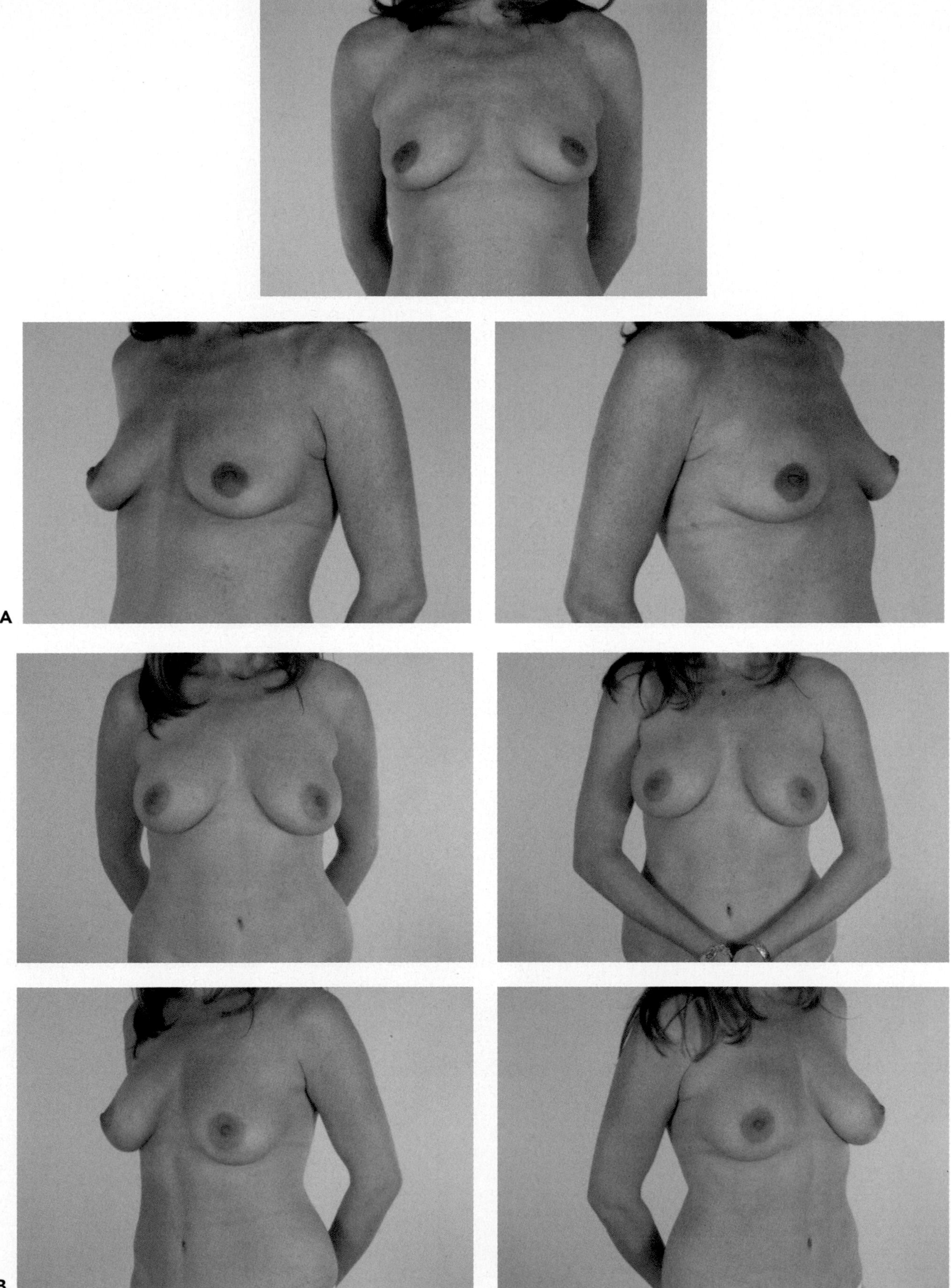

Figure 126.1. Grade I (no animation deformity) in two patients (**A** and **B**).

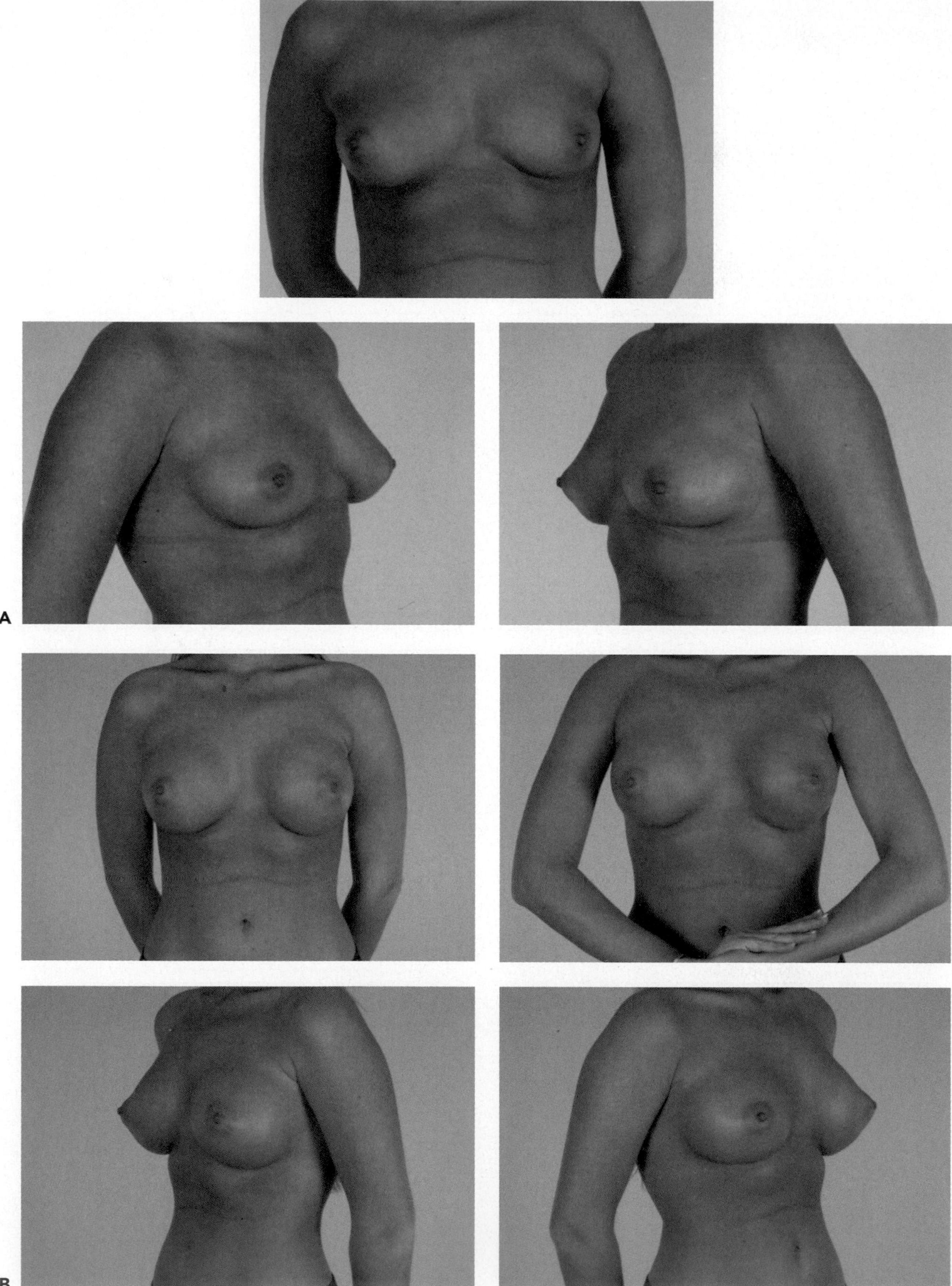

Figure 126.2. Grade II (minimal distortion) in two patients (**A** and **B**).

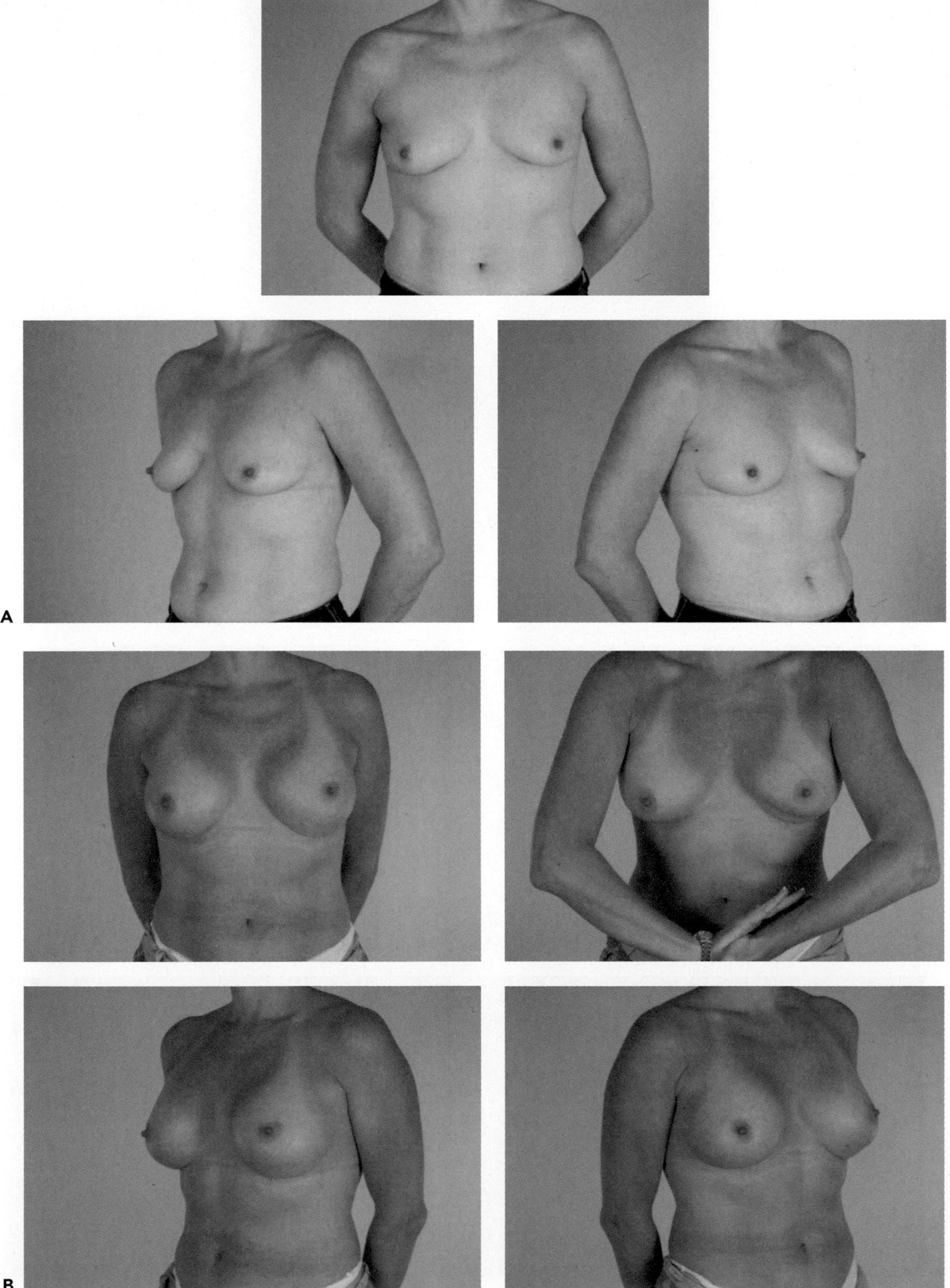

Figure 126.3. Grade III (moderate distortion) in two patients (**A** and **B**).

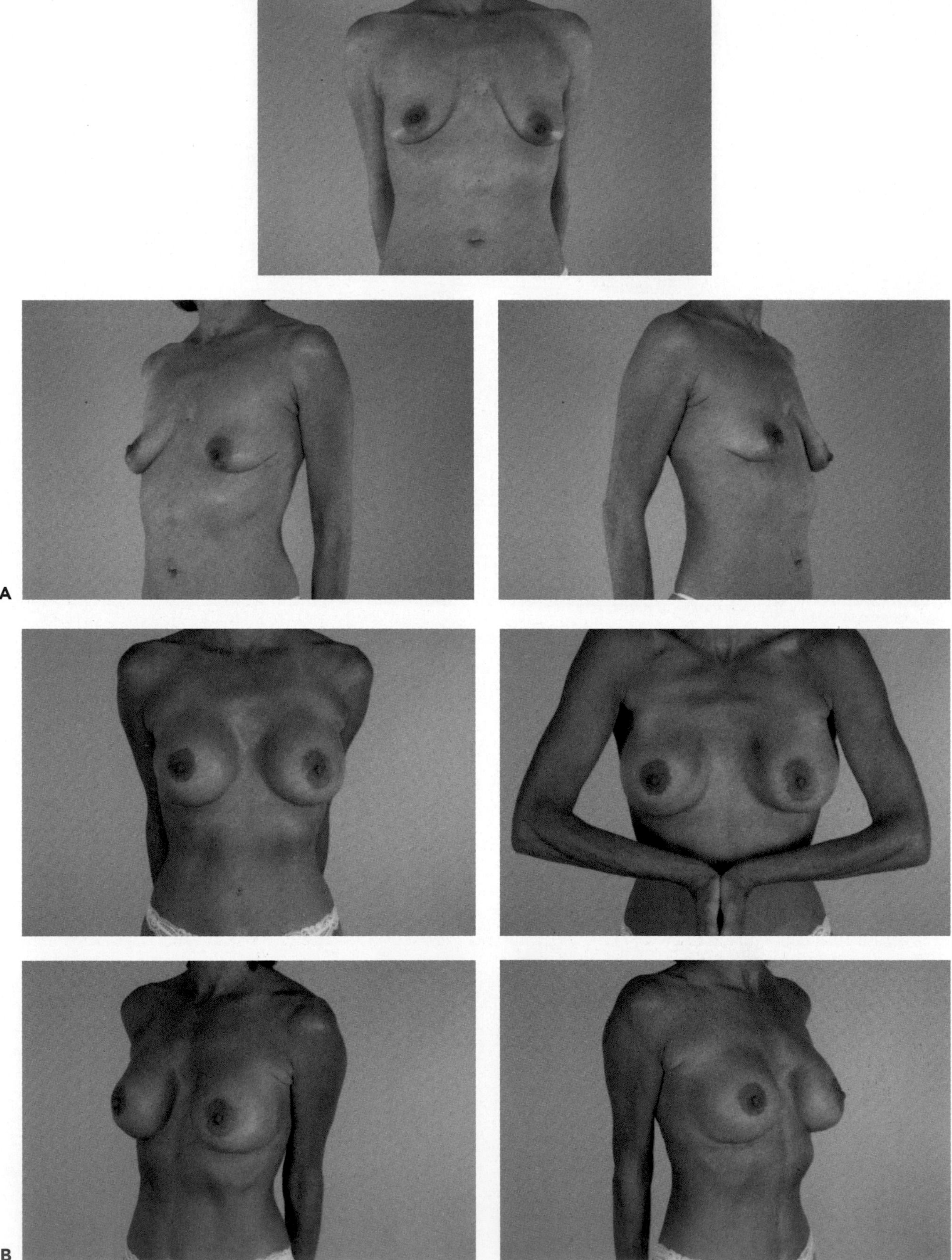

Figure 126.4. Grade IV (severe distortion) in two patients (**A** and **B**).

becomes whether the other benefits of subpectoral positioning are worth the risk of an unattractive animation deformity. The decision regarding subpectoral or subglandular placement requires taking inventory of the pros and cons of both subglandular and subpectoral placement since this sets the stage for the decision. The possible benefits of subglandular placement are little or no animation deformity, improved contour and fill in the superior pole, more natural movement of the breasts when leaning forward, and possibly less postoperative pain. The potential problems with subglandular placement are probably greater risk of capsular contracture, greater visibility of the implant in thin patients, greater incidence of visible rippling, and greater interference with mammography, which is a significant consideration, given the high incidence of breast cancer (6–9).

The benefits of subpectoral positioning include improved upper pole soft tissue camouflage in thin patients, less visible rippling, less visibility of the implant, probably lower rate of capsular contracture (10), and improved visibility of the breast parenchyma on mammogram. Disadvantages to subpectoral placement are the potential for increased animation deformity, possibly somewhat greater postoperative pain, and, in certain patients, less direct control of the upper breast contour. Thus, although some patients might find animation deformity to be a problem, many if not most might still choose subpectoral positioning (6–8). On the basis of the information collected in this study, we recommend that women considering subpectoral breast augmentation be informed of the possibility of animation deformities after positioning an implant behind the pectoralis major muscle. Possible contraindications to subpectoral positioning include women who are bodybuilders or serious upper body athletes.

EDITORIAL COMMENTS

Animation deformities following subpectoral breast augmentation are complex and difficult to treat. Dr Spear and colleagues have studied the incidence of this problem and attempted to provide some preventative and corrective maneuvers. Given that many women choose to have subpectoral or "dual-plane" breast augmentation, some degree of animation deformity is inevitable over time. As the capsule of the breast implant is firmly anchored to the pectoralis major muscle, contraction of that muscle will frequently result in some degree of breast distortion. Once this occurs, it is very difficult to correct if the subpectoral plane is maintained. As the authors point out, conversion to the prepectoral plane is necessary. This then may lead to another set of issues that are discussed in other chapters.

As I read through this chapter, I wondered if there was a way to prevent animation deformities from ever occurring. Like Dr. Spear, most of my breast augmentations are in the dual plane, and these deformities are very infrequent. I typically use smooth, round silicone gel devices and do not use contoured, textured devices. In those patients who have developed animation deformities, it has been my observation that the device itself comprises the majority of the breast mound. There is little natural breast parenchyma, as much of it has been compressed by the device. I agree that prepectoral positioning is a remedy, but the consequences of increased rippling, wrinkling, capsular contracture, and obscured imaging are of concern. Partial remedies such capsulectomy or capsulotomy, autologous fat grafting, and muscle division may have short-term but not long-term success. Thus, as is almost always the case, proper patient and device selection are paramount. During the initial consultation, realistic expectations should be set, and devices should be selected that are less than 50% of the final breast volume. Maintaining good parenchymal coverage over the muscle and implant has been effective in minimizing animation deformities.

M.Y.N.

REFERENCES

1. Spear SL, Schwartz JS, Dayan JH, et al. Outcome assessment of breast distortion following submuscular breast augmentation. *Aesthet Plast Surg* 2009;33(1):44–48.
2. Pelle-Ceravolo M, Del Vescovo A, Bertozzi E, et al. A technique to decrease breast shape deformity during muscle contraction in submuscular augmentation mammaplasty. *Aesthet Plast Surg* 2004;28:288.
3. Maxwell GP. Management of mammary subpectoral breast distortion. *Clin Plast Surg* 1988; 15(4):601.
4. Graf RM, Bernardes A, Rippel R, et al. Subfascial breast implant: a new procedure. *Plast Reconstr Surg* 2003;111(2):904.
5. Spear SL, Carter ME, Ganz J. The correction of capsular contracture by conversion to 'dual-plane' positioning: technique and outcomes. *Plast Reconstr Surg* 2006;118(7 suppl):103S.
6. Spear SL, Bulan EJ, Venturi ML. Breast augmentation. *Plast Reconstr Surg* 2006;118 (7 suppl):188S.
7. Spear SL. Advances in breast augmentation. *Plast Reconstr Surg* 2006;118(7 suppl):197S.
8. Adams WP, Teitelbaum S, Bengston BP, et al. Breast augmentation roundtable. *Plast Reconstr Surg* 2006;118(7 suppl):175S.
9. McCarthy CM, Pusic AL, Disa JJ, et al. Breast cancer in the previously augmented breast. *Plast Reconstr Surg* 2007;119(1):49.
10. Tebbetts JB. Dual plane breast augmentation: optimizing implant-soft-tissue relationships in a wide range of breast types. *Plast Reconstr Surg* 2006;118(7 suppl):81S–98S.

CHAPTER

127

G. Patrick Maxwell
Allen Gabriel

Bioprosthetic Materials for Plastic Surgery of the Breast

INTRODUCTION

Over the last century breast surgery has evolved from a rarely performed surgical venture to a daily occurrence that has become an important part of the rehabilitation process following aesthetic and reconstructive surgeries. The aesthetic quality of breast surgery, fostered by technical advances, has emerged from that of amorphous blobs appearing as breast mounds to nearly normal appearing breasts. Symmetry, which previously was hardly possible and seldom achieved, is now the standard for which we strive.

HISTORY

Controversy regarding the safety of silicone gel–filled breast implants, which were usually placed in a subglandular pocket, resulted in a 1992 moratorium on their use for aesthetic breast augmentation. This forced U.S. surgeons to use saline implants, which were placed under the muscle, thereby gaining extra tissue coverage to conceal the untoward contour irregularities of these implants (1–3). At the same time, the majority of reconstructive surgeons converted to reconstructing breast mounds with saline implants. During the 14 years of the moratorium, surgeons were trained to use saline implants for both reconstructive and aesthetic procedures.

Revisionary breast surgery (secondary or tertiary), which is often performed for the late complications of implant-based breast surgeries, poses a continual challenge to plastic surgeons. These procedures are complex, challenging, and unpredictable. Over the years we have had to deal with thinned breast tissues from large implants that have been placed either in subglandular or subpectoral space or reconstructed with saline implants, leading to long-term complications such as implant extrusion, rupture or deflation, capsular contracture, palpability, rippling, "double-bubble" appearance, "Snoopy breasts," symmastia, and implant malposition (1–3).

For many years capsular contracture has plagued plastic surgery as the most common complication of aesthetic and reconstructive breast surgery (4,5). The majority of revisionary surgeries are performed due to capsular contracture (5,6). Many etiologies have been proposed for this process, and it is clear that its prevention in primary cases includes sound techniques, including precise, atraumatic, bloodless dissection; appropriate triple-antibiotic breast pocket irrigation; and minimization of any points of contamination during the procedure (7,8). Treatment of an established capsule can be more challenging, and multiple techniques have been used for this. The bottom line to any pathophysiologic process is to understand the disease at the cellular level. In this case, it is clear that at the cellular level, capsular contracture is most likely caused by any process that will produce increased inflammation, leading to formation of deleterious cytokines within the periprosthetic pocket. Historically, options for revision and improvement have included replacing saline implants with silicone implants, using capsular flaps to gain additional stability and coverage, or performing a site change operation, which does not allow for complete resolution of some of the implant issues (1,9). Capsular flaps are available, but some patients have extremely thin tissues, and these flaps only allow for subtle improvements. Consequently, in addition to all of the techniques for treating and preventing capsular contracture proposed by others (1,4,7,10–16), we believe that acellular dermal matrix (ADM) is another modality for fighting the evolution of the capsule. ADMs can counteract the inflammatory process, adding additional availability of tissue in-growth and controlling the interface of the pocket.

ACELLULAR DERMAL MATRIX

Use of ADMs has been popularized in both breast and abdominal wall reconstructions and has been reported in a range of clinical settings, including hernia repair, facial and eyelid surgery, cleft palate repair, soft tissue augmentation, tendon repair, ulcer repair, and vaginal sling repair (17–27). In reconstructive cases, they have been used to replace tissue, extend existing tissue, or act as a supplement. In aesthetic cases, they have been used to correct implant rippling and displacement, including symmastia (28–30).

Immediate breast reconstruction using tissue expanders or implants has become one of the most commonly used surgical techniques, which has made visible rippling and contour deformity a more frequently encountered problem (31). The recent use of allogeneic tissue supplements avoids the problems of autologous tissue coverage and provides camouflage, thus decreasing rippling and increasing soft tissue padding (31,43).

The adjunctive use of ADMs in breast reconstruction has been shown to shorten the tissue expansion/implant reconstructive process, avoid mastectomy flap contraction during the latency period of expansion, provide an additional layer of tissue between the skin and implant, and offer an additional option for immediate, single-stage breast implant reconstruction (18,19,44–46).

The rising demand has spurred tremendous growth in the number of available ADMs. Published research regarding the use and efficacy of ADMs in immediate breast reconstruction is growing but has not kept pace with the market explosion. The many features and indications of all ADMs can confound the decision-making process for surgeons who want to incorporate ADMs in their treatment armamentarium.

Acellular dermal matrices can be categorized as either xenograft or allograft in origin. A surgical graft of tissue from one species to an unlike species (or genus or family) is termed a xenograft, whereas the transplant of an organ or tissue from one individual to another of the same species with a different genotype is termed an allograft. All are produced with a similar objective of removing cellular and antigenic components that can cause rejection and infection. The lack of immunogenic epitopes enables the evasion of rejection, absorption, and extrusion (18,19,27). Production processes allow basement membrane and cellular matrix to remain intact. This scaffold is left in place to allow in-growth of the host's fibroblasts and capillaries to eventually incorporate as its own. Much of this scaffold matrix consists of intact collagen fibers and bundles to support tissue in-growth, proteins, intact elastin, hyaluronic acid, fibronectin, fibrillar collagen, collagen VI, vascular channels, and proteoglycan—all of which allow the body to mount its own tissue regeneration process (18,19,26,27,47–50).

All ADMs are cleared by the Food and Drug Administration. Although features and processing may vary among ADMs, the success of the product ultimately depends on its ability to meet the desired characteristics of a model ADM for breast reconstruction or revisionary breast surgery. This discussion focuses on current ADM products used in breast surgery as outlined in Table 127.1. The following is a list of ADMs that are available on the market for a variety of applications: Allograft products are AlloDerm (LifeCell, Branchburg, NJ), NeoForm (RTI Biologics/Tutogen Medical, Alachua, FL, for Mentor, Santa Barbara, CA), AlloMax (Regeneration Technologies/Tutogen Medical, for Bard/Davol, Cranston, RI), and DermaMatrix/FlexHD (Processed by MTF for Synthes CMF, West Chester, PA, and Ethicon, Cornelia, GA). The available xenograft products are SurgiMend (TEI Biosciences, Boston, MA) Enduragen (processed by Tissue Science Laboratories, Hampshire, UK, for Porex, Fairburn, GA), Veritas (Synovis Surgical Innovations, St. Paul, MN), Permacol (Covidien, Mansfield, MA), and Strattice (LifeCell).

PUBLISHED LITERATURE

AlloDerm is clearly in the forefront regarding published literature concerning ADMs for immediate breast reconstruction. A PubMed search using specific brand names and breast reconstruction reveals that a majority of the publications involve AlloDerm. Ten of these papers relate directly to adjunctive ADM treatment of immediate breast reconstruction using AlloDerm (18,19,26,27,31–34), DermaMatrix (35), and NeoForm (36). All of these papers are recent publications, the oldest dating from 2005 (18). All are noncontrolled, retrospective case series. PubMed searches were also performed matching the name of each of the other human and xenograft ADMs—FlexHD, AlloMax, SurgiMend, Enduragen, Synovis, Permacol,

TABLE 127.1 Comparison of Different Commercially Available Acellular Dermal Matrices

Product Name	*Manufacturer*	*Origin*	*Method of Preservation*	*Year Introduced*	*Time to Hydrate*	*Shelf Life*	*Refrigeration Required*
AlloDerm	LifeCell	Donated acellular human dermis	Lyophilized; patented freeze-drying process prevents damaging ice crystals from forming	1994	10–40 min depending on thickness	2 yr	Yes
NeoForm	Manufactured by Regeneration Technologies/ Tutogen Medical for Mentor	Donated acellular human dermis	Solvent dehydrated; gamma irradiated	1997*	5–30 min	5 yr	No
DermaMatrix	Processed by Musculoskeletal Transplant Foundation for Synthes CMF	Donated acellular human dermis	Aseptic processing method (detergent wash), lyophilized	2005	3–10 min	3 yr	No
FlexHD	Processed by Musculoskeletal Transplant Foundation for Ethicon	Donated acellular human dermis	Aseptic processing method (detergent wash), stored in 70% Ethanol	2007	None	Unknown	No
SurgiMend	TEI Biosciences	Fetal bovine dermal collagen	Terminally sterilized with Ethylene Oxide (ETO)	2007	60 sec with room temperature saline	3 yr	No
Strattice	LifeCell	Acellular porcine dermis	Terminally sterilized at low dose e-beam	2008	Minimum of 2 min in sterile saline	2 yr	No
Veritas	Synovis Surgical Innovations	Bovine pericardium collagen	Terminally sterilized via irradiation	2008	None	2 yr	No

*Removed from the market.

and Strattice—with *breast reconstruction* and revealed no listings. It is likely that studies are underway and not yet completed. Most of the articles produced in the search report the use of AlloDerm as a method of providing total coverage of the prosthesis (expander or implant) in the lower pole. The ADM acts as a sling or lower pole support to create an inferior mammary fold, eliminating the typical complication seen with tissue expanders in immediate breast reconstruction.

SCIENCE

As new products are introduced to the marketplace, it is always crucial to understand the science behind each technology. The device industry should be evaluated as critically as the pharmaceutical industry, questioning the science and attempting to understand the mechanism of action.

When evaluating ADMs critically, it is important to understand the differences in how the body responds to the different materials. Not all soft tissue materials elicit the same biologic response. There are three unique processes that can take place with any tissue material that is placed into the body, whether it is a biologic or synthetic material. All products placed into body elicit an inflammatory response with involvement of multiple cytoprotective and cytotoxic cytokines. The continuum of this reaction is controlled by the intrinsic mechanism unique to each scaffold.

REGENERATION

With this process, the product is accepted by the body such that the intact tissue matrix integrates and becomes part of the host through rapid revascularization and cellular repopulation. This is the process that is most beneficial and important for obtaining good outcomes in breast surgery and perhaps the reason why we see less periprosthetic capsular contracture.

RESORPTION

This is the process in which the human body attacks the replaced tissue and breaks it down by completely eliminating it while depositing scar in its place. This is commonly seen with absorbable mesh products.

ENCAPSULATION

During this process, the product is encapsulated through an inflammatory response that is unable to break down the product due to its synthetic nature or in the case of a biologic, due to its having been damaged or denatured in the manufacturing process. Therefore the product is encapsulated and walled off from the host. This process is not unique to synthetic products, but also occurs in relation to any foreign body (e.g., pacemaker, implants) that is placed into the host.

The goal of regenerating tissue is to recapitulate in adult wounded tissue the intrinsic regenerative processes that are involved in normal adult tissue maintenance (37). Scar does not have the native structure, function, and physiology of the original normal tissue. When a wound exceeds a critical deficit it requires a scaffold to organize tissue replacement. Depending on the type of scaffold that is in place, different processes as described earlier will respond. At this point the intrinsic factors of the ADM will be important to aid in each specific regenerative or reparative process. While regenerative healing is characterized by the restoration of the structure, function, and physiology of damaged or absent tissue, reparative healing is characterized by wound closure through scar formation (37). All biologic scaffolds are not the same because of differences in the methods used to process them—materials that encapsulate and scar do not offer the benefits of regenerative healing but lead to suboptimal results.

DISCUSSION

More authors are reporting the use of ADMs in difficult cases to minimize complications. Spear et al. stated that patients with thin mastectomy flaps and/or comorbid conditions that would impair wound healing (smoking, diabetes, steroid use) could benefit from imposition of a layer of material between the tissue expander and inferior mastectomy flap (27). Simulating total muscle coverage may be particularly helpful in stabilizing the implant position and defining the inframammary fold and lateral mammary fold. With this procedure, Spear et al. concluded that total muscle coverage is avoided, and surgery is technically easier, less painful, and more aesthetically pleasing (27). In addition, a recent study showed that tissue expander-implant breast reconstruction with ADM following mastectomy preserves the skin envelope in patients who receive postmastectomy radiation (33). The authors of that study postulated that the ADM hammock may mitigate the deleterious effects seen postradiation. Further investigation in this area is warranted to determine whether ADM can serve as a protective role in this area. A recent animal study showed promise in this area, showing decreased radiation-related periprosthetic inflammation with use of AlloDerm (38). The authors of that study believed that ADM may delay or diminish pseudoepithelium formation and thus may slow progression of capsular formation, fibrosis, and contraction.

The use of ADM in aesthetic surgery is also gaining momentum (39,40,51–53). Figures 127.1 to 127.3 demonstrate the successful use of ADM in challenging revisionary breast surgeries. One obstacle that will continue to arise in aesthetic surgery relates to the cost-benefit ratio, as these products are very expensive, making their surgeries very expensive and at times impossible to finance. No doubt, the coming years will be exciting as we further define all of these issues and continue to advance the science and our understanding for the benefit of our patient population.

As we strive for perfect results, it is important to continue to gather and review data evaluating innovative techniques and devices. Now, we even have more options available for breast augmentation, whether we use them in combination or as stand-alone procedures. We have used combinations of acellular dermal matrix products, silicone implants, and fat grafting successfully in a variety of primary and secondary breast augmentation cases (39). While it is not within the scope of this chapter to discuss fat grafting, we believe that it is important to keep this option in mind (41,42). By combining all of the available options (ADM, silicone implant, fat grafting), we have been able to create "bioengineered breasts" with high patient and surgeon satisfaction (39). As always in plastic surgery, safety is always a concern, and as newer technology and products are introduced, patient education, consent, and follow-up also remain important.

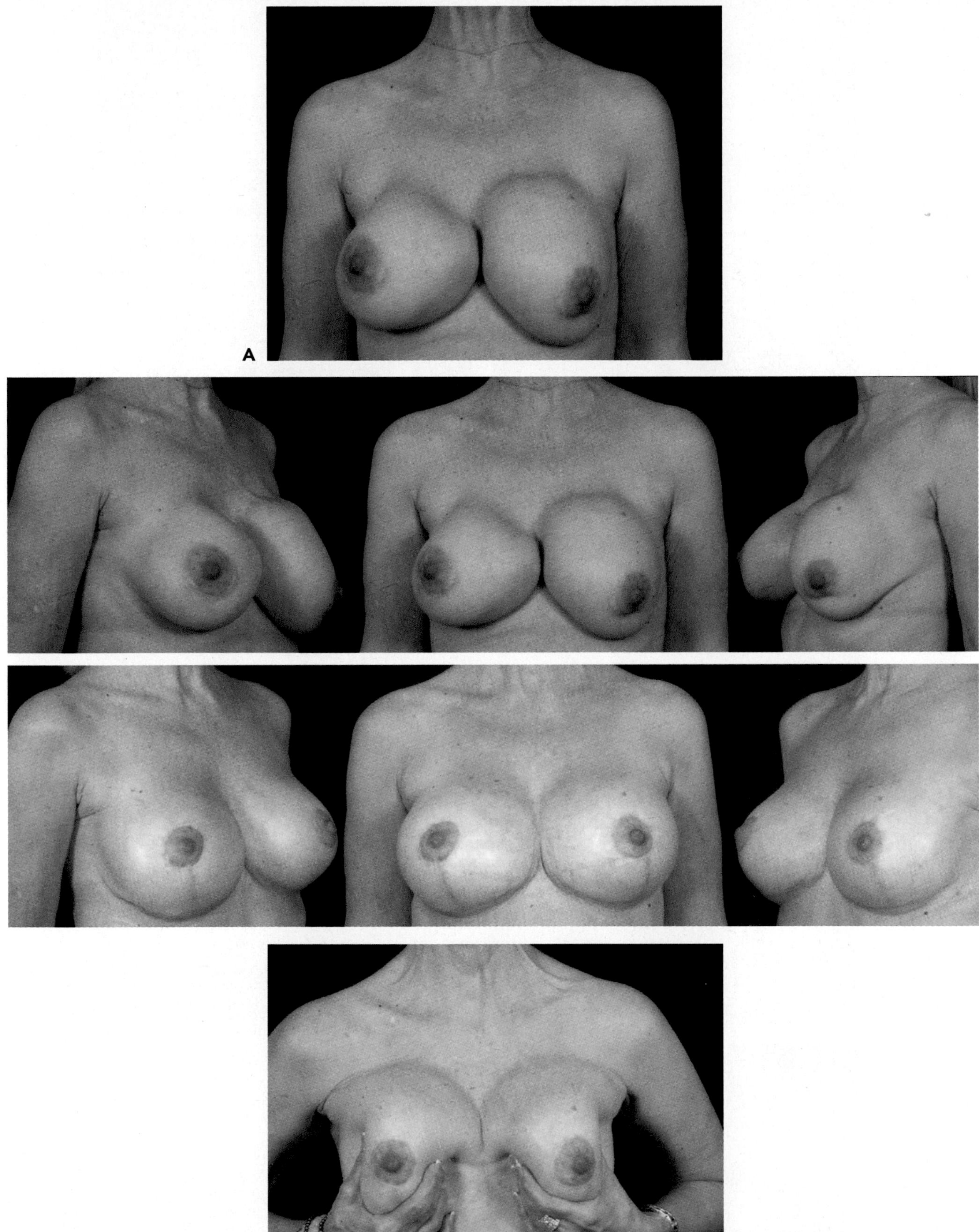

Figure 127.1. **A:** A 42-year-old woman with multiple previous augmentation procedures. Inframammary approach, with exchange, a large implant for a higher-profile, lower-volume, textured silicone gel implant; circumvertical, purse-string mastopexy; use of acellular dermal matrix. **B:** Top row: preoperative views; bottom row: 1-year postoperative views. **C:** Postoperative view.

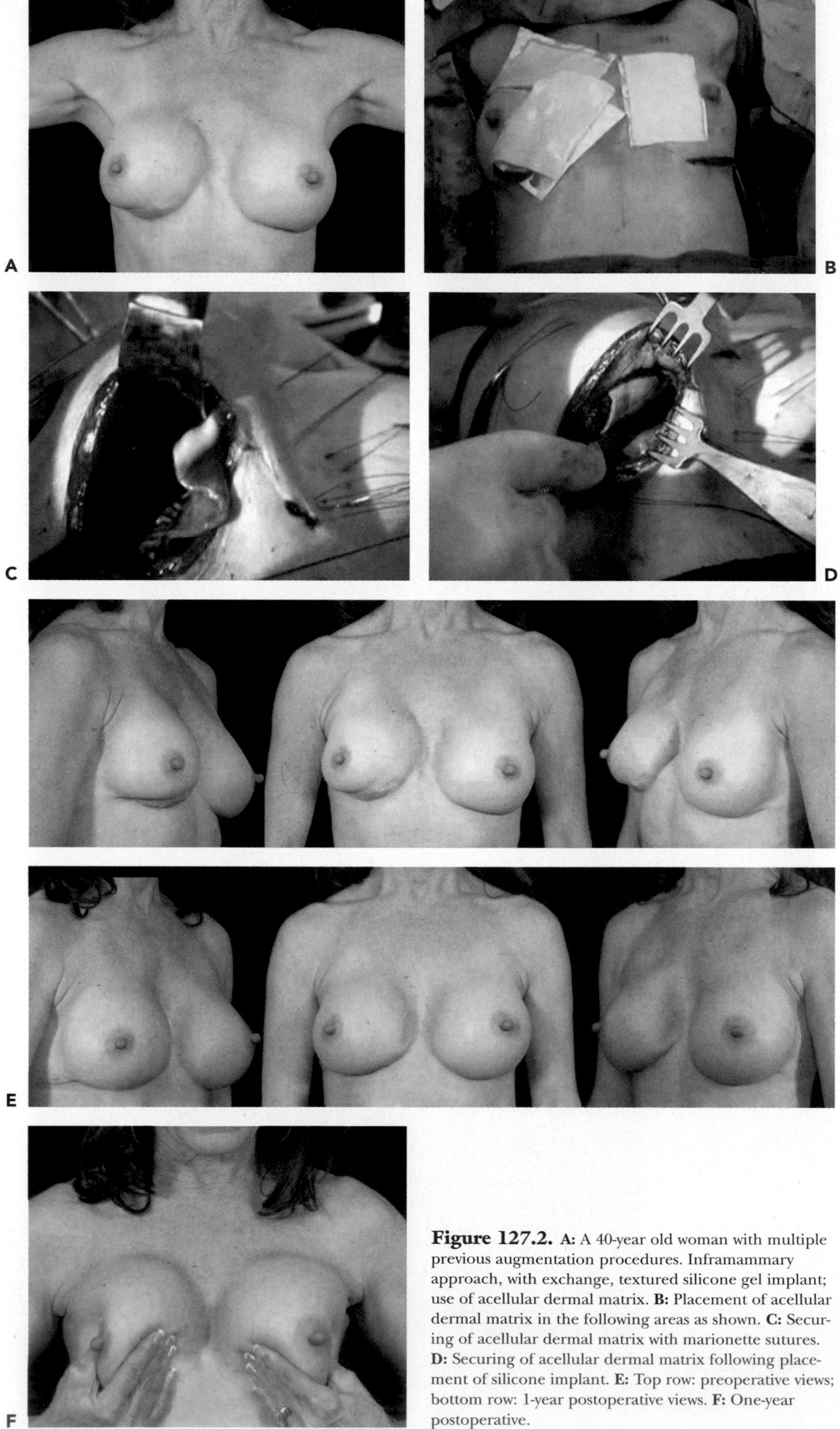

Figure 127.2. **A:** A 40-year old woman with multiple previous augmentation procedures. Inframammary approach, with exchange, textured silicone gel implant; use of acellular dermal matrix. **B:** Placement of acellular dermal matrix in the following areas as shown. **C:** Securing of acellular dermal matrix with marionette sutures. **D:** Securing of acellular dermal matrix following placement of silicone implant. **E:** Top row: preoperative views; bottom row: 1-year postoperative views. **F:** One-year postoperative.

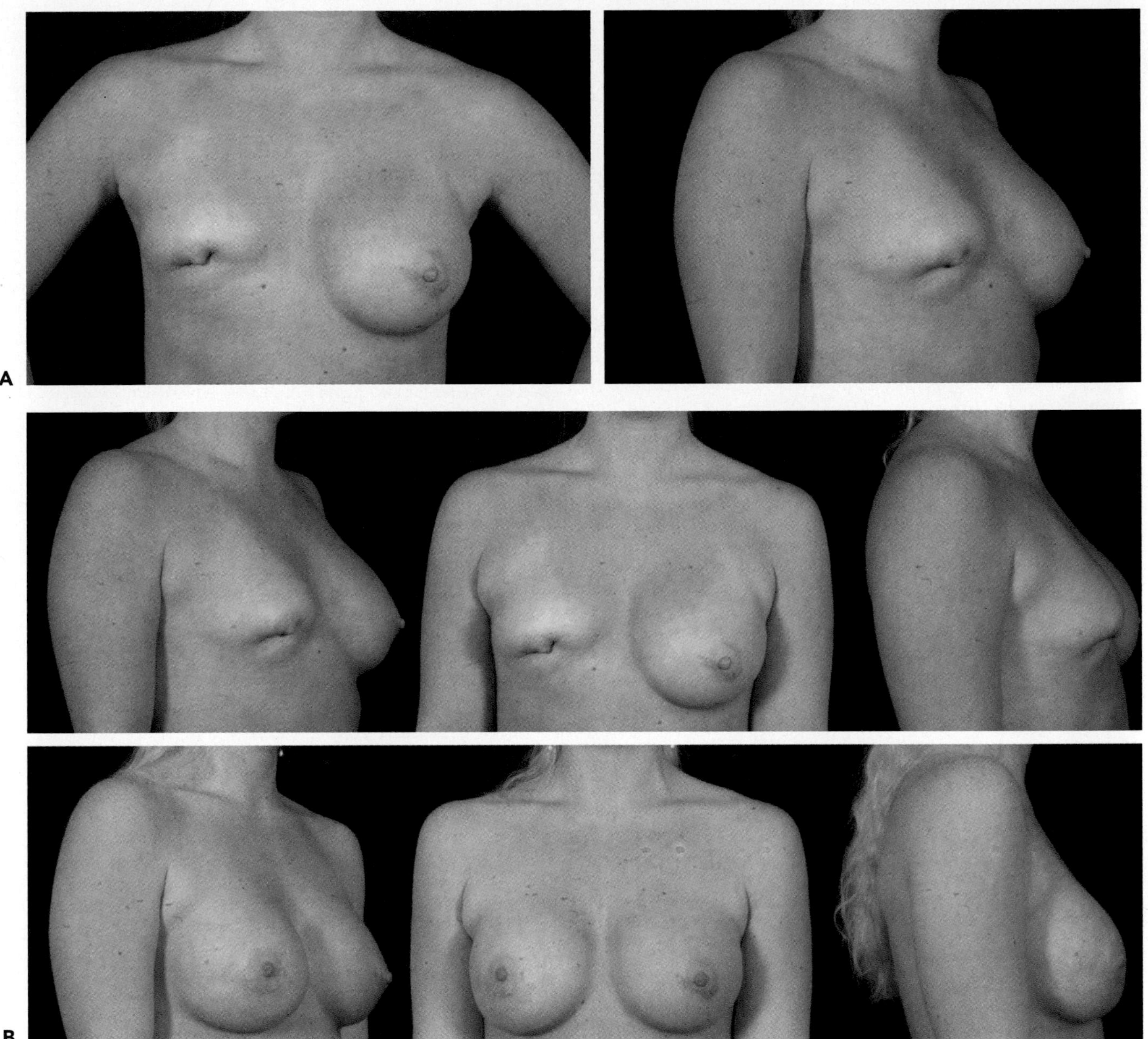

Figure 127.3. **A:** A 35-year-old woman with a history of previous subpectoral augmentation with saline implants with extrusion and lamellar scarring exchanged to a textured silicone implant; use of acellular dermal matrix. **B:** Top row: preoperative views; bottom row: 1-year postoperative views.

CONCLUSION

The use of ADMs in revisionary breast surgery and immediate/delayed reconstructions shows promise in augmenting complications and improving outcomes. In breast reconstructions, their use simplifies and enables the surgeon to achieve complete device coverage at the inferolateral aspect without the need for additional sacrifice of muscle or fascia, therefore decreasing postoperative morbidity. In revisionary breast surgery it offers the surgeon an additional tool for achieving the final aesthetic breast form while minimizing untoward implant complications. Of greatest importance is the role of ADM with its different uses that allow for correction of established capsular contracture and other implant-related issues. We look to the future with optimism that additional research will validate this finding and we will start seeing a decrease in the rate of one of the most common complications (capsular contracture) in both aesthetic and reconstructive breast surgery.

EDITORIAL COMMENTS

Drs. Maxwell and Gabriel provide a nice overview of current bioprosthetic materials for revisional breast surgery. The purpose of this chapter is to introduce the role of ADMs for revision breast augmentation. The authors describe some of the long-term shortcomings of traditional breast augmentation, such as capsular contracture and malpositioning, that have challenged plastic surgeons for years. The discussion of the role of ADMs is nicely prefaced with benefits that include less rippling, correction of symmastia, less capsular contracture, and additional tissue coverage. These benefits are realized not only with the augmentation patient, but also with the reconstructive patient. The various products that are currently available are listed in a very useful table. The only change to this would be that NeoForm will most likely be unavailable, as FlexHD may the sole product marketed by Johnson & Johnson. The various processing methods and their relation to the mechanism of action are described.

ADM is a major advance in breast surgery and will have a clear role in revisional aesthetic breast surgery. These biomaterials have the potential to revascularize and recellularize and will be useful in complex cases. One of the observations regarding ADM is that capsule formation is attenuated. Its use for capsular contracture may be ideal when used to interrupt the spherical nature of the prosthetic capsule. The contractile properties may be attenuated. Clinical trials to investigate this are being considered. Overall, this is a good general overview that sets the stage for future application of bioprosthetic materials in revisional breast augmentation.

M.Y.N.

REFERENCES

1. Maxwell GP, Gabriel A. The neopectoral pocket in revisionary breast surgery. *Aesthet Surg J* 2008;28(4):463–467.
2. Maxwell GP, Gabriel A. Possible future development of implants and breast augmentation. *Clin Plast Surg* 2009;36(1):167–172, viii.
3. Maxwell GP, Gabriel A. The evolution of breast implants. *Clin Plast Surg* 2009;36(1):1–13, v.
4. Spear SL, Carter ME, Ganz JC. The correction of capsular contracture by conversion to "dual-plane" positioning: technique and outcomes. *Plast Reconstr Surg* 2006;118(7 suppl):103S–113S; discussion 114S.
5. Spear SL, Murphy DK, Slicton A, et al. Inamed silicone breast implant core study results at 6 years. *Plast Reconstr Surg* 2007;120(7 suppl 1):8S–16S; discussion 17S–18S.
6. Cunningham B. The Mentor core study on silicone MemoryGel breast implants. *Plast Reconstr Surg* 2007;120(7 suppl 1):19S–29S; discussion 30S–32S.
7. Adams WP Jr, Rios JL, Smith SJ. Enhancing patient outcomes in aesthetic and reconstructive breast surgery using triple antibiotic breast irrigation: six-year prospective clinical study. *Plast Reconstr Surg* 2006;117(1):30–36.
8. Adams WP Jr. Capsular contracture: what is it? What causes it? How can it be prevented and managed? *Clin Plast Surg* 2009;36(1):119–126, vii.
9. Maxwell GP, Tebbetts JB, Hester TR. Site change in breast surgery. Paper Presented at American Association of Plastic Surgeons Annual Meeting, St. Louis, Missouri, May 1994.
10. Gancedo M, Ruiz-Corro L, Salazar-Montes A, et al. Pirfenidone prevents capsular contracture after mammary implantation. *Aesthet Plast Surg* 2008;32(1):32–40.
11. Ma SL, Gao WC. Capsular contracture in breast augmentation with textured versus smooth mammary implants: a systematic review. *Zhonghua Zheng Xing Wai Ke Za Zhi* 2008;24(1): 71–74.
12. Scuderi N, Mazzocchi M, Rubino C. Effects of zafirlukast on capsular contracture: controlled study measuring the mammary compliance. *Int J Immunopathol Pharmacol* 2007;20(3): 577–584.
13. Weintraub JL, Kahn DM. The timing of implant exchange in the development of capsular contracture after breast reconstruction. *Eplasty* 2008;8:e31.
14. Wiener TC. Relationship of incision choice to capsular contracture. *Aesthet Plast Surg* 2008;32(2):303–306.
15. Wong CH, Samuel M, Tan BK, et al. Capsular contracture in subglandular breast augmentation with textured versus smooth breast implants: a systematic review. *Plast Reconstr Surg* 2006;118(5):1224–1236.
16. Zimman OA, Toblli J, Stella I, et al. The effects of angiotensin-converting-enzyme inhibitors on the fibrous envelope around mammary implants. *Plast Reconstr Surg* 2007; 120(7):2025–2033.
17. Bindingnavele V, Gaon M, Ota KS, et al. Use of acellular cadaveric dermis and tissue expansion in postmastectomy breast reconstruction. *J Plast Reconstr Aesthet Surg* 2007;60(11):1214–1218.
18. Breuing KH, Warren SM. Immediate bilateral breast reconstruction with implants and inferolateral AlloDerm slings. *Ann Plast Surg* 2005;55(3):232–239.
19. Breuing KH, Colwell AS. Inferolateral AlloDerm hammock for implant coverage in breast reconstruction. *Ann Plast Surg* 2007;59(3):250–255.
20. Cothren CC, Gallego K, Anderson ED, et al. Chest wall reconstruction with acellular dermal matrix (AlloDerm) and a latissimus muscle flap. *Plast Reconstr Surg* 2004;114(4):1015–1017.
21. Garramone CE, Lam B. Use of AlloDerm in primary nipple reconstruction to improve long-term nipple projection. *Plast Reconstr Surg* 2007;119(6):1663–1668.
22. Glasberg SB, D'Amico RA. Use of regenerative human acellular tissue (AlloDerm) to reconstruct the abdominal wall following pedicle TRAM flap breast reconstruction surgery. *Plast Reconstr Surg* 2006;118(1):8–15.
23. Kim H, Bruen K, Vargo D. Acellular dermal matrix in the management of high-risk abdominal wall defects. *Am J Surg* 2006;192(6):705–709.
24. Nahabedian MY. Secondary nipple reconstruction using local flaps and AlloDerm. *Plast Reconstr Surg* 2005;115(7):2056–2061.
25. Patton JH Jr, Berry S, Kralovich KA. Use of human acellular dermal matrix in complex and contaminated abdominal wall reconstructions. *Am J Surg* 2007;193(3):360–363; discussion 363.
26. Salzberg CA. Nonexpansive immediate breast reconstruction using human acellular tissue matrix graft (AlloDerm). *Ann Plast Surg* 2006;57(1):1–5.
27. Spear SL, Parikh PM, Reisin E, et al. Acellular dermis-assisted breast reconstruction. *Aesthet Plast Surg* 2008;32(3):418–425.
28. Duncan DI. Correction of implant rippling using allograft dermis. *Aesthet Surg J* 2001; 21(1):81–84.
29. Baxter RA. Intracapsular allogenic dermal grafts for breast implant–related problems. *Plast Reconstr Surg* 2003;112(6):1692–1696; discussion 1697–1698.
30. Colwell AS, Breuing KH. Improving shape and symmetry in mastopexy with autologous or cadaveric dermal slings. *Ann Plast Surg* 2008;61(2):138–142.
31. Gamboa-Bobadilla GM. Implant breast reconstruction using acellular dermal matrix. *Ann Plast Surg* 2006;56(1):22–25.
32. Ashikari RH, Ashikari AY, Kelemen PR, et al. Subcutaneous mastectomy and immediate reconstruction for prevention of breast cancer for high-risk patients. *Breast Cancer* 2008;15(3):185–191.
33. Breuing KH, Colwell AS. Immediate breast tissue expander-implant reconstruction with inferolateral AlloDerm hammock and postoperative radiation: a preliminary report. *Eplasty* 2009;9:e16.
34. Zienowicz RJ, Karacaoglu E. Implant-based breast reconstruction with allograft. *Plast Reconstr Surg* 2007;120(2):373–381.
35. Becker S, Saint-Cyr M, Wong C, et al. AlloDerm versus DermaMatrix in immediate expander-based breast reconstruction: a preliminary comparison of complication profiles and material compliance. *Plast Reconstr Surg* 2009;123(1):1–6; discussion 107–108.
36. Losken A. Early results using sterilized acellular human dermis (NeoForm) in post-mastectomy tissue expander breast reconstruction. *Plast Reconstr Surg* 2009;123:1654–1658.
37. Harper JR, McQuillan DJ. A novel regenerative tissue matrix (RTM) technology for connective tissue reconstruction. *Wounds* 2007;(6):20–24.
38. Komorowska-Timek E, Oberg KC, Timek TA, et al. The effect of AlloDerm envelopes on periprosthetic capsule formation with and without radiation. *Plast Reconstr Surg* 2009; 123(3):807–816.
39. Maxwell GP, Gabriel A. Use of acellular dermal matrix (ADM) in revisionary aesthetic breast surgery. *Aesthet Surg J* 2009;29(6):485–493.
40. Mofid MM, Singh NK. Pocket conversion made easy: a simple technique using AlloDerm to convert subglandular breast implants to the dual-plane position. *Aesthet Surg J* 2009;29(1):12–18.
41. Coleman SR. Structural fat grafting: more than a permanent filler. *Plast Reconstr Surg* 2006;118(3 suppl):108S–120S.
42. Coleman SR, Saboeiro AP. Fat grafting to the breast revisited: safety and efficacy. *Plast Reconstr Surg* 2007;119(3):775–785; discussion 786–787.
43. Namnoum, JD. Expander/Implant Reconstruction with AlloDerm: Recent Experience. *PRS* Aug. 2009.
44. Sbitany, H. Acellular Dermis-Assisted Prosthetic Breast Reconstruction versus Complete Submuscular Coverage. *PRS* Dec. 2009.
45. Namnoum, JD. Expander/Implant Reconstruction with AlloDerm: Recent Experience. *PRS* Aug. 2009.
46. Maguina, P. et al. Single-Stage Immediate Breast Reconstruction After Skin-Sparing Mastectomy. *PRS* Dec. 2008.
47. Harper, JR. Extracellular Wound Matrices A Novel Regenerative Tissue Matrix (RTM) Technology for Connective Tissue Recon. *Wounds* 2007.
48. Xu, H. Host response to Human Acellular Dermal Matrix Transplantation in a Primate Model of Abdominal Wall Repair. *Tissue Eng* 2008.
49. Xu, et al. A Porcine-Derived Acellular Dermal Scaffold that Supports Soft Tissue Regen.- *Tissue Engineering* 2009.
50. Connor, J. et al. Retention of structural and biochemical integrity in a biological mesh supports tissue remodeling in a primate abdominal wall model. *Regen Medicine* 2009.
51. Colwell, AS. et al. Improving Shape and Symmetry in Mastopexy with Autologous or Cadaveric Dermal Slings. *Ann Plast Surg* 2008;61(2):138–142.
52. Grabov-Nardini, G. et al. AlloDerm Sling for Correction of Synmastia After Immediate, Tissue Expander, Breast Reconstruction in Thin Women. *Eplasty* 2009;12:9:e54.
53. Duncan, DI. Correction of Implant Rippling Using Allograft Dermis. *Aesthet Surg J* 2001;21(1):81–84.

CHAPTER

128

Scott L. Spear
Mitchel Seruya

Acellular Dermal Matrix for the Treatment and Prevention of Implant-associated Breast Deformities

BRIEF HISTORY

Acellular dermal matrix (ADM) has been increasingly accepted as a useful tool in primary prosthetic breast reconstruction (1–12). Observed benefits include better control of implant position, better implant support and coverage, and the suggestion of a decreased frequency of capsular contracture (1–6,8–11,13–15). In a series of 11 mastectomy patients with poor pectoralis major muscle coverage, Gamboa-Bobadilla placed human acellular dermis matrix (HADM) alongside 13 breast prostheses and found that 92% of patients had a successful reconstruction and 73% had an "excellent" aesthetic outcome (2). Salzberg performed single-stage immediate implant-based reconstruction of 76 breasts in 49 patients using HADM and reported a 0% contracture rate and a 0% "serious" complication rate over a 52-month follow-up period (3). Zienowicz and Karacaoglu observed a 0% rate of contracture, rippling, synmastia, or bottoming out in a study of 30 immediate implant-breast reconstructions with HADM over an 18-month mean folow-up time (6). In a study of 44 primary prosthetic breast reconstructions with HADM, Breuing and Colwell identified a 0% contracture rate, 2.3% extrusion rate, and 4.5% infection rate over a 6-month to 3-year surveillance period (5).

In addition to the growing literature on the applications of ADM for primary prosthetic breast reconstruction, a handful of studies have explored the use of ADM in the treatment of breast implant–associated deformities (5,16–18). Following prosthetic breast surgery, capsular attenuation may develop and manifest as implant malposition or rippling, while capsular contracture may occur in a subset of patients and present as implant firmness or distortion. Duncan described the use of HADM in the correction of 34 patients with implant rippling and observed an improvement in palpable rippling, an average patient satisfaction rate of 85%, a 2.9% rate of capsular contracture, and a 2.9% rate of infection (16). In a case series of 10 patients with breast implant–related problems, including rippling, bottoming out, synmastia, and contracture, Baxter found that 80% of revisions were stable with the use of HADM (17). Finally, Breuing and Colwell reported a 0% recurrence of contracture in 23 breasts treated with capsulectomy and HADM for implant-related contracture (5).

INDICATIONS

Given the low frequency of complications in cases of primary prosthetic breast reconstruction with ADM (1–6,9–11), as well as the encouraging preliminary data on the use of ADM in select cases of secondary prosthetic breast surgery (5,16–18), we believe that ADM may be a useful adjunct in the treatment and prevention of some implant-associated deformities. This is especially significant because many of these problems have proven extraordinarily difficult to consistently correct in the past (19–27). In secondary prosthetic breast surgery, it is hypothesized that ADM may do one or more of the following: offload tension on a capsulorrhaphy suture line to help restore the normal breast boundaries, recreate the implant space to better match an implant's dimensions, interrupt scar formation, and reinforce and essentially thicken thin skin flaps. These properties make ADM a useful adjunct in the correction of recurrent implant malposition, rippling, capsular contracture, and skin flap deficiency, respectively. Furthermore, in primary aesthetic breast implant surgery in the massive-weight-loss population, one could hypothesize that ADM might define the natural breast shape and landmarks by providing inferior pole support. These properties may help prevent loss of inframammary fold definition and implant bottoming out in post-bariatric surgery patients.

CONTRAINDICATIONS

Currently, there are no observed contraindications to ADM use in prosthetic breast surgery. However, there are some drawbacks, specifically the cost of the product. In the United States, 16 × 4 cm sheets of human ADM are priced at $1,878.72 for Alloderm (LifeCell, Branchburg, NJ) and $1,825.00 for DermaMatrix (Synthes, West Chester, PA) (10).

OPERATIVE TECHNIQUE

Techniques to address breast implant–related deformities often include a combination of implant exchange, device position change, capsule modification, and, in select cases, placement of ADM. In general, implants can be exchanged for devices of a different shape, size, or material. When warranted, devices are relocated to a subglandular, prepectoral, subpectoral, or neo-subpectoral pocket. When necessary, capsule modification is performed via capsulotomy, capsulectomy, and/or capsulorrhaphy.

Types of ADM include human- and porcine-derived products. Available human products include AlloDerm (LifeCell), NeoForm (Mentor, Santa Barbara, CA), DermaMatrix (Synthes), and Flex HD (Ethicon, Somerville, NJ). Porcine products include Strattice (LifeCell). Selection of a specific product is based on availability at the time of the procedure. At this time,

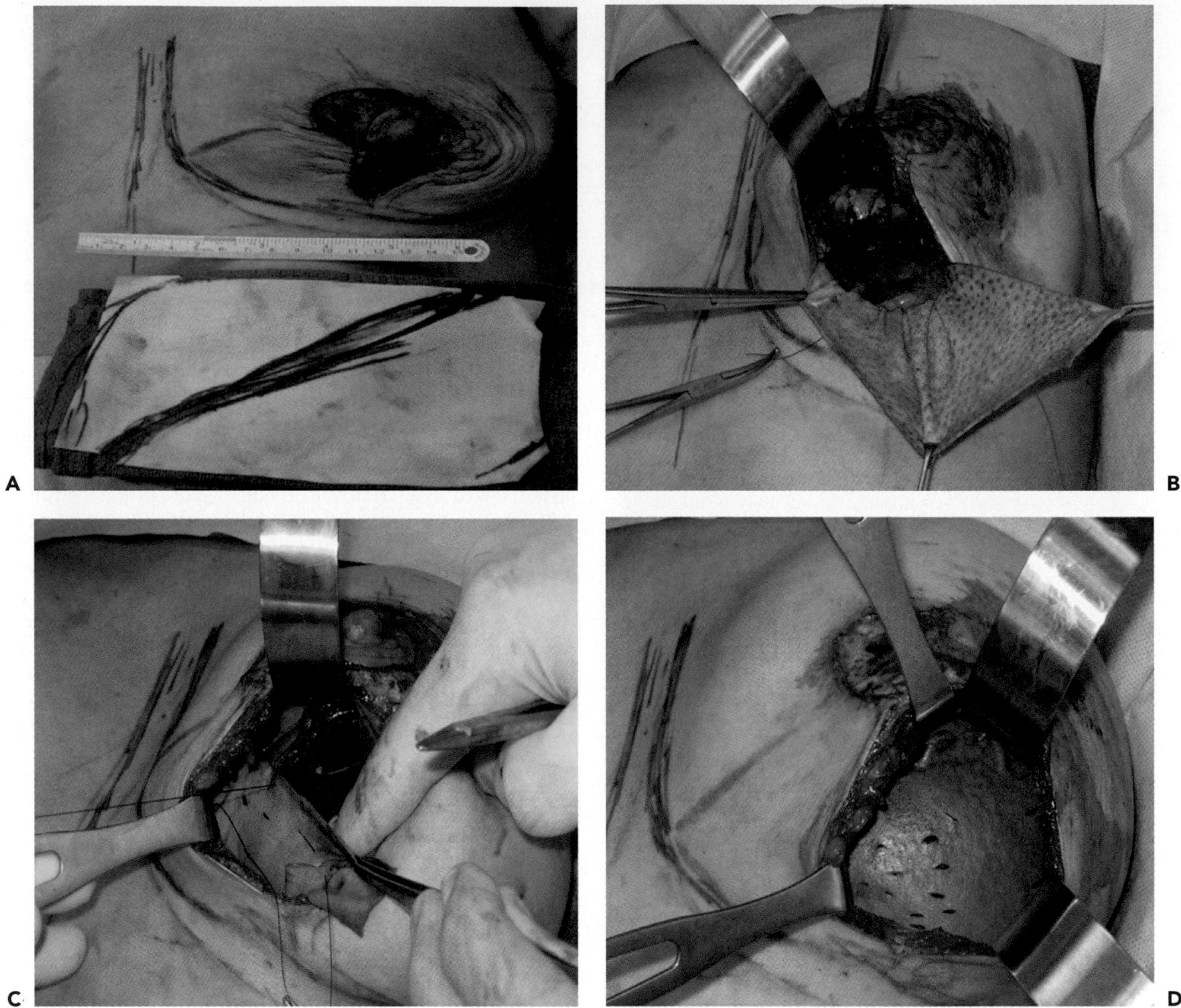

Figure 128.1. **A:** Measurement and shaping of acellular dermal matrix (ADM) for use as an interpositional graft tailored to the preoperatively marked inframammary fold (IMF) and lateral mammary fold (LMF). **B:** Anchoring ADM to the transposed IMF and LMF markings on the chest wall with interrupted or running 2-0 suture. **C:** Closure of the ADM/pectoralis major muscle interface with a running 3-0 suture. **D:** Completed inset of an ADM interpositional graft, functioning as an inferolateral sling.

studies have not shown a clear advantage of one ADM product versus another (10,11).

Depending on the breast implant–associated complication, ADM is placed alongside breast implants as an interpositional (between pectoralis major and chest wall), underlay (between capsule and skin), or overlay (between implant and capsule) graft. In cases of difficult and recurrent capsular contracture, ADM is typically inset as a large interpositional graft. This location serves to interrupt capsule formation beyond the pectoralis major muscle's coverage of the implant, thereby limiting the extent of capsular contracture. For correction of rippling, ADM can also be placed as an interpositional graft. This position provides inferolateral support of the breast device, thereby reducing implant-mediated traction on the breast soft tissue and resultant traction-associated rippling. To correct or prevent loss of inframammary fold definition and implant bottoming out, an interpositional inset is also appropriate. As an inferolateral sling, ADM helps to maintain the natural breast landmarks and provides inferior pole support.

The senior author's technical steps for placement of ADM as an interpositional (between pectoralis major and chest wall) graft have been described previously (8) and are shown in Figure 128.1. Preoperative markings include the patient's midline, desired inframammary fold (IMF), and desired lateral mammary fold (LMF). For total IMF and LMF arc lengths of 18 cm or less, a 12 × 4 cm piece of AlloDerm may be sufficient. For arc lengths greater than 18 cm, a 16 × 4 cm or 16 × 6 cm piece of AlloDerm is more likely appropriate. AlloDerm is reconstituted as necessary, per manufacturer's recommendations.

Depending on the situation, AlloDerm inset can be preceded by device exchange, capsular modification, and/or creation of a neo-subpectoral pocket. For subpectoral placement, the pectoralis major muscle is then identified and isolated. A small portion of the most inferomedial attachment of the pectoralis major muscle is released as necessary to create the desired medial pocket shape. One must be careful not to be overaggressive with the medial release, as it can cause iatrogenic synmastia or "window shading" of the pectoralis muscle.

Using methylene blue, the preoperatively marked IMF and LMF are transposed onto the chest wall muscle. AlloDerm is then placed on the chest wall with its deep dermal surface facing up toward the breast skin flaps. It is inset as an interpositional graft, bordering the inferior aspect of the pectoralis major muscle. The corners of the graft are anchored to the chest wall at the medial and lateral ends of the desired IMF and LMF, respectively, using 2-0 or 3-0 sutures. The remaining central segment of the graft is sutured to the desired IMF and LMF with either interrupted sutures at 1- to 2-cm intervals or as a running stitch. If an interrupted technique is used, the centralmost sutures are left untied and clamped on hemostats. Alternatively, if a running suture is preferred, it is not pulled snug or tied. These measures can access for implant placement and also allow for subsequent tension adjustments.

The breast device is then placed under the pectoralis major muscle and AlloDerm, carefully seating it in the pocket and ensuring that its most inferior and lateral edges lie against the desired IMF and LMF, respectively. In cases of rippling, one must ensure that there is adequate inferolateral support of the implant to avoid rippling. The superior aspect of the AlloDerm is then pulled up toward the inferior border of the pectoralis major muscle, precisely aligning it and cutting any areas of overlap as necessary. The remaining untied interrupted sutures or loosened running suture along the IMF and LMF are then tightened and tied. The AlloDerm is then secured to the pectoralis major muscle with a running 3-0 suture.

It is important to achieve a "hand-in-glove" fit between the breast device, ADM graft, and breast skin flaps. Similar to a skin graft, the ADM should ideally be without folds or wrinkles and should and be in good contact with the breast skin flaps to ensure proper "take" and integration. To reduce the risk of fluid accumulation between the ADM and the breast implant or between the ADM and the breast skin flaps, a drain is often placed in the operative field. Final skin closure is completed with deep dermal, interrupted 3-0 and subcuticular, running 3-0 sutures.

In cases of thin breast skin flaps, an underlay (between capsule and skin) or overlay (between implant and capsule) technique can be used instead. Placement of ADM on the underside of thin breast skin can augment soft tissue coverage of an implant and potentially enhance vascularity to the tenuous flaps via scaffold-mediated angiogenesis. Key operative steps include potential capsule modification and implant exchange, followed by insetting of an ADM underlay graft. With the ADM on stretch, eliminating any wrinkles or folds but avoiding excessive tension, it is secured to the thin regions of the breast skin flaps with interrupted 3-0 sutures.

For correction of recurrent medial malposition, an ADM overlay graft is generally used in combination with a neo-subpectoral pocket (Fig. 128.2) or capsulorrhaphy repair. By reinforcing the capsulorrhaphy suture line, ADM serves to protect the repair while it heals. Key operative steps include first the creation of a neo-subpectoral pocket or performance of a multiple-layer breast capsulorrhaphy, both maneuvers previously described in detail by the senior author (19,28), followed by ADM insetting, breast device placement, and soft tissue closure. Care is taken to ensure that the ADM overlaps the suture line, with generally 1 to 2 cm of overlap. The desired breast implant is then placed, followed by insertion of a single small drain if necessary, closure of the deep breast tissue with 3-0 sutures, and skin closure with deep dermal, interrupted 3-0 and a subcuticular, running 3-0 suture.

POSTOPERATIVE CARE

Generally, patients are discharged on the day of surgery or, in rare cases, on postoperative day 1. Oral antibiotics may be continued until all drains are removed, typically once the output is less than 30 mL per day. Marionette sutures, if used, are usually discontinued 7 to 10 days postoperatively. Key steps to avoid bacterial contamination include using Betadine or alcohol prep of the marionette sutures, cutting one end of the suture flush with the skin, and carefully pulling the other end of the suture to minimize contamination.

CASE EXAMPLES

CORRECTION OF CAPSULAR CONTRACTURE

A 35-year-old woman with a history of several breast augmentation-mastopexy procedures performed at an outside hospital presented with recurrent, bilateral capsular contracture and bilateral inferior pole deficiency (Fig. 128.3). To address these deformities, the patient underwent bilateral periareolar mastopexies, anterior capsulectomies, partial subpectoral placement of smooth, round silicone implants (Allergan 15-234), and insetting of an ADM interpositional graft. Comparison of preoperative and 6-month postoperative photos demonstrated absence of breast distortion and preservation of a natural breast contour. Her correction of bilateral capsular contracture was maintained at 1 year.

CORRECTION OF RIPPLING

A 42-year-old woman with a history of multiple subglandular breast augmentation procedures performed at an outside hospital to address bilateral capsular contracture presented with bilateral breast implant rippling and ptosis (Fig. 128.4). Operative steps to correct these deformities included bilateral circumvertical mastopexies, capsulotomies, repositioning of original smooth, round silicone implants (Allergan 15-457) under a subpectoral pocket, and insetting of ADM interpositional grafts. Six months postoperatively, the patient displayed no evidence of rippling or ptosis. Eleven-month postoperative photos showed stable correction of the implant deformities.

CORRECTION OF INFERIOR MALPOSITION

A 41-year-old woman with a history of multiple breast augmentation procedures presented with inferior malposition of her implants (Fig. 128.5). To treat the deformities, a neo-subpectoral pocket was developed, implants were exchanged for smaller smooth, round silicone implants (Allergan 20-500),

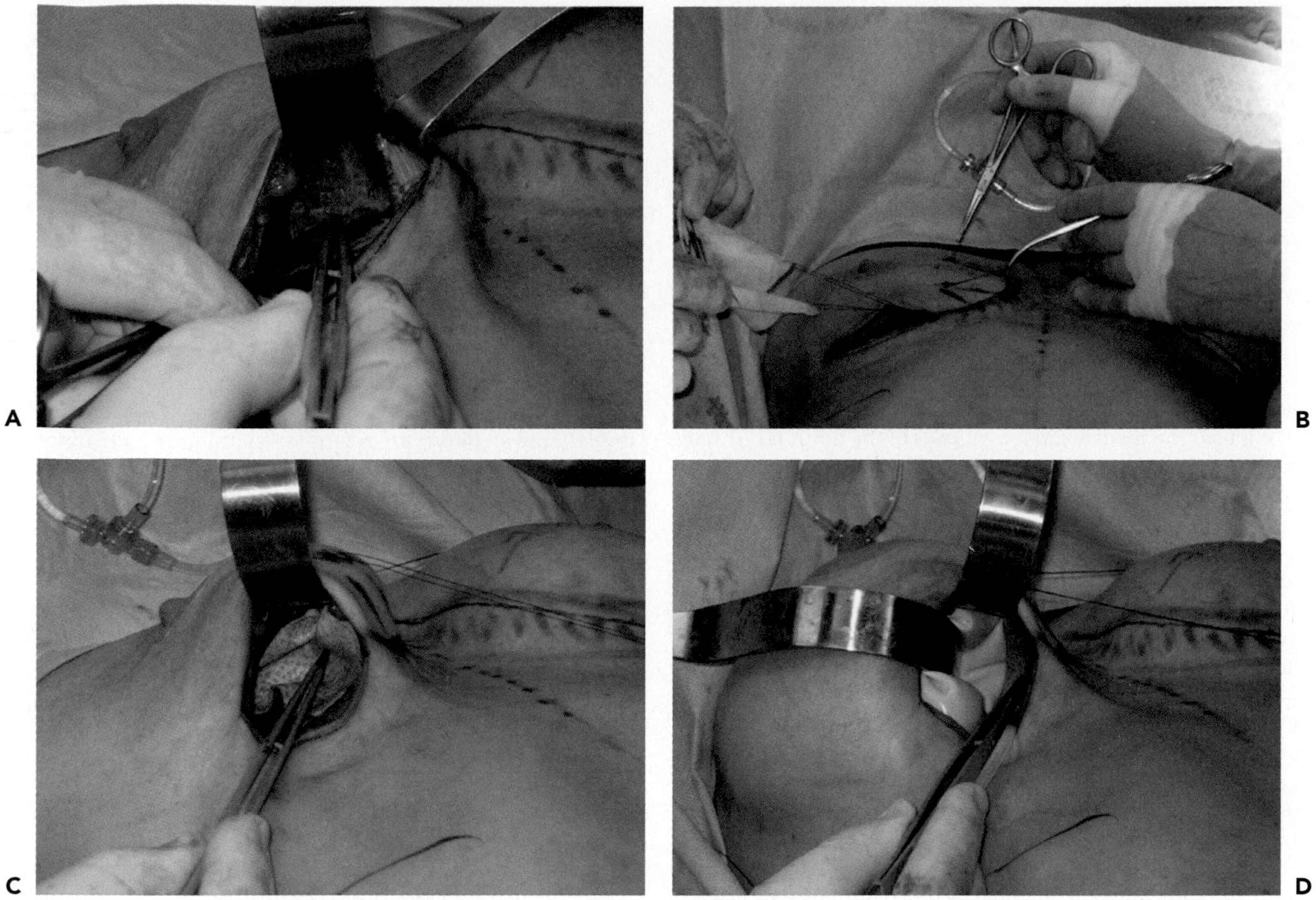

A B C D

Figure 128.2. **A:** Dissection of a neo-subpectoral pocket for correction of recurrent synmastia. **B:** Parachuting an acellular dermal matrix (ADM) overlay graft onto the pectoralis major muscle/capsule interface with 2-0 marionette sutures through the skin. **C:** Careful insetting of ADM along the pectoralis major muscle/capsule junction. **D:** Placement of a breast device in a neo-subpectoral pocket reinforced with an ADM overlay graft.

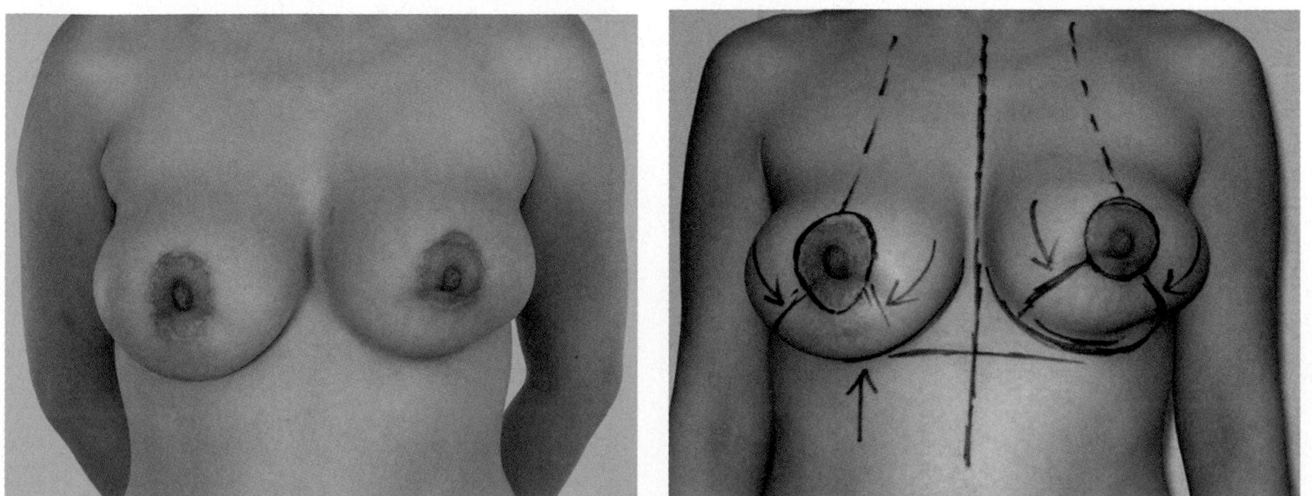

A B

Figure 128.3. **A:** Preoperative view of a 35-year-old patient displaying bilateral capsular contracture and inferior skin flap deficiency after several breast augmentation-mastopexy procedures at an outside hospital. **B:** Operative plan for partial subpectoral placement of smooth, round silicone implants (Allergan 15-234) and insetting of acellular dermal matrix interpositional grafts. (*continued*)

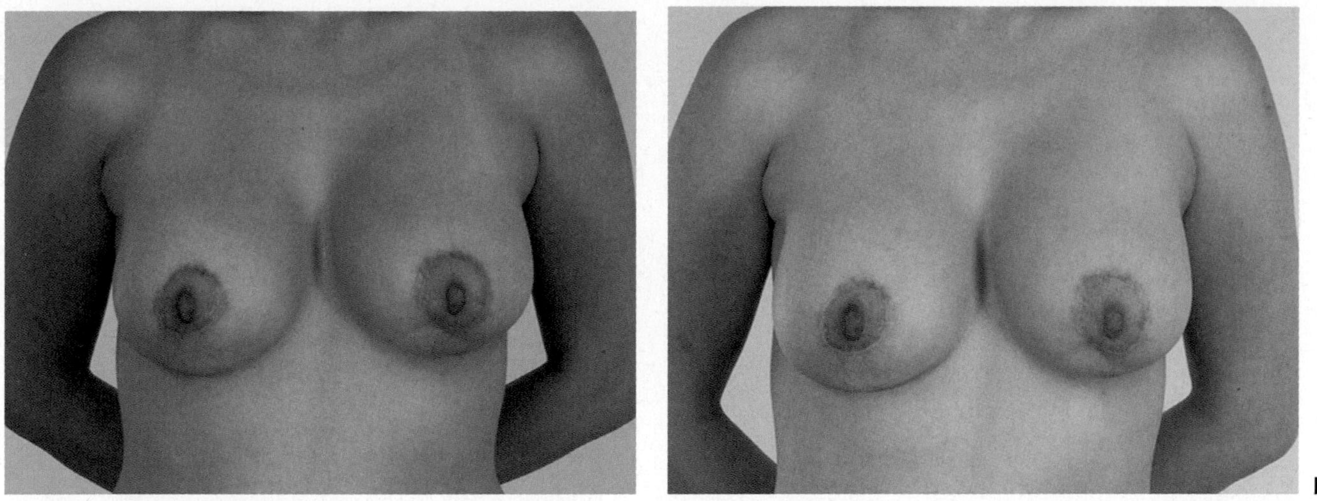

Figure 128.3. (*Continued*) **C:** Postoperative view 6 months after bilateral revision augmentation-mastopexy. **D:** Nine-month postoperative view, showing correction of capsular contracture and absence of breast distortion.

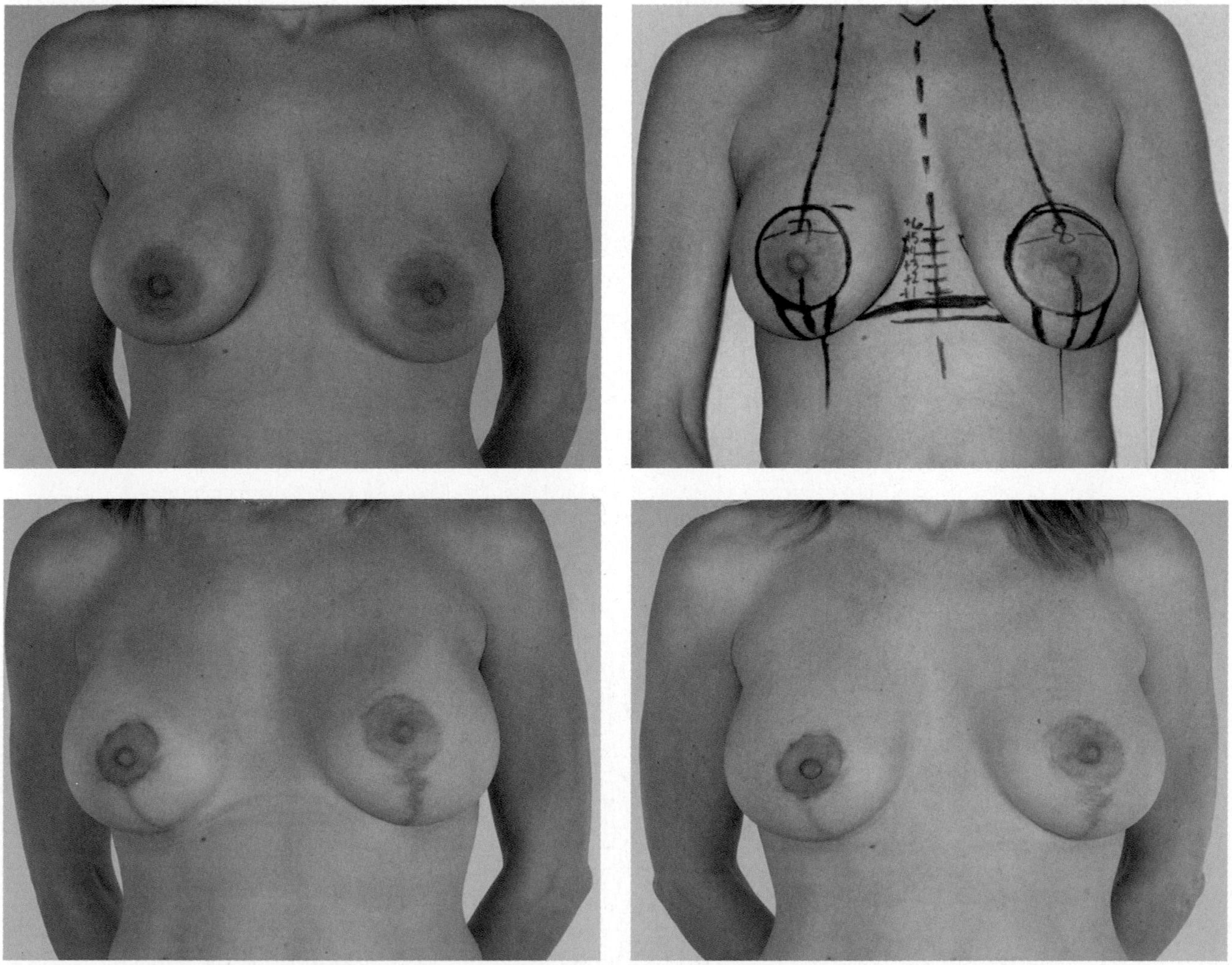

Figure 128.4. **A:** Preoperative view of a 42-year-old patient displaying bilateral breast implant rippling and ptosis after multiple subglandular breast augmentation procedures at an outside hospital. **B:** Operative plan for repositioning of original smooth, round silicone implants (Allergan 15-457) under subpectoral pockets and insetting of acellular dermal matrix interpositional grafts. **C:** Postoperative view 6 months after bilateral revision augmentation-mastopexy. **D:** Eleven-month postoperative view, showing absence of implant rippling and appropriate implant position.

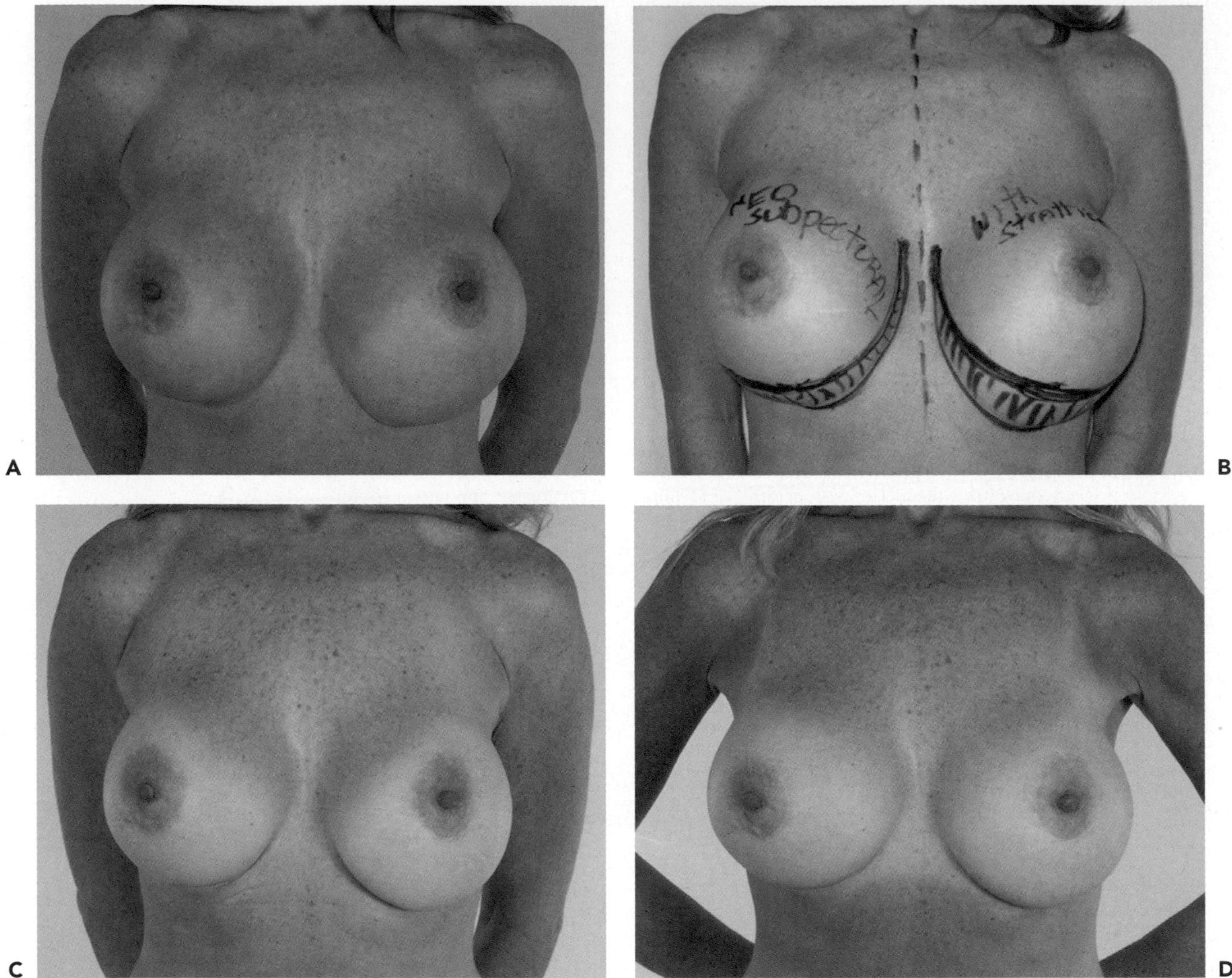

Figure 128.5. **A:** Preoperative view of a 41-year-old patient displaying inferior malposition of bilateral breast implants after multiple breast augmentation procedures. **B:** Operative plan for neo-subpectoral placement of smooth, round silicone implants (Allergan 20-500) and insetting of acellular dermal matrix interpositional grafts. **C:** Postoperative view 9 months after revision augmentation. **D:** Sixteen months postoperatively, showing successful treatment of inferior malposition and stable implant location.

and ADM was placed as an interpositional graft. Postoperative photographs demonstrated successful treatment of implant inferior malposition, which was maintained at 16 months of follow-up.

PREVENTION OF BOTTOMING OUT

A 36-year-old woman with a history of former tobacco use and 117-lb weight loss following bariatric surgery presented for a bilateral breast augmentation-mastopexy procedure (Fig. 128.6). The patient underwent bilateral circumvertical mastopexies, partial subpectoral placement of smooth, round silicone implants (Allergan 15-286, 15-304), and placement of ADM interpositional grafts. Comparison of preoperative and 9-month postoperative photos shows stable and appropriate device position, without signs of soft tissue stretch or implant bottoming out.

SUMMARY

Between November 2003 and August 2008, the senior author used ADM in the treatment and prevention of breast implant deformities in 18 patients with 26 breast prostheses. Indications for ADM use included prevention and treatment of breast implant–related deformities. Specifically, ADM was used for prevention of implant bottoming out ($n = 4$) and correction of capsular contracture ($n = 3$), rippling ($n = 5$), skin flap deficiency ($n = 8$), and malposition ($n = 14$). Depending on availability, different forms of ADM were used, including AlloDerm ($n = 14$), Strattice ($n = 10$), and Flex HD ($n = 2$). On the basis of our experience with 26 breasts, acellular dermal matrix has shown promise in treating and preventing capsular contracture, rippling, implant malposition, and soft tissue thinning. This is especially significant because many of these problems have proven extraordinarily difficult to consistently correct in the past.

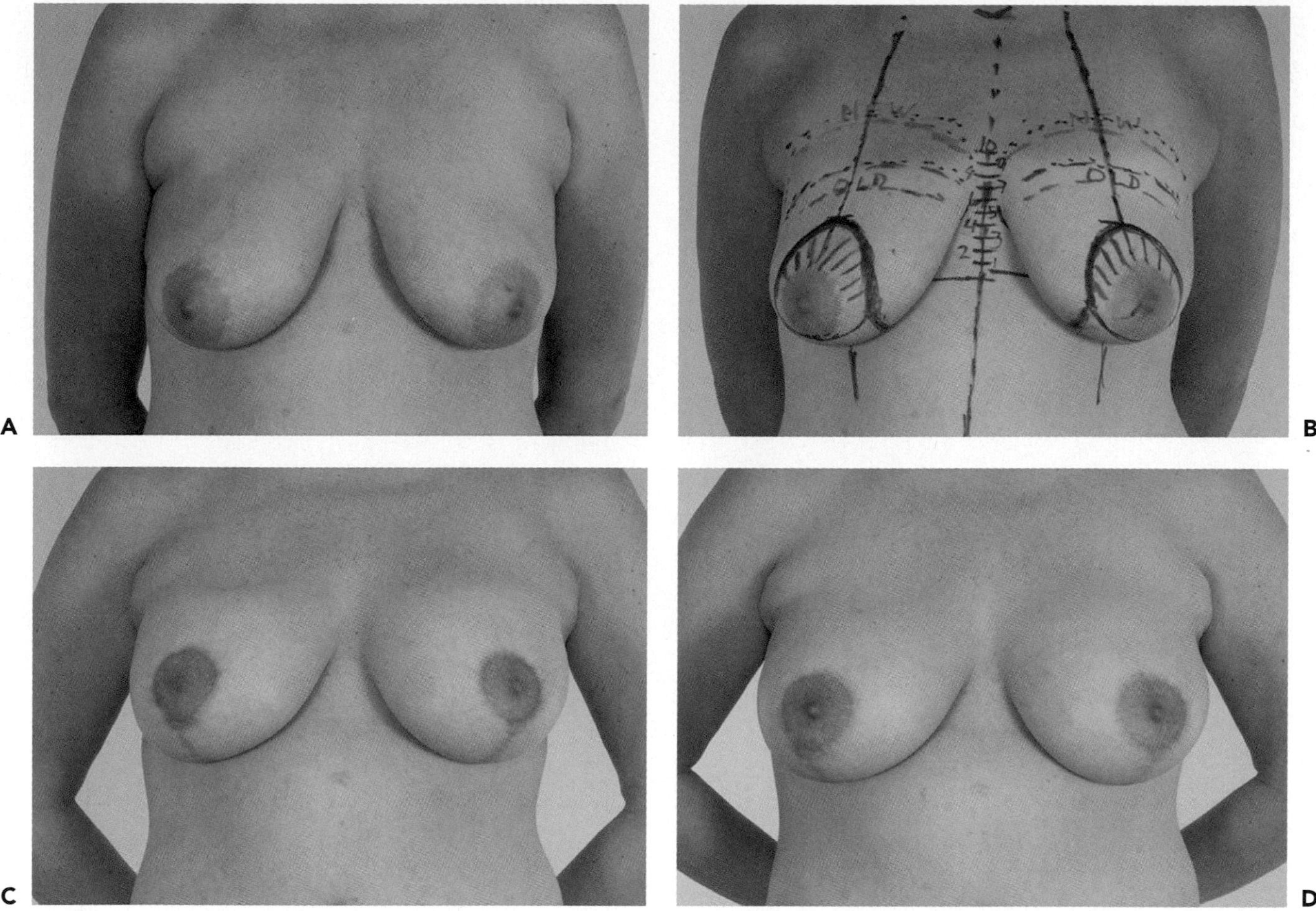

Figure 128.6. **A:** Preoperative view of a 36-year-old patient with a history of former tobacco use and 117-lb weight loss following bariatric surgery presenting for bilateral breast augmentation-mastopexy. **B:** Operative plan for bilateral circumvertical mastopexies, partial subpectoral placement of smooth, round silicone implants (Allergan 15-286, 15-304), and insetting of acellular dermal matrix interpositional grafts. **C:** Postoperative view 5 months after bilateral augmentation-mastopexy. **D:** Nine-month postoperative view with appropriate implant position and no signs of bottoming out.

EDITORIAL COMMENTS

This chapter reviews the indications for ADM in the treatment and prevention of implant-associated breast deformities. The use of ADM as an adjunct for prosthetic breast reconstruction is now well accepted and has been validated by dozens of clinical and experimental studies. The principles and concepts that we have learned from our reconstructive experience are now being applied in the purely aesthetic patient. The authors nicely review the indication for ADM in the aesthetic setting. I have had experience with ADM (AlloDerm) in three different clinical scenarios that warrant comment.

Some of the benefits that have been observed in the reconstructive patient include less capsular contracture and less rippling and wrinkling. In addition, ADM allows for optimal positioning and compartmentalization of the device. Although some of these benefits have not been adequately explained based on the specific mechanism of action, that is, less capsular contracture, there are some theories of how this may work. For a capsule to contract, it must be spherical. Many ADMs have a high elastin component. The advantage of this is that the ratio of elastin to collagen remains unchanged even when the material is integrated into the host tissues. Acellular dermal matrix, when placed along the implant capsule, will disrupt the spherical nature of the device and may prevent the long-term sequelae of contracture. Another theory is that there are cellular feedback mechanisms associated with ADMs that inhibit the deposition of thick collagen along the surface of the ADM.

Correction of rippling and wrinkling has remained a challenge. Traditionally, the plastic surgeon had the option of converting from a saline to silicone gel device, which would afford some degree of correction. The use of autologous fat grafting would also provide some degree of correction. The fat grafts would be placed between the capsule and the skin. Acellular dermis can be used as well. As the authors point out, the ADM can be placed between the capsule and the implant or between the skin and the capsule. Both methods have been useful and successful. The ADM has been observed to revascularize along either plane. The correction can be achieved in the superior, mid, or lower pole of the breast.

Another area for correction is in the situation of implant displacement. This displacement can be medial (synmastia), inferior, or lateral. The edge of the ADM is positioned and sutured to the desired location and then redraped along the capsular surface and tacked down with sutures. I have been impressed with the longevity of the repair, especially since traditional capsulorrhaphy repairs have been associated with a higher recurrence rate.

This is an important chapter that nicely introduces the concept of ADM for the repair of aesthetic breast deformities. The principal limitation for using ADM in aesthetic cases is cost. One can hope that, with streamlined pieces specific for particular problems, the costs will be less.

M.Y.N.

REFERENCES

1. Breuing KH, Warren SM. Immediate bilateral breast reconstruction with implants and inferolateral AlloDerm slings. *Ann Plast Surg* 2005;55:232–239.
2. Gamboa-Bobadilla GM. Implant breast reconstruction using acellular dermal matrix. *Ann Plast Surg* 2006;56:22–25.
3. Salzberg CA. Nonexpansive immediate breast reconstruction using human acellular tissue matrix graft (AlloDerm). *Ann Plast Surg* 2006;57:1–5.
4. Bindingnavele V, Gaon M, Ota KS, et al. Use of acellular cadaveric dermis and tissue expansion in postmastectomy breast reconstruction. *J Plast Reconstr Aesthet Surg* 2007;60:1214–1218.
5. Breuing KH, Colwell AS. Inferolateral AlloDerm hammock for implant coverage in breast reconstruction. *Ann Plast Surg* 2007;59:250–255.
6. Zienowicz RJ, Karacaoglu E. Implant-based breast reconstruction with allograft. *Plast Reconstr Surg* 2007;120:373–381.
7. Preminger BA, McCarthy CM, Hu QY, et al. The influence of AlloDerm on expander dynamics and complications in the setting of immediate tissue expander/implant reconstruction: a matched-cohort study. *Ann Plast Surg* 2008;60:510–513.
8. Spear SL, Parikh PM, Reisin E, et al. Acellular dermis–assisted breast reconstruction. *Aesthet Plast Surg* 2008;32:418–425.
9. Topol BM, Dalton EF, Ponn T, et al. Immediate single-stage breast reconstruction using implants and human acellular dermal tissue matrix with adjustment of the lower pole of the breast to reduce unwanted lift. *Ann Plast Surg* 2008;61:494–499.
10. Becker S, Saint-Cyr M, Wong C, et al. AlloDerm versus DermaMatrix in immediate expander-based breast reconstruction: a preliminary comparison of complication profiles and material compliance. *Plast Reconstr Surg* 2009;123:1–6; discussion, 107–108.
11. Losken A. Early results using sterilized acellular human dermis (NeoForm) in post-mastectomy tissue expander breast reconstruction *Plast Reconstr Surg.* 2009;123(6): 1654–1658.
12. Chun YS, Verma K, Rosen H, et al. Implant-based breast reconstruction using acellular dermal matrix and the risk of post-operative complications. Paper presented at the 88th Annual Meeting of the American Association of Plastic Surgeons, Rancho Mirage, California, March 21–24, 2009.
13. Komorowska-Timek E, Oberg KC, Timek TA, et al. The effect of AlloDerm envelopes on periprosthetic capsule formation with and without radiation. *Plast Reconstr Surg* 2009;123: 807–816.
14. Mofid MM, Singh NK. Pocket conversion made easy: a simple technique using AlloDerm to convert subglandular breast implants to the dual-plane position. *Aesthet Surg J* 2009;29:12–18.
15. Stump A, Holton LH, Connor J, et al. The use of acellular dermal matrix to prevent capsular formation around implants in a primate model. Paper presented at the 25th Annual Meeting of the Northeastern Society of Plastic Surgeons, Philadelphia, Pennsylvania, October 2–5, 2008.
16. Duncan DI. Correction of implant rippling using allograft dermis. *Aesthet Surg J* 2001; 21:81–84.
17. Baxter RA. Intracapsular allogenic dermal grafts for breast implant-related problems. *Plast Reconstr Surg* 2003;112:1692–1696; discussion, 1697–1698.
18. Sultan M, Smith M, Samson W. The correction of significant post augmentation boundary deformities with capsulorrhaphy and AlloDerm. Paper presented at the 25th Annual Meeting of the Northeastern Society of Plastic Surgeons, Philadelphia, Pennsylvania, October 2–5, 2008.
19. Spear SL, Little JW III. Breast capsulorrhaphy. *Plast Reconstr Surg* 1988;81:274–279.
20. Collis N, Platt AJ, Batchelor AG. Pectoralis major "trapdoor" flap for silicone breast implant medial knuckle deformities. *Plast Reconstr Surg* 2001;108:2133–2135; discussion, 2136.
21. Massiha H. Scar tissue flaps for the correction of postimplant breast rippling. *Ann Plast Surg* 2002;48:505–507.
22. Spear SL, Carter ME, Ganz JC. The correction of capsular contracture by conversion to "dual-plane" positioning: technique and outcomes. *Plast Reconstr Surg* 2003;112: 456–466.
23. McGregor JC, Bahia H. A possible new way of managing breast implant rippling using an autogenous fascia lata patch. *Br J Plast Surg* 2004;57:372–374.
24. Becker H, Shaw KE, Kara M. Correction of symmastia using an adjustable implant. *Plast Reconstr Surg* 2005;115:2124–2126.
25. Chasan PE. Breast capsulorrhaphy revisited: a simple technique for complex problems. *Plast Reconstr Surg* 2005;115:296–301; discussion, 302–293.
26. Chasan PE, Francis CS. Capsulorrhaphy for revisionary breast surgery. *Aesthet Surg J* 2008;28:63–69.
27. Foustanos A, Zavrides H. Surgical reconstruction of iatrogenic symmastia. *Plast Reconstr Surg* 2008;121:143e–144e.
28. Spear SL, Dayan JH, Bogue D, et al. The "neosubpectoral" pocket for the correction of symmastia. *Plast Reconstr Surg* 2009;124(3):695–703.

CHAPTER

129

Scott L. Spear
Michael Cohen

Correction of Capsular Contracture After Augmentation Mammaplasty by Conversion to the Subpectoral or "Dual-plane" Position

INTRODUCTION

As the surgical options for correcting capsular contracture and implant malposition have continued to evolve over the last decade, today's surgeon has an increased armamentarium when faced with a patient with this problem (1–4). If the problem is one of capsular contracture, the surgeon may perform a capsulotomy or may attempt to remove as much of the capsule as is necessary. Similarly, if there is implant malposition, capsule may be excised and the implant pocket adjusted in an attempt to reposition the implant (5). All of these techniques, however, are limited by the original choice of implant location. Implants that are placed completely submuscularly will tend to migrate superiorly, whereas implants that are placed completely subglandularly will lose their superior fullness and tend to contract in a more inferior position with rounder shape. Often the solution to these problems is to relocate the implant to a new position entirely.

The dual-plane pocket offers a valuable alternative. Conversion to dual-plane positioning involves creating a subglandular space in the inferior one third of the breast and a confluent subpectoral space in the superior two thirds. This allows the implant to sit in a more appropriate position on the breast while enabling the breast tissue to redrape more naturally.

The purpose of this chapter is to describe a method developed over the last two decades of dealing with established capsular contracture. The method evolved from several years of experience with other procedures, which were not as reliable or consistently successful. By relocating implants to a subpectoral, or dual-plane, position, a more natural breast shape can be obtained with a low risk of capsular contracture or other complications.

TECHNIQUE

To convert a patient from a subglandular or submuscular position to the dual plane, two things must be done. The new dual-plane pocket must be created, and the old pocket must be obliterated. This can be performed through the patient's prior augmentation incision, whether periareolar or inframammary.

For those patients whose original implants were subglandular, a total or near-total capsulectomy is initially performed. The technique of leaving the capsule intact anteriorly to the pectoralis major is not recommended because it restricts the ability of the pectoralis major muscle to redrape over the implant. After removing as much capsule as technically and safely possible, the edge of the pectoralis major muscle is identified (Fig. 129.1) and a pocket dissected beneath the pectoralis major muscle using primarily sharp dissection with fiberoptic lighting and electrocautery and a minimum of blunt dissection (Fig. 129.2). The pectoralis major muscle is released entirely across its inferior origin, and the subpectoral pocket is dissected as far medially as necessary to achieve the desired pocket shape and medial breast border. The initial capsulectomy typically recreates a reasonable approximation of a desirable subglandular breast pocket. The subsequent release of the pectoralis major muscle along its lower border should extend as far medially as the space created by the capsulectomy, unless it is apparent that to do so the breast pocket would extend too far toward the midline. Progressive release of the pectoralis major muscle from inferiorly to superiorly along the sternal border should be done very judiciously if at all. Excessive medial release of the pectoralis major muscle along the sternum risks the creation of symmastia, window shading, or an unnatural medial breast fullness.

Laterally, the pectoralis major should be separated from the pectoralis minor and serratus anterior muscles with the dissection ultimately joining the subpectoral pocket with the space created by the capsulectomy. Any apparent excess space medially, inferiorly, or laterally is closed preferably with internal sutures. The new implant is then placed within the pocket such that the superior two thirds or so is in a subpectoral plane, leaving the inferior one third in the subglandular space (Fig. 129.3). Three to five one-half mattress stabilizing "marionette sutures" are placed between the skin and pectoralis major muscle to stabilize the inferior muscle edge at or near the level of the areola (Fig. 129.4). These marionette sutures are critical in closing off the upper portion of the previous subglandular space to prevent the new implant from dislodging back into the previous purely subglandular pocket.

For those patients whose original implants were primarily or entirely submuscular, the operation is quite different, and in particular capsulectomy is typically more selective. With use of the previous inframammary or periareolar incision, the operation begins by creating the subglandular portion of the new dual-plane, partly subpectoral pocket in a virginal space. Before entering the previous submuscular pocket, dissection thus proceeds in the subglandular plane from the level of the inframammary fold vertically up to the level of the inferior border of the areola. For patients with more soft tissue or ptosis, the dissection may go as far superior as the upper border of the areola. In patients with significant ptosis, a mastopexy may be required. This dissection creates the lowermost portion of a standard subglandular pocket and always exposes the inferior edge of the pectoralis major muscle. After creating this new

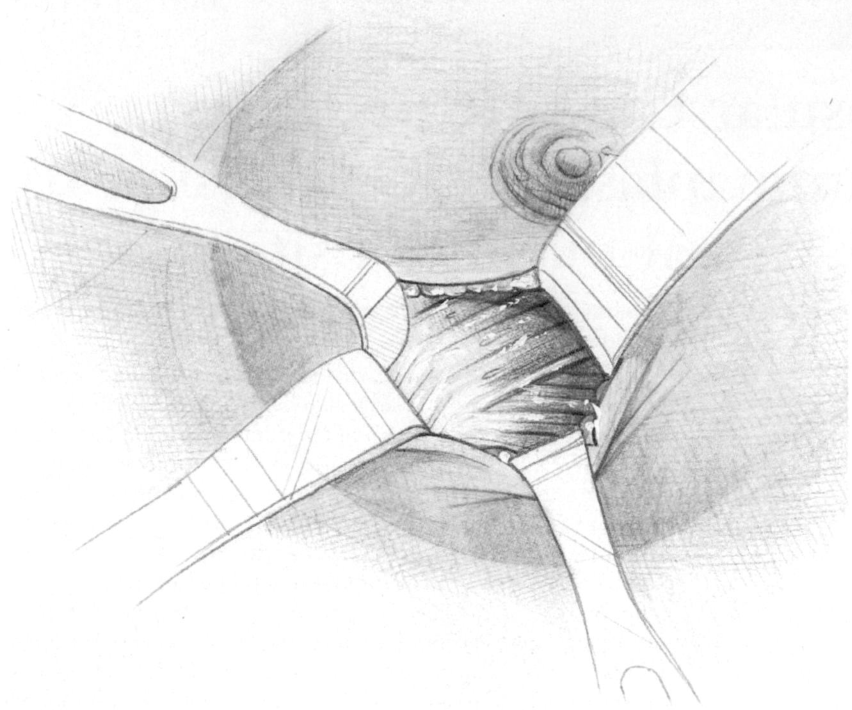

Figure 129.1. Identification of the pectoralis major muscle border.

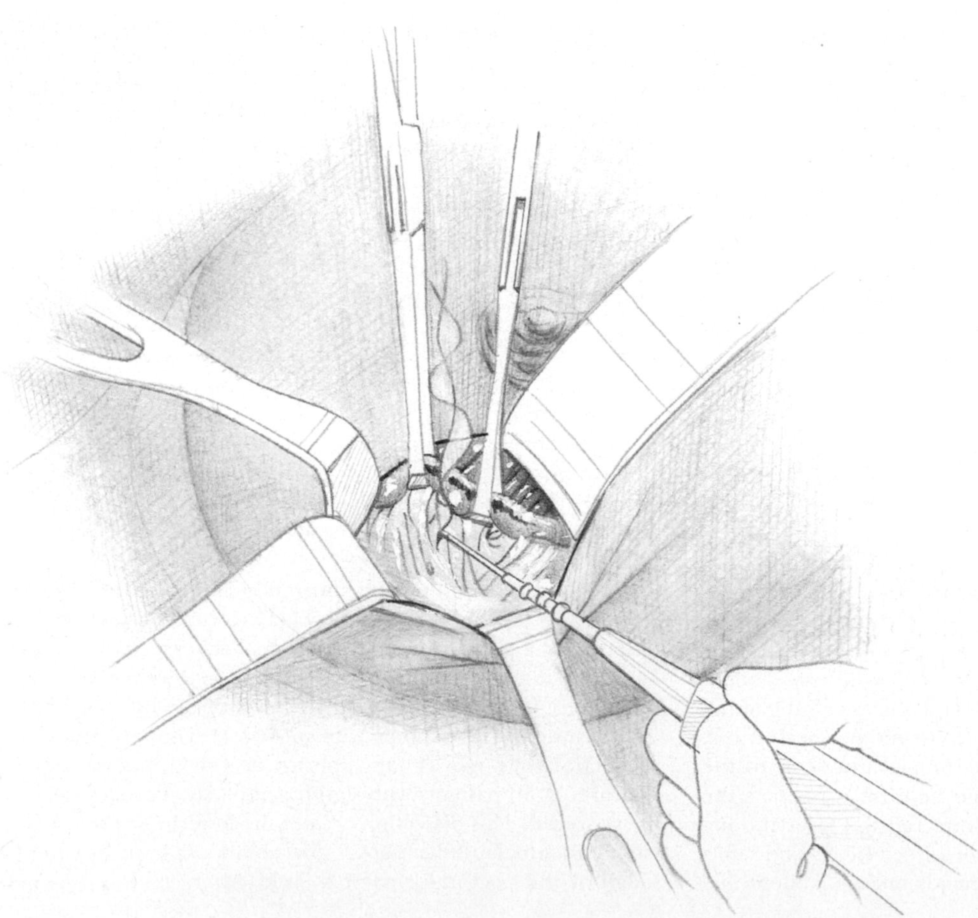

Figure 129.2. Elevation of a submuscular plane beneath the pectoralis major.

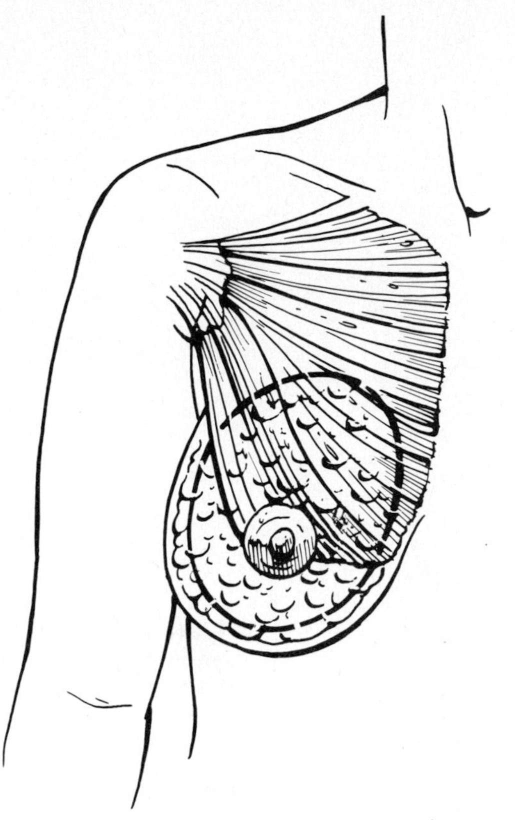

Figure 129.3. Placement of implant in the dual-plane position.

partial subglandular pocket, one identifies the inferior or lowermost border of the pectoralis major muscle. Dissection is begun along the lower border of the pectoralis major, which exposes the capsule of the existing submuscular implant.

Depending on the clinical circumstances of the case, a decision is made at this point regarding which of the three possible operations is performed. With one option, the existing subpectoral space is modified as necessary using capsulotomy and selective capsulectomy while at the same time closing off or removing the inferiormost portion of the capsule. In the second option, a neo-subpectoral plane is developed between the muscle and the underlying capsule, and dissection is carried superiorly between the two to the extent necessary to create the desired superior pocket dimensions. The entire previous pocket formed by capsule deep to the pectoralis major muscle is closed off entirely with sutures, tacking down those tissues to the chest wall to prevent the implant from migrating back into that space. With the third option, a total capsulectomy is done if it is felt to be necessary to prevent recurrence and to allow proper redraping of the soft tissues. In essence, this is a neo-subpectoral pocket with a total capsulectomy. Percutaneous or marionette sutures are not needed when converting from the submuscular to the dual-plane position (Fig. 129.5). The proportion of the implant positioned in the neo-subpectoral plane can vary, and the extent of capsulectomy versus capsule closure can be varied to fit the situation. Total capsulectomy may be useful in cases of severe capsular contracture, particularly early ones. In severe cases, as well as in cases in which the skin and soft tissue of the lower pole are too thin, an acellular

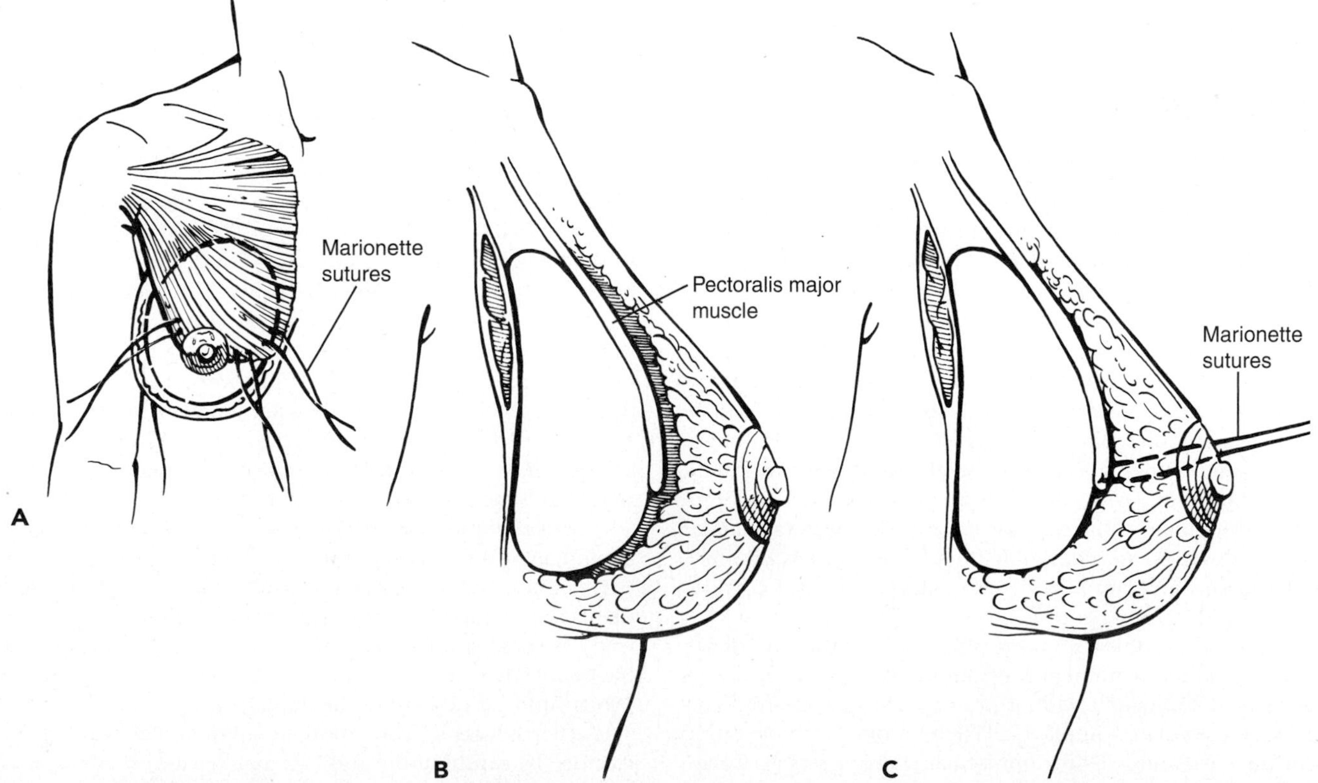

Figure 129.4. **A:** Implant in position with marionette sutures placed at the inferior edge of the pectoralis major muscle. **B:** Implant in position in a previously subglandular patient, before marionette sutures were placed. **C:** Implant in position with residual subglandular space obliterated by marionette sutures.

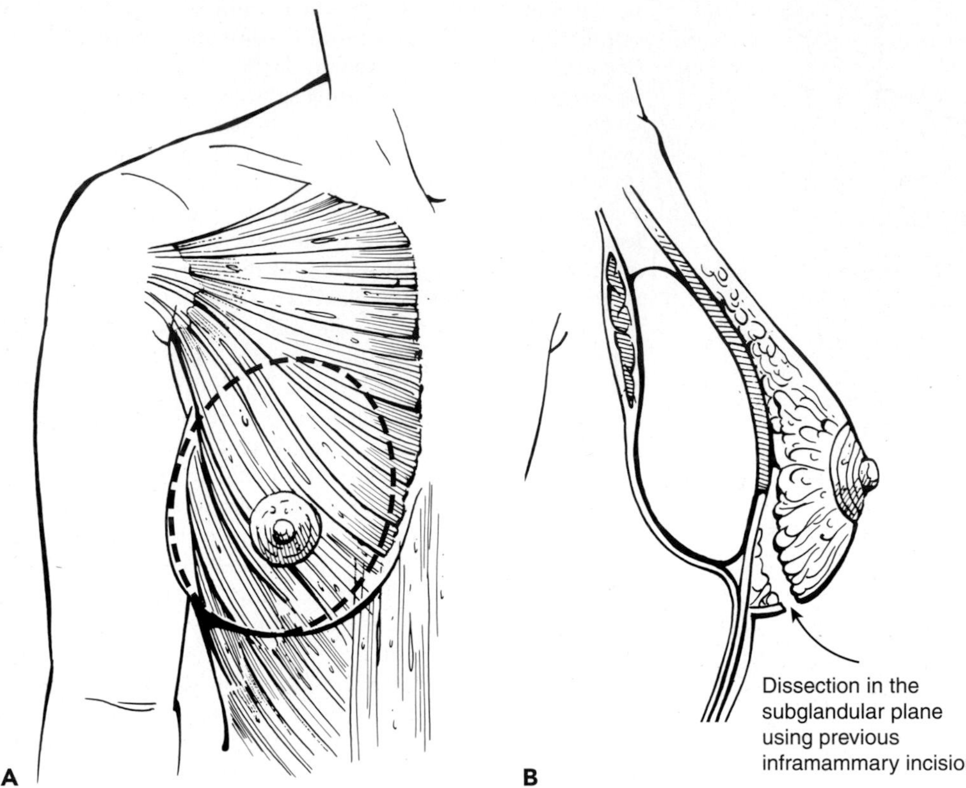

Figure 129.5. **A:** Implant in position in a previously submuscular patient. **B:** Implant in position; note the absence of a subglandular space over the pectoralis major muscle, obviating the need for marionette sutures.

dermis interposition graft can also be used and sutured to the inferior border of the pectoralis major muscle and secured inferiorly to the inframammary fold, as described in Chapter 129 and by other authors (6).

DISCUSSION

Conversion to a dual-plane position allows for correction of established capsular contracture after either previous subglandular or submuscular breast augmentation. The techniques illustrated in this chapter specifically create a fresh, virtually scar tissue–free environment for the placement of the new implant. By creating separate subpectoral and subglandular spaces and then joining them at a customized variable level somewhere between as high as the upper areolar edge to as low as near the inframammary fold, this technique creates a dual-plane position quite similar to that described by Tebbetts in primary breast augmentation (7). Like Tebbetts, we have found that the purposeful dissection in each plane followed by appropriate positioning of the inferior edge of the pectoralis major muscle helps to create a desirable breast shape, avoids a double-bubble deformity, minimizes muscle distortion, and corrects long-standing capsular contracture.

The success of this technique also confirms the experience of others that the removal of previous periprosthetic capsule or scar tissue is compatible with, if not critical to, successfully correcting encapsulated implants. Whether one was converting from the subglandular or submuscular space, a fresh subglandular pocket was created or recreated in the lowermost portion of the breast. In the more ptotic or loose breast, the final implant space might be constructed such that from the upper edge of the areola on down to the inframammary fold, the implant would be in the subglandular position. In the less ptotic or nulliparous breast, only the bottom 10% to 20% of the implant might rest in the subglandular plane.

Subpectoral positioning can be highly successful in achieving results with a low risk of capsular contracture. In a series of 85 patients by Spear et al. (8), all of the patients already had established capsular contracture and thus could rightly be considered at higher risk for capsular contracture at reoperation. At an average of 1 year postoperative, only 2 patients (2%) had a Baker class II capsular contracture, with the remainder being classified as Baker class I (9).

The type of implant used makes no difference in the outcome. Silicone and saline implants, whether textured or smooth, perform equally well in these patients (10,11). The design of silicone implants used today is, in a sense, "postmodern," in that they were designed to withstand Food and Drug Administration scrutiny and thus are made with more durable, thicker, and low-bleed silicone elastomer shells. Similarly, the silicone gel of these devices is more consistent in molecular weight and more cohesive than in earlier devices.

The technique described in this chapter for correcting subglandular capsular contracture was derived from the desire to perform a total or near-total capsulectomy and place the implants subpectorally without the implants either slipping back into the subglandular space or alternatively resulting in a double-bubble deformity from muscle, scar, or fascia restricting the proper inferior descent of the implant.

Earlier efforts at correction of submuscular capsular contracture by capsulotomy and internal release of fascia or scar bands from within the preexisting space were inconsistently successful. The evolution to a dual-plane technique with the purposeful creation of an appropriately sized lower subglandular space before opening the subpectoral space alone was marked

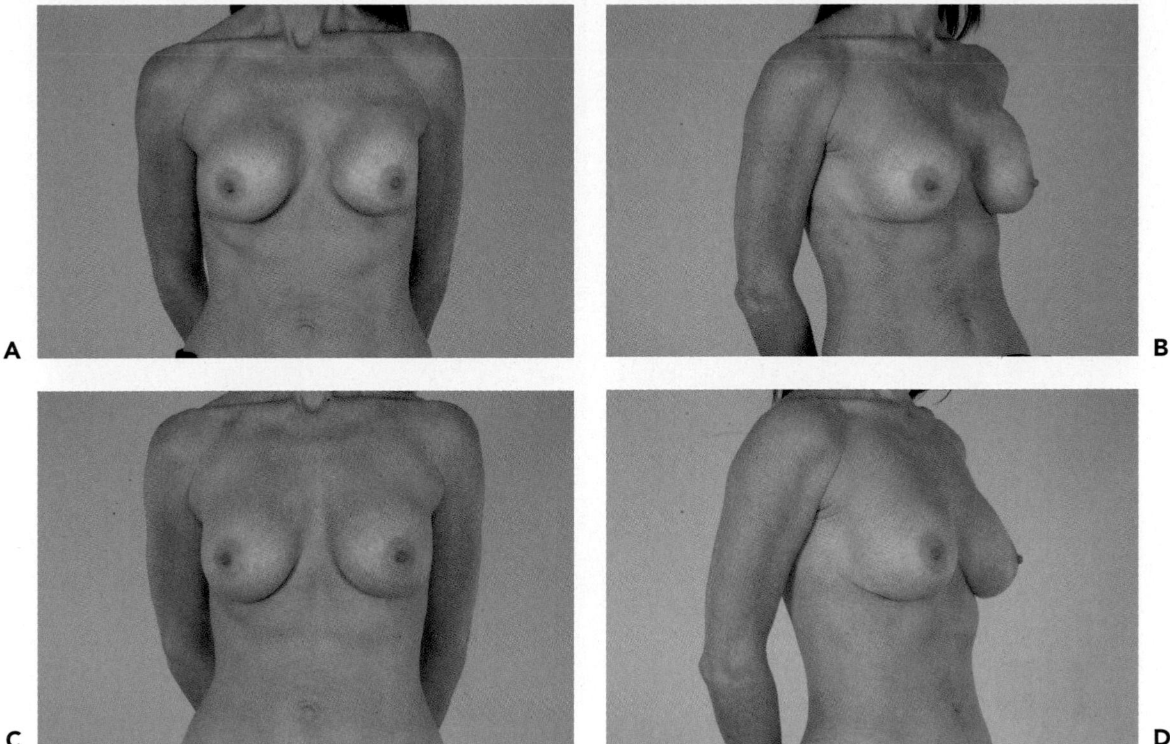

Figure 129.6. A 46-year-old patient 18 years after bilateral subglandular augmentation using silicone implants with a polyurethane cover. **A, B:** Before revision with bilateral Baker grade III capsular contracture. **C, D:** Approximately 1 year after revision with placement of 240-cc smooth silicone implants in the dual-plane position.

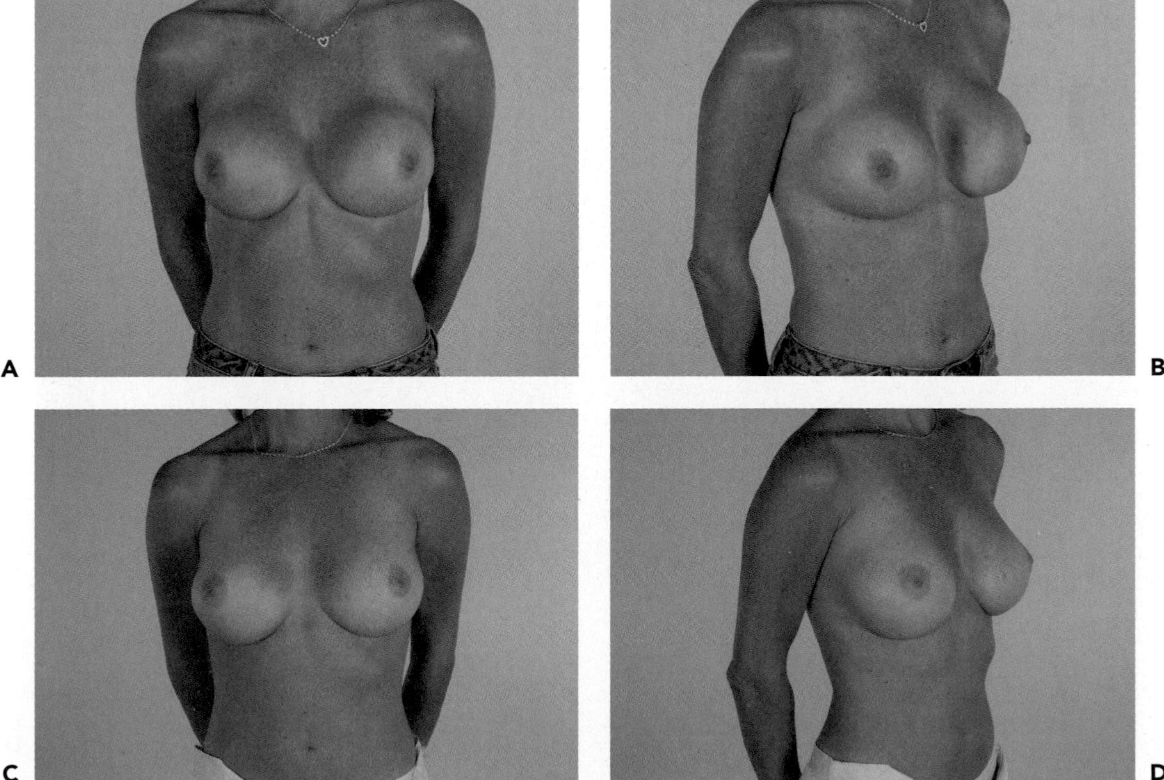

Figure 129.7. A 47-year-old patient 19 years after augmentation with silicone implants via a transaxillary approach in the submuscular plane and 17 years after exchange of implants to the subglandular plane 2 years later. **A, B:** Patient before revision surgery; there is right implant rupture and capsular contracture of Baker grade II. **C, D:** Six-month postoperative views after total capsulectomy and reaugmentation with silicone implants in the neo-subpectoral, dual-plane position.

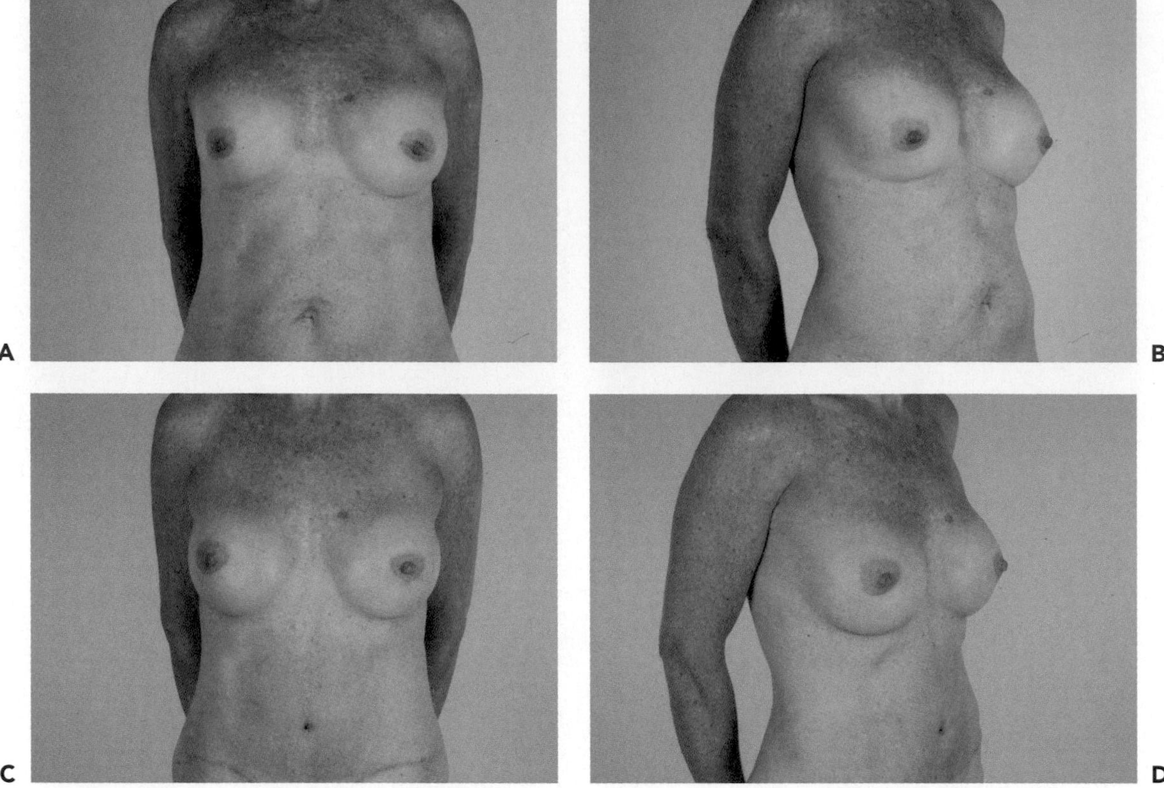

Figure 129.8. A 57-year-old patient 20 years after augmentation with silicone implants in the submuscular position. **A, B:** Patient before revision surgery; there is right implant rupture and capsular contracture of Baker grade II to III. **C, D:** 10-month postoperative views after reaugmentation with silicone implants in partly neo-subpectoral, dual-plane position.

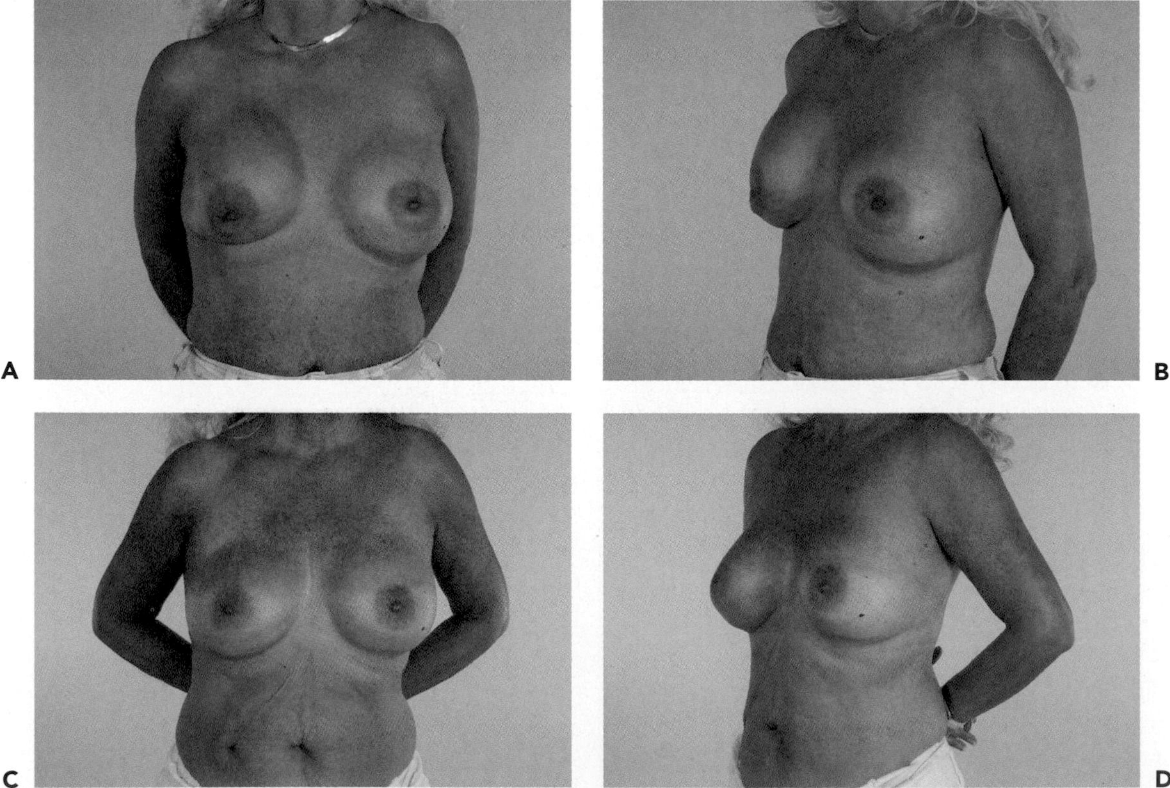

Figure 129.9. This patient underwent breast augmentation with a submuscularly positioned implant approximately 18 years prior to revision surgery. Revision surgery was complicated by a hematoma and resulting capsular contracture on the right. **A, B:** Patient before revision surgery; there is right capsular contracture of Baker grade III on the right. **C, D:** Ten-month postoperative views after capsulectomy and reaugmentation with silicone implants in partly neo-subpectoral, dual-plane position.

by an immediate and dramatic improvement in outcomes with clearer margins for dissection, more recognizable anatomy, and better results with fewer relapses.

Long-established periprosthetic capsular contracture can be confidently and reliably corrected by replacing the existing implants with saline or "postmodern" silicone gel–filled implants in a carefully created dual-plane, partly subpectoral position using the techniques described here. Although other techniques may work in some or even most patients, the technique we describe is straightforward, very anatomic, precise, and highly successful in correcting capsular contracture while avoiding other deformities and complications.

EDITORIAL COMMENTS

Capsular contracture continues to be problematic following breast augmentation, albeit less today with current implant technology than with earlier generations of implants. Management options for women who develop capsular contracture and wish to retain an implant include capsulectomy and replacement of the implant in the same space (subglandular or subpectoral) or replacement of the implant in the alternate space. The conversion from subglandular to subpectoral is more commonly performed primarily because the incidence of capsular contracture is higher when the implant is in the subglandular position. The authors of this chapter have correctly emphasized the importance of obliterating the old space to prevent remigration of the implant into the original pocket, which can at times be more difficult than it seems. Quilting sutures are usually used to obliterate this space but can sometimes result in an aesthetic outcome that is less than expected, especially if there has been significant atrophy and compression of the breast fat. Dimpling of the skin may be observed, but fortunately resolves with time.

I agree with the authors that the dual-plane insertion technique will optimize breast contour and aesthetics. This has been my preferred method of implant insertion for this indication primarily because it allows for better expansion and contouring of the skin envelope. It has been my experience that following excision of the breast capsule, a slightly larger implant may be necessary to recreate the natural breast contour. This is because once the contracted capsule is excised, the skin envelope will expand and require additional volume. Total subpectoral coverage may result in distortion of the skin envelope because optimal fill of the implant may be compromised.

M.Y.N.

REFERENCES

1. Siggelkow W, Lebrecht A, Kolbl H, et al. Dual-plane implant positioning for capsular contracture of the breast in combination with mastopexy. *Arch Gynecol Obstet* 2005;273:79–85.
2. Maxwell PG, Gabriel A. The neopectoral pocket in revisionary breast surgery. *Aesthet Surg J* 2009;28:463–467.
3. Walker PS, Walls B, Murphy DK. Natrelle saline-filled breast implants: a prospective 10-year study. *Aesthet Surg J* 2008;28:19–25.
4. Wong C-H, Samuel M, Tan B-K, et al. Capsular contracture in subglandular breast augmentation with textured versus smooth breast implants: a systematic review. *Plast Reconstr Surg* 2006;118(5):1224–1236.
5. Collis N, Sharpe DT. Recurrence of subglandular breast implant capsular contracture: anterior versus total capsulectomy. *Plast Reconstr Surg* 2000;106:792–794.
6. Mofid MM, Singh NK. Pocket conversion made easy: a simple technique using AlloDerm to convert subglandular breast implants to the dual-plane position. *Aesthet Surg J* 2009;29:12–18.
7. Tebbetts JB. Dual plane breast augmentation: optimizing implant–soft-tissue relationships in a wide range of breast types. *Plast Reconstr Surg* 2001;107(5):1255–1272.
8. Spear SL, Carter ME, Ganz JC. The correction of capsular contracture by conversion to "dual-plane" positioning: technique and outcomes. *Plast Reconstr Surg* 2003;112(2):456–466.
9. Spear SL, Baker JL. Classification of capsular contracture after prosthetic breast reconstruction. *Plast Reconstr Surg* 1995;96(5):1119–1123.
10. Tarpila E, Ghassemifar R, Fagrell D, et al. Capsular contracture with textured versus smooth saline-filled implants for breast augmentation: a prospective clinical study. *Plast Reconstr Surg* 1997;99(7):1934–1939.
11. Collis N, Coleman D, Foo ITH, et al. Ten-year review of a prospective randomized controlled trial of textured versus smooth subglandular silicone gel breast implants. *Plast Reconstr Surg* 2000;106:786–791.

CHAPTER

130

Bradley P. Bengtson

The Inframammary Fold: Histologic and Anatomic Description, Classification and Definitions, and Options for Repair and Reinforcement

The inframammary fold (IMF) is the keystone and most important foundational element of the breast. Prior to 2000, there was a great deal of time, attention, and body of research dedicated to the study of the IMF, and recently there has been resurgence in the recognition of its importance. This chapter presents and discusses the histology and anatomic nuances of the IMF, the terminology and classification of the deformities that may occur surrounding it, and a few techniques for recreating the fold if malposition occurs.

An excellent description of the superficial fascial system of the breast in this area appeared in a review by Nava et al. in a prior edition of this text (1). They described the fascial system of the breast and how it relates to the fold, and they further broke it down anatomically by contour, level, angle, and symmetry (see Fig. 43.1). Histologically, they showed in cross section how the superficial fascial fiber inserted in an oblique vertical position into the chest wall (see Fig. 43.2).

Further histologic and anatomic description is available from Acland's group in Louisville (2) (Fig. 130.1). They showed in detail the region of the IMF and specifically how the fusion of the deep and superficial fascia insert in an oblique fashion from a vertical direction. Why is this important clinically? Every plastic surgeon who has performed a breast reduction with a transverse incision placed originally in the fold has seen the incision ride up to a higher location on the base of the breast postoperatively, particularly if the closure is tight. A similar effect occurs in breast augmentation. If this anatomy is not taken into consideration, an implant may shift down into the slot beneath this vertically oriented fascia, with the incision moving up into a higher location on the breast than originally planned. Furthermore, if these fascial fiber insertions are released either intentionally or unintentionally, the breast or implant can descend even further down onto the chest wall.

I define the IMF anatomically as a resting or sitting fold position and a true fold position where the actual base of the fold resides: where these superficial fascial fibers actually insert into the deeper fascia. This is a minimum of 1 cm, and may be up to 3 cm lower than where the visible, natural, resting skin fold junction is in relation to the chest wall (Figs. 130.2 to 130.5). The resting fold position may also be demonstrated by retracting the fascia of the breast and noting its attachments transmitted through the lower pole of the breast skin (Fig. 130.6). This can also be seen anatomically in every breast augmentation through an IMF incisional approach, and this is why the dissection after the skin incision is made should go directly at a vertical oblique angle of 60–80 deg to avoid disruption of the IMF, preserving the true fold position. In addition I prefer to leave a medial fascial shelf at this true or actual fold at the time of placing a partial submuscular implant, helping to maintain the final fold position in breast surgery. This aids to further support the device and avoid fold malposition (Fig. 130.7).

One further pearl relates to the ideal nipple to inframammary (N-IMF) distance based on certain styles, sizes, and volumes of breast implants. These principles are based on work by Tebbetts and Adams originally described in terms of the TEPID system (tissue characteristics of the breast, envelope, parenchyma, and implant and dimensions and dynamics of the implant relative to the soft tissues) and more recently the "high five" selection system (3,4). We expanded these concepts further and also defined a selector tool that simplifies this relationship and is based on more than 2,000 breast augmentations and measurements (5). For example, If the final implant volume is 300 cc, the N-IMF distance should be approximately 8 cm on maximum stretch. If the skin and tissues are tight, one should add 5 mm; if they are loose, one should subtract 5 mm. Then for each 50 cc one should add or subtract 5 mm, or 1 mm for each 10 cc. So a 400-cc implant should have an ideal fold of 9 cm with normal skin dynamics, and when one is using a 250-cc implant, the ideal N-IMF should be approximately 7.5 cm. This is extremely accurate and is important especially with a shift back to the inframammary incision and for gel devices, particularly future form-stable devices. This is even more critical when a patient has a constricted breast or high IMF. The plastic surgeon needs to be confident about where the new IMF should be set before placing an incision on the breast, and if planned and designed properly, the incision should be directly in or a few millimeters adjacent to the final IMF position (Fig. 130.8A, B). When moving the fold to a new planned or required location, further reinforcement by placing a 2-0 Vicryl from the deep fascia triangulating to the fascia of the upper portion of the incision is important (personal communication, Charles Randquist). This maneuver helps set the fold. It is a less common to lower the fold beyond the true or resting fold except in severely constricted breasts or in revisional breast surgery.

It is key to define and clarify what we are describing, at a minimum, so we can all be sure of speaking the same language. There are many terms and classifications when it comes to the anatomy of this area and subsequent types of deformities that may occur. My goal is not to convert others if they have a specific way to describe these terms, but to make sure that we are using the same semantics, or at least understand what the other person is talking about. The inframammary fold is a

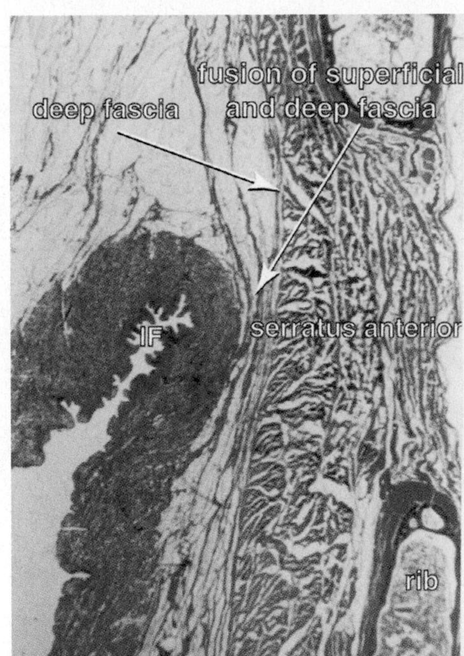

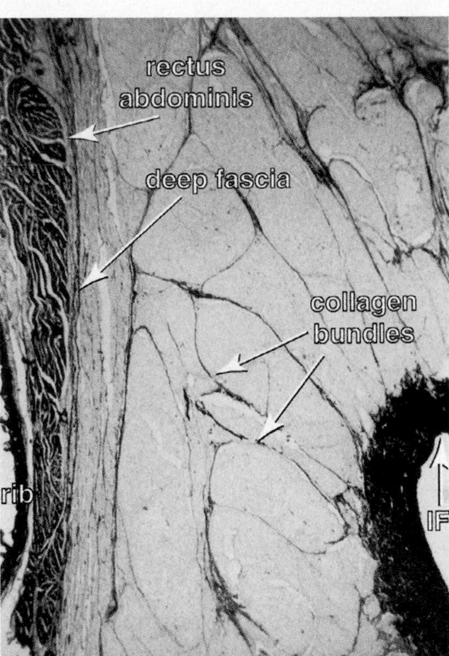

Figure 130.1. **A:** Fusion of superficial and deep fascia with the dermis at the fold level (specimen 350). **B:** Collagen fibers from the superficial fascia inserting into the dermis at, or inferior to, the fold level (specimen 416). Gomori's trichrome stain: collagen 5 green, muscle 5 red, nuclei 5 blue. IF, inframammary fold. (From Muntan CD, Sundine MJ, Rink RD, et al. Inframammary fold: a histologic reappraisal. *Plast Reconstr Surg* 2000;105(2):549–556; with permission.)

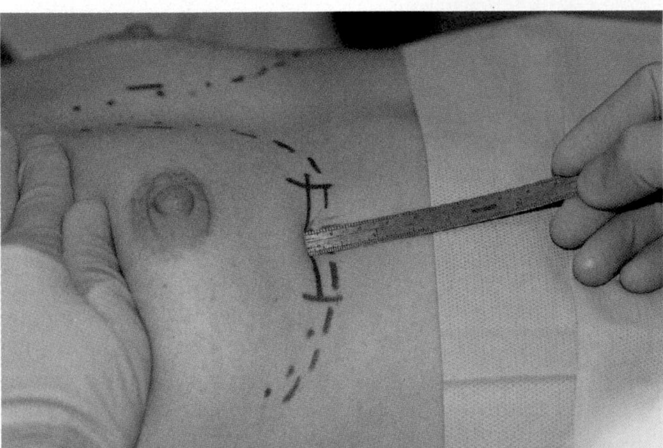

Figure 130.2. The resting fold in the sitting position. When the patient is upright, the breast fascial fibers insert into the skin in this position, creating the skin fold.

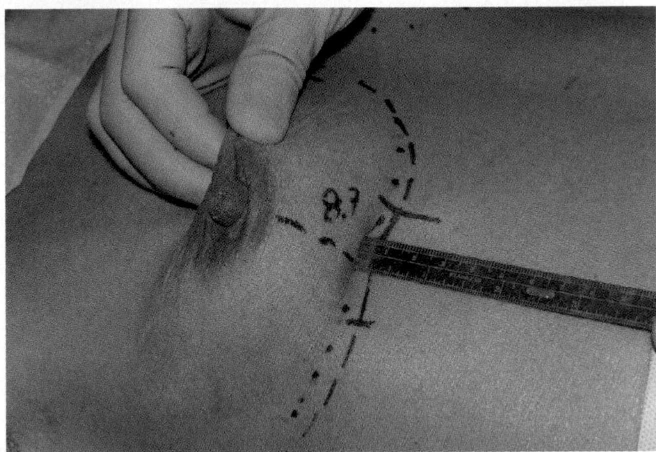

Figure 130.4. Similar to Figure 130.2, this shows the resting fold position 8.7 cm below the nipple on maximal stretch. A 400-cc implant was planned with a 14.5-cm base width and tissue-based planning measurements, so the incision was placed 9.0 cm below the nipple in the area of the true fold.

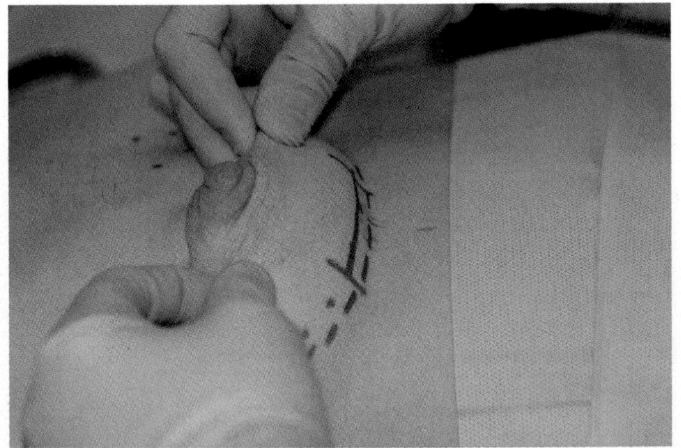

Figure 130.3. This image of the patient in Figure 130.2 shows the position of the true fold where the deeper fascial fibers insert into the chest wall. This position is usually 1 to 2 cm below the resting fold position.

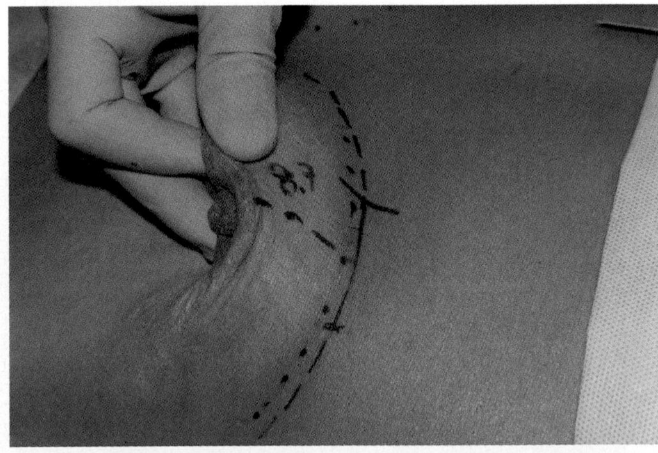

Figure 130.5. The true fold position is demonstrated in the same patient as in Figure 130.4. This is the incision chosen in the new inframammary fold (IMF) location. The IMF was further reinforced at this level just prior to closure.

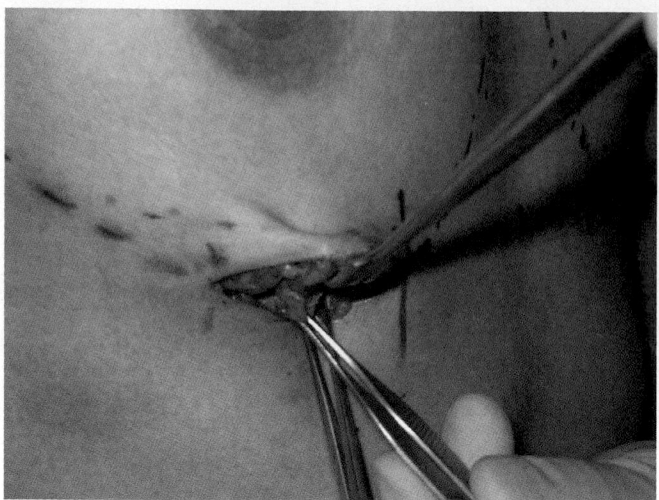

Figure 130.6. The incision shown here is placed in the true fold of the breast. When the breast fascia is grasped and retracted, it shows the insertion into the skin that forms the resting fold when the patient is upright. Determining, maintaining, or setting this fold will help to avoid fold malpositions postoperatively.

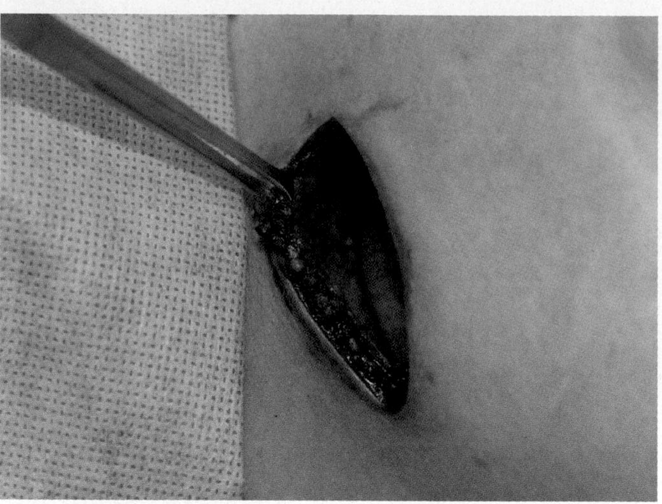

Figure 130.7. The implant rests on the preserved fascial shelf medially in this partial subpectoral implant pocket dissection. From this cranial viewpoint it is easy to see the true fold at the base of the incision which is clearly below the transposed fold to the skin. Setting of this true fold is what determines the final location of the base of the implant.

well-agreed-upon structure. If an IMF incision is planned, the primary surgeon knows accurately where the fold is located and where ideally he or she wants the fold to be placed. The fold is also then measured on maximal stretch from the midnipple point to the fold (N-IMF). Some surgeons also take a measurement from the umbilicus as an additional fixed point of reference. The incision is made and is a reference point for the future. If an implant or breast tissue in the case of a reduction or mastopexy slips below this point with the incision riding up on the breast, by definition I would term this a *fold malposition.*

If, however, the incision and/or fold remains in position but the nipple-to-IMF distance increases in length, I would term this a *stretch deformity.* By contrast, a stretch deformity of the upper pole of the breast with a relatively set IMF is ptosis of the breast: The nipple descends below the IMF, and the upper pole of the breast is stretched. Lower pole stretch occurs when the soft tissues of the breast cannot support either the weight of an implant or residual nascent breast tissue weight, and the bottom or lower pole of the breast stretches. This occurs most frequently in patients with large implants or in breast reduction/mastopexy patients with poor skin tone (i.e., massive-weight-loss patients). Both of these situations—a stretch deformity of the lower pole of the breast or a fold malposition—are often lumped into a broader visual classification of a *bottoming-out deformity.* It is important to know the primary deformity, however, because the treatment options may differ. Often patients will have combinations or portions of both of these problems, either on one breast compared to the contralateral side, or even in the same breast. What follows are some examples of these deformities, malpositions, and problems (Figs. 130.9A, B and 130.10).

There are number of techniques that have been developed using an external approach as championed by Ryan (6,7). These techniques are particularly effective in breast reconstruction surgery where the incisions are already located in the IMF region. For cosmetic revisions, particularly through smaller incisions, reconstruction of the fold may be done internally with high degrees of success (8,9).

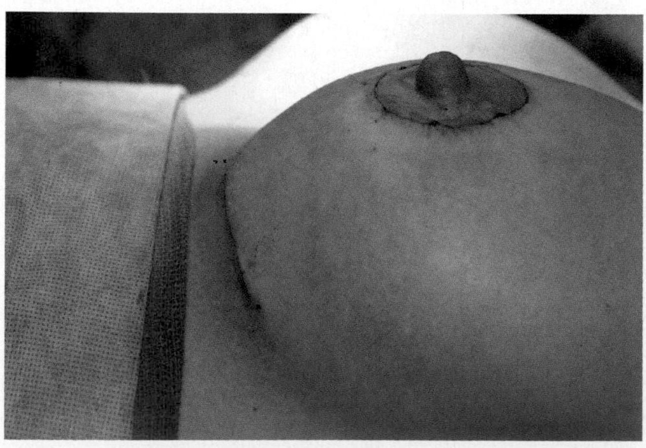

A

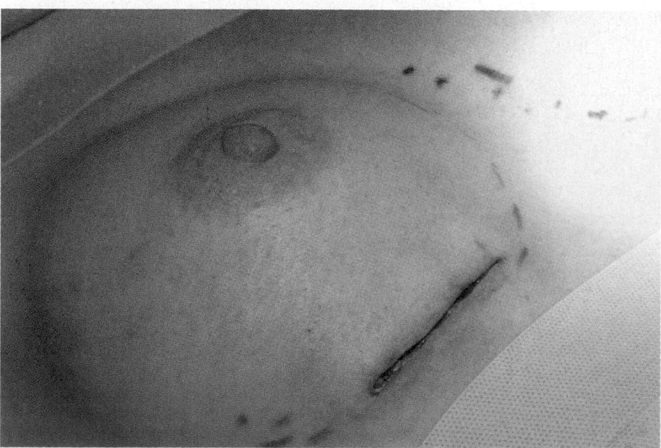

B

Figure 130.8. **A, B:** When appropriate tissue-based planning principles are utilized, the incision lands directly in the new fold position.

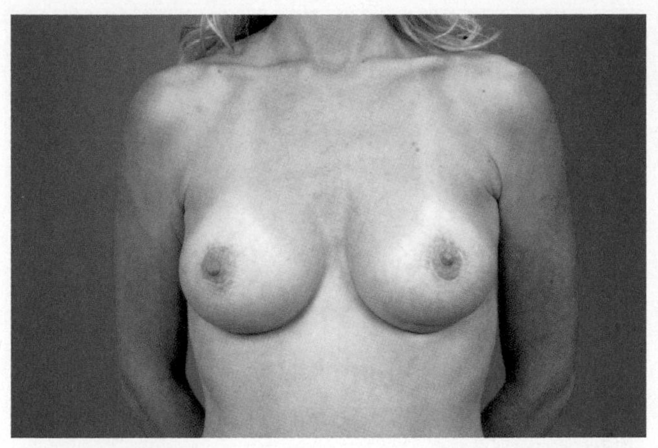

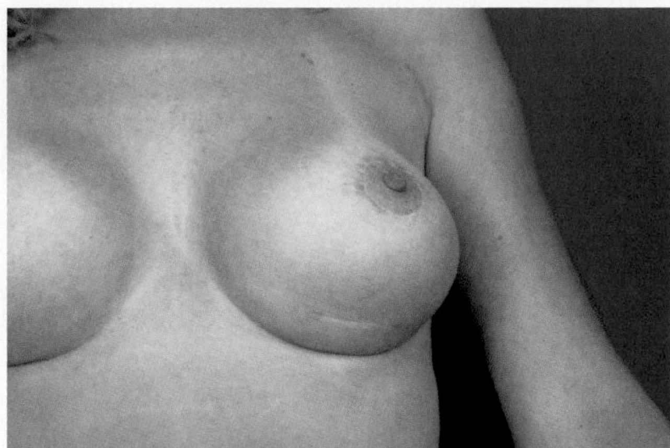

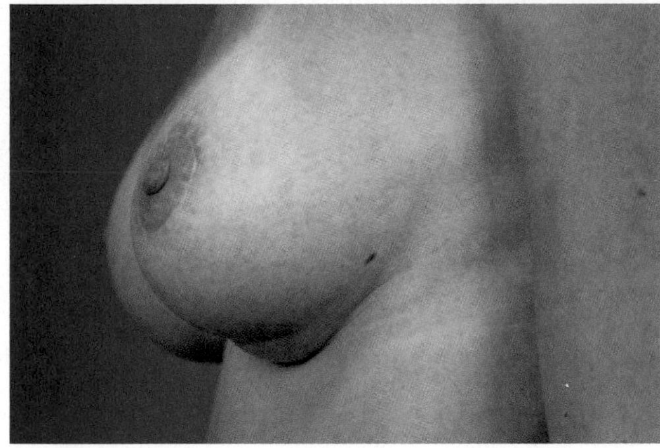

Figure 130.9. A–C: Left inframammary fold (IMF) malposition is shown in multiple views. The prior IMF incision rides up onto the lower pole of the breast, and the nipple appears higher in location on the breast.

Finally, I describe the most recent advance in this arena, using acellular dermal matrices (ADMs) to further reinforce fold malposition deformities and support the lower breast pole. In a prior edition of this text, Spear and colleagues described the problems, as well as a method of closure I use as well but have modified slightly. Either technique may be used, with capsulectomy less important if an ADM is planned in addition to the repair (10) (see Chapter 42, Figs. 42.5 and 42.6).

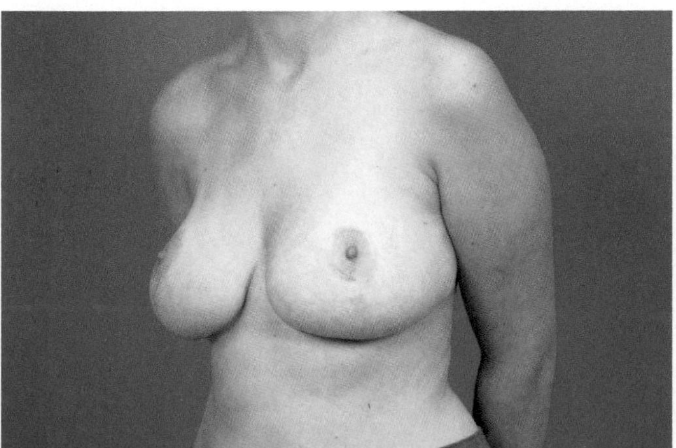

Figure 130.10. Stretch deformity of the lower pole of the breast. The nipple position is stable, so this is not ptosis. The inframammary fold (IMF) is also stable, but the soft tissues from the nipple to the IMF have stretched.

In the cross section view of Fig. 42.6 in Chapter 42, a capsulorrhaphy is performed closing off the prior space and area of pocket malposition. I prefer to excise the redundant capsule in this area of prior fold malposition, both the anterior and deep capsular surface, and suture the fresh soft tissues together to further deter an implant from re-descending back into this pocket (Fig. 130.11A, B). If a dehiscence of these sutures were to occur, the implant could drop back into its prior malposed space. I use currently a nonabsorbable suture such as 3-0 Ethibond to close off the space. Without any concurrent capsular contracture I divide and leave an appropriate amount of capsular tissue to use it as an additional layer of support as a capsular flap further buttressing the implant, suturing the capsule directly into the desired fold layer. I have also found marking this fold with methylene blue helpful. Even with a high degree of measuring and planning, it is critical to sit the patient up prior to final closure to assure fold symmetry.

Recently, ADMs have shown benefits in breast reconstruction and have been making their way into revision breast surgery of prior cosmetic procedures. It is important to view this material as a “both-and” versus an “either-or” material. We should consider doing everything we can to avoid any further revision surgery for these patients. To this end and to limit recurrence, this may include exchange of saline implants for gel, consideration of textured devices, use of smaller devices if extra large volume was a potential contributing cause, and use of standard techniques of repair such as capsulorrhaphy or neosubpectoral pockets and capsular flaps. In addition to these standard techniques, this ADM material may be added as additional support, an internal hammock or a sling, to take additional

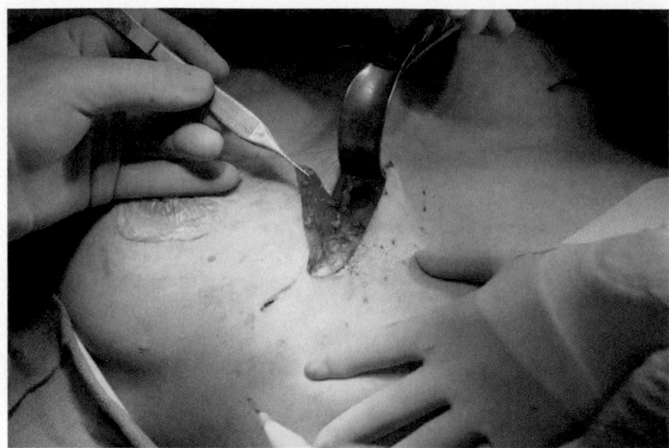

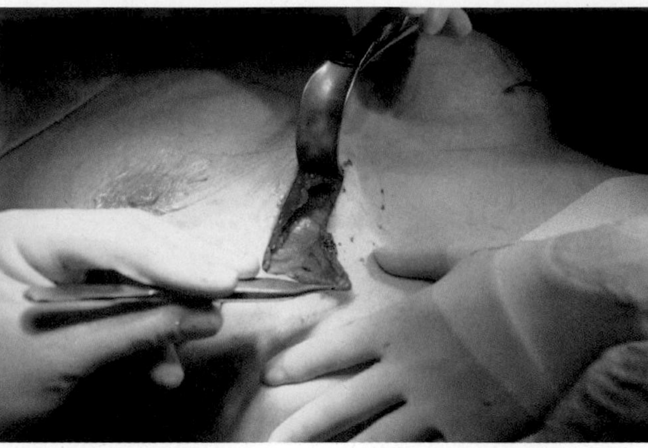

Figure 130.11. **A, B:** Capsulectomy of the redundant capsular tissue. Both the anterior and posterior surfaces are excised and soft tissues closed, reapproximating the anterior abdominal wall skin back down to the chest.

weight off the lower soft tissues of the breast and/or further reinforce a standard fold repair. Techniques vary depending on the specific deformity or problem present. It is also common to have multiple deformities present all at once, such as an IMF and lateral fold malposition. Because this material does so much and is expensive, it is best to focus on the main priority and then use additional material if available and necessary. It is also important to be careful not to create a new complication when correcting another, for example, create a fold malposition when correcting a capsular contracture.

What follows is an example of an IMF malposition reinforced with an ADM tissue. If any portion of a capsular contracture is present, capsulectomy is important to perform as part of this procedure (Fig. 130.12). There is also evidence that no capsular tissue forms on the underneath side of this material or between the implant and the ADM, with the capsule coming to the edge of the ADM and actually stopping at the capsule/ADM junction, thus inhibiting further recurrent capsular contracture (11) (Fig. 130.13). If, however, the capsule is thin and attenuated, which is often the case, the capsule may be used to further support the implant or breast and ADM sandwiched between the superficial side of the capsule and the deep soft tissues of the breast. Multiple methods have been described, from placing this material into the seam of redundant capsule to supporting the lower breast tissue as an internal sling, which I usually prefer for its added benefit of additional thickness and coverage over the lower pole of the breast, which is usually thin. However, the benefit of limiting capsule formation between the implant and soft tissues is lost (Fig. 130.14).

In summary, the IMF is the foundation and keystone of the breast. It is critical for plastic surgeons to understand what is going on at the histologic and anatomic levels, specifically in the fold region. The challenge is to better understand and plan for the desired setting and preservation of the IMF, or, if a planned IMF move is required, to better plan for the final new fold location. Second, we need to have a great deal of respect for the IMF and not disrupt the deeper fascial attachments or cause a descent below the true fold of the breast, creating further work for ourselves and undesirable revisional surgery for the patient. Third, we need to understand the anatomy to better repair, recreate, and reinforce the fold to prevent further

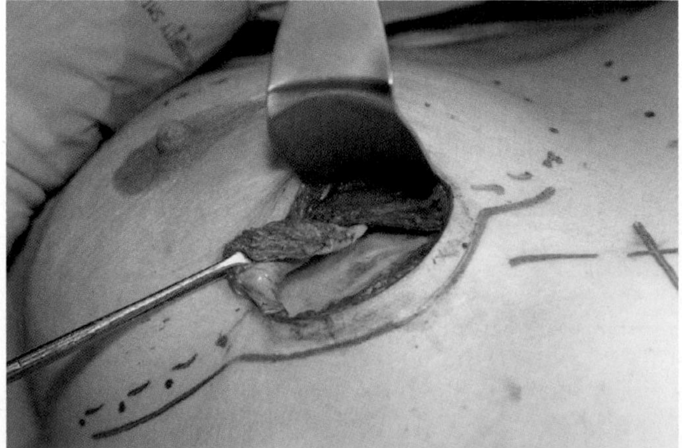

Figure 130.12. Partial capsulectomy being completed maintaining the posterior capsule in position, with this segment of capsule being replaced with acellular dermal matrix.

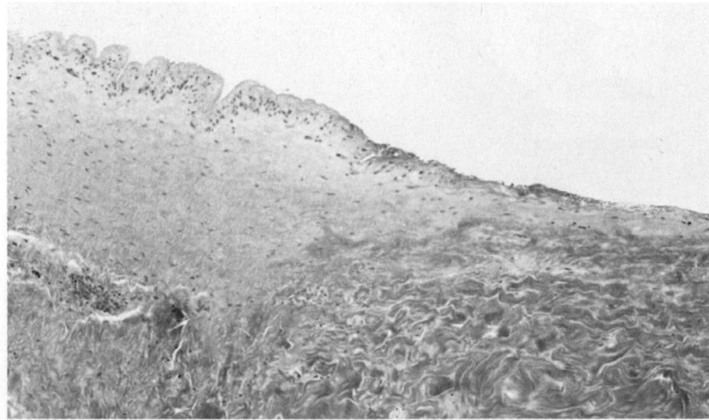

Figure 130.13. Hematoxylin and eosin staining at 100× magnification showing the junction of the undulating breast capsule on the left merging into the acellular dermal matrix (ADM) at the junction, with no capsule formation beneath the ADM.

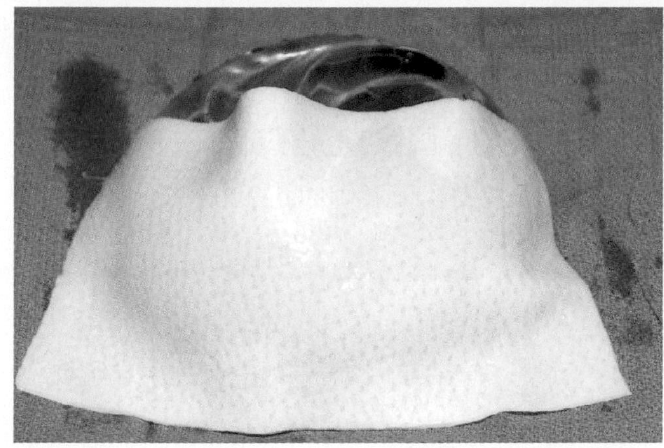

A

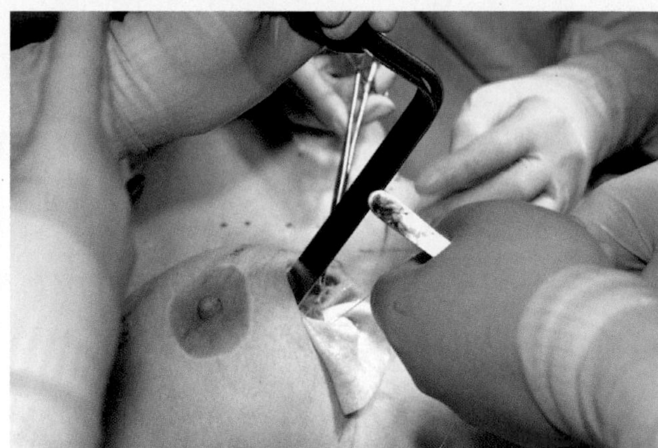

B

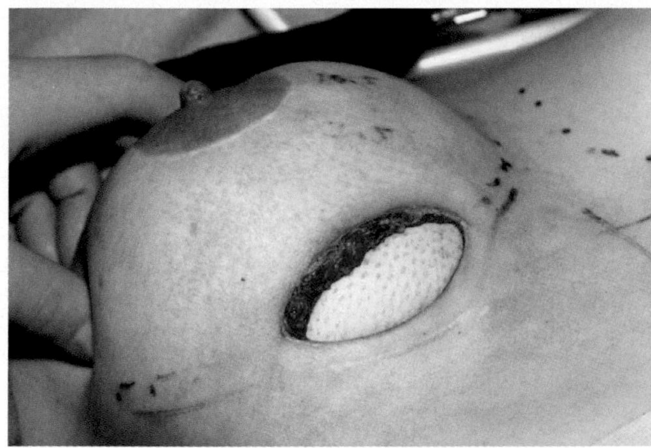

C

Figure 130.14. **A:** Acellular dermal matrix (ADM) shown covering the lower pole of the implant as it will reside in situ. The material will be trimmed into a trapezoidal shape and sutured into position as an extension of the pectoralis major muscle. **B:** ADM being inset, first beginning laterally, then medially into the leading edge of the pectoralis, closing the inframammary fold incision last and setting and supporting the fold. **C:** ADM in final position securing the fold even with firm downward pressure as a internal sling between the device and breast soft tissues.

reoccurrence and preserve our repairs with an even greater degree of success. I hope this chapter will help to better understand, preserve, relocate, and repair the IMF in the future.

EDITORIAL COMMENTS

Dr. Bengtson provides an excellent review of the IMF and its importance in the breast augmentation patient. This chapter reviews the relevance of the IMF when making most measurements related to the choice of device, position of the breast, and symmetry. Dr. Bengtson also reviews the various incisional approaches to breast augmentation and how they can impact the position of the IMF. The chapter also reviews situations in which the location of the IMF can be abnormally affected. Finally, it also deals with the application of acellular dermal matrices and their role and benefit in the correction of these IM-related issues. This important chapter provides the reader with a better understanding of the IMF based on anatomy, histology, and aesthetic importance.

M.Y.N.

REFERENCES

1. Nava M, Ottolenghi J, Egidio R. Re-creating the inframammary fold with the superficial fascial system. In: Spear S, ed. *Surgery of the Breast: Principles and Art.* 2nd ed. Philadelphia: Lippincott Williams & Wilkins; 2006:581–600.
2. Muntan CD, Sundine MJ, Rink RD, et al. Inframammary fold: a histologic reappraisal. *Plast Reconstr Surg* 2000;105(2):549–556.
3. Tebbetts J. A system for breast implant selection based on patient tissue characteristics and implant-soft tissue dynamics. *Plast Reconstr Surg* 2002;109:1306–1409.
4. Tebbetts J, Adams WP. Five critical decisions in breast augmentation using five measurements in 5 minutes: the high five decision support process. *Plast Reconstr Surg* 2005; 116(7):2005–2016.
5. Adams WP Jr, Teitelbaum S, Bengtson BP. Breast implant selector system. U.S. Patent 7685721.
6. Ryan JJ. Recreating the inframammary fold: the external approach. In: Spear S, ed. *Surgery of the Breast: Principles and Art.* 2nd ed. Philadelphia: Lippincott Williams & Wilkins; 2006:560–570.
7. Ryan JJ, Lewis JR. A lower thoracic advancement flap in breast reconstruction after mastectomy. *Plast Reconstr Surg* 1982;70(2):159–160.
8. Versaci AD. Method of reconstructing a pendulous breast utilizing the tissue expander. *Plast Reconstr Surg* 1987;80(3):387–395.
9. Spear S, Little JW. Breast capsulorrhaphy. *Plast Reconstr Surg* 1988;81(2):274–279.
10. Spear SL, Mesbahi AN, Beckenstein M. Recreating the inframammary fold: the internal approach. In: Spear S, ed. *Surgery of the Breast: Principles and Art.* 2nd ed. Philadelphia: Lippincott Williams & Wilkins; 2006:566–580.
11. Bengtson BP. Is capsular contracture a thing of the past? Use of Strattice acellular dermal matrix for prevention of recurrent capsular contracture. Presented at the Atlanta Breast Symposium, Atlanta, Georgia, January 18, 2009.

CHAPTER

131

Mitchell H. Brown

Revision Augmentation With Anatomic Form-stable Silicone Gel Implants

INTRODUCTION

Revision breast augmentation can be a very difficult and challenging undertaking. The normal anatomy that exists in a primary procedure is no longer present. The surgeon must deal with a variety of factors, some predictable and some not predictable. These include external and internal scarring, previously dissected tissue planes, alteration to the deep and superficial blood supply to the breast, alteration to the pectoral muscle, thinning and stretching of the overlying soft tissues, and secondary effects related to the presence of a capsule around the preexisting implant.

There are many possible reasons that a woman presents for secondary implant surgery. The most common seems to be for the management of a capsular contracture (1). Implant malposition is another common presentation and can be divided into malpositions that are superior, inferior, lateral, or medial (Fig. 131.1). Other common indications include management of rippling or implant edge palpability, size change, and the correction of soft tissue changes secondary to hematoma, infection, radiation, or previous surgery. Regardless of the presentation, the management of the secondary implant patient requires a systematic approach to identify the underlying problems, recognize the limitations, and develop a plan that is safe and maximizes the chances for a predictable outcome.

Implant selection in revision augmentation is a key component in achieving a good result. Many options exist, including round saline-filled implants, smooth and textured-surface, round gel implants, and textured, shaped gel implants. The shaped implant is a unique device that offers many potential benefits in the revision patient. Shaped gel implants have been available in one form or another since the 1960s. It was not until the early 1990s, however, that these implants gained widespread acceptance. Their use in primary breast augmentation (2) and in postmastectomy breast reconstruction is well documented (3). Shaped implants are indicated in patients who will benefit from the use of an anatomic device and who require an implant with form stability and are having the implant placed in a pocket that can be precisely controlled with respect to its dimensions.

The benefits of shaped, form-stable cohesive gel implants include their ability to provide a natural and proportionate breast shape (Fig. 131.2); the availability of a wide variety of shapes and sizes to match most breast shapes; maintenance of shape and upper pole fill, which translates into a decreased likelihood of rippling; and a more viscous gel, which is less likely to escape from the implant shell, should the implant lose its integrity (Fig. 131.3) (3). Several studies have demonstrated a low rate of capsular contracture with form-stable anatomic gel implants (3–5). Allergan's core data demonstrate a contracture rate in breast augmentation of 3.3% (5 year) with the Style 410 anatomic gel versus 15.5% (7 year) with round gel implants. In revision patients, the rates are 6.4% (5 year) for the anatomic implant and 20.4% (7 year) using a round device (6). Not only are the contracture rates low, but in addition the form-stable nature of the devices results in less deformation and clinical effect with a contracture compared to less-form-stable devices.

Shaped gel implants are available in a wide selection of shapes and sizes. These vary based upon implant width, height, and projection. The Natrelle 410 by Allergan (Irvine, CA) is one such shaped device. A 3 × 4 matrix based on height and projection provides the surgeon with great flexibility to custom select the implant based on precise patient measurements (Fig. 131.4). The texturing on this implant is designed to promote tissue adherence and implant stability within the breast pocket, a feature that is very helpful in secondary implant patients (Fig. 131.5). With smooth-surface implants, the device behaves as a free-moving object under the breast, which feels distinct and separate from the overlying breast tissue. This may result in unusual displacement of the implant with change in body position. With textured, form-stable gel implants, the resulting more adherent capsule results in a capsule, implant, and breast interface that behaves like a single unified breast mound. This "one breast feel" more closely resembles a normal breast and results in fewer secondary malposition issues (3).

Along with the Natrelle 410, the other anatomic gel implant that is commonly used in North America is the CPG by Mentor Corporation (Santa Barbara, California). This implant comes in three heights and three projections. The textured surface is produced with a negative imprint technique. This surface is less likely to result in tissue integration, therefore stability within the pocket is achieved through precise planning that matches the pocket dissection to the implant dimensions.

INDICATIONS

The decision to proceed with a revision breast augmentation should only be made after careful consideration of the patients concerns and a thorough discussion regarding goals and expectations. It is possible for the primary surgeon to decrease revision rates by committing to basic core principles that include patient education, informed consent, preoperative planning, proper implant selection using tissue-based planning, precise surgical technique, and structured postoperative care. Each indication for a revision can find its roots embedded in one or more of these principles. For example, a patient whose implant was improperly matched to a soft tissue envelope will likely develop implant malposition, rotation, or rippling. A patient who is concerned about an ongoing asymmetry but did not understand that this asymmetry existed preoperatively will not be prepared to accept the continued difference

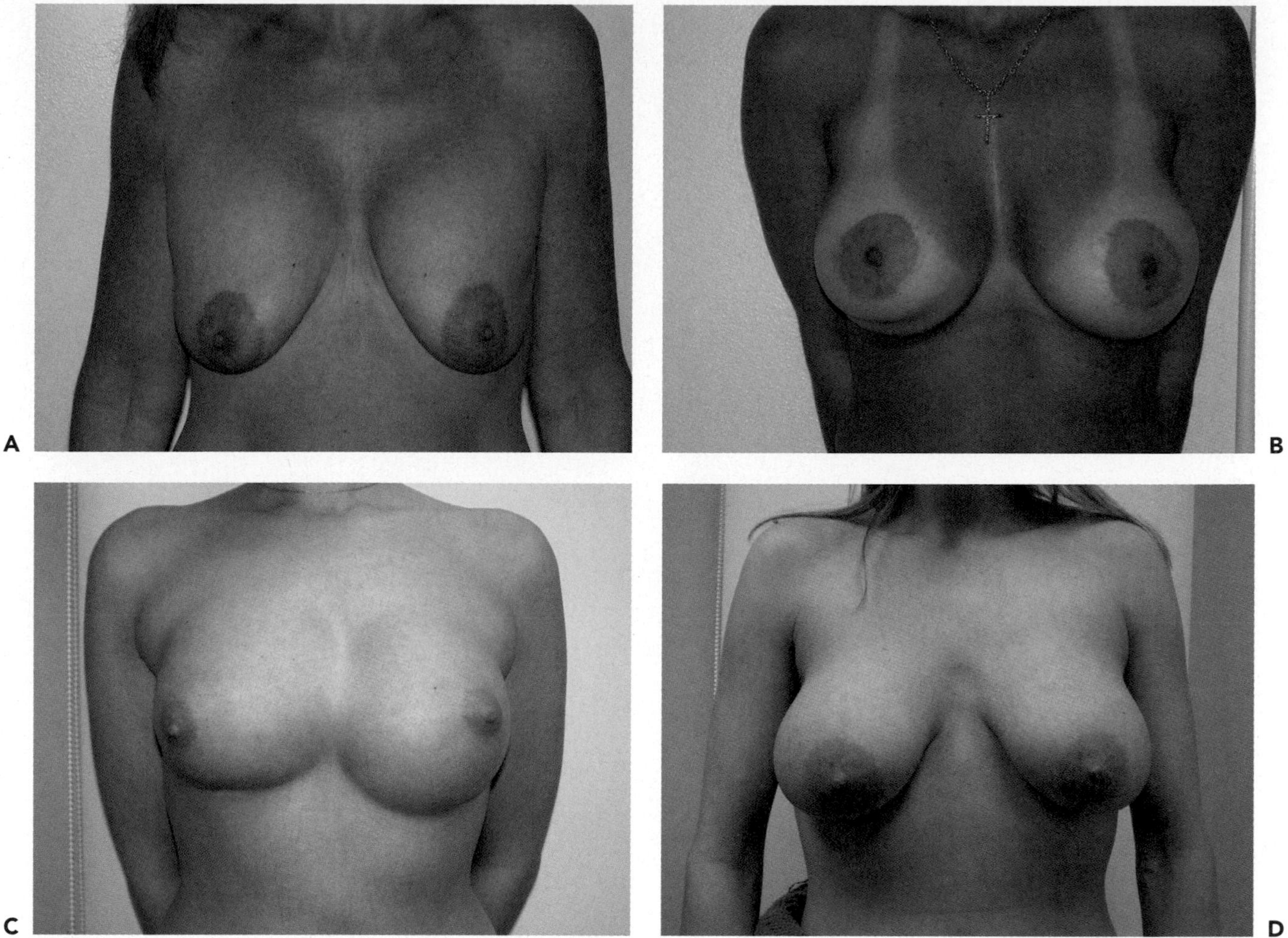

Figure 131.1. Examples of implant malposition. **A:** Superior **B:** Inferior **C:** Medial **D:** Lateral.

in the two breasts. Surgery that uses imprecise technique increases the likelihood of infection, contracture, hematoma, and implant malposition. A device placed through too small an incision will be more likely to fail.

The best way to manage a revision is to have avoided it in the first place. Having said that, it has to be acknowledged that errors do occur, soft tissues do not always behave as planned, well-intentioned decisions do not always turn out to be correct, patient's bodies continue to change. and the principles of gravity continue to exist. For these reasons, the need for revision augmentation surgery will persist.

The first step in evaluating the revision patient is to develop a clear understanding of her concerns and expectations. This may be easier to explain for some patients than for others. Often, patients are abstract in the discussion of their concerns. Phrases such as, "this isn't what I wanted," "I am very unhappy with my breasts," and "my friends tell me this can't be right, it should be fixed" demonstrate displeasure with the outcome but are hardly specific. To correct a problem, one must understand what it is and why it occurred and have a reasonable plan for how to fix it. There is not a solution for every concern, nor is it reasonable to try to correct every outcome that is felt to be less than perfect.

The surgeon and patient should spend time performing a risk-benefit analysis. On one side of the equation are the reasons that the patient wishes a revision. The patient may have symptoms such as pain from a capsular contracture or a tight, poorly healed scar. She may have restriction of movement that affects her ability to do common activities. Other concerns may relate to the effect on quality of life. Asymmetry, improper sizing, malposition, or contracture may limit the wearing of certain clothing styles, and this may affect the patient's self-image, self-esteem, and confidence, all reasons for having the augmentation done in the first place. These concerns must be balanced against the inherent risks and complications of the revision, as well as the likelihood for being able to meet the patient's stated goals. The commonly used phrase, "the enemy of good is better," should be carefully considered and discussed with the patient. There is nothing worse than performing surgery to correct a relatively minor problem only to be left with a major one.

Not all revisions of previous breast augmentations require the use of an implant. Patients who have had multiple previous procedures, painful contractures, implant ruptures, or complex malposition problems may be best served by implant removal with or without capsulectomy. Often, breast reshaping in the form of a mastopexy can be performed simultaneously or at a later date (Fig. 131.6).

When an implant is used for the revision surgery, careful consideration is necessary as to the type of implant to choose. This decision will be dictated by several factors, such as tissue

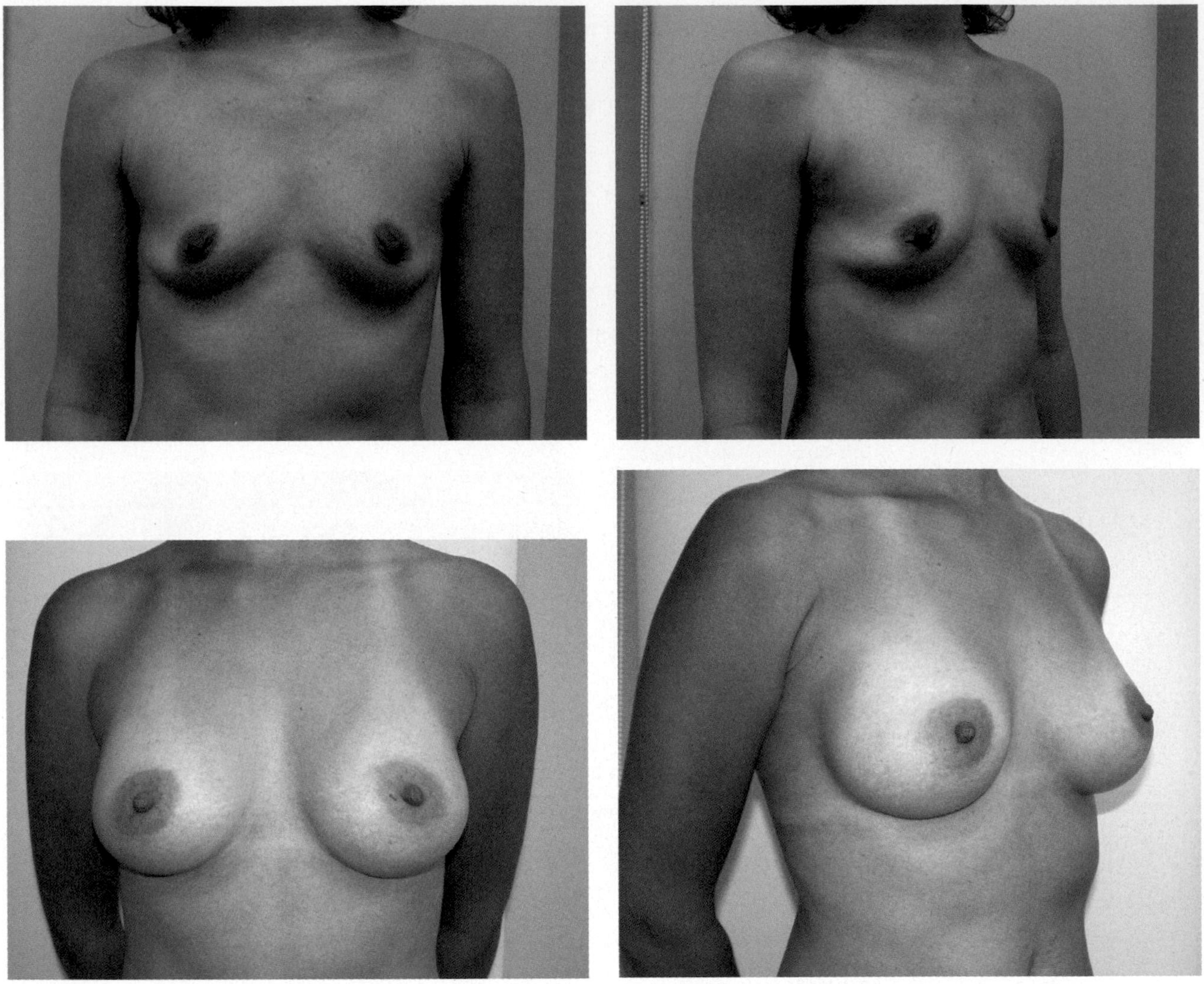

Figure 131.2. Before and 8-month postoperative views of breast augmentation with anatomic gel-filled implants, medium height, full projection, 295 g.

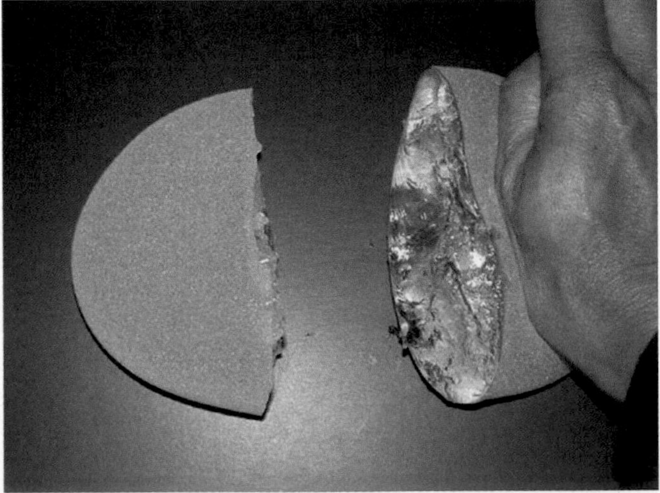

Figure 131.3. Natrelle style 410 implant demonstrating the cohesive nature of the silicone gel.

quantity and quality, desired aesthetic breast shape, need for form stability, ability to control the implant pocket, and patient preference. Shaped gel implants are an excellent choice in many revision cases. The form-stable nature of the gel allows the implant to assist in shaping the breast, a feature that is helpful in many secondary cases. When malposition of the implant is the presenting concern, the use of an implant with texturing will promote stability of the implant within the pocket. The low reported incidence of capsular contracture with the Natrelle 410 implant makes it an excellent choice in patients with problem capsules (3–5).

CONTRAINDICATIONS

As with any procedure, patients undergoing revision breast augmentation must have realistic expectations. There is not a solution for every problem, and in some circumstances it is best not to offer a surgical option.

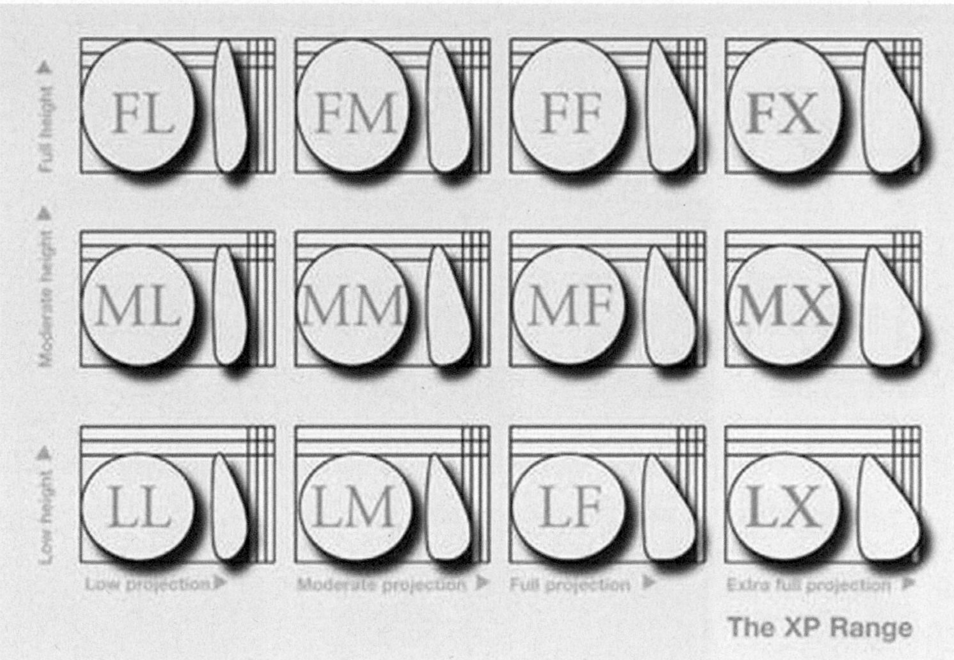

Figure 131.4. Allergan Natrelle style 410 3 × 4 matrix.

Specific contraindications exist when using shaped gel implants in revision surgery. Of course, a patient must be willing to accept the use of a gel device. Outside of North America this is rarely an issue, but there a number of women in Canada and the United States who continue to have a greater comfort level with saline implants. Understanding a woman's goals is key to selecting the best implant. Patients who would like a full-looking upper pole are not good candidates for a shaped implant. The form-stable nature of the gel results in a breast that is slightly firmer than what is seen with more responsive gel devices. Patients who are unwilling to accept this will do better with a softer round gel or saline implant.

The location and length of the surgical scar are important considerations for most implant patients. In revision surgery, there will be a preexisting scar. Surgery should always be performed through an incision that allows for direct access and precise correction of the underlying problem. If that cannot be done through the previous scar, then a new incision should be selected. When using a shaped gel implant, it is critical to have a long enough incision to allow for implant insertion without damaging the device. This is generally in the range of 5 cm. This incision length limits the choice for scar location. Most commonly, the incision will be placed in the inframammary fold or through a large periareolar incision. If an axillary approach is selected, it is imperative that the incision be of adequate length. Patients who are not willing to accept the required scar length and location are not candidates for shaped implants.

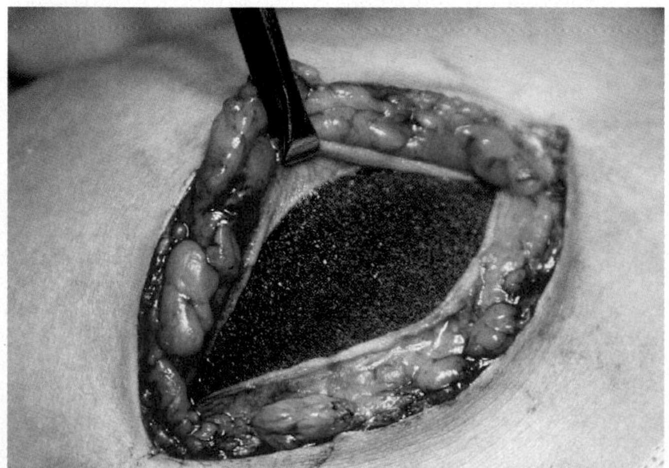

Figure 131.5. Adherence of a capsule to the surface of a Natrelle style 410 implant with Biocell surface. (Photograph courtesy of Dr. Bradley Bengtson.)

One of the greatest advantages of shaped implants is their ability to provide differential fill with a tapered upper pole. Because of their shape, rotation is an issue that is unique to these implants. They must be placed in a pocket that is dissected specifically to match the implant dimensions. When shaped implants are used in revision surgery they must be placed in a new pocket. This can be achieved through a site change or by performing a capsulectomy. If implants are to be placed in a preexisting pocket, then shaped devices are contraindicated.

One of the fundamental principles of using shaped implants is to select a size based upon dimensional planning that pays attention to breast width, breast height, and the soft tissue envelope. This allows for filling out of the soft tissues with minimal risk of rotation. Patients who are not willing to select implant size based on these principles are not well suited for a shaped device.

PREOPERATIVE PLANNING

Careful preoperative planning is a cornerstone of any successful breast augmentation. This statement is especially true in revision surgery. It is absolutely imperative to have a detailed understanding of all previous breast surgeries. Whenever possible, surgical records should be obtained and reviewed. Often,

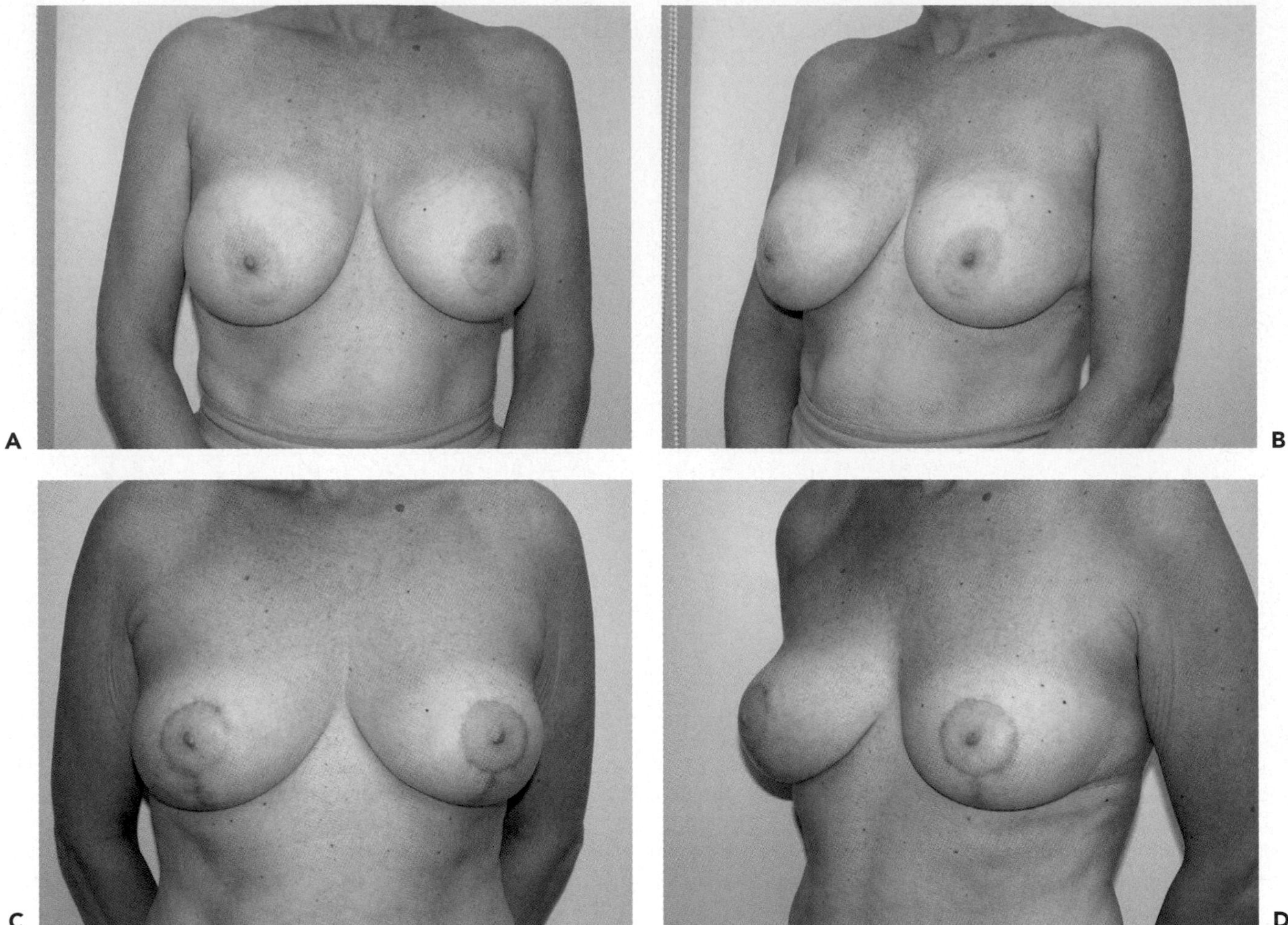

Figure 131.6. **A, B:** A patient with bilateral painful capsule contracture and adequate natural breast tissue. **C, D:** Six weeks following explantation, capsulectomy, and Wise-pattern mastopexy.

women presenting with breast implant problems have had multiple procedures. These may have included mastopexies, reductions, biopsies, or lumpectomies. Each of these surgeries will have left scars and have caused an alteration to the normal blood flow within the breast and to the nipple-areola complex. For each previous breast implant procedure, it is important to know the implant fill, surface, size, pocket, and incision used. Any complications such as infection, contracture, or malposition should be recorded, including the methods by which these complications were treated.

A detailed history should include patient goals and expectations, general health, and an assessment of risk factors for compromised healing, including smoking history, systemic illness, or previous radiation to the breast. Physical examination should focus on three components: the implant, the soft tissues, and the musculoskeletal framework. The implant must be examined for position under the breast tissue and stability within the implant pocket. Malposition should be classified into medial (synmastia), lateral, inferior ("double bubble"), or superior. Implant stability within the pocket should be assessed with the patient in multiple positions, including standing with arms at side and arms over head, lying supine, and leaning forward. The presence of capsular contracture should be noted, along with any areas of rippling or palpable implant edges.

Examination of the soft tissues is very important not only to determine a surgical plan, but also to inform the patient what is realistically achievable with surgical correction. Any asymmetries should be recorded and discussed. Measurements include sternal notch to nipple distance, nipple to inframammary fold (IMF) distance, and breast width. Nipple position on the breast mound should be noted, along with degree of ptosis or glandular ptosis. The quality and quantity of breast tissue in all four quadrants should be assessed to determine adequacy of soft tissue coverage. This may be done by subjective assessment or by more objective measures such as a pinch test. The breast and axilla are examined for abnormal masses, and finally all scars are recorded for both location and quality.

As breast implants require a stable foundation on which to sit, examination of the musculoskeletal anatomy is important. Preexisting scoliosis or chest wall asymmetries should be recorded. When using shaped implants, it is possible to adjust for some of these asymmetries by selecting implants of varying height or projection. Abnormal contour of the sternum either concave or convex will affect medial positioning of implants. The pectoralis muscle should be examined, as it may have been damaged or excessively released with previous surgeries. In rare cases of Poland syndrome, the muscle may be absent or rudimentary.

TABLE 131.1	Options for Implant Pocket
Same pocket	
Open capsulotomy	
Partial capsulectomy	
Same location with complete capsulectomy	
Subglandular to subpectoral	
Subpectoral to subglandular	
Neo-subpectoral	
Convert to dual plane	

The exact surgical plan will be determined by the specifics of the patient. Revision procedures may involve implant removal with or without a mastopexy. When the plan calls for insertion of a new implant, there are several fundamental decisions that need to be made. Pocket selection is a very important consideration. Options for the implant pocket are summarized in Table 131.1. When the capsule around the implant is normal, there is adequate soft tissue coverage, and the implant/soft tissue relationships are acceptable, then the same pocket can be used. This is most common with revisions for size change or minor contractures. In the case of minor contractures, an open capsulotomy or partial capsulectomy is indicated. With Baker III/IV contractures, implant malposition, rippling, or edge palpability, a site change is usually indicated. When revision surgery calls for the use of a shaped gel implant, a pocket change is mandatory to allow for a precise pocket to implant fit. Site change can take the form of a capsulectomy, subglandular to subpectoral conversion, subpectoral to subglandular conversion, or the creation of a new subpectoral pocket on top of a previous subpectoral capsule (7). A variation on site change is the conversion to a dual-plane pocket as described by Spear et al. (8). This approach is helpful in many cases of contracture or superior implant malposition.

A second critical consideration relates to implant type, shape, and size. There is no single formula that can be applied to all cases of revision augmentation, but certain principles can be followed. In cases of contracture, consider the use of a textured surface implant. Several studies suggest that there is a lower capsule contracture rate with textured implants, especially when the implant is placed in the subglandular space (9). Consider the use of smaller implant sizes. Many problems following breast augmentation result from soft tissue changes secondary to a large implant. It is usually better to use a smaller implant size with a skin-tightening procedure rather than fill a skin envelope with larger-volume devices. Shaped gel implants have a central role to play in implant selection for revision augmentation. Although they usually require a new pocket for insertion, they have many benefits, including a lower contracture rate, less rippling, and shape stability. The variety of sizes allows for correction of asymmetries, and the form-stable nature of the gel allows the implant to shape the breast rather than have the breast shape the implant. Selection of the implant size must be based on defined measurements of implant height, width, and projection to ensure stability of the implant under the soft tissues (2,3).

The final preoperative decision relates to the soft tissues. In cases of ptosis, glandular ptosis, asymmetry, or nipple malposition an alteration to the soft tissue envelope may be necessary (Fig. 131.7). Combining a mastopexy with revision of an augmentation is a complex procedure with many variables, some unpredictable. It should be undertaken with caution and only in patients with few risk factors for delayed wound healing. The soft tissues should be handled with extreme care, and all skin undermining should be kept to a minimum to decrease the likelihood of skin flap or nipple loss.

INTRAOPERATIVE AND POSTOPERATIVE CARE

The technical steps required to perform a successful breast augmentation are beyond the scope of this chapter. Many of the principles are shared with revision breast augmentation. Preoperative markings are done with the patient in a standing or sitting position. When shaped implants are used, these markings are critical, as the implant pocket must be dissected just large enough to allow the implant to be inserted. The surgical steps vary depending upon the individual case but usually follow a similar pattern: removal of the old implant, management of the existing capsule,

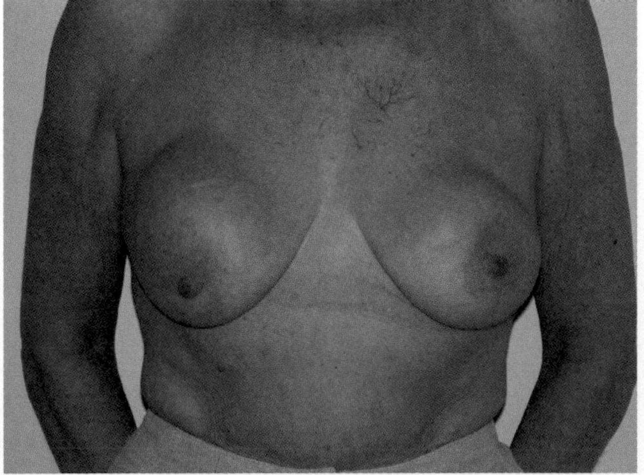

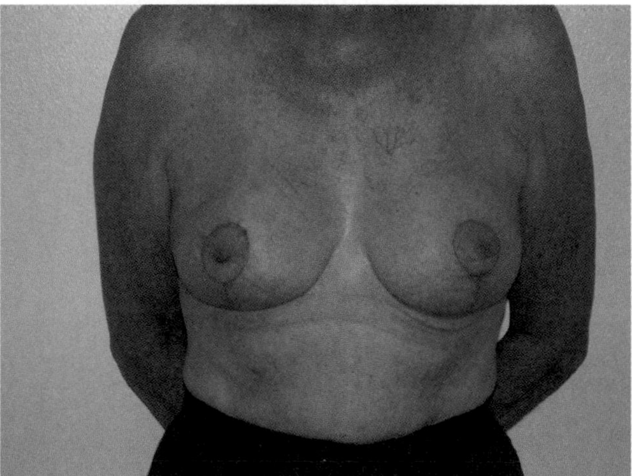

Figure 131.7. Patient with Baker IV contracture and soft tissue ptosis who underwent implant removal, capsulectomy, implant insertion, and overlying mastopexy.

creation or preparation of a pocket for the new implant, insertion of the new implant, and then contouring of the soft tissues. It is always advisable to use precise dissection techniques under direct vision, but this is especially important with shaped devices. In primary augmentation, the use of sizers is rarely indicated, but in revision cases, sizers may be used more frequently. When using a shaped implant, it is important to use a sizer slightly smaller then the anticipated implant size. Too large a sizer will result in overdissection of the pocket and increase the likelihood of rotational problems with the final implant.

Implant insertion is performed using a no-touch or minimal-touch technique. Following insertion, the orientation dots on the implant are palpated to ensure that the implant is sitting in an anatomic position. Closed suction drains are usually necessary in revision procedures, especially when performing a capsulectomy or pocket change. In thin patients with minimal breast tissue, it is important to place the drain in such a way that there is a lengthy subcutaneous tunnel. This will minimize the likelihood of bacterial tracking, especially following drain removal.

Postoperative care protocols vary with procedure and implant type. When correcting implant malposition, bandaging may be desirable to support the implant in a certain position. For example, when correcting synmastia, bandages or a bolster are often placed over the sternum to support the medial repair. Antibiotics are given at least until drain removal. Although displacement massage techniques are routinely used with smooth-surface devices, postoperative massage with shaped implants is contraindicated. Many surgeons place patients in a supportive bra for at least 1 week to encourage implant stability within the implant pocket.

CASES

MALPOSITION

Implant malposition is one of the most common problems that can be treated effectively with the use of a form-stable, shaped gel implant. Several cases will illustrate the principles used for these corrections.

A 26-year-old woman had undergone breast augmentation 6 years earlier through an inframammary-incision, subpectoral placement with 260-cc saline implants. She presented with inferior malposition of the implant and loss of definition of the IMF (Fig. 131.8A, B). An upper pole pinch test revealed less than 2 cm of tissue. It was decided to leave the implants under

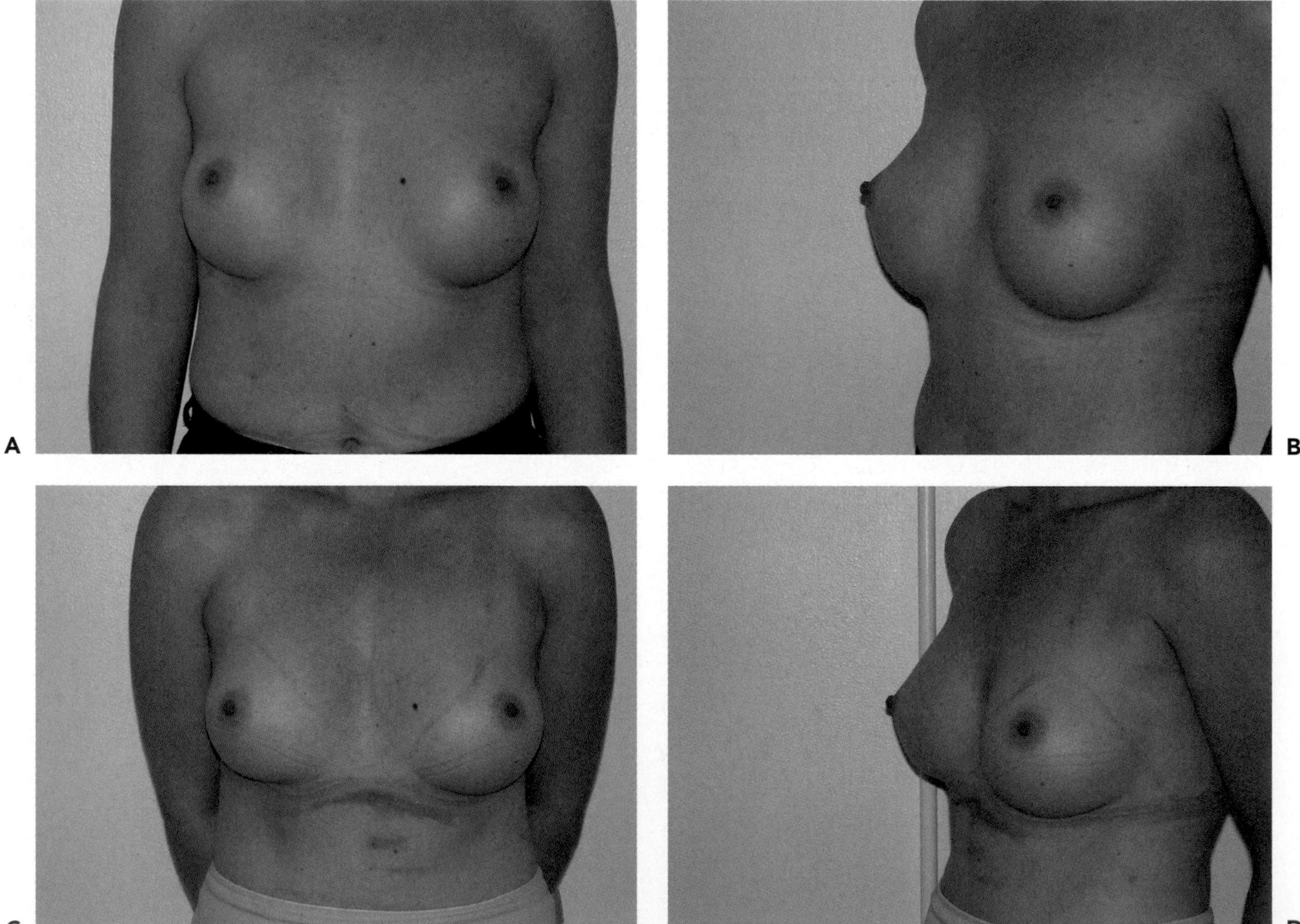

Figure 131.8. Inferior implant malposition treated with explantation, neo-subpectoral pocket, and insertion of a Natrelle style 410 MM280 implant. **A, B:** Preoperative. **C, D:** Six months postoperative.

the pectoral muscle. Explantation was performed together with creation of a new subpectoral pocket anterior to the implant capsule and posterior to the pectoral muscle (7). Care was taken to avoid dissection of the new pocket below the planned IMF. The patient wanted to maintain a similar size. Her breast width was measured at 12 cm, and the sternal notch to nipple distance was 19.5 cm. A Natrelle style 410 MM280 (medium height, moderate projection; Allergan Medical, Irvine CA) implant was selected. This implant has a base width of 12 cm and provides a lower pole projection similar to that of the previous saline device. Six-month postoperative pictures are shown in Figure 8C, D. In this case, a shaped gel implant was selected because the implant was being placed in a new pocket that allowed for precise dissection to the margins of the planned implant. The form-stable and textured characteristics of the device will help in stabilizing the implant in the pocket, making inferior descent of the implant less likely.

A 35-year-old woman presented after attempted correction of breast asymmetry 15 years earlier. She had undergone right breast augmentation with an implant of unknown type and size (Fig. 131.9A, B). Her concerns related to ongoing asymmetry and an abnormal shape of the right breast. Examination revealed a very complicated chest wall with multiple issues including scoliosis, concave deformity of the right chest wall, convex deformity of the left chest wall, lower pectus excavatum, partial absence of the pectoral muscle, and medial displacement of the breast implant. The patient had very reasonable expectations. She wanted to feel more comfortable with the way she looked in clothing. She was prepared to accept some degree of ongoing asymmetry and wanted to be larger on both sides. The surgical plan involved removal of the old implant and insertion of asymmetric implants. Because of the multiple skeletal issues and minimal soft tissue cover, form-stable, shaped implants were selected. On the right side, explantation, partial capsulectomy, suture repair of the medial border, and insertion of a Natrelle style 410 FF375 (full height, full projection) implant were performed. On the left side, a subpectoral Natrelle style 410 LF310 (low height, full projection) implant was used. One-year postoperative results are shown in Figure 131.9C, D.

CONTRACTURE

Perhaps the most common indication for revision surgery is capsular contracture. One option for the treatment of contracture

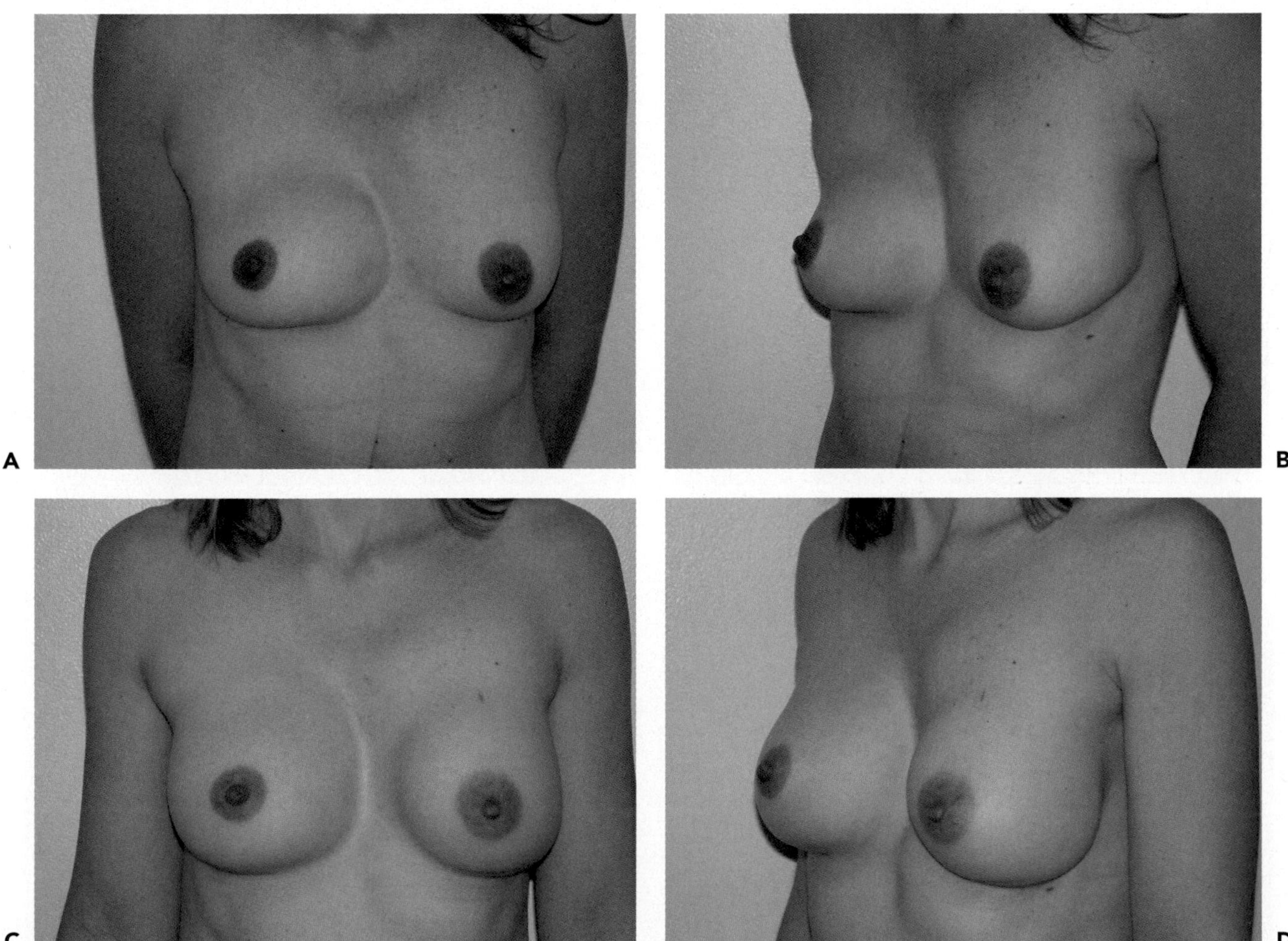

Figure 131.9. Complex chest wall deformity with a medial malposition of a right breast implant treated with implant removal, repair of the medial border, and insertion of a Natrelle style 410 FF375 implant on the right and a Natrelle style 410 LF310 implant on the left. **A, B:** Preoperative. **C, D:** One year postoperative.

is an open capsulotomy. Because the new implant will be placed within an existing capsule, shaped gel implants are not indicated. When changing the pocket through capsulectomy or site change, shaped implants can be very effective. Not only have they been shown to have a low rate of contracture, their form-stable nature makes them more resistant to deformation. This may result in less clinical change to the breast with minor degrees of contracture than is seen with more responsive gel devices.

A 28-year-old woman presented with bilateral Baker IV contractures (Fig. 131.10A–C). She had undergone subpectoral augmentation through an IMF incision with saline implants.

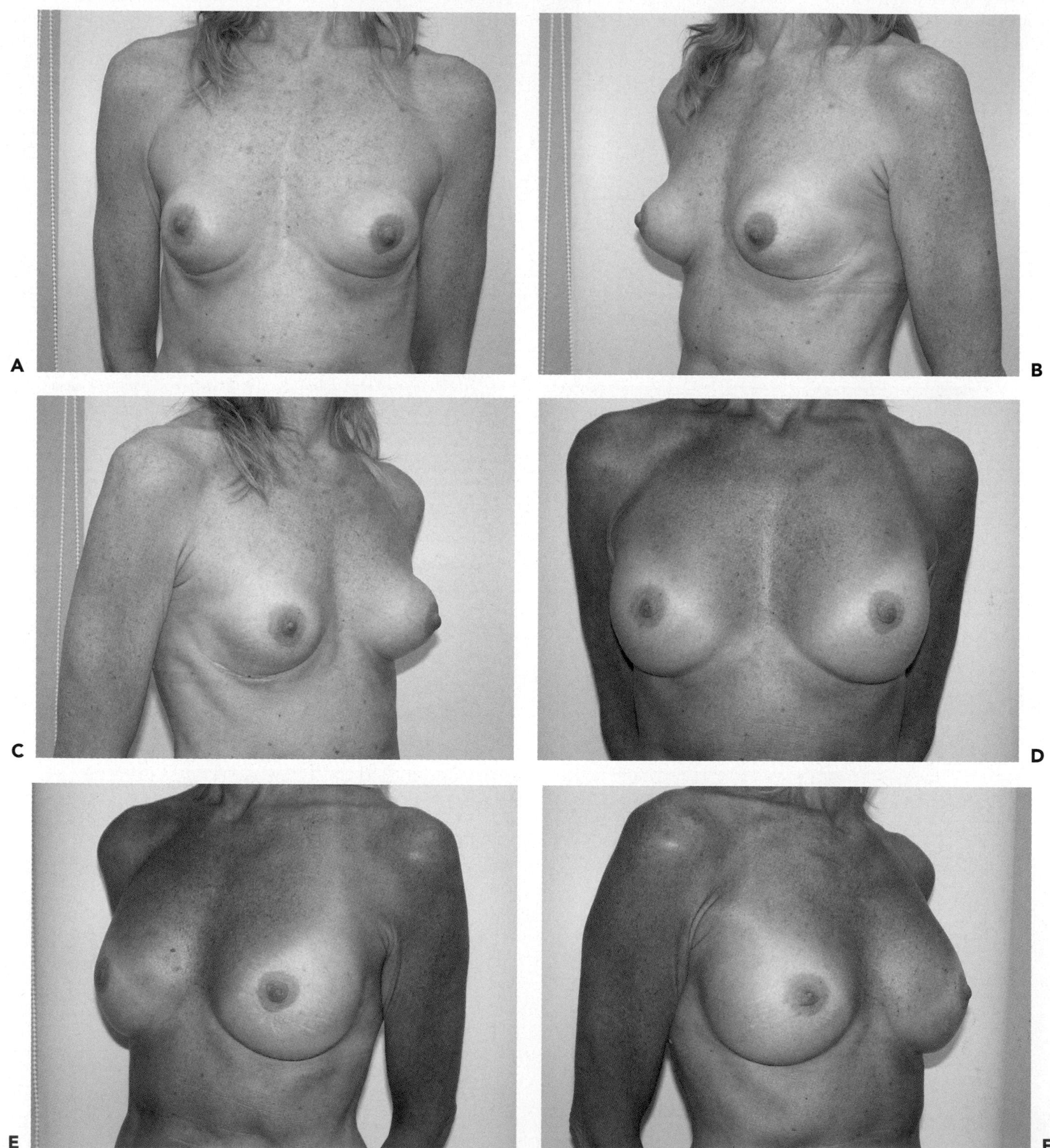

Figure 131.10. Baker IV contracture treated with explantation, neo-subpectoral pocket, and insertion of Natrelle style 410 FM310 implants. **A–C:** Preoperative. **D–F:** Six months postoperative.

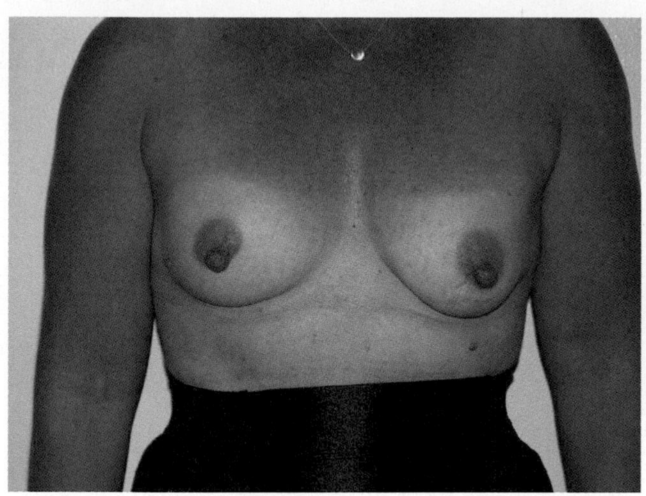
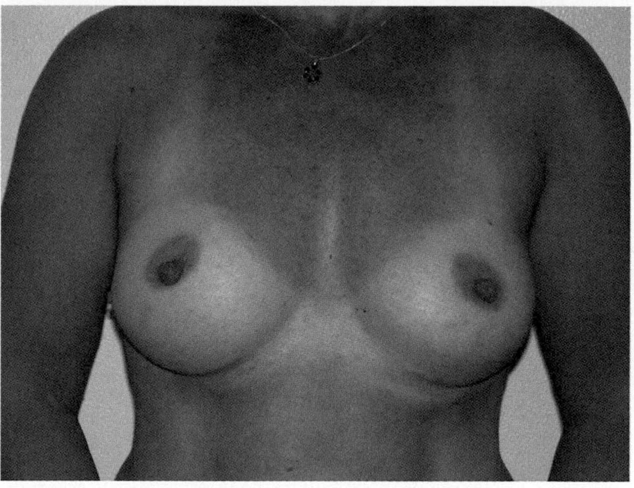

Figure 131.11. Baker III contracture treated with explantation, capsulectomy, and subglandular replacement with a Natrelle style 410 MF295 implant. **A:** Preoperative. **B:** Six months postoperative.

The contractures were described as painful. She desired a softer and larger-appearing breast. At the time of surgery, the implants were removed and the capsule was inspected. It had a smooth wall with no calcifications. There was no fluid within the capsule pocket. It was decided to leave the capsule in situ and create a new subpectoral pocket on top of the capsule. Natrelle style 410 FM310 (full height, moderate projection) implants were inserted along with suction drains in the old capsule space. Results are shown 6 months postoperatively in Fig. 131.10D–F).

A 47-year-old woman presented with Baker III contractures following subglandular augmentation with smooth, round gel implants through an IMF incision (Fig. 131.11A). She had greater than 2 cm of tissue in the upper pole on pinch test. Surgery was carried out to remove the implants. There was calcification in the capsules, and so complete capsulectomies were performed. Care was taken not to dissect a pocket larger than the planned shaped implant. A Natrelle style 410 MF295 (medium height, full projection) implant was inserted into the same subglandular space along with a suction drain. A postoperative view is shown at 6 months in Figure 131.11B.

A 62-year-old woman presented 22 years after breast augmentation with subglandular implants of unknown type or size. She had a bilateral Baker IV contracture with very minimal remaining soft tissue cover. She also had ptosis of the overlying breast tissue (Fig. 131.12A, B). She was in good health and was a nonsmoker. Options were discussed, including explantation only or explantation with a mastopexy. She wanted to maintain her breast size, and so a decision was made to perform an explantation, partial capsulectomy, site change to a subpectoral position, and Wise-pattern mastopexy. Following implant removal, a near-total capsulectomy was performed. A small amount of inferior capsule was saved to act as a hammock to support the implant in the new subpectoral pocket. Other options for managing this issue included suture closure of the subglandular space, percutaneous marionette sutures from the lower edge of the pectoral muscle, and the use of an acellular dermal matrix for added inferolateral support. A Natrelle style 410 MM280 (medium height, moderate projection) implant was selected. Following implant insertion, the mastopexy was shaped around the new breast form. Postoperative results are shown at 6 weeks in Figure 131.12C, D.

RIPPLING

A 39-year-old woman had undergone breast augmentation with saline implants 12 years earlier. The implants were placed through an inferior areola incision and were in a subpectoral position. There was a bilateral Baker III contracture, but the patient's primary concern was visible rippling along the medial border of both breasts, more noticeable on the right. Examination revealed overdissection of the medial pectoral muscle with minimal soft tissue cover in that area (Fig. 131.13A–C). The surgical plan called for correction of the contracture and improvement of the medial rippling. The patient was told that the rippling could not be eliminated but likely could be improved.

There are several methods for the treatment of rippling. If greater soft tissue coverage can be obtained with a site change, then this is an excellent option. If rippling exists even with a subpectoral position, then site change has little to offer. In this case consideration is made for autologous fat grafting or the addition of an acellular dermal matrix to improve coverage in the affected area. A form-stable gel implant can significantly minimize rippling. Although all implants can produce rippling, the form-stable nature of the shaped implants makes rippling much less evident.

The patient underwent implant removal, creation of a new subpectoral pocket, and insertion of a Natrelle style 410 FF375 (full height, full projection) implant. She is shown in Figure 131.13D, E at 6 weeks postoperatively with improvement in both shape and medial rippling. Secondary fat grafting is scheduled.

TUBEROUS BREAST AND POLAND SYNDROME

Although the treatment of tuberous breast deformity and that of Poland syndrome do not represent examples of revision breast implant surgery, they both present special challenges in

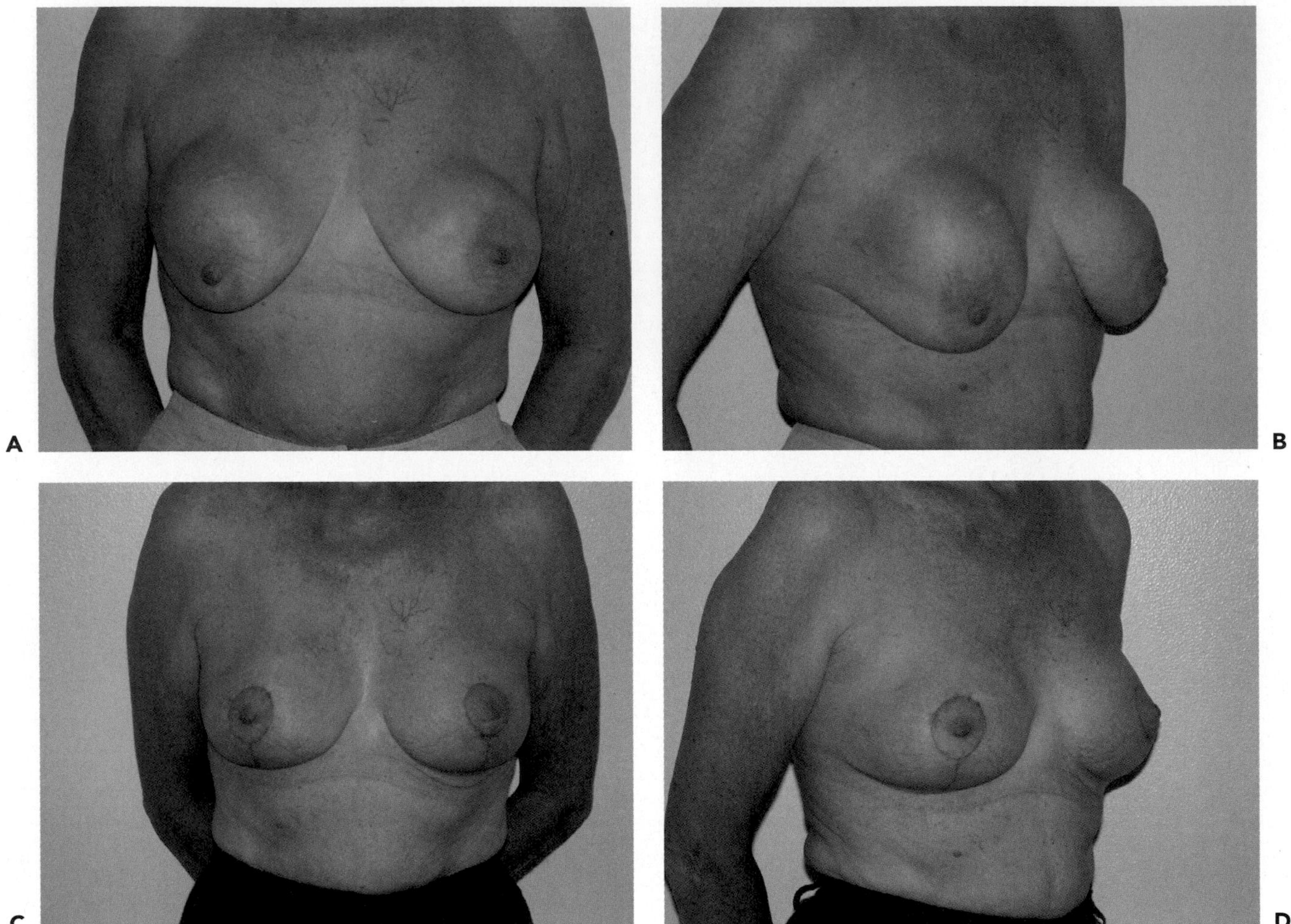

Figure 131.12. Baker IV contracture treated with explantation, subtotal capsulectomy, new subpectoral pocket, Natrelle style 410 MM280 implant insertion, and Wise-pattern mastopexy. **A, B:** Preoperative, **C, D:** Six weeks postoperative.

the use of breast implants that are well addressed with the use of shaped, form-stable gel devices.

The tuberous breast consists of a constellation of findings including hypoplasia, ptosis, constricted base, areola hypertrophy, and pseudoherniation of the areola. Surgical correction is individualized but usually involves the insertion of a breast implant. The most severe forms require two-stage reconstruction with initial expansion of the breast base, but most cases can be corrected in a single stage. The use of a shaped gel implant has been described for this one-stage correction (10). The anatomic implant shape provides more volume in the deficient lower pole and tapers superiorly, where less fullness is required. The form-stable nature of the gel and the texturing of the device help to hold the implant exactly where it is positioned and produce resistance to deformation from the tight lower pole tissues. Patients with tuberous breasts often have asymmetric findings. The matrix of options with these implants assists the surgeon in correcting asymmetry by allowing customized adjustment of implant dimensions. Figure 131.14 shows a 21-year-old woman with type III tuberous breasts. She was treated in a single stage with a circumareolar reduction, radial scoring of the lower pole, and insertion of a Natrelle style 410 MF295 (moderate height, full projection) implant.

Poland syndrome typically presents as a unilateral deformity with absence of the sternal head of the pectoral muscle, loss of the anterior axillary fold, breast hypoplasia, and associated deformities of the nipple-areola complex, thorax, shoulder girdle, and surrounding muscles. Options for correction include both the transfer of autologous tissue and the use of breast implants. When breast implants are used, there is usually a concern with soft tissue coverage due to the absence of the pectoral muscle. Although the addition of a latissimus muscle can add to coverage, this is often avoided due to concern of further weakening the shoulder girdle. Form-stable, shaped implants are an excellent choice in these patients. The anatomic shape will assist in producing a more natural breast form, and the form-stable nature will make rippling less likely. Implant edge palpability is expected due to the minimal soft tissue cover, and this can be dealt with by the use of local flaps or autologous fat transfer. Figure 131.15 shows an 18-year-old woman with right Poland syndrome before and 18 months after a unilateral subglandular augmentation with a Natrelle style 410 LF270 (low height, full projection) implant. Figure 131.16 shows a more difficult case in a 19-year-old

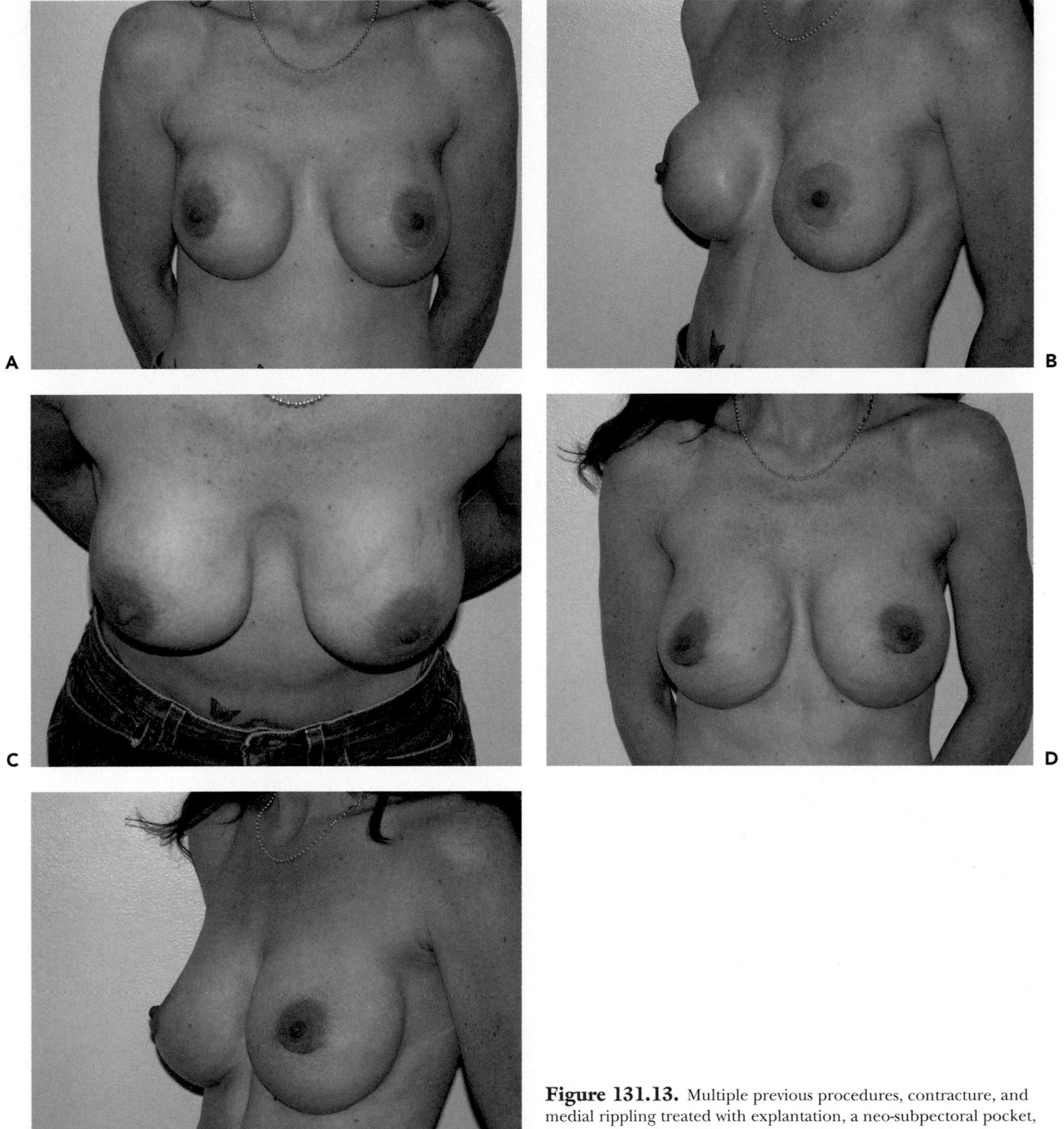

Figure 131.13. Multiple previous procedures, contracture, and medial rippling treated with explantation, a neo-subpectoral pocket, and insertion of a Natrelle style 410 FF375 implant. Secondary fat grafting is scheduled. **A–C:** Preoperative. **D, E:** Six weeks postoperative.

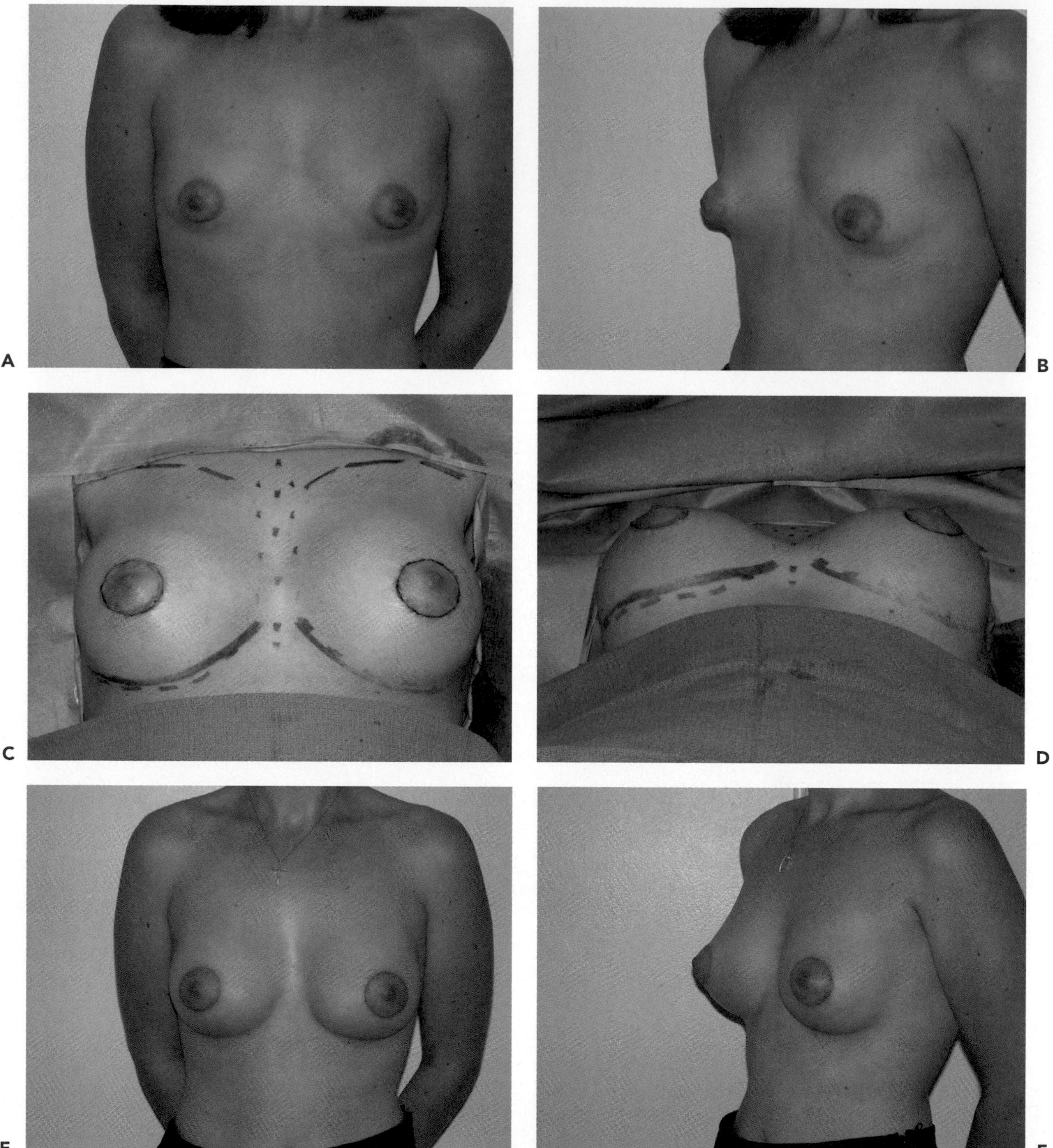

Figure 131.14. Type III tuberous breast deformity treated with areola reduction, radial scoring, and insertion of a Natrelle style 410 MF295 implant. **A, B:** Preoperative. **C, D:** Intraoperative. **E, F:** Six weeks postoperative.

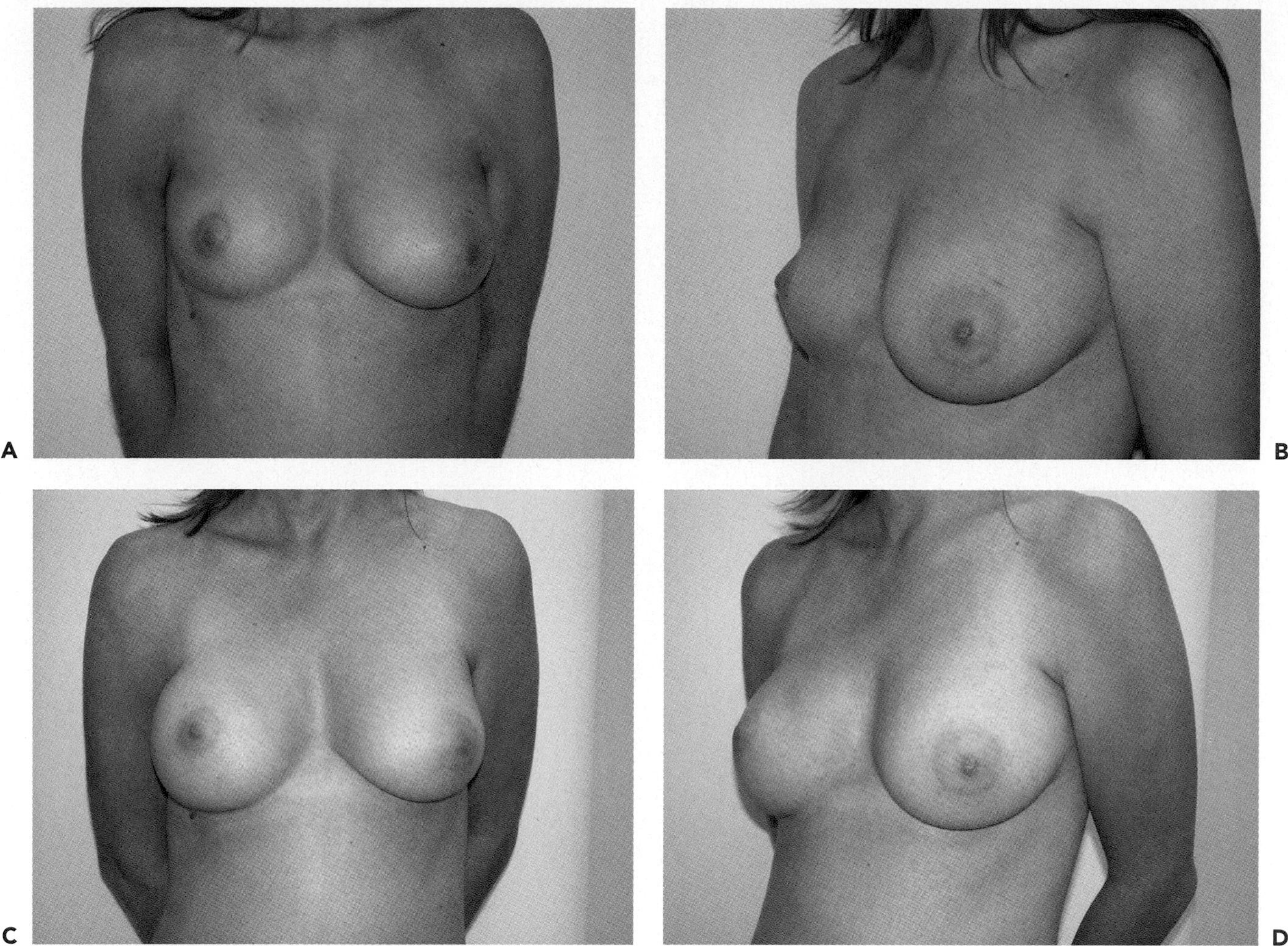

Figure 131.15. Unilateral Poland syndrome with right breast hypoplasia and loss of anterior axillary fold treated with a unilateral subglandular Natrelle style 410 LF270 implant. **A, B:** Preoperative. **C, D:** Six months postoperative.

woman desiring bilateral augmentation. She underwent subglandular implant insertion using a Natrelle style 410 FF220 (full height, full projection) implant on the right and a MM160 (medium height, moderate projection) implant on the left.

RISKS

The risks that are involved with a revision breast augmentation using a shaped, form-stable gel implant are all of the risks associated with primary breast implant surgery and then some. The surgeon is dealing with a breast that has had its normal anatomy and blood supply distorted. There will be preexisting scars both externally and internally. There may be thinning and stretching of the overlying breast tissue. These variables result in an increased risk for infection, exposure, skin flap or nipple necrosis, and delayed wound healing.

The use of a shaped implant dictates the need for an implant pocket that is precisely dissected to fit the new implant. Attempting to place a form stable device in a pocket that it too small will result in buckling of the implant, which may lead to a palpable deformity or shell fracture. If a shaped implant is placed in too large a pocket, rotation and malposition of the device will likely occur. To avoid these problems, the use of shaped implants should be restricted to cases in which the implant will be placed in a newly formed pocket. Precise preoperative planning will determine implant size, and the pocket should then be dissected to match those dimensions. A detailed list of risks associated with revision breast augmentation is given in Table 131.2.

TABLE 131.2	Risks Associated With Revisionary Breast Augmentation
Infection	Implant rupture
Hematoma	Contracture
Seroma	Interference with mammography
Decreased sensation	Rotation
Possible effect on breast-feeding	Malposition
Poor scarring	Asymmetry
Necrosis of tissue	Reoperations for replacement
Skin	Rippling
Nipple-areola	Implant-edge palpability
Fat	Failure to meet patient expectations
Secondary changes to the soft tissues	

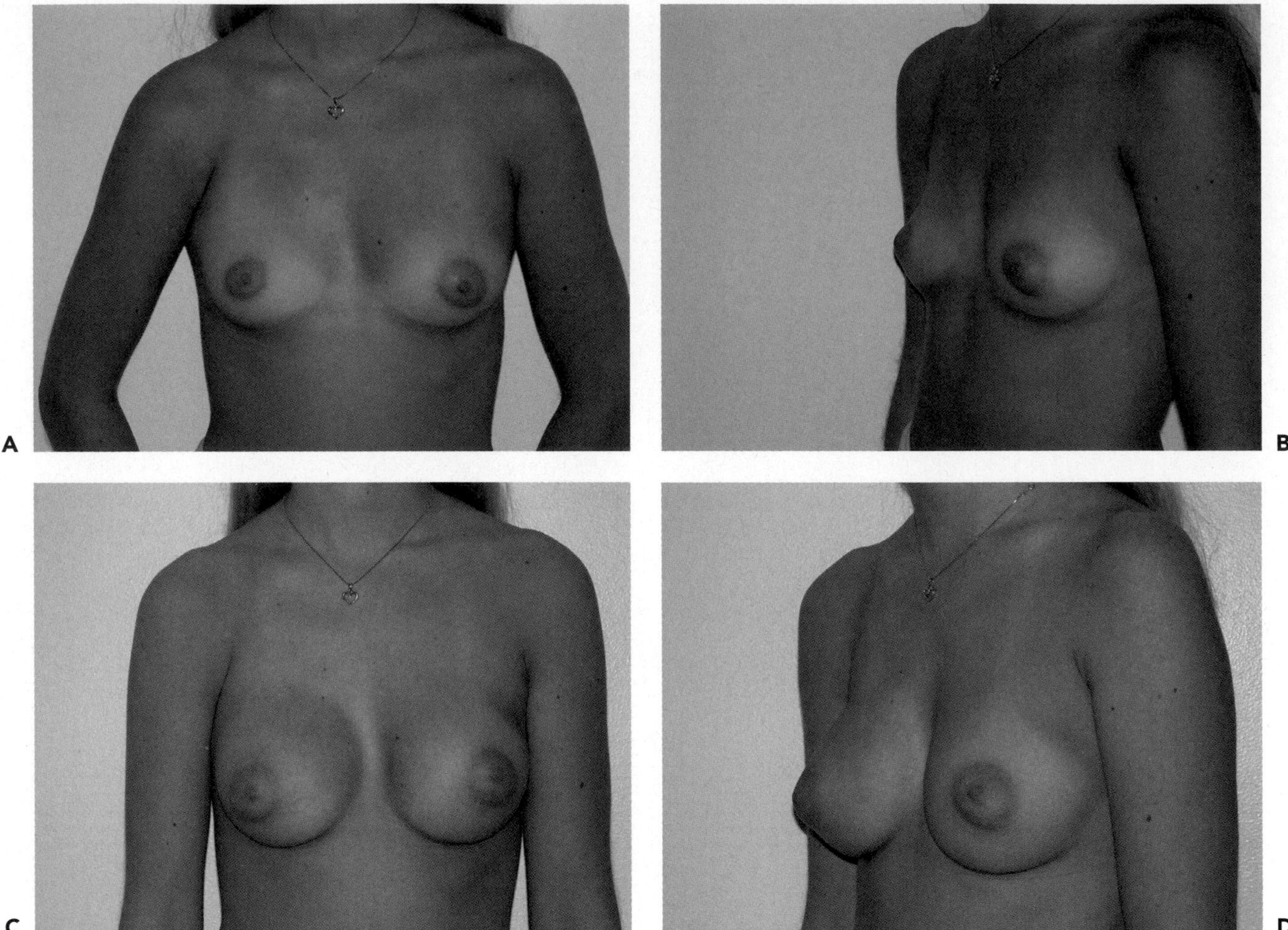

Figure 131.16. Unilateral Poland syndrome treated with bilateral asymmetric subglandular augmentation, Natrelle style 410 FF220 right implant, and Natrelle style 410 MM160 left implant. **A, B:** Preoperative. **C, D:** Six months postoperative.

SUMMARY

Revision augmentation surgery is a more complex and challenging surgery than primary augmentation. These cases are best performed by surgeons who have already developed experience with primary cases. They are also very rewarding procedures. Patients are presenting with concerns that are often making a major impact on their quality of life. In some situations, the patient's outcome can be devastating to them.

It is vital to have a systematic approach in managing these women. This begins with a detailed analysis of the problem, a discussion of expectations, and a review of the risk-benefit equation. Not every problem has a solution, nor should every perceived problem be fixed. When revision involves the use of another breast implant, shaped, form-stable gel devices can be very helpful. Their form-stable nature, tapered upper pole, and low incidence of rupture, contracture, and rippling make them an excellent choice in these patients, who often have abnormal or distorted overlying breast tissue. It is important to remember, however, that it is not all about the implant. The device that is selected is one of many factors that will contribute to success or failure in the revision augmentation patient.

EDITORIAL COMMENTS

Dr. Brown presents an excellent overview of revision breast augmentation. The principal focus of the chapter is breast revision due to capsular contracture, malposition, and palpability. The author emphasizes the importance and advantages of using form-stable anatomic gel implant (style 410). Some of the principal advantages are the lower capsular contracture rate (3.3% vs. 15%) and lack of movement when compared to its smooth, round counterpart. Although capsular contracture is probably reduced, our understanding of this phenomenon is still lacking, especially in light of what we have learned about biofilms and the role that microbes may have in the development of capsular contracture. Perhaps it is the unique texturing of these devices that prevents this long-term sequelae.

The importance of patient selection and patient expectations is properly emphasized. Understanding the nature of the previous operations is critical in order for the plastic surgeon to avoid repeating what was previously performed. A critical observation is that when the revision calls for the use of a form-stable implant, a pocket change is mandatory. The various new pockets are mentioned, including the neosubpectoral pocket. Dr. Brown reviews the salient aspects of implant location, implant size, and breast tissue characteristics. The chapter does not comment on his use of pocket irrigation and use of antibiotics. This is an important consideration especially in revision procedures, where subclinical microbial presence may play a role.

Concerns regarding the use of form-stable implants have been voiced. These include device rotation and the firmness of the device. Dr. Brown details the principles of dimensional planning and the importance of precise pocket dissection. There is clearly a learned component to the use of form-stable devices. Unfortunately, a detailed account regarding technique is beyond the scope of the chapter. I believe that the use of an appropriate implant is the major component when predicting the success of revision breast augmentation. However, there are some other components that may allow plastic surgeons to obtain even better outcomes. The use of acellular dermal matrices has enhanced our ability to better define the breast pocket dimensions, especially in cases of malposition. They may also have a role in reducing the incidence of capsular contracture, as the spherical nature of the capsule is disrupted, which may reduce the contractile forces placed upon the implant. Although evidence is anecdotal, studies are being performed to evaluate this phenomenon. Finally, I feel that it is important to differentiate between elective and necessary revisions when it comes to breast augmentation. Plastic surgeons and the Food and Drug Administration frequently lump all of these together into a revision category that can imply that the revisions were performed because something has gone awry. This is often not the case, as in many instances the revision occurred because the patient changed her mind regarding size, volume, or fill material. Overall, this is an excellent chapter.

M.Y.N.

REFERENCES

1. Spear SL, Murphy DK, Slicton A, et al. Inamed silicone breast implant core study results at 6 years. *Plast Reconstr Surg* 2007;120(7 suppl):8S–16S.
2. Heden P, Jernbeck J, Hober M. Breast augmentation with anatomical cohesive gel implants. *Clin Plast Surg* 2001;28(3):531–552.
3. Brown MH, Shenker R, Silver S. Cohesive silicone gel breast implants in aesthetic and reconstructive breast surgery. *Plast Reconstr Surg* 2005;116(3): 768–779.
4. Heden P, Bone B, Murphy DK, et al. Style 410 cohesive silicone breast implants: safety and effectiveness at 5 to 9 years after implantation. *Plast Reconstr Surg* 2006;118(6):1281–1287.
5. Bengtson BP, Van Natta BW, Murphy DK, et al. Style 410 highly cohesive silicone breast implant core study results at 3 years. *Plast Reconstr Surg* 2007;120(7 suppl):40S–48S.
6. Allergan. Directions for use. Natrelle silicone-filled breast implants. 2009. Available at: http://www.allergan.com/assets/pdf/L034-03_Silicone_DFU.pdf. Accessed July 21, 2010.
7. Maxwell GP, Gabriel A. The neopectoral pocket in revisionary breast surgery. *Aesthet Surg J* 2008;28(4):463–467.
8. Spear SL, Carter ME, Ganz JC. The correction of capsular contracture by conversion to "dual-plane" positioning: technique and outcomes. *Plast Reconstr Surg* 2006;118 (7 suppl):103S–113S; discussion, 114S.
9. Barnsley GP, Sigurdson LJ, Barnsley SE. Textured surface breast implants in the prevention of capsular contracture among breast augmentation patients: a meta-analysis of randomized controlled trials. *Plast Reconstr Surg* 2006;117(7):2182–2190.
10. Panchapakesan V, Brown MH. Management of tuberous breast deformity with anatomic cohesive silicone gel breast implants. *Aesthet Plast Surg* 2009;33(1):49–53.

CHAPTER

132

Neal Handel

Correction of Ptosis in the Previously Augmented Breast

Managing ptosis in the previously augmented patient is an important topic that has not received the attention it deserves. Most women initially undergo breast augmentation in their 20s or early 30s (1). Over time, predictable changes occur in the augmented breast that often lead patients to return for additional surgery (2). Some of these changes are consequences of normal physiologic and aging processes. For example, the breast undergoes involution accompanied by loss of volume, fatty replacement, stretching of skin, diminished elasticity, and progressive ptosis. Pregnancy, breast-feeding, and fluctuations in weight may accelerate these processes. Changes also occur as a direct consequence of the implant, including compression atrophy and thinning of soft tissues, additional skin stretching, acceleration of ptosis, and frequently the development of capsular contracture.

Many augmented patients present requesting correction of ptosis that has occurred gradually over time. These women generally have a similar constellation of findings, including moderate to severe stretching of the skin envelope, atrophy and thinning of the breast tissue, and some degree of contracture (Fig. 132.1) They desire improvement in breast shape and restoration of softness, but few are willing to accept a decrease in breast size. In fact, many patients undergoing secondary surgery want larger implants. The majority of such patients undergo some combination of capsule surgery, mastopexy, and implant exchange. These patients are challenging because consistently good aesthetic results are difficult to achieve, complications are relatively frequent, and disasters occasionally occur.

My interest in this subject was stimulated after observing a high rate of complications and unsatisfactory outcomes in augmented patients undergoing delayed mastopexy. Some were my patients who suffered wound-healing delays, unsatisfactory nipple position, and suboptimal scarring. I have also seen many patients who were referred with severe complications, including extensive skin necrosis, fat necrosis, infections, implant exposure, and partial or full-thickness loss of the nipple and areola (Figs. 132.2 to 132.5).

When these secondary cases result in poor outcomes, it is not only disappointing to the patient, but also worrisome and stressful to the surgeon as well. Such adverse outcomes can also be costly for malpractice carriers. In recent years, litigation stemming from secondary implant surgery has resulted in the greatest monetary losses arising from plastic surgery cases. If patients experience extensive scarring, nipple-areolar loss, or permanent disfigurement of the breast, judgments or settlements are typically in the range of $250,000 to $800,000 (M. Gorney, The Doctors Company, Napa, CA, personal communication, 2003).

There are several reasons why the combination of capsule surgery, mastopexy, and implant exchange is a high-risk procedure. Some of the increased risk arises simply from performing multiple breast procedures simultaneously. For example, it has been reported that when augmentation and mastopexy are combined, the increase in risk is more than just additive. Breast augmentation alone has a relatively low risk of complications, and they are usually not severe. Likewise, when mastopexy alone is performed, the complication rate is relatively low, and the problems quite manageable. However, as Spear (3,4) observed, when the two operations are combined into a single procedure, each operation makes the other more difficult, and each increases the likelihood of complications arising from the other. This occurs because the operations have conflicting goals. The aim of mastopexy is to elevate the nipple and tighten the breast, which is accomplished by reducing the skin envelope. The objective of augmentation is to increase breast volume, which is accomplished by expanding the skin envelope. Thus, concomitant mastopexy and augmentation may result in a relative insufficiency of soft tissue to accommodate the implant, resulting in increased wound tension and devascularization of tissues. The risk of nipple loss is much greater with combined augmentation and mastopexy than with augmentation alone or mastopexy alone (Figs. 132.6 and 132.7). Other adverse consequences arising from combined augmentation-mastopexy include an increased risk of flap necrosis with wound dehiscence and implant exposure, wide or unattractive scars, excessively dilated areolas, unsatisfactory nipple position, diminished skin sensation, fat necrosis, and infection.

When performing surgery to correct ptosis in previously augmented patients, one must contend not only with the increased surgical risk attendant to combined procedures, but also with the significant physiologic and anatomic changes of the breast caused by implants. The most important adverse effect of implants is the thinning and atrophy of breast tissue that inevitably occurs over time.

Plastic surgeons have long been aware that tissue atrophy occurs adjacent to implanted prosthetic devices. In fact, even relatively rigid, nonmalleable tissues are affected; many patients with silicone chin implants have some atrophy of the adjacent mandible (5,6), and erosion and depression of the bony thorax has been described secondary to breast implants. If rigid tissues like bone and cartilage undergo atrophy from implants, it is likely that such changes would be even more dramatic in soft tissues such as the breast. Indeed, it is commonly observed that the soft-tissue envelope surrounding a breast implant becomes extremely attenuated in augmented patients. This finding was emphasized by Tebbetts (7), who observed that the "consequences of excessively large breast implants include ptosis, tissue stretching, tissue thinning, inadequate soft-tissue cover [and] subcutaneous tissue atrophy." As a result of gravity, most of the thinning and tissue atrophy occurs along the inferior pole of the breast. This can be demonstrated on physical examination (Fig. 132.8), and is confirmed on mammograms of the augmented breast (Fig. 132.9).

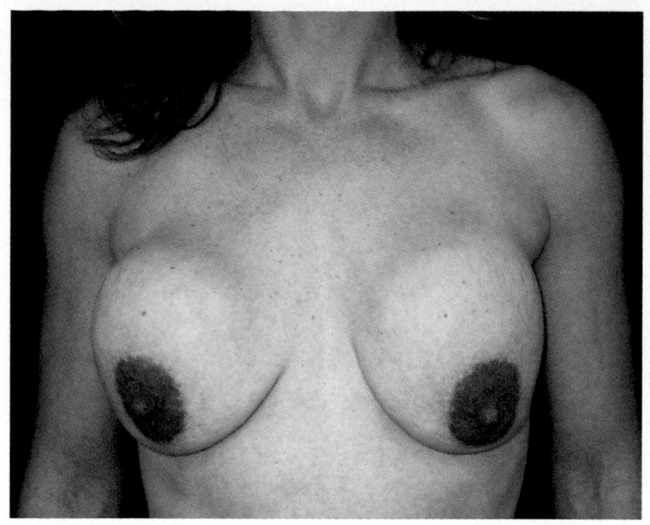

A

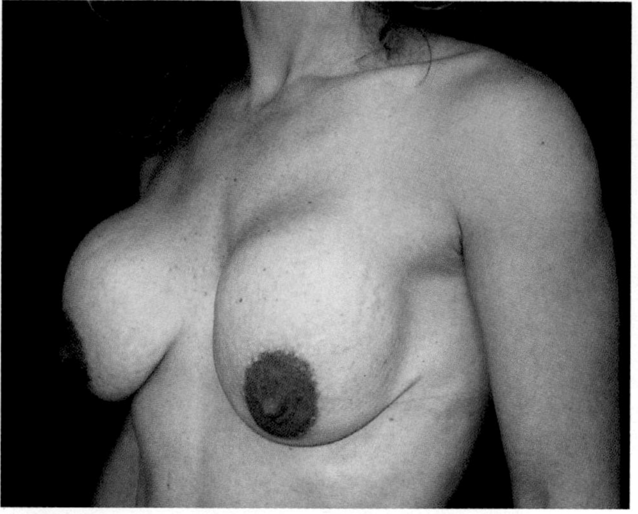

B

Figure 132.1. **A:** Frontal view of a patient with submammary implants for 16 years presenting with ptosis, contracture, and thinning of tissues. **B:** Oblique view confirms ptosis and superior malposition of the implants due to contracture.

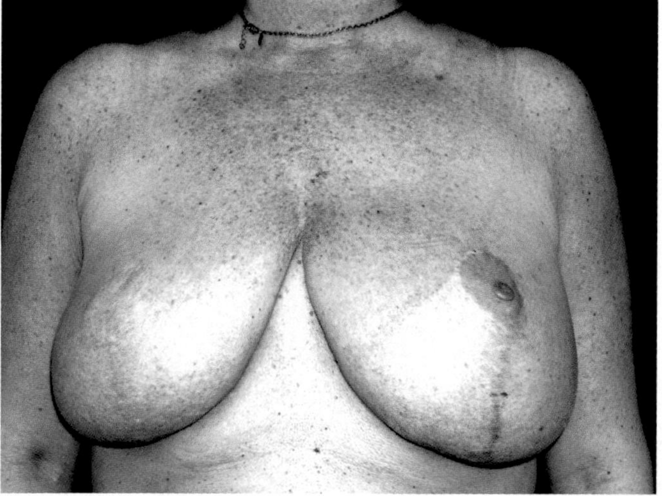

Figure 132.2. A 49-year-old woman sustained complete loss of right nipple-areolar complex after explantation, capsulectomy, mastopexy (Wise skin pattern), and insertion of new implants.

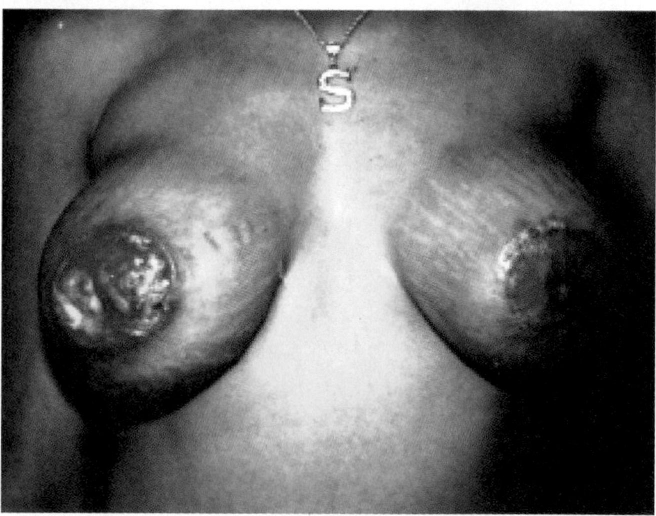

Figure 132.3. A 26-year-old woman with full-thickness loss of nipple-areolar complex and central fat necrosis of the breast after capsulotomy, implant exchange, and periareolar mastopexy.

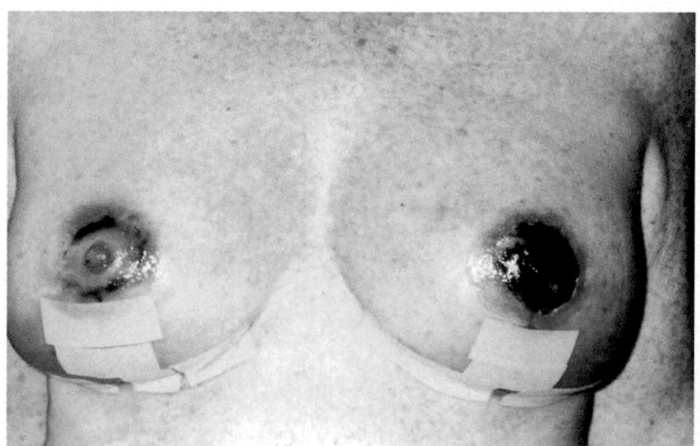

A

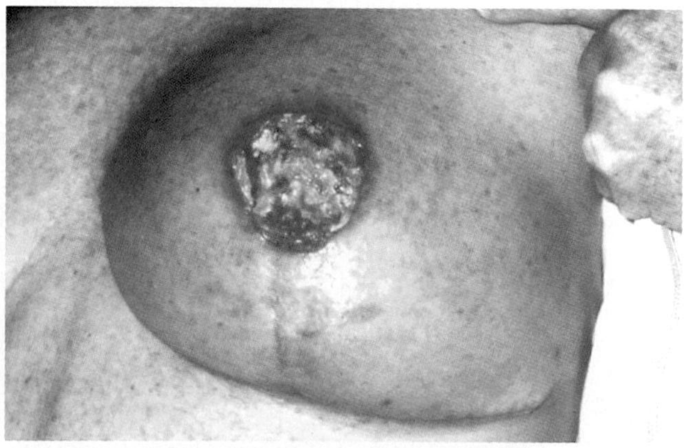

B

Figure 132.4. **A:** A 39-year-old patient at 2 weeks after explantation, capsulectomy, Wise-pattern mastopexy, and insertion of larger implants, with marked ischemic changes of nipples, particularly the left side. **B:** Same patient 1 month postoperatively, with complete loss of left nipple-areolar complex and central fat necrosis of the breast.

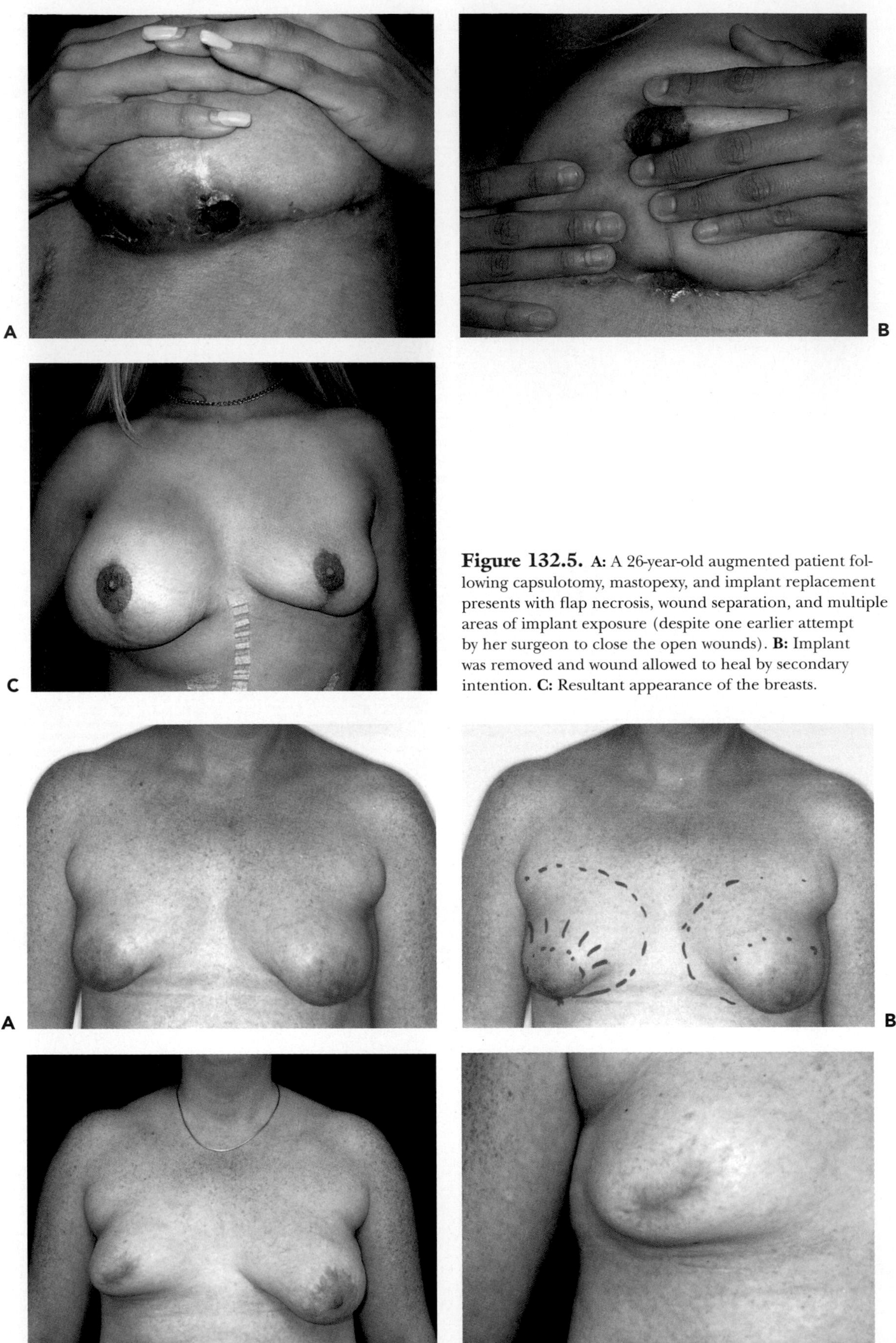

Figure 132.5. **A:** A 26-year-old augmented patient following capsulotomy, mastopexy, and implant replacement presents with flap necrosis, wound separation, and multiple areas of implant exposure (despite one earlier attempt by her surgeon to close the open wounds). **B:** Implant was removed and wound allowed to heal by secondary intention. **C:** Resultant appearance of the breasts.

Figure 132.6. **A:** A 38-year-old patient with ptosis and asymmetry. **B:** Skin markings for right circumareolar mastopexy with augmentation and left crescent mastopexy with augmentation. **C:** The patient sustained complete loss of nipple and areola and central fat necrosis of the right breast, widening of scar, and unsatisfactory correction of the left breast ptosis. **D:** Right breast after excision of necrotic nipple and closure of defect.

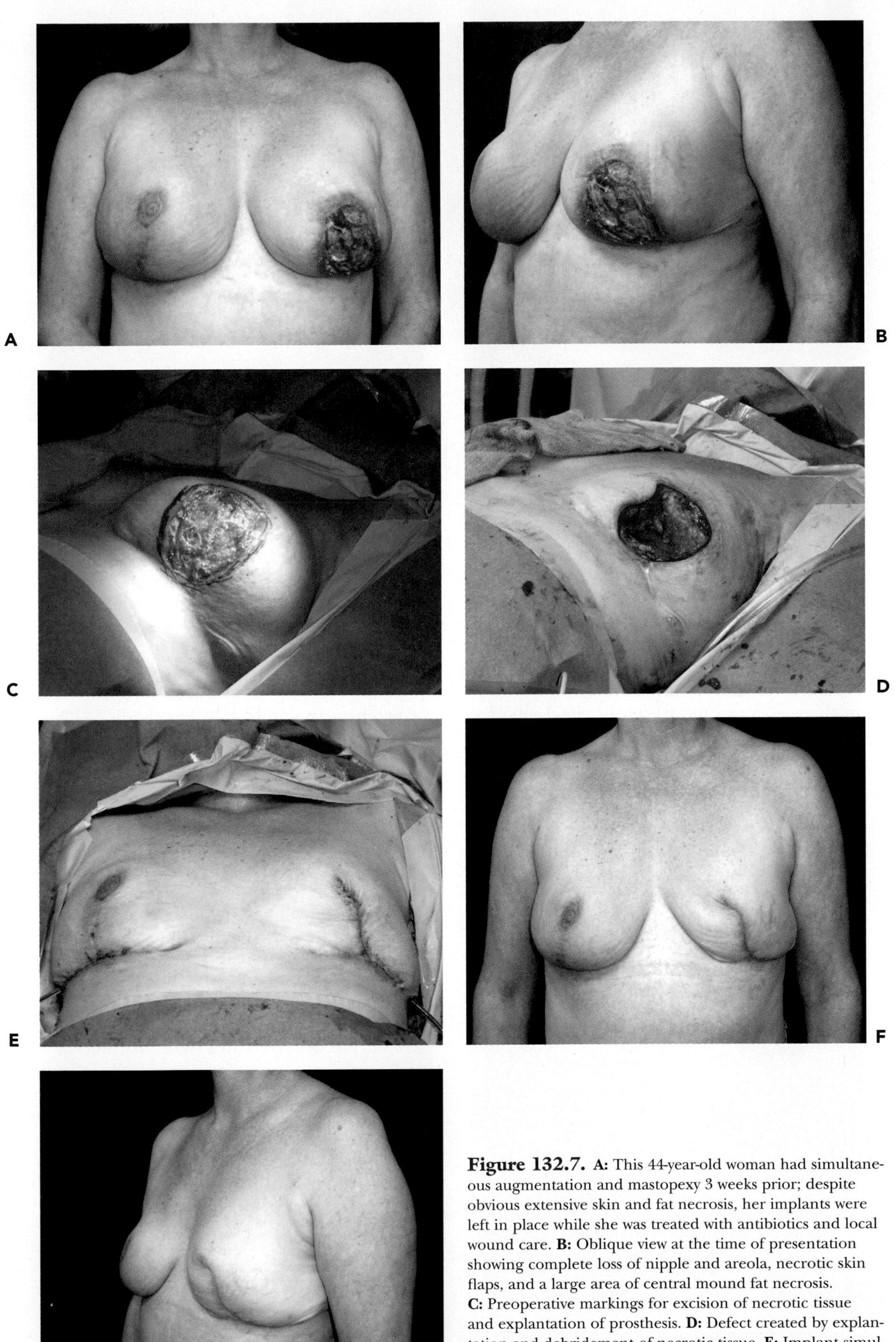

Figure 132.7. **A:** This 44-year-old woman had simultaneous augmentation and mastopexy 3 weeks prior; despite obvious extensive skin and fat necrosis, her implants were left in place while she was treated with antibiotics and local wound care. **B:** Oblique view at the time of presentation showing complete loss of nipple and areola, necrotic skin flaps, and a large area of central mound fat necrosis. **C:** Preoperative markings for excision of necrotic tissue and explantation of prosthesis. **D:** Defect created by explantation and debridement of necrotic tissue. **E:** Implant simultaneously removed from the contralateral side for symmetry. **F, G:** Early (3 weeks postoperative) result.

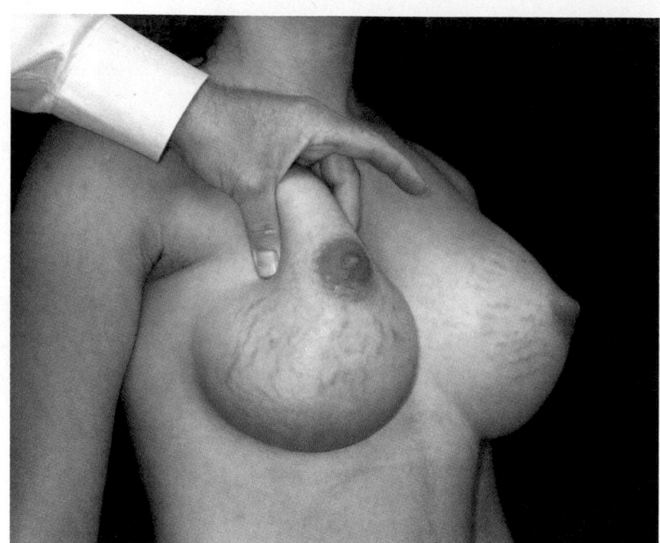

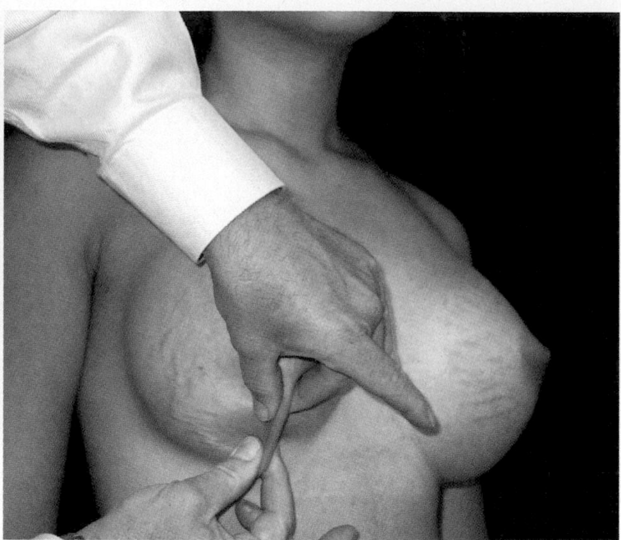

Figure 132.8. **A:** A 22-year-old patient 1 year after augmentation; superior breast parenchyma remains thick. **B:** Pinch test reveals inferior breast tissue that is thin and atrophic and a parenchymal flap only a few millimeters in thickness.

Patients with implants present for prolonged periods not only have tissue thinning and stretching, but also are likely to have a history of previous operations for capsular contracture (8). The surgery performed to relieve contracture, either capsulotomy or capsulectomy, further thins residual breast tissue and compromises blood supply. In addition, with the exception of those who had a transaxillary or transumbilical approach, augmented patients have scars on their breasts from the original procedure; these scars may further impair blood supply to the skin of the breast or nipple-areolar complex.

There is a continuum of risk associated with cosmetic breast operations. The safest operations are primary augmentation alone or primary mastopexy alone. Intermediate in terms of risk is combined augmentation and mastopexy. The highest risk occurs in augmented patients with contracture and ptosis undergoing simultaneous implant exchange, capsule surgery, and mastopexy. The anatomic features of these various groups and their impact on the risk of surgical complications are illustrated in Figure 132.10.

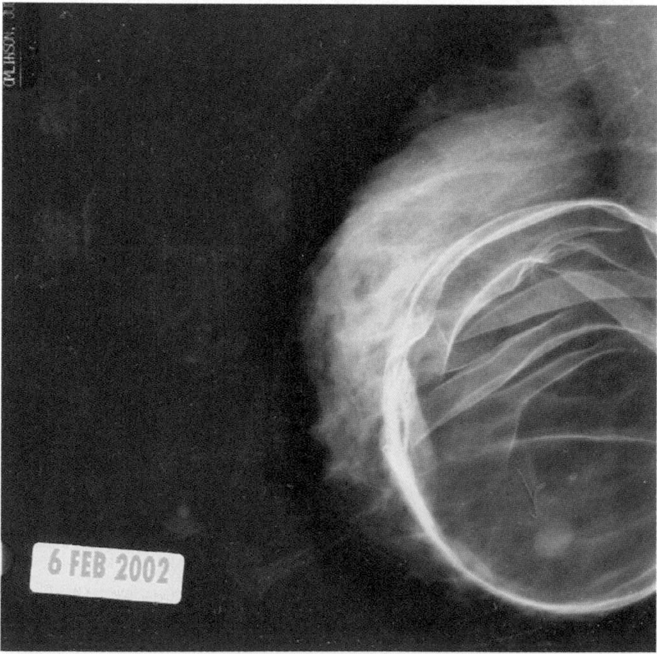

Figure 132.9. Compression mammogram of an augmented breast reveals thick breast parenchyma superiorly but thinned, atrophic tissue inferiorly.

There is a range of treatment options available for augmented patients who have ptosis, with or without contracture. The first is explantation alone, without mastopexy or implant replacement. The second is capsule surgery only, including repositioning of the prosthesis but without mastopexy. A third option is mastopexy alone, without manipulation of the implant. A fourth possibility is explantation with mastopexy. The final option (the riskiest and most frequently performed) is simultaneous explantation, capsule surgery, mastopexy, and insertion of an implant.

Patients who fall into the first category—explantation without mastopexy or reinsertion of an implant—are among the least frequently encountered. However, some individuals with only moderate ptosis and good skin elasticity achieve surprisingly good results simply from explantation. If the surgeon is unsure about how well the skin envelope will contract, mastopexy can always be delayed until a secondary procedure. When performing explantation without immediate reinsertion of an implant, it is advisable to perform a thorough capsulectomy. Usually in patients with a submammary prosthesis, total capsulectomy can be accomplished easily. In those with subpectoral implants, the anterior capsule adjacent to the breast parenchyma can be resected, but excising capsule from the undersurface of the pectoral muscle is tedious and often bloody. One alternative is to score or roughen the capsule with cautery. Likewise, if the posterior capsule is densely adherent to the underlying ribs and intercostal fascia, there is a risk of excessive bleeding and even of a parietal pneumothorax in attempting to resect it. In such cases, roughening of the posterior capsule, either with mechanical abrasion or cautery, will create a raw surface to assure tissue adhesion after the implant is removed. Suction drains in the early postoperative period are mandatory.

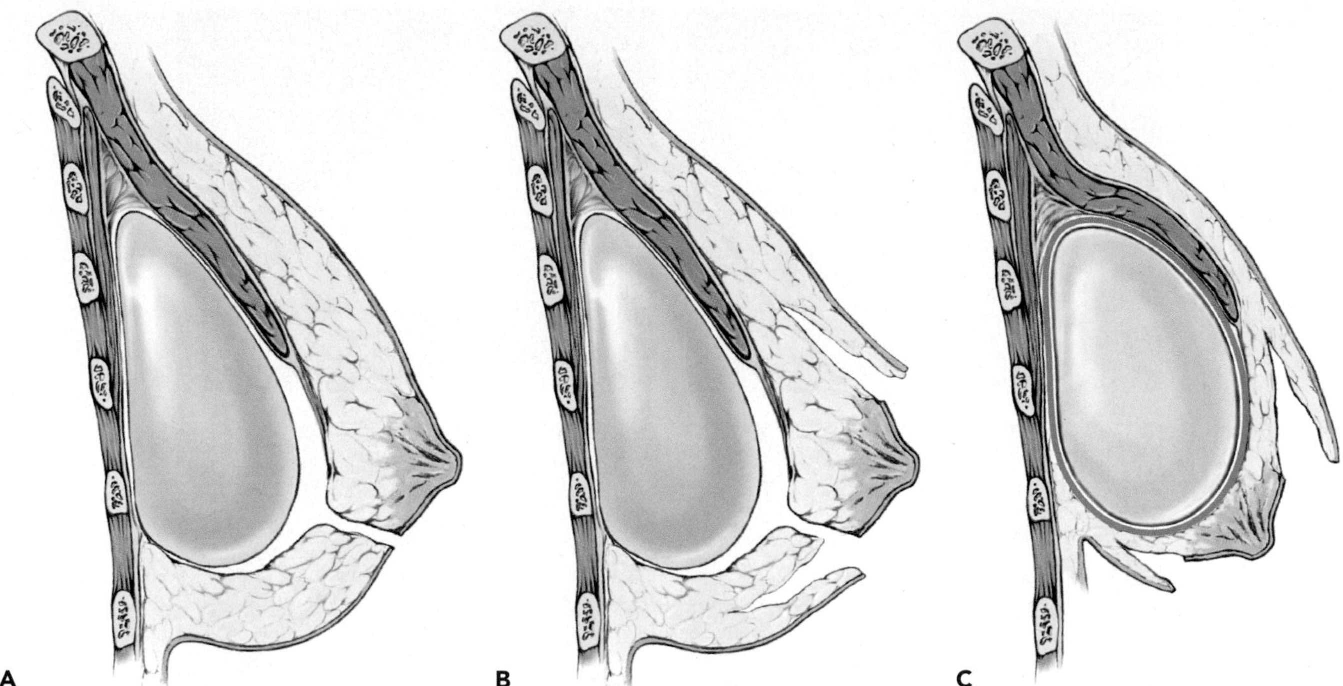

Figure 132.10. **A:** Patients undergoing primary augmentation have thick flaps, no prior incisions on the breast, and little risk of ischemia to skin or nipple. **B:** Patients undergoing combined mastopexy and augmentation are at higher risk of complications because of simultaneous development of mastopexy flaps and undermining of the breast. **C:** Secondary implant patients undergoing capsulectomy, mastopexy, and implant replacement are at high risk for compromised blood supply to mastopexy flaps and nipple-areolar complex.

When substantial portions of the capsule are left in situ, they tend to persist indefinitely. This may contribute to seroma formation and will certainly impair reattachment of the breast to the underlying chest wall. For these reasons, capsulectomy to the greatest degree practical is recommended.

A second and more common category of patients is made up of women who present with "pseudo-ptosis" of the nipple. In these individuals, there often is capsular contracture with superior displacement of the implant. When this occurs in conjunction with laxity of the overlying skin envelope, the nipple-areolar complex can "hang over" the breast mound, pointing downward, giving the appearance of nipple ptosis. In most of these cases the nipple is not actually beneath the inframammary crease, and the appearance of "ptosis" arises as a result of superior malposition of the implant. Often, excellent correction can be achieved with capsulotomy or capsulectomy and modification of the pocket to lower the fold (Fig. 132.11). Sometimes insertion of a larger prosthesis will also help to fill out the redundant skin envelope. If the patient has adequate soft tissue coverage to camouflage the implant, conversion from the submuscular to the submammary or dual-plane position will also often enhance the result by allowing the soft issue to redrape over the implant in a more aesthetically pleasing fashion.

Occasionally one encounters patients who require only mastopexy to achieve the desired improvement. If a patient does not have contracture and the implant is in good condition and in satisfactory position, mastopexy alone is indicated. This circumstance arises frequently in mastectomy patients who were reconstructed with an implant and had contralateral augmentation for symmetry. The augmented breast is much more likely to become ptotic over time than the reconstructed breast, and "touch-up" mastopexy is often necessary to maintain symmetry (Fig. 132.12). The important technical point to bear in mind is that the breast tissue is attenuated, and therefore dissection of the mastopexy flaps must be done in a plane that preserves skin blood supply yet does not interfere with the vascular pedicle to the nipple.

The next option available for augmented patients with ptosis is explantation with mastopexy, without reinsertion of a new prosthesis. This choice appeals to many women, particularly those who have had implants for a long time and no longer wish to be as full breasted, or women who have undergone multiple prior implant operations and wish to eliminate the risk of future implant-related problems (Fig. 132.13). There are also some individuals in whom performing explantation and mastopexy is a useful first stage, with the intention of going back later to insert a new pair of implants. This certainly decreases risk compared to combining all of the procedures into a single operation.

In women undergoing explantation and mastopexy, particularly in combination with capsulectomy, there is a definite increased risk of complications compared to mastopexy in the nonaugmented breast or even mastopexy in conjunction with primary augmentation. As previously noted, the breast tissue is atrophic, the flaps are thin, and capsulectomy as well as the dissection associated with mastopexy further compromise blood supply to the nipple and skin flaps. The relative paucity of breast parenchyma may also change the technical approach to mastopexy. In recent years, there has been an emphasis on parenchymal flaps and internal suturing to enhance results and improve the longevity of mastopexy (9,10). Proponents of these techniques believe that internal suturing or parenchymal slings will decrease the risk of "bottoming out" and prevent

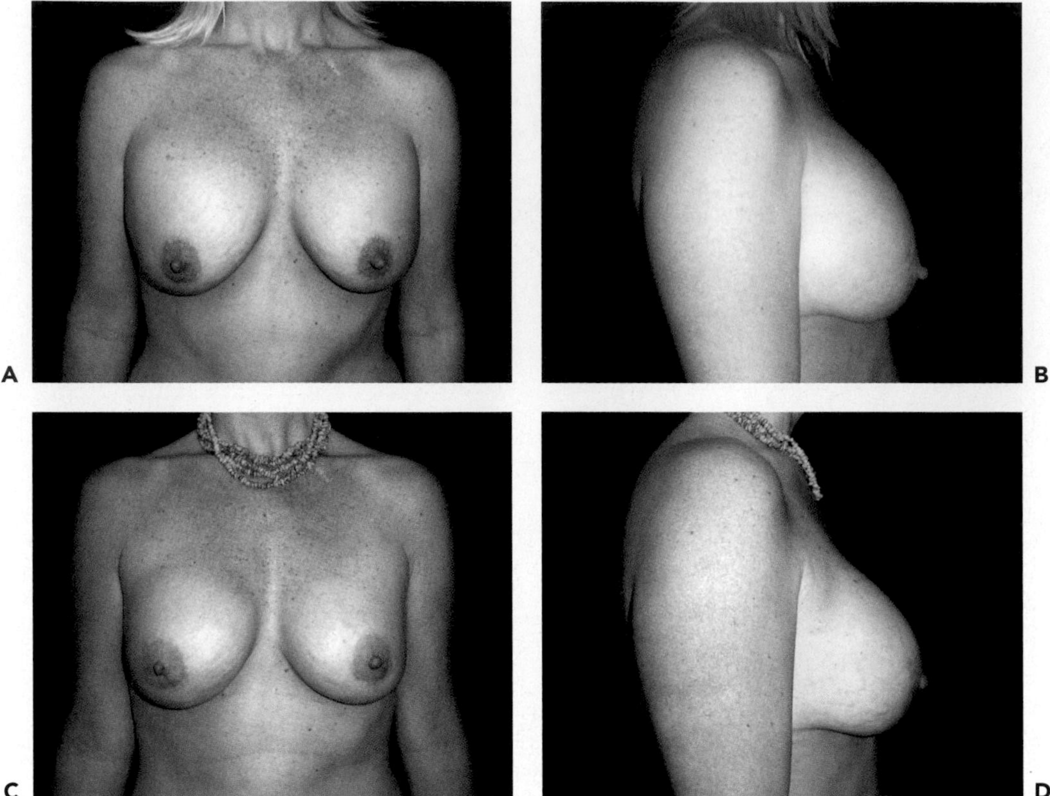

Figure 132.11. **A:** 39-year-old patient augmented 7 years previously, complaining of "droopy" and "unaesthetic" breasts. **B:** Lateral view confirms that the breasts are not truly ptotic but that implants are malpositioned superiorly. **C:** Frontal view after corrective surgery consisting of inferior capsulotomy to the lower pocket. **D:** Lateral view reveals improved breast contour simply from repositioning the implants without the need for any type of "mastopexy."

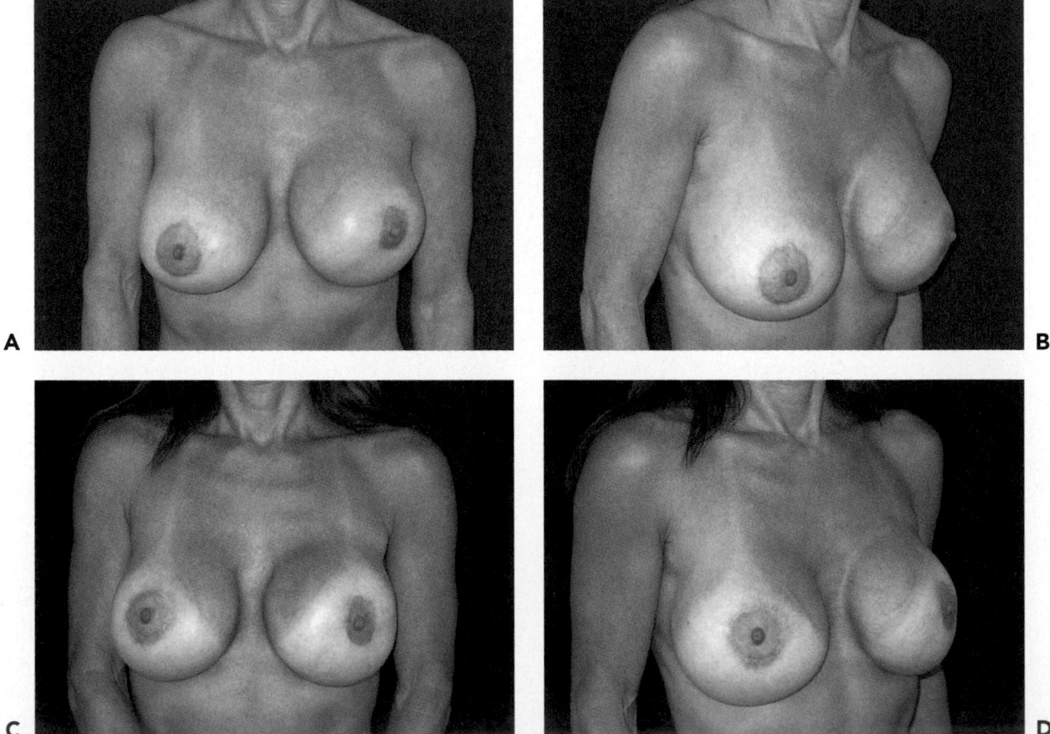

Figure 132.12. **A, B:** Cancer patient, reconstructed with implant on the left and augmented on the right for symmetry, presenting with ptosis of the augmented breast. **C, D:** After periareolar mastopexy of the augmented breast to correct ptosis and improve symmetry with the reconstructed breast; no capsule or implant surgery was necessary.

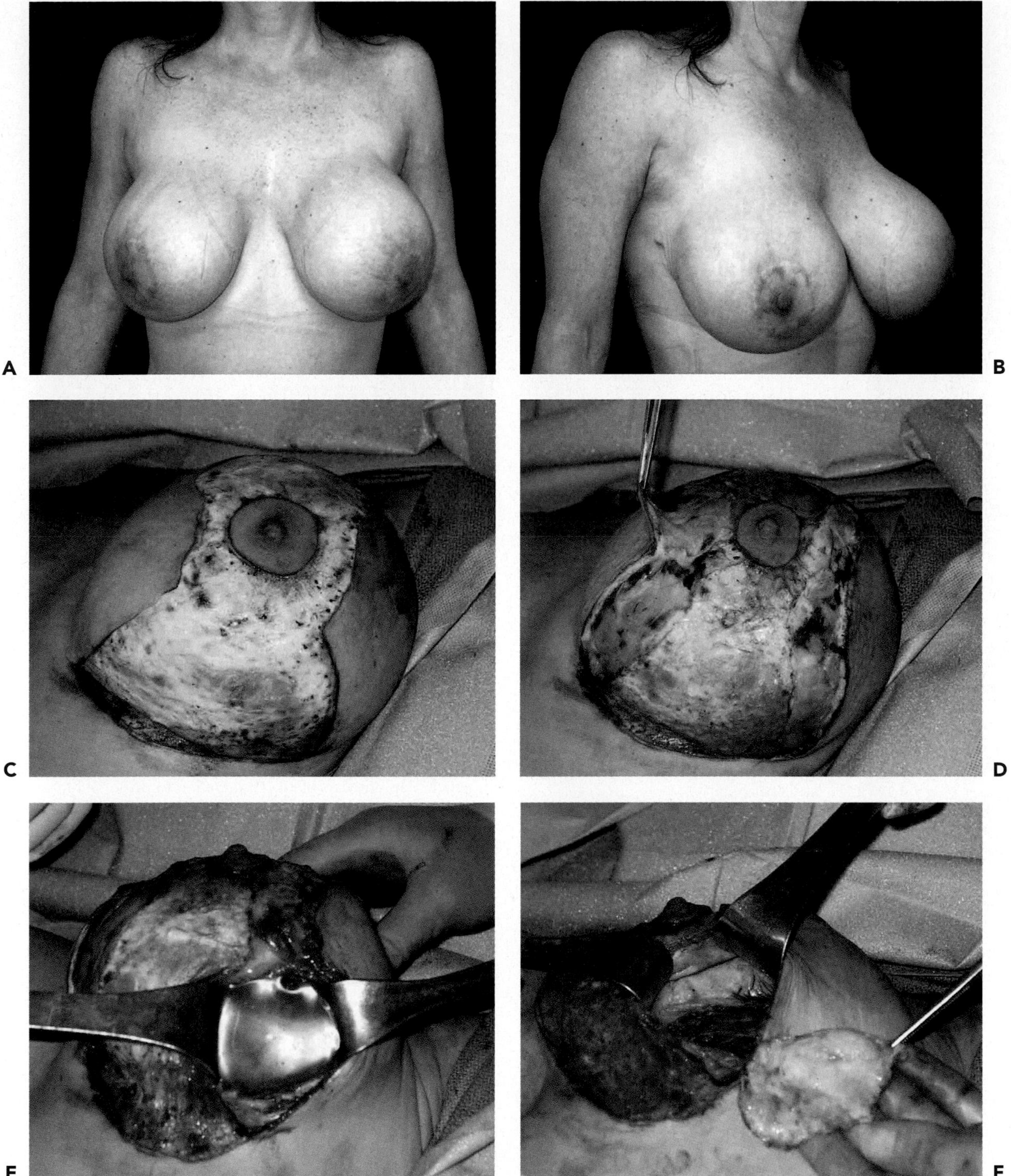

Figure 132.13. **A, B:** Frontal and oblique views of a 37-year-old woman who had initial breast augmentation 15 years previously; she underwent a secondary breast implant procedure including capsulotomy, Benelli mastopexy, and insertion of larger implants. She now complains of ptosis, recurrent contracture, and "heavy" breasts. The patient decided to undergo explantation without new implants in conjunction with mastopexy. **C:** Deepithelialization is performed within confines of the conventional Wise skin pattern. **D:** Mastopexy flaps are elevated only a short distance to preserve blood supply to the skin. **E:** Implant is exposed and removed. **F:** The thickened, contracted posterior capsule is removed. (*continued*)

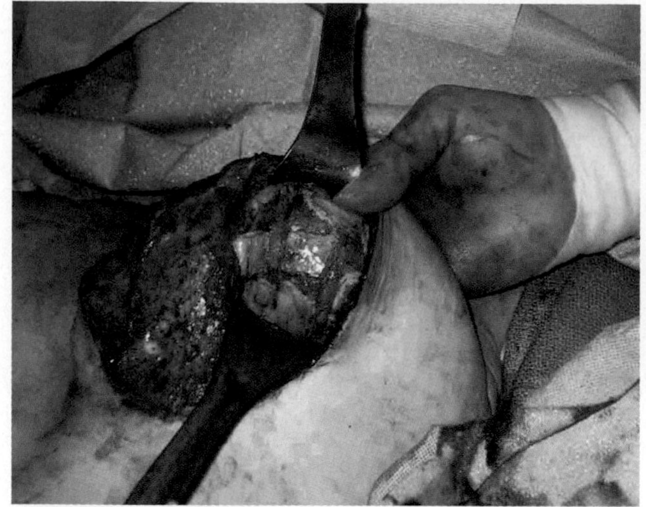

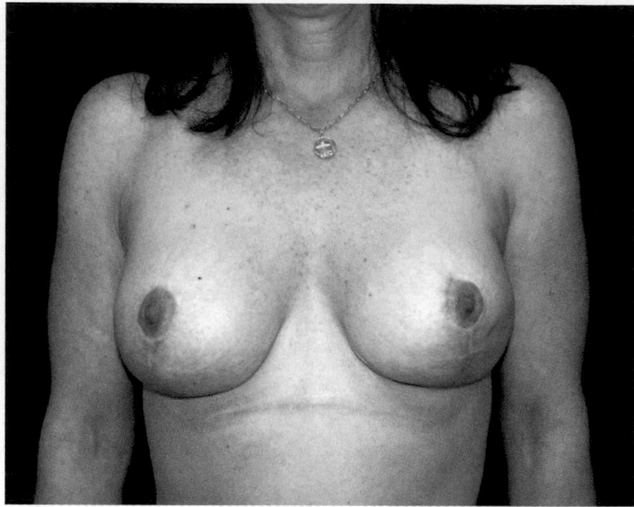

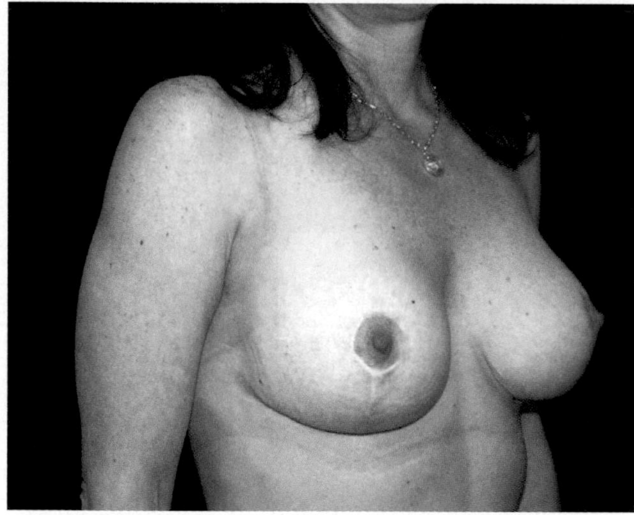

Figure 132.13. (*Continued*) **G:** On the undersurface of the vertical bipedicle flap, the capsule is left attached to preserve blood supply to the nipple; the capsule is scored to encourage reattachment to the underlying chest wall. **H, I:** The postoperative result 6 months after surgery.

recurrent ptosis. In women with implants, however, there frequently is such severe thinning and atrophy of the breast that there simply is not much tissue available for internal rearrangement and suturing. In addition, the parenchyma has largely been detached from the underlying chest wall, resulting in compromised blood supply. These factors combine to make parenchymal suturing technically more difficult and increase the risk of ischemia and fat necrosis. In previously augmented patients undergoing secondary mastopexy, there often is more reliance on skin resection, flap undermining, and dermal adhesion than on parenchymal sutures.

In recent years, "short-scar" techniques, including vertical mastopexy, have increased greatly in popularity. The advantages of such techniques include not only elimination of the scar in the inframammary fold, but also the ability to obtain increased breast projection and improved upper pole fullness (11). This is an excellent approach in many cases, but when performing vertical mastopexy in the previously augmented patient, the surgeon again needs to be aware of changes secondary to implants. Because the tissues of the inferior pole of the breast are generally the most attenuated, techniques that rely on a superior pedicle (Lejour, Lassus) are probably safer (Fig. 132.14), whereas techniques that rely on an inferior pedicle, such as the SPAIR (short-scar periareolar inferior pedicle reduction) mammaplasty (12), may be relatively contraindicated (Fig. 132.15). When selecting the specific operation for ptosis, there is a wide spectrum of procedures among which to choose. These range from a crescent nipple lift to a conventional Wise pattern mastopexy (13). In general, the least aggressive mastopexy that will achieve the desired result is preferred.

The final option available for augmented women seeking correction of ptosis is explantation, capsular surgery, mastopexy, and insertion of breast prosthesis. This is the combination that poses the greatest risk. It is also the combination most frequently requested by patients. Proper planning and surgical execution significantly reduces the risk of ischemic complications. It is critical to avoid excessively long, thin flaps and to minimize tension on closure. In cases in which an implant is being reinserted, it is unnecessary to perform an extensive capsulectomy. Capsulotomy may be safer and equally effective for relieving contracture. It is particularly important not to strip the capsule from the undersurface of thin flaps. In addition, when an implant is being reinserted, it is usually possible to perform a less aggressive mastopexy. In general, the mastopexy that is least disruptive to blood supply should be chosen.

In some cases a simple crescent mastopexy (14) will suffice. Crescent mastopexy is a much more effective operation if a full-thickness wedge of tissue is resected from the level of the skin through the breast parenchyma to the pectoral fascia (Fig. 132.16). When such a full-thickness crescent excision is closed

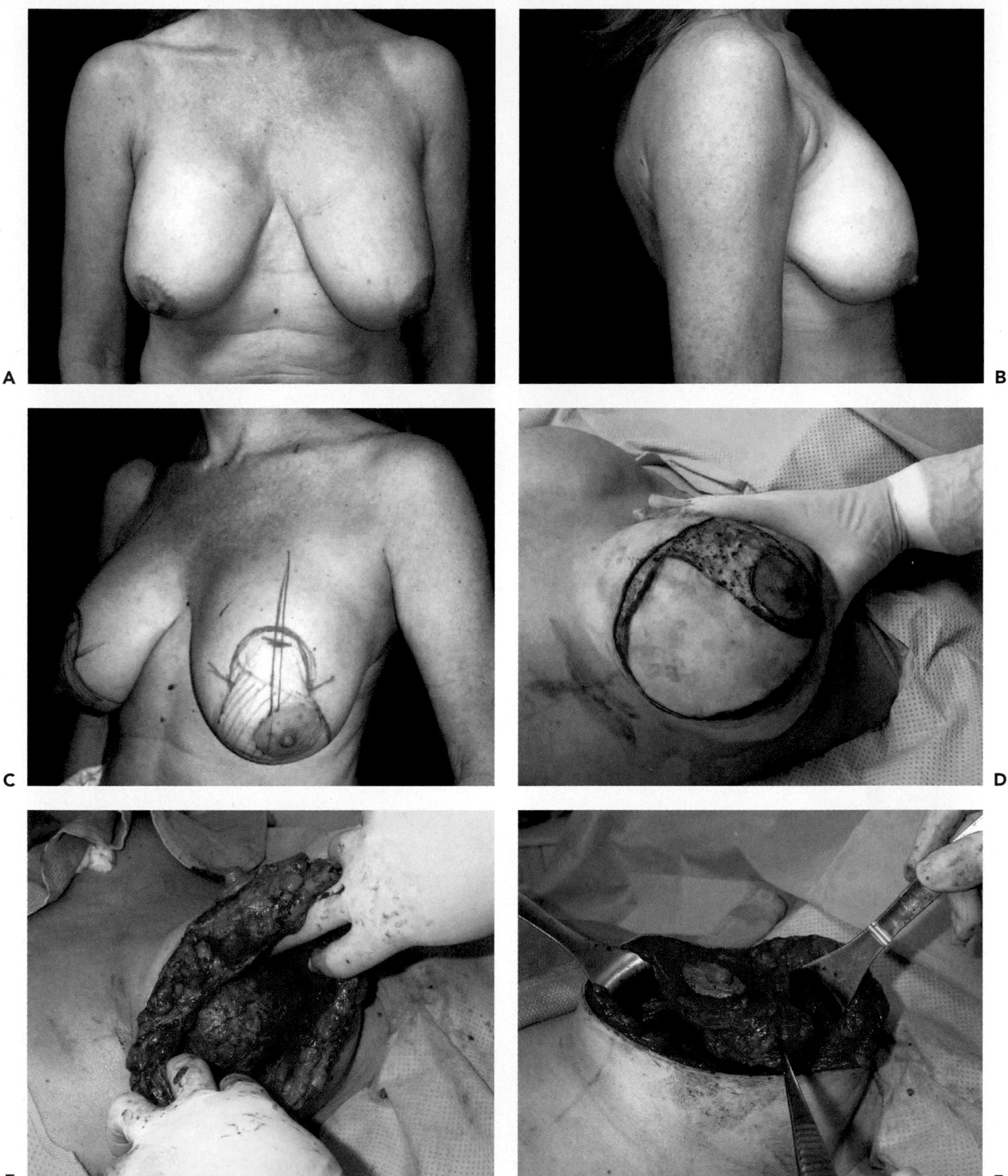

Figure 132.14. **A, B:** Frontal and lateral views of 53-year-old woman with silicone implants for approximately 20 years; she is concerned about ptosis and "leakage" of silicone. Patient desires explantation and mastopexy without insertion of new implants. She specifically wishes to avoid traditional "anchor scar" and requests "vertical mastopexy." **C:** Drawing for vertical mastopexy skin incision and superomedial pedicle to nipple. **D:** Pedicle has been deepithelialized. **E:** The implant (which has significant gel bleed) is removed in continuity with the periprosthetic capsule. **F:** Blood supply and innervation to the nipple are via superomedial pedicle; some extra tissue is left attached to portion of the pedicle, which will be rotated superiorly and provide added upper pole fullness. (*continued*)

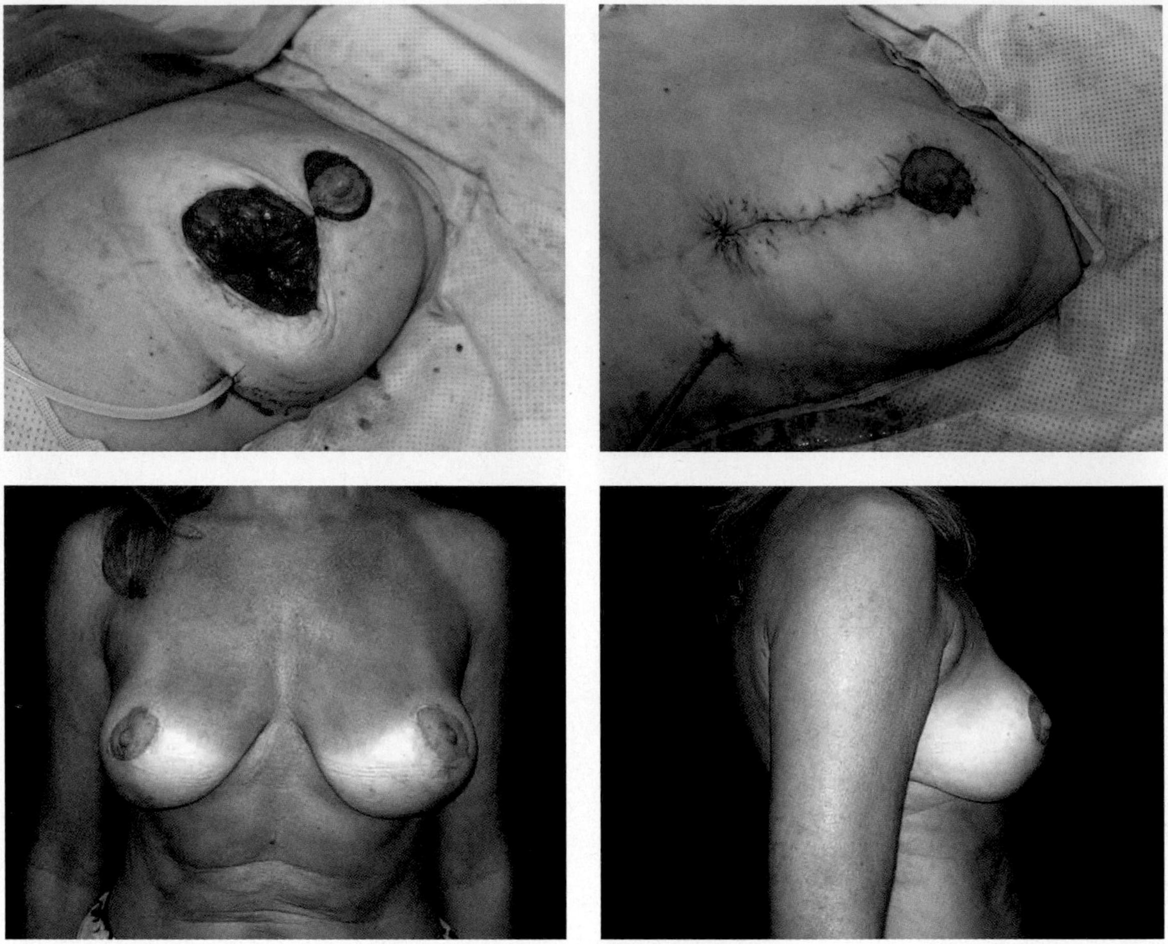

Figure 132.14. (*Continued*) **G:** The nipple has been rotated and inset into the superior portion of a mosque-dome incision; medial and lateral parenchymal pillars are sutured in layers. **H:** Periareolar and vertical skin incisions are closed. **I, J:** Frontal and lateral postoperative views at 6 months.

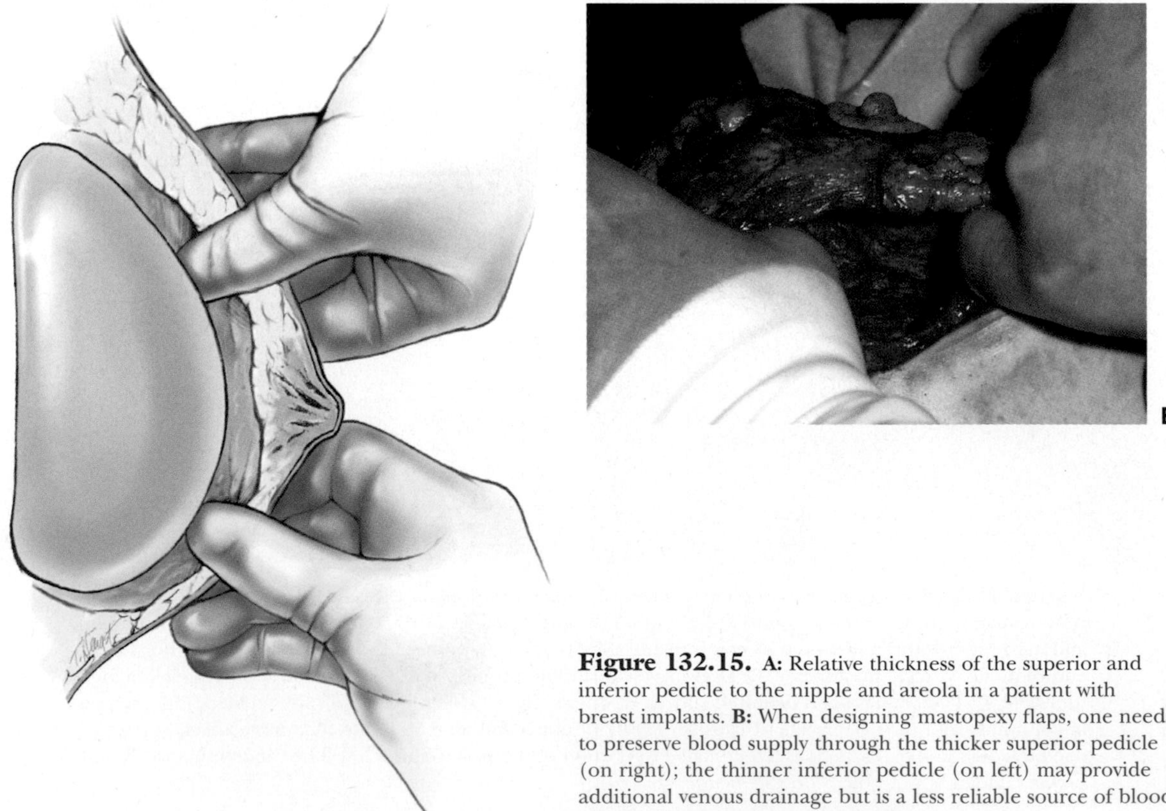

Figure 132.15. **A:** Relative thickness of the superior and inferior pedicle to the nipple and areola in a patient with breast implants. **B:** When designing mastopexy flaps, one needs to preserve blood supply through the thicker superior pedicle (on right); the thinner inferior pedicle (on left) may provide additional venous drainage but is a less reliable source of blood supply to the nipple-areolar complex.

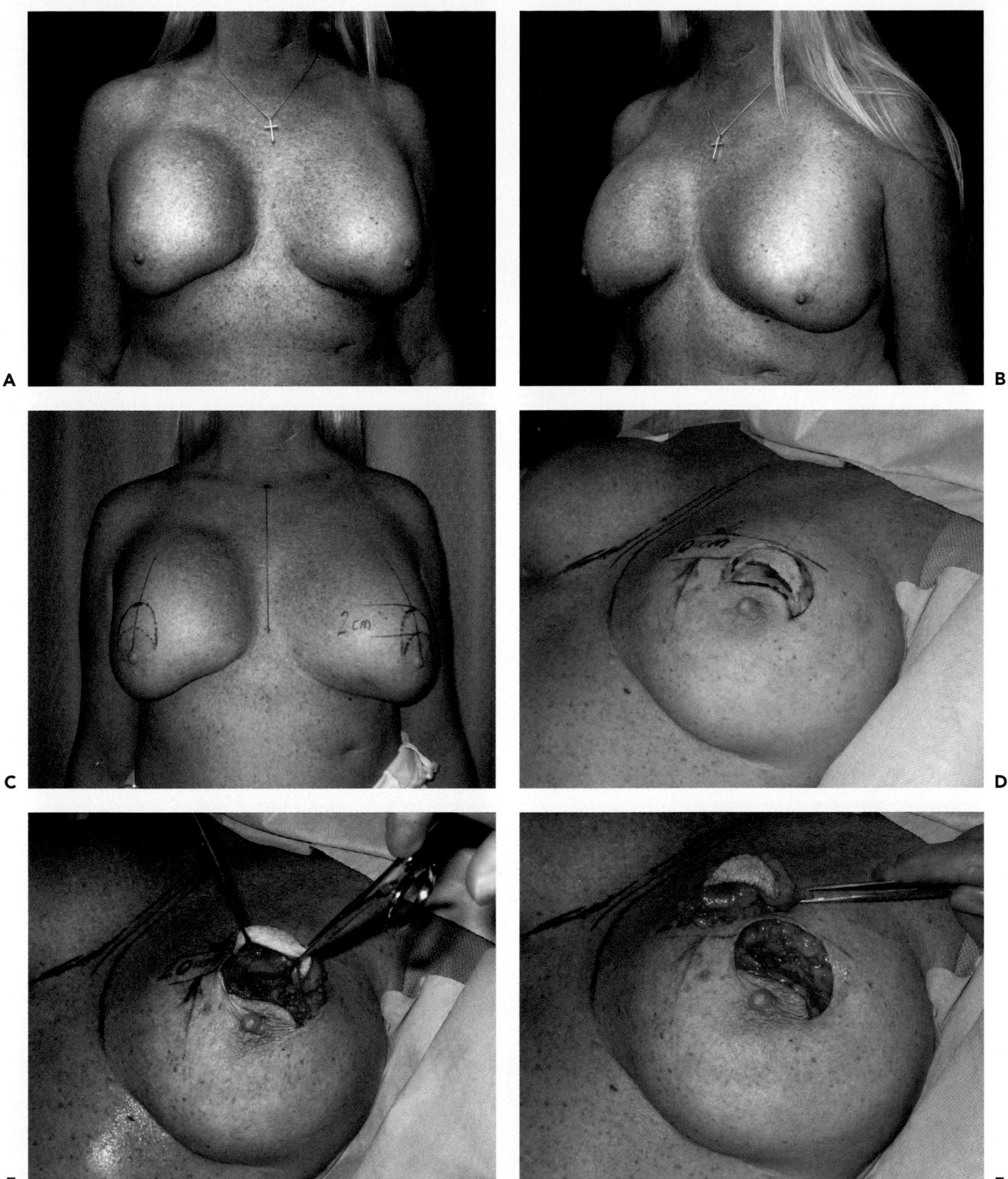

Figure 132.16. **A, B:** Preoperative views of a 47-year-old woman with subpectoral implants present for approximately 20 years; she now complains of ptosis, as well as firmness and implant displacement due to capsular contracture. **C:** Preoperative skin markings for bilateral crescent mastopexy designed to raise the nipple 2 cm on each side. **D:** Skin incision is made and deepened into the underlying breast tissue. **E:** The dissection proceeds through the full thickness of the breast down to the level of the muscle fascia or anterior capsule. **F:** A full-thickness crescent of skin and breast parenchyma is resected. (*continued*)

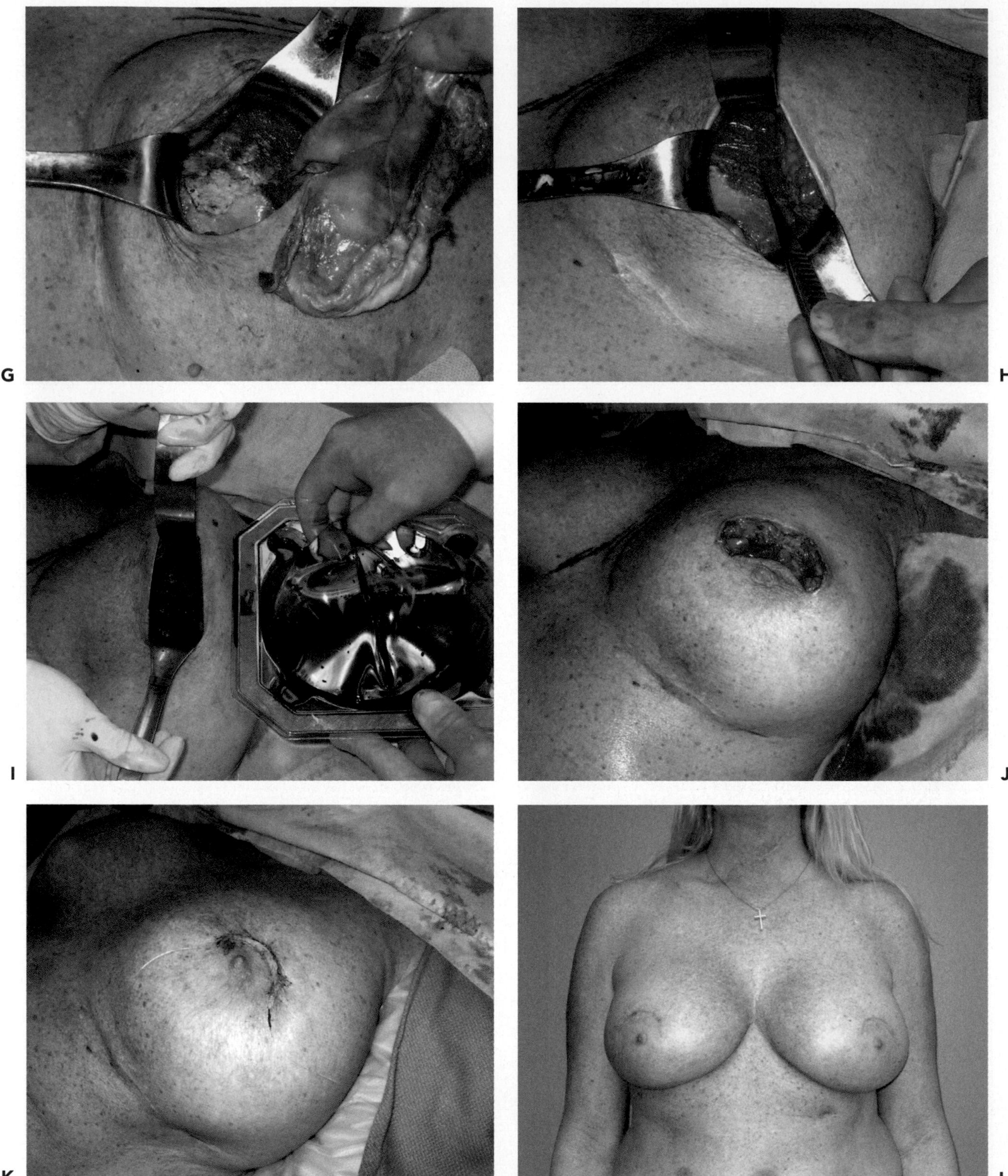

Figure 132.16. (*Continued*) **G**: A subtotal capsulectomy is performed; however, the capsule is not stripped from the posterior aspect (undersurface) of the pectoral muscle. **H**: A new submammary pocket is created, and the anterolateral border of the pectoralis major muscle is reattached to the underlying chest wall. **I**: The new implant is prepared for insertion into the submammary pocket (it is rinsed in Betadine in an effort to discourage formation of a bacterial biofilm in the hope that this will decrease the risk of contracture); in ptotic patients with adequate soft tissue coverage (as in this case), implants are generally converted to the submammary or "dual-plane" pocket because this facilitates redraping of the soft tissues over the implant. **J**: The crescent "defect" is closed in layers to elevate the inferior pole of the breast and to take all tension off the skin closure; this helps to prevent widening of the scar and eliminates unsightly stretching of the upper areola. **K**: Final skin closure. **L, M**: Postoperative views at 4 months. (*continued*)

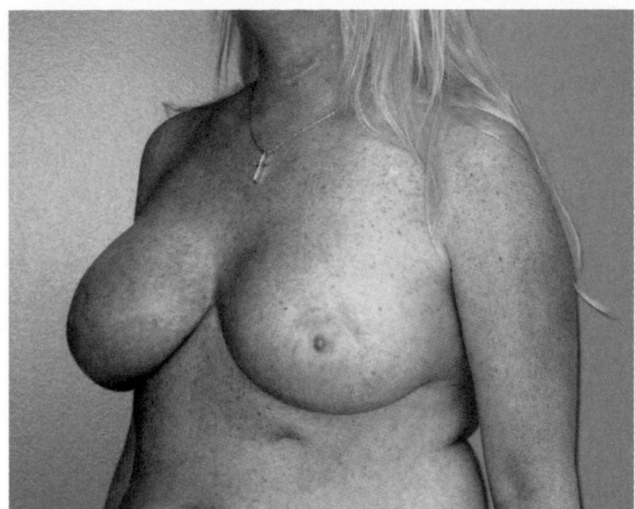

Figure 132.16. (*Continued*)

in layers, it elevates the nipple but also lifts the inferior pole of the breast, reduces tension on the skin closure, minimizes stretching of the superior half of the areola, and prevents spreading of the scar. However, in patients who have had disruption to the nipple blood supply inferiorly and posteriorly (e.g., augmentation through a periareolar incision) it is best to avoid full-thickness excision of superior breast tissue. This may represent the only remaining vascular pedicle to the nipple. In these cases, deepithelialization or full-thickness skin resection only should be performed (Fig. 132.17).

Periareolar mastopexy (15,16) is often useful in secondary implant cases. Although the distance the nipple can be raised is limited to 3 to 4 cm, this operation has great flexibility (Fig. 132.18). The nipple can be elevated vertically (Fig. 132.19), or the skin excision around the nipple can be designed eccentrically to shift the nipple medially or laterally and reposition it on the breast meridian (Figs. 132.20 and 132.21). When the operation is performed using a permanent purse-string suture (Gore-Tex, nylon, or Prolene), the skin-tightening effect is usually permanent, the areola unlikely to spread, and the scar not prone to stretching. One important technical point to remember concerns the angle of beveling when the skin flap is undermined. Because the degree to which the subareolar tissues have been thinned may not be appreciated (particularly with the implant in place), it is easy to bevel the flap too acutely, severely disrupting nipple-areolar blood supply. The dissection should be maintained in a relatively shallow plane to avoid this complication (Fig. 132.22). If the skin excision is concentric, it is usually unnecessary to undermine the peripheral flap at all, and this certainly reduces the risk of nipple ischemia.

Vertical mastopexy may be indicated in patients with a greater degree of glandular ptosis, who require superior repositioning of the nipple and also horizontal reduction of the overly abundant skin brassiere (Fig. 132.23). As noted earlier,

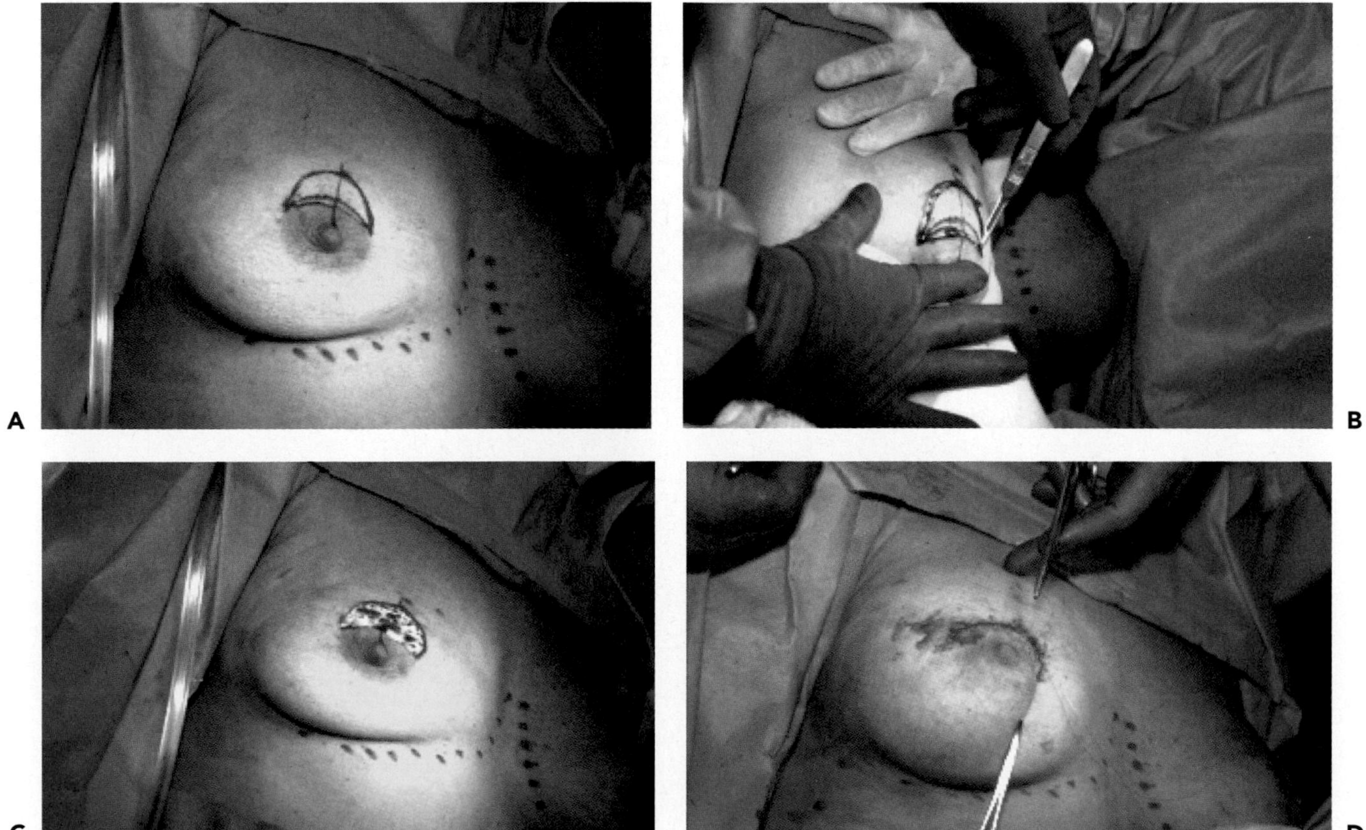

Figure 132.17. In a patient with an implant previously inserted though a periareolar incision, full-thickness resection of breast tissue may jeopardize the blood supply to the nipple and areola; in such cases, only de-deepithelialization or full-thickness skin removal is indicated.

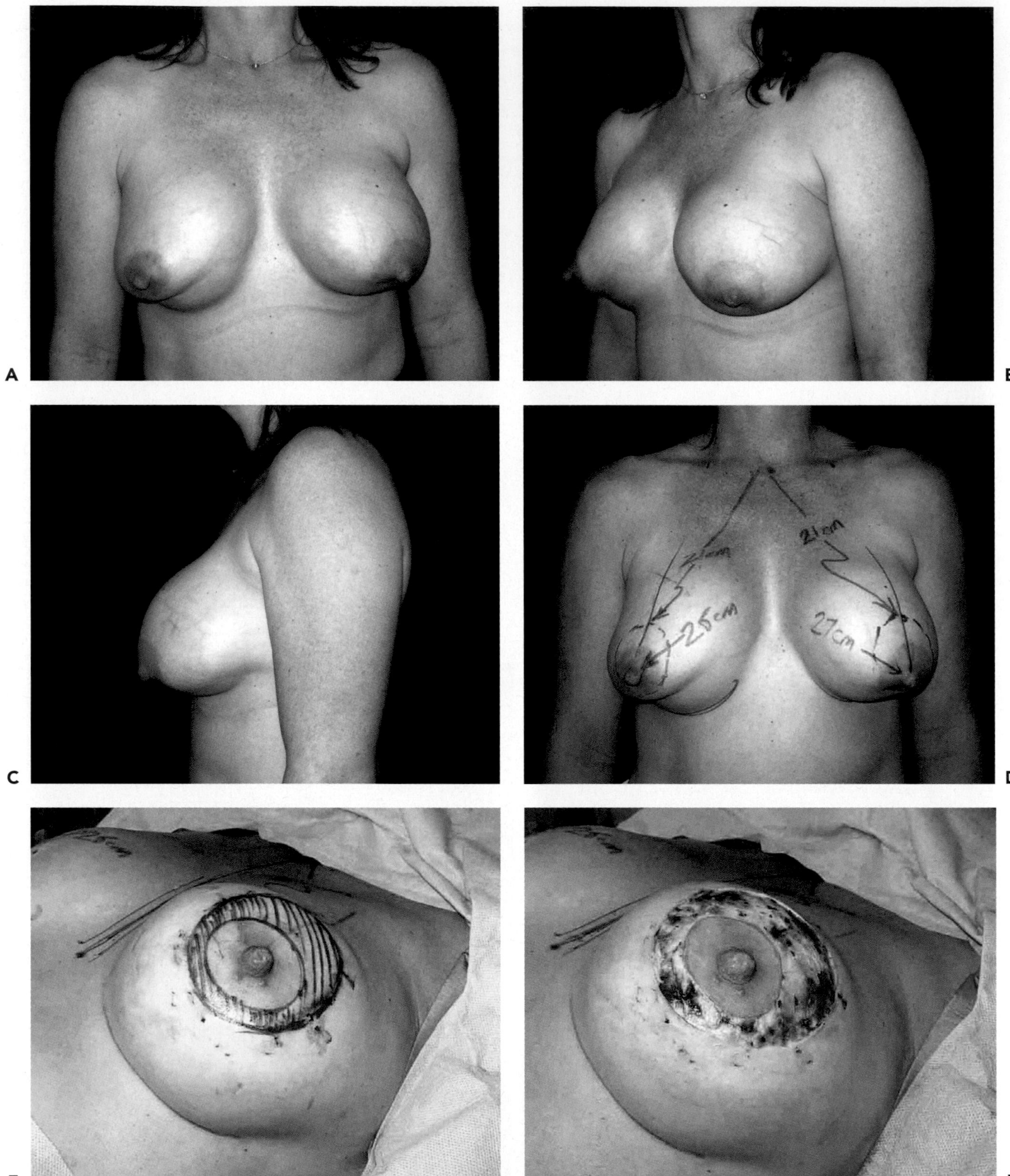

Figure 132.18. **A–C:** Preoperative views of a patient who had subpectoral breast augmentation 15 years earlier. She now has multiple concerns, including ptosis, capsular contracture, "double-bubble" deformity (worse on the right side), excessive upper pole fullness, and asymmetric areolas. **D:** Preoperative measurements and skin markings for asymmetric Benelli mastopexies to be performed in conjunction with capsulectomy, implant exchange, and conversion to the submammary plane. **E:** Area to be deepithelialized is marked and new border of areola circumscribed. **F:** Deepithelialization completed. (*continued*)

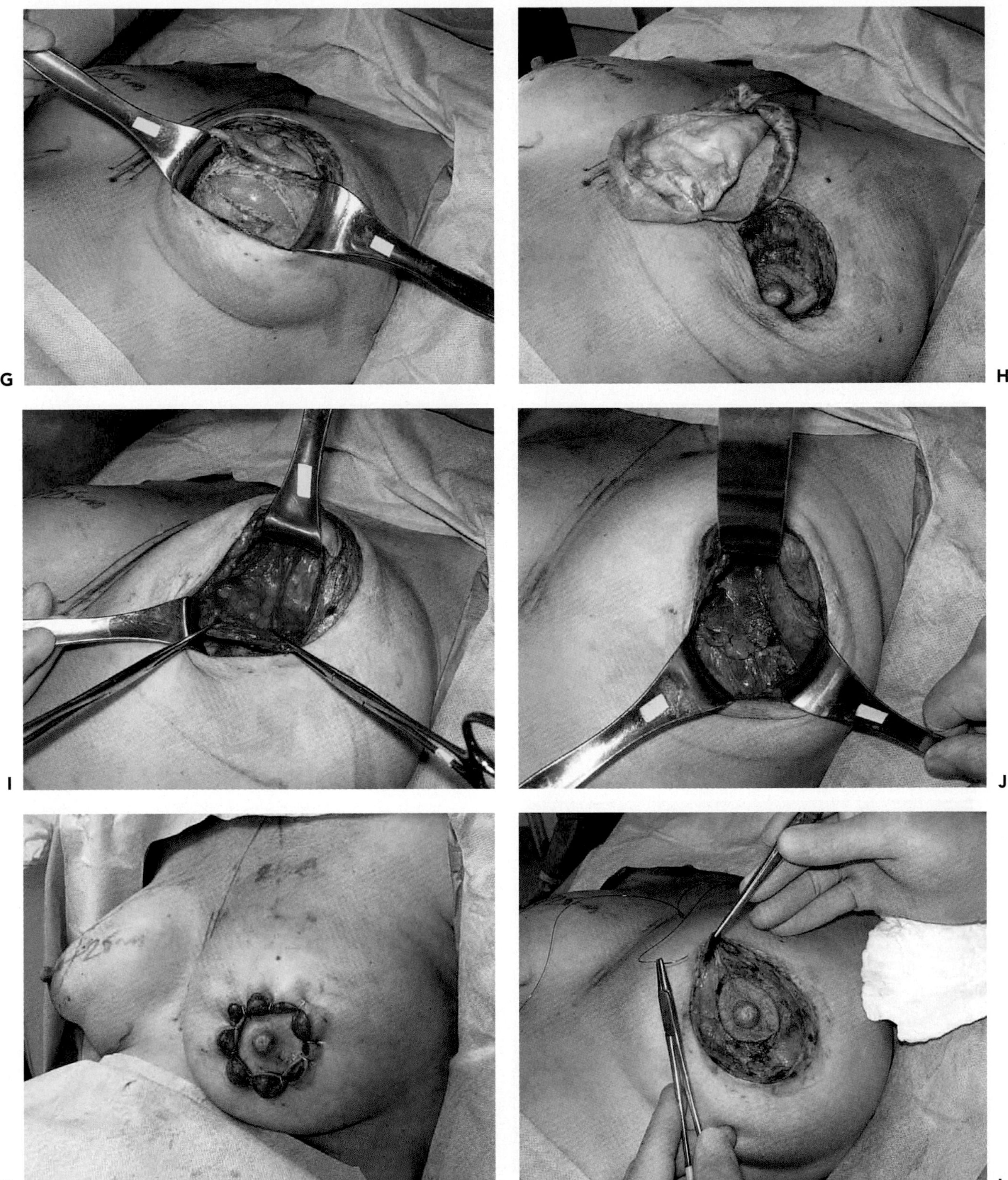

Figure 132.18. (*Continued*) **G:** Access to periprosthetic space is gained inferiorly, where the tissues have already been thinned by the long-term presence of the implant; the superior and medical connections to the nipple are left uninterrupted to ensure adequate blood supply and preserve sensation. **H:** A complete capsulectomy is performed. **I:** The anterolateral border of the pectoralis major muscle is identified and grasped to facilitate dissection of a new submammary pocket. **J:** After the submammary pocket has been created, the pectoralis muscle is reattached to the underlying chest wall with nonabsorbable sutures. **K:** A "sizer" is inserted and the incisions temporarily closed. The patient is placed in a sitting position on the operating table to ensure that the new pocket has been adequately dissected. **L:** The permanent implant is inserted, and the periareolar purse string (usually 0 or #1 Prolene or nylon) is placed in the outer dermal ring. (*continued*)

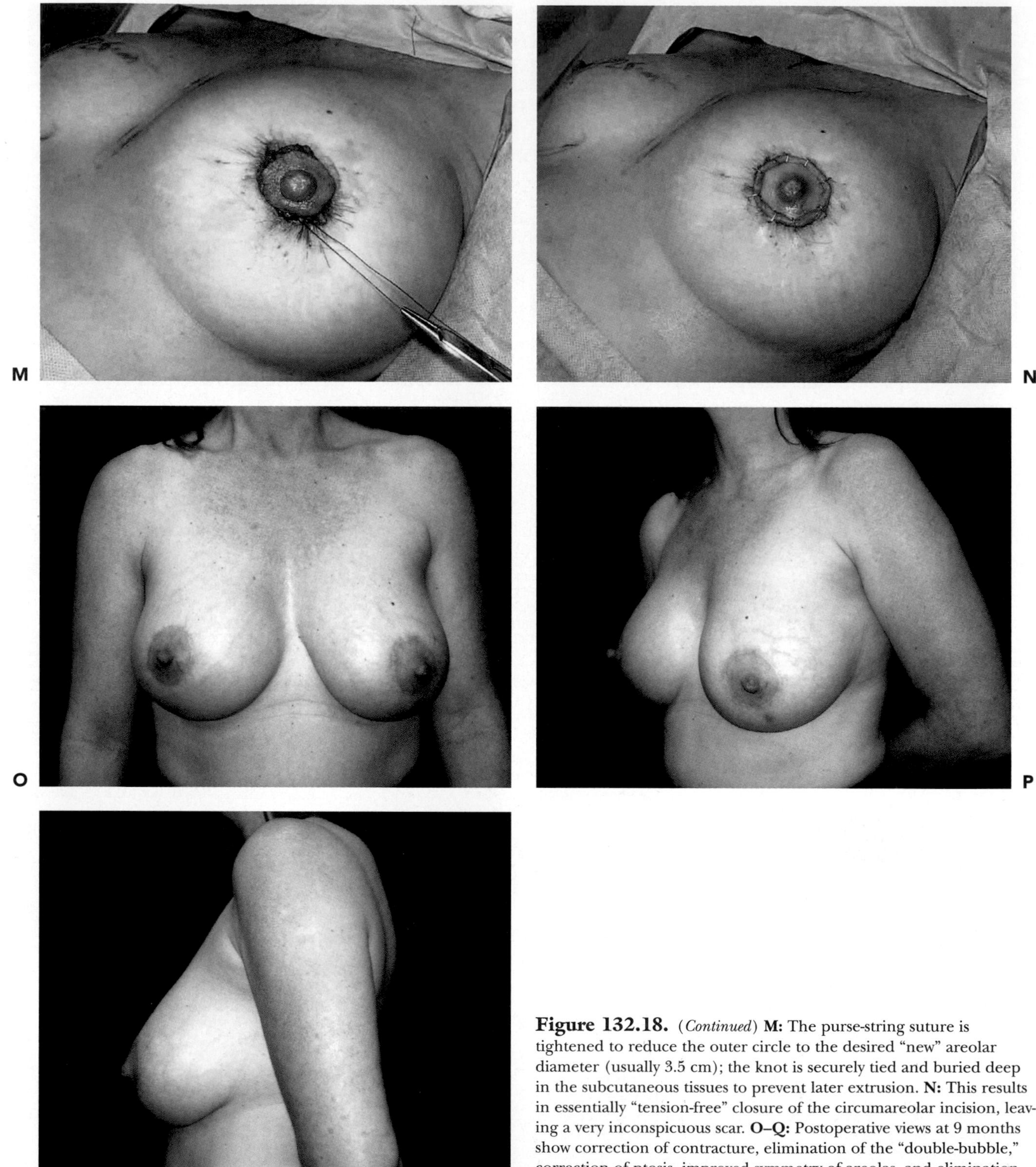

Figure 132.18. (*Continued*) **M:** The purse-string suture is tightened to reduce the outer circle to the desired "new" areolar diameter (usually 3.5 cm); the knot is securely tied and buried deep in the subcutaneous tissues to prevent later extrusion. **N:** This results in essentially "tension-free" closure of the circumareolar incision, leaving a very inconspicuous scar. **O–Q:** Postoperative views at 9 months show correction of contracture, elimination of the "double-bubble," correction of ptosis, improved symmetry of areolas, and elimination of excessive upper pole fullness.

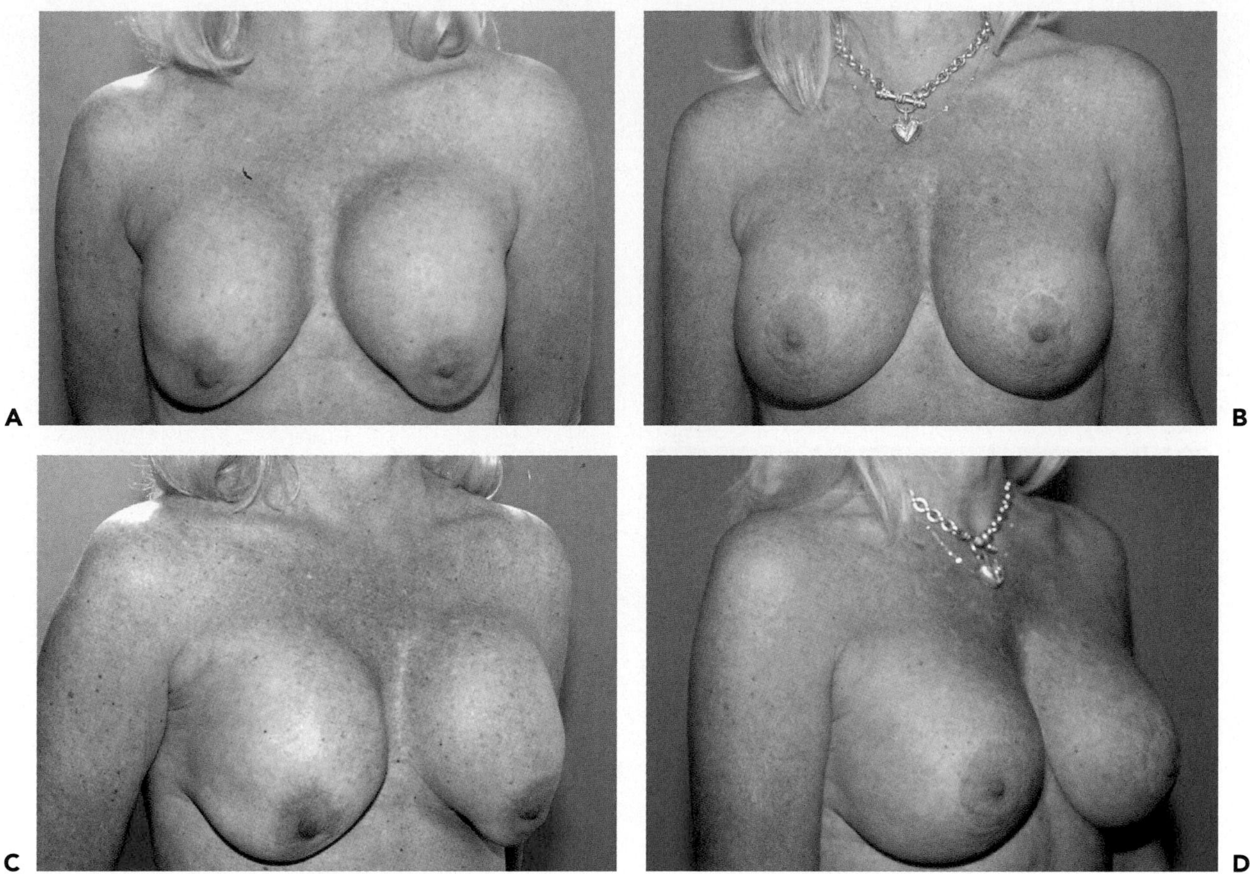

Figure 132.19. Before and after photographs of patient with grade III capsular contracture and moderately severe ptosis, treated with capsulectomy, implant exchange, and periareolar mastopexy.

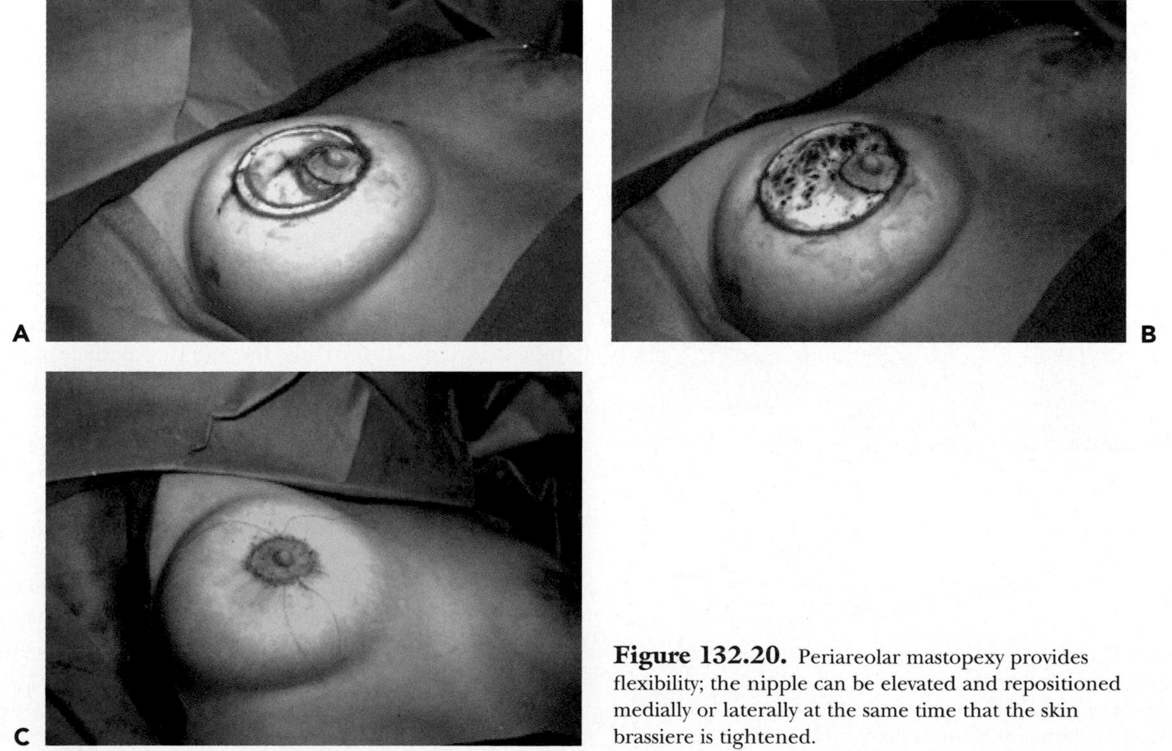

Figure 132.20. Periareolar mastopexy provides flexibility; the nipple can be elevated and repositioned medially or laterally at the same time that the skin brassiere is tightened.

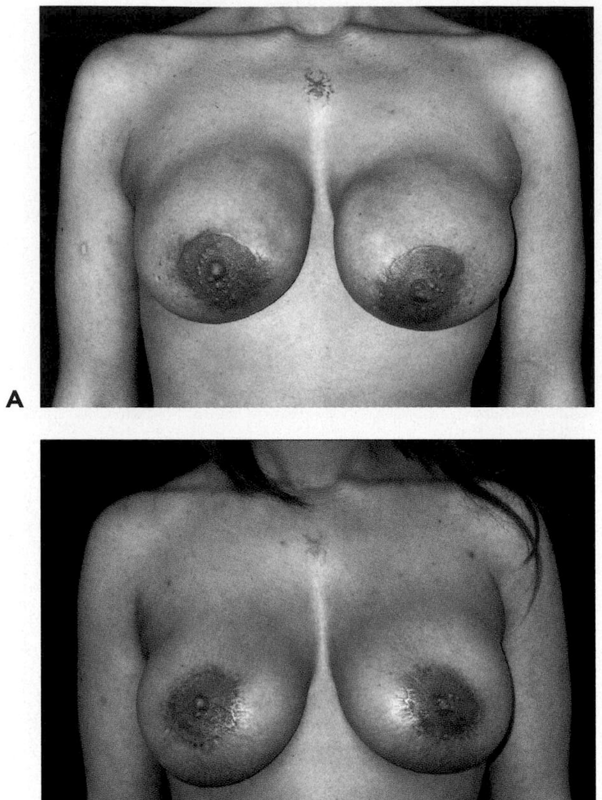

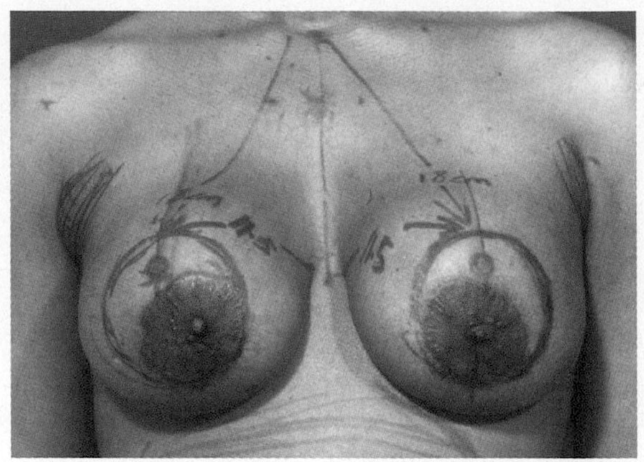

Figure 132.21. **A:** A 26-year-old woman with bilateral Baker grade III contracture, ptosis, and medial malposition of the nipple. **B:** Design for asymmetric eccentric periareolar mastopexy. **C:** After capsulotomy, periareolar mastopexy, and implant replacement.

in designing the flaps for vertical mastopexy it is important to remember that the inferior pole of the breast is the area most likely to be atrophic and thinned secondary to the presence of implants. Thus the pedicle for the nipple and areola should be based primarily superiorly (e.g., Lassus, Lejour), and inferior pedicle techniques (SPAIR) should be avoided. Typically, vertical mastopexy techniques rely upon suturing of the medial and lateral parenchymal "pillars" to support the uplifted breast (17). In the previously augmented patient, there is frequently very little residual parenchyma left in the inferior pole of the breast, so it may be technically difficult to fashion substantial "pillars." It is important, however, to attempt to incorporate breast parenchyma or subcutaneous tissue into the vertical closure and to perform a layered repair. The inferiormost portion of the vertical limb is the most prone to wound breakdown and separation; if there is inadequate tissue covering the breast implant, it may easily become exposed.

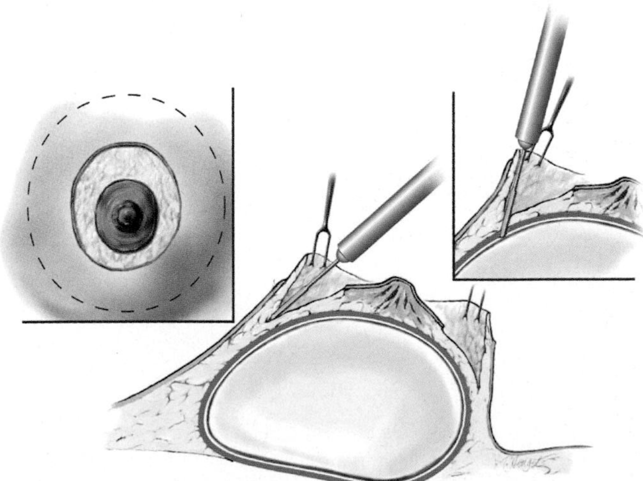

Figure 132.22. In patients with implants, subareolar tissues may have been severely thinned. When performing periareolar mastopexy, care must be taken not to bevel flaps too deeply because of the risk of inadvertent devascularization of the nipple.

Conventional mastopexy, based on the Wise skin pattern excision (18), is useful in many cases as well. This type of skin resection is the most effective in decreasing both the horizontal and vertical dimensions of the skin brassiere (Fig. 132.24). Because the inferior tissues are the most likely to be thin and atrophic, the pedicle to the nipple and areola should be designed so that it relies on a superior, superomedial, or superolateral pedicle. The nipple can also be transferred on a vertical bipedicle flap (19). While the inferior pedicle may be quite thin and atrophic, it may still provide some additional venous drainage for the nipple-areolar complex. Of even greater importance, preservation of the inferior pedicle can provide a protective layer of tissue beneath the skin flaps. Breakdown of the skin at the "T junction" following Wise pattern mastopexy is not infrequent and can lead to exposure of the implant; if the inferior pedicle is preserved, it can serve as a barrier to implant exposure (Fig. 132.25). In some cases, the design of the pedicle and the configuration of the skin flaps must be "customized" to meet the needs dictated by that particular patient's anatomic or physiologic idiosyncrasies (Fig. 132.26).

Regardless of what type of mastopexy is selected, skin resection should be limited initially. It is always best to plan conservatively

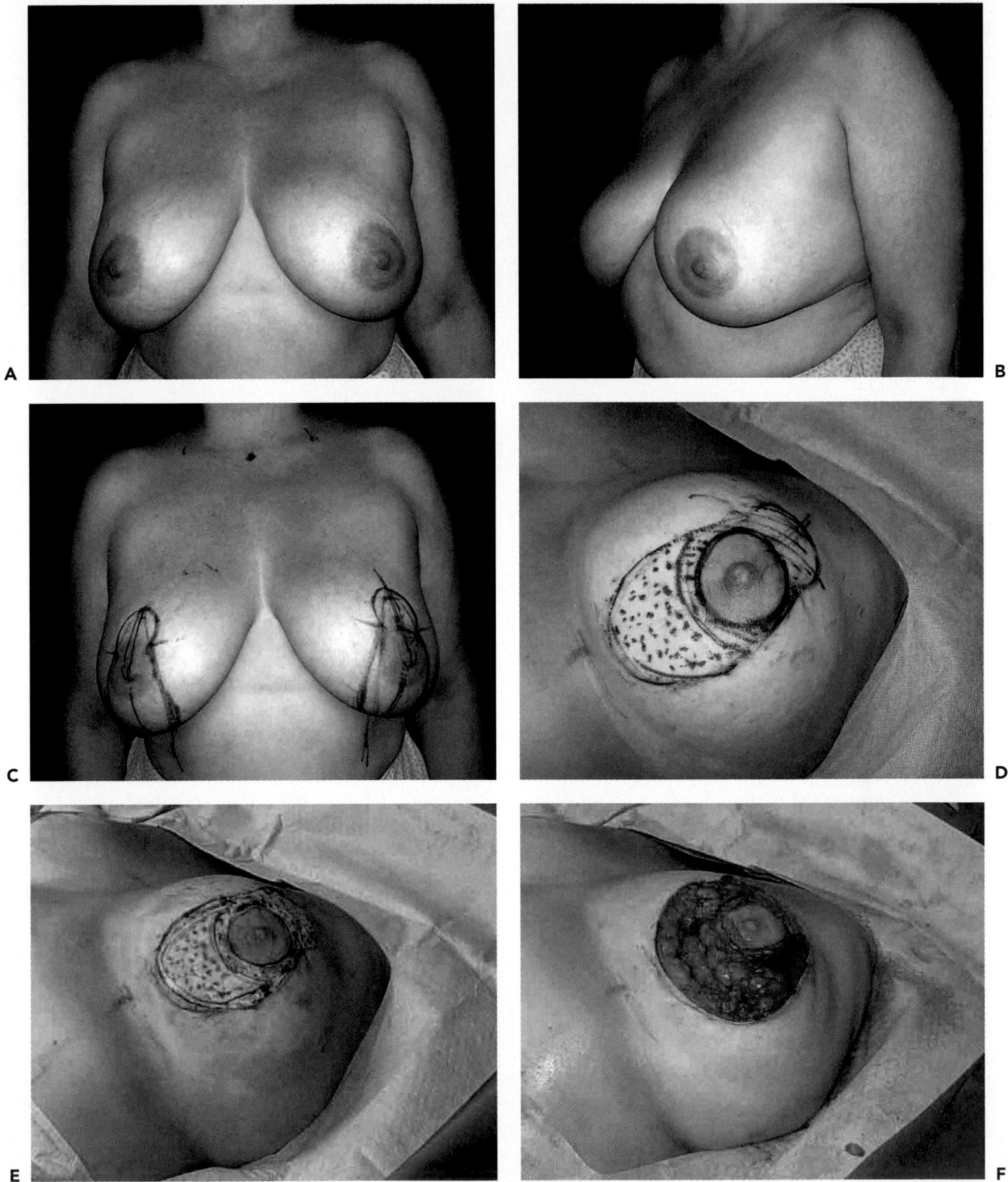

Figure 132.23. **A, B:** A 56-year-old patient with implants and ptosis requests replacement with smaller implants and breast uplift. **C:** Preoperative skin markings for vertical mastopexy with superior pedicle. **D:** Markings during surgery. Full-thickness tissue excision will be performed in the stippled area below the nipple; deepithelialization will be performed in the area of diagonal stripes above the nipple to create a superior pedicle. **E:** Skin incisions completed and deepithelialization of pedicle performed. **F:** Skin and breast tissue resected from central inferior pole, creating the medial and lateral parenchymal "pillars" and giving easy access to the implant. (*continued*)

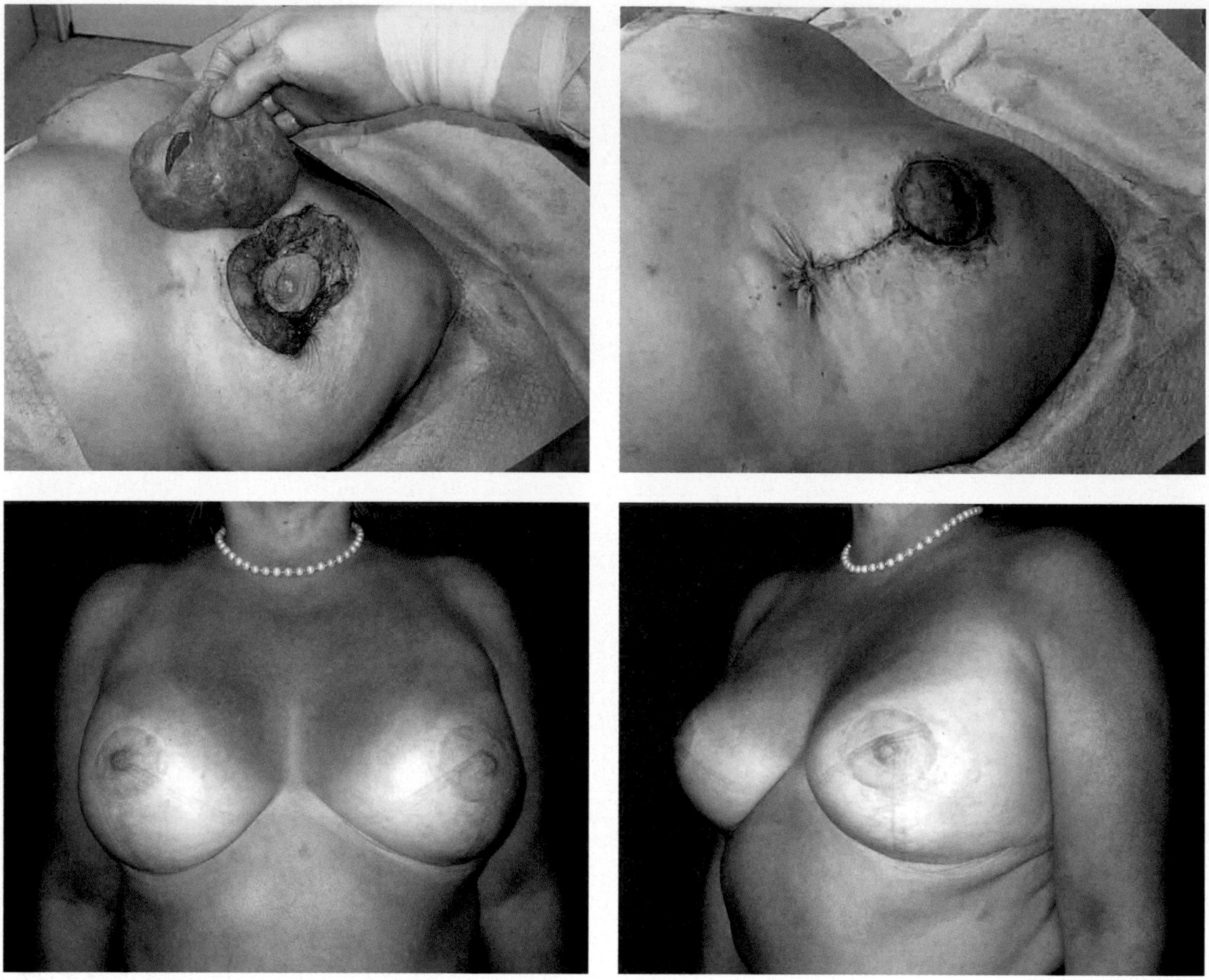

Figure 132.23. (*Continued*) **G:** Old implant and capsule removed in continuity. **H:** New implant inserted and vertical mastopexy incisions closed. **I, J:** Postoperative views 4 months after surgery.

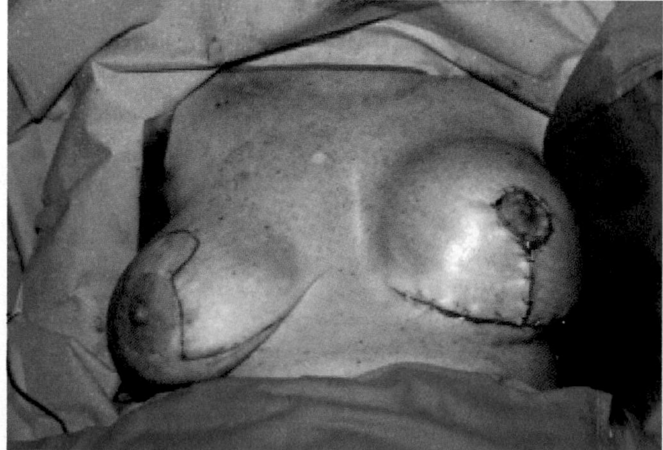

Figure 132.24. Conventional Wise skin-pattern mastopexy in conjunction with capsulotomy effectively reduces vertical and horizontal skin excess.

and then, after the implant has been inserted, to resect additional skin as needed. This will help to reduce the risk of an inadvertent skin shortage and also diminish the likelihood of excessive tension on the closure.

Selection of the properly sized implant is also important. One needs to strike a balance. A large implant will help correct ptosis by filling a deflated skin envelope but will also cause increased tension on the skin flaps and may compress the vascular pedicle to the nipple and areola. It is important to avoid the temptation (or the demand from a patient) to insert an excessively large implant.

During the operation, concern about the viability of the nipple-areolar complex or mastopexy skin flaps may arise. In this situation an implant should not be inserted; it can always be placed at a secondary procedure several months later. If patients are observed to have compromised blood supply postoperatively, there are several measures that can be undertaken to try to improve circulation. Sometimes removing skin sutures around the areola and along the mastopexy incisions

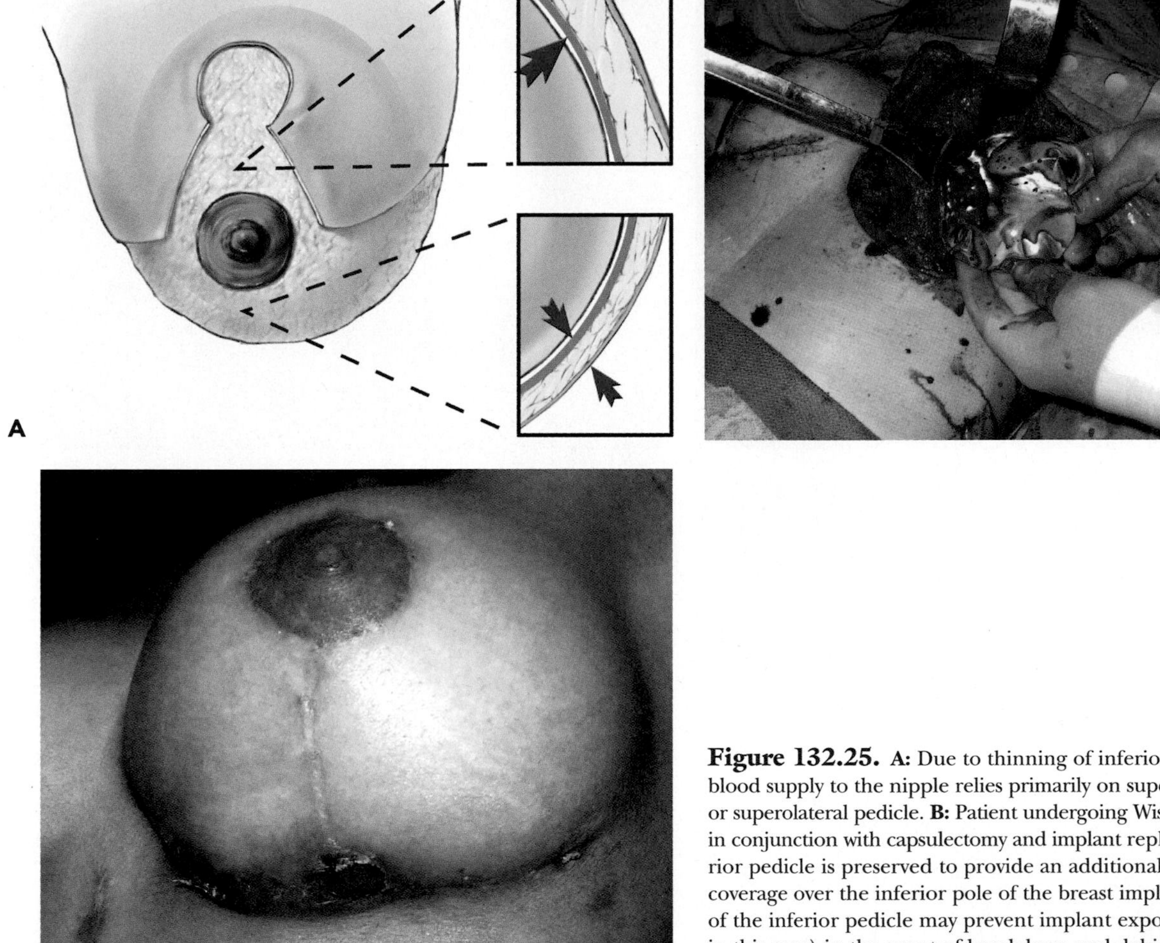

Figure 132.25. **A:** Due to thinning of inferior breast tissue, the blood supply to the nipple relies primarily on superior, superomedial, or superolateral pedicle. **B:** Patient undergoing Wise pattern mastopexy in conjunction with capsulectomy and implant replacement; the inferior pedicle is preserved to provide an additional layer of soft tissue coverage over the inferior pole of the breast implant. **C:** Preservation of the inferior pedicle may prevent implant exposure (as occurred in this case) in the event of breakdown and dehiscence of the mastopexy flaps.

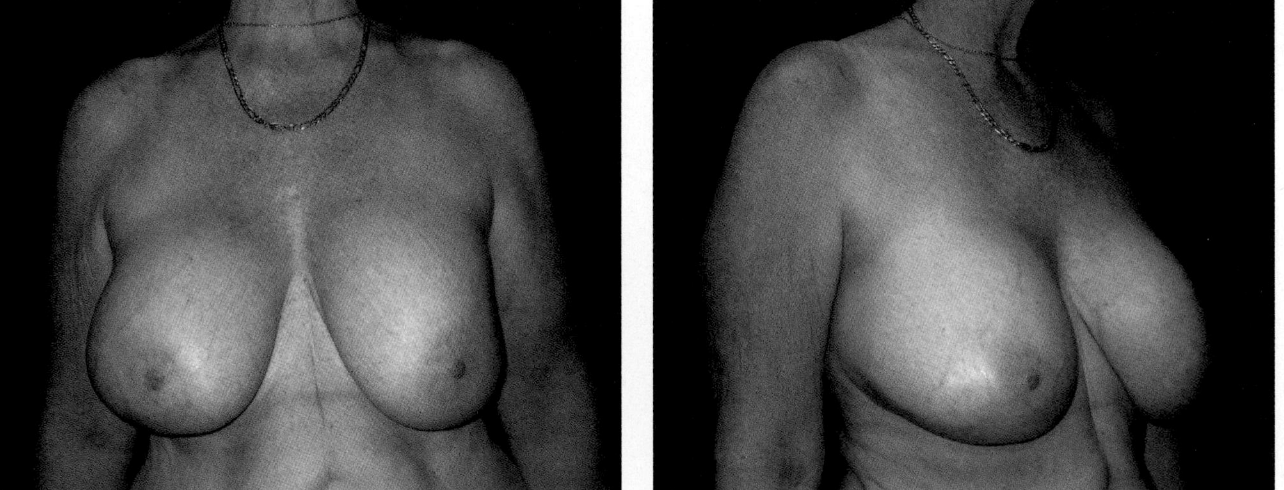

Figure 132.26. **A–C:** Preoperative views of a 64-year-old patient with bilateral ruptured silicone gel implants that have been leaking for a prolonged period of time; on the right side there is extensive infiltration into the breast parenchyma and involvement of the dermis (particularly the lower outer quadrant and lower mid portion of the breast, where the skin is mildly erythematous and very indurated). The patient also has moderately severe ptosis. She wishes to have her leaking implants removed, along with all areas of silicone infiltration, and to have a concomitant breast uplift; the patient wants new implants inserted and is hoping to avoid any "reduction in the size" of her breasts. (*continued*)

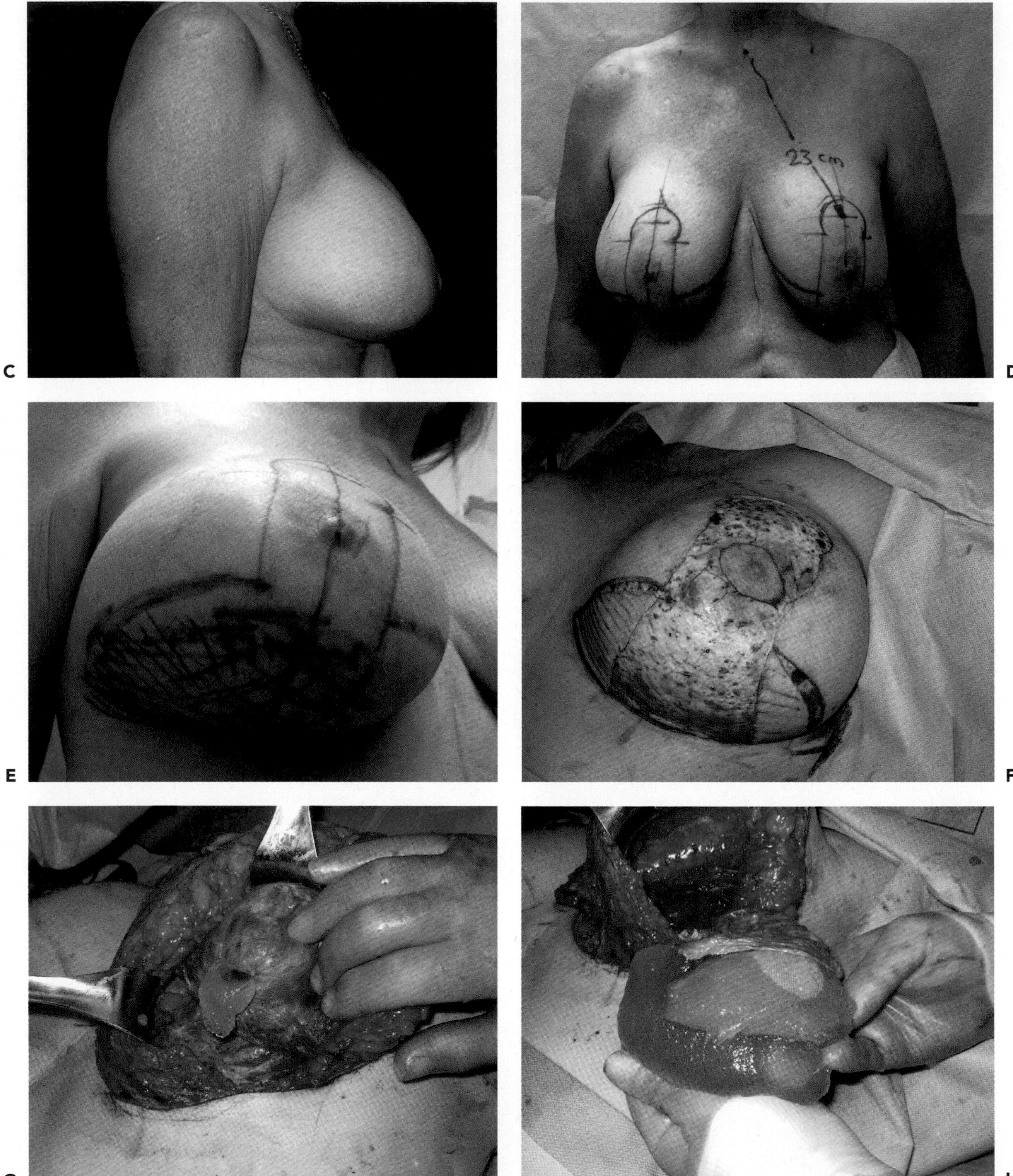

Figure 132.26. (*Continued*) **D:** Preoperative skin marking for Wise pattern mastopexy **E:** Cross-hatched area represents regions where silicone has densely infiltrated into the breast parenchyma and dermis. **F:** On the left side a conventional Wise pattern vertical bipedicle flap is designed and deepithelialized. **G:** When the implant and surrounding capsule are encountered it becomes evident that there is extensive leakage of silicone, but it remains intracapsular. **H:** The free silicone, ruptured elastomer shell with attached Dacron fixation patch (typical of older-generation implants) and scar tissue capsule are removed. (*continued*)

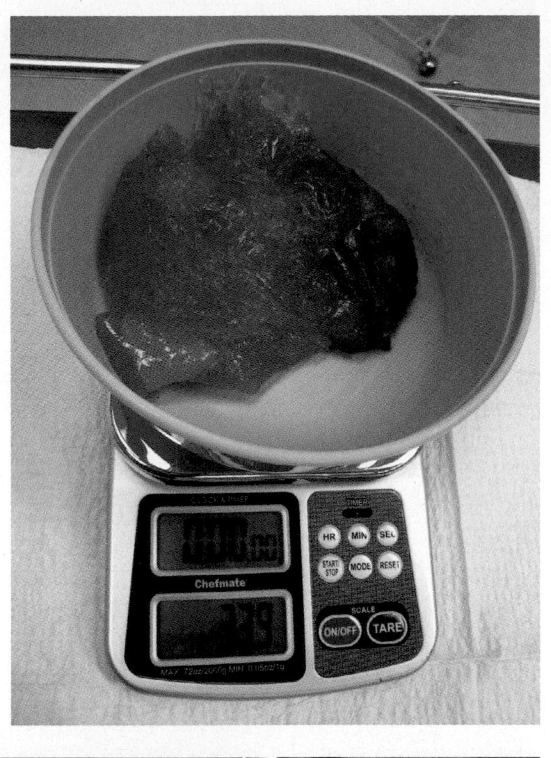

I

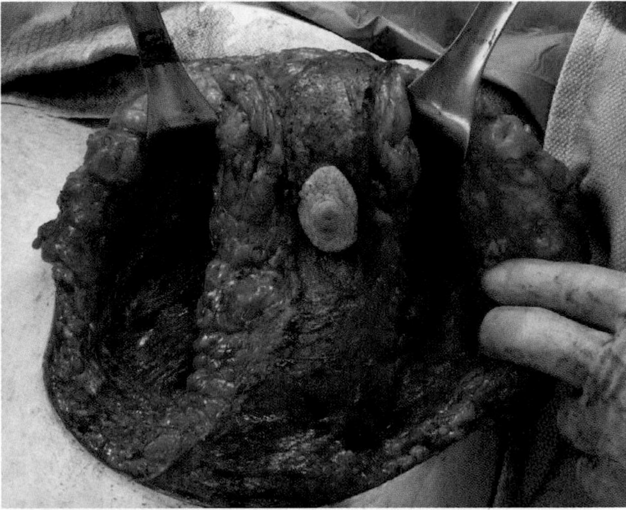

J

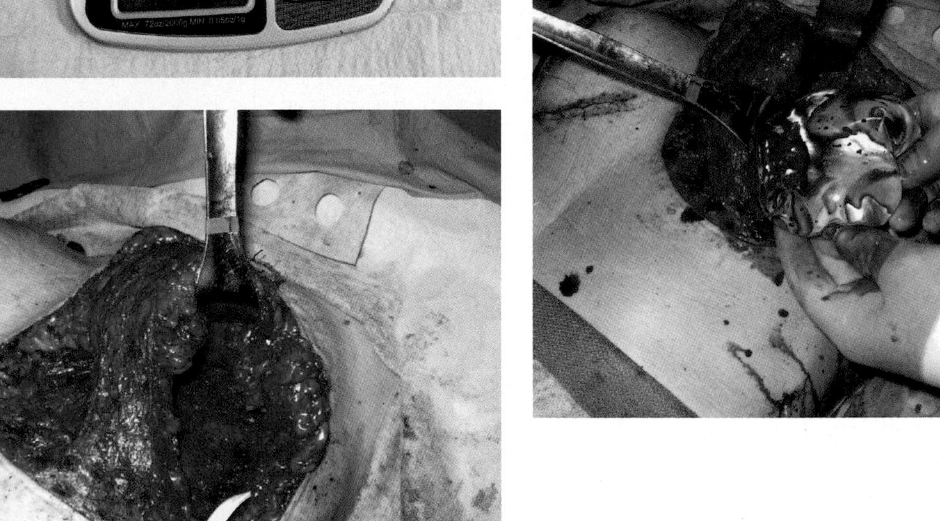

K

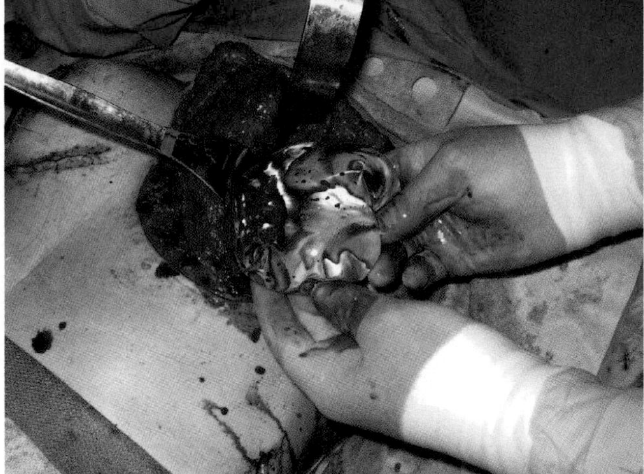

L

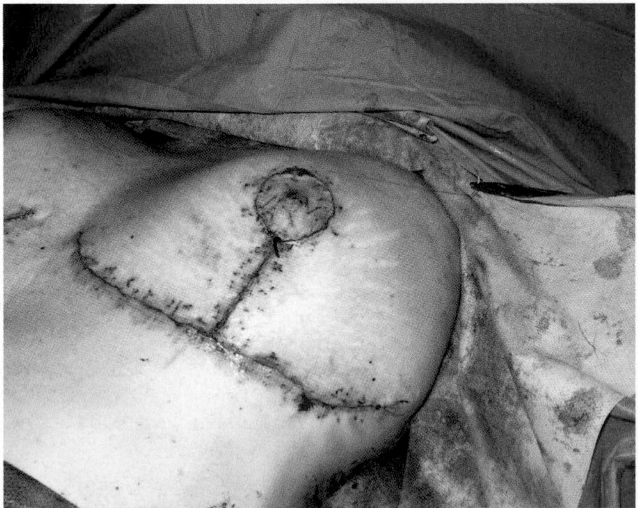

M

Figure 132.26. (*Continued*) **I:** The specimen from the left side weighs 339 g; knowing this helps to determine the appropriate size of implant to insert. **J:** The left nipple and areola have excellent blood supply from the bipedicle flap. **K:** The inferior pedicle will provide an "added" layer of soft tissue over the implant to prevent exposure of the prosthesis in the event of breakdown of the mastopexy flaps. **L:** A 350-cc silicone gel implant is inserted into the pocket; the inferior pedicle drapes over the lower half of the implant. **M:** The mastopexy incisions are closed in layers. (*continued*)

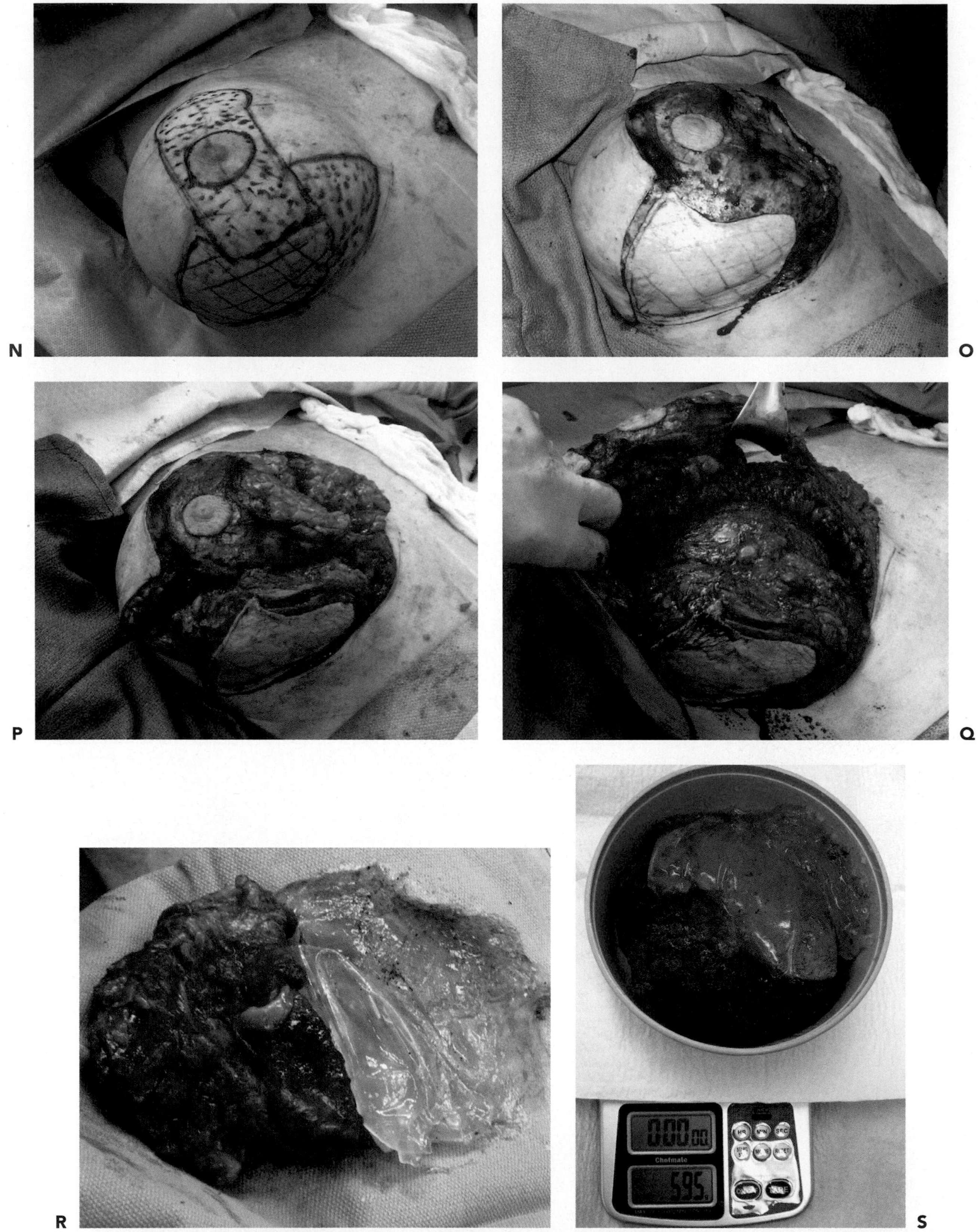

Figure 132.26. (*Continued*) **N:** Skin markings on the right breast for Wise pattern mastopexy; the pedicle to the nipple has been modified to accommodate planned excision of skin and breast parenchyma of the lower lateral and central breast. The stippled area will be deepithelialized to create the superior and "modified" inferior pedicle, while the cross-hatched area represents the area of proposed full-thickness excision of skin and breast parenchyma. **O:** The skin incisions have been made and the pedicles deepithelialized. **P:** The incisions are deepened to create the pedicles and to resect the involved skin and breast tissue in continuity with the underlying capsule and ruptured implant. **Q:** The ruptured implant, capsule, and areas of silicone mastitis and dermatitis are resected en bloc. **R:** The specimen removed from the right breast. **S:** The specimen weighs 595 g; knowing this helps to determine the appropriate size of implant to insert. (*continued*)

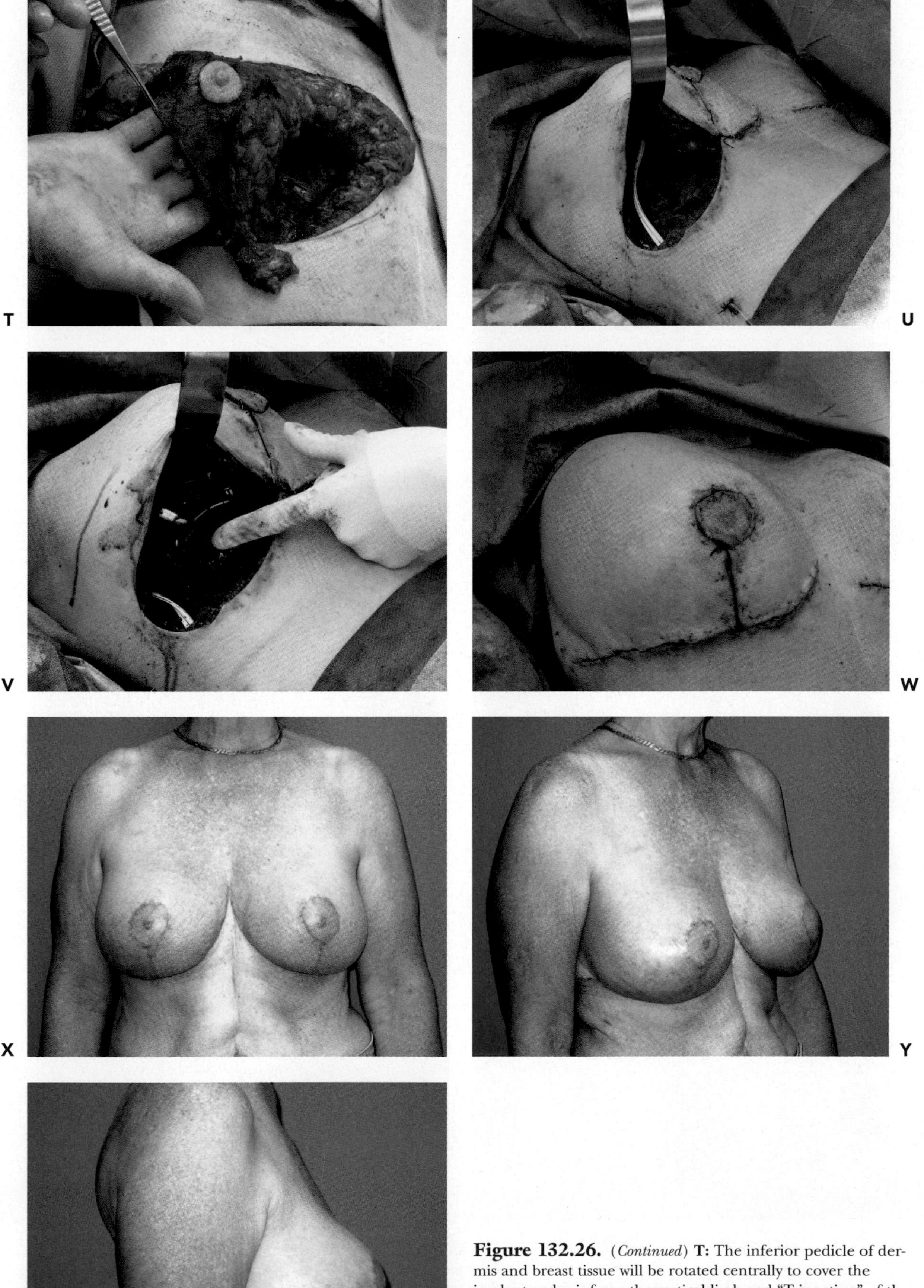

Figure 132.26. (*Continued*) **T:** The inferior pedicle of dermis and breast tissue will be rotated centrally to cover the implant and reinforce the vertical limb and "T junction" of the mastopexy incision. **U:** The "inferior pedicle'" has been sutured in place and the pocket prepared for insertion of the implant. **V:** A 600-cc silicone gel implant is inserted to compensate for the larger amount of tissue resected from the right breast. **W:** Mastopexy incisions approximated. **X–Z:** Postoperative views at 3 months.

will improve venous drainage, relieve congestion, and lead to an immediate improvement in the appearance of the flaps (Fig. 132.27). If a saline implant is present, it can be partially deflated (or removed altogether) to reduce tension on flaps and reverse compression of vascular pedicles. Likewise, removal of a gel-filled implant may dramatically and rapidly improve circulation. Administration of hyperbaric oxygen may also be beneficial. Its role is mediated not as much by increased oxygen tension as by the reduction of free radicals, which helps to reduce the inflammatory response to ischemia and thereby improve perfusion. Nitroglycerine ointment 2% (Nitro-Bid) may also be applied to areas where there is venous congestion in an effort to improve circulation. A suitable regimen is application of 1/2-inch (7.5 mg) of the ointment to the affected area two times daily.

In summary, correction of ptosis in the augmented patient is an increasingly important topic whose complex surgical and medicolegal implications merit careful attention. As the population of augmented women ages, greater numbers will require some combination of breast uplift, capsular surgery, and implant exchange. Such combined surgery is risky, particularly because of the adverse effects of implants on breast anatomy and physiology. These effects include tissue atrophy, thinning and stretching, and reduction of blood supply to the skin and nipple. Caution must be exercised in performing corrective surgery in these individuals. However, with proper planning and attention to detail, most patients will achieve good outcomes, and disastrous results can be avoided (Fig. 132.28).

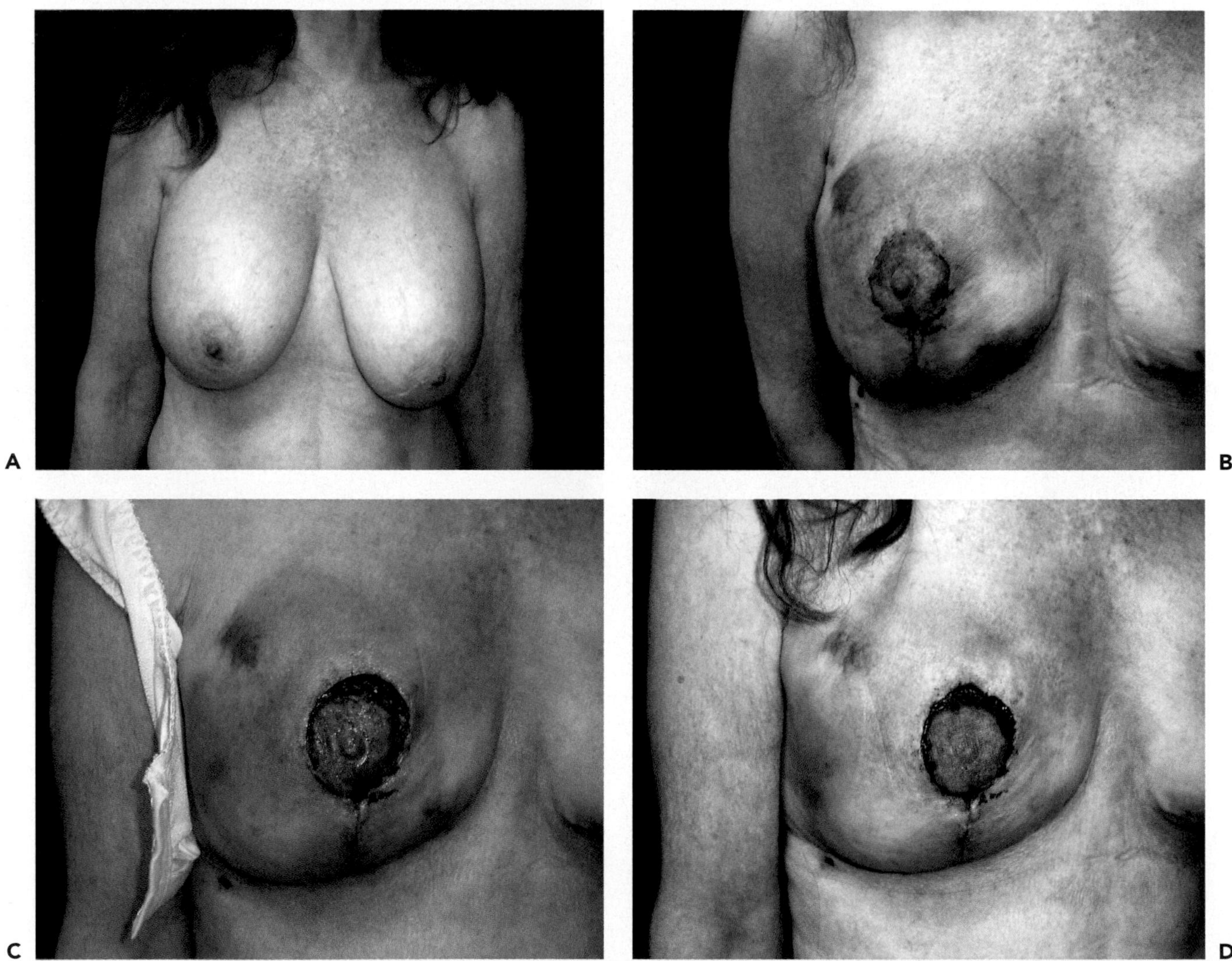

Figure 132.27. **A:** A 57 year-old-woman with implants present for greater than 20 years complaining of large, ptotic, asymmetric breasts; she elects to undergo explantation (without replacement), capsulectomy, and Wise pattern mastopexy. **B:** At 72 hours after surgery the right nipple-areolar complex (NAC) is severely congested, cool to the touch, and without capillary refill; all periareolar sutures are removed and Nitro-Bid cream applied to the areola. **C:** The following day (POD #4), some improvement is noted, with less congestion of the NAC. **D:** By POD #5, there is marked improvement in circulation to the NAC, although patchy areas of venous congestion persist. **E:** At 3 weeks, virtually the entire NAC appears viable. (*continued*)

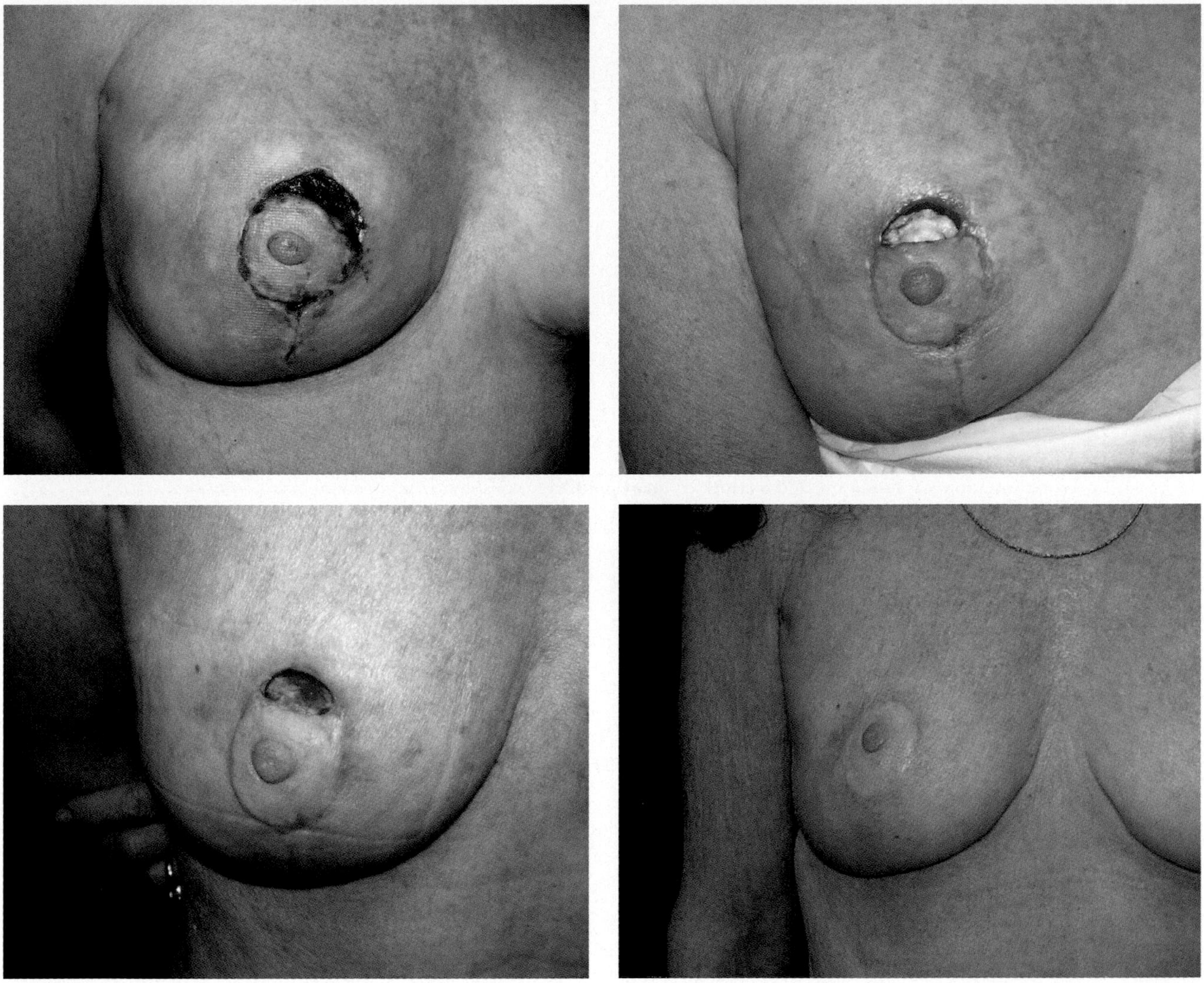

E F

G H

Figure 132.27. (*Continued*) **F:** At 5 weeks, debridement of the eschar reveals underlying fat necrosis; the open wound is treated with conservative debridement and saline wet to dry dressings. **G:** At 7 weeks postoperatively the base of the wound is characterized by healthy granulation tissue; delayed surgical closure is performed. **H:** By 6 months, the area has completely healed, with slight distortion of the areola; this will be corrected with a circumareolar mastopexy.

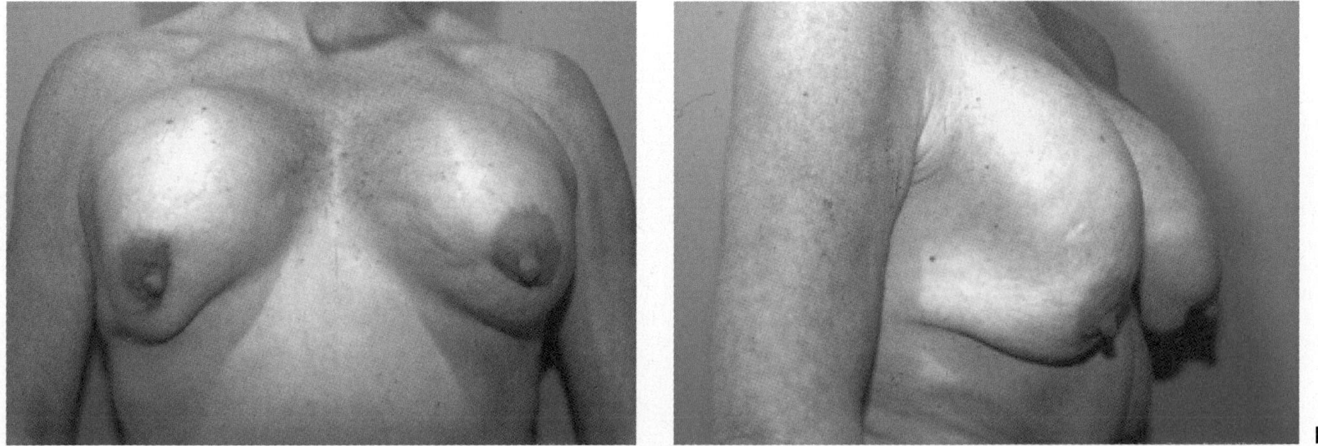

Figure 132.28. **A, B:** Preoperative views of a patient with bilateral Baker grade IV contractures and ptosis. (*continued*)

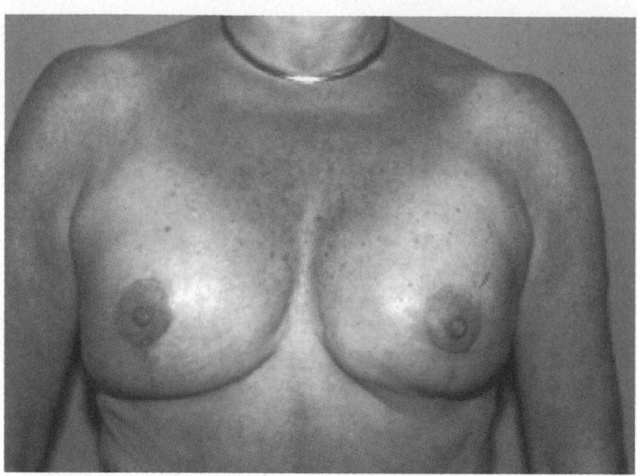

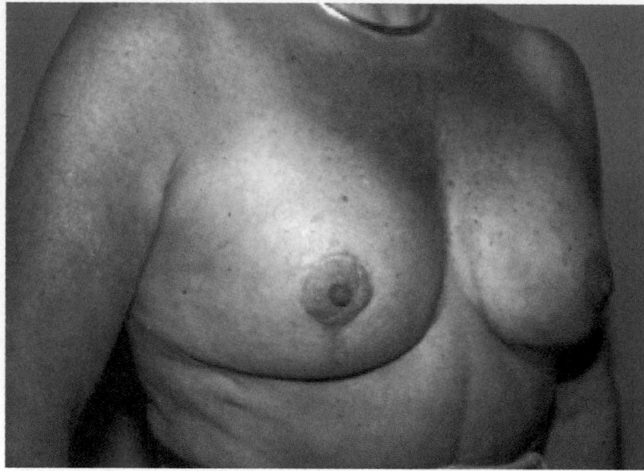

Figure 132.28. (*Continued*) **C, D:** The same patient after two-stage correction. The first stage consisted of explantation, capsulectomy, and mastopexy; the second stage consisted of subpectoral insertion of new implants.

EDITORIAL COMMENTS

This chapter is very important because there is often some degree of uncertainty as to whether a mastopexy should be performed immediately at the time of explantation or at a later date. Dr. Handel correctly emphasizes the important concerns regarding immediate mastopexy in the previously augmented patient. These relate primarily to the residual blood supply to the nipple-areolar complex and the contouring issues in a breast that has undergone some degree of atrophy and compression. In the majority of my cases, the decision has been made not to perform an immediate mastopexy following explanation but rather to wait for several months until some degree of vascular reorganization has occurred and the effects of chronic compression and atrophy on and of the breast have stabilized. It is correctly emphasized that in the setting of explantation with capsulectomy, the incidence of morbidity such as delayed healing and tissue necrosis will be increased. It has also been my observation that some women who have had explantation will be satisfied with the outcome and not proceed with a mastopexy as originally planned. This has generally been the case in younger women in whom smaller implants (less than 250 cc) had been removed.

When a mastopexy is necessary, my preference is to minimize the incisions on the breast to preserve blood supply and reduce scars. I have had the occasion to perform a crescent mastopexy, a periareolar mastopexy, a vertical mastopexy, and an inferior pole excision mastopexy. The final approach was performed in a woman who had pseudoptosis and a long inframammary incision. All have worked well under the appropriate indications. I have not had the need to perform a Wise pattern mastopexy in this setting.

M.Y.N.

REFERENCES

1. American Society of Plastic Surgeons. 2007 Plastic Surgery Statistics. Available at: http://www.plasticsurgery.org/Media/Statistics/2007_Statistics.html. Accessed July 21, 2010.
2. Gabriel SE, Woods JE, O'Fallon M, et al. Complications leading to surgery after breast implantation. *N Engl J Med* 1997;336(10):677–682.
3. Spear SL. Augmentation/mastopexy: "surgeon beware." *Plast Reconstr Surg* 2003;112:905–906.
4. Spear SL, Giese SY. Simultaneous breast augmentation and mastopexy. *Aesthet Surg J* 2002;20:155–164.
5. Pearson DC, Sherris DA. Resorption beneath Silastic mandibular implants: effects of placement and pressure. *Arch Facial Plast Surg* 1999;1:261–265.
6. Matarasso A, Elias AC, Elias RL. Labial incompetence: a marker for progressive bone resorption in Silastic chin augmentation: an update. *Plast Reconstr Surg* 2003;112(2):676–678.
7. Tebbetts JB. The greatest myths in breast augmentation. *Plast Reconstr Surg* 2001;107:1895–1903.
8. McGrath MH, Burkhardt BR. The safety and efficacy of breast implants for augmentation mammaplasty. *Plast Reconstr Surg* 1984;74(4):550–560.
9. Lassus C. Vertical scar breast reduction and mastopexy without undermining. In: Spear SL, ed. *Surgery of the Breast: Principles and Art.* Philadelphia: Lippincott-Raven; 1998:717–734.
10. Lejour M. Vertical mammaplasty for breast reduction and mastopexy. In: Spear SL, ed. *Surgery of the Breast: Principles and Art.* Philadelphia: Lippincott-Raven; 1998:735–747.
11. Spear SL, Howard MA. Evolution of the vertical reduction mammaplasty. *Plast Reconstr Surg* 2003;112(3):855–867.
12. Hammond DC. Short-scar periareolar-inferior pedicle reduction (SPAIR) mammaplasty. *Oper Techn Plast Reconstr Surg* 1999;6:106–118.
13. Handel N. Augmentation mastopexy. In: Spear SL, ed. *Surgery of the Breast: Principles and Art.* Philadelphia: Lippincott-Raven; 1998:921–937.
14. Puckett CL, Meyer VH, Reinisch JF. Crescent mastopexy and augmentation. *Plast Reconstr Surg* 1985;75(4):533–539.
15. Benelli L. A new periareolar mammaplasty: the "round block" technique. *Aesthet Plast Surg* 1990;14:93–98.
16. Brink RR. Management of true ptosis of the breast. *Plast Reconstr Surg* 1993;91(4):657–662.
17. Hall-Findlay EJ. A simplified vertical reduction mammaplasty: shortening the learning curve. *Plast Reconstr Surg* 1999;104(3):748–759.
18. Wise RJ. A preliminary report on a method of planning the mammaplasty. *Plast Reconstr Surg* 1956;17:367–372.
19. McKissock PK. Reduction mammaplasty with a vertical dermal flap. *Plast Reconstr Surg* 1972;49(3):245–252.

Index

Note: Page numbers followed by *f* indicate figure, page numbers followed by *t* indicate tables.

CCS1010